T0074473

EVIDENCE-BASED PHYSICAL THERAPY FOR THE PELVIC FLOOR

THIRD EDITION

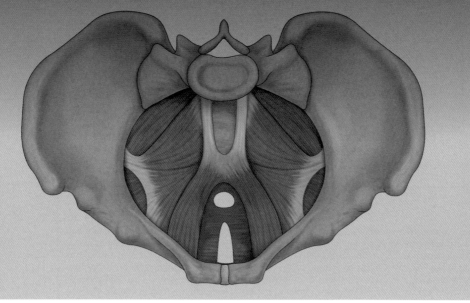

EVIDENCE-BASED PHYSICAL THERAPY FOR THE PELVIC FLOOR
Bridging Science and Clinical Practice

Edited by

Kari Bø, PT, MSc, PhD
Professor
Department of Sports Medicine
Norwegian School of Sports Sciences
Oslo, Norway
Department of Obstetrics and Gynecology
Akershus University Hospital
Lørenskog, Norway

Bary Berghmans, PT, MSc, PhD
Associate Professor
Pelvic care Centre Maastricht
Maastricht University Medical Center+
Maastricht, The Netherlands

Siv Mørkved, PT, MSc, PhD
Professor
Department of Public Health and Nursing
Norwegian University of Science and Technology
Trondheim, Norway

Marijke Van Kampen, PT, MSc, PhD
Professor Emeritus
KU Leuven
Department of Rehabilitation Sciences
Faculty of Kinesiology and Rehabilitation Sciences
Leuven, Belgium

ELSEVIER

First edition 2007
Second edition 2015

Notices

Practitioners and researchers must always rely on their own experience and knowledge in evaluating and using any information, methods, compounds or experiments described herein. Because of rapid advances in the medical sciences, in particular, independent verification of diagnoses and drug dosages should be made. To the fullest extent of the law, no responsibility is assumed by Elsevier, authors, editors or contributors for any injury and/or damage to persons or property as a matter of products liability, negligence or otherwise, or from any use or operation of any methods, products, instructions, or ideas contained in the material herein.

ISBN: 978-0-7020-8308-2

Content Strategist: Andrae Akeh
Content Project Manager: Kritika Kaushik
Design: Brian Salisbury
Marketing Manager: Belinda Tudin

Printed in Great Britain by Bell & Bain Ltd, Glasgow

Last digit is the print number: 9 8 7 6 5 4 3 2 1

Working together to grow libraries in developing countries

www.elsevier.com • www.bookaid.org

CONTENTS

CONTRIBUTORS

The editor(s) would like to acknowledge and offer grateful thanks for the input of all previous editions' contributors, without whom this new edition would not have been possible.

Paul Abrams, MD, FRCS
Professor of Urology
Bristol Urological Institute
Southmead Hospital
Bristol, UK

James Ashton-Miller, PhD
Research Professor, Director, Biomechanics Research
   Laboratory
Department of Mechanical Engineering
University of Michigan
Ann Arbor, MI, USA

Anne Asnong, Dra, Msc
Physiotherapist
Department of Rehabilitation Sciences
KU Leuven, Leuven,
Vlaams-Brabant, Belgium

Matthew D. Barber, MD
Professor of Surgery
Obstetrics, Gynecology and Women's
   Health Institute
Cleveland Clinic
Cleveland, OH, USA

Mohammed Belal, MA, MB B(Chir), FRCS
Consultant Urological Surgeon
Spire South Bank Hospital
Worcester, UK

Bary Berghmans, PT, MSc, PhD
Associate Professor
Health Scientist and Clinical Epidemiologist,
   Pelvic care Centre Maastricht,
   Maastricht University Medical Center+,
   Maastricht, The Netherlands

Nols Bernards, MD
Lecturer
HAN University of Applied Sciences
Institute of Applied Health Studies
Arnhem
The Netherlands

Anna Beurskens, PhD
Professor in Goal Oriented Measurement in Health
   Care
Family Practice
Maastricht University
Maastricht, The Netherlands

Rob de Bie, PhD, MSc, PT
Professor of Physiotherapy Research
Department of Epidemiology
Maastricht University
Maastricht, The Netherlands

Georges Billard, Egnr (Mech Tech)
Chief Executif Officer
Montpellier Physiotherapy Research and Development
   Center VIVALTIS
France

Kari Bø, PhD, PT
Professor
Sports Medicine
Norwegian School of Sports Sciences
Oslo, Norway
Department of Obstetrics and
   Gynecology
Akershus University Hospital
Lørenskog, Norway

Esther Bols, PhD, PT
Senior Lecturer and Researcher
Academy of Physiotherapy
Research Group Autonomy and Participation for
   Persons with a Chronic Illness
Zuyd University
Heerlen, The Netherlands

Robyn Brennan, MPhys
Lecturer, Academic Support and PhD Candidate
Department of Physiotherapy
University of Melbourne
Melbourne, Victoria
Australia

Licia Pazzoto Cacciari, PhD
Postdoctoral Researcher
Centre de Recherche de l'Institut Universitaire de
    Gériatrie de Montréal
Montreal, Canada

Janet Walker Chase, DipPhysio
Physiotherapist
Paediatric Gastroenterology
Victoria
Paediatric Urology Victoria
Royal Children's Hospital
Melbourne, Victoria
Australia

**Pauline Chiarelli, DipPhysio, GradDipHSocSc, M
MedSc, PhD**
Professor (Associate) Physiotherapy
School of Health Sciences
University of Newcastle
New South Wales
Australia

Jacques Corcos, MSC, MD, FRCS
Professor of Urology
Department of Urology
Jewish General Hospital/McGill University
Montreal, Canada

Rebekah Das, PhD
Adjunct Lecturer
School of Health Sciences
University of South Australia
Adelaide, Australia

John O. Delancey, MD
Norman F. Miller Professor of Gynecology
Department of Obstetrics and Gynecology
University of Michigan Medical School
Ann Arbor, MI, USA

Hans Peter Dietz, MD, PhD, FRANZCOG, DDU, CU
Obstetrician/Gynecologist, Urogynecologist
Sydney Urodynamic Centres
Sydney, Australia

Chantale Dumoulin, PT, PhD
Professor
School of Rehabilitation, Faculty of Medicine
Université de Montréal
Montreal, Canada

Sohier Elneil, PhD, FRCOG
Honorary Associate Professor
FPMRS Research Lead
Institute for Women's Health
London, UK

Marieke van Engelenburg-van Lonkhuyzen, PhD
Researcher
Department of Epidemiology
Maastricht University, Faculty of Health, Medicine and
    Life Sciences
Maastricht, The Netherlands

Ruwan Fernando, MD
Consultant, Obstetrician and Urogynaecologist
Department of Urogynaecology
St. Mary's Hospital, Imperial College Health Care NHS
    Trust
London, UK

Cristine Homsi Jorge, PT, PhD
Associate Professor
Department of Health Sciences
Clinics Hospital/Ribeirão Preto Medical School
Ribeirão Preto
Brazil

Helena Frawley, PT, PhD
Associate Professor
Women's Health Physiotherapy Research
School of Health Sciences
The University of Melbourne
Allied Health Research
Royal Women's Hospital Melbourne
Mercy Hospital for Women
Melbourne, Australia

Inge Geraerts, PhD, PT
Assistant Professor
Department of Rehabilitation Sciences
Faculty of Kinesiology and Rehabilitation Sciences
Leuven, Belgium

Sandhya Gupta, MD
Obstetrician and Gynaecologist
Central Gippsland Hospital
Australia

Robert Herbert, PhD
Senior Principal Research Scientist
Neuroscience Research Australia (NeuRA)
Sydney, Australia

Hege H. Johannessen, PT, PhD
Specialist Physiotherapist
Department of Physical Medicine and Rehabilitation
Oestfold Hospital Trust
Sarpsborg, Norway
Associated Professor
Department of Health, Welfare and Organization
Oestfold University College
Fredrikstad, Norway

Gommert van Koeveringe, MD, PhD
Professor of Urology, Section Head of Functional,
    Reconstructive and Neurourology
Department of Urology
Maastricht University Medical Center
Maastricht, The Netherlands

Nucelio Lemos, MD, PhD
Associate Professor
Department of Obstetrics and Gynecology
University of Toronto
Toronto, ON, Canada

Douglas Luchristt, MD, MPH
Fellow, Female Pelvic Medicine and Reconstructive
    Surgery and Clinical Instructor of Obstetrics and
    Gynecology
Obstetrics and Gynecology
Duke University, Durham
NC, USA

Raha Maroyi, MD
Pelvic Trauma Surgeon
Panzi Hospital
Democratic Republic of Congo

Bert Messelink, MD
Urologist
Sexologist Department
Urology Hospital/College Medical Centre
    Leeuwarden City
Leeuwarden, Holland

Mélanie Morin, PT, PhD
Full Professor and Researcher
School of Rehabilitation
Faculty Medicine and Health Sciences
University of Sherbrooke
Director, Urogynecology Research Laboratory
Research Center of the Centre Hospitalier
University of Sherbrooke, Sherbrooke
Canada

Siv Mørkved, PT, MSc, PhD
Professor, Department of Public Health and Nursing
Norwegian University of Science and Technology
Trondheim, Norway

Denis Mukwege, MD, MA, PhD
Professor, Pelvic Trauma Surgeon
Nobel Prize Laureate
Panzi Hospital
Democratic Republic of Congo

Jessica Nargi, MScPT
Registered Physiotherapist
Advanced Pelvic Physiotherapy Centre
Toronto, Canada

Abdallahi N'Dongo, MD
Gynecologist and Obstetrician
Central Hospital Bagnol-sur-Ceze
Bagnol-sur-Ceze
France

Patricia Newmann, PhD
Lecturer
School of Allied Health and Human Movement
University of South Australia
Adelaide, Australia

Patrizia Pelizzo, MD
Second General Surgery Unit
Regional Hospital of Treviso (Ca' Foncello)
University of Padua (DiSCOG)
Italy

Fernanda Pipitone, MD
Urogynecologist
Department of Obstetrics and Gynecology
Hospital das Clinicas/University of Sao Paulo
Sao Paulo, Brazil

Truls Raastad, PhD
Professor
Department of Physical Performance
Norwegian School of Sport Sciences

Ajay Rane, PSM, OAM
Consultant, Urogynaecologist
Head of Obstetrics and Gynaecology
James Cook University
Townsville, Australia

Melita Rotar, MD, DSc
Clinical Institute of Clinical Neurophysiology
University Medical Centre Ljubljana
Ljubljana, SVN

Giulio A. Santoro, MD, PhD
Head, Tertiary Referral Pelvic Floor Center
II°Division of Surgery
AULSS2 Marca Trevigiana, University of Padua
Treviso, Italy

Usama Shahid, MD
Urogynaecology Fellow
James Cook University
Townsville, Australia

Signe Nilssen Stafne, PT, PhD
Physiotherapist, Specialized in Women's Health, MNFF
Department of Clinical Services
St. Olavs Hospital, Trondheim University Hospital
Trondheim, Norway

Abdul Hameed Sultan, FRCOG
Department of Obstetrics and Gynaecology
Croydon University Hospital
Croydon, UK

Merete Kolberg Tennfjord, PhD
Associate Professor
School of Health Sciences
Department of Health and Training
Kristiania University College
Oslo, Norway

Marijke Van Kampen, PT, MSc, PhD
Professor Emeritus, KU Leuven
Department of Rehabilitation Sciences
Faculty of Kinesiology and Rehabilitation Sciences
Leuven, Belgium

Philip EV. Van Kerrebroeck, MD, PhD, MMSc
Professor Emeritus of Urology
University of Maastricht
Maastricht, The Netherlands

David B. Vodušek, MD, PhD, FEAN
Emeritus Professor of Neurology
Consultant, Institute for Clinical Neurophysiology
Division of Neurology
University Medical Centre Ljubljana
Ljubljana, Slovenia

Adrian Wagg, MB, BS
Professor of Healthy Ageing
Department of Medicine
University of Alberta
Edmonton, Alberta
Canada

Jean F. Wyman, PhD
Professor and Cora Meidl Siehl Chair in Nursing
    Research Emerita
University of Minnesota School of Nursing
Minneapolis, MN
USA

Evidence-Based Physical Therapy for the Pelvic Floor is the name of the third edition of this standard in physical therapy.

Pelvic physiotherapy is first-line treatment for most of the pelvic floor disorders, of which most are the result of childbirth trauma in women. Since these female pelvic floor disorders are globally widespread, it is of utmost importance to give women the chance to access this primary care. As president of the International Urogynecological Association (IUGA), it is my task to spread our vision, which is to improve the lives of all women with pelvic floor disorders, at all stages of life, through providing excellent healthcare. This book contributes to our vision. And IUGA's mission is advancement of urogynecological knowledge and patient care through education and promotion of basic and clinical research on disorders of the female pelvic floor globally. This new edition again emphasizes the importance of the evidence-base of physical therapy. The authors did an excellent job and the editor(s) lived up to promise the existing evidence.

This is a very commendable job of all who contributed to this edition. It is only then that we can disseminate knowledge in an ethical manner. This edition covers all aspects of pelvic floor disorders, including stress urinary incontinence, overactive bladder symptoms, pelvic organ prolapse, sexual dysfunction, childbirth trauma, defecatory disorders and pain. Sexual violence and pain are important issues that are addressed in this edition. Though the majority of pelvic floor disorders are seen in females, the authors capture the male pelvic floor as well.

Authors are all key experts in their field, and they have done their work properly. The Editors need no further introduction for their track record in seeking the evidence of research in physical therapy of the pelvic floor.

It is an honor to write this foreword, and I like to thoroughly recommend this new edition!

Alfredo L Milani, MD, PhD
President, International Urogynecological
Association, 2023-24

With pleasure and pride, I write this foreword for the latest edition of this important reference on evidence-based physical therapy for the pelvic floor. This book has been written by many key experts in this field and provides a comprehensive and structured overview of the subject. The basic principles are reviewed — in particular, the important issue of evaluating the evidence through randomized trials and systematic reviews of these data, describing the functional anatomy of the female pelvic floor, the neuroanatomy and neurophysiology of the pelvic floor, and how this interacts with the associated structures in the urinary and colorectal systems.

Accurate assessment of the pelvic floor muscle function is essential, as is defining the anatomical defects; these topics are covered in detail.

The next important aspect, having defined structure and function, is to consider the disorders associated with dysfunction of the pelvic floor in both the male and the female, and how this dysfunction relates to the underlying and associated symptom complex that we see affecting urinary, colorectal, and sexual function.

Pelvic floor dysfunction is of particular importance not only in female patients but also in many male patients with associated pathology, following trauma or after surgery, or after certain neurogenic diseases. In addition, in children, pelvic floor physiotherapy can be very helpful and efficient. It is a particular problem in older patients as well as in patients with neurological disorders and in very fit patients such as elite athletes, in whom the pelvic floor is particularly stressed.

This excellent overview of the subject concludes with the importance of developing clinically meaningful practice guidelines.

I can thoroughly recommend this superb book, which is particularly relevant, not only to those with an interest in sourcing information in this area but also as a reference guide for experts.

Professor John Heesakkers, MD, PhD, MBA
Secretary-General of the International
Continence Society

PREFACE

It is with great pleasure and excitement that we present the third edition of our book Evidence-based Physical Therapy for the Pelvic Floor: Bridging Science and Clinical Experience. We are very happy to introduce several new chapters and also new authors in this edition: Electromyography, Pudendal Neuralgia and Other Intrapelvic Nerve Entrapments, Obstetric Anal Sphincter Injuries, Evidence for Pelvic Floor Muscle Training for Pelvic Organ Prolapse Related to the Peripartum, Evidence for Pelvic Floor Muscle Training for Anal Incontinence Related to the Peripartum Period, Female Genital Fistula, Constipation: Prevalence, Causes and Pathophysiology, Pain Physiology, Conservative Therapies to Treat Pelvic Floor Pain in Males, The Prevalence and Consequences of Sexual Violence to the Pelvic Floor, Gynaecological Cancer and Pelvic Floor Dysfunction, and Evidence of Mobile Apps: Where Do We Stand and Where Should We Go? We are especially proud to welcome Nobel Peace Prize Laureate Dr. Dennis Mukwege and his team among our new authors, bringing important, thought-provoking and necessary attention to this very sad and devastating area of women's health.

It is our hope this new updated edition again will attract all physical therapists and other health professions interested in the broad area of function and dysfunction of the pelvic floor. The editors of this book have more than 30 years of experience in clinical practice and clinical research in the prevention, assessment and treatment of symptoms of pelvic floor dysfunctions. Between us, our experience covers most areas of physical therapy for the pelvic floor, from children, women and men to special groups such as pregnant and postpartum women, athletes, the elderly and patients with special health problems. In addition, we have extensive background in other areas of physical therapy, such as sports physiotherapy, neurology, rehabilitation, musculo-skeletal, ergonomics, exercise science, health promotion, biomechanics, motor control and learning, and implementation of guidelines.

Management of pelvic floor dysfunctions is truly a multidisciplinary field in which every (health) profession should play its own evidence-based role for the highest benefit of patients. With this in mind, we are very proud that so many leading international clinicians, researchers and opinion leaders from different professions have participated in the realization of this book. Our sincere and warmest thanks to all of you for your unique contribution and the time and effort you have put in to making this book a truly evidence-based and up-to-date textbook.

We sincerely hope to have created a special and important book for the physical therapy profession for pelvic floor dysfunction. We anticipate that it will be useful for physical therapy schools and will be found in scientific libraries worldwide. Moreover, it is our hope that this book will become the base for postgraduate studies in pelvic floor physical therapy. In addition, it is our hope that the multidisciplinary nature of the authorship of this book will be reflected in the readership, serving all relevant health professionals, such as gynaecologists, urologists, proctologists, rehabilitation doctors, nurses, midwives and others working in conservative treatment and pelvic floor muscle training, as well as those in the physical therapy field.

As in the medical profession, clinical practice of physical therapy for pelvic floor dysfunctions has built up from a base of clinical experience, through small experimental studies to clinical trials. Today, clinicians can build on protocols from high-quality randomized clinical trials (RCTs) showing sufficient effect size (the difference between the change in the intervention group and the change in the control group). A quick search on PEDro (the Physiotherapy Evidence Database, Sydney, Australia, https://pedro.org.au) shows that physical therapy has changed rapidly from being a non-scientific field to a profession with a strong scientific platform. In November 2022, there were more than 56,000 RCTs, systematic reviews and evidence-based clinical practice guidelines in different areas of physical therapy listed in the database. Although this book recognizes that much more research is needed in the prevention, assessment and treatment of many conditions in the pelvic floor area, there are already more than 100 RCTs evaluating the effect of pelvic floor muscle training for stress, mixed and urgency urinary incontinence. Hence, in good clinical practice, the physical therapist should adapt individual patient training programmes according to the protocols from these studies rather than using theories or models which are not backed by clinical data. In addition, good clinical practice should always be individualized and should be based on a combination of clinical experience, knowledge from high-quality RCTs and patient preferences. However, the strongest and first direction is always to search and use protocols that have proven to be effective. Next to this, good clinical practice should always be based on respect, empathy and strong ethical grounding.

In 2001, Lewis Wall, professor of urogynecology, wrote an editorial in the International Urogynecology Journal describing seven stages in the life of medical innovations:

1. Promising report, clinical observation, case report, short clinical series
2. Professional and organizational adoption of the innovation
3. The public accepts the innovation—state or third party pays for it
4. Standard procedure—into textbooks (still no critical evaluation)
5. **RCT!**
6. Professional denunciation
7. Erosion of professional support, discredit

He stated that by the time stage 7 is concluded, or even before the RCT has started, the procedure may already have given way to a new procedure or method which has grown in its wake. This cycle continues with these new methods and procedures being prescribed to patients without patients being informed about the effect, risk factors or complications. It is also noteworthy that, in most cases, patients are unaware of the fact that there is no scientific base for the proposed treatment. Although Wall's description of the lifecycle applies specifically to medical innovations, we are subject to the same scrutiny and criticism in physical therapy.

Physical therapy modalities, in comparison with surgery, rarely produce serious side effects or complications; however, we suggest that Wall's seven stages may also be very useful to show how different theories, and not science, impact on physical therapy practice. We are keenly aware and concerned that in the long run such unscientific evolution of practice will damage patients, the physical therapy profession itself and parties responsible for compensation. In particular, the use of such untested models and theories as a background for implementing new interventions when there is proven evidence available for treatment strategies must be considered bad clinical practice—and may even be considered unethical. Hence, it is our hope that this book will be a big step towards evidence-based practice in all symptom areas of pelvic floor dysfunction.

This does not mean that we should not treat conditions for which there are no or only few/weak controlled studies to support clinical practice. However, we sincerely believe that all physical therapists should be aware of the different levels and value of statements, theories, clinical experience, knowledge from research designs other than RCTs and knowledge from high-quality research. It is a duty to openly explain to patients and other parties that the proposed treatment is not based on high-quality studies, but only on the best available knowledge and/or experience at that time. The profession should never confuse statements, clinical experience and theories with evidence from high-quality RCTs, and optimally, we should not use new modalities in regular clinical practice until they have proved to be effective in RCTs. In this book, we have tried our best to differentiate between the different levels of knowledge and evidence and to be very clear about the limitations of the research underlying the recommendations for practice. In line with this, we have left out those areas that were not convincing because of lack of evidence. These areas include:

- The role or effect of pelvic floor muscle training on core stability to prevent/treat low back and pelvic girdle pain
- The effect of 'functional training' on pelvic floor dysfunctions
- The role of motor control training as the sole treatment of pelvic floor dysfunction
- The definition, assessment and treatment for hypertone/overactive pelvic floor
- The effect of body posture on the pelvic floor
- The effect of breathing on the pelvic floor

Our aim is to continue updating the evidence in all areas of research in pelvic floor physical therapy. Therefore, it is our hope that the next edition will already include more areas because of the continuing growth of knowledge based on high-quality research.

The evidence presented in this book is based on reviews from the Cochrane Library, the International

Consensus Meetings on Incontinence (ICI), the National Institute for Health and Care Excellence (NICE) guidelines, other systematic reviews and updated searches on newer RCTs. However, the conclusions of these high-quality systematic reviews can differ because they are a product of how the authors have posed their research questions, what type of studies they have included, what choice of outcome measures they have made and how they have classified the studies. Therefore, not all conclusions in this book are in line with other conclusions. The goal of the editors of this book is to evaluate only clinically relevant research questions. Moreover, our selection procedure and strategy for the inclusion and exclusion of studies should be transparent and easy to understand for the readers of the book.

Active exercise is the core of physical therapy interventions. Passive treatments may be used to stimulate non-functioning muscles and to manage pain so that active exercise becomes possible. The following is a quote from Hippocrates (460-377 BC) which elegantly lends itself to the philosophy of physical therapy:

All parts of the body which have a function, if used in moderation and exercised in labors in which each is accustomed, become thereby healthy, well-developed and age more slowly, but if unused and left idle they become liable to disease, defective in growth, and age quickly.

It is the role of the physical therapist to motivate patients and to facilitate exercise and adapted physical activity throughout the lifespan.

It is our hope that new students in this exciting and interesting field will find enough guidance in this book to begin to prevent, assess and treat pelvic floor dysfunction effectively in their clients/patients, but they must also learn to be critical of new theories and modalities that have not yet been tested sufficiently. For experienced physical therapists, it is our hope that providing contemporary scientific evidence to support or contradict clinical practice will effect changes in clinical practice and will push for more high-quality clinical research projects. Hopefully, you will enjoy reading the book just as much as we have enjoyed working with it. Through working on the book, we have certainly become aware of many unanswered questions, and we have identified many new research areas that need to be addressed in this challenging area. We encourage the readers interested in research to continue with formal education in research methodology (MSc and PhD programs) and join us in trying to make high-quality clinical research in the future. We appreciate any constructive feedback for chapters to be changed or included for the next edition.

Kari Bø, Professor, PhD, PT, Exercise Scientist
Bary Berghmans, Associate Professor, Researcher, PhD, PT, Clinical Epidemiologist, Health Scientist
Marijke Van Kampen, Professor Emeritus, PhD, PT
Siv Mørkved, Professor, PhD, PT

Overview of Physical Therapy for Pelvic Floor Dysfunction

Kari Bø

PELVIC FLOOR DYSFUNCTION

The framework of this book is based on the approach to disorders of the pelvic floor in women described by Wall and DeLancey (1991), who stated that 'pelvic floor dysfunction, particularly as manifested by genital prolapse and urinary or faecal incontinence, remains one of the largest unaddressed issues in women's health care today' (p. 486). In their opinion, lack of success in treating patients with pelvic floor dysfunction is due to a professional 'compartmentalization' of the pelvic floor.

Each of the three outlets in the pelvis has had its own medical specialty, with the urethra and bladder belonging to the urologist, the vagina and female genital organs belonging to the gynaecologist, and the colon and rectum belonging to the gastroenterologist and the colorectal surgeon (Fig. 1.1).

Wall and DeLancey (1991) argue that instead of concentrating on the three 'holes' in the pelvis, one should look at the 'whole pelvis', with the pelvic floor muscles (PFMs), ligaments and fasciae as the common supportive system for all of the pelvic viscera.

The interaction between the PFMs and the supportive ligaments was later elaborated by DeLancey (1993) and Norton (1993) as the 'boat in dry dock theory'. The ship is analogous to the pelvic organs, the ropes

to the ligaments and fasciae, and the water to the supportive layer of the PFMs (Fig. 1.2). DeLancey (1993) argues that as long as the PFMs function normally, the pelvic floor is supportive and the ligaments and fascia are under normal tension. When the PFMs relax or are damaged, the pelvic organs must be held in place by the ligaments and fasciae alone. If the PFMs cannot actively support the organs, over time the connective tissue also will become stretched and damaged.

Bump and Norton (1998) used this theoretical framework in their overview of the epidemiology and natural history of pelvic floor dysfunction. They suggested that pelvic floor dysfunction may lead to conditions such as:
- urinary incontinence (stress, urge and mixed incontinence),
- faecal incontinence,
- pelvic organ prolapse (POP),
- sensory and emptying abnormalities of the lower urinary tract,
- defecatory dysfunction,
- sexual dysfunction, and
- chronic pain syndromes.

Bump and Norton (1998) described three stages in the development of pelvic floor dysfunction:
1. A perfect pelvic floor that is anatomically, neurologically and functionally normal.

2. A less than perfect but well-compensated pelvic floor in an asymptomatic patient.
3. A functionally decompensated pelvic floor in the patient with end-stage disease, with urinary incontinence, anal incontinence or POP.

A model describing aetiological factors possibly leading to or causing pelvic floor dysfunction in women has been developed, classifying the factors into:

- predisposing factors (e.g., gender, genetic, neurological, anatomical, collagen, muscular, cultural and environmental),

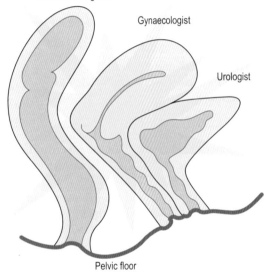

Fig. 1.1 Gynaecologists, urologists and colorectal surgeons concentrate on their areas of interest and tend to ignore the pelvic floor common to them all.

- inciting factors (e.g., childbirth, nerve damage, muscle damage, radiation, tissue disruption, radical surgery),
- promoting factors (e.g., constipation, occupation, recreation, obesity, surgery, lung disease, smoking, menstrual cycle, infection, medication, menopause), and
- decompensating factors (e.g., ageing, dementia, debility, disease, environment, medications).

In 2008 DeLancey et al. further developed this model to what they named the *integrated lifespan model*. They described a graphical tool to integrate pelvic floor function related to pelvic floor disorders in three major phases: (1) development of functional reserve during an individual's growth, (2) variations in the amount of injury and potential recovery that occur during and after vaginal birth, and (3) deterioration occurring with advancing age. The authors suggest that this model should be used to focus on more refined preventive strategies of pelvic floor dysfunction risk in an individual woman as opposed to more general recommendations for all women (DeLancey et al., 2008).

Wall and DeLancey (1991) argued that progress in the treatment of pelvic floor dysfunction in women would occur more rapidly if a unified, cross-disciplinary approach to disorders of the pelvic support was developed. Wall and DeLancey (1991) mentioned only the different medical professions as part of a multidisciplinary team. In this book we will argue that physical therapists (PTs), having assessment and treatment of the musculoskeletal system in general as their specialty, should be core professionals in a multidisciplinary approach to pelvic floor dysfunction.

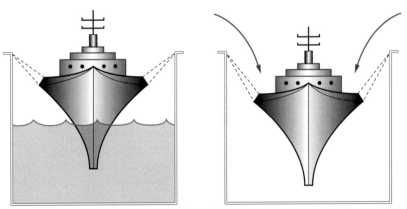

Fig. 1.2 The 'boat in dry dock' analogy. *(Reproduced with permission from Norton, 1993.)*

PHYSICAL THERAPY FOR THE PELVIC FLOOR

The Nature of Physical Therapy

In May 1999, at the 14th General Meeting of the World Confederation for Physical Therapy (WCPT), a position statement describing the nature and process of physical therapy/physiotherapy was approved by all member nations (WCPT, 1999). This description will be used as a foundation and framework to give an overview of physical therapy/physiotherapy in pelvic floor dysfunction. The term *physical therapy* will be used throughout this book in accordance with the guidelines of the WCPT Europe.

According to the WCPT, physical therapy is 'providing services to people and populations to develop, maintain and restore maximum movements and functional ability throughout the lifespan'. The main area of practice for PTs is musculoskeletal pain and dysfunction. However, many PTs also specialize in other areas, such as the cardiorespiratory field, neurology and coronary disease. In all areas, PTs aim to improve functional capacity and improve patients' ability to maintain or increase their physical activity level.

The PFMs are not responsible for gross motor movements alone but work in synergy with other trunk muscles. Therefore, pelvic floor dysfunction may lead to symptoms during movement and perceived restriction in the ability to stay physically active (Bø et al., 1989; Nygaard et al., 1990). For example, several studies have shown that urinary incontinence may lead to a change in movement patterns during physical activities (Bø et al., 1989; Nygaard et al., 1990), withdrawal from regular fitness activities and troublesome difficulties when being active (Brown and Miller, 2001; Nygaard et al., 1990).

Lifelong participation in regular moderate physical activity is important in the prevention of several diseases and is an independent factor in the prevention of osteoporosis, obesity, diabetes mellitus, high blood pressure, coronary heart disease, breast and colon cancer, depression and anxiety (Bouchard et al., 1993; Pedersen and Saltin, 2015; Physical Activity Guidelines Advisory Committee, 2018).

In addition, limitations in the ability to move or conduct activities of daily living either due to age or injuries may also lead to other problems, such as secondary incontinence. Physical therapy for pelvic floor dysfunction may therefore also include physical activities for increasing general function and fitness level.

> *Physical therapy includes the provision of services in circumstances where movement and function are threatened by the process of ageing or that of injury or disease.*
>
> *WCPT (1999)*

Hippocrates (5th to 4th centuries BC) claimed that 'all parts of the body which have a function, if used in moderation and exercised in labours in which each is accustomed, become thereby healthy, well-developed and age more slowly, but if unused and left idle they become liable to disease, defective in growth, and age quickly'.

The PFMs are subject to continuous strain throughout the lifespan. In particular, the pelvic floor of women is subject to tremendous strain during pregnancy and childbirth (DeLancey et al., 2008; Mørkved, 2003). In addition, hormonal changes may influence the pelvic floor and pelvic organs, and a decline in muscle strength may occur due to ageing. Hence, the PFMs may need regular training to stay healthy throughout life.

> *Physical therapy is concerned with identifying and maximizing movement potential, within the spheres of health promotion, prevention, treatment and rehabilitation.*
>
> *WCPT (1999)*

PTs may promote PFM training (PFMT) by writing about the issue in newspapers, in women's magazines and on social media, and by informing their regular patients about PFMT, including PFMT in regular exercise classes and particularly in antenatal and postnatal training, as well as before and after pelvic surgery in men and women. PTs who treat pelvic floor dysfunction should be fully trained in this specialty or should refer to colleagues who have thorough knowledge to treat patients according to the principles of evidence-based physical therapy (Frawley et al., 2018).

> *Physical therapy is an essential part of the health services delivery system. PTs practice independently of other healthcare providers and also within interdisciplinary rehabilitation/habilitation programmes for the restoration of optimal function and quality of life in individuals with both loss and disorders of movement.*
>
> *WCPT (1999)*

Physical therapy work is usually set up by referral from medical practitioners, but in many countries PTs themselves are primary contact practitioners. Both systems require good collaboration between the medical and physical therapy professions.

The referral system implies that the medical practitioner is aware of what the PT can offer, and has PTs available to send referrals to. One of the weaknesses of this system is that medical practitioners who are not motivated or who have insufficient knowledge about the evidence for different physical therapy interventions will not send suitable patients to physical therapy. The patients will more likely be offered traditional medical treatment options such as medication or surgery. These treatments may have adverse effects and are more expensive than exercise therapy (Black and Downs, 1996; Smith et al., 2002). In addition, the referral system is expensive because it involves an extra consultation.

The argument against PTs as primary contact practitioners has been that PTs do not have enough education to make differential diagnoses and may therefore not detect more serious diseases such as cancer or neurological disease underlying the symptoms. With no active referral from the medical professions, there has also been concern that fewer patients would be aware that modalities offered by a physiotherapist are evidence-based treatment options. In addition, since PTs in general have little knowledge of branding and marketing, patients may be more attracted to other parties advocating their practices.

The editors of this book do not take a stand for either system of physical therapy service. We believe that prevention and treatment of pelvic floor dysfunction needs a multidisciplinary approach and would encourage collaboration between physicians and PTs at all levels of assessment and treatment. However, the essence of our approach, as shown in the title of this book, is that in the best interest of patients, only practitioners who work within evidence-based modalities should be part of this collaboration.

Physical therapy involves . . . using knowledge and skills unique to physical therapists and is the service only provided by or under the direction and supervision of a physical therapist.

WCPT (1999)

The educational standard of PTs differs between countries throughout the world. However, in most countries PTs can continue with a master's degree and a doctoral degree.

Physical therapy schools are within the university in many countries, but in other countries physical therapy is taught in polytechnic schools or colleges below university level.

There can be different educational requirements for entry into undergraduate programmes within one country and from country to country. In most countries, however, physical therapy is a professional education and the entry level for physical therapy undergraduate studies is quite high, in some countries being at the same level as medicine. In the area of pelvic floor dysfunction, traditionally the level of scientific background has been quite high, with several academic professors of physical therapy and many practitioners and researchers with master and doctoral degrees.

However, the emphasis on pelvic floor dysfunction in undergraduate physical therapy curricula varies between countries at both the undergraduate and postgraduate physical therapy level. The broad knowledge of anatomy and physiology, pathophysiology, medical science, clinical assessment and treatment modalities learned by all PTs can be applied to the pelvic floor. Several countries also have postgraduate education programmes for PTs specializing either in women's health or pelvic floor physical therapy with the education level and content varying between countries (Frawley et al., 2018).

The physical therapy process includes assessment, diagnosis, planning, intervention, and evaluation (WCPT, 1999).

Assessment

Assessment includes both the examination of individuals or groups with actual or potential impairments, functional limitations, disabilities or other conditions of health by history taking, screening and the use of specific tests and measures, and evaluation of the results of examination through analysis and synthesis within a process of clinical reasoning.

WCPT (1999)

In patients with pelvic floor dysfunction, after thorough history taking, the PT will assess the function of the pelvic floor by visual observation, vaginal palpation and/or measurement of muscle activity (measurement of vaginal or urethral squeeze pressure using evaluation modalities like manometry, dynamometry, electromyography

[EMG] and ultrasound/magnetic resonance imaging [MRI]) (Bø and Sherburn, 2005).

Diagnosis

In carrying out the diagnostic process, physical therapists may need to obtain additional information from other professionals.

WCPT (1999)

Most PTs in private practice obtain referrals of patients from general practitioners. These medical practitioners themselves seldom have access to urodynamics, EMG or ultrasound/MRI.

A diagnosis of stress or urgency incontinence or pelvic pain syndrome can often not be based on history taking alone (Abrams et al., 2002; Haylen et al., 2010). Therefore, interdisciplinary collaborations with other professionals with access to urodynamic testing such as urogynaecologists and urologists are highly recommended. In real life, most PTs in private practice treat patients who have not undergone a thorough diagnostic investigation.

DeLancey (1996) has suggested that the cure and improvement rates of PFMT would be higher for stress urinary incontinence (SUI) if more detailed knowledge about the pathophysiology of each patient was available.

Planning

A plan of intervention includes measurable outcome goals negotiated in collaboration with the patient/client, family or caregiver. Alternatively, it may lead to referral to another agency in cases which are inappropriate for physical therapy.

WCPT (1999)

It is extremely important that the patient decides the final goal of the treatment. For example, not all women need to be totally dry during jumping because they may never perform this activity.

One goal for an elderly woman might be to be able to lift her grandchild without leaking or feeling heaviness or bulging from a POP. If she is able to contract the PFMs with a certain degree of strength, this may be quite easy to accomplish with proper instruction of pre-contraction of the PFMs before and during lifting.

Another woman may have the goal of being totally dry or having good organ support while playing tennis (Bø, 2004a). To achieve this, she may need much more

intensive PFMT because she needs to build up muscle volume and stiffness of the pelvic floor to prevent opening and excessive downward movement during increase in intra-abdominal pressure or a high ground reaction force (Bø, 2004b).

Considering that most PTs treat patients with pelvic floor dysfunction without a full diagnosis, it is of utmost importance that they communicate with other medical professions if they discover discrepancies between expected outcomes or suspect other underlying conditions to be the cause of the patient's complaints. For example, urgency and urgency incontinence may be the first signs of neurological diseases such as multiple sclerosis.

Intervention

In general, physical therapy intervention is implemented and modified to reach agreed goals and may include manual handling; movement enhancing; physical, electro-therapeutic and mechanical agents; functional training (muscle strength and endurance, coordination, motor control, body awareness, flexibility, relaxation, cardiorespiratory fitness); provision of aids and appliances; patient/client related instruction and counseling; documentation and coordination; and communication.

WCPT (1999)

In treating pelvic floor dysfunction, the mainstay of physical therapy is education about the dysfunction, information regarding lifestyle interventions, manual techniques and PFMT (Bø et al., 2017).

PFMT can be taught with or without the use of biofeedback or other adjunctive therapies, such as electrical stimulation or mechanical agents. It includes teaching of the correct contraction, muscle and body awareness, coordination and motor control, muscle strength and endurance, and relaxation.

The PT will choose different treatment programmes for different conditions and different patients. In some cases the PT will also provide preventive devices to the patients and teach them how to use them. Interventions may also be aimed at preventing impairments, functional limitations, disability and injury, and include the promotion and maintenance of health, quality of life, and fitness in all ages and populations. To prevent urinary incontinence, teaching pelvic floor exercises in pregnancy and after childbirth is essential.

The choice of interventions should always be based on the highest level of evidence available. Ideally, the PT will choose the protocol from a randomized controlled trial (RCT) where the intervention has been shown to be effective and adjust this to the patient's needs and practical requirements (Bø and Herbert, 2009). Unfortunately, not all exercise protocols have been explained with sufficient details enabling clinicians to use them directly. There are attempts to improve the details in reporting the interventions, and hopefully this will change to the better in future publications (Slade et al., 2016).

In the area of SUI, there is sufficient knowledge from RCTs to choose an effective training protocol. However, in other conditions that may be caused by pelvic floor dysfunction such knowledge is not yet available. The PT then has to develop a programme on the basis of clinical experience (his or her own, or that of other experts), small experimental studies or theories. It is essential that such experience or theories are quickly developed into research hypotheses and tested in RCTs by trained researchers to see if there is a clinically worthwhile effect (Bø and Herbert, 2009). It is important that the PT is honest and informs the patient about the evidence level of the treatment offered. To be a health professional implies only to market evidence-based practices.

Collaboration between experienced clinicians and researchers is extremely important in planning clinical research. Experienced clinicians should not jump at new theories and ideas or change their practice based on theories and small experimental studies alone. Ideally, the only information that should lead to a drastic change of clinical practice is results (positive or negative) from RCTs (Bø and Herbert, 2009).

When undertaking research and deciding on a physical therapy intervention, the PT must be aware that the 'quality of the intervention', particularly the intensity of the physical therapy intervention, will affect the outcome. Ineffective (low-dose) or even harmful treatments can be used in an RCT that has high-quality methodology (Hoogeboom et al., 2020). These research challenges are the same when conducting RCTs that include both surgery and PFMT, and the methodological quality of studies of both surgery and PFMT has been variable (Dmochowski et al., 2013; Dumoulin et al., 2018; Hay-Smith et al., 2011).

When participating in research led by other professionals, it is important that the physical therapy intervention meets quality standards (Hoogeboom et al., 2020). No drug company would dream of conducting a study with a non-optimal dosage of the drug. In published RCTs, there are several PFMT programmes with low dosage showing little or no effect (Hay-Smith et al., 2011; Herbert and Bø, 2005).

Evaluation

Evaluation necessitates re-examination for the purpose of evaluating outcomes.

WCPT (1999)

Using the same outcome measures before and after treatment is mandatory for the purpose of evaluating outcomes in clinical practice.

In treating symptoms of pelvic floor dysfunction, the PT uses different forms of PFMT (independent variable in experimental research) to change the condition (named *dependent variable* in experimental research, e.g., stage of POP, pelvic pain or SUI).

It is mandatory that PTs use the concept of the International Classification of Impairments, Disabilities and Handicaps (ICIDH) (1997), later changed to the International Classification of Functioning, Disability and Health (ICF) (2002), to evaluate efficacy of the intervention. The ICF is a World Health Organization (WHO)-approved system designed to classify health and health-related states. According to this system, different health components are related to specific diseases and conditions:

- body functions: physiological and psychological functions of body systems (e.g., delayed motor latency of the nerves to the PFM),
- body structures: anatomical parts (e.g., rupture or atrophy of the PFM),
- impairments: problems in body function or structure such as significant deviation or loss (e.g., weak or non-coordinated PFM),
- activity: execution of a task or action by an individual (e.g., to stay continent during increase in abdominal pressure),
- participation: involvement in a life situation (being able to participate in social situations like playing tennis or aerobic dancing without fear or embarrassment of leaking), and
- environment (e.g., easy access to the bathroom).

Physical therapy aims to improve factors involving all of these components. Therefore we need to select different outcome measures for different components. For example,

PFMT may improve timing of the co-contraction during cough (ICF: body functions, neurophysiology). This may be measured by wire or needle EMG.

One of the aims for PFMT in treating POP is to alter the length/stiffness of the PFMs so that they sit at a higher anatomical location inside the pelvis (ICF: body structure, anatomy). This may be measured using MRI or ultrasound.

Impairment of the PFMs can result from inability to produce optimal strength (force) or possessing a low tonicity. Muscle strength can be measured by manometers or dynamometers during attempts of maximal contraction. Resting muscle tone can be measured with surface EMG.

Ambulatory urodynamics of urethral pressure during physical activities may be developed as a future measure of automatic co-contraction during activity.

Urinary leakage could be classified as disability in the ICIDH and as activity in the new ICF system. The actual leakage can be measured by the number of leakage episodes (self-report) or pad tests.

Physical therapy also aims at, for example, reducing urinary leakage to a point where this is no longer restricting the patient from participation in social activities (ICF: participation). This can be measured by quality-of-life questionnaires. PTs can also work politically to improve the environment, such as advocating for easy access to toilets in public buildings.

Ideally, PTs should assess the effect of the physical therapy intervention in all of these components using outcome measures with high responsiveness (measurement tools that can detect small differences), reliability (intra- and inter-tester reproducibility) and validity (to what degree the measurement tool measures what it is meant to measure). The WCPT states that PTs should 'use terminology that is widely understood and adequately defined' and 'recognize internationally accepted models and definitions'.

In the area of pelvic floor dysfunction, we are fortunate to have international committees working on standardization and terminology. The International Continence Society (ICS) constantly revises its standardization of terminology (Abrams et al., 2002), and the Clinical Assessment Group within the same society has also delivered a standardization document (https://www.ics.org). There are many working group documents from the International Urogynecological Association (IUGA) and the ICS (e.g., Bø et al. [2017], D'Ancona et al. [2019], Rogers et al. [2018] and more on the way; see webpages of the ICS and IUGA for further information on published and upcoming standardization documents).

PTs must refer to definitions and terminology from the WHO, WCPT, ICS and IUGA and for definitions and standards developed in exercise science and motor learning and control to be able to communicate effectively with other professions.

Linking Research and Practice

Emphasise the need for practice to be evidence-based whenever possible . . . [and] appreciate the interdependence of practice, research and education within the profession.

WCPT (1999)

Sackett et al. (2000) defined evidence-based medicine as 'the conscientious, explicit and judicious use of current best evidence in making decisions about care of individual patients'. Neither the best available external clinical evidence (RCTs) nor clinical expertise alone is good enough for decision making in clinical practice. Without clinical experience, 'evidence' can ignore the individual's needs and circumstances, and without evidence, 'experience' can become old-fashioned/out of date.

Evidence-based physical therapy practice has a theoretical body of knowledge, uses the best available scientific evidence in clinical decision making and uses standardized outcome measures to evaluate the care provided (Herbert et al., 2005).

Herbert et al. (2005) stated that research conducted as part of routine clinical practice can be prone to bias because there is often a lack of comparison of outcomes with outcomes of randomized controls. In such studies, it may be difficult to distinguish between effects of intervention and natural recovery or statistical regression. In addition, self-reported outcomes may be biased because patients may feel obliged to the therapist. There may be no record or follow-up of drop-outs, outcome measures may be distorted by assessors' expectations of intervention, adherence to the training protocol is seldom reported and long-term results are often not available. The best evidence of effects of an intervention comes from randomized trials with adequate follow-up and blinding of assessors and, where possible, blinding of patients.

Our understanding of the mechanisms of therapies is often incomplete, and it is unknown whether the effects of some physical therapy interventions are large enough to be worthwhile (effect size).

Only high-quality clinical research (RCTs) potentially provides unbiased estimates of the effect size (Herbert, 2000a,b). This provides several challenges in clinical practice.

To increase their level of knowledge in clinical practice, PTs need to:

- stay updated in pathophysiology;
- use interventions for which we have evidence-based knowledge of dose–response issues;
- if possible, use interventions/protocols based on results/protocols from high-quality RCTs with positive results (clinically relevant effect size);
- use pre- and post-treatment tests that are responsive, reliable and valid; and
- measure adherence and adverse effects.

ROLE OF THE PHYSICAL THERAPIST IN PELVIC FLOOR DYSFUNCTION

The PT has multiple roles:

- working in a team with other health professionals (e.g., general practitioner, urologist, gynaecologist, urogynaecologist, radiologist, midwife and nurse),
- evaluating the degree of pelvic floor dysfunction symptoms and complaints and overall condition by covering all components of the ICF,
- fully evaluating PFM performance, including ability to contract, resting condition and strength,
- setting individual treatment goals and plan treatment programmes in collaboration with the patient,
- treating the condition individually and/or conduct PFM exercise classes, and
- teaching preventive PFM exercises individually or in classes during pregnancy and postnatally.

Clinicians without a research background can participate in high-standard research as deliverers of high-quality physical therapy and conduct evaluation of the intervention. They should, however, refuse to be involved in studies with low-quality methodology and/or low-quality intervention (e.g., inadequate dosage).

PTs with a research background should:

- conduct basic research on tissue adaptation to different treatment modalities;
- participate in the development of responsive, reliable and valid tools to assess PFM function and strength and outcome measures; and
- conduct high-quality methodological and interventional RCTs to evaluate effect of different physical therapy interventions.

REFERENCES

Abrams, P., Cardozo, L., Fall, M., et al. (2002). The standardization of terminology of lower urinary tract function: report from the standardization sub-committee of the International Continence Society. *Neurourology and Urodynamics, 21*, 167–178.

Black, N. A., & Downs, S. H. (1996). The effectiveness of surgery for stress urinary incontinence in women: A systematic review. *British Journal of Urology, 78*, 487–510.

Bø, K. (2004a). Urinary incontinence, pelvic floor dysfunction, exercise and sport. *Sports Medicine, 34*(7), 451–464.

Bø, K. (2004b). Pelvic floor muscle training is effective in treatment of stress urinary incontinence, but how does it work? *International Urogynecology Journal and Pelvic Floor Dysfunction, 15*, 76–84.

Bø, K., Frawley, H. C., Haylen, B. T., et al. (2017). An International Urogynecological Association (IUGA)/International Continence Society (ICS) joint report on the terminology for the conservative and nonpharmacological management of female pelvic floor dysfunction. *Neurourology and Urodynamics, 36*, 221–244.

Bø, K., & Herbert, R. (2009). When and how should new therapies become routine clinical practice? *Physiotherapy, 95*, 51–57.

Bø, K., Mæhlum, S., Oseid, S., et al. (1989). Prevalence of stress urinary incontinence among physically active and sedentary female students. *Scandinavian Journal of Sports Science, 11*(3), 113–116.

Bø, K., & Sherburn, M. (2005). Evaluation of female pelvic-floor muscle function and strength. *Physical Therapy, 85*(3), 269–282.

Bouchard, C., Shephard, R. J., & Stephens, T. (1993). *Physical activity, fitness, and health. Consensus Statement.* Champaign, IL: Human Kinetics Publishers.

Brown, W., & Miller, Y. (2001). Too wet to exercise? Leaking urine as a barrier to physical activity in women. *Journal of Science and Medicine in Sport, 4*(4), 373–378.

Bump, R. C., & Norton, P. A. (1998). Epidemiology and natural history of pelvic floor dysfunction. *Obstetrics and Gynecology Clinics of North America, 25*(4), 723–746.

D'Ancona, C. D., Haylen, B. T., Oelke, M., et al. (2019). An International Continence Society (ICS) report on the terminology for adult male lower urinary tract and pelvic floor symptoms and dysfunction. *Neurourology and Urodynamics, 38*(2), 433–477.

DeLancey, J. O. (1993). Anatomy and biomechanics of genital prolapse. *Clinical Obstetrics and Gynecology, 36*(4), 897–909.

DeLancey, J. O. (1996). Stress urinary incontinence: where are we now, where should we go? *American Journal of Obstetrics and Gynecology, 175*, 311–319.

DeLancey, J. O. L., Low, L. K., Miller, J. M., et al. (2008). Graphic integration of causal factors of pelvic floor disorders: an integrated life span model. *American Journal of Obstetrics and Gynecology, 199*(6), 610.

Dmochowski, R., Athanasiou, S., Reid, F., et al. (2013). Committee 14. Surgery for urinary incontinence in women. In P. Abrams, L. Cardozo, S. Khoury, et al. (Eds.), *Incontinence: Fifth international consultation on incontinence* (pp. 1307–1376). Netherlands: European Association of Urology, Arnheim.

Dumoulin, C., Cacciari, L. P., & Hay-Smith, E. J. C. (2018). Pelvic floor muscle training versus no treatment, or inactive control treatments, for urinary incontinence in women. *Cochrane Database of Systematic Reviews.* 10, Art. No. CD005654.

Frawley, H. C., Neumann, P., & Delany, C. (2018). An argument for competency-based training in pelvic floor physiotherapy practice. *Physiotherapy Theory and Practice, 35*(12), 1117–1130.

Haylen, B. T., de Ridder, D., Freeman, R. M., et al. (2010). An International Urogynecological Association (IUGA)/ International Continence Society (ICS) joint report on terminology for female pelvic floor dysfunction. *International Urogynecology Journal and Pelvic Floor Dysfunction, 21*, 5–26.

Hay-Smith, E. J. C., Herderschee, R., Dumoulin, C., et al. (2011). Comparisons of approaches to pelvic floor muscle training for urinary incontinence in women. *Cochrane Database of Systematic Reviews.* 12, Art. No. CD009508.

Herbert, R. D. (2000a). Critical appraisal of clinical trials. I: estimating the magnitude of treatment effects when outcomes are measured on a continuous scale. *The Australian Journal of Physiotherapy, 46*, 229–235.

Herbert, R. D. (2000b). Critical appraisal of clinical trials. II: estimating the magnitude of treatment effects when outcomes are measured on a dichotomous scale. *The Australian Journal of Physiotherapy, 46*, 309–313.

Herbert, R. D., Jamtvedt, G., Mead, J., et al. (2005). *Practical Evidence-Based Physiotherapy.* Oxford: Elsevier.

Herbert, R. D., & Bø, K. (2005). Analysis of quality of interventions in systematic reviews. *BMJ, 331*, 507–509.

Hoogeboom, T. J., Kousemaker, M. C., van Meeteren, N. L. U., et al. (2020). The i-CONTENT tool for assessing therapeutic quality of exercise programs employed in randomised clinical trials. *British Journal of Sports Medicine, 55*(20), bjsports-2019-101630.

Mørkved, S. (2003). *Urinary incontinence during pregnancy and after childbirth. Effect of pelvic floor muscle training in prevention and treatment.* Trondheim, Norway: Doctoral thesis. NTNU.

Norton, P. (1993). Pelvic floor disorders: The role of fascia and ligaments. *Clinical Obstetrics and Gynecology, 36*(4), 926–938.

Nygaard, I., DeLancey, J. O. L., Arnsdorf, L., et al. (1990). Exercise and incontinence. *Obstetrics and Gynecology, 75*, 848–851.

Pedersen, B. K., & Saltin, B. (2015). Exercise as medicine— evidence for prescribing exercise as therapy in 26 different chronic diseases. *Scandinavian Journal of Medicine & Science, 25*(Suppl. 3), 1–72.

Physical Activity Guidelines Advisory Committee. (2018). *2018 Physical Activity Guidelines Advisory Committee Scientific Report.* Washington, DC: US Department of Health and Human Services.

Rogers, R. G., Pauls, R. N., Thakar, R., et al. (2018). An International Urogynecological Association (IUGA)/ International Continence Society (ICS) joint report on the terminology for the assessment of sexual health of women with pelvic floor dysfunction. *Neurourology and Urodynamics, 37*(4), 1220–1240.

Sackett, D., Straus, S., Richardson, W., et al. (2000). *Evidence-Based Medicine: How to Practice and Teach EBM* (second ed.). London: Churchill Livingstone.

Slade, S. C., Dionne, C. E., Underwood, M., et al. (2016). Consensus on Exercise Reporting Template (CERT): modified delphi study. *Physical Therapy, 96*(10), 1514–1524.

Smith, T., Daneshgari, F., Dmochowski, R., et al. (2002). Surgical treatment of incontinence in women. In P. Abrams, L. Cardozo, S. Khoury, et al. (Eds.), *Incontinence: Second international consultation on incontinence* (pp. 823–863). Plymouth, UK: Health Publication/Plymbridge Distributors.

Wall, L., & DeLancey, J. (1991). The politics of prolapse: a revisionist approach to disorders of the pelvic floor in women. *Perspectives in Biology and Medicine, 34*(4), 486–496.

World Conference of Physical Therapy (WCPT). (1999). *Description of physical therapy. 14th general meeting.* Yokohama, Japan: World Confederation of Physical Therapy.

World Health Organization. (1997). *International classification of impairments, disabilities and handicaps (ICIDH).* Zeist, Netherlands: World Health Organization.

World Health Organization. (2002). *International classification of functioning, disability and health (ICF).* Geneva: World Health Organization.

2

Critical Appraisal of Randomized Trials and Systematic Reviews of the Effects of Physical Therapy Interventions for the Pelvic Floor

Rob Herbert

OUTLINE

In Chapter 1, Kari Bø described her vision of physical therapy for the pelvic floor. A core part of that vision is that practice should be guided by evidence in the form of high-quality clinical research. This chapter develops that theme by considering one specific sort of evidence: evidence about the effects of interventions. The chapter begins by identifying the sorts of evidence that tell us about the effects of intervention. It then explores how readers of the research literature can differentiate between high- and low-quality evidence. The chapter concludes by briefly considering how high-quality evidence of the effects of intervention can be used to assist clinical decisions.

RANDOMIZED TRIALS AND SYSTEMATIC REVIEWS

Randomized Trials

Randomized trials (also called randomized *clinical* trials or randomized *controlled* trials [RCTs]) are used to estimate the effects of interventions. They involve sampling people (trial 'subjects' or 'participants') from clinical populations who either have a health disorder (in studies of treatment) or are at risk of a health disorder (in studies of prevention). The key feature of randomized trials is that each participant in the trial is randomly allocated either to a group that receives the intervention of interest or a group that does not receive the intervention. The group of participants that does not receive the intervention is often called the *control group*. The effect of the intervention is determined by comparing the outcomes of participants in the intervention and control groups.

There are several variations of this broad approach (Herbert et al., 2022). In some trials, participants in both groups receive standard care but participants in one group additionally receive the intervention of interest. In another variation, one group receives the intervention of interest and the other group receives a different intervention. All of these variations can be referred to as randomized trials.

Randomized trials differ from other types of studies of the effects of intervention because in randomized trials there is comparison between outcomes of people randomized to groups that do and do not receive a particular intervention. Randomization makes it possible to separate out the effects of intervention from other factors that influence clinical outcomes, such as the natural history of a condition, or statistical phenomena such as statistical regression. A simple way of thinking of the logic of randomized trials is as follows (see Herbert [2020a] for a more nuanced rationale): randomization generates groups that are likely to have similar characteristics, especially when the groups are large. So when we give the intervention of interest to one group and not the other, differences in the outcomes of the two groups cannot be attributable to differences in the groups' characteristics but must instead be attributable to the intervention. A complication is that, because randomization produces groups with similar but not identical characteristics, small differences in outcomes could be due to differences in the groups' characteristics at baseline. (This is true even if methods such as stratified random allocation are used [Herbert, 2005].) The difference between the outcomes of the two groups in a randomized trial provides an estimate of the effect of intervention. Statistical methods can be used to assess how much the estimated effect of intervention could be distorted by chance differences between groups at baseline.

Importantly, randomization is the *only* completely satisfactory way to generate two groups that we can know are comparable (have similar characteristics). For this reason, only randomized trials can ensure a 'fair comparison' between intervention and control groups. (Some empirical evidence suggests that well-conducted non-randomized trials often produce results similar to randomized trials [Benson and Hartz, 2000; Concato et al., 2000; but see Kunz and Oxman, 1998], but there is no reason we should *expect* that to be so.)

Systematic Reviews

Many physical therapy interventions, including several interventions for the pelvic floor, have been subjected to multiple randomized trials. Where more than one trial has examined the effects of the same intervention, we can potentially learn more from a careful examination of the totality of evidence provided by all relevant randomized trials than from any individual trial. Potentially we can get more information about the effects of an intervention from literature reviews than from individual studies.

Until a few decades ago, reviews of the literature were conducted in an unsystematic way. Authors of reviews would find what they considered to be relevant trials, read them carefully and write about the findings of those trials. The authors of the best reviews were able to differentiate between high- and low-quality trials to bring together a balanced synthesis that fairly reflected what existing trials said about the effects of the intervention.

Traditional (narrative) reviews have always had one important shortcoming: their methods are inscrutable. It is difficult for readers of narrative reviews to know if the review was carried out optimally. Readers cannot determine, without specific knowledge of the literature under review, whether the reviewer identified all of the relevant trials and properly weighted the findings of high- and low-quality studies. In addition, readers usually cannot know how the reviewer went about drawing together the findings of the relevant trials to synthesize the review's conclusions. There must always be some concern that the evidence provided in narrative reviews is biased by selective reporting of studies, unbalanced assessment of trial quality or partial interpretations of what the best trials mean.

The method of *systematic* reviews was developed in the late 1970s to overcome some of the shortcomings of narrative reviews (Hunt, 1997). The most important characteristic of systematic reviews is that they explicitly describe the methods used to conduct the review. Systematic reviews typically have a Methods section that describes how the search was conducted, how trials were selected, how data were extracted and how the data were used to synthesize the findings of the review. Thus, in systematic reviews, the methods are transparent. This means that the reader can make judgements about how well the review was conducted. Most systematic reviews attempt to minimize bias by attempting to find all relevant trials, or at least a representative subset of the relevant trials. In addition, predetermined criteria are used to assess the quality of trials, and to draw together the findings of individual trials to generate an overall conclusion (Box 2.1).

What Can't Randomized Trials and Systematic Reviews Tell Us?

Theoretically, randomized trials could provide us with estimates of the effects of every physical therapy intervention and every component of every physical therapy intervention. In practice, we are a long way from that position, and it is likely that we will never get there. That is because randomized trials are cumbersome instruments. They are able to provide unbiased estimates of the effects of interventions, but they do so at a cost. Many trials enroll hundreds or even thousands of participants and follow them for months or years. The magnitude of this undertaking means that it is not possible to conduct trials to examine the effects of every permutation of every component of every intervention for every patient group.

In practice, therefore, the best that randomized trials can provide us with is indicative estimates of the average effects of typical interventions administered in a small subset of reasonable ways to typical populations, even though we usually expect that when the intervention is applied in clinical settings its effects will vary depending on precisely how the intervention is administered and precisely who the intervention is administered to.

Randomized trials can suggest treatment approaches, but the fine detail of how interventions are implemented will always have to be informed by clinical experience, by our understandings of how the intervention works and by common sense.

In recent years, attempts have been made to develop research methods that allow researchers to 'personalize' estimates of treatment effect (see Nguyen et al. [2020] and Künzel et al. [2019] for good examples) and to generalize the findings of trials to other contexts (Bareinboim and Pearl, 2016; Dahabreh and Hernán, 2019). However, these methods are still in their infancy and have not yet been widely adopted by clinical trialists.

Randomized trials and systematic reviews of randomized trials are suited to answering questions about the effects of interventions but are not able to answer other sorts of questions. For example, different sorts of designs are required to answer questions about the prognosis of a particular condition or about the interpretation of a diagnostic test (Herbert et al., 2022).

A major limitation of randomized trials is that the methods developed for analysing randomized trials can only be applied to quantitative measures of outcomes. But it is not possible to quantify the full complexity of people's thoughts and feelings with quantitative measures (Herbert and Higgs, 2004). If we want to understand how people experience an intervention we need to consult studies that employ qualitative methods, such as focus groups or in-depth interviews, rather than randomized trials. In general, qualitative methods cannot tell us about the effects of intervention, but because they can tell us about people's experiences of intervention, they can inform decisions about whether or not to intervene in a particular way.

How Can the Evidence Be Located, and How Much Evidence Is There?

Several databases can be used to locate randomized trials and systematic reviews of the effects of intervention.

PubMed indexes the general health literature and can be accessed free of charge at https://www.pubmed.gov. A particularly helpful subsite—PubMed Clinical Queries (https://pubmed.gov/clinical/)—provides an efficient way to find randomized trials and systematic reviews.

CENTRAL (https://www.cochranelibrary.com/central), a resource produced by the Cochrane Collaboration, specifically indexes randomized trials and is free in many countries. (To see a list of countries from which

CENTRAL can be accessed free of charge, click on the Help tab and follow the link to Access Options.)

The only database that specifically indexes randomized trials and systematic reviews of physical therapy interventions is PEDro. It is freely available at https://www.pedro.org.au. In December 2020 a quick search of the PEDro database for records indexed as relevant to the 'perineum or genitourinary system' yielded 1373 randomized trials and 331 systematic reviews.

Dimensions of Quality of Randomized Trials and Systematic Reviews

Randomized trials and systematic reviews vary greatly in quality. There are high-quality studies that have been carefully designed, meticulously conducted and rigorously analysed, and there are low-quality studies that have not! Physical therapists must be able to differentiate between high- and low-quality studies if they are to be able to discern the real effects of intervention.

A key characteristic of high-quality randomized trials and systematic reviews is that they are relatively *unbiased*. In other words, they do not systematically underestimate or overestimate effects of intervention. Another important characteristic of trials and reviews is their *relevance* to clinical practice. If trial and reviews are to be useful, they must tell us about the effects of interventions when administered well to appropriate patients, and about the effects of the intervention on outcomes that are important. Finally, we would like trials and reviews to provide us with *precise estimates* of the size of treatment effects. The precision of the estimates is primarily a function of the sample size (the number of subjects in a trial or the number of subjects in all studies in a review). Thus the highest-quality trials and reviews, those that best support clinical decision making, are large, unbiased and relevant.

The following sections consider how readers of trials and reviews can assess these aspects of quality in randomized trials and systematic reviews.

DETECTING BIAS IN TRIALS AND REVIEWS

Detecting Bias in Randomized Trials

When we read reports of randomized trials we would like to know if the trials are biased or not. Another way of saying this is that we need to assess the 'internal validity' of the trials.

One way to assess internal validity is to see how well the trial has been designed. Over the past 50 years, methodologists have refined the methods used to conduct randomized trials to the extent that there is now consensus, at least with regard to the main features of trial design, about what constitutes best practice in the design of clinical trials (Moher et al., 2001; Pocock, 1984). This suggests that we could assess internal validity of individual trials by examining how well their methods correspond to what is thought to be best practice in trial design.

Alternatively, we could base judgements about the validity of trials on empirical evidence of bias. Several studies have shown that, all else being equal, certain design features are associated with larger estimates of the effects of intervention (e.g., Chalmers et al., 1983; Colditz et al., 1989; Moher et al., 1998; Page et al., 2016; Schulz et al., 1995). This has been interpreted as indicating that these design features are markers of bias, although there are alternative interpretations (Herbert, 2020b).

Potentially we could use either of these approaches: we could base decisions about the validity of trials either on expert opinion or empirical evidence. There is much debate about which is the best way to assess validity. But fortunately both approaches suggest that trial validity should be assessed by looking for the presence of similar features of trial design (Box 2.2).

Random Allocation

There are theoretical reasons to believe that true random allocation reduces the possibilities for bias (Berger, 2005; Rubin, 1974), and some empirical evidence supports this position (Kunz and Oxman, 1998). It is important that a random, as distinct from haphazard, process is used. In practice, random allocation sequences are almost always computer generated.

If the random allocation sequence is to result in true random allocation of trial participants to groups, it is necessary that any person who recruits patients into the

---

BOX 2.2 **Key Features Conferring Validity to Clinical Trials**

- True (concealed) random allocation of participants to groups
- Blinding of participants and assessors
- Adequate follow-up

trial is unaware, at the time he or she makes decisions about whether or not to admit a patient into the trial, which group the patient would subsequently be allocated to. Similarly, it is important that patients do not know, prior to choosing to participate in the trial, which group they would be allocated to if they were to participate in the trial. This is referred to *concealment* of the allocation schedule.

Failure to conceal allocation potentially distorts randomization because experimenters might be reluctant to let patients with the most serious symptoms into the trial if they know that the next-recruited patient is to be allocated to the control group, and patients may be less likely to agree to participate in the trial if they know that they will subsequently be allocated to the control group. This would generate groups that are not comparable at baseline with regard to disease severity, so it introduces potential for serious bias. For this reason, concealment is desirable and is thought to protect against bias in randomized trials.

Of the trials of physical therapy for the pelvic floor listed on the PEDro database, only 32% explicitly conceal the allocation schedule.

Blinding

A second key design feature is blinding. The process of blinding implies that the allocation of each trial participant (whether the participant is in the intervention group or the control group) is hidden from people associated with the trial (including trial participants, the physical therapists administering the intervention and the people assessing trial outcomes).

Blinding of the *participants* in a trial is achieved by giving a sham intervention to subjects in the control group. Sham interventions are interventions that resemble the intervention of interest but which are thought to have no specific therapeutic effect. An example of the use of a sham condition is in the trial by Chang et al. (2011) of acupressure for stress urinary incontinence (SUI). In that trial, participants in the intervention group received conventional acupressure to acupoints, whereas participants in the control (sham) group received light acupressure to sites other than acupoints.

By providing a sham intervention, all trial participants can appear to receive intervention even though only the intervention group receives active intervention. Consequently, trial participants can be 'kept in the dark' about whether they are receiving the intervention or control condition.

The usual justification for blinding trial participants is that this makes it possible to determine if an intervention has more of an effect than just a placebo effect. In other words, it becomes possible to determine if the effect of intervention is due to the specific action of the intervention or effects of non-specific procedures involved in administration of intervention. In so far as placebo effects occur, they are expected to occur to an equal degree in intervention and sham intervention groups, so it is thought that in sham-controlled trials the estimated effect of intervention—the difference between group outcomes—is not influenced by placebo effects.

An additional and perhaps more important justification is that in trials with self-reported outcomes, blinding of participants removes the possibility of bias created by patients misreporting their outcomes. In unblinded trials, patients in the intervention group could exaggerate improvements in their outcomes and patients in the control group could understate improvements in their outcomes, perhaps because they believe that this is what assessors want to hear. When participants are blinded (when they do not know if they received the intervention or control conditions), there should be no difference in reporting tendencies of the two groups, so it is thought that estimates of the effect of intervention (the difference between groups) cannot be biased by differential reporting.

In most trials of physical therapy interventions for the pelvic floor, it is difficult to administer a sham intervention that is both credible and inactive. For example, it is difficult to conceive of a sham intervention for training pelvic floor muscles. In that case the best alternative may be to deliver an inactive intervention to the control group, even if the inactive intervention does not exactly resemble the active intervention. An example is the trial by Dumoulin et al. (2004) that compared pelvic floor rehabilitation (electrical stimulation of pelvic floor muscles plus pelvic floor muscle exercises) with biofeedback. These authors gave the control group relaxation massage to the back and extremities in the belief that this would control, to some degree, the effects of placebo (including the attention paid to trial participants by the therapists) and misreporting of outcomes. Such trials provide some control, but perhaps not complete control, of the confounding effects of placebo and misreporting of outcomes.

The difficulties of providing an adequate sham intervention preclude participant blinding in most trials of physical therapy interventions for the pelvic floor. Only 9% of these trials truly blind participants.

It is also desirable that the *person assessing trial outcomes* is blinded. Blinding of assessors ensures that assessments are not biased by the assessor's expectations of the effects of intervention. When objective outcome measures are used, blinding of assessors is easily achieved by using assessors who are not otherwise involved in the study and are not told about which patients are in the intervention and control groups. However, blinding of assessors is more difficult when trial outcomes are self-reported (e.g., as in studies that ask women whether they 'leak'). In that case the assessment is conducted by the participant, so the assessment is only blinded if the participant is blind.

Theoretically, blinding can provide some protection, but not complete protection, from the bias that arises from beliefs of trial participants or outcome assessors about the allocation of particular trial participants. However, even when blinding is implemented perfectly, beliefs about allocation may still bias the trial's findings (Mathieu et al., 2014).

Follow-Up

A third feature of trial design that is likely to determine a trial's validity is the completeness of follow-up.

In most trials, participants are randomized to groups but, for various reasons, outcome measures are not subsequently obtained from all participants. Such 'loss to follow-up' occurs, for example, when subjects become too ill to be measured, or they die, go on holiday or have major surgery, or because the researchers lose contact with the participant. Loss to follow-up potentially 'unrandomizes' allocation and can produce systematic differences in the characteristics of the two groups, so it potentially biases estimates of the effects of intervention.

How much loss to follow-up is acceptable in a randomized trial? When is loss to follow-up so extreme that it potentially causes serious bias? There is no simple and universally applicable answer to these questions. However, losses to follow-up of less than 10% of randomized subjects are usually considered unlikely to produce serious bias, and losses to follow-up of greater than 20% are often thought be a potential source of serious bias. Fortunately, most trials of physical therapy interventions for the pelvic floor have adequate follow-up: 62% of the relevant trials have less than 15% loss to follow-up.

A related but more technical issue concerns problems with deviations from the trial protocol. Protocol deviations occur when, for example, people do not receive the intervention as allocated (e.g., if participants in an exercise group do not adhere to their exercise programs) or if outcome measures are not measured at the allocated times. This presents a dilemma for the person analysing the data: should data from these subjects be excluded? Should data from subjects who did not receive the intervention be analysed as if those subjects had been allocated to the control group? In most cases the answer to both questions is no!

Most methodologists believe that the best way to deal with protocol violations in randomized trials is to analyse the data as if the protocol violation did not occur (for a nice summary of the arguments, see Fisher et al. [1990], and for a discussion of alternatives, see Schrier et al. [2014]). In this approach, called *analysis by intention to treat* (Hollis and Campbell, 1999), all subjects' data are analysed, regardless of whether the subjects received the intervention as allocated or not, and each subject's data are analysed in the group to which the subject was allocated. (Some researchers also stipulate that an 'analysis by intention to treat' must involve imputation of missing data so that even trial participants with missing data can be included in the analysis. Wood et al. [2004] discuss how this can be done.) Analysis by intention to treat is thought to be the least biased way to analyse trial data in the presence of protocol violations. Of the relevant trials on PEDro, 27% explicitly analyse by intention to treat.

Detecting Bias in Systematic Reviews
The Search Strategy

Systematic reviewers attempt to provide an unbiased summary of the findings of relevant trials. Ideally, systematic reviews would summarize the findings of all relevant trials that had ever been conducted. That would achieve two ends: it would ensure that the reviewer had taken full advantage of all of the information available from all extant trials, and it would mean that the summary of the findings of the trials was not biased by selective retrieval of only those trials with atypical estimates of the effects of the intervention.

Unfortunately, it is usually not possible to find complete reports of all relevant trials: reports of some trials are published in obscure journals, others are published in obscure languages, many are published only in abstract format and some are not published at all. Consequently, even the most diligent reviewers will fail to find some trial reports.

Given that it is usually not possible to find reports of all relevant trials, the next best thing is for reviewers to obtain reports of *nearly all* trials. To this end, most reviewers conduct quite thorough literature searches. For a Cochrane systematic review of pelvic floor muscle training (PFMT) for urinary incontinence in women, Dumoulin et al. (2018) searched, among other sources, the Cochrane Incontinence Group trials register, CENTRAL, Medline and ClinicalTrials.gov (a register of clinical trials), and conducted a page-by-page 'handsearch' of selected journals and conference proceedings. Some reviewers include trials published only as abstract form, whereas others include only full papers on the grounds that most abstracts have not been peer reviewed and often contain too little information to be useful.

Occasionally systematic reviewers conduct limited searches, such as by searching only Medline. This is potentially problematic: even though Medline is the largest database of medical literature, such searches are likely to miss much of the relevant literature. It has been estimated that Medline only indexes between 17% and 89% of all relevant trials (Dickersin et al., 1994; Michaleff et al., 2011).

When reading a systematic review, it is important to check that the literature search in the review is reasonably recent. If a report of a systematic review is more than a few years old, it is likely that several trials will have been conducted since the search was conducted, and the review may provide an out-of-date summary of the literature.

Assessment of Trial Quality and Risk of Bias

Systematic reviewers typically find more than one trial that investigates the effects of a particular intervention, and often the quality of the trials is varied. Obviously it is not appropriate to weight the findings of all trials without regard to trial quality. Particular attention should be paid to the highest-quality trials because these trials are likely to be least biased; the poorest-quality trials should be ignored. Systematic reviews should assess the quality of the trials in the review, and quality assessments should be taken into account when drawing conclusions from the review.

A range of methods have been used to assess the quality of trials in systematic reviews. The most common approach is to use a quality scale to assess quality and then to ignore the findings of trials with low-quality scores. Commonly used scales include the PEDro scale (Maher et al., 2003) and the Cochrane risk of bias tool. A copy of the PEDro scale is shown in Box 2.3. These scales assess quality based on the presence or absence of design features thought to influence validity, including true concealed randomization, blinding of participants and assessors, adequate follow-up and intention-to-treat analysis.

This approach sounds sensible, but there are some reasons to believe that it may discriminate inappropriately between trials. The available evidence suggests that there is only moderate agreement between the ratings obtained with different quality scales (Colle et al., 2002). Nonetheless, it is not known how better to assess trial quality, so these rudimentary procedures must suffice for now. For the time being we should expect systematic reviews to take into account the quality of trials, but we cannot be too discerning about how quality is assessed (Box 2.4).

BOX 2.3   The PEDro Scale

1. Eligibility criteria were specified.
2. Subjects were randomly allocated to groups.
3. Allocation was concealed.
4. The groups were similar at baseline.
5. There was blinding of all subjects.
6. There was blinding of all therapists.
7. There was blinding of all assessors.
8. Measures of outcome were obtained from >85% of subjects.
9. Data were analysed by 'intention to treat'.
10. Between-group statistical comparisons are reported.
11. Point measures and measures of variability are reported.

   More details on this scale are available from https://pedro.org.au/english/learn/faq/.

BOX 2.4   Key Features Conferring Validity to Systematic Reviews

- An adequate search strategy that finds an unbiased subset of nearly all relevant trials.
- The review considers trial quality when drawing conclusions about the effects of intervention.

DETECTING 'SPIN' AND SLOPPY ANALYSIS

Readers of reports of randomized trials and systematic reviews rely on authors to provide an accurate and objective report of their studies. Unfortunately, that does not always occur. Some authors 'spin' the findings of their trials or reviews (e.g., Nascimento et al., 2019; Nascimento et al., 2020)—that is, they make exaggerated claims about the effectiveness of interventions that are not supported by an objective analysis of the data. Another problem is that some researchers lack the statistical expertise needed to analyse their data in a rigorous way, so their statistical analyses are poorly conducted.

There are two ways that the authors of trials and reviews can reassure readers that they have provided an accurate and objective account of their research. The first is by registering the study protocol on a trial registry. (A list of major clinical trial registries is provided at https://www.who.int/clinical-trials-registry-platform/network/primary-registries. The primary registry for systematic reviews is PROSPERO at https://www.crd.york.ac.uk/PROSPERO/.) Registering a study involves specifying, before the study is conducted, the question that the study is designed to answer and the methods that the study will use. Often a link is provided from the registry to the full study protocol. After a study report has been published, it is possible for journal reviewers and careful readers to cross-check the published report against the registered study protocol. Discrepancies between the protocol and the report, such as change to primary outcomes, or changes to statistical methods used to analyse the primary outcome, may be suggestive of spin.

A second way that the authors of trials and reviews can reassure readers of the probity of their research is to provide access to the study data (Herbert, 2008; Taichman et al., 2017). This allows journal reviewers and statistically capable readers to re-analyse the data. The potential to re-analyse data provides a mechanism for detecting poor analyses. Replication of the results in a trial report provides reassurance.

Readers of clinical trial and systematic review reports may not have the time, expertise or inclination either to cross-check study reports against registered protocols or re-analyse study data. Nonetheless, all readers can be reassured by transparent reporting: registered studies which make their data available are generally more trustworthy than studies that are not registered and which do not make their data available for scrutiny.

ASSESSING RELEVANCE OF TRIALS AND SYSTEMATIC REVIEWS

Not all valid trials are useful trials. Some provide valid tests of poorly administered interventions, others provide valid tests of the effects of intervention on inappropriate samples of patients and yet others provide valid tests of the effect of intervention on meaningless outcomes. The following sections consider how the quality of the intervention, the selection of patients and outcomes can influence the *relevance* of randomized trials and systematic reviews.

Quality of Intervention

Randomized trials are most easily applied to pharmacological interventions. In one sense, pharmacological interventions are relatively simple: they involve the delivery of a drug to a patient. Because pharmacological interventions are quite simple, they tend to be administered in quite similar ways in all trials. (One possible exception is the dose of the drug, but toxicity studies, pharmacokinetic studies and dose-finding studies often constrain the range of doses before definitive trials are carried out, so even this parameter is often fairly consistent across studies.) In contrast, many physical therapy interventions are complex. In trials of physical therapy interventions, the intervention is often tailored to the individual patient based on specific examination findings, and sometimes the intervention consists of multiple components, perhaps administered in a range of settings by a range of health professionals. Consequently, a single intervention (e.g., PFMT) may be administered in quite different ways across trials.

Wherever there is the possibility of administering the intervention in a range of ways, we need to consider whether, in a particular trial, the intervention was administered well (Herbert and Bø, 2005). It is reasonable to be suspicious of the findings of trials where the intervention was administered in a way that would appear to be suboptimal.

Criticisms have been leveled against trials because the interventions were administered by unskilled therapists (e.g., Brock et al., 2002) or because the intervention was administered in a way that was contrary to the way in which the intervention is generally administered (e.g., Clare et al., 2004), or because the intervention was not sufficiently intense to be effective (e.g., Ada, 2002; Herbert and Bø, 2005). Such criticisms are sometimes reasonable and sometimes not.

Recently, Hoogeboom et al. (2020) described a new tool, the i-CONTENT tool, for appraising the quality of exercise programs evaluated in randomized trials. The i-CONTENT tool could be used to appraise the quality of exercise programs implemented in randomized trials of PFMT.

Of course, it is impossible to know with any certainty how an intervention should be administered before first knowing how effective the intervention is. Trials must necessarily be conducted before good information is available about how to administer the intervention. Consequently, a degree of latitude ought to be offered to clinical trialists: we should be prepared to trust the findings of trials that test interventions that are applied in ways other than the ways we might choose to apply the intervention, as long as the application of the intervention in the trial was not obviously suboptimal.

Patients

Trials of a particular intervention may be carried out on quite different patient groups. Readers need to be satisfied that the trial was applied to an appropriate group of patients. It could be reasonable to ignore the findings of a trial if the intervention was administered to a group of patients for whom the intervention was generally considered inappropriate. An example might be the application of pelvic floor exercises to reverse prolapse in women who already have complete prolapse of the internal organs. Most therapists would agree that once prolapse is complete, conservative intervention is no longer appropriate and surgical intervention is necessary.

The same caveat applies here: it is impossible to know with certainty, at the time a trial is conducted, for whom an intervention will be most effective. Again we must be prepared to give trialists some latitude: we should be prepared to trust the findings of trials that test interventions on patients other than the patients we might choose to apply the intervention to as long as the patient group was not obviously inappropriate.

Outcomes

The last important dimension of the relevance of a clinical trial concerns the outcomes that are measured. Ultimately, if an intervention for the pelvic floor is to be useful, it must improve quality of life. For example, there is arguably little value in an intervention that increases the strength of pelvic floor muscles if it does not also increase quality of life.

Studies of variables such as muscle strength can help us understand the mechanisms by which interventions work, but they cannot tell us if the intervention is worth doing. The trials that best help us to decide whether or not to apply an intervention are those that determine the effect of intervention on quality of life.

Many trials do not measure quality of life directly, but instead they measure variables that are thought to be closely related to quality of life. For example, Bø et al. (2000) determined the effect of PFMT for women with SUI on the risk of incontinence-related problems with social life, sex life and physical activity. It would appear reasonable to expect that problems with social life, sex life and physical activity directly influence quality of life, so this trial provides useful information with which to make decisions about PFMT for women with SUI.

USING ESTIMATES OF EFFECTS OF INTERVENTION TO MAKE DECISIONS ABOUT INTERVENTION

The most useful piece of information a clinical trial can give us is an estimate of the size of the effects of the intervention. We can use estimates of the effect of intervention to help us decide if an intervention does enough good to make it worth its expense, risks and inconvenience (Herbert, 2000a,b).

Obtaining Estimates of the Effects of Intervention From Randomized Trials and Systematic Reviews

Most people experience an improvement in their condition over the course of any intervention. But the magnitude of the improvement only partly reflects the effects of intervention. People get better, often partly because of intervention, but usually also because the natural course of the condition is one of gradual improvement or because apparently random fluctuations in the severity of the condition tend to occur in the direction of an improvement in the condition. (The latter is called *statistical regression*; for an explanation, see Herbert et al. [2022].) In addition, part of the recovery may be due to placebo effects or to patients politely overstating the magnitude of the improvements in their condition.

As several factors contribute to the improvements that people experience over time, the improvement in the condition of treated patients cannot provide a measure of the effect of intervention. A far better way to estimate the effects of intervention is to determine the magnitude of the difference in outcomes of the intervention and control groups. This is most straightforward when outcomes are measured on a continuous scale. Examples of continuous outcome measurements are pad test weights, measures of global perceived effect of intervention or duration of labour. These variables are continuous because it is possible to measure the amount of the variable on each subject.

An estimate of the mean effects of intervention on continuous variables is obtained simply by taking the difference between the mean outcomes of the intervention and control groups. For example, a study by Bø et al. (1999) compared pelvic floor exercises with a no-exercise control condition for women with SUI. The primary outcome was urine leakage measured using a stress pad test. Over the 6-month intervention period, women in the control group experienced a mean reduction in leakage of 13 g, whereas women in the PFMT group experienced a mean reduction of 30 g. Thus the mean effect of exercise, compared to controls, was to reduce leaking by about 17 g, or about 50% of the initial leakage.

Other outcomes are dichotomous. Dichotomous outcomes cannot be quantified on a scale; they are events that either happen or not. An example comes from the trial by Chiarelli and Cockburn (2002) of a program of interventions designed to prevent postpartum incontinence. Three months postpartum, women were classified as being continent or incontinent. This outcome (incontinent/continent) is dichotomous because it can have only one of two values.

When outcomes are measured on a dichotomous scale we would not normally talk about the mean outcome. Instead, we talk about the risk (or probability) of the outcome; our interest is in how much intervention changes the risk of the outcome.

Chiarelli et al. (2002) found that 125 of the 328 women in the control group were still incontinent at 3 months, and 108 of 348 women in the intervention group were still incontinent at 3 months. Thus the risk of being incontinent at 3 months was 125/328 (38.1%) for women in the control group, and the risk was reduced to 108/348 (31%) in the intervention group. So the effect of the 3-month intervention was to reduce the risk of incontinence at 3 months postpartum by 7.1% (i.e., 38.1%–31%). This figure, the difference in risks, is sometimes called the *absolute risk reduction*. An absolute risk reduction of 7.1% is equivalent to preventing incontinence in one in every 14 women treated with the intervention.

Using Estimates of the Effects of Intervention

Estimates of the effects of intervention can be used to inform the single most important clinical decision: whether or not to apply a particular intervention for a particular patient.

Decisions about whether to apply an intervention need to weigh the potential benefits of intervention against all negative consequences of intervention. So, for example, when deciding whether or not to undertake a program of PFMT, a woman with SUI has to decide if the expected reduction in leakage of about one-half warrants the inconvenience of daily exercise. And when deciding whether to embark on a program to prevent postpartum incontinence, a woman needs to decide whether she is prepared to undertake the program for a 1 in 14 chance of being continent when she otherwise would not be.

USING GRADE TO EVALUATE EVIDENCE AND RECOMMENDATIONS FOR PRACTICE

The preceding pages describe how evidence about the effects of interventions obtained from randomized trials and systematic reviews of randomized trials can be used to support clinical decisions about intervention. Specific consideration was given to how to distinguish between high- and low-quality evidence, how to decide if the evidence is relevant to the clinical decision and how to decide if the effects of an intervention are large enough to make the intervention worthwhile.

The GRADE tool (GRADE Working Group 2005; Guyatt et al., 2008) formalizes these processes. GRADE was initially developed to assist the developers of clinical practice guidelines, but it provides a useful framework for anyone who wants to rigorously evaluate whether a particular health intervention should be recommended for use in clinical practice. The GRADE tool begins by rating the *quality of evidence* of the effect of intervention on each relevant outcome. The quality of evidence is determined by risk of bias, the precision and relevance ('indirectness') of estimates of effect and, when more than one source of evidence is being evaluated, the consistency of the evidence and the likelihood that the evidence is representative of all evidence. In addition, GRADE can be used to rate the strength of recommendations for clinical practice. Recommendations are strongest when there is high-quality evidence, when most patients would judge that the expected benefits outweigh any likely harm and the intervention is cost effective. You can find out more about GRADE at https://www.gradeworkinggroup.org/.

REFERENCES

Ada, L., Commentary on Green, J., Forster, A., Bogle, S. et al., (2002). Physiotherapy for patients with mobility problems more than 1 year after stroke: A randomized controlled trial. (Lancet 359:199–203). *Australian Journal of Physiotherapy*, 48, 318.

Bareinboim, E., & Pearl, J. (2016). Causal inference and the data-fusion problem. *Proceedings of the National Academy of Sciences of the United States of America*, 113, 7345–7352.

Benson, K., & Hartz, A. J. (2000). A comparison of observational studies and randomized, controlled trials. *The New England Journal of Medicine*, 342, 1878–1886.

Berger, V. W. (2005). *Selection bias and covariate imbalances in randomized clinical trials*. Chichester: Wiley.

Bø, K., Talseth, T., & Holme, I. (1999). Single blind, randomized controlled trial of pelvic floor exercises, electrical stimulation, vaginal cones, and no treatment in management of genuine stress incontinence in women. *British Medical Journal*, 318, 487–493.

Bø, K., Talseth, T., & Vinsnes, A. (2000). Randomized controlled trial on the effect of pelvic floor muscle training on quality of life and sexual problems in genuine stress incontinent women. *Acta Obstetricia et Gynecologica Scandinavica*, 79, 598–603.

Brock, K., Jennings, K., Stevens, J., & Picard, S. (2002). The Bobath concept has changed [comment on critically appraised paper, Australian Journal of Physiotherapy 48:59]. *Australian Journal of Physiotherapy*, 48(2), 156.

Chalmers, T. C., Celano, P., Sacks, H. S., et al. (1983). Bias in treatment assignment in controlled clinical trials. *The New England Journal of Medicine*, 309, 1358–1361.

Chang, K. K., Wong, T. K., Wong, T. H., et al. (2011). Effect of acupressure in treating urodynamic stress incontinence: A randomized controlled trial. *The American Journal of Chinese Medicine*, 39, 1139–1159.

Chiarelli, P., & Cockburn, J. (2002). Promoting urinary continence in women after delivery: Randomized controlled trial. *British Medical Journal*, 324, 1241.

Clare, H. A., Adams, R., & Maher, C. G. (2004). A systematic review of efficacy of McKenzie therapy for spinal pain. *Australian Journal of Physiotherapy*, 50, 209–216.

Colditz, G. A., Miller, J. N., & Mosteller, F. (1989). How study design affects outcomes in comparisons of therapy. I: Medical. *Statistics in Medicine*, 8, 441–454.

Colle, F., Rannou, F., Revel, M., et al. (2002). Impact of quality scales on levels of evidence inferred from a systematic review of exercise therapy and low back pain. *Archives of Physical Medicine and Rehabilitation*, 83, 1745–1752.

Concato, J., Shah, N., & Horwitz, R. I. (2000). Randomized controlled trials, observational studies, and the hierarchy of research designs. *The New England Journal of Medicine*, 342, 1887–1892.

Dahabreh, I.J., & Hernan, M.A. (2019). Extending inferences from a randomized trial to a target population. *European Journal of Epidemiology*, 34, 719–722.

Dickersin, K., Scherer, R., & Lefebvre, C. (1994). Systematic reviews: Identifying relevant studies for systematic reviews. *British Medical Journal*, 309, 1286–1291.

Dumoulin, C., Cacciari, L. P., & Hay-Smith, E. J. C. (2018). Pelvic floor muscle training versus no treatment, or inactive control treatments, for urinary incontinence in women. *Cochrane Database of Systematic Reviews*. (10), Art. No. CD005654.

Dumoulin, C., Gravel, D., Bourbonnais, D., et al. (2004). Reliability of dynamometric measurements of the pelvic floor musculature. *Neurourology Urodynamics*, 23, 134–142.

Fisher, L. D., Dixon, D. O., Herson, J., et al. (1990). Intention to treat in clinical trials. In K. E. Peace (Ed.), *Statistical issues in drug research and development* (pp. 331–350). New York.

GRADE Working Group. (2004). Grading quality of evidence and strength of recommendations. *British Medical Journal*, 328, 1490.

Guyatt, G. H., Oxman, A. D., & Vist, G. E. (2008). GRADE: an emerging consensus on rating quality of evidence and strength of recommendations. *British Medical Journal*, 336, 924–926.

Herbert, R. D. (2000a). Critical appraisal of clinical trials. I: Estimating the magnitude of treatment effects when outcomes are measured on a continuous scale. *Australian Journal of Physiotherapy*, 46, 229–235.

Herbert, R. D. (2000b). Critical appraisal of clinical trials. II: Estimating the magnitude of treatment effects when outcomes are measured on a dichotomous scale. *Australian Journal of Physiotherapy*, 46, 309–313.

Herbert, R. D. (2005). Randomisation in clinical trials. *Australian Journal of Physiotherapy*, 51, 58–60.

Herbert, R. D. (2008). Researchers should make data freely available. *Australian Journal of Physiotherapy*, 54, 3.

Herbert, R. D. (2020a). Causal inference: an introduction. *Journal of Physiotherapy*, 66, 273–277.

Herbert, R. D. (2020b). Meta-epidemiological studies of bias may themselves be biased. *Journal of Clinical Epidemiology*, 123, 127–130.

Herbert, R. D., & Bø, K. (2005). Analysing effects of quality of interventions in systematic reviews. *British Medical Journal*, 331, 507–509.

Herbert, R. D., & Higgs, J. (2004). Complementary research paradigms. *Australian Journal of Physiotherapy*, 50, 63–64.

Herbert, R. D., Jamtvedt, G., Mead, J., et al. (2022). *Practical Evidence-Based Physiotherapy* (3rd ed.). Oxford: Elsevier.

Hollis, S., & Campbell, F. (1999). What is meant by intention to treat analysis? Survey of published randomized trials. *British Medical Journal*, 319, 670–674.

Hoogeboom, T. J., Kousemaker, M. C., van Meeteren, N. L., et al. (2020). i-CONTENT tool for assessing therapeutic quality of exercise programs employed in randomised clinical trials. *British Journal of Sports Medicine*, 55(20).

Hunt, M. M. (1997). *How science takes stock: The story of meta-analysis*. New York: Sage.

Kunz, R., & Oxman, A. D. (1998). The unpredictability paradox: review of empirical comparisons of randomized and non-randomized clinical trials. *British Medical Journal*, 317, 1185–1190.

Künzel, S. R., Sekhon, J. S., Bickel, P. J., et al. (2019). Metalearners for estimating heterogeneous treatment effects using machine learning. *Proceedings of the National Academy of Sciences of the United States of America*, 116, 4156–4165.

Maher, C. G., Sherrington, C., Herbert, R. D., et al. (2003). Reliability of the PEDro scale for rating quality of randomized controlled trials. *Physical Therapy*, 83, 713–721.

Mathieu, E., Herbert, R. D., McGeechan, K., et al. (2014). A theoretical analysis showed that blinding cannot eliminate potential for bias associated with beliefs about allocation in randomised clinical trials. *Journal of Clinical Epidemiology*, 67, 667–671.

Michaleff, Z. A., Costa, L. O. P., Moseley, A. M., et al. (2011). CENTRAL, PEDro, PubMed and EMBASE are the most comprehensive databases indexing randomised controlled trials of physiotherapy interventions. *Physical Therapy*, 91, 190–197.

Moher, D., Pham, B., Cook, D., et al. (1998). Does quality of reports of randomized trials affect estimates of intervention efficacy reported in meta-analyses? *Lancet*, 352, 609–613.

Moher, D., Schulz, K. F., & Altman, D. G. (2001). The CONSORT statement: revised recommendations for improving the quality of reports of parallel group randomized trials. *BMC Medical Research Methodology*, 1, 2.

Nascimento, D. P., Costa, L. O. P., Gonzalez, G. Z., et al. (2019). Abstracts of low back pain trials are poorly reported, contain spin of information and are inconsistent with the full text: an overview study. *Archives of Physical Medicine and Rehabilitation*, 100, 1976–1985.

Nascimento, D. P., Gonzalez, G. Z., Araujo, A. C., et al. (2020). Eight out of every ten abstracts of low back pain systematic reviews presented spin and inconsistencies with the full text: an analysis of 66 systematic reviews. *Journal of Orthopaedic & Sports Physical Therapy*, 50, 17–23.

Nguyen, T. L., Collins, G. S., Landais, P., & Le Manach, Y. (2020). Counterfactual clinical prediction models could help to infer individualized treatment effects in randomized controlled trials—an illustration with the International Stroke Trial. *Journal of Clinical Epidemiology*, 125, 47–56.

Page, M. J., Higgins, J. P., Clayton, G., et al. (2016). Empirical evidence of study design biases in randomized trials: systematic review of meta-epidemiological studies. *PLoS One*, 11 e0159267.

Pocock, S. J. (1984). *Clinical trials: A practical approach*. New York: Wiley.

Rubin, D. B. (1974). Estimating causal effects of treatments in randomized and nonrandomized studies. *Journal of Educational Psychology*, 66, 688–701.

Schulz, K., Chalmers, I., Hayes, R., et al. (1995). Empirical evidence of bias: dimensions of methodological quality associated with estimates of treatment effects in controlled trials. *Journal of the American Medical Association*, 273, 408–412.

Shrier, I., Steele, R. J., Verhagen, E., et al. (2014). Beyond intention to treat: what is the right question? *Clinical Trials*, 11, 28–37.

Taichman, D. B., Sahni, P., Pinborg, A., et al. (2017). Data sharing statements for clinical trials—a requirement of the International Committee of Medical Journal Editors. *The New England Journal of Medicine*, 376(23), 2277–2279.

Wood, A. M., White, I. R., & Thompson, S. G. (2004). Are missing data adequately handled? A review of published randomized controlled trials in major medical journals. *Clinical Trials*, 1, 368–376.

3

Functional Anatomy of the Female Pelvic Floor

James A. Ashton-Miller and John O.L. DeLancey

INTRODUCTION

The anatomic structures that prevent incontinence during elevations in abdominal pressure are primarily sphincteric, augmented secondarily by musculofascial supportive systems. In the urethra, for example, the action of the vesical neck and urethral sphincteric mechanisms at rest constrict the urethral lumen and keep urethral closure pressure higher than bladder pressure. The striated urogenital sphincter, the smooth muscle sphincter in the vesical neck and the circular and longitudinal smooth muscle of the urethra all contribute to this closure pressure. In addition, the mucosal and vascular tissues that surround the lumen provide a hermetic seal via coaptation, aided by the connective tissues in the urethral wall. Decreases in the number of striated muscle sphincter fibres occur with age and parity, but changes in the other tissues are not well understood.

A supportive hammock under the urethra and vesical neck provides a firm backstop against which the urethra is compressed during increases in abdominal pressure to maintain urethral closure pressures above the rapidly increasing bladder pressure. This supporting layer consists of the anterior vaginal wall and the connective tissue that attaches it to the pelvic bones through the pubovaginal portion of the levator ani muscle and the uterosacral and cardinal ligaments comprising the tendinous arch of the pelvic fascia.

At rest the levator ani acts to maintain the urogenital hiatus closed in the face of hydrostatic pressure due to gravity and slight abdominal pressurization. During the dynamic activities of daily living the levator ani muscles are additionally recruited to maintain hiatal closure in the face of inertial loads related to having to decelerate caudal movements of the viscera as well as the additional load related to increases in abdominal pressure resulting from activation of the diaphragm and abdominal wall musculature.

Urinary incontinence is a common condition in women, with prevalence ranging from 8.5% to 38% depending on age, parity and definition (Thomas et al., 1980; Herzog et al., 1990). Most women with incontinence have stress urinary incontinence (SUI), not infrequently with urge incontinence (Diokno et al., 1987). Both types of incontinence are primarily due to an inadequate urethral sphincter which develops too little urethral closure pressure to prevent urine leakage (DeLancey et al., 2008, 2010). Usually this is treated using conservative therapy or, if that fails, then surgery. Despite the common occurrence of SUI, there have been few advances in our understanding of its cause in the past 40 years. Most of the many surgical procedures for alleviating SUI involve the principle of improving bladder neck support (Colombo et al., 1994; Bergman & Elia, 1995). Treatment selection based on specific anatomic abnormalities has awaited identification, in each case, of the muscular, neural and/or connective tissues involved.

Understanding how the pelvic floor structure/function relationships provide bladder neck support can help guide treatment selection and effect. For example if, while giving vaginal birth, a woman sustains a partial tear of a portion of her pelvic muscles that influence her continence, then pelvic muscle exercises may be effective.

On the other hand, if portions of those muscles are irretrievably lost, for example due to complete and permanent denervation, then no amount of exercising will restore them; pelvic muscle exercises may well lead to agonist muscle hypertrophy, but whether or not this will restore continence will depend upon whether the agonist muscles can compensate for the lost muscle function.

This chapter reviews the functional anatomy of the pelvic floor structures and the effects of age on urethral support and the urethral sphincter, and attempts to clarify what is known about the different structures that influence stress continence. This mechanistic approach should help guide research into pathophysiology, treatment selection and prevention of SUI. In addition, we also review the structures that resist genital prolapse because vaginal delivery confers a 4- to 11-fold increase in risk of developing pelvic organ prolapse (Mant et al., 1997).

HOW IS URINARY CONTINENCE MAINTAINED?

Urethral closure pressure must be greater than bladder pressure, both at rest and during increases in abdominal pressure, to retain urine in the bladder and prevent leakage. The resting tone of the urethral muscles maintains a

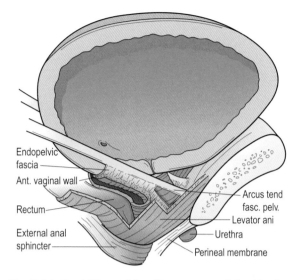

Fig. 3.1 Lateral View of the Components of the Urethral Support System. Note how the levator ani muscles support the rectum, vagina and urethrovesical neck. Also note how the endopelvic fascia beside the urethra attaches to the levator ani muscle; contraction of the levator muscle leads to elevation of the urethrovesical neck. Puborectalis muscle is removed for clarity. (Redrawn from DeLancey 1994, with permission of C V Mosby Company, St Louis. DeLancey)

favorable pressure relative to the bladder when urethral pressure exceeds bladder pressure. The primary factor that determines continence is the maximum urethral closure pressure developed by the urethral sphincter (DeLancey et al., 2008, 2010).

During activities such as coughing, when bladder pressure increases several times higher than urethral pressure, a dynamic process increases urethral closure pressure to enhance urethral closure and maintain continence (Enhörning 1961). Both the magnitude of the resting closure pressure in the urethra and the increase in abdominal pressure generated during a cough determine the pressure at which leakage of urine occurs (Kim et al., 1997).

Although analysis of the degree of resting closure pressure and pressure transmission provides useful theoretical insights, it does not show how specific injuries to individual component structures affect the passive or active aspects of urethral closure. A detailed examination of the sphincteric closure and the urethral support subsystems (Fig. 3.1) is required to understand these relationships.

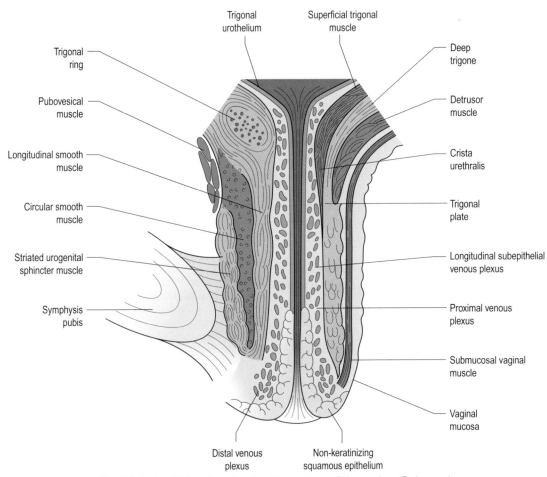

Fig. 3.2 Midsagittal section showing the anatomy of the urethra. (DeLancey)

The dominant element in the urethral sphincter is the striated urogenital sphincter muscle, which contains a striated muscle in a circular configuration in the middle of the urethra and strap-like muscles distally. In its sphincteric portion, the urogenital sphincter muscle surrounds two orthogonally-arranged smooth muscle layers and a vascular plexus that helps to maintain closure of the urethral lumen.

THE URINARY SPHINCTERIC CLOSURE SYSTEM

Sphincteric closure of the urethra is normally provided by the urethral striated muscles, the urethral smooth muscle and the vascular elements within the submucosa (Figs 3.2 and 3.3) (Strohbehn et al., 1996; Strohbehn &

DeLancey, 1997). Each is believed to contribute equally to resting urethral closure pressure (Rud et al., 1980).

Anatomically, the urethra can be divided longitudinally into percentiles, with the internal urethral meatus representing point 0 and the external meatus representing the 100th percentile (Table 3.1). The urethra passes through the wall of the bladder at the level of the vesical neck where the detrusor muscle fibres extend below the internal urethra meatus to as far as the 15th percentile.

The striated urethral sphincter muscle begins at the termination of the detrusor fibres and extends to the 64th percentile. It is circular in configuration and completely surrounds the smooth muscle of the urethral wall.

Starting at the 54th percentile, the striated muscles of the urogenital diaphragm, the compressor urethrae and

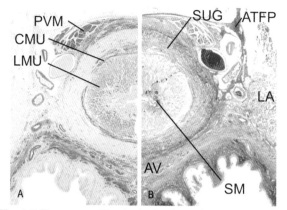

Fig. 3.3 Transverse Histologic Section of the Mid-Urethra of a 21-Year-Old Woman. (A) Structures are visualized using a sigma-actin smooth muscle stain, which shows the pubovesical muscle (PVM), the circumferential smooth muscle (CMU) layer, and the longitudinal smooth muscle (LMU) layer. (B) The contralateral side is stained with Masson's trichrome to show the arcus tendineus fascia pelvis (ATFP), the striated urogenital sphincter (SUG), the levator ani (LA), the anterior vaginal wall (AV), and the submucosa of the urethra (SM). (From Strohbehn et al., 1996, with permission of Lippincott Williams & Wilkins, Baltimore, MD.)

TABLE 3.1   Urethral topography and urethral and paraurethral structures

Percentile of urethral length	Location: Region of the urethra	Structures
0–20	Intramural	Internal urethral meatus Detrusor loop
20–60	Mid-urethra	Striated urethral sphincter muscle Smooth muscle
60–80	Urogenital diaphragm	Compressor urethrae muscle Urethrovaginal sphincter Smooth muscle
80–100	Distal urethra	Bulbocavernosus muscle

the urethrovaginal sphincter can be seen. They are continuous with the striated urethral sphincter and extend to the 76th percentile. Their fibre direction is no longer circular. The fibres of the compressor urethrae pass over the urethra to insert into the urogenital diaphragm near the pubic ramus.

The urethrovaginal sphincter surrounds both the urethra and the vagina (Fig. 3.4). The distal terminus of the urethra runs adjacent to, but does not connect with, the bulbocavernosus muscles (DeLancey 1986).

Functionally, the urethral muscles maintain continence in various ways. The U-shaped loop of the detrusor smooth muscle surrounds the proximal urethra, favoring its closure by constricting the lumen.

The striated urethral sphincter is composed mainly of type 1 (slow-twitch) fibres, which are well suited to maintaining constant tone as well as allowing voluntary increases in tone to provide additional continence protection (Gosling et al., 1981). Distally, the recruitment of the striated muscle of the urethrovaginal sphincter and the compressor urethrae compress the lumen.

The smooth muscle of the urethra may also play a role in determining stress continence. The lumen is surrounded by a prominent vascular plexus that is believed to contribute to continence by forming a watertight seal

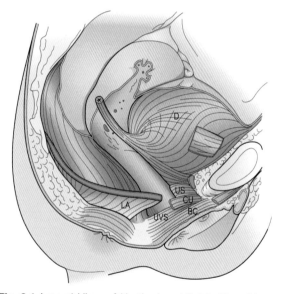

Fig. 3.4 Lateral View of Urethral and Pelvic Floor Muscular Anatomy. BC, bulbocavernosus; CU, compressor urethrae; D, detrusor; LA, levator ani; US, urethral sphincter; UVS, urethrovaginal sphincter. Puborectalis muscle is removed for clarity. (DeLancey)

via coaptation of the mucosal surfaces. Surrounding this plexus is the inner longitudinal smooth muscle layer. This in turn is surrounded by a circular layer, which itself lies inside the outer layer of striated muscle.

The smooth muscle layers are present throughout the upper four-fifths of the urethra. The circular configuration of the smooth muscle and outer striated muscle layers suggests that the contraction of these layers has a role in constricting the lumen. The mechanical role of the inner longitudinal smooth muscle layer is presently unresolved. Contraction of this longitudinal layer may help to open the lumen to initiate micturition rather than to constrict it.

CLINICAL CORRELATES OF URETHRAL ANATOMY AND EFFECTS OF AGING

There are several important clinical correlates of urethral muscular anatomy. Perhaps the most important is that SUI is caused by problems with the urethral sphincter mechanism as well as with urethral support. Although this is a relatively new concept, the supporting scientific evidence is strong.

The usual argument for urethral support playing an important role in SUI is that urethral support operations cure SUI without changing urethral function. Unfortunately, this logic is just as flawed as suggesting that obesity is caused by an enlarged stomach because gastric stapling surgery, which makes the stomach smaller, is effective in alleviating obesity. The fact that urethral support operations cure SUI does not implicate urethral hypermobility as the cause of SUI.

Most studies have shown not only that there is substantial variation in resting urethral closure pressures in normal women compared with those with SUI, but also that the severity of SUI correlates quite well with resting urethral closure pressure.

Loss of urethral closure pressure probably results from age-related deterioration of the urethral musculature as well as from neurologic injury (Hilton & Stanton, 1983; Snooks et al., 1986; Smith et al., 1989a, 1989b). For example, the total number of striated muscle fibres within the ventral wall of the urethra has been found to decrease seven-fold as women progress from 15 to 80 years of age, with an average loss of 2% per year (Fig. 3.5) (Perucchini et al., 2002a).

Because the mean fibre diameter does not change significantly with age, the cross-sectional area of striated muscle in the ventral wall decreases significantly with age; however, nulliparous women seemed relatively protected (Perucchini et al., 2002b). This 65% age-related loss in the number of striated muscle fibres found *in vitro* is consistent with the 54% age-related loss in closure pressure found *in vivo* by Rud et al., 1980,

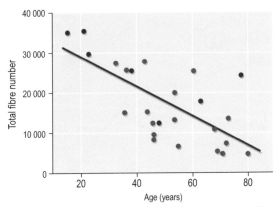

Fig. 3.5 Decrease in Total Number of Striated Muscle Fibres in the Ventral Wall with Age. The red circles denote data from nulliparous women, and the blue circles denote data from parous women. (From Perucchini et al., 2002a, with permission of Lippincott Williams & Wilkins, Baltimore, MD.)

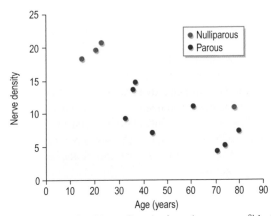

Fig. 3.6 Decreasing Nerve Density (number per mm²) in the Ventral Wall of the Urethra with Age. This is a subgroup of the data in Fig. 3.5 (Perucchini et al., 2002a). The red circles denote data from nulliparous women and the blue circles denote data from parous women. (From Pandit et al., 2000, with permission of Lippincott Williams & Wilkins, Baltimore, MD.)

suggesting that it may be a contributing factor. However, prospective studies are needed to directly correlate the loss in the number of striated muscle fibres with a loss in closure pressure *in vivo*.

It is noteworthy that in our *in vitro* study thinning of the striated muscle layers was particularly evident in the proximal vesical neck and along the dorsal wall of the urethra in older women (Perucchini et al., 2002b). The concomitant seven-fold age-related loss of nerve fibres in these same striated urogenital sphincters (Fig. 3.6) directly correlated with the loss in striated muscle fibres

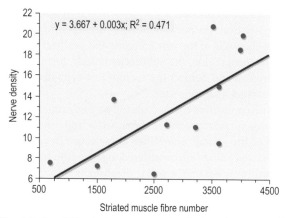

$$y = 3.667 + 0.003x; R^2 = 0.471$$

Fig. 3.7 Correlation between nerve density (number per mm²) and total fibre number in the ventral wall of the urethra. No distinction is made between nulliparous and parous women (Perucchini et al., 2002a). In the equation given for the regression line, y denotes the ordinate, x the abscissa and R^2 the coefficient of variation. (From Pandit et al., 2000, with permission of Lippincott Williams & Wilkins, Baltimore, MD.)

(Fig. 3.7) in the same tissues (Pandit et al., 2000); and the correlation supports the hypothesis of a neurogenic source for SUI and helps to explain why faulty innervation could affect continence.

We believe that the ability of pelvic floor exercise to compensate for this age-related loss in sphincter striated muscle may be limited under certain situations. Healthy striated muscle can increase its strength by about 30% after an intensive 8–12 weeks of progressive resistance training intervention (e.g. Skelton et al., 1995). For example, suppose an older woman had a maximum resting urethral closure pressure of 100 cmH₂O when she was young but it is now 30 cmH₂O due to loss of striated sphincter muscle fibres. If she successfully increases her urethral striated muscle strength by 30% through an exercise intervention and there is a one-to-one correspondence between urethral muscle strength and resting closure pressure, she will only be able to increase her resting closure pressure by 30%, from 30 cmH₂O to 39 cmH₂O, an increment less than one-tenth of the 100 cmH₂O increase in intravesical pressure that occurs during a hard cough. It remains to be determined whether pelvic floor muscle exercise is as effective in alleviating SUI in women with low resting urethral pressures as it can be in women with higher resting pressures, especially for women participating in activities with large transient increases in abdominal pressure.

URETHRAL (AND ANTERIOR VAGINAL WALL) SUPPORT SYSTEM

Support of the urethra and vesical neck is determined by the endopelvic fascia of the anterior vaginal wall through their fascial connections to the arcus tendineus fascia pelvis and connection to the medial portion of the levator ani muscle.

It is our working hypothesis that both urethral constriction and urethral support contribute to continence. Active constriction of the urethral sphincter maintains urine in the bladder at rest. During increases in abdominal pressure, the vesical neck and urethra are compressed to a closed position when the raised abdominal pressure surrounding much of the urethra exceeds the fluid pressure within the urethral lumen (see Fig. 3.1). The stiffness of the supportive layer under the vesical neck provides a backstop against which abdominal pressure compresses the urethra. This anatomic division mirrors the two aspects of pelvic floor function relevant to SUI: urethral closure pressure at rest and the increase in urethral closure caused by the effect of abdominal pressure.

Support of the urethra and distal vaginal wall are inextricably linked. For much of its length the urethra is fused with the vaginal wall, and the structures that determine urethral position and distal anterior vaginal wall position are the same.

The anterior vaginal wall and urethral support system consists of all structures extrinsic to the urethra that provide a supportive layer on which the proximal urethra and mid-urethra rest (DeLancey 1994). The major components of this supportive structure are the vaginal wall, the endopelvic fascia, the arcus tendineus fasciae pelvis and the levator ani muscles (see Fig. 3.1).

The endopelvic fascia is a dense, fibrous connective tissue layer that surrounds the vagina and attaches it to each arcus tendineus fascia pelvis laterally. Each arcus tendineus fascia pelvis in turn is attached to the pubic bone ventrally and to the ischial spine dorsally.

The arcus tendineus fasciae pelvis are tensile structures located bilaterally on either side of the urethra and vagina. They act like the catenary-shaped cables of a suspension bridge and provide the support needed to suspend the urethra on the anterior vaginal wall. Although it is well defined as a fibrous band near its origin at the pubic bone, the arcus tendineus fascia pelvis becomes a broad aponeurotic structure as it passes dorsally to insert into the ischial spine. It therefore appears as a sheet of fascia as it fuses with the endopelvic fascia, where it merges with the levator ani muscles (see Fig. 3.1).

Levator Ani Muscles

The levator ani muscles also play a critical role in supporting the pelvic organs (Halban & Tandler, 1907; Berglas & Rubin, 1953; Porges et al., 1960). Not only has evidence of this been seen in magnetic resonance scans (Kirschner-Hermanns et al., 1993; Tunn et al., 1998) but histological evidence of muscle damage has been found (Koelbl et al., 1998) and linked to operative failure (Hanzal et al., 1993).

There are three basic regions of the levator ani (Kearney et al., 2004) (Figs 3.8 and 3.9):

- the first region is the iliococcygeal portion, which forms a relatively flat, horizontal shelf spanning the potential gap from one pelvic sidewall to the other;

- the second portion is the pubovisceral muscle, which arises from the pubic bone on either side and attaches to the walls of the pelvic organs and perineal body;

- the third region, the puborectal muscle, forms a sling around and behind the rectum just cephalad to the external anal sphincter.

The connective tissue covering on both superior and inferior surfaces are called the superior and inferior fasciae of the levator ani. When these muscles and their associated fasciae are considered together, the combined structures make up the pelvic diaphragm.

The opening within the levator ani muscle through which the urethra and vagina pass (and through which prolapse occurs), is called the urogenital hiatus of the levator ani. The rectum also passes through this opening, but because the levator ani attaches directly to the anus it is not included in the name of the hiatus. The hiatus, therefore, is supported ventrally (anteriorly) by the pubic bones and the levator ani muscles, and dorsally (posteriorly) by the perineal body and external anal sphincter.

The normal baseline activity of the levator ani muscle keeps the urogenital hiatus closed by compressing the

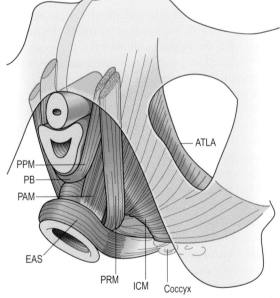

Fig. 3.8 Schematic view of the levator ani muscles from below after the vulvar structures and perineal membrane have been removed showing the arcus tendineus levator ani (ATLA); external anal sphincter (EAS); puboanal muscle (PAM); perineal body (PB) uniting the two ends of the puboperineal muscle (PPM); iliococcygeal muscle (ICM); puborectal muscle (PRM). Note that the urethra and vagina have been transected just above the hymenal ring. (DeLancey)

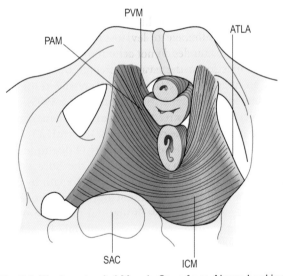

Fig. 3.9 The Levator Ani Muscle Seen from Above Looking Over the Sacral Promontory (SAC) Showing the Pubovaginal Muscle (PVM). The urethra, vagina and rectum have been transected just above the pelvic floor. PAM, puboanal muscle; ATLA, arcus tendineus levator ani; ICM, iliococcygeal muscle. (The internal obturator muscles have been removed to clarify levator muscle origins.) (From Kearney et al., 2004, with permission of Elsevier North Holland, New York. DeLancey)

vagina, urethra and rectum against the pubic bone, the pelvic floor and organs in a cephalic direction (Taverner 1959). This constant activity of the levator ani muscle is analogous to that in the postural muscles of the spine. This continuous contraction is also similar to the continuous activity of the external anal sphincter muscle, and closes the lumen of the vagina in a manner similar to that by which the anal sphincter closes the anus. This constant action eliminates any opening within the pelvic floor through which prolapse could occur.

A maximal voluntary contraction of the levator ani muscles causes the pubovisceral muscles and the puborectalis muscles to further compress the mid-urethra, distal vagina and rectum against the pubic bone distally and against abdominal hydrostatic pressure more proximally. It is this compressive force and pressure that one feels if one palpates a pelvic floor muscle contraction intravaginally. Contraction of the bulbocavernosus and the ventral fibres of the iliococcygeus will only marginally augment this compression force developed by the puboviseral and puborectalis muscles because the former develops little force and the latter is located too far dorsally to have much effect intravaginally.

Finally, maximal contraction of the mid and dorsal iliococcygeus muscles elevates the central region of the posterior pelvic floor, but likely contributes little to a vaginal measurement of levator strength or pressure because these muscles do not act circumvaginally.

When injury to the levator ani occurs it is usually caused by vaginal birth (DeLancey et al., 2003). Biomechanical computer simulations suggest this injury most likely occurs when stretch and tension in the muscle nearest the pubic bone peak near the end of the second stage of labour (Jing et al., 2012). Injuries to the levator ani are associated with genital prolapse (DeLancey et al., 2007) and in the next section we shall discuss why.

Interactions Between the Pelvic Floor Muscles and the Endopelvic Fasciae

The levator ani muscles play an important role in protecting the pelvic connective tissues from excess load. Any connective tissue within the body may be stretched by subjecting it to a tensile force. Skin expanders used in plastic surgery stretch the dense and resistant dermis to extraordinary degrees, and flexibility exercises practised by dancers and athletes elongate leg ligaments. Both these observations underscore the adaptive nature of connective tissue when subjected to repeated tension over time.

If the ligaments and fasciae within the pelvis were subjected to continuous stress imposed on the pelvic floor by the great force of abdominal pressure, they would stretch. This stretching does not occur because the constant tonic activity of the pelvic floor muscles (Parks et al., 1962) closes the urogenital hiatus and carries the weight of the abdominal and pelvic organs, preventing constant strain on the ligaments and fasciae within the pelvis.

The interaction between the pelvic floor muscles and the supportive ligaments is critical to pelvic organ support. As long as the levator ani muscles function to properly maintain closure of the genital hiatus, the ligaments and fascial structures supporting the pelvic organs are under minimal tension. The fasciae simply act to stabilize the organs in their position above the levator ani muscles.

When the pelvic floor muscles relax or are damaged, the pelvic floor opens thereby placing the distal vagina between a zone of high abdominal pressure and the lower atmospheric pressure outside the body. The resulting pressure differential, which acts across the distal vaginal wall much like the wind on a sail, causes it to cup thereby increasing tension in the vaginal wall. This tension pulls the cervix caudally placing the uterine suspensory ligaments under tension and allowing the distal anterior vaginal wall to further cup (Chen et al., 2009). Although the ligaments can sustain these loads for short periods of time, if the pelvic floor muscles do not close the pelvic floor then the connective tissue will eventually fail, resulting in pelvic organ prolapse.

The support of the uterus has been likened to a ship in its berth floating on the water attached by ropes on either side to a dock (Paramore, 1918). The ship is analogous to the uterus, the ropes to the ligaments and the water to the supportive layer formed by the pelvic floor muscles. The ropes function to hold the ship (uterus) in the centre of its berth as it rests on the water (pelvic floor muscles). If, however, the water level falls far enough that the ropes are required to hold the ship without the supporting water, the ropes would break.

The analogous situation in the pelvic floor involves the pelvic floor muscles supporting the uterus and vagina, which are stabilized in position by the ligaments and fasciae. Once the pelvic floor musculature becomes damaged and no longer holds the organs in place, the supportive connective tissue is placed under stretch until it fails.

While the attachment of the levator ani muscles into the perineal body is important, it is uni- or bilateral damage to the pubic origin of this ventral part of the levator ani muscle during delivery that is one of the irreparable injuries to the pelvic floor. Recent magnetic resonance imaging (MRI) has vividly depicted these defects and it has been shown that up to 20% of primiparous women have a visible defect in the levator ani muscle on MRI (DeLancey et al., 2003), with a concomitant loss in levator muscle strength (DeLancey et al., 2007).

It is likely that this muscular damage is an important factor associated with recurrence of pelvic organ prolapse after initial surgical repair. Moreover, these defects were found to occur more frequently in those individuals complaining of SUI (DeLancey et al., 2003). An individual with muscles that do not function properly has a problem that is not surgically correctable.

PELVIC FLOOR FUNCTION RELEVANT TO STRESS URINARY INCONTINENCE

Functionally, the urethral sphincter is primarily responsible for maintaining urinary continence, aided secondarily by interactions between the levator ani muscle and the endopelvic fascia which help maintain continence and provide pelvic support. Impairments usually become evident when the system is stressed.

One such stressor is a hard cough that, driven by a powerful contraction of the diaphragm and abdominal muscles, can cause a transient increase of 150 cmH_2O, or more, in abdominal pressure. This transient pressure increase causes the proximal urethra to undergo a downward (caudodorsal) displacement of about 10 mm in the midsagittal plane that can be viewed on ultrasonography (Howard et al., 2000b). This displacement is evidence that the inferior abdominal contents are forced to move caudally during a cough.

Because the abdominal contents are essentially incompressible, the pelvic floor and/or the abdominal wall must stretch slightly under the transient increase in abdominal hydrostatic pressure, depending on the level of neural recruitment. The ventrocaudal motion of the bladder neck that is visible on ultrasonography indicates that it and the surrounding passive tissues have acquired momentum in that direction. The pelvic floor then needs to decelerate the momentum acquired by this mass of abdominal tissue.

The resulting inertial force causes a caudal-to-cranial pressure gradient in the abdominal contents, with the greatest pressure arising nearest the pelvic floor. While the downward momentum of the abdominal contents is being slowed by the resistance to stretch of the pelvic floor, the increased pressure compresses the proximal intra-abdominal portion of the urethra against the underlying supportive layer of the endopelvic fasciae, the vagina, and the levator ani muscles.

We can estimate the approximate resistance of the urethral support layer to this displacement. The ratio of the displacement of a structure in a given direction to a given applied pressure increase is known as the compliance of the structure.

If we divide 12.5 mm of downward displacement of the bladder neck (measured on ultrasonography) during a cough by the transient 150 cmH_2O increase in abdominal pressure that causes it, the resulting ratio (12.5 mm divided by 150 cmH_2O) yields an average compliance of 0.083 mm/cmH_2O in healthy nullipara (Howard et al., 2000b). In other words, the cough displaces the healthy intact pelvic floor 1 mm for every 12 cmH_2O increase in abdominal pressure. (Actually, soft tissue mechanics teaches us to expect ever smaller displacements as the abdominal pressure increments towards the maximum value.)

The increase in abdominal pressure acts transversely across the urethra, altering the stresses in the walls of the urethra so that the anterior wall is deformed toward the posterior wall, and the lateral walls are deformed towards one another, thereby helping to close the urethral lumen and prevent leakage due to the concomitant increase in intravesical pressure.

If pelvic floor exercises lead to pelvic floor muscle hypertrophy, then the resistance of the striated components of the urethral support layer can be expected to also increase. This is because the longitudinal stiffness and damping of an active muscle are linearly proportional to the tension developed in the muscle (e.g. Blandpied & Smidt, 1993); for the same muscle tone, the hypertrophied muscle contains more cross-bridges in the strongly-bound state (across the cross-sectional area of the muscle) and these provide greater resistance to stretch of the active muscle.

If there are breaks in the continuity of the endopelvic fascia (Richardson et al., 1981) or if the levator ani muscle is damaged, the supportive layer under the urethra will be more compliant and will require a smaller pressure increment to displace a given distance.

Howard et al., (2000b) showed that compliance increased by nearly 50% in healthy primipara to 0.167 mm/cmH$_2$O and increased even further in stress-incontinent primipara by an additional 40% to 0.263 mm/cmH$_2$O. Thus, the supportive layer is considerably more compliant in these incontinent patients than in healthy women; it provides reduced resistance to deformation during transient increases in abdominal pressure so that closure of the urethral lumen cannot be ensured and SUI becomes possible.

An analogy that we have used previously is attempting to halt the flow of water through a garden hose by stepping on it (DeLancey, 1990). If the hose was lying on a noncompliant trampoline, stepping on it would change the stress in the wall of the hose pipe, leading to a deformation and flattening of the hose cross-sectional area, closure of the lumen and cessation of water flow, with little indentation or deflection of the trampoline. If, instead, the hose was resting on a very compliant trampoline, stepping on the hose would tend to accelerate the hose and underlying trampoline downward because the resistance to motion (or reaction force) is at first negligible, so little flattening of the hose occurs as the trampoline begins to stretch. While the hose and trampoline move downward together, water would flow unabated in the hose. As the resistance of the trampoline to downward movement increasingly decelerates the downward movement of the foot and hose, flow will begin to cease. Thus, an increase in compliance of the supporting tissues essentially delays the effect of abdominal pressure on the transverse closure of the urethral lumen, allowing leakage of urine during the delay.

Additionally, the constant tone maintained by the pelvic muscles relieves the tension placed on the endopelvic fascia. If the nerves to the levator ani muscle are damaged (such as during childbirth) (Allen et al., 1990), the denervated muscles would atrophy and leave the responsibility of pelvic organ support to the endopelvic fascia alone. Over time, these ligaments gradually stretch under the constant load and this viscoelastic behaviour leads to the development of prolapse.

There are several direct clinical applications for this information. The first concerns the types of damage that can occur to the urethral support system. An example is the paravaginal defect, which causes separation in the endopelvic fascia connecting the vagina to the pelvic sidewall and thereby increases the compliance of the fascial layer supporting the urethra. When this occurs, increases in abdominal pressure can no longer effectively compress the urethra against the supporting endopelvic fascia to close it during increases in abdominal pressure. When present, this paravaginal defect can be repaired surgically and normal anatomy can thus be restored.

Normal function of the urethral support system requires contraction of the levator ani muscle, which supports the urethra through the endopelvic fascia. During a cough, the levator ani muscle contracts simultaneously with the diaphragm and abdominal wall muscles to build abdominal pressure. This levator ani contraction helps to tense the suburethral fascial layer, as evidenced by decreased vesical neck motion on ultrasonographic evaluation (Miller et al., 2001), thereby enhancing urethral compression. It also protects the connective tissue from undue stresses. Using an instrumented speculum (Ashton-Miller et al., 2002), the strength of the levator ani muscle has been quantified under isometric conditions (Sampselle et al., 1998), the maximum levator force available to close the distal vagina has been shown to differ in the supine and standing postures (Morgan et al., 2005), and racial differences have been found in the levator muscle contractile properties (Howard et al., 2000a).

Striated muscle takes 35% longer to develop the same force in the elderly as in young adults, and its maximum force is also diminished by about 35% (Thelen et al., 1996a). These changes are due not to alterations in neural recruitment patterns, but rather to age-related changes in striated muscle contractility (Thelen et al., 1996b) due to the age-related loss of fast-twitch fibres (Claflin et al., 2011). Happily, and unlike that in the adjacent obturator internus muscle, the decrease in levator ani cross-sectional area or volume is not significant with older age (Morris et al., 2012), presumably due to the levator being comprised of slow-twitch muscle fibres. If the striated muscle of the levator ani becomes damaged or if its innervation is impaired, the muscle contraction will take even longer to develop the same force. This decrease in levator ani strength, in turn, is associated with decreased stiffness, because striated muscle strength and stiffness are directly and linearly correlated (Sinkjaer et al., 1988).

Alternatively, if the connection between the muscle and the fascia is broken (Klutke et al., 1990), then the normal mechanical function of the levator ani during a cough is lost. This phenomenon has important implications for clinical management. Recent evidence from

TABLE 3.2 Effects of changes in cough pressure and pressure transmission ratio on urethral closure pressure and the potential leakage of urine

Example	$Pves_R$	$Pura_R$	UCP_R (Pura – Pves)	Cough	PTR (%)	$\Delta Pura_C$	$Pves_C$	$Pura_C$	UCP_C	Status
1	10	60	+50	200	100	200	210	260	+50	C
2	10	60	+50	200	70	140	210	200	–10	I
3	10	30	+20	100	70	70	110	100	–10	I
4	10	60	+50	100	70	70	110	130	+20	C
5	10	30	+20	50	70	35	60	55	–5	I

Parameters that have been varied are italicized to show how changes in specific parameters can change continence status. All pressures are expressed as cmH_2O. C, continent; $\Delta Pura$, change in urethral pressure; I, incontinent; PTR, pressure transmission ratio; $Pura_C$, urethral pressure during cough; $Pura_R$, urethral pressure at rest; $Pves_C$, bladder pressure during cough; $Pves_R$, vesical pressure at rest; UCP_C, urethral closure pressure during cough; UCP_R, urethral closure pressure at rest.

MRI scans, reviewed in a blinded manner shows the levator ani can be damaged unilaterally or bilaterally in certain patients (DeLancey et al., 2003). This damage, which most often occurs in the pubovisceral muscle near its pubic enthesis (Kim et al., 2011), has been shown to be associated with vaginal birth (Miller et al., 2010). Injury to the levator ani may also be related to urethral sphincter dysfunction (Miller et al., 2004).

URETHROVESICAL PRESSURE DYNAMICS

The anatomical separation of sphincteric elements and supportive structures is mirrored in the functional separation of urethral closure pressure and pressure transmission. The relationship between resting urethral pressure, pressure transmission and the pressure needed to cause leakage of urine are central to understanding urinary continence. These relationships have been described in what we have called the 'pressuregram' (Kim et al., 1997). The constrictive effect of the urethral sphincter deforms the wall of the urethra so as to maintain urethral pressure above bladder pressure, and this pressure differential keeps urine in the bladder at rest. For example, if bladder pressure is 10 cmH_2O while urethral pressure is 60 cmH_2O, a closure pressure of 50 cmH_2O prevents urine from moving from the bladder through the urethra (Table 3.2, Example 1).

Bladder pressure often increases by 200 cmH_2O or more during a cough, and leakage of urine would occur unless urethral pressure also increases. The efficiency of this pressure transmission is expressed as a percentage. A pressure transmission of 100% means, for example, that during a 200 cmH_2O increase in bladder pressure

(from 10 cmH_2O to 210 cmH_2O), the urethral pressure would also increase by 200 cmH_2O (from 60 to 260 cmH_2O) (see Table 3.2, Example 1).

The pressure transmission is less than 100% for incontinent women. For example, abdominal pressure may increase by 200 cmH_2O while urethral pressure may only increase by 140 cmH_2O, for a pressure transmission of 70% (see Table 3.2, Example 2).

If a woman starts with a urethral pressure of 30 cmH_2O, resting bladder pressure of 10 cmH_2O and her pressure transmission is 70%, then with a cough pressure of 100 cmH_2O her bladder pressure would increase to 110 cmH_2O while urethral pressure would increase to just 100 cmH_2O and leakage of urine would occur (see Table 3.2, Example 3).

In Table 3.2, Example 4 shows the same elements, but with a higher urethral closure pressure; and similarly, Example 5 shows what happens with a weaker cough.

According to this conceptual framework, resting pressure and pressure transmission are the two key continence variables. What factors determine these two phenomena? How are they altered to cause incontinence? Although the pressuregram concept is useful for understanding the role of resting pressure and pressure transmission, it has not been possible to reliably make these measurements because of the rapid movement of the urethra relative to the urodynamic transducer during a cough.

CLINICAL IMPLICATIONS OF LEVATOR FUNCTIONAL ANATOMY

Pelvic muscle exercise has been shown to be effective in alleviating SUI in many, but not all, women

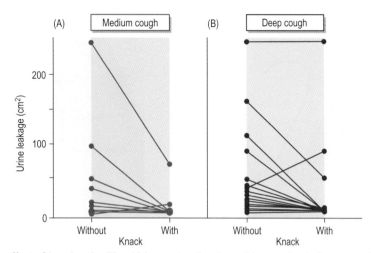

Fig. 3.10 The effect of learning the 'Knack' (precontracting the pelvic muscles before a cough) on reducing the total amount of urine leaked during three separate medium-intensity coughs (left panel) and during three separate deep coughs (right panel) measured 1 week after the women had learned the skill. Each line joins the wet area on one trifold paper towel for each of the 27 women observed coughing without the Knack (denoted by 'Without') with that observed on a second paper towel when the same women used the Knack (denoted 'With') (Miller et al., 1998b). With regard to the units on the ordinate, a calibration test showed that every cm^2 of wetted area was caused by 0.039 ml urine leakage. (From Miller et al., 1998b, with permission of Blackwell Science, Malden, MA.)

(Bø & Talseth, 1996). Having a patient cough with a full bladder and measuring the amount of urine leakage is quite simple (Miller et al., 1998a). If the muscle is normally innervated and is sufficiently attached to the endopelvic fascia, and if by contracting her pelvic muscles before and during a cough a woman is able to decrease that leakage (Fig. 3.10) (Miller et al., 1998b), then simply learning when and how to use her pelvic muscles may be an effective therapy. If this is the case, then the challenge is for the subject to remember to use this skill during activities that transiently increase abdominal pressure.

If the pelvic floor muscle is denervated as a result of substantial nerve injury, then it may not be possible to rehabilitate the muscle sufficiently to make pelvic muscle exercise an effective strategy. In order to use the remaining innervated muscle, women need to be told **when** to contract the muscles to prevent leakage, and they need to learn to strengthen pelvic muscles.

A stronger muscle that is not activated during the time of a cough cannot prevent SUI. Therefore, teaching proper timing of pelvic floor muscles would seem logical as part of a behavioural intervention involving exercise. The efficacy of this intervention is currently being tested in a number of ongoing randomized controlled trials.

In addition, if the muscle is completely detached from the fascial tissues, then despite its ability to contract, the contraction may no longer be effective in elevating the urethra or maintaining its position under stress.

ANATOMY OF THE POSTERIOR VAGINAL WALL SUPPORT AS IT APPLIES TO RECTOCELE

The posterior vaginal wall is supported by connections between the vagina, the bony pelvis and the levator ani muscles (Smith et al., 1989b). The lower one-third of the vagina is fused with the perineal body (Fig. 3.11), which is the attachment between the perineal membranes on either side. This connection prevents downward descent of the rectum in this region.

If the fibres that connect one side with the other rupture then the bowel may protrude downward resulting in a posterior vaginal wall prolapse (Fig. 3.12).

The midposterior vaginal wall is connected to the inside of the levator ani muscles by sheets of endopelvic fascia (Fig. 3.13). These connections prevent ventral movement of the vagina during increases in abdominal pressure. The medial most aspect of these paired sheets is referred to as the rectal pillars.

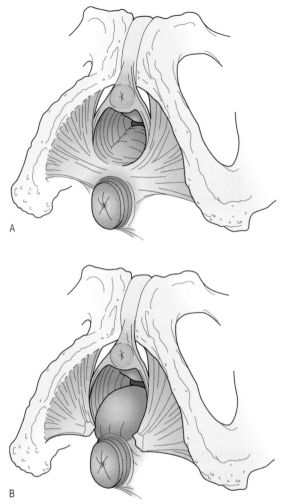

A

B

Fig.3.11 (A) The perineal membrane spans the arch between the ischiopubic rami with each side attached to the other through their connection in the perineal body. (B) Note that separation of the fibres in this area leaves the rectum unsupported and results in a low posterior prolapse. (DeLancey)

In the upper one-third of the vagina, the vaginal wall is connected laterally by the paracolpium. In this region there is a single attachment to the vagina, and a separate system for the anterior and posterior vaginal walls does not exist. Therefore when abdominal pressure forces the vaginal wall downward towards the introitus, attachments between the posterior vagina and the levator muscles prevent this downward movement.

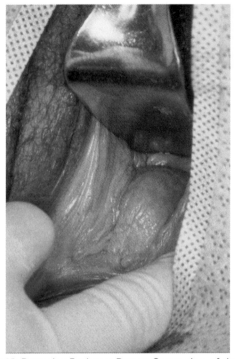

Fig. 3.12 Posterior Prolapse Due to Separation of the Perineal Body. Note the end of the hymenal ring, which lies laterally on the side of the vagina, is no longer united with its companion on the other side. (DeLancey)

The uppermost area of the posterior vagina is suspended, and descent of this area is usually associated with the clinical problem of uterine and/or apical prolapse. The lateral connections of the midvagina hold this portion of the vagina in place and prevent a midvaginal posterior prolapse (Fig. 3.14). The multiple connections of the perineal body to the levator muscles and the pelvic sidewall (Figs 3.15 and 3.16) prevent a low posterior prolapse from descending downward through the opening of the vagina (the urogenital hiatus and the levator ani muscles). Defects in the support at the level of the perineal body most frequently occur during vaginal delivery and are the most common type of posterior vaginal wall support problem.

ACKNOWLEDGEMENT

Supported by Public Health Service grants R01 DK 47516 and 51405, P30 AG 08808 and P50 HD 44406.

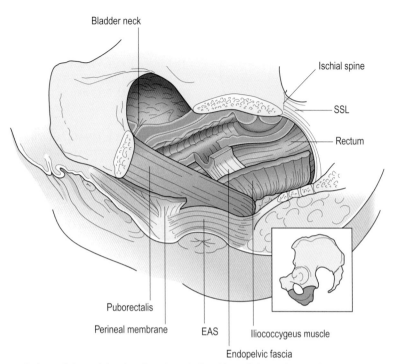

Bladder neck

Ischial spine

SSL

Rectum

Puborectalis

Perineal membrane

EAS

Iliococcygeus muscle

Endopelvic fascia

Fig. 3.13 Lateral view of the pelvis showing the relationships of the puborectalis, iliococcygeus and pelvic floor structures after removal of the ischium below the spine and sacrospinous ligament (SSL) (EAS, external anal sphincter). The bladder and vagina have been cut in the midline, yet the rectum left intact. Note how the endopelvic fascial 'pillars' hold the vaginal wall dorsally, preventing its downward protrusion. (DeLancey)

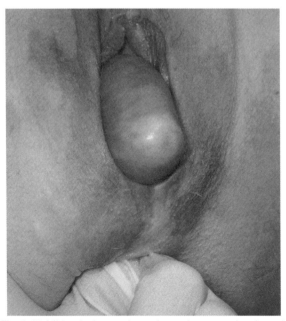

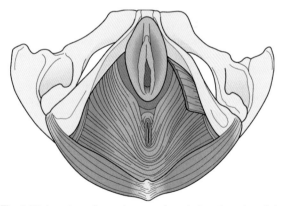

Fig. 3.15 Levator ani muscles seen from below the edge of the perineal membrane (urogenital diaphragm) can be seen on the left of the specimen. (DeLancey)

Fig. 3.14 Midvaginal posterior prolapse that protrudes through the introitus despite a normally supported perineal body. (DeLancey)

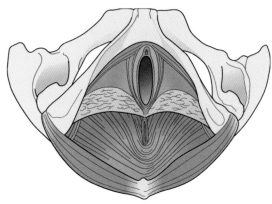

Fig. 3.16 Position of the perineal membrane and its associated components of the striated urogenital sphincter, the compressor urethrae and the urethrovaginal sphincter. (DeLancey)

REFERENCES

Allen, R. E., Hosker, G. L., Smith, A. R. B., et al. (1990). Pelvic floor damage and childbirth: A neurophysiological study. *British Journal of Obstetrics and Gynaecology*, *97*(9), 770–779.

Ashton-Miller, J. A., DeLancey, J. O. L., & Warwick, D. N. (2002). *Method and apparatus for measuring properties of the pelvic floor muscles.* US Patent 6468232 B1.

Berglas, B., & Rubin, I. C. (1953). Study of the supportive structures of the uterus by levator myography. *Surgery Gynecology & Obstetrics*, *97*, 677–692.

Bergman, A., & Elia, G. (1995). Three surgical procedures for genuine stress incontinence: Five-year follow-up of a prospective randomized study. *American Journal of Obstetrics and Gynecology*, *173*(1), 66–71.

Blandpied, P., & Smidt, G. L. (1993). The difference in stiffness of the active plantarflexors between young and elderly human females. *Journal of Gerontology*, *48*(2), M58–M63.

Bø, K., & Talseth, T. (1996). Long-term effect of pelvic floor muscle exercise 5 years after cessation of organized training. *Obstetrics & Gynecology*, *87*(2), 261–265.

Chen, L. C., Ashton-Miller, J. A., & DeLancey, J. O. (2009). A 3-D finite element model of anterior vaginal wall support to evaluate mechanisms underlying cystocele formation. *Journal of Biomechanics*, *42*, 1371–1377.

Claflin, D. S., Larkin, L. M., Cederna, P. S., et al. (2011). Effects of high- and low-velocity resistance training on the contractile properties of skeletal muscle fibers from young and older humans. *Journal of Applied Physiology*, *111*(4), 1021–1030.

Colombo, M., Scalambrino, S., Maggioni, A., et al. (1994). Burch colposuspension versus modified marshal–marchetti–Krantz urethropexy for primary genuine stress

urinary incontinence: A prospective, randomized clinical trial. *American Journal of Obstetrics and Gynecology*, *171*(6), 1573–1579.

DeLancey, J. O. L. (1986). Correlative study of paraurethral anatomy. *Obstetrics & Gynecology*, *68*(1), 91–97.

DeLancey, J. O. L. (1990). Anatomy and physiology of urinary continence. *Clinical Obstetrics and Gynecology*, *33*(2), 298–307.

DeLancey, J. O. L. (1994). Structural support of the urethra as it relates to stress urinary incontinence: The hammock hypothesis. *American Journal of Obstetrics and Gynecology*, *170*(6), 1713–1723.

DeLancey, J. O. L. (1999). Structural anatomy of the posterior pelvic compartment as it relates to rectocele [Comment]. *American Journal of Obstetrics and Gynecology*, *180*(4), 815–823.

DeLancey, J. O. L., Fenner, D. E., Guire, K., et al. (2010). Differences in continence system between community-dwelling black and white women with and without urinary incontinence in the EPI study. *American Journal of Obstetrics and Gynecology*, *202*(6), 584.e1–584.e12.

DeLancey, J. O. L., Kearney, R., Chou, Q., et al. (2003). The appearance of levator ani muscle abnormalities in magnetic resonance images after vaginal delivery. *Obstetrics & Gynecology*, *101*(1), 46–53.

DeLancey, J. O. L., Morgan, D. M., Fenner, D. E., et al. (2007). Comparison of levator ani muscle defects and function in women with and without pelvic organ prolapse. *Obstetrics & Gynecology*, *109*(2 Pt. 1), 295–302.

DeLancey, J. O. L., Trowbridge, E. R., Miller, J. M., et al. (2008). Stress urinary incontinence: Relative importance of urethral support and urethral closure pressure. *Journal Urology*, *179*(6), 2286–2290.

Diokno, A. C., Wells, T. J., & Brink, C. A. (1987). Urinary incontinence in elderly women: Urodynamic evaluation. *Journal of the American Geriatrics Society*, *35*(10), 940–946.

Enhörning, G. (1961). Simultaneous recording of intravesical and intraurethral pressure. *Acta Chirurgica Scandinavica*, *276*(Suppl. l.), 1–68.

Gosling, J. A., Dixon, J. S., Critchley, H. O. D., et al. (1981). A comparative study of the human external sphincter and periurethral levator ani muscles. *British Journal of Urology*, *53*(1), 35–41.

Halban, J., & Tandler, I. (1907). *Anatomie und Aetiologie der Genitalprolapse beim Weibe.* Vienna: Wilhelm Braumuller.

Hanzal, E., Berger, E., & Koelbl, H. (1993). Levator ani muscle morphology and recurrent genuine stress incontinence. *Obstetrics & Gynecology*, *81*(3), 426–429.

Herzog, A. R., Diokno, A. C., Brown, M. B., et al. (1990). Two-year incidence, remission, and change patterns of urinary incontinence in noninstitutionalized older adults. *Journal of Gerontology*, *45*(2), M67–M74.

Hilton, P., & Stanton, S. L. (1983). Urethral pressure measurement by microtransducer: The results in symptom-free women and in those with genuine stress incontinence. *British Journal of Obstetrics and Gynaecology, 90*(10), 919–933.

Howard, D., DeLancey, J. O. L., Tunn, R., et al. (2000a). Racial differences in the structure and function of the stress urinary continence mechanism in women. *Obstetrics & Gynecology, 95*(5), 713–717.

Howard, D., Miller, J. M., DeLancey, J. O. L., et al. (2000b). Differential effects of cough, Valsalva, and continence status on vesical neck movement. *Obstetrics & Gynecology, 95*(4), 535–540.

Jing, D., Ashton-Miller, J. A., & DeLancey, J. O. L. (2012). A subject-specific anisotropic visco-hyperelastic finite element model of female pelvic floor stress and strain during the second stage of labor. *Journal of Biomechanics, 45*(3), 455–460.

Kearney, R., Sawhney, R., & DeLancey, J. O. L. (2004). Levator ani muscle anatomy evaluated by origin–insertion pairs. *Obstetrics & Gynecology, 104*(1), 168–173.

Kim, J., Ramanah, R., DeLancey, J. O. L., et al. (2011). On the anatomy and histology of the pubovisceral muscle enthesis in women. *Neurourology and Urodynamics, 30*(7), 1366–1370.

Kim, K.-J., Ashton-Miller, J. A., Strohbehn, K., et al. (1997). The vesicourethral pressuregram analysis of urethral function under stress. *Journal of Biomechanics, 30*(1), 19–25.

Kirschner-Hermanns, R., Wein, B., Niehaus, S., et al. (1993). The contribution of magnetic resonance imaging of the pelvic floor to the understanding of urinary incontinence. *British Journal of Urology, 72*(5 Pt. 2), 715–718.

Klutke, G. C., Golomb, J., Barbaric, Z., et al. (1990). The anatomy of stress incontinence: Magnetic resonance imaging of the female bladder neck and urethra. *Journal Urology, 43*(3), 563–566.

Koelbl, H., Saz, V., Doerfler, D., et al. (1998). Transurethral injection of silicone microimplants for intrinsic urethral sphincter deficiency. *Obstetrics & Gynecology, 92*(3), 332–336.

Mant, J., Painter, R., & Vessey, M. (1997). Epidemiology of genital prolapse: Observations from the oxford planning association study. *British Journal of Obstetrics and Gynaecology, 104*(5), 579–585.

Miller, J. M., Ashton-Miller, J. A., & DeLancey, J. O. L. (1998a). Quantification of cough-related urine loss using the paper towel test. *Obstetrics & Gynecology, 91*(5 Pt. 1), 705–709.

Miller, J. M., Ashton-Miller, J. A., & DeLancey, J. O. L. (1998b). A pelvic muscle precontraction can reduce cough-related urine loss in selected women with mild SUI. *Journal of the American Geriatrics Society, 46*(7), 870–874.

Miller, J. M., Brandon, C., Jacobson, J. A., et al. (2010). MRI findings in patients considered high risk for pelvic floor injury studied serially after vaginal childbirth. *American Journal of Roentgenology, 195*(3), 786–791.

Miller, J. M., Perucchini, D., Carchidi, L. T., et al. (2001). Pelvic floor muscle contraction during a cough and decreased vesical neck mobility. *Obstetrics & Gynecology, 97*(2), 255–260.

Miller, J. M., Umek, W. H., Delancey, J. O. L., et al. (2004). Can women without visible pubococcygeal muscle in MR images still increase urethral closure pressures? *American Journal of Obstetrics and Gynecology, 191*(1), 171–175.

Morgan, D. M., Kaur, G., Hsu, Y., et al. (2005). Does vaginal closure force differ in the supine and standing positions? *American Journal of Obstetrics and Gynecology, 192*, 1722–1728.

Morris, V. C., Murray, M. P., DeLancey, J. O. L., et al. (2012). A comparison of the effect of age on levator ani and obturator internus muscle cross-sectional areas and volumes in nulliparous women. *Neurourology and Urodynamics, 31*(4), 481–486.

Pandit, M., DeLancey, J. O. L., Ashton-Miller, J. A., et al. (2000). Quantification of intramuscular nerves within the female striated urogenital sphincter muscle. *Obstetrics & Gynecology, 95*(6 Pt. 1), 797–800.

Paramore, R. H. (1918). The uterus as a floating organ. In *The statics of the Female pelvic viscera* (p. 12). London: HK Lewis & Company.

Parks, A. G., Porter, N. H., & Melzak, J. (1962). Experimental study of the reflex mechanism controlling the muscle of the pelvic floor. *Diseases of the Colon & Rectum, 5*, 407–414.

Perucchini, D., DeLancey, J. O. L., Ashton-Miller, J. A., et al. (2002a). Age effects on urethral striated muscle: I. Changes in number and diameter of striated muscle fibers in the ventral urethra. *American Journal of Obstetrics and Gynecology, 186*(3), 351–355.

Perucchini, D., DeLancey, J. O. L., Ashton-Miller, J. A., et al. (2002b). Age effects on urethral striated muscle: II. Anatomic location of muscle loss. *American Journal of Obstetrics and Gynecology, 186*(3), 356–360.

Porges, R. F., Porges, J. C., & Blinick, G. (1960). Mechanisms of uterine support and the pathogenesis of uterine prolapse. *Obstetrics & Gynecology, 15*, 711–726.

Richardson, A. C., Edmonds, P. B., & Williams, N. L. (1981). Treatment of stress urinary incontinence due to paravaginal fascial defect. *Obstetrics & Gynecology, 57*(3), 357–362.

Rud, T., Andersson, K. E., Asmussen, M., et al. (1980). Factors maintaining the intraurethral pressure in women. *Investigative Urology, 17*(4), 343–347.

Sampselle, C. M., Miller, J. M., Mims, B., et al. (1998). Effect of pelvic muscle exercise on transient incontinence during pregnancy and after birth. *Obstetrics & Gynecology, 91*(3), 406–412.

Sinkjaer, T., Toft, E., Andreassen, S., et al. (1988). Muscle stiffness in human ankle dorsiflexors: Intrinsic and reflex components. *Journal of Neurophysiology, 60*(3), 1110–1121.

Skelton, D. A., Young, A., Greig, C. A., et al. (1995). Effects of resistance training on strength, power, and selected functional abilities of women aged 75 and older. *Journal of the American Geriatrics Society, 43*(10), 1081–1087.

Smith, A. R. B., Hosker, G. L., & Warrell, D. W. (1989a). The role of partial denervation of the pelvic floor in the aetiology of genitourinary prolapse and stress incontinence of urine: A neurophysiological study. *British Journal of Obstetrics and Gynaecology, 96*(1), 24–28.

Smith, A. R. B., Hosker, G. L., & Warrell, D. W. (1989b). The role of pudendal nerve damage in the aetiology of genuine stress incontinence in women. *British Journal of Obstetrics and Gynaecology, 96*(1), 29–32.

Snooks, S. J., Swash, M., Henry, M. M., et al. (1986). Risk factors in childbirth causing damage to the pelvic floor innervation. *International Journal of Colorectal Disease, 1*(1), 20–24.

Strohbehn, K., & DeLancey, J. O. L. (1997). The anatomy of stress incontinence. *Operating Technology Gynecology Surgery, 2*, 15–16.

Strohbehn, K., Quint, L. E., Prince, M. R., et al. (1996). Magnetic resonance imaging anatomy of the female urethra: A direct histologic comparison. *Obstetrics & Gynecology, 88*(5), 750–756.

Taverner, D. (1959). An electromyographic study of the normal function of the external anal sphincter and pelvic diaphragm. *Diseases of the Colon & Rectum, 2*, 153–160.

Thelen, D. G., Ashton-Miller, J. A., Schultz, A. B., et al. (1996a). Do neural factors underlie age differences in rapid ankle torque development? *Journal of the American Geriatrics Society, 44*(7), 804–808.

Thelen, D. G., Schultz, A. B., Alexander, N. B., et al. (1996b). Effects of age on rapid ankle torque development. *The Journals of Gerontology Series A Biological Sciences and Medical Sciences, 51*(5), M226–M232.

Thomas, T. M., Plymat, K. R., Blannin, J., et al. (1980). Prevalence of urinary incontinence. *British Medicine Journal, 281*(6250), 1243–1245.

Tunn, R., Paris, S., Fischer, W., et al. (1998). Static magnetic resonance imaging of the pelvic floor muscle morphology in women with stress urinary incontinence and pelvic prolapse. *Neurourology and Urodynamics, 17*(6), 579–589.

4

Neuroanatomy and Neurophysiology of Pelvic Floor Muscles

Melita Rotar and David B. Vodušek

INTRODUCTION

The pelvic floor is composed of three interconnected layers of muscle and connective tissue which function as a unit. The muscles are the levator ani (muscle) which consists of iliococcygeus, puborectalis and pubococcygeus muscles, and the coccygeus muscle. The pelvic floor muscles (PFMs) support pelvic organs and contribute to normal bladder, bowel and sexual function. PFM support should not be considered as passive but as an active support mechanism through coordinated contraction and relaxation of the muscles which are controlled by the nervous system.

PFM activity is closely coordinated with perineal striated muscles (the transverse perineal, bulbospongiosus [previously bulbocavernosus] and ischiocavernosus) and the striated sphincters (urethral and anal).

INNERVATION OF PELVIC FLOOR MUSCLES

Somatic Motor Pathways

Striated muscles of the perineum are innervated by the pudendal nerve. Its fibres originate from alpha motor neurons in a localized column of cells in the sacral spinal cord called *Onuf's nucleus* (Mannen et al., 1982), expanding in humans from the second to third sacral segment (S2–S3) and occasionally into S1 (Schroder, 1985) on the ventrolateral border of the ventral horn in the sacral cord. Within Onuf's nucleus there is some spatial separation between motor neurons concerned with the control of the urethral and anal sphincters. Sphincter alpha motor neurons are uniform in size and smaller than the other alpha motor neurons. They also differ with respect to their high concentrations of amino acid, neuropeptide, noradrenaline (norepinephrine), serotonin and dopamine containing terminals, which represent the substrate for the distinctive neuropharmacological responses of these neurons, and differ from those of limb muscles, the bladder and the PFMs.

The somatic motor fibres (axons from alpha motor neurons) leave the spinal cord in the anterior roots and fuse with the posterior roots to constitute the spinal nerve. After passing through the intravertebral foramen, the spinal nerve divides into a posterior and an anterior ramus (Bannister, 1995). Somatic fibres from the anterior rami of S1–S4 form the sacral plexus. Traditionally

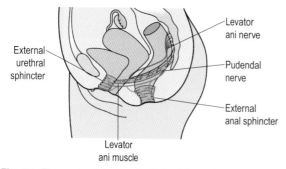

Fig. 4.1 The pudendal nerve is derived from the anterior rami of roots S1–S4. It continues through the greater sciatic foramen and enters in a lateral direction into the ischiorectal fossa. Its muscular branches innervate the external anal sphincter and the external urethral sphincter. There may be muscular branches for the levator ani, which is, as a rule, innervated by direct branches from the sacral plexus (from above)—the levator ani nerve.

the pudendal nerve is described as being derived from the S2–S4 anterior rami, but there may be some contribution from S1, and possibly little or no contribution from S4 (Marani et al., 1993).

The pudendal nerve continues through the greater sciatic foramen and enters in a lateral direction through the lesser sciatic foramen into the ischiorectal fossa (Alcock's canal). In the posterior part of Alcock's canal the pudendal nerve gives off the inferior rectal nerve, then it branches into the perineal nerve and the dorsal nerve of the penis/clitoris.

Spinal motor neurons for the levator ani group of muscles originate from S3 to S5 segments and show some overlap with sphincter motor neurons (Barber et al., 2002). It is generally accepted that the main innervation for the PFMs is through direct branches from the sacral plexus ('from above') rather than predominantly by branches of the pudendal nerve ('from below') (Fig. 4.1).

Significant variability of normal human neuroanatomy is probably the source of remaining controversies originating from anatomical studies of peripheral innervation of the pelvis, which have so far been performed in only a small number of cases.

Higher nervous system regions control spinal cord motor nuclei by descending pathways; these inputs to PFM motor neurons are manifold, and mostly 'indirect' (through several interneurons). More direct connections to Onuf's nucleus are from some nuclei in the brainstem (raphe, ambiguous) and from

paraventricular hypothalamus. The representation of PFMs in the motor cortex is not well characterized, but it has been shown to include supplementary motor area and primary motor cortex (M1) in two different activation patterns: activation of PFMs independently of synergists and activation of PFMs prior to and in coordination with synergists (Yani et al., 2018).

In the past decades the insight into supraspinal control of bladder and bowel control as well as PFM function has become possible using functional imaging techniques: single-photon emission computed tomography, positron emission tomography (PET) and functional magnetic resonance imaging (fMRI). Single-photon emission computed tomography is a nuclear medicine tomographic imaging technique which can identify the activated area but, in contrast to PET, is unable to measure the degree of activation.

PET relies on the intravenous application of a radioactive isotope that accumulates in metabolically active brain regions. Brain areas that control a particular activity during a particular manoeuvre (e.g., pelvic floor contraction) are more metabolically active than other 'non-active' brain areas. The increase in metabolism is accompanied by an increase in blood flow through the particular area, and this can be recorded. PET, however, cannot detect rapid changes in metabolism but is able to render enough anatomical detail to be useful for functional anatomical studies. Using radioisotope techniques, brain regions involved in voluntary control of PFMs were identified (Blok et al., 1997) as well as neural control of micturition (Fukuyama et al., 1996), followed by many studies of neural control in health and disease (Dasgupta et al., 2005; Herzog et al., 2006; Nour et al., 2000).

Using a different recording principle (but based on similar physiological facts), fMRI is even better for providing detailed functional anatomical data. (These techniques can also demonstrate brain areas with 'less activity', as in the 'resting state', thus indicating inhibition of certain brain areas during execution of some manoeuvres.) fMRI can detect rapid changes in brain metabolism by measuring the changing proportion of oxygenated and deoxygenated haemoglobin in brain areas without exposing individuals to radiation. Its spatial and temporal resolution is much greater compared to other imaging techniques; however, imaging requires many repeated captures of the same frame to increase the signal-to-noise ratio (Catana et al., 2012).

Brain activation during voluntary PFM contraction was extensively analysed using 1.5 Tesla (T) or 3T magnets. It revealed that many different areas were activated in healthy volunteers (Krhut et al., 2014; Kuhtz-Buschbeck et al., 2007; Zhang et al., 2005), and that the activations differ in patients with pelvic floor disorders (Kutch et al., 2015; Seseke et al., 2013). Dynamic brain imaging with 1.5T and 3T magnets requires additional smoothing and is of little use as a diagnostic tool. With high-resolution 7T fMRI, however, single-subject imaging is possible (Dumoulin et al., 2018; Van der Zwaag et al., 2009). Thus, neural representations of the pelvic floor in the whole brain can be visualized (Groenendijk et al., 2020).

PET studies have revealed activation of the (right) ventral pontine tegmentum (in the brainstem) during holding of urine in human subjects (Blok et al., 1997). This finding is consistent with the location of the 'L region' in cats, proposed to control PFM nuclei. In addition, periaqueductal grey (PAG) was found to be activated in many studies (Dasgupta et al., 2005; Griffiths et al., 2007; Kuhtz-Buschbeck et al., 2005; Seseke et al., 2006). PAG can be described as a relay for ascending visceral input from pelvic organs to higher brain regions (amygdala, hypothalamus, thalamus), as well as a relay from forebrain regions to the sacral spinal cord through the pontine micturition centre (PMC) (Blok and Holstege, 1994; Craig, 2003). The PAG and hypothalamus are the only structures with direct connections to the PMC (Kuipers et al., 2006).

The connections described serve the coordinated inclusion of PFM into 'sacral' (lower urinary tract [LUT]; anorectal and sexual) functions. Individual PFMs and sphincters need not only be neurally coordinated 'within' a particular function (e.g., with bladder activity), but the single functions need to be neurally coordinated with each other (e.g., voiding and defaecation, voiding and erection).

The sacral function control system is proposed to be a part of the 'emotional motor system' derived from brain or brainstem structures belonging to the limbic system. It consists of the medial and a lateral component (Holstege, 1998). The medial component represents diffuse pathways originating in the caudal brainstem and terminating on (almost all) spinal grey matter, using serotonin in particular as its neurotransmitter. This system is proposed to 'set the threshold' for overall changes in muscle activity, such as in muscle tone under different physiological conditions (e.g., sleeping).

The lateral component of the emotional motor system consists of discrete areas in the hemispheres and the brainstem responsible for specific motor activities such as micturition and mating. The pathways belonging to the lateral system use spinal premotor interneurons to influence motor neurons in somatic and autonomic spinal nuclei, thus allowing for confluent interactions of various inputs to modify the motor neuron activity.

PFM nuclei also receive descending corticospinal input from the cerebral cortex. PET studies have revealed activation of the superomedial precentral gyrus during voluntary PFM contraction, and of the right anterior cingulate gyrus during sustained PFM straining (Blok et al., 1997). Not surprisingly, PFM contraction can be obtained by electrical or magnetic transcranial stimulation of the motor cortex in man (Brostrom, 2003; Vodušek, 1996).

Afferent Pathways

Because PFM function is intimately connected to pelvic organ function, it is proposed that all sensory information from the pelvic region is relevant for PFM neural control.

The sensory neurons are bipolar. Their cell bodies are in spinal ganglia. They send a long process to the periphery and a central process into the spinal cord where it terminates segmentally or—after branching for reflex connections—ascends in some cases as far as the brainstem (Bannister, 1995).

The afferent pathways from the anogenital region and pelvic region are divided into somatic and visceral. Somatic afferents derive from touch, pain and thermal receptors in skin and mucosa and from proprioceptors in muscles and tendons. (Proprioceptive afferents arise particularly from muscle spindles and Golgi tendon organs.) The visceral afferents accompany both parasympathetic and sympathetic efferent fibres. The somatic afferents accompany the pudendal nerves and the levator ani nerve, and direct somatic branches of the sacral plexus. The different groups of afferent fibres have different reflex connections and transmit, at least to some extent, different afferent information.

The terminals of pudendal nerve afferents in the dorsal horn of the spinal cord are found ipsilaterally, but also bilaterally, with ipsilateral predominance (Ueyama et al., 1984).

The proprioceptive afferents form synaptic contacts in the spinal cord and have collaterals ('primary afferent collaterals') which run ipsilaterally in the dorsal spinal columns to synapse in the gracilis (dorsal column) nuclei in the brainstem. This pathway transmits information about innocuous sensations from the PFMs.

The lateral columns of the spinal cord transmit information concerning pain sensations from perineal skin, as well as sexual sensations. In humans, this pathway is situated superficially just ventral to the equator of the cord and is probably the spinothalamic tract (Torrens and Morrison, 1987).

The spinal pathways that transmit sensory information from the visceral afferent terminations in the spinal cord to more rostral structures can be found in the dorsal, lateral and ventral spinal cord columns.

NEURAL CONTROL OF SACRAL FUNCTIONS

Neural Control of Continence

At rest, continence is assured by an adequate bladder storage function and a competent sphincter mechanism, including not only the striated and smooth muscle sphincter but also the PFMs.

Bladder control has two modes: storage and emptying. Switching between these two is accomplished at the level of brainstem with the assistance of two regions: the lateral (L region) and the medial (M region). The L region in the brainstem has also been called the *storage centre* (Blok et al., 1997). This area was active in PET studies of those volunteers who could not void but contracted their PFMs. The L region is thought to exert a continuous exciting effect on the Onuf's nucleus and thereby on the striated urinary sphincter during the storage phase; in humans, it is probably part of a complex set of 'nerve impulse pattern generators' for different coordinated motor activities, such as breathing, coughing and straining.

When the bladder volume reaches a critical level, afferent signals increase. If the timing for voiding is appropriate, the activity switches from the L region to the M region and the bladder empties.

The M region is also called the *pontine micturition centre* or *Barrington's nucleus*, which was shown to be associated with micturition in cats and rats (Barrington, 1925) decades before functional imaging revealed such a structure in man by PET and fMRI (Athwal et al., 2001; Griffiths et al., 2005).

Normal kinesiological sphincter electromyography (EMG) recordings show continuous activity of motor units at rest (as defined by continuous firing of motor unit potentials), which as a rule increases with increasing bladder fullness. Reflexes mediating excitatory outflow to the sphincters are organized at the spinal level (the guarding reflex). During physical stress (e.g., coughing, sneezing), the pressure in the abdominal cavity (and hence within the bladder and lower rectum) rises. Activation of the PFMs is mandatory to prevent leakage and may be perceived as occurring in two steps by two different activation processes. Coughing and sneezing are thought to be generated by individual pattern generators within the brainstem, and thus activation of PFM is a preset coactivation—and not primarily a 'reflex' reaction—to increased intra-abdominal pressure. In addition, there is an auxiliary reflex PFM response to increased abdominal pressure due to distension of muscle spindles within PFMs. The PFMs can of course also be voluntarily activated anticipating an increase in abdominal pressure. Such timed voluntary activity may be learned (the 'Knack') (Miller et al., 1998; Miller et al., 2008). PFM contraction increases the urethral pressure and reflexly decreases detrusor activity, and thus micturition, helping to maintain continence (Shafik and Shafik, 2003).

Neural Control of Micturition

Centres in the pons (brainstem) coordinate micturition as such, but areas rostral to the pons (the hypothalamus and other parts of the brain including the frontal cortex) are responsible for the timing of the start of micturition. The PMC coordinates the activity of motor neurons of the urinary bladder and the urethral sphincter (both nuclei located in the sacral spinal cord), receiving afferent input via the PAG matter. The central control of LUT function is organized as an on–off switching circuit (or a set of circuits, rather) that maintains a reciprocal relationship between the urinary bladder and urethral outlet.

Without the PMC and its spinal connections, coordinated bladder/sphincter activity is not possible, thus patients with lesions of the PMC or its spinal connections demonstrate bladder sphincter discoordination (dyssynergia). Functional imaging studies have shown that activation of brainstem centres in patients with detrusor sphincter dyssynergia differs from normal subjects (Seseke et al., 2019). Patients with lesions above the pons do not show detrusor sphincter dyssynergia but have urge incontinence (due to bladder overactivity). Furthermore, they demonstrate non-inhibited sphincter relaxations and an inability to delay voiding to an appropriate place and time.

Voluntary micturition is a behaviour pattern that starts with relaxation of the striated urethral sphincter and PFMs. Voluntary PFM contraction during voiding can lead to a stop of micturition; this is thought to be a consequence of collateral connections of PFM control to detrusor control nuclei. Descending inhibitory pathways for the detrusor have been demonstrated (De Groat et al., 2001). Bladder contractions are also inhibited by reflexes, activated by afferent input from the PFMs, perineal skin and anorectum (Sato et al., 2000).

Neural Control of Anorectal Function

Faeces stored in the colon are transported past the rectosigmoid 'physiological sphincter' into the normally empty rectum, which can store up to 300 mL of contents. Rectal distension causes regular contractions of the rectal wall, which is affected by the intrinsic nervous (myenteric) plexus, and prompts the desire to defaecate (Bartolo and MacDonald, 2002). Stool entering the rectum is also detected by stretch receptors in the rectal wall and PFMs; their discharge leads to the urge to defaecate. It starts as an intermittent sensation, which becomes more and more constant. Contraction of the PFMs may interrupt the process, probably by concomitant inhibitory influences to the defaecatory neural 'pattern generator', but also by 'mechanical' insistence on sphincter contraction and the propelling of faeces back to the sigmoid colon (Bartolo and MacDonald, 2002).

Bowel function is controlled by the medial prefrontal cortex and the anterior cingulate gyrus. Information is conveyed along spinal cord tracts to motor neurons in Onuf's nucleus. Tonic contraction of internal and external anal sphincters prevents bowel contents to pass through and thereby contribute to continence (Kaiser and Ortega, 2002).

With passage of faeces, the rectum distends and triggers the rectoanal inhibitory reflex, mediating a short relaxation of the internal anal sphincter with concomitant contraction of the external anal sphincter. Thus bowel contents can pass into the anal canal and come in contact with anal mucosa, where the receptors differentiate between gas, liquid or solid stool (Hoffman et al., 2016; Sagar and Pemberton, 1996). Such

'sampling' normally occurs seven times in an hour, but the frequency is lower in incontinent patients (Palit et al., 2012).

The PFMs are thus intimately involved in anorectal function. Apart from the 'sensory' role of the PFMs and the external anal sphincter function, the puborectalis muscle is thought to maintain the 'anorectal' angle, which facilitates continence, and has to be relaxed to allow defaecation. Current concepts suggest that defaecation requires increased rectal pressure coordinated with relaxation of the anal sphincters and PFM—that is, defaecation is best performed when an urge to defaecate is combined with the voluntary decision to 'let go' (relaxation of PFMs and the anal sphincter). This may be combined with a voluntary increase in the abdominal pressure by activating the diaphragm and abdominal muscles.

Pelvic floor relaxation allows opening of the anorectal angle and perineal descent, facilitating faecal expulsion. Puborectalis and external anal sphincter activity during evacuation is generally inhibited. However, observations by EMG and defaecography in healthy subjects suggest that the puborectalis may not always relax during defaecation (Fucini et al., 2001).

NEURAL CONTROL OF THE SEXUAL RESPONSE

Sexual arousal is a multifactorial response which comprises emotional as well as physical and behavioural aspects. fMRI studies reveal that there are many brain areas involved in the processing of sexual information, such as the orbitofrontal cortex, cuneus, precuneus, globus pallidus, putamen and thalamus (Seok et al., 2016). During ejaculation in men and orgasm in women, activation of the dorsolateral pontine tegmentum was demonstrated using PET (Huynh et al., 2013); the authors postulate that the area controls the parasympathetic output, whereas the ventrolateral pontine area mediates PFM contractions through direct projections to pelvic floor motor neurons.

Climax in humans (in both sexes, and in experimental animals) elicits rhythmic contractions of the pelvic floor/perineal muscles, which in the male drives the ejaculate from the urethra (assisted by a coordinated bladder neck closure). PFM activity in males during ejaculation, as recorded by EMG, is a repetitive contraction over several seconds (Petersen et al., 1955).

However, PFMs are assumed to present specific activation throughout the sexual encounter. Apart from general changes in muscle tone set by the emotional motor system, the sacral reflex circuitry behaviour, as known from studies (Vodušek, 2002a), would allow for reflex activation of the PFMs during genital stimulation. Tonic stimulation of the reflex is postulated to hinder venous outflow from the penis/clitoris, thus helping erection. Reflex contraction of the PFMs should conceivably contribute to the achievement of the 'orgasmic platform' (contraction of the levator ani and, in the female, the circumvaginal muscles). Muscle activity measured with surface EMG confirmed that PFMs responded to sexual stimuli (Gentilcore-Saulnier et al., 2010; Hannan-Leith et al., 2019).

The role of PFMs in sexuality is mirrored in results of studies demonstrating improvement of sexual function after PFM training (Lowenstein et al., 2010; Lúcio et al., 2014).

NEUROPHYSIOLOGY OF PELVIC FLOOR MUSCLES

Muscle activity is thoroughly dependent on neural control. 'Denervated' muscle atrophies and turns into fibrotic tissue. Muscle, like every tissue, consists of cells (muscle fibres). But the functional unit within striated muscle is not a single muscle cell but a motor unit. A motor unit consists of one alpha (or 'lower') motor neuron (from the motor nuclei in the spinal cord), and all of the muscle cells that this motor neuron innervates. In other words the motor unit is the basic functional unit of the somatic motor system; control of a muscle means control of its motor units. Thus, in discussing neural control of muscle, we really only need to consider the motor neurons in the spinal cord and all of the influences they are exposed to.

The function of pelvic floor and sphincter lower motor neurons is organized quite differently from other groups of motor neurons. In contrast to the reciprocal innervation that is common in limb muscles, the neurons innervating each side of the PFMs have to work in harmony and synchronously. Sphincters indeed may be morphologically considered to constitute 'one' muscle, which is innervated by two nerves (left and right)!

By concomitant activity, the PFM acts as the 'closure unit' of the excretory tracts, the 'support unit' for pelvic viscera and an 'effector unit' in the sexual response. In general, muscles involved in these functions from both sides of the body act in a strictly unified fashion as 'one muscle': this has been demonstrated for the pubococcygei muscles but has not really been documented for the whole group of PFMs and sphincters (Deindl et al., 1993). However, as each muscle in the pelvis has its own unilateral peripheral innervation, dissociated activation patterns are possible and have been reported between the two pubococcygei (Deindl et al., 1994), and between the levator ani and urethral sphincter (Kenton and Brubaker, 2002).

The differences in the evolutionary origin of the sphincter muscles and levator ani furthermore imply that unilateral activation may be less of an impossibility for the PFMs than for sphincters. It can be postulated that the neural mechanisms controlling the different muscles involved in sphincter mechanisms and pelvic organ support may not be as uniform as has been assumed. How much variability there is in normal activation patterns of PFMs is not yet clarified. It is clear, however, that the coordination between individual PFMs can definitively be impaired by disease or trauma.

TONIC AND PHASIC PELVIC FLOOR MUSCLE ACTIVITY

The normal striated sphincter muscles demonstrate some continuous motor unit activity at rest as revealed by kinesiological EMG (Fig. 4.2). This differs between individuals and continues also after subjects fall asleep during the examination (Chantraine, 1973). This physiological spontaneous activity may be called *tonic* and depends on prolonged activation of certain tonic motor units (Vodušek, 1982).

The 'amount' of tonic motor unit activity can, in principle, be assessed by counting the number of active motor unit potentials or analysing the interference pattern by EMG; this has so far not been much studied. Thus little is known about the variability and the normal range of tonic activity in normal subjects, and the reproducibility of findings; this makes it difficult to assess the validity of results from the few studies reporting activity changes accompanying LUT, anorectal or sexual dysfunction.

As a rule, tonic motor unit activity increases with bladder filling, while at the same time being dependent on the rate of filling. Any reflex or voluntary activation is mirrored first in an increase of the firing frequency

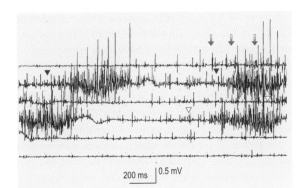

Fig. 4.2 Kinesiological electromyography recording from anal sphincter muscle. Concentric needle electrode recording in a 40-year-old continent woman. Note ongoing sparse firing of motor unit potentials, which is called the *tonic activity* (on this time scale the motor unit potentials/MUP are just thin perpendicular lines, as seen in the uppermost ray—before the thin arrows indicate reflex excitation). Tonic motor units as a rule have small amplitudes (small thin perpendicular lines). Tonic activity can also be seen after the voluntary contraction (last two rays). Recruitment of additional motor units can be seen on reflex manoeuvres (thin arrows: pinpricks at anal wedge; full arrows: strong cough), and on command to contract (empty arrows). The additionally recruited motor units have larger phosphomonoesters.

of these motor units. Conversely, inhibition of firing is apparent on initiation of voiding.

With any stronger activation manoeuvre (e.g., contraction, coughing), and only for a limited length of time, new motor units are recruited (see Fig. 4.2). These may be called *phasic* motor units. Increase of muscle activity is required to improve continence control (Ashton-Miller and DeLancey, 2007). As a rule they have potentials of higher amplitudes and their discharge rates are higher and irregular. A small percentage of motor units with an 'intermediate' activation pattern can also be encountered (Vodušek, 1982). It has to be stressed that this typing of motor units is electrophysiological, and no direct correlation to histochemical typing of muscle fibres has so far been achieved.

With regard to tonic activity, sphincters differ from some perineal muscles; tonic activity is encountered in many but not all detection sites for the levator ani muscle (Deindl et al., 1993; Vodušek, 1982) and is practically never seen in the bulbocavernosus muscle (Vodušek, 1982). In the pubococcygeus of the normal female, there is some increase of activity during bladder filling, and reflex increases in activity during any activation

manoeuvre performed by the subject (e.g., talking, deep breathing, coughing).

On voiding, inhibition of the tonic activity of the external urethral sphincter, as well as the PFMs, leads to relaxation. This can be detected as a disappearance of all EMG activity, which precedes detrusor contraction. Similarly, the striated anal sphincter relaxes with defaecation and also micturition (Read, 1990).

Reflex Activity of Pelvic Floor Muscles

The human urethral and anal striated sphincters seem to have no muscle spindles; their reflex reactivity is thus intrinsically different from the levator ani muscle complex, in which muscle spindles and Golgi tendon organs have been demonstrated (Borghi et al., 1991). Thus PFMs have the intrinsic proprioceptive 'servo-mechanism' for adjusting muscle length and tension, whereas the sphincter muscles depend on afferents from skin and mucosa. Both muscle groups are integrated in reflex activity, which incorporates pelvic organ function.

The reflex activity of PFMs is clinically and electrophysiologically evaluated by eliciting the bulbocavernosus and anal reflex. The bulbocavernosus reflex is evoked on non-painful stimulation of the glans (or electrically, the dorsal penile/clitoral nerve). As recorded electromyographically, it is a complex response: its first component is thought to be an oligosynaptic reflex and the later component a polysynaptic reflex (Vodušek and Janko, 1990). The polysynaptic anal reflex is elicited by painful (pinprick) stimulation in the perianal region.

The constant tonic activity of sphincter muscles is thought to result from the characteristics of their 'low-threshold' motor neurons and the constant 'inputs' (either of reflex segmental or suprasegmental origin). It is supported by cutaneous stimuli, by pelvic organ distension and by intra-abdominal pressure changes.

Sudden increases in intra-abdominal pressure as a rule lead to brisk PFM (reflex) activity, which has been called the *guarding reflex*; it is organized at the spinal level and is a viscero-muscular reflex (Chancellor et al., 2005). It needs to be considered that 'sudden increases in intra-abdominal pressure', if caused by an intrinsically driven manoeuvre (i.e., coughing), include feed-forward activation of the PFMs as part of the complex muscle activation pattern. The observed PFM activation in the normal subject (e.g., during coughing) is thus a compound 'feed-forward' and 'reflex' muscle activation.

Another common stimulus leading to an increase in PFM activity is pain. The typical phasic reflex response to a nociceptive stimulus is the anal reflex. It is commonly assumed that prolonged pain in pelvic organs is accompanied by an increase in 'reflex' PFM activity, which would indeed be manifested as 'an increased tonic motor unit activity'. This has so far not been much formally studied. Whether such chronic PFM overactivity might itself generate a chronic pain state and even other dysfunctions may be a tempting hypothesis but has not been well demonstrated so far.

There is some evidence that PFM activity is modulated by various other reflex mechanisms associated with increase in intra-abdominal, bladder, urethral and anal pressures (Shafik et al., 2006a; Shafik et al., 2006b; Shafik et al., 2007; Shafik et al., 2008).

PFMs adapt their activity to the amount of stress that is performed on the pelvic floor, and therefore their activity is greater when running compared to standing (Luginbuehl et al., 2016), and the activity further increases with increasing speed. It has been shown that running triggers preactivation before and reflex activation after heel strike (Leitner et al., 2016).

To correspond to their functional (effector) role as pelvic organ supporters (e.g., during coughing, sneezing), sphincters for the LUT and anorectum, and as an effector in the sexual arousal response, orgasm and ejaculation, PFMs also have to be involved in very complex involuntary activity, which coordinates the behaviour of pelvic organs (smooth muscle) and several different groups of striated muscles. This activity is to be understood as originating from so-called pattern generators within the central nervous system, particularly the brainstem. These pattern generators ('reflex centres') are genetically inbuilt.

AWARENESS OF MUSCLE

The sense of position and movement of one's body (mostly dependent on muscle activity) is referred to as proprioception and is particularly important for sensing limb position (stationary proprioception) and limb movement (kinaesthetic proprioception).

Proprioception relies on special mechanoreceptors in muscles, muscle tendons and joint capsules. In muscles there are specialized stretch receptors (muscle spindles) and in tendons there are Golgi tendon organs, which sense the contractile force. In addition,

stretch-sensitive receptors signaling postural information are in the skin. This cutaneous proprioception is particularly important for controlling movements of muscles without bony attachment (lips, anal sphincter). By these means of afferent input, the functional status of a striated muscle (or rather a certain movement) is represented in the brain. Indeed, muscle awareness reflects the amount of sensory input from various sites. Typically, feedback to awareness on limb muscle function (acting at joints) is derived not only from input from muscle spindles, and receptors in tendons, but also from the skin, and from visual input, and so forth. The concept of 'awareness' thus, in fact, overlaps with the ability to voluntarily change the state of a muscle (see the following).

As opposed to the somatic nervous system, the visceral sensation (informing on the state of inner organs) does not reach consciousness, unless some activity is required (e.g., full bladder).

The PFMs (and sphincters) are on one hand intimately involved in visceral functions (mostly acting in the extraconscious realm), and on the other hand, lack several of the preceding sensory input mechanisms available to other striated muscles, and therefore the brain is not 'well informed' on their status. In addition, there may be a gender difference, inasmuch as PFM awareness in females seems to be, in general, less compared to males. (The authors conclude this on the basis of long personal experience with PFM EMGs in both genders; there seems to be no formal study on PFM activation patterns in men apart from ejaculation.)

Healthy males have no difficulties in voluntarily contracting the pelvic floor, but up to 30% of healthy women cannot do it readily on command. The need for 'squeezing out' the urethra at the end of voiding and the close relationship of penile erection and ejaculation to PFM contractions may be the origin of this gender difference. The primarily weak awareness of PFMs in women may be further jeopardized by vaginal delivery.

Voluntary Activity of Pelvic Floor Muscles

Skilled movement of distal limb muscles requires individual motor units to be activated in a highly focused manner by the primary motor cortex. By contrast, activation of axial muscles (necessary to maintain posture, etc.), while also under voluntary control, depends particularly on vestibular nuclei and reticular formation to create predetermined 'motor patterns'.

The PFMs are not, strictly speaking, axial muscles, but several similarities to axial muscles can be proposed regarding their neural control. In any case, PFMs are under voluntary control (i.e., it is possible to voluntarily activate or inhibit the firing of their motor units). EMG studies have shown that the activity of motor units in the urethral sphincter can be extinguished at both low and high bladder volumes even without initiating micturition (Sundin and Petersen, 1975; Vodušek, 1994).

To voluntarily activate a striated muscle we have to have the appropriate brain 'conceptualization' of that particular movement, which acts as a rule within a particular complex 'movement pattern'. This evolves particularly through repeatedly executed commands and represents a certain 'behaviour'.

Proprioceptive information is crucial for striated muscle motor control both in the 'learning' phase of a certain movement and for later execution of overlearned motor behaviours. It is passed to the spinal cord by fast-conducting, large-diameter myelinated afferent fibres and is influenced not only by the current state of the muscle but also by the efferent discharge the muscle spindles receive from the nervous system via gamma efferents. To work out the state of the muscle, the brain must take into account these efferent discharges and make comparisons between the signals it sends out to the muscle spindles along the gamma efferents and the afferent signals it receives from the primary afferents.

Essentially, the brain compares the signal from the muscle spindles with the copy of its motor command (the 'corollary discharge' or 'efferents copy') which was sent to the muscle spindle intrafusal muscle fibres by the CNS via gamma efferents. The differences between the two signals are used in deciding on the state of the muscle. The experiments were carried out in limb muscles (McCloskey, 1981), but it has been suggested (Morrison, 1987) that similar principles rule in bladder neurocontrol.

NEUROMUSCULAR INJURY TO THE PELVIC FLOOR DUE TO VAGINAL DELIVERY

Many studies using different techniques have demonstrated neurogenic and structural damage to the PFMs and sphincter muscles as a consequence of vaginal delivery (Blomquist et al., 2020; De Araujo et al., 2018; Vodušek, 2002b), but not in caesarean delivery

(Blomquist et al., 2018). Other lesion mechanisms, such as muscle ischaemia, may also be operative during vaginal childbirth. As a consequence, the PFMs would become weak; such weakness has indeed been demonstrated (Verelst and Leivseth, 2004). The sphincter mechanisms and pelvic organ support become functionally impaired, with stress urinary incontinence and prolapse being a logical consequence.

Although muscle weakness may be a common consequence of childbirth injury, there seem to be further pathophysiological possibilities for deficient PFM function; it is not only the strength of muscle contraction that defines its functional integrity.

Normal neural control of muscle activity leads to coordinated and timely responses to ensure appropriate muscle function as required. Muscular 'behavioural' patterns have been studied by kinesiological EMG recording (Deindl et al., 1993). Changes in muscular behaviour may originate from minor and repairable neuromuscular pelvic floor injury (Deindl et al., 1994).

In nulliparous healthy women, two types of behavioural patterns, named *tonic pattern* and *phasic pattern*, respectively, can be found:

- The tonic pattern consists of a crescendo–decrescendo type of activity (probably derived from grouping of slow motor units) that may be the expression of constant ('tonic') reflex input parallel to the breathing pattern.
- The phasic pattern, probably related to fast-twitch motor unit activation, is motor unit activity seen only during activation manoeuvres, either voluntary contraction or coughing.

With respect to these muscle activation patterns, parous women with stress urinary incontinence are subject to several possible changes (Deindl et al., 1994), such as a significant reduction of duration of motor unit recruitment, unilateral recruitment of reflex response in the pubococcygeal muscle and paradoxical inhibition of continuous firing of motor units in PFM activation on coughing.

The reasons for such persisting abnormalities are not clear and are difficult to explain by muscle denervation (which has been amply studied) alone. Although not directly proven in studies, it is reasonable to assume that motor denervation is accompanied also by sensory denervation of the PFMs. In addition to denervation injury, there may be some further temporary 'inhibitors' of PFM activity, such as periods of pain and discomfort after childbirth (e.g., perineal tears, episiotomy), increased by attempted PFM contraction.

All of the preceding factors may lead to a temporary disturbance of PFM activation patterns after childbirth. This, in combination with a particularly vulnerable pelvic floor neural control (which only evolved in its complexity phylogenetically after the attainment of the upright stance), might become persistent, even if the factors originally leading to the problem disappear.

CONCLUSION

The PFMs are a deep muscle group that have some similarities in their neural control with axial muscles. They are under prominent reflex and relatively weak voluntary control, with few and poor sensory data contributing to awareness of these muscles. Furthermore, their neural control mechanism is fragile due to its relative phylogenetic recency, and is exposed to trauma and disease due to its expansive anatomy (from the frontal cortex to the most caudal part of the spinal cord, and extensive peripheral innervation, both somatic and autonomic).

Vaginal delivery may lead to structural and denervation changes in the PFMs, but also to secondary changes in their activation patterns. Dysfunctional neural control induced by trauma, disease or purely functional causes may manifest itself by over- or underactivity, and/or by discoordination of PFM activity. Often these disturbances are not 'hardwired' into the nervous system, but only a problem of neural control 'software' (which can be 're-programmed'). Therefore, physical therapy should in many patients provide an appropriate, and even best available, treatment.

REFERENCES

Ashton-Miller, J. A., & DeLancey, J. O. L. (2007). Functional anatomy of the female pelvic floor. *Annals of the New York Academy of Sciences, 1101*, 266–296.

Athwal, B. S., Berkley, K. J., Hussain, I., et al. (2001). Brain responses to changes in bladder volume and urge to void in healthy men. *Brain, 124*, 369–377.

Bannister, L. H. (1995). *Gray's anatomy: The anatomical basis of medicine and surgery* (38th ed.). New York: Churchill Livingstone.

Barber, M. D., Bremer, R. E., Thor, K. B., et al. (2002). Innervation of the female levator ani muscles. *American Journal of Obstetrics and Gynecology, 187*, 64–71.

Barrington, F. J. F. (1925). The effect of lesions of the hind- and mid-brain on micturition in the cat. *Experimental Physiology, 15*, 81–102.

Bartolo, D. C. C., & MacDonald, A. D. H. (2002). Fecal continence and defecation. In J. H. Pemberton, M. Swash, & M. M. Henry (Eds.), *The pelvic floor: Its function and disorders* (pp. 77–83). London: W. B. Saunders.

Blok, B. F., & Holstege, G. (1994). Direct projections from the periaqueductal gray to the pontine micturition center (M-region). An anterograde and retrograde tracing study in the cat. *Neuroscience Letters, 166*, 93–96.

Blok, B. F. M., Sturms, L. M., & Holstege, G. (1997). A PET study on cortical and subcortical control of pelvic floor musculature in women. *The Journal of Comparative Neurology., 389*, 535–544.

Blomquist, J. L., Caroll, M., Munoz, A., et al. (2018). Association of delivery mode with pelvic floor disorders after childbirth. *Journal of the American Medical Association., 320*, 2438–2447.

Blomquist, J. L., Caroll, M., Munoz, A., et al. (2020). Pelvic floor muscle strength and the incidence of pelvic floor disorders after vaginal and cesarean delivery. *American Journal of Obstetrics and Gynecology, 222*, 62e1–62e8.

Borghi, F., Di Molfetta, L., Garavoglia, M., et al. (1991). Questions about the uncertain presence of muscle spindles in the human external anal sphincter. *Panminerva Medica, 33*, 170–172.

Brostrom, S. (2003). Motor evoked potentials from the pelvic floor. *Neurourology and Urodynamics, 22*, 620–637.

Catana, C., Drzezga, A., Heiss, W.-D., et al. (2012). PET/MRI for neurologic applications. *Journal of Nuclear Medicine, 53*, 1916–1925.

Chancellor, M. B., Perkin, H., & Yoshimura, N. (2005). Recent advances in the neurophysiology of stress urinary incontinence. *Scandinavian Journal of Urology and Nephrology, 39*, 21–24.

Chantraine, A. (1973). Examination of the anal and urethral sphincters. In J. E. Desmedt (Ed.), *New developments in electromyography and clinical neurophysiology. Vol. 2.* (pp. 421–432). Basel: Karger.

Craig, A. D. (2003). Interoception: The sense of the physiological condition of the body. *Current Opinion in Neurobiology, 13*, 500–505.

Dasgupta, R., Critchley, H. D., Dolan, R. J., et al. (2005). Changes in brain activity following sacral neuromodulation for urinary retention. *The Journal of Urology, 174*, 2268–2272.

De Araujo, C. C., Coelho, S. A., Stahlsmidt, P., et al. (2018). Does vaginal delivery cause more damage to the pelvic floor than cesarean section as determined by 3D ultrasound evaluation? A systematic review. *International Urogynecology Journal., 29*, 639–645.

De Groat, W. C., Fraser, M. O., Yoshiyama, M., et al. (2001). Neural control of the urethra. *Scandinavian Journal of Urology & Nephrology - Supplementum, 207*, 35–43 discussion 106–125.

Deindl, F. M., Vodušek, D. B., Hesse, U., et al. (1993). Activity patterns of pubococcygeal muscles in nulliparous continent women. *British Journal of Urology, 72*, 46–51.

Deindl, F. M., Vodušek, D. B., Hesse, U., et al. (1994). Pelvic floor activity patterns: Comparison of nulliparous continent and parous urinary stress incontinent women. A kinesiological EMG study. *British Journal of Urology, 73*, 413–417.

Dumoulin, S. O., Fracasso, A., van der Zwaag, W., et al. (2018). Ultra–high field MRI: Advancing systems neuroscience towards mesoscopic human brain function. *NeuroImage, 168*, 345–357.

Fucini, C., Ronchi, O., & Elbetti, C. (2001). Electromyography of the pelvic floor musculature in the assessment of obstructed defecation symptoms. *Diseases of the Colon & Rectum, 44*, 1168–1175.

Fukuyama, H., Matsuzaki, S., Ouchi, Y., et al. (1996). Neural control of micturition in man examined with single photon emission computed tomography using 99mTc-HM-PAO. *NeuroReport, 7*(18), 3009–3012.

Gentilcore-Saulnier, E., McLean, L., Goldfinger, C., et al. (2010). Pelvic floor muscle assessment outcomes in women with and without provoked vestibulodynia and the impact of physical therapy program. *The Journal of Sexual Medicine, 7*, 1003–1022.

Griffiths, D., Derbyshire, S., Stenger, A., et al. (2005). Brain control of normal and overactive bladder. *The Journal of Urology, 174*, 1862–1867.

Griffiths, D., Tadic, S. D., Schaefer, W., et al. (2007). Cerebral control of the bladder in normal and urge-incontinent women. *NeuroImage, 37*, 1–7.

Groenendijk, I. M., Luijten, S. P. R., de Zeeuw, C. I., et al. (2020). Whole brain 7T–fMRI during pelvic floor muscle contraction in male subjects. *Neurourology and Urodynamics, 39*, 382–392.

Hannan-Leith, M. N., Dayan, M., Hatfield, G., et al. (2019). Is pelvic floor sEMG a measure of women's sexual response? *The Journal of Sexual Medicine, 16*, 70–82.

Herzog, J., Weiss, P. H., Assmus, A., et al. (2006). Subthalamic stimulation modulates cortical control of urinary bladder in parkinson's disease. *Brain, 129*, 3366–3375.

Hoffman, B. L., Schorge, J. O., Bradshaw, K. D., et al. (2016). In *Williams gynecology*(3rd ed.) (pp. 561–576). New York: McGraw-Hill Education.

Holstege, G. (1998). The emotional motor system in relation to the supraspinal control of micturition and mating behavior. *Behavioural Brain Research, 92*, 103–109.

Huynh, H. K., Willemsen, A. T. M., Lovick, T. A., et al. (2013). Pontine control of ejaculation and female orgasm. *The Journal of Sexual Medicine, 10*, 3038–3048.

Kaiser, A. M., & Ortega, A. E. (2002). Anorectal anatomy. *Surgical Clinics of North America, 6*, 1125–1138.

Kenton, K., & Brubaker, L. (2002). Relationship between levator ani contraction and motor unit activation in the urethral sphincter. *American Journal of Obstetrics and Gynecology, 187*, 403–406.

Krhut, J., Holy, P., Tintera, J., et al. (2014). Brain activity during bladder filling and pelvic floor muscle contractions: A study using functional magnetic resonance imaging and synchronous urodynamics. *International Journal of Urology, 21*, 169–174.

Kuhtz-Buschbeck, J. P., van der Horst, C., Pott, C., et al. (2005). Cortical representation of the urge to void: A functional magnetic resonance imaging study. *The Journal of Urology, 174*, 1477–1481.

Kuhtz–Buschbeck, J. P., van der Horst, C., Wolff, S., et al. (2007). Activation of the supplementary motor area (SMA) during voluntary pelvic floor muscle contractions—an fMRI study. *NeuroImage, 35*, 449–457.

Kuipers, R., Mouton, L. J., & Holstege, G. (2006). Afferent projections to the pontine micturition center in the cat. *The Journal of Comparative Neurology., 494*, 36–53.

Kutch, J. J., Yani, M. S., Asavasopon, S., et al. (2015). Altered resting state neuromotor connectivity in men with chronic prostatitis/chronic pelvic pain syndrome: A MAPP research network neuroimaging study. *NeuroImage Clinical, 8*, 493–502.

Leitner, M., Moser, H., Eichelberger, P., et al. (2016). Evaluation of pelvic floor muscle activity during running in continent and incontinent women: An exploratory study. *Neurourology and Urodynamics, 36*, 1570–1576.

Lowenstein, L., Gruenwald, I., Gartman, I., et al. (2010). Can stronger pelvic muscle floor improve sexual function? *International Urogynecology Journal., 21*, 553–556.

Lúcio, A., D'Ancona, C., Lopes, M., et al. (2014). The effect of pelvic floor muscle training alone or in combination with electrostimulation in the treatment of sexual dysfunction in women with multiple sclerosis. *Multiple Sclerosis Journal., 20*, 1761–1768.

Luginbuehl, H., Naeff, R., Zahnd, A., et al. (2016). Pelvic floor muscle electromyography during different running speeds: An exploratory and reliability study. *Archives of Gynecology and Obstetrics, 293*, 117–124.

Mannen, T., Iwata, M., Toyokura, Y., et al. (1982). The Onuf's nucleus and the external anal sphincter muscles in amyotrophic lateral sclerosis and shy–drager syndrome. *Acta Neuropathologica, 58*, 255–260.

Marani, E., Pijl, M. E., Kraan, M. C., et al. (1993). Interconnections of the upper ventral rami of the human sacral plexus: A reappraisal for dorsal rhizotomy in neurostimulation operations. *Neurourology and Urodynamics*, *12*, 585–598.

McCloskey, D. I. (1981). Corollary changes: Motor commands and perception. In J. M. Brookhart, & V. B. Mountcastle (Eds.), *Handbook of physiology, section I: The nervous system Vol. 2.* (pp. 1415–1447). Bethesda, MD: American Physiological Society (part 2).

Mier, W., & Mier, D. (2015). Advantages in functional imaging of the brain. *Frontiers in Human Neuroscience*, *9*, 249.

Miller, J. M., Ashton-Miller, J. A., & DeLancey, J. O. (1998). A pelvic muscle precontraction can reduce cough-related urine loss in selected women with mild SUI. *Journal of the American Geriatrics Society*, *46*, 870–874.

Miller, J. M., Sampselle, C., Ashton-Miller, J., et al. (2008). Clarification and confirmation of the knack maneuver: The effect of volitional pelvic floor muscle contraction to preempt expected stress incontinence. *International Urogynecology Journal and Pelvic Floor Dysfunction*, *19*, 773–782.

Morrison, J. F. B. (1987). Reflex control of the lower urinary tract. In M. Torrens, & J. F. Morrison (Eds.), *The Physiology of the Lower Urinary Tract* (pp. 193–235). London: Springer Verlag.

Nour, S., Svarer, C., Kristensen, J., et al. (2000). Cerebral activation during micturition in normal men. *Brain*, *123*, 781–789.

Palit, S., Lunniss, P. J., & Scott, S. M. (2012). The physiology of human defecation. *Digestive Diseases and Sciences*, *57*, 1445–1464.

Petersen, I., Franksson, C., & Danielson, C. O. (1955). Electromyographic study of the muscles of the pelvic floor and urethra in normal females. *Acta Obstetricia et Gynecologica Scandinavica*, *34*, 273–285.

Read, N. W. (1990). Functional assessment of the anorectum in fecal incontinence. In G. Bock, & J. Whelan (Eds.), *Neurobiology of incontinence: Ciba foundation symposium 151* (pp. 119–138). Chichester: John Wiley.

Sagar, P. M., & Pemberton, J. H. (1996). Anorectal and pelvic floor function. Relevance of continence, incontinence, and constipation. *Gastroenterology Clinics of North America*, *25*, 163–182.

Sato, A., Sato, Y., & Schmidt, R. F. (2000). Reflex bladder activity induced by electrical stimulation of hind limb somatic afferents in the cat. *Journal of the Autonomic Nervous System*, *1*, 229–241.

Schroder, H. D. (1985). Anatomical and pathoanatomical studies on the spinal efferent systems innervating pelvic structures. 1. Organization of Spinal Nuclei in Animals. 2. The nucleus X-pelvic motor system in man. *Journal of the Autonomic Nervous System*, *14*, 23–48.

Seok, J. W., Sohn, J. H., & Cheong, C. (2016). Neural substrates of sexual arousal in heterosexual males: Event-related fMRI investigation. *Journal of Physiological Anthropology*, *35*, 8.

Seseke, S., Baudewig, J., Kallenberg, K., et al. (2006). Voluntary pelvic floor muscle control—an fMRI study. *NeuroImage*, *31*, 1399–1407.

Seseke, S., Baudewig, J., Ringert, R. H., et al. (2013). Monitoring brain activation changes in the early postoperative period after radical prostatectomy using fMRI. *NeuroImage*, *78*, 1–6.

Seseke, S., Leitsman, C., Hijazi, S., et al. (2019). Functional MRI in patients with detrusor sphincter dyssynergia: Is the neural circuit affected? *Neurourology and Urodynamics*, *38*(8), 2104–2111.

Shafik, A., & Shafik, I. A. (2003). Overactive bladder inhibition in response to pelvic floor exercises. *World Journal of Urology*, *20*, 374–377.

Shafik, A., Shafik, I., El Sibai, O., et al. (2006a). Role of the perineal muscles in micturition. *Journal of Pelvic Medicine and Surgery.*, *12*(1), 19–24.

Shafik, A., Shafik, I. A., El Sibai, O., et al. (2007a). Effect of urethral stimulation on vesical contractile activity. *The American Journal of the Medical Sciences*, *334*, 240–243.

Shafik, A., Shafik, A. A., El Sibai, O., et al. (2007b). The response of the corporal tissue and cavernosus muscles to urethral stimulation: An effect of penile buffeting of the vaginal introitus. *Journal of Andrology*, *28*, 853–857.

Shafik, A., Shafik, I. A., El Sibai, O., et al. (2008). A study of the effect of straining on the cavernosus muscles: Identification of "straining-cavernosus reflex" and its clinical significance. *Andrologia*, *40*, 23–28.

Shafik, A., Shafik, I., Shafik, A. A., et al. (2006b). The caverno-so-anal reflex: Response of the anal sphincters to cavernosus muscles' stimulation. *Asian Journal of Andrology*, *8*, 331–336.

Sundin, T., & Petersen, I. (1975). Cystometry and simultaneous electromyography from the striated urethral and anal sphincters and from levator ani. *Investigative Urology*, *13*, 40–46.

Torrens, M., & Morrison, J. F. B. (1987). In *The physiology of the lower urinary tract*. London: Springer-Verlag.

Ueyama, T., Mizuno, N., Nomura, S., et al. (1984). Central distribution of afferent and efferent components of the pudendal nerve in cat. *The Journal of Comparative Neurology.*, *222*, 38–46.

Van der Zwaag, W., Francis, S., Head, K., et al. (2009). fMRI at 1.5, 3 and 7 T: characterising BOLD signal changes. *NeuroImage*, *47*, 1425–1434.

Verelst, M., & Leivseth, G. (2004). Are fatigue and disturbances in preprogrammed activity of pelvic floor muscles associated with female stress urinary incontinence? *Neurourology and Urodynamics*, *23*, 143–147.

Vodušek, D. B. (1982). *Neurophysiological study of sacral reflexes in man [in Slovene]*. Master's thesis. Ljubljana: Institute of Clinical Neurophysiology. University E Kardelj in Ljubljana, 55.

Vodušek, D. B. (1994). Electrophysiology. In B. Schuessler, J. Laycock, P. Norton, et al. (Eds.), *Pelvic floor re-education, principles and practice* (pp. 83–97). London: Springer-Verlag.

Vodušek, D. B. (1996). Evoked potential testing. *Urologic Clinics of North America, 23*, 427–446.

Vodušek, D. B. (2002a). Sacral reflexes. In J. H. Pemberton, M. Swash, & M. M. Henry (Eds.), *Pelvic floor: Its functions and disorders* (pp. 237–247). London: Saunders.

Vodušek, D. B. (2002b). The role of electrophysiology in the evaluation of incontinence and prolapse. *Current Opinion in Obstetrics and Gynecology, 14*, 509–514.

Vodušek, D. B., & Janko, M. (1990). The bulbocavernosus reflex. a single motor neuron study. *Brain, 113*(3), 813–820.

Yani, M. S., Wondolowski, J. H., Eckel, S. P., et al. (2018). Distributed representation of pelvic floor muscles in human motor cortex. *Scientific Reports, 8*, 7213.

Zhang, H., Reitz, A., Kollias, S., et al. (2005). An fMRI study of the role of suprapontine brain structures in the voluntary voiding control induced by pelvic floor contraction. *NeuroImage, 24*, 174–180.

5

Measurement of Pelvic Floor Muscle Function and Strength

CHAPTER CONTENTS

52

5.1 Introduction

Kari Bø

CLASSIFICATION AND DEFINITIONS

The International Classification of Impairments, Disabilities and Handicaps (ICIDH) (World Health Organization, 1997), later changed to the International Classification of Functioning, Disability and Health (ICF) (World Health Organization, 2002), is a World Health Organization approved system for classification of health and health-related states in rehabilitation science, with the latest update completed in 2018. According to this system, the causes of a non-optimally functioning pelvic floor (e.g., muscle and nerve damage after vaginal birth, a wide levator hiatus or a sagging pelvic floor) can be classified as the *pathophysiological* component. Non-functioning pelvic floor muscles (PFMs; reduced force generation, inadequate timing or coordination) are the *impairment* component, and the symptom of pelvic floor dysfunction (e.g., urinary leakage, faecal incontinence or pelvic organ prolapse) is a *disability*. How the symptoms and conditions affect the woman's quality of life and participation in fitness activities is an *activity* or *participation* component.

Physical therapists (PTs) working to prevent or treat pelvic floor dysfunction aim to improve disability and activity/participation components by improving PFM function. Hence it is important to measure all ICF components. In this chapter, we deal only with the pathophysiological and impairment component, with a focus on assessment of the ability to contract the PFMs and measurement of PFM strength and endurance, resting activity and ability to relax.

The main reasons for PTs to conduct high-quality assessment of the ability to contract the PFMs and different aspects of PFM function are as follows:

1. Without proper instruction, many women are unable to volitionally contract PFMs on demand. This may be because the muscles are situated at the floor of the pelvis and are not visible from the outside. In addition, the muscles are seldom used consciously. Low levels of knowledge about the PFMs have been found in several studies (De Freitas et al., 2019; Gram and Bø, 2019; Neels et al., 2016). Neels et al. (2016) found that 8% of nulliparous women thought that the PFMs were located in the abdomen or at the caput femoris. Several studies have shown that more than 30% of women do not contract their PFMs correctly at their first consultation, even after thorough individual instruction (Benvenuti et al., 1987; Bø et al., 1988; Bump et al., 1991; Kegel, 1948). In a sample of 998 women with pelvic floor dysfunction (urinary incontinence, anal incontinence and pelvic organ prolapse), Tibaek and Dehlendorff (2014) found that 70% were unable to contract at baseline. The most common errors are contracting the gluteal, hip adductor or abdominal muscles instead of the PFMs (Bø et al., 1988; Neels et al., 2018). Some women also stop breathing or try to exaggerate inspiration instead of contracting the PFMs. Some studies have

demonstrated that many women also strain, causing PFM descent, instead of actively squeezing and lifting the PFMs upward (Bø et al., 1990; Bump et al., 1991). More recently, in a study of 212 nulliparous women, 75 (37%) answered that the PFMs also involve an outward pushing movement (Neels et al., 2016). Furthermore, Uechi et al. (2020) found that in 81 women with a mean age of 46.8 years (SD: 17.9), only 33% had a correct self-perception of the strength of their contraction. No agreement ($\kappa = 0.139$, $p = 0.087$) was found between the examiner's classification and the women's estimation of their PFM contraction. Therefore, proper assessment of the ability to contract with feedback to the patient on the performance (ability and strength) of the contraction is of utmost importance before commencing a PFM training program.

2. In intervention studies evaluating the effect of PFM training, whether this would be for strength/tone or relaxation, the training is the independent variable meant to cause a change in the dependent variable (e.g., stress urinary incontinence, pelvic organ prolapse or pelvic floor pain) (Thomas et al., 2015). Thus measurement of different aspects of PFM function before and after training is important to determine whether the intervention has made significant changes. Even in the presence of tissue pathology (e.g., neuropathy), if there is no change in PFM function after a training program commensurate with that pathology, the training program may not have been of insufficient dosage (intensity, frequency or duration of the training period) or the participants have had inadequate adherence (Bouchard et al., 1994). No effect may be due to untrainable underlying pathology, but it is also likely that such programs have not followed exercise science recommendations.

In this chapter we describe different measurement tools such as clinical observation, vaginal palpation, electromyography, vaginal squeeze pressure measurement (manometry), urethral pressure measurement (stationery and ambulatory), dynamometry, ultrasonography and magnetic resonance imaging in use for assessment of the PFMs. This can be either assessment of unconscious co-contraction of the PFMs during an increase in abdominal pressure or the ability to volitionally perform a correct contraction. A correct voluntary contraction is described as an elevation and squeeze around the pelvic openings (Kegel, 1948). For definitions related to muscle function, see the work of Bø et al. (2017) and Frawley et al. (2021).

In theory, one can measure different stages of a PFM contraction. The first is the constant state of contraction always present except before and during voiding and defaecation (resting activity). The second is increased tone as the bladder and bowel fills. Neither of these two stages include a conscious, voluntary PFM contraction. The third is a voluntary contraction (the Knack). The fourth is automatic, unconscious pre- or co-contraction of the PFMs during increase in intra-abdominal pressure or ground reaction forces. The latter is extremely difficult to measure with sufficient validity as measurement during, for example, running or jumping is prone to measurement flaws due to difficulties separating the measures from intra-abdominal pressure or cross-talk from nearby muscles and movement of the measurement device during physical activity (Bø and Nygaard, 2020).

Muscle strength measurement may be considered an indirect measure of PFM function in real-life activities. Women with no leakage do not contract voluntarily before coughing or jumping. Their PFM contraction is considered to be an automatic co-contraction occurring as a quick and effective activation of an intact neural system.

Other important factors for a quick and effective contraction are the location of the pelvic floor within the pelvis, the muscle bulk, stiffness/elasticity of the pelvic floor and intact connective tissue. If the pelvic floor is well positioned and stable, it may therefore not be necessary with a contraction of the PFMs during increases in intra-abdominal pressure or ground reaction forces.

A stretched and weak pelvic floor may be positioned lower within the pelvis compared with a well-trained or non-injured pelvic floor (Bø, 2004). The time for stretched muscles to reach an optimal contraction may be too slow to be effective in preventing descent against increased abdominal pressure (e.g., sneeze), thereby allowing leakage to occur.

In general, when measuring muscle strength, it can be difficult to isolate the muscles to be tested, and many test subjects need adequate time and instruction in how to perform the test. In addition, the test situation may not reflect the whole function of the muscles, and the generalizability from the test situation to real-world activity (external validity) must be established (Thomas et al., 2015). Therefore, when reporting results from muscle testing, it is important to specify the equipment used, position during testing, testing procedure, instruction and motivation given, and what parameters are tested (e.g., ability to contract, maximum strength, endurance) (Frawley et al., 2021). When testing the PFM, additional challenges are present because muscle action and location are not easily observable.

In the early 1980s Feinstein introduced the term *clinimetrics*, which is the practice of assessing or describing symptoms, signs and laboratory findings by means of scales, indices and other quantitative instruments (Fava et al. 2012). More recent information and tutorials about clinimetrics can be found at https://www.cosmin.nl and the PEDro database. We also recommend reading the Canadian Physiotherapy Association's Guide to Enhanced Clinical Decision Making (Finch et al., 2002) for a deeper understanding of measurement properties. In general, whether a measurement tool should be used in clinical practice or in research depends on its *responsiveness*, *reliability* and *validity*. These terms are used slightly differently in different research areas and have somewhat different definitions in different textbooks of research methodology. The definitions given next are the ones we have chosen to use in this textbook:

- *Responsiveness*: the degree or amount of variation that the device is capable of measuring; the ability of a tool to detect small differences or small changes (Currier, 1990).
- *Reliability*: consistency or repeatability of a measure. The most common way to establish the stability of a test is to perform a test–retest. *Intra-test* reliability is conducted by one researcher measuring the same procedure in the same subjects twice. *Inter-test* reliability is conducted when two or more clinicians or researchers are conducting measurement of the same subjects (Currier, 1990).
- *Validity*: degree to which a test or instrument measures what it is supposed to measure. The relationship between reliablity and validity is illustrated in Fig. 5.1.1.

- *Logical (face) validity*: condition that is claimed when the measure obviously involves the performance being measured (e.g., squeeze and elevation of the PFMs can be felt by vaginal palpation).
- *Content validity*: condition that is claimed when a test adequately samples what it should cover (few methods measure both squeeze pressure and elevation of the PFMs).
- *Criterion validity*: the degree to which the scores on a test are related to some recognized standard, or criterion (e.g., clinical observation of inward movement of the perineum during attempts to contract the PFMs compared with ultrasonography).
- *Concurrent validity*: involves a measuring instrument being correlated with some criterion administered at the same time or concurrently (e.g., simultaneous observation of inward movement during measurement of PFM strength with manometers and dynamometers).
- *Predictive validity*: degree to which scores of predictor variables can accurately predict criterion scores.
- *Diagnostic validity*: ability of a measure to detect differences between those having a diagnosis/problem/condition/symptom with those who do not.
- *Sensitivity*: the proportion of positives that are correctly identified by the test.
- *Specificity*: the proportion of negatives that are correctly identified by the test (Altman, 1997; Currier, 1990; Thomas et al., 2015).

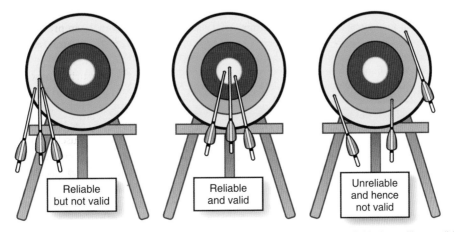

Fig. 5.1.1 Relationship between reliability and validity. A measurement can be reliable but still not valid (not assessing what it is meant to measure). However, it cannot be valid without being reliable.

It is important for PTs who treat patients with pelvic floor dysfunction to understand the qualities and limitations of the measurement tools they use (Bø and Sherburn, 2005). This chapter will provide the information needed for PTs to understand the application of each tool to the measurement of the PFMs. In many instances the PT may need thorough supervised instruction from other professionals before starting to use new equipment, such as ultrasonography and invasive electromyography (concentric needle and wire). In many cases, when available, receiving results from assessment of the PFMs from other professionals with special competence (e.g., radiologists) provides the best results.

REFERENCES

Altman, D. G. (1997). *Practical statistics for medical research* (9th ed.). London: Chapman & Hall.

Benvenuti, F., Caputo, G. M., Bandinelli, S., et al. (1987). Re-educative treatment of female genuine stress incontinence. *American Journal of Physical Medicine, 66*, 155–168.

Bø, K. (2004). Pelvic floor muscle training is effective in treatment of stress urinary incontinence, but how does it work? *International Urogynecology Journal and Pelvic Floor Dysfunction, 15*, 76–84.

Bø, K., Frawley, H., Haylen, B., et al. (2017). An International Urogynecological Association (IUGA)/International Continence Society (ICS) joint report on the terminology for the conservative and nonpharmacological management of female pelvic floor dysfunction. *Neurourology and Urodynamics, 36*, 221–244.

Bø, K., Kvarstein, B., Hagen, R., et al. (1990). Pelvic floor muscle exercise for the treatment of female stress urinary incontinence. II: Validity of vaginal pressure measurements of pelvic floor muscle strength and the necessity of supplementary methods for control of correct contraction. *Neurourology and Urodynamics, 9*, 479–487.

Bø, K., Larsen, S., Oseid, S., et al. (1988). Knowledge about and ability to correct pelvic floor muscle exercises in women with urinary stress incontinence. *Neurourology and Urodynamics, 7*, 261–262.

Bø, K., & Nygaard, I. E. (2020). Is physical activity good or bad for the pelvic floor? *Sports Medicine, 50*(3), 471–484.

Bø, K., & Sherburn, M. (2005). Evaluation of female pelvic floor muscle function and strength. *Physiotherapy, 85*(3), 269–282.

Bouchard, C., Shephard, R. J., & Stephens, T. (1994). *Physical activity, fitness, and health: International proceedings and consensus statement.* Champaign, IL: Human Kinetics.

Bump, R., Hurt, W. G., Fantl, J. A., et al. (1991). Assessment of Kegel exercise performance after brief verbal instruction. *American Journal of Obstetrics and Gynecology, 165*, 322–329.

Currier, D. P. (1990). *Elements of research in physiotherapy* (3rd ed.). Baltimore, MD: Williams & Wilkins.

De Freitas, L. M., Bø, K., Fernandes, A. C. N. L., et al. (2019). Pelvic floor muscle knowledge and relationship with muscle strength in Brazilian women: A cross-sectional study. *International Urogynecology Journal, 30*(11), 1903–1909.

Fava, G. A., Tomba, E., & Sonino, N. (2012). Clinimetrics: The science of clinical measurements. *International Journal of Clinical Practice, 66*(1), 11–15.

Finch, E., Brooks, D., Stratford, P., et al. (2002). *Physical rehabilitation outcome measures: A guide to enhanced clinical decision making* (2nd ed.). Toronto, Canada: Canadian Physiotherapy Association.

Frawley, H. E., Morin, M., Shelly, E., et al. (2021). Terminology for pelvic floor muscle function and dysfunction. *Neurourology and Urodynamics.* In manuscript.

Gram, M. D., & Bø, K. (2019). High level rhythmic gymnasts and urinary incontinence: Prevalence, risk factors, and influence on performance. *Scandinavian Journal of Medicine & Science in Sports, 30*(1), 159–165.

Kegel, A. H. (1948). Progressive resistance exercise in the functional restoration of the perineal muscles. *American Journal of Obstetrics and Gynecology, 56*, 238–249.

Neels, H., de Wachter, S., Wyndaele, J.-J., et al. (2018). Common errors made in attempt to contract the pelvic floor muscles in women early after delivery: A prospective observational study. *European Journal of Obstetrics & Gynecology and Reproductive Biology, 220*, 113–117.

Neels, H., Wyndaele, J.-J., Tjalma, W. A. A., et al. (2016). Knowledge of the pelvic floor in nulliparous women. *Journal of Physical Therapy Science, 28*(5), 1524–1533.

Thomas, J. R., Nelson, J. K., & Silverman, S. J. (2015). *Research methods in physical activity* (7th ed.). Champaign, IL: Human Kinetics.

Tibaek, S., & Dehlendorff, C. (2014). Pelvic floor muscle function in women with pelvic floor dysfunction: A retrospective chart review, 1992–2008. *International Urogynecology Journal, 25*(5), 663–669.

Uechi, N., Fernandes, A. C. N. L., Bø, K., et al. (2020). Do women have an accurate perception of their pelvic floor muscle contraction? A cross-sectional study. *Neurourology and Urodynamics, 39*(1), 361–366.

World Health Organization. (1997). *International Classification of Impairments, Disabilities and Handicaps (ICIDH).* Zeist, Netherlands: World Health Organization.

World Health Organization. (2002). *International Classification of Functioning, disability, and health (ICF).* Geneva: World Health Organization.

5.2 Visual Observation and Palpation

Kari Bø

VISUAL OBSERVATION

A correct contraction can be observed clinically (Kegel, 1948), by ultrasound (Beco et al., 1987; Dietz et al., 2002; Petri et al., 1999) or with dynamic magnetic resonance imaging (MRI) (Bø et al., 2001; Stoker et al., 2001).

In 1948, Kegel described a correct pelvic floor muscle (PFM) contraction as a squeeze around the urethral, vaginal and anal openings, and an inward lift that could be observed at the perineum (Kegel, 1948, 1952). He estimated the inward movement in the lying position to be 3 to 4 cm (Kegel, 1952). However, newer research visualizing lifting distance inside the body with MRI and ultrasound has not supported his estimation, which was based on visual observation. Bø et al. (2001) demonstrated a mean inward lift during PFM contraction to be 10.8 mm (SD: 6) in 16 women using dynamic MRI in a sitting position. This corresponded with an inward lift of 11.2 mm (95% CI: 7.2–15.3) measured with suprapubic ultrasound in a supine position (Bø et al., 2003).

Most physical therapists (PTs) would use visual observation of the PFM contraction as a starting point for measurement of the ability to contract. Despite this, there is a paucity of research on responsiveness, reliability and validity of this method.

Bø et al. (1990) used observation of movement of a vaginal catheter, vaginal palpation and vaginal squeeze pressure to measure PFM function and strength. They registered the ability to contract from visual observation as:

- correct (inward movement of the catheter),
- no contraction (no movement), and
- straining (outward movement).

There was 100% agreement between observation and the vaginal palpation test in women who either contracted correctly or were not able to contract according to the palpation test. The observation classified six who were straining and were not detected on the palpation test. Hence observation of movement may be more sensitive to straining and the Valsalva manoeuvre than palpation.

Responsiveness

No studies have been found evaluating the responsiveness of visual observation.

Intra- and Inter-Rater Reliability

Devreese et al. (2004) developed an inspection scale for the PFMs and abdominal muscles to be used in the crook lying, sitting and standing positions. Contractions were inspected during both voluntary contraction and reflex contraction during coughing. They classified the contraction of the PFMs as either 'coordinated' (inward movement of 1 cm of the perineum and a visible contraction of the deep abdominal muscle) or 'not coordinated' (downward movement of the pelvic floor and/ or an outward movement of the abdominal wall). The results of inter-tester reliability showed kappa coefficients between 0.94 and 0.97. Contrary to these findings, Slieker-ten Hove et al. (2009) tested intra- and inter-observer reliability of observation and found inter-rater weighted kappa (Kw) values of only 0.33 during coughing and 0.013 during straining. Kw for inter-rater reliability for visible co-contraction was 0.52. Intra- and inter-observer reliability for visible co-contraction were 0.48 and 0.52, respectively. There was high intra- and inter-observer reliability in observation of incontinence, relaxation and inward movement during PFM contraction. In a newer study, Pena et al. (2021) found an intra-tester reliability of k = 0.73 and a significant association between visual observation and vaginal palpation. Inter-tester reliability was not tested.

Validity

Shull et al. (2002) stated that by visual observation, one is generally observing superficial perineal muscles. From this observation, researchers assume that the levator ani is responding similarly. It may, however, not be the case.

Observing the inward movement of a correct PFM contraction is the starting point for measurement of PFM function and has the advantage of being a simple, noninvasive method. However, the inward lift may be created by contraction of superficial muscle layers only and have no influence on urethral closure mechanism. Conversely, there may be palpable PFM contraction with no visible outside movement. A correct lift can be difficult to observe from the outside, particularly in obese women. In addition, it is questionable whether it is possible to grade centimetres or millimetres of inward movement from the outside of the body. In the future, ultrasound may take over the role of visual observation and would also serve as a biofeedback and teaching tool.

Whether the muscle action observed by visual observation or ultrasound is sufficiently strong to increase urethral closure pressure can only be measured by urodynamic assessment in the urethra and bladder. Interestingly, Bump et al. (1991) found that, although contracting correctly, only 50% of a population of continent and incontinent women were able to voluntarily contract the PFMs with enough force to increase urethral pressure.

Sensitivity and Specificity

Devreese et al. (2004) found that continent women exhibited significantly better coordination between the pelvic floor and lower abdominal muscles during coughing and in crook lying, sitting and standing. Amaro et al. (2005) compared 50 women with stress urinary incontinence (SUI) and 50 continent women. They found that there was a negative visual observation of the ability to contract in 25.5% of the SUI group compared to 0 in the non-incontinent group.

Conclusion

Intra-tester reliability can be high, but inter-tester reliability is low in visual observation. Hence, the method should only be used when one tester is involved. Visual observation can be used in clinical practice to give a first impression about the ability to contract. Further estimation about the amount of the inward movement is not recommended. Visual observation should not be used for scientific purposes because MRI and especially ultrasound are more responsive, reliable and valid methods to assess movement during contraction, straining and physical exertion.

CLINICAL RECOMMENDATIONS

Pelvic Floor Muscle Assessment Using Observation

- Inform and explain the procedure to the patient.
- Teach the patient how to contract the PFMs by use of models, anatomical drawings and imagery.
- After the patient has undressed, ask the patient to lie down on the bench with the hips and knees bent and shoulder width apart (crook lying). Cover the pelvic area with a towel. Support the legs of the patient (one leg against the wall, the other leg supported with one hand).
- Allow some time for the patient to practice before observing the contraction.
- Ask the patient to breathe normally and then lift the perineum inwards and squeeze around the openings without any movement of the pelvis or visible co-contraction of the gluteal or hip adductor muscles. A small drawing in of the lower abdomen at maximum PFM contraction is accepted. Observe the patient's attempt to contract and register how the contraction was performed (correct, no contraction, inconclusive, straining).
- If there is an observable contraction, give positive feedback and explain that you will palpate to register action of the deeper muscles, and coordination and strength of the contraction. If you are not able to observe inward movement, explain that this is common at the first attempt, that it is not always easy to assess from the outside, and that you need to conduct a vaginal palpation to be sure whether there is a contraction or not.

Vaginal Palpation

Vaginal palpation (Fig. 5.2.1) is used to:
1. assess the ability of the patient to contract and relax the PFMs correctly;
2. measure PFM muscle strength via a maximal occlusive and lifting force (assessing the person's attempt to conduct a maximum voluntary contraction [MVC]), ability to sustain a contraction (endurance) or perform repeated contractions (endurance); and
3. assess other elements of PFMs, such as resting tension/muscle activity, the ability to fully relax after a contraction, coordination with lower abdominal muscles, symmetry of right and left PFM contraction, scarring and adhesions, and the presence of pain, major PFM injuries, speed and sequence of recruitment of the levator ani with the perineal muscles, and transverse and anteroposterior diameters of the urogenital hiatus (Bø et al., 2017; Frawley et al., 2021).

The International Continence Society (ICS) Clinical Assessment Group (see https://www.ics.org) has proposed qualitative scales (absent, partial, full) of measurement for some of these parameters. Slieker-ten Hove et al. (2009) assessed the reliability of trained PTs

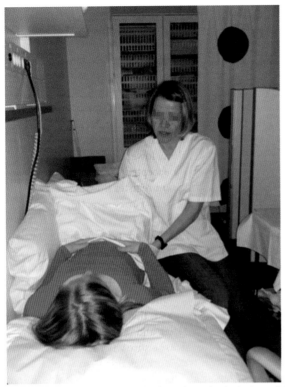

Fig. 5.2.1 During vaginal palpation the physical therapist instructs the patient about how to perform a contraction correctly ('Squeeze around my finger and try to lift the finger inwards') and tells her how well she is able to do it and also about coordination skills and strength. With encouragement, most patients are able to contract harder.

using these scales and found that in general, the intra-rater reliability was much higher than the inter-rater reliability. Moderate to substantial inter-rater reliability was found for palpation of pain, levator closure and voluntary contraction. However, endurance and fast contraction had a Kw value of 0.47 and 0.17, respectively. Palpation of involuntary contraction during coughing and movement of the perineum had an inter-rater reliability of 0.33 and 0.03, respectively. Kegel (1948, 1952) described vaginal palpation as a method to evaluate the ability to perform a correct contraction. He placed one finger in the distal one-third of the vagina and asked the woman to lift inwards and squeeze around the finger. Kegel did not use this method to measure PFM strength. He classified the contraction qualitatively as correct or not. In addition, he developed the 'perineometer', a pressure manometer, to measure PFM strength through vaginal squeeze pressure (Kegel, 1948). Pena et al. (2021)

> **BOX 5.2.1 The Modified Oxford Grading Scale**
>
> The modified Oxford grading scale is a 6-point scale where half numbers of + and − can be added when a contraction is considered to fall between two full grades, so it expands to a 15-point scale when both + and − are used:
>
> 0 = no contraction
> 1 = flicker
> 2 = weak
> 3 = moderate (with lift)
> 4 = good (with lift)
> 5 = strong (with lift)
>
> *Adapted from* Newman, 2008.

found substantial intra-rater reliability (k = 0.74) of assessment of the ability to perform a correct contraction.

Van Kampen et al. (1996) reported that after Kegel first described vaginal palpation as a method to evaluate PFM function, more than 25 different palpation methods have been developed. Some examiners use one finger, and others use two fingers.

Worth et al. (1986) and Brink et al. (1989) have evaluated pressure, duration, muscle 'ribbing' and displacement of the examiner's finger in a specific scoring system. This system has mainly been used by American nurses. There has been no systematic research to determine the best method of palpation to assess the ability to contract or any of the parameters of muscle strength, endurance or power.

Laycock developed the modified Oxford grading system (Box 5.2.1) to measure PFM strength (British Medical Research Council, 1943; Laycock, 1994), and this seems to be the system mostly used by PTs to assess PFM strength in clinical practice.

Responsiveness in Grading of Pelvic Floor Muscle Strength

The Oxford grading system has been modified from the Medical Research Council scale (1943), which suffers from poor responsiveness and non-linearity (Beasley, 1961).

One of the difficulties of measurement using the modified Oxford scale is that it produces one value for two elements (occlusion and lift) in the one scale. The palpating fingers may not be sensitive enough to differentiate the proportions of occlusion versus lift. To separate these two elements, manometers or dynamometers can be used to evaluate occlusion, and ultrasound to measure the lift component. When the responsiveness of the modified Oxford scale is tested against vaginal squeeze pressure, it should be recognized that only one element, occlusion, is being compared.

Bø and Finckenhagen (2001) questioned the responsiveness of the modified Oxford scale (without + and −) because they did not find that the scale could separate between weak, moderate, good or strong when comparing measurement of vaginal squeeze pressure. This was supported by Morin et al. (2004) comparing vaginal palpation and dynamometry in continent and incontinent women. They found that important overlaps were observed between each category of vaginal palpation. Mean force values differed significantly only between non-adjacent levels in palpation assessment (e.g., between 1 and 3, 1 and 4, 1 and 5, 2 and 4, and 2 and 5 [p < 0.05]).

Frawley et al. (2006) found that the Oxford grading scale using + and − had lower kappa values in intra-test reliability testing and recommended using the original 6-point scale in research.

Intra- and Inter-Rater Reliability of Vaginal Palpation to Assess Pelvic Floor Muscle Strength

The results from studies evaluating intra- and inter-rater reliability of vaginal palpation for strength measurement are conflicting (Bø and Finckenhagen, 2001; Ferreira et al., 2011; Frawley et al., 2006; Hahn et al., 1996; Isherwood and Rane, 2000; Jean-Michel et al., 2010; Jeyaseelan et al., 2001; Laycock and Jerwood, 2001; McKey and Dougherty, 1986).

Isherwood and Rane (2000) found high inter-rater reliability, whereas Jeyaseelan et al. (2001) concluded that inter-tester reliability should not be assumed and needs to be established when two or more clinicians are involved in pre- and post-treatment assessment.

Bø and Finckenhagen (2001) using the 6-point scale and Laycock and Jerwood (2001) using the 15-point scale found agreement between testers in only 45% and 46.7% of the tested cases, respectively. The latter was supported by Jean-Michel et al. (2010) reporting that test–retest values for the Oxford muscle grading system were unacceptably poor within and between examiners. However, no data were reported in the study. Ferreira et al. (2011) found only fair inter-rater reliability

of vaginal palpation (k = 0.33, 95% CI: 0.09–057) and conferred that palpation did not separate between weak, moderate, good or strong compared with manometry.

Devreese et al. (2004) developed a new vaginal palpation system assessing muscle 'tone', endurance, speed of contraction, strength, lift (inward movement) and coordination, and evaluated both superficial and deep PFMs. They found reliability coefficients between 0.75 and 1.00 for measurements of the preceding parameters. The scoring system developed is qualitative and open to personal interpretation, but it was a first step towards standardizing a measurement system for observation and palpation.

Frawley et al. (2006) found 79% complete agreement in both crook lying and supine using the 6-point scale, but this dropped to 53% and 58%, respectively, using the 15-point scale. They tested intra-tester reliability of vaginal digital assessment and found good to very good kappa values of 0.69, 0.69, 0.86 and 0.79 for crook lying, supine, sitting and standing positions, respectively. In addition, they compared vaginal palpation with vaginal squeeze pressure measurement (Peritron) and found that the Peritron was more reliable than vaginal palpation (Frawley et al., 2006). However, V3lløyhaug et al. (2016) found that palpation correlated with manometry (rs = 0.74) and with proportional change in the hiatal area (rs = 0.67) and anteroposterior diameter (rs = 0.69) on ultrasound.

PELVIC FLOOR MUSCLE RESTING ACTIVITY/TONE/STIFFNESS

Muscle 'tone' requires a universally acceptable definition to establish a reliable measurement system. The International Urogynecological Association (IUGA)/ICS joint report on the terminology for the conservative and non-pharmacological management of female pelvic floor dysfunction (Bø et al., 2017) defined muscle tone as state of the muscle, usually defined by its resting tension, clinically determined by resistance to passive movement. Muscle tone has two components: the contractile component, created by the low frequency activation of a small number of motor units, and the viscoelastic component, which is independent of neural activity and reflects the passive physical properties of the elastic tension of the muscle fiber elements and the osmotic pressure of the cells. Hypertonicity is defined as an increase in muscle tone related to the contractile or viscoelastic components that can be associated with either elevated contractile activity and/or passive stiffness in the muscle. Hypotonicity is defined as a decrease in muscle tone related to the contractile or viscoelastic components that can be associated with either reduced contractile activity and/ or passive stiffness in the muscle. Neurogenic hyper- or hypotonicity and non-neurogenic hyper- or hypotonicity are recommended to describe the diagnosis and inform management. Stiffness is defined as resistance to deformation. Passive elastic stiffness is the ratio of the change in the passive resistance or passive force (ΔF) to the change in the length displacement (ΔL) or $\Delta F/\Delta L$.24. The term should only be used if stiffness is measured quantitatively, such as with the use of instruments such as dynamometry or myotonometry (Bø et al., 2017). The elastic component or 'elastic stiffness' is measured qualitatively by pressing or squeezing a muscle. However, measurement of the viscoelastic component is more complex and is dependent on the speed at which the muscle is moved using pendular, oscillatory and resonant frequency measurements (Simons and Mense, 1998). These viscoelastic measurements are not possible for the PFMs because the PFMs do not pass over a joint to allow elongation and then shortening. If the PFMs are elongated using vaginal palpation to stretch the muscle fibres, the muscle belly is being compressed by the examining digit and elastic stiffness is again being measured. Tension may be a better terminology than tone.

One can also discuss how one can assess that there is no motor unit activity. At least for the PFMs, there is always electromyographic activity, except before and during voiding (Fowler et al., 2002). Slieker-ten Hove et al. (2009) found that voluntary relaxation had an inter-rater Kw value of 0.37 and palpation of involuntary relaxation during straining had a Kw value of 0.15 only. In contrast, Devreese et al. (2004) found high agreement in inter-observer reliability in tone (95%–100% agreement) assessed with their score system. Dietz and Shek (2008a) proposed a new scale for resting tone from 0 (muscle not palpable) to 5 (hiatus very narrow, no distension possible, 'woody' feel, possibly with pain: vaginismus) and found a Kw value of 0.55 (CI: 0.44–0.66). A low resting tone was associated with pelvic organ prolapse (POP). Importantly, Davidson et al. (2020) did a prospective observational study involving 125 musculoskeletal and pelvic floor physiotherapists. A novel device was developed that replicates the haptic feedback

that clinicians assess as muscle stiffness. Measurements of displacement, force and stiffness were recorded. The results showed wide overlap between each scale category assigned to the stiffness values, from low stiffness at −3 (119 [106,132] N/m), to moderate stiffness at 0 (462 [435,489] N/m) to high stiffness at +3 (897 [881,913] N/m). Consistency in applying the scale was poor, and the probability of a similar value of stiffness being assigned to the same scale category by different PTs was low. The authors concluded that palpation of muscle tone should be used with caution in diagnosing and defining patient care.

PALPATION OF PELVIC FLOOR MUSCLE INJURIES

MRI and ultrasound are commonly used to assess injuries to the PFMs. Dietz et al. (2006) compared vaginal palpation and 4D pelvic floor ultrasound and concluded that palpation of the pubovisceral muscle correlated poorly with 3/4D ultrasound in detecting levator ani trauma. Dietz and Shek (2008b) in a study of 110 women concluded that palpatory detection of major levator trauma was less repeatable than identification by ultrasound. In another study (Dietz et al., 2012), vaginal palpation was compared with 3/4D ultrasound analysed with either render or multislice imaging, and kappa values between 0.35 and 0.56 were found. Kruger et al. (2013) assessed 72 women age 60 years and older and found that the predictive ability of the digital assessment varied from poor to moderate. The variable 'width between insertions' performed best. Palpation could not distinguish between uni- and bilateral trauma. Van Delft et al. (2015) found that the correlation between vaginal palpation and transperineal and endovaginal ultrasound was only fair with Cohen's kappa of 0.34 and 0.37, respectively. In contradiction, Nyhus et al. (2020) investigating 195 women scheduled for either SUI or POP surgery found moderate correlation between ultrasound measurements and modified Oxford grading score with 0.52 for 2D anterior-posterior diameter, 0.62 for 3D anterior-posterior diameter and 0.47 for hiatal area ($p < 0.001$ for all). The prevalence of major levator injury was 22.6%. On the ultrasound contraction scale, proportional change in 2D levator hiatal anterior-posterior diameter of less than 1% corresponded to absent, 2% to 14% to weak, 15% to 29% to normal and greater than 30% to strong contraction.

Validity

Several investigators have studied criterion validity of vaginal palpation comparing vaginal palpation and vaginal squeeze pressure (Bø and Finckenhagen, 2001; Hahn et al., 1996; Isherwood and Rane, 2000; Jarvis et al., 2001; Kerschan-Schindel et al., 2002; McKey and Dougherty, 1986).

Isherwood and Rane (2000) compared vaginal palpation using the Oxford grading system and compared it with an arbitrary scale on a perineometer from 1 to 12. They found a high kappa of 0.73. In contrast, Bø and Finckenhagen (2001) found a kappa of 0.37 comparing the Oxford grading system with vaginal squeeze pressure. Heitner (2000) concluded that lift was most reliably tested with palpation, and that all other measures of muscle function were better tested with electromyography.

Hahn et al. (1996) found that there was a better correlation of vaginal palpation and pressure measurement in continent than in incontinent women (r = 0.86 and 0.75, respectively). This was supported by Morin et al. (2004) comparing vaginal palpation with dynamometry, finding r = 0.73 in continent and r = 0.45 in incontinent women, respectively.

Lying, Sitting or Standing?

PFM function and strength are often measured in a supine position, even though urinary leakage is more common in the upright position with gravity acting on the PFMs. Very few studies have addressed measurement in different positions.

Devreese et al. (2004) investigated inter-rater reliability of clinical observation and vaginal palpation in crook lying, sitting and standing positions. They found high inter-tester reliability in all positions but did not report whether there were differences in measurement values in the different positions.

Frawley et al. (2006) found that vaginal palpation of PFM contraction had moderate to high intra-test reliability in crook lying, supine, sitting and standing positions. Both Bø and Finckenhagen (2003) and Frawley et al. (2006) found that PTs and patients preferred testing using vaginal palpation and vaginal squeeze pressure in lying positions. Bø and Finckenhagen (2003) found that the testing procedure was easiest to standardize when the patient was supine and therefore recommend this in clinical practice.

For scientific purposes, the position of the patient should be chosen according to the research question, and the test position must be reported to allow comparison between studies (Bo et al., 2017; Frawley et al., 2021).

One or Two Fingers?

There is a discussion whether one or two fingers should be used for vaginal palpation (Bø et al., 2005; Shull et al., 2002), and this may depend on factors such as whether the patient is nulliparous and has a narrow vaginal introitus and urogenital hiatus, or whether there is introital discomfort or pain.

Hoyte et al. (2001) reported increased diameters from non-symptomatic parous women to parous women with POP. In parous women, vaginal birth may have stretched the PFMs and its investing fascia. However, time and PFM training may normalize this in many women.

When palpating, the anterior and posterior vaginal walls are always in apposition and in contact with the finger. The lateral vaginal walls expand in the upper vagina at the level of the fornices and above the level of the levator ani. At the PFM level, the lateral diameter of the urogenital hiatus marks the medial borders of the levator ani, and these borders may be palpated through the intervening vaginal mucosa.

Ghetti et al. (2005) stated that intra- and inter-rater reliability of vaginal palpation to assess the diameter of the hiatus needs to be done. In addition, criterion validity between MRI/ultrasound and vaginal palpation of the hiatus must be established.

Putting a muscle on stretch makes it more difficult to perform a maximal contraction (Frontera and Meredith, 1989). Therefore the aim of palpation should be to gain maximum sensation for the palpation with no stretch. This must not be confused with the fact that a quick stretch can be used to facilitate the stretch reflex. Quick stretch is one technique used by PTs to facilitate a correct PFM contraction if the patients are unable to contract (Brown, 2001).

Sensitivity and Specificity

There are few studies comparing measurement of PFM function in continent and incontinent women using vaginal palpation.

Hahn et al. (1996) compared 30 continent and 30 incontinent women using vaginal palpation and found that the group of incontinent women had lower scores on the palpation test (1.0 ± 0.1) compared to the group of continent women (1.9 ± 0.1) (p < 0.001).

Devreese et al. (2004) found a significant difference in favour of continent women in speed of contraction, maximum strength and coordination of both superficial and deep PFMs, and inward movement of the superficial, but not the deep, PFMs assessed with vaginal palpation. Amaro et al. (2005) found normal function assessed by palpation in 18% of incontinent women versus 90% in the continent group. Thompson et al. (2006a,b) also confirmed stronger PFMs in continent compared to incontinent women.

CONCLUSION

Today most PTs use vaginal palpation to evaluate PFM function because both squeeze pressure and lift can be registered, although with poor discrimination. It is a low-cost method and is relatively easy to conduct.

Vaginal palpation of PFM contraction is recommended as a good technique for PTs to understand, teach and give feedback to patients about correctness of the contraction. Position of the patient, instruction given and the use of one or two fingers must be standardized and reported. However, whether palpation is robust enough to be used as an outcome measure before and after treatment and for scientific purposes to measure muscle strength or other muscle functions is questionable. Palpation as a method to detect morphological abnormalities remains under discussion.

CLINICAL RECOMMENDATIONS

Palpation Procedure

Following perineal observation, with the patient in the crook lying position:

- Explain the palpation procedure to the patient and obtain consent.
- Prepare examination gloves, gel and tissues, and check with the patient for latex and gel allergy. Use vinyl gloves for preference.
- Wash hands, put on gloves and apply a little gel on the palpating gloved finger(s).
- Gently part the labia and insert one finger in the outer one-third of the vagina.
- Ask the patient whether she feels comfortable.
- If appropriate, insert the second finger.

- Ask the patient to lift in and squeeze around the finger(s) and observe or control the action so that the pelvis is not moving, or the hip adductor or gluteal muscles are not contracted.
- Give feedback of correctness, performance and strength.
- Record whether PFM contraction is:
  - correct
  - only possible with visible co-contraction of other muscles
  - not present
  - in the opposite direction (straining or Valsalva)
- To record the MVC, request a 3- to 5-second maximum effort PFM contraction after one or two submaximal 'practice' contractions. If you do not have a sensitive, reliable and valid tool to measure strength, use the Oxford grading scale to record the MVC. Separately record the lift component as absent, partial or complete.
- Note the voluntary relaxation after these contractions, and record this as absent, partial or full.
- If no further vaginal measurements are to be made, discard the examination gloves into the appropriate waste disposal and allow the patient privacy for dressing.

REFERENCES

Amaro, J. L., Moreira, E. C. H. M., Gameiro, M. O. O., et al. (2005). Pelvic floor muscle evaluation in incontinent patients. *International Urogynecology Journal and Pelvic Floor Dysfunction*, 16, 352–354.

Beasley, W. C. (1961). Quantitative muscle testing: Principles and applications to research and clinical services. *Archives of Physical Medicine and Rehabilitation*, 42, 398–425.

Beco, J., Sulu, M., Schaaps, J. P., et al. (1987). A new approach to urinary continence disorders in women: Urodynamic ultrasonic examination by the vaginal route [in French]. *Journal de Gynecologie Obstetrique et Biologie de la Reproduction*, 16, 987–998.

Bø, K., & Finckenhagen, H. B. (2001). Vaginal palpation of pelvic floor muscle strength: Inter-test reproducibility and the comparison between palpation and vaginal squeeze pressure. *Acta Obstetricia et Gynecologica Scandinavica*, 80, 883–887.

Bø, K., & Finckenhagen, H. B. (2003). Is there any difference in measurement of pelvic floor muscle strength in supine and standing position? *Acta Obstetricia et Gynecologica Scandinavica*, 82, 1120–1124.

Bø, K., Frawley, H., Haylen, B., et al. (2017). An International Urogynecological Association (IUGA)/International Continence Society (ICS) joint report on the terminology for the conservative and nonpharmacological management of female pelvic floor dysfunction. *Neurourology and Urodynamics, 36*, 221–244.

Bø, K., Kvarstein, B., Hagen, R., et al. (1990). Pelvic floor muscle exercise for the treatment of female stress urinary incontinence. II: Validity of vaginal pressure measurements of pelvic floor muscle strength and the necessity of supplementary methods for control of correct contraction. *Neurourology and Urodynamics, 9*, 479–487.

Bø, K., Lilleås, F., Talseth, T., et al. (2001). Dynamic MRI of pelvic floor muscles in an upright sitting position. *Neurourology and Urodynamics, 20*, 167–174.

Bø, K., Raastad, R., & Finckenhagen, H. B. (2005). Does the size of the vaginal probe affect measurement of pelvic floor muscle strength? *Acta Obstetricia et Gynecologica Scandinavica, 84*, 129–133.

Bø, K., Sherburn, M., & Allen, T. (2003). Transabdominal ultrasound measurement of pelvic floor muscle activity when activated directly or via transversus abdominis muscle contraction. *Neurourology and Urodynamics, 22*, 582–588.

Brink, C., Sampselle, C. M., Wells, T., et al. (1989). A digital test for pelvic muscle strength in older women with urinary incontinence. *Nursing Research, 38*(4), 196–199.

British Medical Research Council. (1943). Aid to the investigation of peripheral nerve injuries. In *War memorandum* (pp. 11–46). London: Her Majesty's Stationery Office.

Brown, C. (2001). Pelvic floor re-education: A practical approach. In J. Corcos, & E. Schick (Eds.), *The urinary sphincter* (pp. 459–473). New York: Marcel Dekker.

Bump, R., Hurt, W. G., Fantl, J. A., et al. (1991). Assessment of Kegel exercise performance after brief verbal instruction. *American Journal of Obstetrics and Gynecology, 165*, 322–329.

Davidson, M. J., Nielsen, P. M. F., Taberner, A. H., et al. (2020). Is it time to rethink using digital palpation for assessment of muscle stiffness? *Neurourology and Urodynamics, 39*, 279–285.

Devreese, A., Staes, F., De Weerdt, W., et al. (2004). Clinical evaluation of pelvic floor muscle function in continent and incontinent women. *Neurourology and Urodynamics, 23*, 190–197.

Dietz, H. P., Hyland, G., & Hay-Smith, J. (2006). The assessment of levator trauma: A comparison between palpation and 4D pelvic floor ultrasound. *Neurourology and Urodynamics, 25*, 424–427.

Dietz, H. P., Jarvis, S., & Vancaillie, T. (2002). The assessment of levator muscle strength: A validation of three ultrasound techniques. *International Urogynecology Journal and Pelvic Floor Dysfunction, 13*, 156–159.

Dietz, H. P., Moegni, H., & Shek, K. L. (2012). Diagnosis of levator avulsion injury: A comparison of three methods. *Ultrasound in Obstetrics and Gynecology, 40*(6), 693–698.

Dietz, H. P., & Shek, K. L. (2008a). The quantification of levator muscle resting tone by digital assessment. *International Urogynecology Journal and Pelvic Floor Dysfunction, 19*(11), 1489–1493.

Dietz, H. P., & Shek, C. (2008b). Validity and reproducibility of the digital detection of levator trauma. *International Urogynecology Journal and Pelvic Floor Dysfunction, 19*(8), 1097–1101.

Ferreira, C. H., Barbosa, P. B., de Oliveira Souza, F., et al. (2011). Inter-rater reliability study of the modified Oxford grading scale and the Peritron manometer. *Physiotherapy, 97*(2), 132–138.

Fowler, C. J., Benson, J. T., Craggs, M. D., et al. (2002). Clinical neurophysiology. In P. Abrams, L. Cardozo, S. Khourhy, et al. (Eds.), *Incontinence: Second international consultation on incontinence* (pp. 389–424). Plymouth, UK: Health Publication/Plymbridge Distributors.

Frawley, H. C., Galea, M. P., Philips, B. A., et al. (2006). Reliability of pelvic floor muscle strength assessment using different test positions and tools. *Neurourology and Urodynamics, 25*(3), 236–242.

Frawley, H. E., Morin, M., Shelly, E., et al. (2021). An International Continence Society (ICS) report on the terminology for pelvic floor muscle assessment. *Neurourology and Urodynamics, 40*(5), 1217–1260.

Frontera, W., & Meredith, C. (1989). Strength training in the elderly. In R. Harris, & S. Harris (Eds.), *Physical activity, aging and sports. Vol 1: Scientific and medical research* (pp. 319–331). Albany, NY: Center for the Study of Aging.

Ghetti, C., Gregory, W. T., Edwards, S. R., et al. (2005). Severity of pelvic organ prolapse associated with measurements of pelvic floor function. *International Urogynecology Journal and Pelvic Floor Dysfunction, 16*(6), 432–436.

Hahn, I., Milsom, I., Ohlson, B. L., et al. (1996). Comparative assessment of pelvic floor function using vaginal cones, vaginal digital palpation and vaginal pressure measurement. *Gynecologic and Obstetric Investigation, 41*, 269–274.

Heitner, C. (2000). *Valideringsonderzoek naar palpatie en myofeedback bij vrouwen met symptomen van stress urineincontinentie*. Netherlands: Master's thesis. University of Maastricht.

Hoyte, L., Schierlitz, L., Zou, K., et al. (2001). Two- and 3-dimensional MRI comparison of levator ani structure, volume, and integrity in women with stress incontinence and prolapse. *American Journal of Obstetrics and Gynecology, 185*(1), 11–19.

Isherwood, P., & Rane, A. (2000). Comparative assessment of pelvic floor strength using a perineometer and digital examination. *British Journal of Obstetrics and Gynaecology, 107*, 1007–1011.

Jarvis, S., Dietz, H., & Vancaillie, T. (2001). A comparison between vaginal palpation, perineometry and ultrasound in the assessment of levator function. *International Urogynecology Journal and Pelvic Floor Dysfunction, 12*(Suppl. 3), 31.

Jean-Michel, M., Biller, D. H., Bena, J. F., et al. (2010). Measurement of pelvic floor muscular strength with the colpexin pull test: A comparative study. *International Urogynecology Journal and Pelvic Floor Dysfunction, 21*, 1011–1017.

Jeyaseelan, S., Haslam, J., Winstanley, J., et al. (2001). Digital vaginal assessment: An inter-tester reliability study. *Physiotherapy, 87*(5), 243–250.

Kegel, A. H. (1948). Progressive resistance exercise in the functional restoration of the perineal muscles. *American Journal of Obstetrics and Gynecology, 56*, 238–249.

Kegel, A. H. (1952). Stress incontinence and genital relaxation. *Ciba Clinical Symposia, 4*(2), 35–51.

Kerschan-Schindl, K., Uher, E., Wiesinger, G., et al. (2002). Reliability of pelvic floor muscle strength measurement in elderly incontinent women. *Neurourology and Urodynamics, 21*, 42–47.

Kruger, J. A., Dietz, H. P., Budgett, S. C., et al. (2013). Comparison between transperineal ultrasound and digital detection of levator ani trauma. Can we improve the odds? *Neurourology and Urodynamics, 33*(3), 307–311.

Laycock, J. (1994). Clinical evaluation of the pelvic floor. In B. Schussler, J. Laycock, P. Norton, et al. (Eds.), *Pelvic floor Re-education* (pp. 42–48). London: Springer-Verlag.

Laycock, J., & Jerwood, D. (2001). Pelvic floor muscle assessment: The perfect scheme. *Physiotherapy, 87*(12), 631–642.

McKey, P. L., & Dougherty, M. C. (1986). The circumvaginal musculature: Correlation between pressure and physical assessment. *Nursing Research, 35*(5), 307–309.

Morin, M., Dumoulin, C., Bourbonnais, D., et al. (2004). Pelvic floor maximal strength using vaginal digital assessment compared to dynamometric measurements. *Neurourology and Urodynamics, 23*, 336–341.

Newman, D. K., Laycock, J. (2008). Clinical Evaluation of the Pelvic Floor Muscles. In: Baessler, K., Burgio, K. L., Norton, P. A., Schüssler, B., Moore, K. H., Stanton, S. L. (eds) Pelvic Floor Re-education. Springer, London.

Nyhus, M. Ø., Oversand, S. H., Salvesen, Ø., et al. (2020). Ultrasound assessment of pelvic floor muscle contraction: Reliability and development of an ultrasound-based contraction scale. *Ultrasound in Obstetrics and Gynecology, 55*(1), 125–131.

Pena, C. C., Bø, K., de la Ossa, A. M. P., Fernandes, A. C. N. L., et al. (2021). Are visual inspection and digital palpation reliable methods to assess ability to perform a pelvic floor muscle contraction? An intra-rater study. *Neurourology and Urodynamics, 40*(2), 680–687.

Petri, E., Koelbl, H., & Schaer, G. (1999). What is the place of ultrasound in urogynecology? A written panel. *International Urogynecology Journal and Pelvic Floor Dysfunction, 10*, 262–273.

Shull, B., Hurt, G., Laycock, J., et al. (2002). Physical examination. In P. Abrams, L. Cardozo, S. Khoury, et al. (Eds.), *Incontinence: Second international consultation on incontinence* (pp. 373–388). Plymouth, UK: Health Publication/Plymbridge Distributors.

Simons, D. G., & Mense, S. (1998). Understanding and measurement of muscle tone as related to clinical muscle pain. *Pain, 75*, 1–17.

Slieker-ten Hove, M. C., Pool-Goudzwaard, A. L., Eijkemans, M. J., et al. (2009). Face validity and reliability of the first digital assessment scheme of pelvic floor muscle function confirm the new standardized terminology of the International Continence Society. *Neurourology and Urodynamics, 28*(4), 295–300.

Stoker, J., Halligan, S., & Bartram, C. (2001). Pelvic floor imaging. *Radiology, 218*, 621–641.

Thompson, J. A., O'Sullivan, P., Briffa, N. K., et al. (2006a). Altered muscle activation patterns in symptomatic women during pelvic floor muscle contraction and valsalva manoeuvre. *Neurourology and Urodynamics, 25*, 268–276.

Thompson, J. A., O'Sullivan, P. B., Briffa, N. K., et al. (2006b). Assessment of voluntary pelvic floor muscle contraction in continent and incontinent women using transperineal ultrasound, manual muscle testing and vaginal squeeze pressure. *International Urogynecology Journal and Pelvic Floor Dysfunction, 17*, 624–630.

Van Delft, K. W. M., Sultan, A. H., Thakar, R., et al. (2015). Agreement between palpation and transperineal and endovaginal ultrasound in the diagnosis of levator ani avulsion. *International Urogynecology Journal, 26*, 33–39.

Van Kampen, M., De Weerdt, W., Feys, H., et al. (1996). Reliability and validity of a digital test for pelvic muscle strength in women. *Neurourology and Urodynamics, 15*, 338–339.

Volløyhaug, I., Mørkved, S., Salvesen, Ø., et al. (2016). Assessment of pelvic floor muscle contraction with palpation, perineometry and transperineal ultrasound: A cross-sectional study. *Ultrasound in Obstetrics and Gynecology, 47*(6), 768–773.

Worth, A., Dougherty, M., & McKey, P. (1986). Development and testing of the circumvaginal muscles rating scale. *Nursing Research, 35*(3), 166–168.

5.3 Manometry: Vaginal Squeeze Pressure Measurement

Kari Bø

Measurement of squeeze pressure is the most commonly used method to measure pelvic floor muscle (PFM) maximum strength and endurance. The patient is asked to contract the PFMs either as hard as possible—maximum voluntary contraction or maximum strength—to sustain a contraction (endurance) or repeat as many contractions as possible (endurance). The measurement can be done either in the urethra, vagina or rectum.

Kegel (1948) developed the perineometer, which is a vaginal pressure device connected to a manometer, showing the pressure in millimetres of mercury (mmHg) as a measure of PFM strength. He did not report any data about responsiveness, reliability or validity for his method. The term *perineometer* is somewhat misleading because the pressure-sensitive region of the probe of the manometer is not placed at the perineum, but in the vagina at the level of the levator ani. Currently, several types of vaginal pressure devices are available to measure vaginal squeeze pressure, all with different device sizes and technical parameters (Bø et al., 1990a; Dougherty et al., 1986; Laycock and Jerwood, 1994; Sigurdardottir et al., 2009) (Figs 5.3.1–5.3.3). The tools measure pressure in units of mmHg, cmH_2O or hPa. For terminology and definitions, see the work of Bø et al. (2017) and Frawley et al. (2021).

RESPONSIVENESS

In most studies describing measurement tools, data on responsiveness are not reported. However, some apparatuses applying a specialized balloon catheter connected to a fibreoptic microtip and strain gauge pressure transducer have shown high responsiveness (Abrams et al., 1986; Bø et al., 1990a; Dougherty et al., 1986; Kvarstein et al., 1983; Svenningsen and Jensen, 1986). In the apparatus of

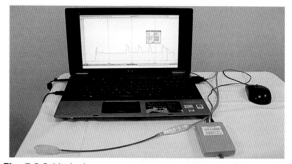

Fig. 5.3.2 Vaginal squeeze pressure measured with a vaginal balloon connected to a microtip pressure transducer. *(Camtech AS, Sandvika, Norway.)*

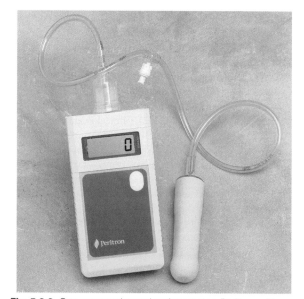

Fig. 5.3.3 One commonly used perineometer: Peritron with vaginal probe. *(Cardio Design Pty Ltd, Oakleigh VIC 3166, Australia.)*

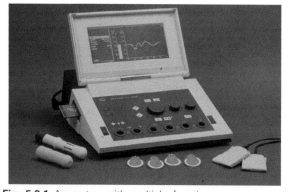

Fig. 5.3.1 Apparatus with multiple functions: measurement of pelvic floor muscle function with surface electromyography and vaginal and rectal squeeze pressure. *(Enraf Nonius International, 2600 AV Delft, Netherlands.)*

Bø et al. (1990a) (Camtech AS, Sandvika, Norway), the transducer's measurement range is 0 to 400 cmH$_2$O, with linearity of 0.5% to 1%, hysteresis less than 0.5%, thermal baseline drift less than 0.5% (typically 0.2 cmH$_2$O per °C) and thermal sensitivity drift less than 0.1% per °C (Kvarstein et al., 1983; Svenningsen and Jensen, 1986).

Intra- and Inter-Tester Reliability

Several authors (Bø et al., 1990a; Dougherty et al., 1986; Ferreira et al., 2011; Frawley et al., 2006; McKey and Dougherty, 1986; Sigurdardottir et al., 2009; Tennfjord et al., 2017; Wilson et al., 1991) have shown that vaginal squeeze pressure can be measured with satisfactory reliability. However, Dougherty et al. (1991) reported a within-subjects mean of 15.5 mmHg (SD: 3.9) and a between-subjects mean of 132.4 mmHg (SD: 11.5) in healthy subjects with an age range from 19 to 61 years. A significant variation was confirmed by Bø et al. (1990a), who also showed that at the first attempt some women needed some time to find and recruit motor units, whereas other women fatigued, causing the strength to drop considerably after only a few attempts. However, comparing the results of the whole group of women on two different occasions 14 days apart, reproducible results were found. Wilson et al. (1991) also found a significant difference between first and last contractions. They did not find a significant difference between measurements obtained with a full or empty bladder or during the menstrual cycle. Dougherty et al. (1991) did not find a significant difference when muscle strength was measured on different days, at different times of the day or during stress.

Kerschan-Schindl et al. (2002) tested intra-tester reliability of the Peritron perineometer and found that the absolute difference in maximal contraction force and mean contraction force within 5 seconds was less than 5.3 mmHg and 4.5 mmHg, respectively. Frawley et al. (2006) tested intra-tester reliability of the Peritron perineometer and found intra-class correlation (ICC) values for squeeze pressure readings to be 0.95, 0.91, 0.96 and 0.92 for crook lying, supine, sitting and standing positions, respectively. The ICC values for endurance testing in the same positions were much lower: 0.05, 0.42, 0.13 and 0.35. ICC values for resting pressure were 0.74, 0.77, 0.47 and 0.29. They concluded that there were high values of reliability of maximal voluntary contraction measured by the Peritron. However, endurance testing was unreliable, and so was resting pressure in the sitting and

standing positions. High intra-tester reliability of strength measurement was also confirmed by Chehrehrazi et al. (2009), whereas Rahmani and Mohseni-Bandpei (2011) found high intra-tester ICC values for both strength and endurance of the Peritron of 0.95 for strength and 0.94 for endurance with somewhat lower values for between-day comparisons of 0.88 and 0.83, respectively. Sigurdardottir et al. (2009) found an inter-rater ICC value of 0.97, p < 0.001 and a coefficient of variation of 11.1% testing maximum voluntary contraction by the Myomed 932. Ferreira et al. (2011) found moderate inter-rater reliability for the Peritron manometer; the difference between examiners was less than 10 cmH$_2$O in 11 of the 19 (58%) cases. Tennfjord et al. (2017) found that ICC values were very good (ICC >0.90) for all measurements, but considerable inter-variation of scores and outliers were seen for measurements representing the highest values. Agreement with mean differences (bias) and minimal detectable change for the intra-rater assessment for vaginal resting pressure was −0.44 ± 8.7 cmH$_2$O, for PFM strength −0.22 ± 7.6 cmH$_2$O and for muscular endurance 0.75 ± 59.5 cmH$_2$O/s. The interrater agreement for vaginal resting pressure was 1.36 ± 9.0 cmH$_2$O, for PFM strength 2.24 ± 9.0 cmH$_2$O and for muscular endurance 15.89 ± 69.7 cmH$_2$O/s. They concluded that in clinical practice, significant improvement in PFM variables needs to exceed the minimal detectable change to be above the error of measurement.

Validity

For urinary incontinent women, measurement within the urethra has the best face and content validity for measuring urethral closure pressure caused by the force of muscle contraction, for pelvic organ prolapse it would be the vagina and for bowel problems it would be the anal canal. Because of the risk of infection and the lack of availability of equipment in most physical therapy clinics, measurement in the urethra has mostly been used for research purposes (Benvenuti et al., 1987; Lose, 1992). Rectal pressure may not be a valid measure of the PFMs in relation to urinary incontinence because it also includes contraction of the anal sphincter muscle. However, in men, rectal pressure is the only practical option. In contrast to men, most women would have little sense of where the urethra is located, and most women probably would have the optimal sense of PFM contraction in the vagina. Therefore vaginal squeeze pressure is the most used method clinically.

PLACEMENT OF THE DEVICE

Size of the vaginal probe differs between devices. Some devices cover the full length of the vagina, and placement of the probe is therefore not a problem. Using smaller devices (Bø et al., 1990a; Dougherty et al., 1986), the location of the probe in the vagina creates both a reliability and validity problem because the balloon may be located outside the anatomical location of the PFMs. The balloon or transducer must be placed at the same anatomical level and at the level where the PFMs are located. Kegel (1948, 1952) suggested that the PFMs were located in the distal one-third of the vagina, and Bø (1992) found that most women had the highest pressure rise when the balloon was placed with the middle of the balloon 3.5 cm inside the introitus. However, individual differences were found.

SIZE AND SHAPES OF THE DEVICE

Results reported from different squeeze pressure and electromyography (EMG) apparatus cannot be compared due to differences in the diameter of the vaginal devices. There is discussion regarding the optimum diameter of vaginal devices (Schull et al., 2002). It is unknown whether a wide-diameter vaginal device stretches the PFMs, inhibiting its activity or, conversely, increasing activity by providing firm proprioceptive feedback. In a study by Bø et al. (2005), measurement of PFM maximum strength was compared using two commonly used apparatuses with a different size of the vaginal probe. Significant differences were found, and it was concluded that measurements obtained with different methods cannot be compared. The validity of larger probes, also for dynamometers, can be questioned as they open the vagina and stretch the PFMs. This does not mirror a normal situation where the vagina is closed and when we are training the PFMs.

INFLUENCE FROM INCREASED ABDOMINAL PRESSURE

Squeeze pressure measurements obtained from all three canals can be invalid because an increase in abdominal pressure will increase the measured pressures. The PFMs form one wall of the abdominopelvic cavity, and all rises in abdominal pressure will increase the pressure measured in the urethra, vagina and rectum.

Both Bø et al. (1988) and Bump et al. (1991) have shown that straining is a common error when women attempt to contract their PFMs, and therefore an erroneous measurement can be registered. However, because a correct contraction involves an observable inward movement of the perineum or the instrument, and straining creates a downward movement, some authors (Bø et al., 1990b; Bump et al., 1996) have suggested that a valid measurement can be ensured by simultaneous observation of inward movement of the perineum.

Some researchers (Cammu and Van Nylen, 1998) have tried to avoid co-contraction of the abdominal muscles interfering with measurement of PFM strength by use of surface EMG on the rectus abdominis muscle to train subjects to relax their abdominal muscles or by simultaneous abdominal pressure measurement. Performance of a near-maximal PFM contraction is important to achieve the best training effect (Komi, 1992; Wilmore and Costill, 1999). Several researchers (Bø et al., 1990b; Dougherty et al., 1991; Neumann and Gill, 2002; Sapsford et al., 2001), however, have shown that there is a co-contraction of the deep abdominal muscles (lower transversus abdominis and internal oblique) during attempts at a correct, maximal contraction. Neumann and Gill (2002) also reported that during a maximum PFM contraction the mean abdominal pressure was 9 mmHg (range: 2–19). The abdominal pressure rose to a mean of 27 mmHg (range: 11–34) with a head and leg lift from supine while performing a PFM contraction, and 36 mmHg (range: 33–52) during forced expiration and PFM contraction when supine—two activities that require diaphragmatic and outer abdominal muscle (external oblique and rectus abdominis) activity. A normal co-contraction of the lower abdominal wall therefore can be allowed because abdominal pressure rise is small with this co-contraction.

Dougherty et al. (1991) allowed an increase in abdominal pressure of 5 mmHg only to ensure the least abdominal pressure interference with the measurement results. Bø et al. (1990b) standardized the testing by not allowing any movement of the pelvis during measurement. Further investigation is required to assess how subtle changes in postural activity might affect vaginal pressure measurements.

Contraction of other muscles, such as the hip adductor and external rotator muscles and gluteals, also alters intravaginal pressure measurement (Bø et al., 1990b; Peschers et al., 2001). Bø and Stien (1994) showed with concentric needle EMG in women without urinary incontinence that contraction of these other muscles increased muscle activity in both the striated urethral wall muscle and the PFMs. However, when analysing the whole group of women, contraction of the other pelvic muscles did not give a higher-pressure response than contraction of the PFMs alone. However, caution must be exercised, because for some individuals this may occur. Kruger et al. (2019) compared a PFM contraction with contraction of internal rotation of the hips, external rotation of the hips, abduction of the hips, adduction of the hips, contraction of the gluteal muscles, pelvic tilt (primarily the rectus abdominis muscle), indrawing (primarily the transversus abdominis muscle), abdominal crunch (primarily the rectus abdominis muscle), deep inspiration and deep expiration with a device measuring intra-abdominal pressure and pressure at the location of the PFMs. They found that the squeeze pressure at the PFM location was higher during a PFM contraction than all other muscle contractions, except during a cough and abdominal curl-up. However, very importantly: during cough and curl-up, the intra-abdominal pressure was very high, and the targeted PFM contractions developed higher pressures compared to abdominal pressure than any other exercise tested. It was concluded that the Femfit® device was able to distinguish between abdominal and PFM pressures simultaneously. Because the gross motor pattern of gluteal and adductor activity is not part of the normal neuromuscular action of the PFM and lower transversus abdominis synergy, co-contractions of the outer pelvic muscles are discouraged when measuring PFM action and strength.

Jean-Michel et al. (2010) developed an interesting new device: the Colpexin pull test. This instrument measures the pull-out resistance or force required to remove the sphere from the vagina during active contraction, which represents the strength of the PFMs. This is a promising new device measuring eccentric contraction of the PFMs with no influence of abdominal pressure. However, testing is required of responsiveness, reliability and validity. A new device has also been developed (Arora et al., 2015; Kruger et al., 2013) (Fig. 5.3.4). The Femfit® is a pressure sensor array designed to measure the pressure profile along the length of the vagina. Thus this device aims to assess simultaneous intra-abdominal pressure and PFM contraction. It contains eight pressure sensors mounted onto a flexible printed circuit board which is encapsulated in soft biocompatible

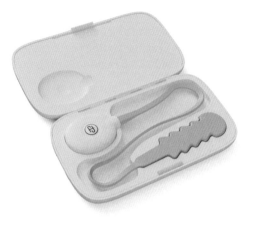

Fig. 5.3.4 The FemFit® is developed to measure simultaneous intra-abdominal pressure and pressure at the location of the pelvic floor muscles.

silicone. The Femfit® has a total length of 80 mm and a maximal width of 24 mm, and is only 4 mm thick. A test–retest study by Cacciari et al. (2020) indicated excellent reliability for PFM contraction and straining manoeuvre both in lying and standing positions, within and between sessions. For straining manoeuvres while standing, increased variability was found by a wider limit of agreement on Bland–Altman plots (spanning 31.3–43.3 mmHg). A significant moderate to strong correlation was found between measurements of PFM contraction using the Femfit® and dynamometry or palpation (Pearson's coefficient = 0.72, p = 0.006; Spearman's rho = 0.68, p = 0.005, respectively). This is promising, as the slim and flexible nature of the device means that it could be used in future studies to determine the vaginal pressure profile and thus pelvic floor function during physical activity. Further studies are needed to assess validity during more strenuous exercise over time (e.g., running, jumping and lifting).

Sensitivity and Specificity

Several case–control studies comparing PFM strength with vaginal squeeze pressure in continent and incontinent women have demonstrated that continent women have better strength than incontinent women (Amaro et al., 2005; Borin et al., 2013; Hahn et al., 1996; Hilde et al., 2012; Mørkved et al., 2004; Thompson et al., 2006), and that there is an association between improvement in muscle function or strength and reduction in urinary incontinence (Bø, 2003). However, some studies have not found an association between increase in muscle strength and improvement in incontinence (Elser et al., 1999), which may be explained by the fact that there was no improvement in muscle strength following the low-dosage exercise protocol.

CONCLUSION

Because all increases in abdominal pressure will affect urethral, vaginal and rectal pressures, squeeze pressure cannot be used alone. With simultaneous observation of inward movement of the perineum, it is likely that a correct contraction is measured. Cautious teaching of the patient, standardization of instruction and motivation, and standardization of the patient's position and performance are mandatory. If the aim is to measure the ability to close the urethra, urethral pressure should be measured. If overall PFM strength is the aim of the investigation, vaginal squeeze pressure (pressure manometry or dynamometric force) is preferred because this is the least invasive method with a low risk of infection in women.

CLINICAL RECOMMENDATIONS

Measurement of vaginal squeeze pressure using manometers is difficult, and clinical skills and experience are important factors in achieving reliable and valid results. The method must be used with caution. However, when used in accordance with knowledge from research in this area, measurement of PFM contraction can give important information and feedback to both the patient and therapist (Fig. 5.3.5). The method is as follows:
- Fully inform the patient about the test procedure and gain consent.
- Give the patient privacy to undress and a drape to place over herself on the examination couch.
- Always start the instruction with observation and palpation of PFM contraction.
- If the patient is unable to contract, strains or uses other muscles instead of the PFMs, valid pressure measurement is not possible.
- The patient can be supine, crook lying, sitting or standing. Use the same position for each assessment for that patient.

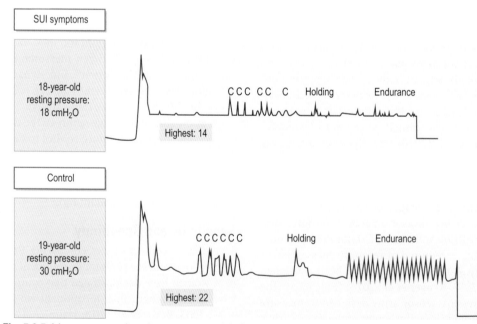

Fig. 5.3.5 Measurement of resting pressure, pelvic floor muscle maximal strength, attempts of holding and repeated contractions at first-time consultation in two nulliparous female sports students. Both were able to contract the pelvic floor muscles as assessed by vaginal palpation. The first had proven urodynamic stress urinary incontinence (SUI) with 43 g of leakage on ambulatory urodynamics. The second had no symptoms of pelvic floor dysfunction.

- The physical therapist should be in a position to be able to observe the perineum.
- Prepare the measuring device before washing hands and putting on examination gloves.
- Follow local infection control guidelines regarding covering the probe, or use a single-use apparatus.
- Gently insert the probe, or ask the patient to do it.
- Once the probe is comfortably in place, instruct the patient to relax and breathe normally before the PFM contraction.
- Gently support the device to keep it in the same intravaginal position.
- Instruct the patient to contract the PFMs as hard as possible with no visible co-contraction of hip adductor, gluteal or rectus abdominis muscles (pelvic tilt) and then to relax without pressing the perineum downwards.
- A small indrawing or 'hollowing' using the internal abdominals with maximum contraction and no tilting of the pelvis is allowed.
- Resting pressure, holding time and repeated contractions can also be registered depending on the device parameters.
- Only contractions with simultaneous visible inward movement of the perineum or the measurement device can be considered valid measurements of PFM strength.
- Register at least three contractions, and use the maximum or mean of the three contractions.
- Other aspects of muscle performance, such as holding time and number of repeated contractions (endurance), onset of contraction, slope and area under the curve, and resting pressure (relaxation) can be measured if the equipment used provides for this.
- Gently remove the probe, and either dispose of the intravaginal component or wash it according to local guidelines before sterilization.
- Allow the patient privacy to dress before discussing the results.

REFERENCES

Abrams, R., Batich, C., Dougherty, M., et al. (1986). Custom-made vaginal balloons for strengthening circumvaginal musculature. *Biomaterials Medical Devices and Artificial Organs, 14*(3–4), 239–248.

Amaro, J. L., Moreira, E. C. H. M., Gameiro, M. O. O., et al. (2005). Pelvic floor muscle evaluation in incontinent patients. *International Urogynecology Journal and Pelvic Floor Dysfunction, 16*, 352–354.

Arora, A. S., Kruger, J. A., Budgett, D. M., et al. (2015). Clinical evaluation of a high-fidelity wireless intravaginal pressure sensor. *International Urogynecology Journal, 26*, 243–249.

Benvenuti, F., Caputo, G. M., Bandinelli, S., et al. (1987). Re-educative treatment of female genuine stress incontinence. *American Journal of Physical Medicine, 66*, 155–168.

Bø, K. (1992). Pressure measurements during pelvic floor muscle contractions: The effect of different positions of the vaginal measuring device. *Neurourology and Urodynamics, 11*, 107–113.

Bø, K. (2003). Pelvic floor muscle strength and response to pelvic floor muscle training for stress urinary incontinence. *Neurourology and Urodynamics, 22*, 654–658.

Bø, K., Frawley, H., Haylen, B., et al. (2017). An International Urogynecological Association (IUGA)/International Continence Society (ICS) joint report on the terminology for the conservative and nonpharmacological management of female pelvic floor dysfunction. *Neurourology and Urodynamics, 36*, 221–244.

Bø, K., Kvarstein, B., Hagen, R., et al. (1990a). Pelvic floor muscle exercise for the treatment of female stress urinary incontinence. I: Reliability of vaginal pressure measurements of pelvic floor muscle strength. *Neurourology and Urodynamics, 9*, 471–477.

Bø, K., Kvarstein, B., Hagen, R., et al. (1990b). Pelvic floor muscle exercise for the treatment of female stress urinary incontinence. II: Validity of vaginal pressure measurements of pelvic floor muscle strength and the necessity of supplementary methods for control of correct contraction. *Neurourology and Urodynamics, 9*, 479–487.

Bø, K., Larsen, S., Oseid, S., et al. (1988). Knowledge about and ability to correct pelvic floor muscle exercises in women with urinary stress incontinence. *Neurourology and Urodynamics, 7*, 261–262.

Bø, K., Raastad, R., & Finckenhagen, H. B. (2005). Does the size of the vaginal probe affect measurement of pelvic floor muscle strength? *Acta Obstetricia et Gynecologica Scandinavica, 84*, 129–133.

Bø, K., & Stien, R. (1994). Needle EMG registration of striated urethral wall and pelvic floor muscle activity patterns during cough, Valsalva, abdominal, hip adductor, and gluteal muscle contractions in nulliparous healthy females. *Neurourology and Urodynamics, 13*, 35–41.

Borin, L. C. M. S., Nunes, F. R., & Guirro, E. C. O. G. (2013). Assessment of pelvic floor muscle pressure in female athletes. *Physical Medicine and Rehabilitation, 5*, 189–193.

Bump, R., Hurt, W. G., Fantl, J. A., et al. (1991). Assessment of Kegel exercise performance after brief verbal instruction. *American Journal of Obstetrics and Gynecology, 165*, 322–329.

Bump, R., Mattiasson, A., Bø, K., et al. (1996). The standardization of terminology of female pelvic organ prolapse and pelvic floor dysfunction. *American Journal of Obstetrics and Gynecology, 175*, 10–17.

Cacciari, L. P., Kruger, J., Goodman, J., et al. (2020). Reliability and validity of intravaginal pressure measurements with a new intravaginal pressure device: The FemFit®. *Neurourology and Urodynamics, 39*, 253–260.

Cammu, H., & Van Nylen, M. (1998). Pelvic floor exercises versus vaginal weight cones in genuine stress incontinence. *European Journal of Obstetrics & Gynecology and Reproductive Biology, 77*, 89–93.

Chehrehrazi, M., Arab, A. M., Karimi, N., et al. (2009). Assessment of pelvic floor muscle contraction in stress urinary incontinent women: Comparison between transabdominal ultrasound and perineometry. *International Urogynecology Journal and Pelvic Floor Dysfunction, 20*, 1491–1496.

Dougherty, M. C., Abrams, R., & McKey, P. L. (1986). An instrument to assess the dynamic characteristics of the circumvaginal musculature. *Nursing Research, 35*, 202–206.

Dougherty, M., Bishop, K., Mooney, R., et al. (1991). Variation in intravaginal pressure measurement. *Nursing Research, 40*, 282–285.

Elser, D., Wyman, J., McClish, D., et al. (1999). The effect of bladder training, pelvic floor muscle training, or combination training on urodynamic parameters in women with urinary incontinence. *Neurourology and Urodynamics, 18*, 427–436.

Ferreira, C. H. J., Barbosa, P. B., de Oliveira Souza, F., et al. (2011). Inter-rater reliability study of the modified Oxford grading scale and the Peritron manometer. *Physiotherapy, 97*, 132–138.

Frawley, H. C., Galea, M. P., Phillips, B. A., et al. (2006). Reliability of pelvic floor muscle strength assessment using different test positions and tools. *Neurourology and Urodynamics, 25*(3), 236–242.

Frawley, H. E., Morin, M., Shelly, E., et al. (2021). An International Continence Society (ICS) report on the terminology for pelvic floor muscle assessment. *Neurourology and Urodynamics, 40*(5), 1217–1260.

Hahn, I., Milsom, I., Ohlson, B. L., et al. (1996). Comparative assessment of pelvic floor function using vaginal cones, vaginal digital palpation and vaginal pressure measurement. *Gynecologic and Obstetric Investigation, 41*, 269–274.

Hilde, G., Stær-Jensen, J., Engh, M. E., et al. (2012). Continence and pelvic floor status in nulliparous women at midterm pregnancy. *International Urogynecology Journal, 23*, 1257–1263.

Jean-Michel, M., Biller, D. H., Bena, J. F., et al. (2010). Measurement of pelvic floor muscular strength with the Colpexin pull test: A comparative study. *International Urogynecology Journal and Pelvic Floor Dysfunction, 21*, 1011–1017.

Kegel, A. H. (1948). Progressive resistance exercise in the functional restoration of the perineal muscles. *American Journal of Obstetrics and Gynecology, 56*, 238–249.

Kegel, A. H. (1952). Stress incontinence and genital relaxation; a nonsurgical method of increasing the tone of sphincters and their supporting structures. *Ciba Clinical Symposia, 4*(2), 35–51.

Kerschan-Schindl, K., Uher, E., Wiesinger, G., et al. (2002). Reliability of pelvic floor muscle strength measurement in elderly incontinent women. *Neurourology and Urodynamics, 21*, 42–47.

Komi, P. V. (1992). In *Strength and power in sport: The encyclopaedia of sports medicine* (Vol. 3). Oxford: Blackwell Science.

Kruger, J., Goodman, J., Budgett, D., et al. (2019). Can you train the pelvic floor muscles by contracting other related muscles? *Neurourology and Urodynamics, 38*(2), 677–683.

Kruger, J., Hayward, L., Nielsen, P., et al. (2013). Design and development of a novel intra-vaginal pressure sensor. *International Urogynecology Journal, 24*, 1715–1721.

Kvarstein, B., Aase, O., Hansen, T., et al. (1983). A new method with fiberoptic transducers used for simultaneous recording of intravesical and urethral pressure during physiological filling and voiding phases. *Journal of urology, 130*, 504–506.

Laycock, J., & Jerwood, D. (1994). Development of the bradford perineometer. *Physiotherapy, 80*, 139–142.

Lose, G. (1992). Simultaneous recording of pressure and cross-sectional area in the female urethra: A study of urethral closure function in healthy and stress incontinent women. *Neurourology and Urodynamics, 11*, 54–89.

McKey, P. L., & Dougherty, M. C. (1986). The circumvaginal musculature: Correlation between pressure and physical assessment. *Nursing Research, 35*, 307–309.

Mørkved, S., Salvesen, K. Å., Bø, K., et al. (2004). Pelvic floor muscle strength and thickness in continent and incontinent nulliparous pregnant women. *International Urogynecology Journal and Pelvic Floor Dysfunction, 15*, 384–390.

Neumann, P., & Gill, V. (2002). Pelvic floor and abdominal muscle interaction: EMG activity and intra-abdominal pressure. *International Urogynecology Journal and Pelvic Floor Dysfunction, 13*, 125–132.

Peschers, U., Gingelmaier, A., Jundt, K., et al. (2001). Evaluation of pelvic floor muscle strength using four different techniques. *International Urogynecology Journal and Pelvic Floor Dysfunction, 12*, 27–30.

Rahmani, N., & Mohseni-Bandpei, M. A. (2011). Application of perineometer in assessment of pelvic floor muscle strength and endurance: A reliability study. *Journal of Bodywork and Movement Therapies, 15*, 209–214.

Sapsford, R., Hodges, P., Richardson, C., et al. (2001). Co-activation of the abdominal and pelvic floor muscles during voluntary exercises. *Neurourology and Urodynamics, 20*, 31–42.

Schull, B., Hurt, G., Laycock, J., et al. (2002). Physical examination. In P. Abrams, L. Cardozo, S. Khoury, et al. (Eds.), *Incontinence: Second international consultation on incontinence* (pp. 373–388). Plymouth, UK: Health Publication/Plymbridge Distributors.

Sigurdardottir, T., Steingrimsdottir, T., Arnason, A., et al. (2009). Test–retest intra-rater reliability of vaginal measurement of pelvic floor muscle strength using Myomed 932. *Acta Obstetricia et Gynecologica Scandinavica, 88*, 939–943.

Svenningsen, L., & Jensen, Ø. (1986). Application of fiberoptics to the clinical measurement of intra-uterine pressure in labour. *Acta Obstetricia et Gynecologica Scandinavica, 65*, 551–555.

Tennfjord, M. K., Engh, M. E., & Bø, K. (2017). An intra-and interrater reliability and agreement study of vaginal resting pressure, pelvic floor muscle strength and muscular endurance, using a manometer. *International Urogynecology Journal, 28*, 1507–1514.

Thompson, J. A., O'Sullivan, P. B., Briffa, N. K., et al. (2006). Assessment of voluntary pelvic floor muscle contraction in continent and incontinent women using transperineal ultrasound, manual muscle testing and vaginal squeeze pressure. *International Urogynecology Journal and Pelvic Floor Dysfunction, 17*, 624–630.

Wilmore, J., & Costill, D. (1999). *Physiology of sport and exercise* (2nd ed.). Champaign, IL: Human Kinetics.

Wilson, P., Herbison, G., & Heer, K. (1991). Reproducibility of perineometry measurements. *Neurourology and Urodynamics, 10*, 399–400.

5.4 Pelvic Floor Dynamometry

Chantale Dumoulin and Licia P Cacciari

INTRODUCTION

Precise, quantitative measurements of pelvic floor muscle (PFM) function (i.e., passive strength (tone), active strength, contraction speed, endurance and coordination) are critical for documenting the clinical progression of neuromuscular dysfunctions and assessing a patient's response to a PFM physical therapy intervention.

Dynamometers accurately, and independent of an evaluator's subjective judgement, measure muscle power and force (Bø et al., 2017). Although dynamometers came into general use at the end of the 19th century to evaluate trunk as well as upper- and lower-extremity muscles (Mafi et al., 2012), dynamometric technology has only been applied to PFM assessment in the past three decades. Up until now, it has been reserved for the female anatomy. According to Bø et al. (2017), PFM dynamometry is defined as 'the measurement of PFM resting and contractile forces using strain gauges mounted on a speculum (a dynamometer), which is inserted into the vagina. Dynamometry measures force in Newton units'.

A total of 13 dynamometers, with varying shapes and technical properties, have been described in the literature (Ashton-Miller et al., 2014; Bérubé et al., 2018; Castro-Pardiñas et al., 2017; Constantinou and Omata, 2007; Dumoulin et al., 2003; Kruger et al., 2015; Martinho et al., 2015; Nunes et al., 2011; Parezanović-Ilić et al., 2009; Romero-Cullerés et al., 2017; Rowe, 1995; Saleme et al., 2009; Verelst and Leivseth, 2004). Some do not correspond to the definition of Bø et al. (2017) with regard to their shape and sensor type, but all are designed to measure PFM resting and contractile forces.

Caufriez et al. (1993, 1998) were the first to report the use of dynamometers to measure PFM function; however, their work was only reported in non–peer-reviewed manuscripts at the time. Caufriez's dynamometer (known as the *pince tonimétrique*) was initially designed to assess PFM passive and active tone and consists of two speculum branches that can be opened anteroposteriorly, in an angular excursion like scissors to increase the vaginal aperture, by pressing on two handles. It was commercialized as 'the Pelvimetre' by a French company and has been the object of peer review–published PFM dynamometry research since 2017, starting with an article by

Castro-Pardiñas et al. (2017) on the reliability and known group validity (continent/incontinent).

Rowe (1995) were the second to report the use of a dynamometer to measure PFM function; however, it was mentioned only later in a brief conference abstract in 2015. Rowe's dynamometer comprised a probe with a movable rigid-window section against which the PFMs pressed during a contraction to record forces. No further publication was found after the original abstract.

The study by Sampselle et al. (1998) at Michigan University was the first to report the use of a PFM dynamometer in a clinical trial. A patent document published in 2002 described the aluminum dual-branch speculum with manual adjustment from 0 to 10 cm used in these trials in more detail (Ashton-Miller et al., 2002). In 2014, the same group proposed a modified version of the handheld dynamometer design to minimize the effect of intra-abdominal pressure (IAP) on the measurement of PFM strength (Ashton-Miller et al., 2014).

In 2003, Dumoulin et al. designed and developed the Montreal dynamometric speculum (Fig. 5.4.1) (Dumoulin et al., 2003). The speculum comprises two aluminum branches: the upper branch is fixed, and the other branch can be slowly opened by an adjustable screw allowing the PFM forces to be measured at different introital vaginal anteroposterior diameters. The distance between the two branches can be adjusted from a minimum of 5 mm to 40 mm. PFM forces are measured by strain gauges glued on each side of the movable lower branch of the speculum. Since its initial design, several of the dynamometer's functionalities have been improved: for example, (1) the base supporting the speculum now enables insertion to follow the natural angle of the vagina (Morin et al., 2008b; Morin et al., 2010b); (2) the mechanism that widens the vaginal opening was modified to create a smoother opening, and a numerical linear-position transducer was incorporated to provide real-time measurement of the distance between the two branches during a dynamic stretch (Morin et al. 2008b; Morin et al., 2010b); (3) a third branch, distally positioned in the vagina, was added to verify whether the recorded PFM forces are being influenced by IAP (Morin et al., 2006); and (4) the size of the branches was reduced to that of a paediatric speculum to enable the assessment of women with vaginal atrophy and vulvovaginal pain (Mercier et al., 2019; Morin et al., 2010a) (Fig. 5.4.2). In 2013, a small cylindrical handheld dynamometer was developed to measure PFM function anteroposteriorly without its fixed base, thus allowing measurements to be taken in a standing position (Dumoulin, 2014). Further development in 2019 advanced the dynamometer to allow measurement without the evaluator having to hold the instrument during use (El-Sayegh et al., 2020).

Another PFM dynamometer was developed by Verelst and Leivseth (2004). The specificity of this handheld instrument lies in its ability to measure PFM forces in the transverse direction of the urogenital hiatus, for the first time. The Verelst and Leivseth dynamometer comprises two semirounded parallel branches; one branch contains a metal plate to which a strain gauge is affixed. During a PFM contraction the metal plate is deformed and the resulting forces are measured. Both branches can be opened, enabling 30- to 50-mm-width measurements. The sensor is also connected to a signal-processing system.

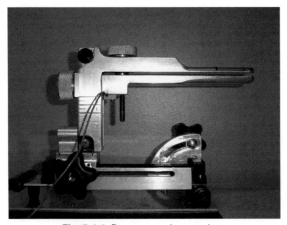

Fig. 5.4.1 Dynamometric speculum.

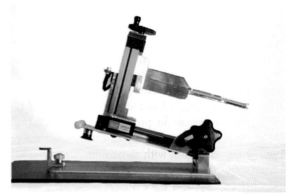

Fig. 5.4.2 The latest version of the Montreal dynamometer.

In 2007, Constantinou and co-workers designed a four-sensor probe (Constantinou and Omata, 2007; Constantinou et al., 2007). Each sensor is mounted on a leaf spring that, when inserted, can be expanded from 23 to 70 mm to make counter-resistance with the vaginal wall and then retracted for ease of removal. This configuration enables assessment of the spatial distribution of forces as well as the positioning of the sensors in each quadrant (anterior, posterior, left and right) during a PFM contraction. A positioning system was added to the probe handle to track the orientation/angulation of the probe during a PFM assessment (Peng et al., 2007).

Similarly, Saleme et al. (2009) designed a multidirectional PFM measuring tool to evaluate the spatial distribution of PFM forces; however, the sensors are not mounted on extractible leaf springs but directly on the probe instead, allowing anteroposterior and laterolateral measurement simultaneously at a fixed 35-mm opening. No further publication about this tool was found after the initial one.

Three additional dynamometric prototypes were then developed; all of them use a conventional gynaecological two-branch speculum to which strain gauges are affixed and connected to a computer (Nunes et al., 2011; Parezanović-Ilić et al., 2009; Romero-Cullerés et al., 2017). The support system for Nunes' stainless steel speculum can be adjusted to evaluate the PFM forces in both the anteroposterior and transverse directions from 10 to 28 mm (Nunes et al., 2011). The Parezanović-Ilić speculum evaluates PFM forces in the anteroposterior direction and at an angle (opening of the branch of the speculum in the vagina) corresponding to contact between the speculum and vaginal mucosa (Parezanović-Ilić et al., 2009). The Romero-Cullerés speculum involves two pivoting branches, each with a handle and a frontal area in which an inductive displacement sensor is attached to a spring of known stiffness allowing force measurement in an anteroposterior direction via a linear regression equation (Romero-Cullerés et al. 2017).

New Zealand's elastometer, developed by Kruger et al. (2015), was designed to assess PFM passive forces to investigate their role in predicting delivery-related trauma. It consists of a handheld device comprising two aluminum branches with detachable acetyl-plastic speculum tips (Fig. 5.4.3). A load-cell amplifier and a displacement transducer have been integrated into the

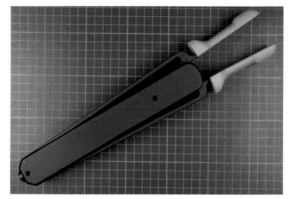

Fig. 5.4.3 Elastometer. *(Courtesy J Kruger, P Nielsen and A Taberner.)*

handpiece, providing force and branch separation measurements to a central computerized unit. The elastometer is innovative because the two branches can be separated by pressing a button that activates a motor incorporated into the speculum. This enables the evaluator to apply a controlled stretch, at a constant speed, to the PFMs in a transverse direction to assess PFM passive properties.

First in an abstract in 2014 and then in a manuscript, Martinho et al. (2015) reported on the intra and interrater reliability of measurements taken from a PFM dynamometer commercialized by a Brazilian company. The vaginal dynamometer is cylindrical in shape (9.5 cm in length and 3.3 cm in diameter), made externally from plastic, made internally with steel structures and equipped with a load cell 2 cm from its base, which can measure anteroposterior unidirectional compressive strength in kilogram/force units (Martinho et al., 2015).

Bérubé et al. (2018) introduced another dynamometer. It consists of two 3D printed, single-participant use, saddle-shaped arms which open parallel to each other with a force transducer mounted on the posterior arm to allow measurement of PFM properties in an anteroposterior direction. Opening and closing of the dynamometer arms is automatically controlled up to 55 mm. The unit is portable, allowing for use in a supine position (Bérubé et al., 2018).

Finally, we also found three commercial PFM dynamometers (Elvie, 2013; PeriCoach, 2014; Fizimed, 2018) which will not be discussed in this section as their main use is giving biofeedback to women with PFM dysfunction rather than measuring PFM function.

ACCEPTANCE

One patent and six studies (Ashton-Miller et al., 2002; Bérubé et al., 2018; Dumoulin et al., 2004; Kruger et al., 2015; Morin et al., 2010a; Morin et al., 2017; Verelst and Leivseth, 2004) reported on the acceptance/comfort of the dynamometric procedures in different populations of women. Ashton-Miller et al. (2002), in the patent of the dynamometer, report: 'In tests it was found that blade separation distances, for example, of 5 mm, 2.0 cm and 4.5 cm, were acceptable'. Dumoulin et al. (2004) evaluated the acceptance of passive and active force measurements among young and middle-aged women with stress urinary incontinence (SUI) during the course of their test–retest reliability study. Study participants found the dynamometer acceptable and the measuring procedures not painful (Dumoulin et al., 2004). Morin et al. (2010b) also confirmed the acceptance of the procedures, but this time in relation to the passive properties assessment, including dynamic stretches (lengthening/shortening cycles) among young and middle-aged continent women. Verelst and Leivseth (2004) reported that the diameter used was well tolerated by healthy parous women. Bérubé et al. (2018) reported that women, in their sample of nulliparous women with no history of vulvar pain, did not have significant discomfort during, after or between sessions. Finally, Kruger et al. (2015) found, in their reliability study with 20 female volunteers, that elastometer measurements of stiffness at apertures of up to 50 mm are well tolerated by this population.

PSYCHOMETRIC ASSESSMENT

Reliability Studies: Intra- and Inter-Rater, Within- and Between-Visits

Nine of the 13 dynamometers have shown reliability in one or more of their dynamometric measurements in populations with and without PFM dysfunctions (Table 5.4.1). Most have presented *intra-rater reliability* either *within-visit* (n = 9 studies: Bérubé et al., 2018; Czyrnyj et al., 2019; Dumoulin et al., 2004; Kruger et al., 2015; Miller et al., 2007; Passaro et al., 2014; Romero-Cullerés et al., 2013; Romero-Cullerés et al., 2017; Romero-Cullerés et al., 2020) or *between-visits* (n = 14 studies: Ashton-Miller et al., 2014; Bérubé et al., 2018; Czyrnyj et al., 2019; dos Reis Nagano et al., 2018; Dumoulin et al., 2004; Kruger et al., 2011; Passaro et al., 2014; Martinho et al., 2015; Miller et al., 2007; Morin et al., 2007;

Morin et al., 2008b; Navarro-Brazález et al., 2018; Nunes et al., 2011; Verelst and Leivseth, 2004). Only five studies have presented *inter-rater reliability in three dynamometers* (dos Reis Nagano et al., 2018; Martinho et al., 2015; Navarro-Brazález et al., 2018; Romero-Cullerés et al., 2020; Romero-Cullerés et al., 2013). Inter-rater reliability is more relevant when the dynamometer is not attached to a base but rather handheld, in which case measurement can be influenced by the evaluator.

Forces during PFM maximal voluntary contractions (maximal strength) were the most studied parameter (n = 14 studies: Ashton-Miller et al., 2014; Bérubé et al., 2018; Czyrnyj et al., 2019; dos Reis Nagano et al., 2018; Dumoulin et al., 2004; Martinho et al., 2015; Miller et al., 2007; Navarro-Brazález et al., 2018; Nunes et al., 2011; Passaro et al., 2014; Romero-Cullerés et al., 2013; Romero-Cullerés et al., 2017; Romero-Cullerés et al., 2020; Verelst and Leivseth, 2004). In nine studies the assessment of PFM function was extended to study the reliability of other parameters such as passive muscle properties, contraction speed, fatigue and endurance (Bérubé et al., 2018; Czyrnyj et al., 2019; dos Reis Nagano et al., 2018; Dumoulin et al., 2004; Kruger et al., 2011; Kruger et al., 2015; Morin et al., 2007; Morin et al., 2008b; Passaro et al., 2014).

Overall, the reliability of dynamometric measurements has been extensively studied for various PFM functions and in different populations. The results suggest good to excellent reliability, which makes them a good assessment tool to assess PFM function. It should be pointed out, however, that the inter-rater reliability of dynamometric measurements has been evaluated in only three of the nine handheld dynamometers, and it therefore deserves further investigation, especially as inter-rater reliability is always lower than intra-rater reliability.

VALIDITY STUDIES

Criterion Validity

To date, there is no recognized gold standard for evaluating PFM function, so it is impossible to evaluate the validity criterion of individual dynamometric instruments. Consequently, validation of PFM dynamometers must rely on the construct validity, which Dunn et al. (1989) has defined as 'the extent to which a test can be proven to measure a hypothetical construct'—in this case, the PFM function. Various studies need to be performed to support the construct's validity, specifically convergent validity (i.e., correlation with another instrument) and the Known Groups Method (Nunnally and Bernstein, 1994; Portney and Watkins, 2000).

Convergent validity studies were conducted for six dynamometers: the Montreal dynamometer (Morin et al., 2004; Morin et al., 2006), Constantinou's four-sensor probe (Yoshimura et al., 2004), Ashton-Miller's instrumented speculum (Ashton-Miller et al., 2014; Brincat et al., 2011; Morgan et al., 2005; Morgan et al., 2009), Parezanović-Ilić's speculum (Parezanović-Ilić et al., 2009), Romero-Cullerés's speculum (Romero-Cullerés et al., 2013; Romero-Cullerés et al., 2017; Romero-Cullerés et al., 2020) and the Pelvimetre (Navarro-Brazález et al., 2018).

TABLE 5.4.1	Reliability of PFM functional measurements using different dynamometers		
Dynamometer	**Sample**	**Method**	**Results**
Bérubé, 2018	20 nulliparous women No UI or POP risk factors (mean age 35 ± 15 years)	Number of evaluators: 1 Number of visits: 2 Time between visits: 1 week Task 1: 3 rest at a dynamometer opening of 0 to 40 mm and at two speeds (25 mm/s and 50 mm/s) Outcomes: baseline force, peak force, rate of force development (RFD), relative peak force, stiffness and absolute and relative stress relaxation responses Task 2: 3 MVC at two different anteroposterior dynamometer openings (25 mm, 35 mm) Outcomes: baseline force, peak force, relative peak force and RFD	**Within-visit reliability** Passive PFM properties Φ 0.74 - 0.98 for all measures except Stiffness Φ 0.56 - 0.93 or absolute and relative normalized stress relaxation response at 5s Φ 0.19 - 0.95 Active PFM properties Φ 0.89 - 0.96 for all measures **Between-visit reliability** Passive PFM properties Stiffness Φ 0.77 RPF Φ 0.75 - 0.76 all absolute and relative stress relaxation responses Φ 0.24 - 0.86 Active PFM properties RFD and relative peak force during MVC Φ 0.89 - 0.93 Baseline and peak force Φ 0.11 - 0.85
Czyrnyj, 2019	Twenty nulliparous women (mean age = 35 ± 15 years)	Number of evaluators: 1 Number of visits: 3 Time between visits: 1 week Task 1: 3 rest at a dynamometer opening of 0 to 40 mm and at two speeds (25 mm/s and 50 mm/s) Outcomes: peak force, rate of force development, relative peak force and stiffness Task 2: 3 MVC at two different anteroposterior dynamometer openings (25 mm, 35 mm) Outcomes: baseline force, peak force, relative peak force, rate of force development	1) **Within-visit reliability** Φ 0.45 - 0.98 for all measures 2) **Between-visit reliability:** Φ 0.57 - 0.94 for all measures

Continued

TABLE 5.4.1   Reliability of PFM functional measurements using different dynamometers—cont'd

Dynamometer	Sample	Method	Results
Navarro Brazález, 2018	20 women, with pelvic floor dysfunction symptoms (mean age = 40 ± 10 years)	Number of evaluators: 2 Number of visits: 3 Time between visits: 7 days intra-rater and 1-2 days inter-raters Task: 3 MVCs Outcomes: mean relative peak force	Inter-rater Between-visit reliability Lin's Concordance Correlation Coefficient (CCC) 0.93 Intra-rater Between-visit reliability CCC = 0.96 Bland–Altman plot showed good inter and intra-rater agreement with little random variability for all instruments
Miller, 2007	12 nulliparous continent women (mean age = 25, between 21- 44 years)	Number of evaluators: 1 Number of visits: 3 Time between visits: ±1 week apart Task: 2 MVCs Outcomes: mean/best of the two relative peak force	Within-visit reliability CR: ±3.8 to ±4.2 N Corresponding ICC for measures repeated twice in any single day CR: 0.83, SEM: 0.86 (CV 13.9%) Between-visit reliability CR: ±5.5 N to ±8.2 N
Ashton Miller, 2014	40 incontinent women (mean age 54 ± 13 years)	Number of evaluators: 1 Number of visits: 2 Time between visits: 1 month Task: 1 MVC Outcomes: relative peak force	Between-visit reliability CR: ±3.1 N
Dumoulin, 2004	29 parous women with SUI (between 27 - 42 years)	Number of evaluators: 1 Number of visits: 3 Time between visits: ±4 weeks Task 1: 3 MVC in 3 vaginal apertures (19, 24, 29mm) (anteroposterior diameter) Outcomes: relative peak force Task 2: 1 sustained MVC (1min) at 24mm vaginal aperture Outcomes: maximum rate of force development (MRFD), % loss in strength after 10 and 60 sec relative to the peak force	Within-visit reliability one trial 19 mm: Φ 0.69, SEM 1.30 N (CV 33%) 24 mm: Φ 0.86, SEM 1.62 N (CV 23%) 29 mm: Φ 0.74, SEM 2.78 N (CV 33%) Within-visit reliability (mean of three trials) 19 mm: Φ 0.71, SEM 1.22 N (CV 30%) 24 mm: Φ 0.88, SEM 1.49 N (CV 21%) 29 mm: Φ 0.76, SEM 2.11 N (CV 24%) Between-visit reliability MRFD at 24 mm: Φ 0.86 % loss of strength: Φ 0.10-0.38
Morin, 2007	19 parous women with SUI (mean age = 36 ± 4 years)	Number of evaluators: 1 Number of visits: 2 Time between visits: 8 weeks Task 1: speed contraction (contract maximally and relax as quickly as possible during a 15s) Outcomes: rate of force development, number of contractions, peak force Task 2: sustained MVC (90s) Outcomes: normalized area under the curve between 10-60s	Between-visit reliability Φ 0.79 - 0.92

TABLE 5.4.1	Reliability of PFM functional measurements using different dynamometers—cont'd		
Dynamometer	**Sample**	**Method**	**Results**
Morin, 2008b	32 SUI postmenopausal (mean age = 56 ± 6 years)	Number of evaluators: 1 Number of visits: 2 Time between visits: ±2 weeks Task 1: 2 rest at minimal (15mm) vaginal aperture Outcomes: mean force Task 2: 2 rest at maximal tolerated vaginal aperture Outcomes: mean force Task 3: 2 rest at lengthening and shortening cycles Outcomes: (a) forces at minimal, maximal, mean and common aperture of 20mm; (b) passive elastic stiffness (PES) minimal, maximal, mean and common aperture of 20 mm; (c) aperture at a common force of 0.5 N; (d) hysteresis Task 4: 2 sustained stretch (1min) Outcomes: % of loss in passive forces after 1min	Between-visit reliability (2 trials) 1. Passive resistance at minimal aperture Φ 0.57, SEM 0.34 N (CV 88%) 2. Passive resistance at maximal aperture Φ 0.82 SEM 0.57 N (CV 25%) 3. Lengthening and shortening cycles (a) Φ 0.51 - 0.91, SEM 0.28 - 0.73 N (CV 18% - 150%) (b) Φ 0.74 - 0.93, SEM 0.03 - 0.10 N/mm (CV 13 - 23%) (c) Φ 0.35, SEM 1.4 mm (CV 7.5%) (d) Φ 0.88, SEM 2.2 N.mm (CV 28%) 4. % of loss in passive forces Φ 0.66, SEM 6.4 N (CV 20%)
Passaro, 2014	10 nulliparous women (mean age = 28 ± 5 years)	Number of evaluators: 1 Number of sessions: 2 Time between sessions: 1 month Task: 3 MVC (10s) Outcomes: baseline, peak force, 1st peak, endurance (area under the curve 8s window), strength loss (complementary area under the curve), rate of force development, rate of force decline	Within visit reliability Φ 0.89 – 1 for all except strength loss (Φ 0.75) and rate of force decline (Φ 0.51) Between-visit reliability Φ 0.86 – 0.96 for all except strength loss (Φ 0.73)
Martinho 2015	18 nulliparous women, no urogynecological symptoms (mean age = 25 ± 4 years)	Number of evaluators: 2 Number of sessions: 3 (2 on same day) and 1 the next day Time between session: 1 day Task: 3 MVC Outcomes: maximum strength, average strength, endurance (duration of a 60% plateau)	Intra-rater reliability: Φ 0.94 – 0.96 for all except endurance (Φ 0.88 - 0.86) Inter-rater reliability: Φ 0.80 – 0.91 for all except endurance (Φ 0.59 - 0.81)
Reis Nagano, 2018	20 healthy women (mean age = 31 ± 6 years)	Number of evaluators: 2 Number of sessions: 3 Time between sessions: 1 week Task: MVC (anteroposterior and transverse diameters) Outcomes: baseline, peak force, peak time, average force and impulse (area under the curve from baseline to 1st peak)	Intra-rater, between-visit reliability Anteroposterior: Φ 0.60 - 0.89 Transverse: Φ 0.40 - 0.89 Inter-rater, within-visit reliability Anteroposterior: Φ 0.77 - 0.95 Transverse: Φ 0.38 - 0.86 Inter-rater, between-visit reliability Anteroposterior: Φ 0.71 - 0.97 Transverse: Φ 0.54 - 0.95

Continued

TABLE 5.4.1		Reliability of PFM functional measurements using different dynamometers—cont'd	
Dynamometer	**Sample**	**Method**	**Results**
Verelst, 2004	20 parous women, continent (median age = 39 years)	Number of evaluators: 1 Number of visits: 2 Time between visits: 2 to 4 days Task 1: MVC at 30, 35, 40, 45 and 50 mm (transverse diameter) Outcomes: peak force	Between-visit reliability Coefficient of variation: 30 mm = 22%; 35 mm = 15%; 40 mm = 11%; 45 mm = 10%; 50 mm = 8%
Nunes, 2011	17 nulliparous women, continent (mean age = 25 ± 4 years)	Number of evaluators: 1 Number of visits: 3 Time between visits: ±3 weeks Tasks: 3 MVC at an aperture corresponding to a common passive force of 4.9 N	Between-visit reliability Anteroposterior: Φ 0.71 - 0.89, SEM: 1.96 N (CV 70%) Transverse: Φ 0.46 - 0.72, SEM: 1.86 N (CV 44%)
Romero-Culleres, 2013	122 women with SUI (mean age = 55, between 33-78 year)	Number of evaluators: 3 Number of visits: not reported Time between visits: not reported Tasks: 3 MVC Outcomes: peak force	Intra-rater physician Φ 0.93 (95% CI: 0.90 - 0.95) Inter-rater Φ 0.92 (95% CI: 0.89 - 0.97)
Romero-Culleres, 2017	102 women with SUI (mean age = 56 ± 10 years)	Number of evaluators: 1 Number of visits: 1 Task: 2 MVC Outcomes: relative peak force	Within-visit reliability Φ 0.98 (95% CI: 0.97 - 0.99)
Romero-Culleres, 2020	122 women with SUI (mean age = 56 ± 10 years) and 30 continent women (mean age = 36 ± 10 years)	Number of evaluators: 3 Number of visits: 1 Tasks: 4 MVC (2 by physiatrist, 1 by physio and 1 by midwife) Outcomes: relative peak force	Within-visit, intra-rater reliability Φ 0.94 (95% CI, 0.92 - 0.96) Within-visit, inter-rater reliability Φ 0.94 (95% CI, 0.91 - 0.95)
Kruger, 2011	12 continent women (mean age = 44, between 26-58 years)	Number of evaluators: 1 Number of visits: 2 Time between visits: ±3–5 days Task: 3 rest during stretch (20 stepwise increments) Outcomes: passive stiffness	Between-visit variability Trial 2 (visit 1 vs 2) Φ 0.92 (95%CI 0.89 - 0.93), Trial 3 (visit 1 vs 2) Φ 0.86 (95% CI 0.82 - 0.89)
Kruger, 2015	12 and 20 women (mean age not reported)	Number of evaluators: 1 Number of visits: 1 Time between visits: not clear Task: 3 stretch-release cycles 30-50mm in 20mm/sec Outcomes: passive stiffness	Within-visit reliability elastometer held in situ during the procedure Φ 0.99 (95% CI 0.96 - 0.99, n=20) elastometer removed and then re-inserted 5min later Φ 0.93 (95% CI 0.78 - 0.98, n=12)

CR, coefficient of repeatability; CV, coefficient of variation; ICC, intra-class correlation coefficient; SEM, standard error of mean; SUI, stress urinary incontinence, PES, passive elastic stiffness; SUI, stress urinary incontinence; CI, confidence interval; MVC, maximal voluntary contraction.

Most studies compared dynamometry outcomes with digital assessment scores of PFM strength (Ashton-Miller et al., 2014; Morin et al., 2004; Navarro-Brazález et al., 2018; Parezanović-Ilić et al., 2009; Romero-Cullerés et al., 2013; Romero-Cullerés et al., 2017; Romero-Cullerés et al., 2020; Yoshimura et al., 2004). Furthermore, dynamometry outcomes were compared with electromyography (EMG; Morin et al., 2006; Navarro-Brazález et al., 2018), intravaginal manometry (Navarro-Brazález et al., 2018), IAP (Ashton-Miller et al., 2014; Morgan et al., 2005; Morin et al., 2006) and PFM morphometry on magnetic resonance images (Morgan et al., 2009).

In studies comparing dynamometry outcomes with the digital assessment scores of PFM strength, the sample size varied from 12 in one study (Yoshimura et al., 2004) to more than 100 women in four studies (Navarro-Brazález et al., 2018; Romero-Cullerés et al., 2013; Romero-Cullerés et al., 2017; Romero-Cullerés et al., 2020). All included women with urinary incontinence. Three studies also included asymptomatic controls (Morin et al., 2004; Parezanović-Ilić et al., 2009; Romero-Cullerés et al., 2020), and one woman with anal incontinence and pelvic organ prolapse (POP; Navarro-Brazález et al., 2018). Digital assessment procedures were similar between studies. For all, assessment was performed with women in a supine position and the PFM strength was graded according to similar 0 to 5 palpation scales. Six studies (Morin et al., 2004; Navarro-Brazález et al., 2018; Romero-Cullerés et al., 2013; Romero-Cullerés et al., 2017; Romero-Cullerés et al., 2020; Yoshimura et al., 2004) used the modified Oxford grading system (Laycock, 1992). Parezanović-Ilić et al. (2009) used the 0 to 5 Digital Pelvic Assessment rating scale (Guerette et al., 2004), Navarro-Brazález et al. (2018) used both the modified Oxford grading system and Levator Ani testing (a scale frequently used in this field of study), and Ashton-Miller et al. (2014) classified women into two categories (good/excellent and poor/fair strength) based on the Brink scale (Brink et al., 1994).

Dynamometric assessment conditions were similar between studies. Only two studies specified the vaginal aperture, and both used minimal dynamometric openings (19 mm in the work of Morin et al. [2004] and 24 mm in the work of Navarro-Brazález et al. [2018]). According to Morin et al. (2004), this would be the closest to the vaginal aperture in palpation assessments. All studies acquired maximum forces during two to five trials of maximal PFM voluntary contractions. Five studies calculated the delta force from the peak force minus baseline (Ashton-Miller et al., 2014; Morin et al., 2004; Navarro-Brazález et al., 2018; Romero-Cullerés et al., 2017; Romero-Cullerés et al., 2020). Most studies reported forces in Newtons (N), with the exception of Navarro-Brazález et al. (2018), who reported it in grams. In four studies, dynamometric forces were compared to each palpation grade. For all, mean peak forces increased significantly across palpation assessment categories, although with substantial overlapping between adjacent palpation categories. In addition, mean peak forces varied largely across studies for each of the palpation grades: 1, 2, 3, 4, and 5 respectively:

- 1.8 N, 2.6 N, 3.9 N, 5.0 N, 6.5 N (Morin et al., 2004)
- 0.4 N, 0.7 N, 1.0 N, 1.3 N, 1.8 N (Parezanović-Ilić et al. 2009)
- 0.1 N, 0.3 N, 0.6 N, 0.9 N, 1.2 N (Romero-Cullerés et al., 2017)
- 0.5 N, 0.4 N, 0.6 N, 0.8 N, 1.0 N (Romero-Cullerés et al., 2020)

Finally, Ashton-Miller et al. (2014) divided women into only two categories as per digital palpation, good/excellent and poor/fair, and found a significant difference in force outputs between groups (3.8 ± 1.8 N vs 2.0 ± 0.8 N, p = 0.01). Four studies reported on the correlation between force and palpation grades, with results ranging from moderate (Spearman's ϱ (r_s) = 0.56 [Morin et al., 2004], linear regression (r^2) = 0.52 for the modified Oxford grading system and r^2 = 0.47 for Levator Ani testing [Navarro-Brazález et al., 2018]) to strong (r_s = 0.89 [Yoshimura et al., 2004], r^2 = 0.85 [Parezanović-Ilić et al., 2009]). Finally, three studies reported on areas under receiver operating characteristic curves as a diagnostic accuracy indicator of force measurements with respect to palpation grades (Romero-Cullerés et al., 2013; Romero-Cullerés et al., 2017; Romero-Cullerés et al., 2020), with values ranging from 0.79 (95% CI: 0.71–0.88 [Romero-Cullerés et al., 2013]) to 0.87 (95% CI: 0.81–0.92) [Romero-Cullerés et al., 2020]).

In an effort to validate PFM dynamometric measurements, Morin et al. (2006) attached four pairs of EMG electrodes along the lower branch of the dynamometer. The location of the highest EMG amplitude corresponded to the location of the resultant force applied to the dynamometer, confirming that forces recorded by the dynamometer were in fact originating from PFMs. Navarro-Brazález et al. (2018) also used surface EMG, this time overlying both sides of the anus during maximal and sustained PFM contractions. However, they only found a very weak positive correlation between EMG and dynamometric outcomes. Lastly, Navarro-Brazález et al. (2018) compared dynamometry with pressure outcomes from a balloon-type intravaginal manometer (Peritron, Melbourne, Australia), finding moderate correlation between peak forces and pressures on maximal PFM contractions ($r^2 = 0.75$) and further supporting the validity of dynamometric measurements.

How much IAP influenced dynamometric measurements was also assessed in three studies (Ashton-Miller et al., 2014; Morgan et al. 2005; Morin et al., 2006). Morgan et al. (2005) assessed 39 asymptomatic women using a dynamometer and a microtip catheter placed in the bladder to monitor IAP at rest and during a maximum PFM contraction in supine and standing positions. IAP measurements did not correlate with dynamometric outputs ($r^2 = 0.01$), suggesting that the vaginal closure force was influenced by but not entirely dependent on IAP. Morin et al. (2006) assessed 10 continent women using dynamometry and an intra-rectal balloon to monitor changes in IAP. IAP influence on dynamometric forces was considered small both on maximal PFM contraction (7%) and straining (14%), standardized to 50 and 100 cmH_2O. Finally, Ashton-Miller et al. (2014) reported evidence for cross-talk between IAP signals and dynamometric outputs with an improved instrumented speculum specifically designed to distinguish the vaginal closure force from IAP variations. Overall, IAP influence on dynamometric forces is minimal but increases with straining.

Morgan et al. (2009) assessed PFM function and morphometry in 103 women with SUI and 108 asymptomatic controls using dynamometry and magnetic resonance imaging. Significant correlations were found between the vaginal rest force and the length of the bladder neck or the length/area index of the striated urogenital sphincter (SUS; −0.27 and 0.18, respectively). Correlations were also significant for maximum PFM contraction and SUS length, area and length/area index (−0.27, 0.15 and 0.28, respectively), suggesting that a smaller SUS is associated with a poorer PFM dynamometric function. Overall, convergent validity studies support PFM dynamometry as a valid measurement of PFM function.

Known Groups Validity

This type of construct validity focuses on the ability of a new instrument to discriminate between groups that are known to be different (Dunn, 1989; Portney and Watkins, 1993; Portney and Watkins, 2000). In other words, if a dynamometer proved to be capable of differentiating between the PFM function of continent and incontinent women, this capacity would support its construct validity. The following section presents Known Groups validity studies in SUI versus continent women, POP versus controls, provoked vestibulodynia versus controls, and women with levator ani avulsion/defect versus controls.

Pelvic Floor Muscle Functional Differences Between Continent and Stress Urinary Incontinent Women

Four research groups presented data on continent and incontinent women. In the study by Morin et al. (2004), 30 continent women and 59 women with SUI, aged between 21 and 44 years, were recruited. The Montreal dynamometer was used to assess multiple PFM parameters. An analysis of covariance was used to control for the confounding variables of age and parity during comparisons of PFM function in continent and incontinent women. The incontinent women demonstrated both lower passive force and absolute endurance than the continent women ($p \leq 0.05$). The rate-of-force development and number of rapid contractions were both lower among the SUI participants ($p = 0.01$) (Morin et al., 2004).

In another study, Morin et al. (2007) investigated the involuntary PFM response during coughing in 31 continent women and 30 women with symptoms of SUI. Participants were instructed to perform two maximal coughs. There was a significant difference, favoring continent women, for the maximal rate-of-force development (rapidity to contract prior to a cough) ($p = 0.032$) and a strong tendency for PFM peak force prior to a cough.

Finally, Morin et al. (2008a) compared PFM passive properties in 34 postmenopausal continent and 34 SUI women. SUI women demonstrated lower passive forces at minimal, mean and maximal apertures ($p < 0.05$) as well as lower passive elastic stiffness at maximal aperture ($p = 0.038$). The lower initial passive resistance and higher contribution of passive forces to total voluntary strength in incontinent women support the role of passive properties in maintaining continence (Morin et al., 2008a). These three studies with the Montreal dynamometer suggest that PFM dynamometric parameters differ between continent and incontinent women at rest, during maximal voluntary contraction and during a cough.

Verelst and Leivseth (2004) used their intravaginal probe to determine whether there is a difference between continent and SUI women. Twenty-six continent and twenty SUI parous women were examined. Fatigue was measured with the intravaginal device and the time-to-fatigue was defined as the time it took for a 10% decline in the initial maximal reference force. Time-to-fatigue was identical in the two groups (10.5 seconds in the continent group and 11.5 seconds in the incontinent group). Only normalized maximal force was significantly different between the groups, being lower in the incontinent group ($p = 0.013$). It is likely, according to Verelst and Leivseth (2004), that reduced normalized maximal force, as found in the incontinent group, is an important contributing factor to urinary incontinence. In a second study, Verelst and Leivseth (2007) compared passive and active forces as measured in continent and incontinent parous women. Twenty-four parous continent and 21 parous incontinent women were examined using their intravaginal device. Passive and active force/stiffness were measured by increasing the transverse diameter of the vagina. To allow a more accurate comparison between groups, measured forces were normalized with respect to body weight. No difference was found between the groups according to passive force, but the active force was significantly higher ($p = 0.030$) in the continent group when normalized for body weight. Further, normalized active stiffness was significantly reduced in the incontinent group ($p = 0.021$). Both active force development and active stiffness in the PFMs were significantly reduced in SUI women. Peng and colleagues (Peng et al. 2007; Shishido et al. 2008), using the Constantinou four-sensor probe, studied the vaginal pressure profile along the vaginal wall between 23 continent women and 10 women with symptoms of SUI. The continent group had significantly greater maximum pressure than the stress SUI group on the posterior vaginal side at rest (mean $3.4 + 0.3$ vs $2.01 + 0.36$ N/cm^2) and during PFM contraction ($4.18 + 0.26$ vs $2.25 + 0.41$ N/cm^2). The activity pressure difference between the posterior and anterior vaginal walls in the continent women's group was significantly increased when the PFMs contracted compared to that at rest ($3.29 + 0.21$ vs $2.45 + 0.26$ N/cm^2). However, the change observed in the SUI group was not significant ($1.85 + 0.38$ vs $1.35 + 0.27$ N/cm^2). The authors concluded that voluntary PFM contraction imposes significant closure forces along the vaginal wall of continent women but not in SUI women and discriminates between these two groups. In contrast, Delancey et al. (2008) compared 103 women with SUI and 108 asymptomatic controls in groups matched for age, race, parity and hysterectomy, and found no differences either in the vaginal closure force during a maximal pelvic muscle contraction or at rest. Of interest, some of the previous studies showed that the difference between SUI and continent PFM function was mostly related to PFM parameters other than maximal forces. However, Parezanović-Ilić (2009), in a case–control study, compared two groups of women aged 20 to 58 years (continent women or women with urinary incontinence) with regard to PFM strength measured with a vaginal dynamometer and found that the mean PFM force of healthy women was significantly higher than in incontinent women (1.44 ± 0.38 daN vs 0.78 ± 0.31 daN ($t = 8.89$, $df = 88$, $p < 0.001$). Finally, Chamochumbi et al. (2012), using the Nunes speculum, studied active and passive PFM forces in 16 continent and 16 SUI middle-aged women. Evaluation of PFM passive and active forces was done in the anteroposterior and left–right directions. The anteroposterior active strength was significantly higher in the continent women ($0.3 + 0.2$ N) compared to the SUI women ($0.1 + 0.1$ N), implying that SUI women had a lower anteroposterior active strength than continent women (Chamochumbi et al., 2012).

In conclusion, the ability of most of the preceding dynamometers to discriminate different aspects of PFM function among SUI and continent women confirmed further aspects of their construct validity.

Pelvic Floor Muscle Functional Differences Between Women With and Without Provoked Vestibulodynia

Two studies used the Montreal dynamometer to assess women suffering from provoked vestibulodynia (Fontaine et al., 2018; Morin et al., 2017), but in only one (Morin et al., 2017) were cases compared to controls. To minimize discomfort in this population with known pain at the vaginal entry, the dynamometer branches were reduced to a paediatric speculum size. Passive and active properties of the PFMs were assessed in 56 women with provoked vestibulodynia and 56 controls at rest, on repeated lengthening and shortening cycles and during different PFM contraction tasks. Overall, women with provoked vestibulodynia showed higher tone, lower strength and endurance, less speed of contraction, and higher resistance at maximal aperture. This supports the hypothesis that provoked vestibulodynia is related to PFM dysfunction and confirms the capacity of dynamometric assessments to detect those differences.

Pelvic Floor Muscle Functional Differences Between Women With and Without Pelvic Organ Prolapse

Two studies (Berger et al., 2018; DeLancey et al., 2007) compared PFM function among women with and without POP using Ashton-Miller's instrumented speculum. DeLancey et al. (2007) assessed 151 women with prolapse and 135 with normal pelvic organ support as controls matched for age, race and hysterectomy status. Results showed that women with POP presented less vaginal closure force on PFM contraction than controls (2.0 N compared with 3.2 N, p < 0.001). Berger et al. (2018) assessed 60 women with posterior prolapse, 90 with anterior prolapse and 103 controls with normal support. Similarly, there were significant differences in generated vaginal closure forces across the three groups, with the prolapse groups generating weaker vaginal closure forces than the control group (p = 0.004). No differences were found between the two prolapse groups after controlling for prolapse size (p = 0.43). Together, these results suggest that pelvic organ support is related to PFM function and confirm the capacity of dynamometric instruments to detect those differences.

Pelvic Floor Muscle Function in Women With and Without Levator Ani Defect

Two studies compared PFM function in primiparous women with and without levator ani defects. Brincat et al. (2011) compared 29 women with levator ani defects to 128 women without levator ani defects with regard to intravaginal resting closure force (rest), vaginal closure force during a PFM contraction, and the difference between rest and vaginal closure force. Women with levator ani defects showed significantly lower rest force and less ability to augment their vaginal closure force with MVC compared to women with no levator ani defects (2.04 [1.0] vs 1.6 [0.2] N and 2.28 [1.6] vs 1.3 [0.8] N, respectively). In another study from Cyr et al. (2017), 22 primiparous women diagnosed with puborectalis avulsion injury were compared to 30 without at 3 months postpartum for PFM function, using the Montreal dynamometric speculum. Passive properties (passive forces and stiffness) during dynamic stretches, maximal strength, speed of contraction and endurance were measured. Women with avulsion showed lower passive forces at maximal and 20-mm vaginal apertures as well as lower stiffness at 20-mm aperture (p = 0.048). Significantly lower strength, speed of contraction and endurance were also found in women with avulsion (p = 0.005). Together, both studies confirm that PFM function is impaired in primiparous women with puborectalis defect/avulsion. Moreover, it highlights specific muscle parameters that are altered in this population, such as passive properties, strength, speed of contraction and endurance.

Predicting Outcomes of Pelvic Floor Muscle Rehabilitation

PFM dynamometry has also been shown to be useful in predicting PFM treatment outcomes. Dumoulin et al. (2010) evaluated, in the secondary analysis of a randomized controlled trial on PFM rehabilitation in young postpartum women, the relationship between pre–physical therapy PFM function and treatment outcome. The relationship between potential predictive PFM function variables, as measured by a PFM dynamometer, and physical therapy success was studied using forward stepwise multivariate logistic regression analysis. Forty-two women (74%) were classified as treatment successes; 15 (26%) were not. Treatment success was associated with lower pre-treatment PFM passive force and greater PFM endurance ($p < 0.05$), although the association with the latter was barely statistically significant. These results, the first using dynamometry, contribute new information on predictors of success for an 8-week PFM physical therapy program in women with persistent postpartum SUI. More research is needed in this area, using dynamometry, to identify for pre-treatment those women with PFM dysfunction (urinary incontinence, POP or pain) who are more likely to respond to physical therapy.

CONCLUSION

PFM dynamometers are reliable, valid and responsive instruments that can directly measure PFM passive forces, active forces and forces during effort, such as a Valsalva manoeuvre or a cough. Different dynamometric units allow for the evaluation of PFM forces in different directions (anteroposteriorly and laterally); at different vaginal apertures; during rest, maximal PFM contraction and effort; and using a multitude of parameters (strength, endurance, rapidity of contraction, etc.). In addition, measurements can be taken in the supine position and, with some units, in sitting or standing positions.

Clearly, dynamometry has multiple clinical applications: firstly, it can inform clinicians about a patient's specific PFM dysfunction in terms of passive strength, maximum strength, rapidity of contraction, coordination and endurance. These PFM dysfunctions need to be rehabilitated and their progress monitored. Secondly, although fairly recent and, as of yet, reported in only one trial, dynamometry has been used to predict treatment outcomes.

Although dynamometers appear to be a highly promising tool for assessing PFM function, commercial units are only starting to be available. Furthermore, although the development and psychometric evaluation of the PFM dynamometer have substantially progressed over the past 20 years, inter-rater reliability studies of hand-held dynamometers are still required. Most importantly, measurement protocols including dynamometer size, dynamometer opening and task description need to be standardized to advance our understanding of PFM dysfunctions in different populations. Right now, each dynamometer has its own procedure. Normative data on the PFM function are still relatively rare and require further study. Finally, dynamometers measure force but not displacement of the PFMs. Other measurements tools such as imaging instruments are needed to inform on PFM lift.

CLINICAL RECOMMENDATIONS (Based on the Montreal Dynamometer)

- Explain the tool and the procedures to the patient.
- After the patient has undressed, ask her to adopt a supine position, hips and knees flexed and supported, feet flat on a treatment table.
- Prior to the insertion of the dynamometer's probe/speculum, give detailed instructions about contracting the PFMs using anatomical models, drawings and vaginal palpation.
- Confirm correct contraction of the PFMs.
- Prepare the dynamometer by covering each branch of the probe/speculum with a condom lubricated with a hypoallergenic gel.
- Bring the two branches of the measuring device to their minimum aperture and gently insert the dynamometer into the vaginal cavity in an anteroposterior axis to a depth of 5 cm. Note the angle of dynamometer on insertion to ensure repeating the same testing situation from one measurement to the next.
- Gently separate the two branches to obtain the appropriate aperture.
- Allow some time for the woman to adjust to the sensation of the probe/speculum inside her vagina—time that can be used for practicing the required manoeuvre before recording a task (e.g., PFM maximal contraction).
- For a PFM maximal contraction, ask the patient to breathe normally and then to squeeze and lift the PFMs as if to prevent the escape of flatus and urine.
- Standardize the commands and provide encouragement.
- Give positive feedback while taking measurements such as strength, endurance and coordination during active tasks, or encourage relaxation during passive force measurements.
- Record the results.
- After the evaluation session, discard the condoms and disinfect the dynamometer.

REFERENCES

Ashton-Miller, J. A., Delancey, J. O., & Warnick, D. N. (2002). *Method and apparatus for measuring properties of the pelvic floor muscles.* US Patent 6468232B1.

Ashton-Miller, J. A., Zielinski, R., Miller, J., et al. (2014). Validity and reliability of an instrumented speculum designed to minimize the effect of intra-abdominal pressure on the measurement of pelvic floor muscle strength. *Clinical Biomechanics (Bristol, Avon), 29*(10), 1146–1150.

Berger, M. B., Kolenic, G. E., Fenner, D. E., et al. (2018). Structural, functional, and symptomatic differences between women with rectocele versus cystocele and normal support. *American Journal of Obstetrics and Gynecology, 218,* 510.e1–510.e8.

Bérubé, M., Czyrnyj, C. S., & McLean, L. (2018). An automated intravaginal dynamometer: Reliability metrics and the impact of testing protocol on active and passive forces measured from the pelvic floor muscles. *Neurourology and Urodynamics, 37,* 1875–1888.

Bø, K., Frawley, H. C., Haylen, B. T., et al. (2017). An International Urogynecological Association (IUGA)/ International Continence Society (ICS) joint report on the terminology for the conservative and nonpharmacological management of female pelvic floor dysfunction. *International Urogynecology Journal, 28,* 191–213.

Brincat, C. A., DeLancey, J. O. L., & Miller, J. M. (2011). Urethral closure pressures among primiparous women with and without levator ani muscle defects. *International Urogynecology Journal, 22,* 1491–1495.

Brink, K. H., LaCasce, J. H., & Irish, J. D. (1994). The effect of short-scale wind variations on shelf currents. *Journal of Geophysical Research-Oceans, 99,* 3305–3314.

Castro-Pardiñas, M. A., Torres-Lacomba, M., & Navarro-Brazález, B. (2017). Muscle function of the pelvic floor in healthy, puerperal women with pelvic floor dysfunction. *Actas Urológicas Españolas, 41,* 249–257.

Caufriez, M. (1993). Postpartum: Rééducation urodynamique. In *Approche globale et technique analytique* (pp. 36–44). Brussels: Collection Maïte.

Caufriez, M. (1998). *Thérapies manuelles et instrumentales en uro-gynécologie.* Brussels: Collection Maïte.

Chamochumbi, C. C. M., Nunes, F. R., Guirro, R. R. J., et al. (2012). Comparison of active and passive forces of the pelvic floor muscles in women with and without stress urinary incontinence. *Revista Brasileira de Fisioterapia, 16,* 314–319.

Constantinou, C. E., & Omata, S. (2007). Direction sensitive sensor probe for the evaluation of voluntary and reflex pelvic floor contractions. *Neurourology and Urodynamics, 26,* 386–391.

Constantinou, C. E., Omata, S., Yoshimura, Y., et al. (2007). Evaluation of the dynamic responses of female pelvic floor using a novel vaginal probe. *Annals of the New York Academy of Sciences, 1101,* 297–315.

Cyr, M.-P., Kruger, J., Wong, V., et al. (2017). Pelvic floor morphometry and function in women with and without puborectalis avulsion in the early postpartum period. *American Journal of Obstetrics and Gynecology, 216,* 274.e1–274.e8.

Czyrnyj, C.S., Lanteigne, E., Boucher, S., et al. (2019). Speed and force validation of an improved intravaginal dynamometer design. *CMBES Proceedings, 42,* 1–5.

DeLancey, J. O. L., Morgan, D. M., Fenner, D. E., et al. (2007). Comparison of levator ani muscle defects and function in women with and without pelvic organ prolapse. *Obstetrics & Gynecology, 109,* 295–302.

DeLancey, J., Trowbridge, E., Miller, J., et al. (2008). Stress urinary incontinence: Relative importance of urethral support and urethral closure pressure. *Journal of Urology, 179,* 2286–2290.

Dos Reis Nagano, R. C., Biasotto-Gonzalez, D. A., da Costa, G. L., et al. (2018). Test–retest reliability of the different dynamometric variables used to evaluate pelvic floor musculature during the menstrual cycle. *Neurourology and Urodynamics, 37,* 2606–2613.

Dumoulin, C., Bourbonnais, D., & Lemieux, M. C. (2003). Development of a dynamometer for measuring the isometric force of the pelvic floor musculature. *Neurourology and Urodynamics, 22,* 648–653.

Dumoulin, C., Gravel, D., Bourbonnais, D., et al. (2004). Reliability of dynamometric measurements of the pelvic floor musculature. *Neurourology and Urodynamics, 23,* 134–142.

Dumoulin, C., Bourbonnais, D., Morin, M., et al. (2010). Predictors of success for physiotherapy treatment in women with persistent postpartum stress urinary incontinence. *Archives of Physical Medicine and Rehabilitation,* 91(7), 1059–1063.

Dumoulin, C., Dumoulin, A. Dynamometer for measurement of soft tissue forces such as pelvic floor muscle. International Patent number WO 2014/176689.

Dunn, W. (1989). Reliability and validity. In L. J. Miller (Ed.), *Developing norm-referenced standardized tests* (pp. 149–168). New York: Haworth Press.

El-Sayegh, B., Dumoulin, C., Ali, M., et al. (2020). A dynamometer-based wireless pelvic floor muscle force monitoring. In *42nd annual international conference of the IEEE engineering in medicine and biology society (EMBC)* (pp. 6127–6130).

Elvie. (2013). *Elvie trainer [online].* Available: https://www.elvie.com/en-us/shop/elvie-trainer. (Accessed 08.12.20).

Fizimed. (2018). *Emy: Kegel training with biofeedback.* Available: https://www.fizimed.com/en/emy-device. (Accessed 08.12.20).

Fontaine, F., Dumoulin, C., Bergeron, S., et al. (2018). Pelvic floor muscle morphometry and function in women with primary and secondary provoked vestibulodynia. *The Journal of Sexual Medicine, 15,* 1149–1157.

Guerette, N., Neimark, M., Kopka, S. L., et al. (2004). Initial experience with a new method for the dynamic assessment of pelvic floor function in women: The kolpexin pull test. *International Urogynecology Journal and Pelvic Floor Dysfunction*, 15, 39–43.

Kruger, J., Nielsen, P., Budgett, S., et al. (2015). An automated hand–held elastometer for quantifying the passive stiffness of the levator ani muscle in women. *Neurourology and Urodynamics*, 34, 133–138.

Kruger, J., Nielsen, P., Dietz, H. P., et al. (2011). Test-retest reliability of an instrumented elastometer for measuring passive stiffness of the levator ani muscle. *Neurourology and Urodynamics*, 30, 865–867.

Laycock, J. (1992). *Assessment and treatment of pelvic floor dysfunction: Physiotherapy in the management of pelvic floor dysfunction in relation to female urinary incontinence.* Bradford, UK: Doctoral thesis. University of Bradford.

Mafi, P., Mafi, R., Hindocha, S., et al. (2012). A systematic review of dynamometry and its role in hand trauma assessment. *The Open Orthopaedics Journal*, 6, 95–102.

Martinho, N. M., Marques, J., Silva, V. R., et al. (2015). Intra and inter-rater reliability study of pelvic floor muscle dynamometric measurements. *Brazilian Journal of Physical Therapy*, 19, 97–104.

Martinho, N. M., Silva, V. R., Marques, J., et al. (2016). The effects of training by virtual reality or gym ball on pelvic floor muscle strength in postmenopausal women: A randomized controlled trial. *Brazilian Journal of Physical Therapy*, 20, 248–257.

Mercier, J., Morin, M., Zaki, D., et al. (2019). Pelvic floor muscle training as a treatment for genitourinary syndrome of menopause: A single-arm feasibility study. *Maturitas*, 125, 57–62.

Miller, J. M., Ashton-Miller, J. A., Perruchini, D., et al. (2007). Test–retest reliability of an instrumented speculum for measuring vaginal closure force. *Neurourology and Urodynamics*, 26, 858–863.

Morgan, D. M., Kaur, G., Hsu, Y., et al. (2005). Does vaginal closure force differ in the supine and standing positions? *American Journal of Obstetrics and Gynecology*, 192, 1722–1728.

Morgan, D. M., Umek, W., Guire, K., et al. (2009). Urethral sphincter morphology and function with and without stress incontinence. *Journal of Urology*, 182, 203–209.

Morin, M., Bergeron, S., Khalifé, S., et al. (2010a). Dynamometric assessment of the pelvic floor muscle function in women with and without provoked vestibulodynia. *International Urogynecology Journal*, 29, 1140–1141.

Morin, M., Binik, Y. M., Bourbonnais, D., et al. (2017). Heightened pelvic floor muscle tone and altered contractility in women with provoked vestibulodynia. *The Journal of Sexual Medicine*, 14, 592–600.

Morin, M., Bourbonnais, D., Gravel, D., et al. (2004). Pelvic floor muscle function in continent and stress urinary incontinent women using dynamometric measurements. *Neurourology and Urodynamics*, 23, 668–674.

Morin, M., Dumoulin, C., Gravel, D., et al. (2007). Reliability of speed of contraction and endurance dynamometric measurements of the pelvic floor musculature in stress incontinent parous women. *Neurourology and Urodynamics*, 26, 397–403.

Morin, M., Gravel, D., Bourbonnais, D., et al. (2008a). Comparing pelvic floor muscle tone in postmenopausal continent and stress urinary incontinent women. *Neurourology and Urodynamics*, 27, 610–611.

Morin, M., Gravel, D., Bourbonnais, D., et al. (2008b). Reliability of dynamometric passive properties of the pelvic floor muscles in postmenopausal women with stress urinary incontinence. *Neurourology and Urodynamics*, 27, 819–825.

Morin, M., Gravel, D., Bourbonnais, D., et al. (2010b). Application of a new method in the study of pelvic floor muscle passive properties in continent women. *Journal of Electromyography and Kinesiology*, 20, 795–803.

Morin, M., Gravel, D., Dumoulin, C., et al. (2006). *Influence of increased cough intensity on the activation timing and contractile force of associated pelvic floor muscle contraction in continent women.* Christchurch, New Zealand: International Continence Society Annual Meeting.

Navarro-Brázález, B., Lacomba, M. T., de la Villa, P., et al. (2018). The evaluation of pelvic floor muscle strength in women with pelvic floor dysfunction: A reliability and correlation study. *Neurourology and Urodynamics*, 37, 269–277.

Nunes, F. B., Martins, C. C., de Oliveira Guirro, E. C., et al. (2011). Reliability of bidirectional and variable-opening equipment for the measurement of pelvic floor muscle strength. *Physical Medicine and Rehabilitation*, 3, 21–26.

Nunnally, J. C., & Bernstein, I. H. (1994). *Psychometric theory* (3rd ed.). New York: McGraw Hill.

Passaro, A., Cacciari, L., Amorim, A., et al. (2014). Intrarater reliability of strength assessment of pelvic floor muscles. *Neurourology and Urodynamics*, 33(6), 982–983.

Parezanović-Ilić, K., Jevtić, M., Jeremić, B., et al. (2009). Muscle strength measurement of pelvic floor in women by vaginal dynamometer. *Srpski Arhiv Za Celokupno Lekarstvo*, 137, 511–517.

Peng, Q., Jones, R., Shishido, K., et al. (2007). Spatial distribution of vaginal closure pressures of continent and stress urinary incontinent women. *Physiological Measurement*, 28, 1429–1450.

PeriCoach. (2014). *PeriCoach: The best kegel exerciser.* Available: https://www.pericoach.com/. (Accessed 08.12.20).

Portney, L. G., & Watkins, M. P. (1993). *Foundations of clinical research: Applications to practice.* Boston: Prentice Hall.

Portney, L. G., & Watkins, M. P. (2000). *Foundations of clinical research: Applications to practice* (2nd ed.). Boston: Prentice Hall.

Romero-Cullerés, G., Peña-Pitarch, E., Jané-Feixas, C., et al. (2013). Reliability and validity of a new vaginal dynamometer to measure pelvic floor muscle strength in women with urinary incontinence. *Neurourology and Urodynamics, 32*, 658–659.

Romero-Cullerés, G., Peña-Pitarch, E., Jané-Feixas, C., et al. (2020). Reliability and diagnostic accuracy of a new vaginal dynamometer to measure pelvic floor muscle strength. *Female Pelvic Medicine & Reconstructive Surgery, 26*, 514–519.

Romero–Cullerés, G., Peña–Pitarch, E., Jané–Feixas, C., et al. (2017). Intra–rater reliability and diagnostic accuracy of a new vaginal dynamometer to measure pelvic floor muscle strength in women with urinary incontinence. *Neurourology and Urodynamics, 36*, 333–337.

Rowe, P. (1995). A new system for the measurement of pelvic floor muscle strength in urinary incontinence. In *12th international congress of the world confederation for physical therapy*.

Saleme, C. S., Rocha, D. N., Del Vecchio, S., et al. (2009). Multidirectional pelvic floor muscle strength measurement. *Annals of Biomedical Engineering, 37*, 1594–1600.

Sampselle, C. M., Miller, J. M., Mims, B. L., et al. (1998). Effect of pelvic muscle exercise on transient incontinence during pregnancy and after birth. *Obstetrics & Gynecology, 91*, 406–412.

Shishido, K., Peng, Q., Jones, R., et al. (2008). Influence of pelvic floor muscle contraction on the profile of vaginal closure pressure in continent and stress urinary incontinent women. *Journal of Urology, 179*, 1917–1922.

Verelst, M., & Leivseth, G. (2004). Force–length relationship in the pelvic floor muscles under transverse vaginal distension: A method study in healthy women. *Neurourology and Urodynamics, 23*, 662–667.

Verelst, M., & Leivseth, G. (2007). Force and stiffness of the pelvic floor as function of muscle length: A comparison between women with and without stress urinary incontinence. *Neurourology and Urodynamics, 26*, 852–857.

Yoshimura, Y., Yamaguchi, O., Omata, S., et al. (2004). The assessment of pelvic floor muscle function using a novel and directionally sensitive intra-vaginal sensor probe. *Neurourology and Urodynamics*. https://www.ics.org/Abstracts/Publish/42/000560.pdf.

5.5 Electromyography

Mélanie Morin

INTRODUCTION

Electromyography (EMG) is the recording of electrical potentials generated by the depolarization of muscle fibre membranes (Bø et al., 2017; Frawley et al., 2021). This assessment tool can be useful for different clinical and research purposes, which can be broadly divided into two categories (Vodušek, 2015). The first is the use of EMG in neurophysiology for the diagnosis of denervation/reinnervation or myopathy (Bianchi et al., 2017). To this end, muscle constituents (e.g., muscle fibres and motor units) are investigated using intra-muscular electrodes (Bianchi et al., 2017). This approach, also referred to as the motor unit EMG technique, will be briefly presented. This chapter will mainly cover the second category: the use of EMG for assessing the behaviour or pattern of activity of the muscle. Also called *kinesiological EMG* (or *surface EMG* [sEMG], this widespread approach in pelvic floor physical therapy uses surface electrodes of various forms (e.g., surface perineal electrode, probe and catheter [anal, vaginal, urethral]). Proper interpretation of the EMG while acknowledging its inherent limitations and clinometric properties will be discussed in agreement with current evidence and internationally accepted guidelines.

MUSCLE FIBRES AND MOTOR UNIT

Understanding the EMG signal implies a good grasp of muscle physiology and how bioelectrical current is generated. Motor control relies on the activation of motor units, not the recruitment of single muscle fibres (Enoka and Duchateau, 2016). A motor unit consists of alpha motor neuron located in the spinal cord and the pool of muscle fibres it innervates. When a muscle is activated, either voluntarily or through reflex arcs, the electrical current travels from the motor neuron, through its axon and to its end (the neuromuscular junction) (Enoka and Duchateau, 2016). This results in the generation of action potentials in all muscle fibres belonging to the motor unit.

The action potential propagates along all muscle fibres in both directions away from the neuromuscular junction. The action potential corresponds more specifically to depolarization of the muscle fibre due to the influx of Na+ followed by repolarization related to the efflux of K+. The recorded EMG signal represents the bioelectrical activity generated by a single motor unit (i.e., motor unit potential [MUP]) up to the summation of the activity arising from the muscle fibres of several motor units (Enoka and Duchateau, 2016). As muscle force is produced, the EMG signal amplitude increases by two main mechanisms, namely the recruitment of additional motor units and the increase in the firing rate of the already active motor units (i.e., rates at which they discharge action potentials) (Kukulka and Clamann, 1981; van Bolhuis et al., 1997). The recruitment order of motor units is usually organized to progressively activate the smallest units that can generate slow and low force and end with the largest, most powerful and strong motor units (Farina et al., 2016).

MOTOR UNIT ELECTROMYOGRAPHY FOR NEUROPHYSIOLOGY ASSESSMENT

Intra-muscular EMG can be used in clinical neurophysiology to selectively assess the activity of individual MUPs. This assessment focuses on muscle constituents (muscle fibres and motor units) to investigate motor unit physiology and pathophysiology. This technique was shown to be valid for differentiating between normal, denervated, and reinnervated and myopathic muscle (Bianchi et al., 2017; Vodušek, 2015). Other neurophysiological tests, including pudendal nerve terminal motor latency, sacral reflex and pudendal somatosensory evoked potentials, are often used along with intra-muscular EMG to assess involvement of the neuromuscular system by trauma or disease (Bianchi et al., 2017; Olsen and Rao, 2001). To obtain the level of selectivity needed to record the MUP, needle or wire electrodes are used. The electrodes can be inserted to assess the urethral sphincter, the superficial pelvic floor muscles (PFMs) (e.g., bulbocavernosus) and the deep layers (e.g., levator ani) (Bø and Stien, 1994), but the external anal sphincter remains the most routinely evaluated muscle because of the ease of the evaluation and the availability of normative data (Podnar and Vodušek, 2001). The EMG examination is usually initiated with a qualitative observation of spontaneous activity elicited by the insertion of the intra-muscular electrode. In normally innervated muscle a short burst of activity can be observed due to the mechanical stimulation of excitable membranes, whereas in the absence of insertion activity, a complete denervation atrophy can be suspected (Podnar and Vodušek, 2001). Examination of resting activity can also be performed as a constant discharge of low-threshold motor units is observed in the normally innervated external anal sphincter (Podnar et al., 2002a) and some parts of the levator ani muscle (Deindl et al., 1993). Normal MUPs are stable with a similar shape repeated following a regular and constant pattern (Podnar and Vodušek, 2001). In contrast, pathological spontaneous activity is characterized by fibrillation and irregular wave shapes such as positive sharp peaks (Podnar and Vodušek, 2001). Quantitative analysis of the electrical activity of motor units can be performed using two different approaches (Bianchi et al., 2017). The first considers the overall activity of intermingled MUPs in which an interference pattern with turn and amplitude is analysed (Bianchi et al., 2017). The second is the analysis of individual MUP waveforms including the amplitude, the duration and the number of phases (or times the signal crosses the baseline). These parameters are calculated using one of the three MUP analysis techniques described (multi-MUP, manual-MUP, single-MUP) (Bianchi et al., 2017; Podnar et al., 2002b). The values obtained from both approaches—the interference pattern and the individual MUP—are compared to the standardized normative data, using both mean (± standard deviation) and outlier limits criteria to diagnose neuropathic/myopathic signs (Bianchi et al., 2017; Podnar and Vodušek, 2001; Podnar et al., 2002b). In a recent systematic review by Bianchi et al. (2017), analysis of individual MUPs was stated as the most recommended approach (level B evidence), given its highest sensitivity and specificity, to detect denervation/reinnervation and neuropathic changes relative to diverse conditions (e.g., medullar lesion, multiple system atrophy, Parkinson's, progressive supranuclear palsy). Specific diagnosis criteria are beyond the scope of this chapter.

KINESIOLOGICAL SURFACE ELECTROMYOGRAPHY

As opposed to needle EMG employed for neurophysiological diagnosis purposes, kinesiological sEMG aims to characterize the muscle behaviour at rest and during voluntary contraction, reflex activation or functional activities (Frawley et al., 2021). Different types of surface electrodes have been used, such as electrodes positioned on an intra-vaginal probe to capture the PFMs globally or specific/selected portions depending on the configuration (Aljuraifani et al., 2019a; Voorham-van der Zalm et al., 2013), electrodes integrated into an intra-anal probe to examine the external anal sphincter and the posterior portion/aspect of the PFMs (Peng et al., 2016), external electrodes stuck to the perineum to evaluate the superficial layer of the PFMs (Gentilcore-Saulnier et al., 2010), as well as electrodes mounted on a catheter that can adhere by suction on the urethral wall to assess the urethral sphincter (Stafford et al., 2010; Stafford et al., 2012; Stafford et al., 2015) or on the vaginal wall to assess the levator ani muscle (Keshwani and McLean, 2013; Morin et al., 2020). The most common configuration that has been used so far is the conventional electrode pairs (Auchincloss and McLean, 2009; Aukee et al., 2002; Engman et al., 2004; Grape et al., 2009; Keshwani and McLean, 2013; Loving et al., 2014; Romanzi et al., 1999; Thompson et al., 2006; Thorp et al., 1996), but other sophisticated arrangements have been used with multi-electrodes (Besomi et al., 2019). More specifically, linear array or matrix surface electrodes (also known as electrode arrays or grids, multichannel sEMG, high-density sEMG) equally spaced along the circumference of an intra-anal probe have been used to assess the external anal sphincter (Enck et al., 2004; Peng et al., 2016). The organization of these electrodes reached a high level of selectivity enabling the investigation of an action potential travelling along muscle fibre and identification of the innervation zone (Enck et al., 2004; Peng et al., 2016). Likewise, a similar multi-electrode configuration using the Multiple Array Probe Leiden (MAPLe) allowed the intra-anal/intra-vaginal assessment of different depths and locations to record the activity arising from different PFMs (i.e., pubococcygeus, puborectalis, external anal sphincter) (Voorham-van der Zalm et al., 2013).

sEMG can be used for different types of evaluation including the estimation of the level of muscle activation, assessment of timing and pattern of activation, measurement of frequency content, and evaluation of evoked activation (Besomi et al., 2019; McLean and Brooks, 2017).

Estimation of the Level of Muscle Activation

The estimation of the level of muscle activation is the most common applications of sEMG recordings. It is

estimated by measuring the amplitude of the sEMG signal, which refers to the number of microvolts a muscle generates (Bø et al., 2017; Frawley et al., 2021). The sEMG system can provide a measure of the actual amount of sEMG activity in microvolts or an average microvolt value (i.e., average rectified value or root mean square) (Clancy et al., 2016). sEMG can be used to reflect the activity of the muscle at rest (also known as baseline or tonic activity) (Enck and Vodušek, 2006; Frawley et al., 2021; Podnar et al., 2002a). Unlike most skeletal muscles that are normally electrically silent at rest (Basmajian, 1957; Clemmesen, 1951), the PFMs were shown to have a level of constant EMG activity to maintain urinary and anal continence and support of pelvic/abdominal contents. Such activity was recorded in many, but not all, sites of the levator ani (Deindl et al., 1993) and the deeper external anal sphincter muscle (Podnar et al., 2002a). The level of activation at rest was found to be influenced by bladder fullness (McLean et al., 2016), respiratory function (Aljuraifani et al., 2019b; Hodges et al., 2007) and posture (Hodges et al., 2007). It was also found to be modulated by sexual stimuli, such as the visualization of a sexually explicit video (Hannan-Leith et al., 2019). In addition to normal resting activity, a pathogenic increase in resting activity has also been described (Morin et al., 2017; Simons and Mense, 1998). sEMG offers the unique advantage of specifically assessing and discriminating the active electrogenic component of tone related to the neural drive, given that the passive component (i.e., the viscoelastic properties of the muscle tissues) is not captured by EMG (Thibault-Gagnon and Morin, 2015). This has contributed to enhancing our understanding of the pathophysiology of pelvic floor disorders related to increased tone (Morin et al., 2017; Thibault-Gagnon and Morin, 2015), but it has also been used for relaxation training as this pathological activity is amenable to voluntary control (Glazer et al., 1995; McKay et al., 2001). Furthermore, the assessment of the sEMG amplitude during PFM maximal voluntary contraction or contraction at different intensities is probably the most widely spread application of sEMG in pelvic floor disorders. It has been used for assessment purposes to reflect the contractile properties of the muscle (see the section on discriminant validity) and as a treatment tool or biofeedback to assist/guide PFM training (Kannan et al., 2018; Norton and Cody, 2012). Evaluation of the amplitude of sEMG was also shown to be relevant for the assessment of the involuntary response of the PFMs in functional activities such as incontinence provocative activities (Moser et al., 2018). For instance, increase in the sEMG amplitude of the urethral sphincter and the PFMs was observed in both women and men during coughing and during postural challenges, especially those related to rise in intra-abdominal pressure (Aljuraifani et al., 2019b; Hodges et al., 2007; Luginbuehl et al., 2016a; Smith et al., 2007; Stafford et al., 2012). Likewise, to ensure proper occlusion and support of the urethra during exertion, increase in the sEMG amplitude was also found during impact activities such as running (Leitner et al., 2017; Luginbuehl et al., 2016b; Moser et al., 2018). However, it should be highlighted that the assessment of sEMG during functional tasks has its load of technical considerations including crosstalk and artefacts (see the section on technical considerations and interpretation of sEMG).

Assessment of Timing and Pattern of Activation

The assessment of temporal events, which refers to the detection of the time at which specific events occur, is yet another advantage of sEMG (Besomi et al., 2019). More specifically, it encompasses the time to peak muscle activation of the PFMs, the time to return to baseline muscle activity and the reaction time (i.e., latency between a stimulus/command and activation onset) (Frawley et al., 2021). The timing of PFM activity can also be quantified by assessing the onset of the PFMs relative to other muscles, provocative activities or other aspects of a task (Frawley et al., 2021). The PFMs were shown to prepare and preactivate prior to a rise of intra-abdominal pressure (i.e., coughing) and postural challenges (e.g., arm movement, stepping) in both men and women, which could be relevant for continence (Aljuraifani et al., 2019a; Smith et al., 2007; Stafford et al., 2012; Stafford et al., 2014). In addition to the assessment of timing, incorrect patterns of activation such as dyssynergia can also be evaluated using sEMG. Paradoxical PFM or sphincter contraction when relaxation is functionally required, such as in miction and defaecation, is part of the diagnosis criteria for PFM dyssynergia (Frawley et al., 2021).

Measurement of Frequency Content

Analysis of the sEMG signal frequency content (also known as the power spectrum) is useful to assess the myoelectrical manifestation of fatigue (Besomi et al., 2019; Frawley et al., 2021). It consists in extracting information about the power spectrum of the sEMG (i.e., mean and median frequency using a Fourier or autoregressive approach) during sustained or repeated intermittent contractions (Clancy et al., 2016). When muscle fatigues, the median frequency shifts to lower frequencies due to altered muscle fibre recruitment and other changes in the contractile properties (Frawley et al., 2021). Although this application has been widely used in skeletal muscle (Mohseni Bandpei et al., 2014), it is still rarely found in investigations of the PFMs. Only a few studies evaluating PFM fatigue during running (Koenig et al., 2020) and the involvement in vulvodynia (Glazer et al., 1998) have been published.

Evaluation of Evoked Activation

An emergent application of sEMG is the assessment of evoked potential recordings to gain insight in neural control of the PFMs (Enck and Vodušek, 2006). A magnetic stimulation can be applied to the motor cortex involved in the control of the PFMs and the resultant activity of the PFMs is recorded (Yani et al., 2018). Using this setting in combination with functional magnetic resonance imaging, cortical areas responsible for motor control of the PFMs have been investigated (Asavasopon et al., 2014). The synergy between the PFMs and the gluteal muscle was also demonstrated (Asavasopon et al., 2014). Furthermore, high and low frequencies of repetitive transcranial magnetic stimulation were suggested to have an excitatory and inhibitory effect, respectively, on PFM tonic activity (Yani et al., 2019).

TECHNICAL CONSIDERATIONS AND INTERPRETATION OF SURFACE ELECTROMYOGRAPHY

It should be stressed that not all EMG recordings are the same. The characteristics and technical considerations of the recordings setup and analysis procedures directly influence the quality of the EMG recordings and clinometric properties of the measurements. EMG has a good logical (face) validity as it measures electrical activity arising from the skeletal muscle (Besomi et al., 2019). However, technical expertise with a thorough understanding of the principles underlying EMG measurements is required to interpret EMG signals. Several guidelines have been published to assist in proper interpretation of the signals and selection of optimal parameters (Besomi et al., 2019; Besomi et al., 2020; Enoka and Duchateau, 2015; Vigotsky et al., 2018). Key factors in sEMG measurements including the complex anatomy of the PFMs, cross-talk, artefact/noise and confounding factors will be presented followed by technical specifications influencing the signal such as the characteristics of the electrode and signal acquisition and processing.

Key Factors in Surface Electromyography Measurements

The complex anatomy of the PFMs, with various origins/insertions, different layers and fibre orientations, is a main challenge in sEMG recording. sEMG electrodes should be located along the fibres to capture the action potential travelling from one electrode to the other (Besomi et al., 2019). The electrodes should be located away from the innervation zone, the end-fibre region and tendinous/connective tissues (e.g., perineal body) (Besomi et al., 2019). Consequently, most of the commercially available probes offer a suboptimal design with wrong orientation of the electrodes (Keshwani and McLean, 2015). A reason for this is that the probes are most frequently designed for both delivering electrical stimulation and recording sEMG as a biofeedback tool. This adds to the complexity of interindividual variations and changes in fibre orientation during contraction (Besomi et al., 2019).

Also to be considered is *cross-talk*, which corresponds to muscle activity from nearby muscles such as the hip rotators and/or deep abdominal muscles that can contaminate the recorded sEMG signal. Cross-talk can lead to misinterpretation of PFM sEMG activity (Bø et al., 2017). Obtaining a signal completely exempt of unwanted signals from muscles lying in the vicinity of the muscle of interest is not a simple task (Farina et al., 2016). Non-selective recordings carry the risk of cross-talk, whereas selective recordings may fail to detect activity in all parts of the source muscle (Farina et al., 2016). The risk of cross-talk is increased especially when evaluating the PFMs during concomitant contraction of the abdominal and hip muscles (Keshwani and McLean, 2013, 2015). The magnitude of cross-talk within a detected sEMG signal can be quantified using different techniques such as cross-correlation coefficients (Disselhorst-Klug et al., 2009; Farina et al., 2016). However, as highlighted by Flury et al. (2017) in a scoping review with a systematic search, the assessment

of cross-talk in PFM assessment has been rarely studied. Concern was also expressed that because the PFMs have synergic activation with neighbouring muscle like the transverse abdominis and gluteal muscles (Asavasopon et al., 2014; Bø and Stien, 1994; Sapsford et al., 2001), it is quite challenging to discriminate synergy from cross-talk (Flury et al., 2017).

Artefact is another aspect to take into consideration and is defined as extraneous information in the sEMG signal from sources other than the target muscle, such as the environment (e.g., electromagnetic radiation) or other body functions (Frawley et al., 2021). Artefact examples include movement or contact quality artefact, heart rate, skin electrode shear and electrode bridging (Frawley et al., 2021). Artefacts are likely to occur when assessing PFM sEMG during movements such as jumping and running (Keshwani and McLean, 2013, 2015). The recording of resting activity is particularly susceptible to artefact or contamination by ambient noise. A low proportion of noise in the signal (or higher signal-to-noise ratio) is required to ensure validity of the measurement (Frawley et al., 2021).

A plethora of *confounding factors* can influence the sEMG signal. For instance, in EMG guidelines non-specific to PFM assessment the importance of skin preparation is emphasized, as it is suggested to be a major source of noise (Besomi et al., 2019; Hermens et al., 2000). Hence to ensure an optimal skin–electrode interface, the skin should be hairless, cleaned using abrading paste and dried, and the electrodes should be securely adhered to the skin surface using adhesive (Besomi et al., 2019). This is not achievable with intra-cavity probes. Moreover, several individual/patient characteristics are also known to influence the sEMG recordings, including the temperature, the humidity/lubrication, the cutaneous/mucosal tissue thickness, the amount of fat tissue and the positioning/direction of electrodes with respect to the muscle fibres (Clancy et al., 2016; Enoka and Duchateau, 2015; Vigotsky et al., 2018). The technical considerations presented in the following section are also part of the confounding factors influencing the signal. These factors preclude comparison between individuals of raw amplitude and the establishment of normative or cut-off values. Normalization of the sEMG amplitude is therefore considered critical when comparing data across individuals (Besomi et al., 2020; Disselhorst-Klug et al., 2009). It makes it possible to control for the confounding variables that would influence the amplitude of the sEMG signal and thus alter the nature of its relationship to muscle activation (Besomi et al., 2020). Concretely, the normalized sEMG amplitude value provides information about the degree of muscle activation present in a specific task context, expressed relative to a reference value used for normalization (Besomi et al., 2020). Various methods have been described in a consensus document about skeletal muscle assessment (Besomi et al., 2020). Among these, the normalization relative to a voluntary contraction was studied for assessing PFMs and was found reliable (Pereira-Baldon et al., 2020).

Technical Considerations

The International Continence Society in agreement with the International Society of Electrophysiology and Kinesiology (Merletti, 2017) formulated recommendations for reporting technical considerations for EMG assessment (see the work of Frawley et al. [2021] for more details). Key elements are presented next.

The relevance of the *electrode characteristics* has been investigated in a recent systematic review of the electrodes commercially available for assessing PFMs (Keshwani and McLean, 2015):

- *Different shapes or geometries of intra-vaginal probes* were found, including cylindrical, dumbbell and pear shapes. As opposed to cylindrical probes, it was proposed that enlarged probes at the level of the PFMs and tapered at the introitus may limit movement of the probe relative to the vaginal wall and hence reduced motion artefacts (Keshwani and McLean, 2015). The main disadvantage of these enlarged probes is that they may be uncomfortable upon insertion and distort the anatomy. Although sparsely studied, the shape of the probe should be taken into account in regard to its positioning relative to the PFMs. A cylindrical electrode with ring electrodes and a pear-shaped probe were shown located 3 cm and 6 cm cranial to the musculature, respectively, whereas a cylindrical multi-electrode probe was correctly aligned with the PFMs given the multitude of recording surfaces (Voorham-van der Zalm et al., 2006; Voorham-van der Zalm et al., 2013).
- A wide variety of *electrode recording surfaces (size and spacing)* mounted on an intra-vaginal probe is reported in the literature (Keshwani and McLean, 2015). Larger, widely spaced electrodes capture the signal from a larger pool of motor units (Besomi et al., 2019; Keshwani and McLean, 2015). This enhances the representativity of the activity originating from the whole muscle and may increase the measurement reliability as a similar pool of active motor units is more consistently assessed between trials (Auchincloss and McLean, 2009; Keshwani and McLean, 2015). However, the disadvantage is that they are more prone to cross-talk contamination (Auchincloss and McLean, 2009; Keshwani and McLean, 2015). In contrast, smaller closer electrodes have a reduced likelihood of cross-talk but pick up fewer MUPs and are therefore less generalizable to the entire muscle (Farina et al., 2016). They are also more susceptible to baseline noise (Huigen et al., 2002). With small interelectrode distances, attention should be paid to the application of gel to avoid the creation of conductive bridges between electrodes (Besomi et al., 2019).

- Different *arrangements of electrodes* are also available on the market. Suboptimal designs have circumferential electrodes (i.e., ring electrodes) and electrodes recording differential amplification on one side relative to the other. Probes with electrodes aligned with the muscle fibre direction should be privileged. These include intra-vaginal probes with pairs of electrodes positioned on each side that can assess the right and left separately (Aljuraifani et al., 2019a; Keshwani and McLean, 2015). In addition to complying with the principle of recording action potential travelling along the muscle fibres, it enables the assessment of asymmetry. Regarding surface-adhesive electrodes placed externally on the perineum, although part of routine anorectal and urodynamic examination (Rosier et al., 2017; Sultan et al., 2017), they have been criticized for their lack of specificity since they are far from the musculature of interest.

- Regarding the *electrode configuration* to assess PFMs, a differential amplification, in which the amplifier suppresses the common noise signals to both electrodes relative to a ground reference and then amplifies the difference, is generally preferable as it is less prone to noise and cross-talk (Besomi et al., 2019). However, high-quality monopolar electrodes (i.e., common noise detected by a single electrode and the ground is subtracted) can offer a good performance (Voorham-van der Zalm et al., 2013).

sEMG signal acquisition and processing have a significant impact on the data collected, including the signal amplitude, timing and spectral content. Commercially available EMG biofeedback units usually incorporate unadjustable, and often unknown, presets pertaining to signal acquisition and processing/conditioning.

When using a customable EMG device, the inspection of raw and unprocessed sEMG signals is the first recommended step to high-quality acquisition because the source of error/noise can be more easily identified (Merletti, 2017). The signal can then be filtered, smoothed and averaged using various processing techniques. These techniques require advanced knowledge and understanding for optimizing sEMG data (see the work of Merletti et al. [2016] for more information). However, they are beyond the scope of this chapter.

RELIABILITY OF SURFACE ELECTROMYOGRAPHY

As presented in the previous section, the reliability of sEMG depends strongly on the quality and characteristics of the sEMG setting/system used. Using various types of intra-vaginal probes (e.g., FemiScan, Periform, Thought Technology sensor T6050, MAPLe, suction electrode) for assessing the signal amplitude during maximal voluntary contraction, intra-session reliability was generally shown to be excellent (according to the standards proposed by Portney and Watkins [2000] to interpret intra-class correlation coefficients [ICCs]) (Auchincloss and McLean, 2009; Grape et al., 2009; Keshwani and McLean, 2012; Koenig et al., 2017; Oleksy et al., 2021). This suggests that when the probe is not removed, changes in sEMG amplitude may reflect true improvement in PFM activation. When assessing between-session (or between-day) reliability, inconsistent results are observed with studies showing a poor reliability (high coefficients of variation observed) (Thorp et al., 1991) and, based on ICCs, a fair reliability (Auchincloss and McLean, 2009), good reliability (Auchincloss and McLean, 2009; Keshwani and McLean, 2012; Oleksy et al., 2021) and excellent reliability (Keshwani and McLean, 2012; Voorham-van der Zalm et al., 2013). The challenge consists in controlling, as much as possible, the factors that bias the measurements, including the probe positioning. Although some authors have raised concerns regarding the between-session reliability (Auchincloss and McLean, 2009; Thorp et al., 1991), the most recent and sophisticated systems, with the advances in knowledge and technology, appear to show better reliability (Keshwani and McLean, 2012; Voorham-van der Zalm et al., 2013). It should be highlighted that some authors assess reliability using correlation coefficients and t-tests (Aukee et al., 2002; Engman et al., 2004; Glazer et al., 1999;

Gunnarsson and Mattiasson, 1994; Loving et al., 2014; Romanzi et al., 1999), which are not recommended in isolation to assess reliability (Portney and Watkins, 2000). The reliability of baseline resting activity has been assessed in only a few studies. Similarly to maximal voluntary contraction, intra-session reliability was shown to be excellent (Grape et al., 2009; Koenig et al., 2017), whereas between-session reliability was lower, ranging from good to excellent (Grape et al., 2009; Oleksy et al., 2021; Voorham-van der Zalm et al., 2013). Regarding the assessment of muscle activation during running, only within-session reliability was assessed, and excellent ICCs were obtained (Luginbuehl et al., 2016b). Interestingly, the assessment of spectral content showed good to excellent between-session reliability (Oleksy et al., 2021). Furthermore, Enck et al. (2010) showed that a linear-array/high-density electrode was reliable for assessing the location of the innervation zone, which opens up new possibilities for preventing neuronal trauma during vaginal delivery.

CONCURRENT VALIDITY

It is important to reaffirm that the amplitude of the signal cannot be interpreted as a direct force measurement (Clancy et al., 2016; Enoka and Duchateau, 2015; Vigotsky et al., 2018). As studied in the field of musculoskeletal sEMG assessment, the relation between sEMG amplitude and force output is patient- and muscle dependent and mainly non-linear (Clancy et al., 2016). Very few data are available regarding this relationship specifically for PFMs. For instance, Stafford et al. (2015) showed a strong significant but non-linear relationship between the striated linear sphincter activity and the displacement of pelvic structures measured concomitantly during contraction of the PFMs in men. In contrast, Morin et al. (2020) showed a strong linear relationship between the activity of the puborectalis measured with an intra-vaginal suction electrode and the stiffness evaluated simultaneously with shear wave elastography in women. Other studies have mainly looked into correlation coefficients between the sEMG amplitude during maximal voluntary contraction and other strength measures taken at different moments and obtained inconsistent results (Botelho et al., 2013; Júnior et al., 2014; Macêdo et al., 2018; Navarro-Brazález et al., 2018; Pereira et al., 2014; Yang et al., 2019). For instance, regarding the association with ultrasound, non-significant correlations were found with bulbocavernosus thickness

(Pereira et al., 2014), hiatus diameter and levator thickness (Júnior et al., 2014). Correlations with palpation (modified Oxford scale) ranged from weak (Navarro-Brazález et al., 2018) to good (Botelho et al., 2013; Pereira et al., 2014; Yang et al., 2019). Correlations with manometry were fair (Navarro-Brazález et al., 2018), good (Pereira et al., 2014) and excellent (Macêdo et al., 2018). Overall, it is difficult to judge whether these conflicting results are explained by the non-linear relationships between sEMG and other tools or by the different qualities in the sEMG measures.

RESPONSIVENESS

As recognized in a recent consensus statement, a technically good EMG recording is capable of detecting even small differences in sEMG related to increasing muscle activation (Besomi et al., 2019). The ability of sEMG measurement to detect changes after treatment has been investigated mainly for sEMG amplitude during maximal voluntary contraction. For instance, several prospective studies (Dannecker et al., 2005; Liu et al., 2018; Marques et al., 2013; Rett et al., 2007; Segal et al., 2016; Stüpp et al., 2011) and randomized clinical trials (Alves et al., 2015; Aukee et al., 2002; Bertotto et al., 2017) have shown a significant increase in signal amplitude following PFM training in women with prolapse and urinary incontinence. Similarly, a significant increase in sEMG amplitude during maximal voluntary contraction was found in prospective studies in women with an overactive bladder (Segal et al., 2016) and with anal incontinence (Segal et al., 2018). Very few studies found non-significant changes (Batista et al., 2011; Nyhus et al., 2020), which could be explained by their low dose of treatment. It should, however, be emphasized that EMG does not capture all strength gains relative to strength training (Rainoldi et al., 2016). Early gains, mainly related to an increase in motor unit recruitment and optimization of frequency of discharge, result in a higher signal amplitude (Rainoldi et al., 2016). However, strength gains related to hypertrophy, generally occurring at a later stage of training, are not reflected or captured in increased sEMG amplitude (Rainoldi et al., 2016). Regarding the responsiveness of sEMG to detect changes in resting sEMG, conflicting results are found in the literature. Some prospective studies found significant reduction in resting sEMG after PFM exercise with biofeedback and manual therapy (Chmielewska et al., 2016; Glazer et al., 1995; Jantos, 2008; Weiss, 2001), whereas others found non-significant changes (Gentilcore-Saulnier et al., 2010; McKay et al., 2001). Given that the assessment of resting sEMG is highly influenced by confounding factors and is subject to noise, it is not clear if these inconsistencies are due to variability in treatment effectiveness or lack of responsiveness of sEMG.

KNOWN-GROUP/DISCRIMINANT VALIDITY

When applied and interpreted properly, sEMG may provide useful insight for characterizing PFM differences between women with or without pelvic floor disorders. Inconsistencies are found, however, in the current literature when comparing groups, which can be explained by the multiple factors affecting the sEMG signal and interfering with between-group comparisons (see the section on technical considerations and interpretation of sEMG) (Besomi et al., 2020). In a recent systematic review and meta-analysis conducted by Falah-Hassani et al. (2021), 16 studies were found comparing sEMG amplitude in women with and without incontinence. They reported conflicting results for amplitude at rest, during maximal voluntary contraction and during functional activities (e.g., running). They explained that the interpretation of findings from the included studies was limited, as none presented convincing data to rule out cross-talk or artefacts, and most did not report normalized sEMG amplitudes. One study suggested a difference in activation timing between women with and without stress incontinence (Smith et al., 2007); it showed a delayed activation of the PFMs in a postural challenge, which provides insight into the potential role of motor control in incontinence.

As discussed in Chapter 9.2, in some studies, the multiple factors affecting the sEMG amplitude at rest may also have interfered with the capacity of sEMG to detect a difference between women with and without chronic pelvic pain. Most studies found higher resting activity in women and men with chronic pelvic pain (Engman et al., 2004; Frasson et al., 2009; Gammoudi et al., 2016; Glazer et al., 1998; Hetrick et al., 2006; Loving et al., 2014; Morin et al., 2017; Polpeta et al., 2012; Shafik and El-Sibai, 2002), whereas no differences between groups were found in three studies (Naess and Bo, 2015; Reissing et al., 2004; van der Velde and Everaerd, 1999). When accounting for factor bias affecting the sEMG signal by using normalization or ratio values, women with pain showed higher activation of the PFMs during dynamic stretching (Morin et al., 2017) and higher response of the superficial PFMs related to vulvar pain stimuli (Gentilcore-Saulnier et al., 2010) in comparison to asymptomatic controls. Furthermore, for the same reasons, findings regarding reduced contractility of the PFMs have been mixed when evaluating women with chronic pelvic pain. Some studies found lower sEMG amplitude during maximal voluntary contraction (Glazer et al., 1998; Reissing et al., 2004), whereas others reported non-significant differences (Engman et al., 2004; Naess and Bo, 2015; Polpeta et al., 2012; Tu et al., 2008). However, endurance was found to be lower in several studies when assessing mean sEMG amplitude during 40- to 60-second contractions (Engman et al., 2004; Naess and Bo, 2015; Polpeta et al., 2012; Reissing et al., 2004). Interestingly, this is in line with the study of Glazer et al. (1998) reporting differences in the power spectrum between women with and without vulvodynia. Overall, further research, using high-quality sEMG and proper interpretation of the signals, is required to further advance our understanding of the sEMG clinometric properties and to elucidate the inconsistencies in the literature regarding pelvic floor disorder pathophysiology.

CLINICAL RECOMMENDATIONS

Like all assessment tools, sEMG presents advantages and limitations for evaluating the PFMs (Frawley et al., 2021):

- It provides a valuable and objective measure of muscle activation during PFM contraction.
- It is the only tool that can directly assess the active/neurogenic component of tone.
- It allows evaluation of specific and precise features related to timing and fatigue.
- The comparison of raw sEMG between individuals is challenging because of confounding factors affecting the signal. A normalization process is required.
- Interpretation of sEMG should rely on an in-depth understanding of the signal generation process, and technical skills are needed. Caution is required when assessing sEMG during concomitant hip/abdominal contractions or during movements (e.g., jumping, running), as confounding factors such as cross-talk and artefacts should be taken into account.
- sEMG measurements are not all equivalent. The clinometric properties of sEMG, including the validity of the measures, are dependent on the quality of the signals. Advances in technology and improvement in the quality of measurements are seen in recent studies, which will likely provide new insight into pelvic floor function.

REFERENCES

Aljuraifani, R., Stafford, R. E., Hall, L. M., et al. (2019a). Activity of deep and superficial pelvic floor muscles in women in response to different verbal instructions: A preliminary investigation using a novel electromyography electrode. *The Journal of Sexual Medicine, 16*, 673–679.

Aljuraifani, R., Stafford, R. E., Hall, L. M., et al. (2019b). Task-specific differences in respiration-related activation of deep and superficial pelvic floor muscles. *Journal of Applied Physiology, 126*, 1343–1351.

Alves, F. K., Riccetto, C., Adami, D. B., et al. (2015). A pelvic floor muscle training program in postmenopausal women: A randomized controlled trial. *Maturitas, 81*, 300–305.

Asavasopon, S., Rana, M., Kirages, D. J., et al. (2014). Cortical activation associated with muscle synergies of the human male pelvic floor. *Journal of Neuroscience, 34*, 13811–13818.

Auchincloss, C. C., & McLean, L. (2009). The reliability of surface EMG recorded from the pelvic floor muscles. *Journal of Neuroscience Methods, 182*, 85–96.

Aukee, P., Immonen, P., Penttinen, J., et al. (2002). Increase in pelvic floor muscle activity after 12 weeks' training: A randomized prospective pilot study. *Urology, 60*, 1020–1023; discussion 1023–1024.

Basmajian, J. V. (1957). New views on muscular tone and relaxation. *Canadian Medical Association, 77*, 203–205.

Batista, R. L., Franco, M. M., Naldoni, L. M., et al. (2011). Biofeedback and the electromyographic activity of pelvic floor muscles in pregnant women. *Revista Brasileira de Fisioterapia, 15*, 386–392.

Bertotto, A., Schvartzman, R., Uchôa, S., et al. (2017). Effect of electromyographic biofeedback as an add-on to pelvic floor muscle exercises on neuromuscular outcomes and quality of life in postmenopausal women with stress urinary incontinence: A randomized controlled trial. *Neurourology and Urodynamics, 36*, 2142–2147.

Besomi, M., Hodges, P. W., Clancy, E. A., et al. (2020). Consensus for Experimental Design in Electromyography (CEDE) project: Amplitude normalization matrix. *Journal of Electromyography and Kinesiology, 53*, 102438.

Besomi, M., Hodges, P. W., Van Dieën, J., et al. (2019). Consensus for Experimental Design in Electromyography (CEDE) project: Electrode selection matrix. *Journal of Electromyography and Kinesiology, 48*, 128–144.

Bianchi, F., Squintani, G. M., Osio, M., et al. (2017). Neurophysiology of the pelvic floor in clinical practice: A systematic literature review. *Functional Neurology, 32*, 173–193.

Bø, K., Frawley, H. C., Haylen, B. T., et al. (2017). An International Urogynecological Association (IUGA)/International Continence Society (ICS) joint report on the terminology for the conservative and nonpharmacological management of female pelvic floor dysfunction. *Neurourology and Urodynamics, 36*, 221–244.

Bø, K., & Stien, R. (1994). Needle EMG registration of striated urethral wall and pelvic floor muscle activity patterns during cough, Valsalva, abdominal, hip adductor, and gluteal muscle contractions in nulliparous healthy females. *Neurourology and Urodynamics, 13*, 35–41.

Botelho, S., Pereira, L. C., Marques, J., et al. (2013). Is there correlation between electromyography and digital palpation as means of measuring pelvic floor muscle contractility in nulliparous, pregnant, and postpartum women? *Neurourology and Urodynamics, 32*, 420–423.

Chmielewska, D., Stania, M., Smykla, A., et al. (2016). Bioelectrical activity of the pelvic floor muscles after 6-week biofeedback training in nulliparous continent women. *Acta of Bioengineering and Biomechanics, 18*, 105–113.

Clancy, E. A., Negro, F., & Farina, D. (2016). Single-channel techniques for information extraction from the surface EMG signal. In R. Merletti, & D. Farina (Eds.), *Surface electromyography: Physiology, engineering and applications* (pp. 91–125). Hoboken, NJ: John Wiley & Sons.

Clemmesen, S. (1951). Some studies on muscle tone. *Proceedings of the Royal Society of Medicine, 44*, 637–646.

Dannecker, C., Wolf, V., Raab, R., et al. (2005). EMG-Biofeedback assisted pelvic floor muscle training is an effective therapy of stress urinary or mixed incontinence: A 7-year experience with 390 patients. *Archives of Gynecology and Obstetrics, 273*, 93–97.

Deindl, F. M., Vodušek, D. B., Hesse, U., et al. (1993). Activity patterns of pubococcygeal muscles in nulliparous continent women. *British Journal of Urology, 72*, 46–51.

Disselhorst-Klug, C., Schmitz-Rode, T., & Rau, G. (2009). Surface electromyography and muscle force: Limits in sEMG-force relationship and new approaches for applications. *Clinical biomechanics, 24*, 225–235.

Enck, P., Franz, H., Azpiroz, F., et al. (2004). Innervation zones of the external anal sphincter in healthy male and female subjects. Preliminary results. *Digestion, 69*, 123–130.

Enck, P., Franz, H., Davico, E., et al. (2010). Repeatability of innervation zone identification in the external anal sphincter muscle. *Neurourology and Urodynamics, 29*, 449–457.

Enck, P., & Vodušek, D. B. (2006). Electromyography of pelvic floor muscles. *Journal of Electromyography and Kinesiology, 16*, 568–577.

Engman, M., Lindehammar, H., & Wijma, B. (2004). Surface electromyography diagnostics in women with partial vaginismus with or without vulvar vestibulitis and in asymptomatic women. *Journal of Psychosomatic Obstetrics and Gynaecology, 25*, 281–294.

Enoka, R. M., & Duchateau, J. (2015). Inappropriate interpretation of surface EMG signals and muscle fiber characteristics impedes understanding of the control of neuromuscular function. *Journal of Applied Physiology, 119*, 1516–1518.

Enoka, R. M., & Duchateau, J. (2016). Physiology of muscle activation and force generation. In R. Merletti, & D. Farina (Eds.), *Surface electromyography: Physiology, engineering and applications* (pp. 1–29). Hoboken, NJ: John Wiley & Sons.

Falah-Hassani, K., Reeves, J., Shiri, R., et al. (2021). The pathophysiology of stress urinary incontinence: A systematic review and meta-analysis. *International Urogynecology Journal, 32*, 501–552.

Farina, D., Stegeman, D. F., & Merletti, R. (2016). Biophysics of the generation of EMG signals. In R. Merletti, & D. Farina (Eds.), *Surface electromyography: Physiology, engineering and applications* (pp. 30–53). Hoboken, NJ: John Wiley & Sons.

Flury, N., Koenig, I., & Radlinger, L. (2017). Crosstalk considerations in studies evaluating pelvic floor muscles using surface electromyography in women: A scoping review. *Archives of Gynecology and Obstetrics, 295*, 799–809.

Frasson, E., Graziottin, A., Priori, A., et al. (2009). Central nervous system abnormalities in vaginismus. *Clinical Neurophysiology, 120*, 117–122.

Frawley, H., Shelly, B., Morin, M., et al. (2021). An International Continence Society (ICS) report on the terminology for pelvic floor muscle assessment. *Neurourology and Urodynamics, 40*(5), 1217–1260.

Gammoudi, N., Affes, Z., Mellouli, S., et al. (2016). The diagnosis value of needle electrode electromyography in vaginismus. *Sexologies, 25*, E57–E60.

Gentilcore-Saulnier, E., McLean, L., Goldfinger, C., et al. (2010). Pelvic floor muscle assessment outcomes in women with and without provoked vestibulodynia and the impact of a physical therapy program. *The Journal of Sexual Medicine, 7*, 1003–1022.

Glazer, H. I., Jantos, M., Hartmann, E. H., et al. (1998). Electromyographic comparisons of the pelvic floor in women with dysesthetic vulvodynia and asymptomatic women. *Journal of Reproductive Medicine, 43*, 959–962.

Glazer, H. I., Rodke, G., Swencionis, C., et al. (1995). Treatment of vulvar vestibulitis syndrome with electromyographic biofeedback of pelvic floor musculature. *Journal of Reproductive Medicine, 40*, 283–290.

Glazer, H. I., Romanzi, L., & Polaneczky, M. (1999). Pelvic floor muscle surface electromyography. Reliability and clinical predictive validity. *Journal of Reproductive Medicine, 44*, 779–782.

Grape, H. H., Dedering, A., & Jonasson, A. F. (2009). Retest reliability of surface electromyography on the pelvic floor muscles. *Neurourology and Urodynamics, 28*, 395–399.

Gunnarsson, M., & Mattiasson, A. (1994). Circumvaginal surface electromyography in women with urinary incontinence and in healthy volunteers. *Scandinavian Journal of Urology and Nephrology, 157*, 89–95.

Hannan-Leith, M. N., Dayan, M., Hatfield, G., et al. (2019). Is pelvic floor sEMG a measure of women's sexual response? *The Journal of Sexual Medicine, 16,* 70–82.

Hermens, H. J., Freriks, B., Disselhorst-Klug, C., et al. (2000). Development of recommendations for SEMG sensors and sensor placement procedures. *Journal of Electromyography and Kinesiology, 10,* 361–374.

Hetrick, D. C., Glazer, H., Liu, Y.-W., et al. (2006). Pelvic floor electromyography in men with chronic pelvic pain syndrome: A case–control study. *Neurourology and Urodynamics, 25,* 46–49.

Hodges, P. W., Sapsford, R., & Pengel, L. H. (2007). Postural and respiratory functions of the pelvic floor muscles. *Neurourology and Urodynamics, 26,* 362–371.

Huigen, E., Peper, A., & Grimbergen, C. A. (2002). Investigation into the origin of the noise of surface electrodes. *Medical, & Biological Engineering & Computing, 40,* 332–338.

Jantos, M. (2008). Vulvodynia: A psychophysiological profile based on electromyographic assessment. *Applied Psychophysiology and Biofeedback, 33,* 29–38.

Júnior, E. A., Jármy-Di Bella, Z. I., Diniz Zanetti, M. R., et al. (2014). Assessment of pelvic floor of women runners by three-dimensional ultrasonography and surface electromyography. A pilot study. *Medical ultrasound, 16,* 21–26.

Kannan, P., Winser, S. J., Fung, B., et al. (2018). Effectiveness of pelvic floor muscle training alone and in combination with biofeedback, electrical stimulation, or both compared to control for urinary incontinence in men following prostatectomy: Systematic review and meta-analysis. *Physical Therapy, 98,* 932–945.

Keshwani, N., & McLean, L. (2012). Development of a differential suction electrode for improved intravaginal recordings of pelvic floor muscle activity: Reliability and motion artifact assessment. *Neurourology and Urodynamics, 31,* 1272–1278.

Keshwani, N., & McLean, L. (2013). A differential suction electrode for recording electromyographic activity from the pelvic floor muscles: Crosstalk evaluation. *Journal of Electromyography and Kinesiology, 23,* 311–318.

Keshwani, N., & McLean, L. (2015). State of the art review: Intravaginal probes for recording electromyography from the pelvic floor muscles. *Neurourology and Urodynamics, 34,* 104–112.

Koenig, I., Eichelberger, P., Leitner, M., et al. (2020). Pelvic floor muscle activity patterns in women with and without stress urinary incontinence while running. *Annals of Physical and Rehabilitation Medicine, 63,* 495–499.

Koenig, I., Luginbuehl, H., & Radlinger, L. (2017). Reliability of pelvic floor muscle electromyography tested on healthy women and women with pelvic floor muscle dysfunction. *Annals of Physical and Rehabilitation Medicine, 60,* 382–386.

Kukulka, C. G., & Clamann, H. P. (1981). Comparison of the recruitment and discharge properties of motor units in human brachial biceps and adductor pollicis during isometric contractions. *Brain Research, 219,* 45–55.

Leitner, M., Moser, H., Eichelberger, P., et al. (2017). Evaluation of pelvic floor muscle activity during running in continent and incontinent women: An exploratory study. *Neurourology and Urodynamics, 36,* 1570–1576.

Liu, Y. J., Wu, W. Y., Hsiao, S. M., et al. (2018). Efficacy of pelvic floor training with surface electromyography feedback for female stress urinary incontinence. *International Journal of Nursing Practice, 24,* e12698.

Loving, S., Thomsen, T., Jaszczak, P., et al. (2014). Pelvic floor muscle dysfunctions are prevalent in female chronic pelvic pain: A cross-sectional population-based study. *European Journal of Pain, 18,* 1259–1270.

Luginbuehl, H., Baeyens, J. P., Kuhn, A., et al. (2016a). Pelvic floor muscle reflex activity during coughing—an exploratory and reliability study. *Annals of Physical and Rehabilitation Medicine, 59,* 302–307.

Luginbuehl, H., Naeff, R., Zahnd, A., et al. (2016b). Pelvic floor muscle electromyography during different running speeds: An exploratory and reliability study. *Archives of Gynecology and Obstetrics, 293,* 117–124.

Macêdo, L. C., Lemos, A., Vasconcelos, D. A., et al. (2018). Correlation between electromyography and perineometry in evaluating pelvic floor muscle function in nulligravidas: A cross-sectional study. *Neurourology and Urodynamics, 37,* 1658–1666.

Marques, J., Botelho, S., Pereira, L. C., et al. (2013). Pelvic floor muscle training program increases muscular contractility during first pregnancy and postpartum: Electromyographic study. *Neurourology and Urodynamics, 32,* 998–1003.

McKay, E., Kaufman, R. H., Doctor, U., et al. (2001). Treating vulvar vestibulitis with electromyographic biofeedback of pelvic floor musculature. *Journal of Reproductive Medicine, 46,* 337–342.

McLean, L., & Brooks, K. (2017). What does electromyography tell us about dyspareunia? *Sexual Medicine Reviews, 5,* 282–294.

McLean, L., Normandeau, C., & Hodder, J. (2016). The impact of state of bladder fullness on tonic and phasic activation of the pelvic floor muscles in women. *Journal of Electromyography and Kinesiology, 27,* 60–65.

Merletti, R. (2017). Standards for reporting EMG data. *Journal of Electromyography and Kinesiology, 34,* I–II.

Merletti, R., Botter, A., & Barone, U. (2016). Detection and conditioning of surface EMG signals. In R. Merletti, & D. Farina (Eds.), *Surface electromyography: Physiology, engineering and applications* (pp. 54–90). Hoboken, NJ: John Wiley & Sons.

Mohseni Bandpei, M. A., Rahmani, N., Majdoleslam, B., et al. (2014). Reliability of surface electromyography in the assessment of paraspinal muscle fatigue: An updated systematic review. *Journal of Manipulative and Physiological Therapeutics*, 37, 510–521.

Morin, M., Binik, Y. M., Bourbonnais, D., et al. (2017). Heightened pelvic floor muscle tone and altered contractility in women with provoked vestibulodynia. *The Journal of Sexual Medicine*, 14, 592–600.

Morin, M., Salomoni, S. E., Stafford, R. E., et al. (2022). Validation of shear wave elastography as a noninvasive measure of pelvic floor muscle stiffness. *Neurology and Urodynamics*, 41, 1620–1628.

Moser, H., Leitner, M., Baeyens, J. P., et al. (2018). Pelvic floor muscle activity during impact activities in continent and incontinent women: A systematic review. *International Urogynecology Journal*, 29, 179–196.

Naess, I., & Bø, K. (2015). Pelvic floor muscle function in women with provoked vestibulodynia and asymptomatic controls. *International Urogynecology Journal*, 26, 1467–1473.

Navarro-Brazález, B., Torres Lacomba, M., de la Villa, P., et al. (2018). The evaluation of pelvic floor muscle strength in women with pelvic floor dysfunction: A reliability and correlation study. *Neurology and Urodynamics*, 37, 269–277.

Norton, C., & Cody, J. D. (2012). Biofeedback and/or sphincter exercises for the treatment of faecal incontinence in adults. *Cochrane Database of Systematic Reviews*, 7, CD002111.

Nyhus, M., Mathew, S., Salvesen, Ø., et al. (2020). Effect of preoperative pelvic floor muscle training on pelvic floor muscle contraction and symptomatic and anatomical pelvic organ prolapse after surgery: Randomized controlled trial. *Ultrasound in Obstetrics and Gynecology*, 56, 28–36.

Oleksy, Ł., Mika, A., Sulowska-Daszyk, I., et al. (2021). The reliability of pelvic floor muscle bioelectrical activity (sEMG) assessment using a multi-activity measurement protocol in young women. *International Journal of Environmental Research and Public Health*, 18(2), 765.

Olsen, A. L., & Rao, S. S. (2001). Clinical neurophysiology and electrodiagnostic testing of the pelvic floor. *Gastroenterology Clinics of North America*, 30, 33–54, v–vi.

Peng, Y., He, J., Khavari, R., et al. (2016). Functional mapping of the pelvic floor and sphincter muscles from high-density surface EMG recordings. *International Urogynecology Journal*, 27, 1689–1696.

Pereira-Baldon, V. S., de Oliveira, A. B., Padilha, J. F., et al. (2020). Reliability of different electromyographic normalization methods for pelvic floor muscles assessment. *Neurology and Urodynamics*, 39, 1145–1151.

Pereira, V. S., Hirakawa, H. S., Oliveira, A. B., et al. (2014). Relationship among vaginal palpation, vaginal squeeze pressure, electromyographic and ultrasonographic variables of female pelvic floor muscles. *Brazilian Journal of Physical Therapy*, 18, 428–434.

Podnar, S., Mrkaić, M., & Vodušek, D. B. (2002a). Standardization of anal sphincter electromyography: Quantification of continuous activity during relaxation. *Neurourology and Urodynamics*, 21, 540–545.

Podnar, S., & Vodušek, D. B. (2001). Protocol for clinical neurophysiologic examination of the pelvic floor. *Neurourology and Urodynamics*, 20, 669–682.

Podnar, S., Vodušek, D. B., & Stalberg, E. (2002b). Comparison of quantitative techniques in anal sphincter electromyography. *Muscle & Nerve*, 25, 83–92.

Polpeta, N. C., Giraldo, P. C., Juliato, C. R., et al. (2012). Electromyography and vaginal pressure of the pelvic floor muscles in women with recurrent vulvovaginal candidiasis and vulvodynia. *Journal of Reproductive Medicine*, 57, 141–147.

Portney, L. G., & Watkins, M. P. (2000). *Foundations of clinical research: Applications to practice*. Boston: Prentice Hall.

Rainoldi, A., Moritani, T., & Boccia, G. (2016). EMG in exercise physiology and sports. In R. Merletti, & D. Farina (Eds.), *EMG in exercise physiology and sports* (pp. 501–539). Hoboken, NJ: John Wiley & Sons.

Reissing, E. D., Binik, Y. M., Khalife, S., et al. (2004). Vaginal spasm, pain, and behavior: An empirical investigation of the diagnosis of vaginismus. *Archives of Sexual Behavior*, 33, 5–17.

Rett, M. T., Simoes, J. A., Herrmann, V., et al. (2007). Management of stress urinary incontinence with surface electromyography-assisted biofeedback in women of reproductive age. *Physical Therapy*, 87, 136–142.

Romanzi, L. J., Polaneczky, M., & Glazer, H. I. (1999). Simple test of pelvic muscle contraction during pelvic examination: Correlation to surface electromyography. *Neurourology and Urodynamics*, 18, 603–612.

Rosier, P., Schaefer, W., Lose, G., et al. (2017). International Continence Society good urodynamic practices and terms 2016: Urodynamics, uroflowmetry, cystometry, and pressure-flow study. *Neurourology and Urodynamics*, 36, 1243–1260.

Sapsford, R. R., Hodges, P. W., Richardson, C. A., et al. (2001). Co-activation of the abdominal and pelvic floor muscles during voluntary exercises. *Neurourology and Urodynamics*, 20, 31–42.

Segal, S., Morse, A., Sangal, P., et al. (2016). Efficacy of FemiScan pelvic floor therapy for the treatment of urinary incontinence. *Female Pelvic Medicine & Reconstructive Surgery*, 22, 433–437.

Segal, S., Morse, A., Sangal, P., et al. (2018). Efficacy of FemiScan pelvic floor therapy for the treatment of anal incontinence. *Female Pelvic Medicine & Reconstructive Surgery*, 24, 367–370.

Shafik, A., & El-Sibai, O. (2002). Study of the pelvic floor muscles in vaginismus: A concept of pathogenesis. *European Journal of Obstetrics & Gynecology and Reproductive Biology, 105,* 67–70.

Simons, D. G., & Mense, S. (1998). Understanding and measurement of muscle tone as related to clinical muscle pain. *Pain, 75,* 1–17.

Smith, M. D., Coppieters, M. W., & Hodges, P. W. (2007). Postural activity of the pelvic floor muscles is delayed during rapid arm movements in women with stress urinary incontinence. *International Urogynecology Journal and Pelvic Floor Dysfunction, 18,* 901–911.

Stafford, R. E., Ashton-Miller, J. A., Sapsford, R., et al. (2012). Activation of the striated urethral sphincter to maintain continence during dynamic tasks in healthy men. *Neurourology and Urodynamics, 31,* 36–43.

Stafford, R. E., Coughlin, G., Lutton, N. J., et al. (2015). Validity of estimation of pelvic floor muscle activity from transperineal ultrasound imaging in men. *PLoS One, 10*(12), e0144342.

Stafford, R. E., Mazzone, S., Ashton-Miller, J. A., et al. (2014). Dynamics of male pelvic floor muscle contraction observed with transperineal ultrasound imaging differ between voluntary and evoked coughs. *Journal of Applied Physiology, 116,* 953–960.

Stafford, R. E., Sapsford, R., Ashton-Miller, J., et al. (2010). A novel transurethral surface electrode to record male striated urethral sphincter electromyographic activity. *Journal of Urology, 183,* 378–385.

Stüpp, L., Resende, A. P., Oliveira, E., et al. (2011). Pelvic floor muscle training for treatment of pelvic organ prolapse: An assessor-blinded randomized controlled trial. *International Urogynecology Journal, 22,* 1233–1239.

Sultan, A. H., Monga, A., Lee, J., et al. (2017). An International Urogynecological Association (IUGA)/International Continence Society (ICS) joint report on the terminology for female anorectal dysfunction. *Neurourology and Urodynamics, 36,* 10–34.

Thibault-Gagnon, S., & Morin, M. (2015). Active and passive components of pelvic floor muscle tone in women with provoked vestibulodynia: A perspective based on a review of the literature. *The Journal of Sexual Medicine, 12,* 2178–2189.

Thompson, J. A., O'Sullivan, P. B., Briffa, N. K., et al. (2006). Assessment of voluntary pelvic floor muscle contraction in continent and incontinent women using transperineal ultrasound, manual muscle testing and vaginal squeeze pressure measurements. *International Urogynecology Journal and Pelvic Floor Dysfunction, 17,* 624–630.

Thorp, J. M., Jones, L. H., Wells, E., et al. (1996). Assessment of pelvic floor function: A series of simple tests in nulliparous women. *International Urogynecology Journal and Pelvic Floor Dysfunction, 7,* 94–97.

Thorp, J. M., Jr., Bowes, W. A., Jr., Droegemueller, W., et al. (1991). Assessment of perineal floor function: Electromyography with acrylic plug surface electrodes in nulliparous women. *Obstetrics & Gynecology, 78,* 89–92.

Tu, F. F., Holt, J., Gonzales, J., & Fitzgerald, C. M. (2008). Physical therapy evaluation of patients with chronic pelvic pain: A controlled study. *American Journal of Obstetrics and Gynecology, 198*(3), 272.e1–272.e7.

Van Bolhuis, B. M., Medendorp, W. P., & Gielen, C. C. (1997). Motor unit firing behavior in human arm flexor muscles during sinusoidal isometric contractions and movements. *Experimental Brain Research, 117,* 120–130.

Van der Velde, J., & Everaerd, W. (1999). Voluntary control over pelvic floor muscles in women with and without vaginistic reactions. *International Urogynecology Journal and Pelvic Floor Dysfunction, 10,* 230–236.

Vigotsky, A. D., Halperin, I., Lehman, G. J., et al. (2018). Interpreting signal amplitudes in surface electromyography studies in sport and rehabilitation sciences. *Frontiers in Physiology, 8,* 985.

Vodušek, D. B. (2015). Measurement of pelvic floor muscle function and strength, and pelvic organ prolapse. In K. Bø, B. Berghmans, S. Mørkved, et al. (Eds.), *Evidence-based physical therapy for the pelvic floor: Bridging science and clinical practice* (2nd ed.) (pp. 43–109). Edinburgh: Churchill Livingstone.

Voorham-van der Zalm, P. J., Pelger, R. C., van Heeswijk-Faase, I. C., et al. (2006). Placement of probes in electrostimulation and biofeedback training in pelvic floor dysfunction. *Acta Obstetricia et Gynecologica Scandinavica, 85,* 850–855.

Voorham-van der Zalm, P. J., Voorham, J. C., van den Bos, T. W., et al. (2013). Reliability and differentiation of pelvic floor muscle electromyography measurements in healthy volunteers using a new device: The Multiple Array Probe Leiden (MAPLe). *Neurourology and Urodynamics, 32,* 341–348.

Weiss, J. M. (2001). Pelvic floor myofascial trigger points: Manual therapy for interstitial cystitis and the urgency-freqslruency syndrome. *Journal of Urology, 166,* 2226–2231.

Yang, X., Zhu, L., Li, W., et al. (2019). Comparisons of electromyography and digital palpation measurement of pelvic floor muscle strength in postpartum women with stress urinary incontinence and asymptomatic parturients: A cross-sectional study. *Gynecologic and Obstetric Investigation, 84,* 599–605.

Yani, M. S., Fenske, S. J., Rodriguez, L. V., et al. (2019). Motor cortical neuromodulation of pelvic floor muscle tone: Potential implications for the treatment of urologic conditions. *Neurourology and Urodynamics, 38,* 1517–1523.

Yani, M. S., Wondolowski, J. H., Eckel, S. P., et al. (2018). Distributed representation of pelvic floor muscles in human motor cortex. *Scientific Reports, 8,* 7213.

5.6 Urethral Pressure Measurements

Mohammed Belal and Paul Abrams

Continence depends on the intramural and extramural forces that maintain urethral closure while the bladder is filling. Stress leakage may occur if the urethral resistance is overcome by abdominal forces, therefore resulting in a vesical pressure that is higher than urethral pressure (Barnes, 1961). An understanding of urethral function is vital in incontinence.

Urethral pressure measurements are a common method of measuring urethral function. They assess the ability of the urethra to prevent urinary incontinence. They can be measured at single points in the urethra or most commonly over the entire length of the urethra (urethral pressure profile [UPP]). We begin with the definitions of urethral pressure parameters, followed by the different methods and techniques used to obtain urethral pressures. The advantages and disadvantages of the different methods and techniques will be discussed.

DEFINITIONS

Urethral pressure is defined as 'the fluid pressure needed to just open a closed (collapsed) urethra' (Griffiths, 1985). This definition implies that the urethral pressure is similar to an ordinary fluid pressure (i.e., is a scalar [does not have a direction] quantity with a single value at each point along the length of the urethra; Lose et al., 2002).

From the definition, it is apparent that the introduction of catheters changes the properties of the closed urethra, but the effect on the urethral pressure measurement was considered to be small (Griffiths, 1985). Urethral pressure measures the intra- and extramural forces that cause apposition of the urethral walls, and associated definitions are as follows (Fig. 5.6.1):

- The *urethral pressure profile* is a graph indicating the intraluminal pressure along the length of the urethra.
- The *urethral closure pressure profile* is given by the subtraction of intravesical pressure from urethral pressure.
- *Maximum urethral pressure* (MUP) is the maximum pressure of the measured profile.
- *Maximum urethral closure pressure* (MUCP) is the maximum difference between the urethral pressure and the intravesical pressure. This is the reserve

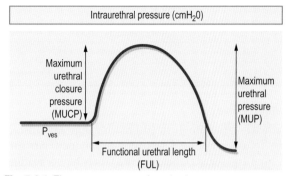

Fig. 5.6.1 The measurement of urethral pressure parameters.

pressure of the urethra to prevent leakage. The calculation of MUCP (p_{ucp}) requires the simultaneous recording of both intraurethral (p_{ura}) and intravesical (p_{ves}) pressure. The calculation is as follows: $p_{ucp} = p_{ura} - p_{ves}$.

- *Functional urethral length* is the length of the urethra along which the urethral pressure exceeds intravesical pressure in women.

METHODS OF MEASURING URETHRAL PRESSURE PROFILOMETRY

There are currently three methods of measuring urethral pressure profilometry:

- the fluid perfusion technique or the Brown Wickham technique (Brown and Wickham, 1969),
- microtip/fibreoptic catheters, and
- balloon catheters.

A summary of the advantages and disadvantages of the different methods is shown in Table 5.6.1.

Fluid Perfusion Technique

The fluid perfusion technique measures the pressure needed to perfuse the catheter, which is withdrawn at a constant speed, at a constant rate. The constant rate of infusion is usually provided by a syringe driver. The measured quantity can be quite close to the local urethral pressure, provided that the urethra is highly distensible (Griffiths, 1980). Several factors affect the technique, as discussed in the following.

TABLE 5.6.1   Advantages and disadvantages of the different methods of measuring urethral pressures

	Fluid Perfusion Technique	Microtip/Fibreoptic Catheters	Balloon Catheters
Advantages	Less prone to movement artefacts Cheap	Measure rapid pressure changes	No orientation dependence
Disadvantages	Slow response to pressure changes	Influenced by transducer shape and orientation Stiffness of the catheter can lead to further artefacts, so a flexible catheter is required Expensive and fragile	Dilating effect on urethra Expensive

Catheter Size

Catheter sizes from 4- to 10-French gauge are satisfactory to use in the fluid perfusion technique (Harrison, 1976). Large-sized catheters give a falsely higher reading because they record urethral elasticity as well as the urethral closure pressure (Lose, 1992).

Catheter Eyeholes

Two opposing side holes 5 cm from the tip of the catheter are satisfactory (Abrams et al., 1978). A larger number of holes does not improve accuracy. The orientation is not important.

Perfusion Rate

A perfusion rate of 2 to 10 mL/min will give an accurate measurement of closure pressure (Abrams et al., 1978). A syringe driver is preferable to a peristaltic pump.

Catheter Withdrawal Speed

The catheter should preferably be withdrawn continuously with the optimal withdrawal speed of less than 7 mm/s (Hilton, 1982). The usual rate of withdrawal is between 1 and 5 mm/s.

Response Time

Response time is dependent on the rate of perfusion and the rate of catheter withdrawal. The perfusion method is able to record a maximum rate of change between 34 and 50 cmH_2O/s.

Microtip/Fibreoptic Catheters

Microtransducer catheters have the ability to measure rapid changes in pressure. However, they appear to have several disadvantages. Firstly, there is a significant degree of positional dependence (Hilton and Stanton, 1983a). For example, if the catheter microtransducer is facing anteriorly, then the MUP is greater and the functional urethral length is shorter than posteriorly

(Abrams et al., 1978). Secondly, bending in urethral wall tissue may lead to a superimposition of local urethral tissue and transducer interactions on the urethral pressure: this requires the catheters to be quite flexible. If used, it is recommended that the transducer faces laterally (Anderson et al., 1983).

A new urodynamic method using a novel microtip catheter called *high-definition urethral pressure profilometry* has been suggested. This method combines a novel microtip catheter with advanced signal processing to enable spatial data location and the reconstruction of a pressure image inside the urethra (Klünder et al., 2016). However, this has only been used in animal models and appears to be reproducible but has not been translated from animal models into humans (Klünder et al., 2017).

Balloon Catheters

The advantages of balloon catheters in measuring urethral pressures are that they avoid orientation dependence. However, in the past, technical problems meant that the balloons were too large, causing a dilatation effect on the urethra. This results in an overestimation of the urethral pressure. In addition, the length of the balloon is important. If the balloon is too long, this averages out the pressure variations along the length of the urethra. Recent balloon catheters have overcome these difficulties (Pollak et al., 2004).

Air-Filled Catheters

Air-filled catheters have been actively marketed for the past few years and in some geographical areas are widely used. However, as the scientific basis for introduction of this technology for pressure measurement in urodynamics was not clear, a study group examined the evidence and concluded that further systematic laboratory and clinical research is necessary before air-filled catheters can be recommended for routine clinical use (Abrams et al., 2017).

FACTORS AFFECTING MAXIMUM URETHRAL CLOSURE PRESSURES

Urethral pressure measurement can be carried out at different bladder volumes and in different subject positions at rest, during coughing or straining, and during voiding.

Bladder Volume

Urethral closure pressure measurement in women depends on bladder volume. In continent women, the urethral closure pressure increases with increasing volume. However, in women with stress incontinence, it tends to decrease with increasing volume (Awad et al., 1978).

Patient Position

Position also has an effect on urethral closure pressure: continent women show an increase in urethral closure pressure on standing, whereas women with stress incontinence show a decrease in pressure on standing (Henriksson et al., 1977; Hendriksson et al., 1979). However, there is poor reproducibility of the urethral closure pressure in the standing position, thus limiting clinical use (Dorflinger et al., 2002).

Pelvic Floor Activity

Pelvic floor muscle (PFM) activity is always active except before and during voiding. However, a failure of relaxation of the voluntary pelvic floor contraction increases urethral closure pressure. This can usually be overcome by repeating the urethral pressure profilometry twice more or until a reproducible pattern is obtained, and if need be, over a longer period of time. Conversely, the effect of pelvic floor activity on the urethra can be assessed during measurement of urethral pressure. The catheter is placed at the point of MUP, and the patient is asked to contract the pelvic floor voluntarily as if trying to stop themselves from passing urine. In normal women an increment above the MUCP is seen. A value of less than 10 cmH$_2$O

above the MUCP denotes a poor pelvic floor squeeze in the fluid perfusion technique (Table 5.6.2).

The variation of urethral closure pressures depends on the method used and the position, and to facilitate reliable recordings, recommendations on the standardization of urethral pressure measurements have been made. Some of the recommendations of the International Continence Society subcommittee on the standardization of urethral pressure measurements are presented next (Lose et al., 2002).

STANDARDIZATION OF URETHRAL PRESSURE MEASUREMENTS

The investigator is asked to specify:
1. type of measurement (point–profilometry–ambulatory);
2. period of time over which the measurement was recorded;
3. constant (given by the probe) or variable cross-sectional area of the urethra (i.e., inflation of a balloon);
4. patient position;
5. bladder volume;
6. manoeuvres (coughing, Valsalva, other);
7. withdrawal speed (for profilometry);
8. infusion medium and rate of infusion (for fluid-perfused catheters);
9. type of catheter;
10. size of catheter;
11. catheter material/flexibility;
12. orientation of a directional sensor;
13. sensor position fixation (for point pressures or during coughing/straining);
14. zeroing of pressure sensors:
    – external transducers (and fluid-filled catheters): superior edge of the symphysis pubis (piezometric) for pressure reference height, and to correct for viscous pressure losses within the catheter,

TABLE 5.6.2 **Comparison of clinical PFM strength assessment by experienced clinicians and urethral pressure assessment (fluid perfusion technique)**			
PFM Strength as Assessed by Urologist/Urogynaecologist	Normal	Reduced	Absent
Number of patients	2757	3399	485
Urethral pressure assessment (cmH$_2$O)	18.1	8.8	3.6
(SD)	(15.5)	(11.1)	(7.5)

A large series from the Bristol Urological Institute over a period of 15 years.
PFM, pelvic floor muscle.

zero of pressure should be set as the reading in air when the fluid is flowing (zero reference point is atmospheric pressure)

- microtip transducers calibrated to atmospheric pressure, but no pressure reference height is needed for catheter-mounted transducers, and when calculating closure pressure using multi-sensor microtips, any difference in vertical height between the 'bladder' transducer and urethral transducer(s) should be taken into account; and

15. recording apparatus:

- describe the type of recording apparatus: the frequency response of the total system should be stated; equipment with a sampling rate of 18 Hz can satisfactorily record cough-produced pressure changes in the urethra (Thind et al., 1994).

NORMAL URETHRAL PRESSURE PROFILES

There are sex differences between men and women in the range of normal urethral pressure values. In men, MUP does not significantly decrease with age (Abrams, 1997), whereas in women, after menopause, MUP decreases. Prostatic length tends to increase with age in men; however, urethral length tends to decrease in women. A rough guide to MUP in women is a value of 92 – age (cmH$_2$O) using values obtained from the fluid perfusion technique (Edwards and Malvern, 1974).

Urethral Pressure Profile Shape
Men
Certain features are seen in the male UPP; there are two peaks: the presphincter peak followed by the prostatic plateau and then the sphincter peak (Fig. 5.6.2). Abnormalities in the presphincteric prostatic plateau can be due to bladder neck hypertrophy or prostatic enlargement. The sphincter peak in men can be too high, as

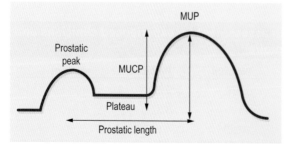

Fig. 5.6.2 MUP profile measurements, demonstrating the prostatic peak, plateau and length. *MUCP,* Maximum urethral closure pressure; *MUP,* maximum urethral pressure.

seen in some neurogenic patients, or too low in male patients with iatrogenic causes of stress incontinence, such as after prostate surgery.

Women
The female UPP tends to symmetrical in shape, as seen in Fig. 5.6.1.

Normal and abnormal UPPs are shown in Figs. 5.6.3 and 5.6.4, respectively. Women can also have low or high urethral pressures. A high urethral pressure sometimes denotes Fowler's syndrome, a condition in which idiopathic sphincter overactivity causes voiding difficulties (Fowler et al., 1988). A low urethral pressure may denote intrinsic sphincter deficiency, which usually results from childbirth and may lead to stress urinary incontinence (SUI). A biphasic pressure wave may suggest a urethral diverticulum.

The measurement of resting UPPs has several uses
- In post-prostatectomy incontinence; there is a close association between sphincter damage and a reduction in the MUCP (Hammerer and Huland, 1997).
- There is some evidence that a low MUCP is associated with a poor outcome with surgery in women for SUI (Hilton and Stanton, 1983b).
- Urethral pressure measurements may provide an answer to unexplained incontinence in women.
- In female patients with a non-relaxing sphincter, the UPP may guide treatment success with sacral neuromodulation.
- When considering patients for urinary diversion surgery, the MUCP gives an indication as to whether an artificial sphincter is necessary. An MUCP greater than 50 cmH$_2$O would not require a sphincter if a good-volume, low-pressure reservoir is created (Abrams, 1997).

Urethral Pressure Profile and Incontinence Surgery
Several studies have suggested that female patients with a low urethral closure pressure and urethral length have a worse outcome after incontinence surgery (Bhatia and Ostergard, 1982; Hilton, 1989; Hilton and Stanton, 1983b). Some have not shown any difference (Harris et al., 2011; Sand et al., 2000).

RESTING URETHRAL PRESSURE PROFILES
Responsiveness
Microtip catheters have a high frequency response greater than 2000 Hz, which is more than adequate to

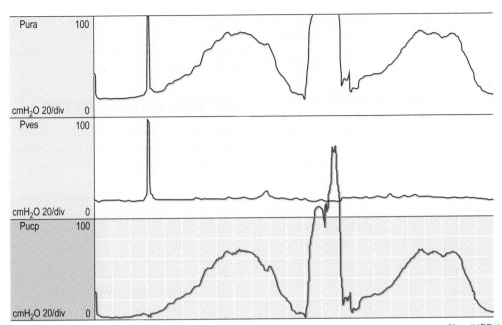

Fig. 5.6.3 Normal urethral pressures in women. The diagram shows two urethral pressure profiles (UPPs) with the shorter higher peak being the artefact recorded when the catheter is passed though the sphincter area to perform the second UPP seen on the right. *Pucp,* Urethral closure pressure; *Pura,* intraurethral pressure; *Pves,* intravesical pressure.

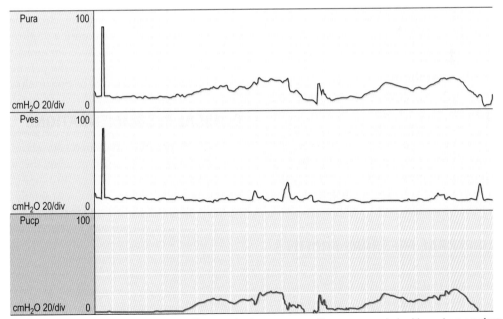

Fig. 5.6.4 Reduced urethral pressures. Two urethral pressure profiles are recorded with a short artefact between them (see Fig. 5.6.3). *Pucp,* Urethral closure pressure; *Pura,* intraurethral pressure; *Pves,* intravesical pressure.

record physiological events in the lower urinary tract. The fluid perfusion technique has a reduced responsiveness in comparison.

Reliability

The reproducibility and repeatability of the fluid perfusion technique and the microtip catheter have been shown to be reasonable (Abrams et al., 1978; Hilton, 1982; Wang and Chen, 2002). The standard deviation of measurements made in a single occasion of the fluid perfusion technique and the microtip catheter is shown to be approximately 5 and 3 cmH$_2$O, respectively (Abrams et al., 1978; Hilton and Stanton, 1983a). The inter-test measurements show a standard deviation of 3.5 to 5 cmH$_2$O depending on menstrual status (Hilton, 1982; van Geelen et al., 1981). Recently, balloon catheters have shown reasonable correlations with microtip catheters (Pollak et al., 2004).

Validity

The validity of the measurements of resting urethral pressure profilometry depends on the technique used. The measured quantity can be very close to the local urethral pressure, provided that the urethra is highly distensible (Griffiths, 1980) in the case of the fluid perfusion technique.

Microtip catheters measure the stress of the urethral wall, not the pressure. The validity of urethral pressure measurements in assessing PFM strength is high.

Sensitivity and Specificity

Female patients with SUI generally have significantly lower mean values of MUP than continent women (Hilton and Stanton, 1983a). The MUP is lowest in those women (and men) with increasingly severe SUI. However, there is a large overlap between the MUPs of normal and incontinent patients. Urethral pressure profilometry therefore does not have the diagnostic accuracy for SUI to be used alone (Versi, 1990).

STRESS URETHRAL PRESSURE PROFILES

This method assesses the pressure transmission from the abdominal cavity to the proximal urethra. Decreased conductance of abdominal pressure is associated with stress incontinence. Essentially a UPP is performed, preferably with a microtip catheter with the patient coughing. If the urethral closure pressures become negative on coughing, then leakage is likely and represents a positive test. Ideally the stress UPP should be carried out in the erect position with a full bladder. This poses practical issues. A lack of specificity with the test has limited its use (Versi, 1990). Stress UPPs are no longer used regularly in clinical practice.

URETHRAL REFLECTOMETRY

There has been interest in urethral reflectometry. The technique involves placing a thin polyurethane bag in the urethra. A pump applies preselected pressures stepwise to the bag. For every step, the cross-sectional area is measured by acoustic reflectometry. Measurements are made both during inflation and deflation (Klarskov and Lose, 2007a). The initial results are comparable to urethral pressure profilometry (Klarskov and Lose, 2007b). Urethral reflectometry is not commercially available and has only been used for research purposes in three university departments and two phase I clinical trial units (Khayyami et al., 2016).

CONCLUSION

Resting urethral pressure measurements can be made using several techniques, and the results are influenced by the technique used and biological factors. Urethral pressure measurements are static measurements that do not reflect the forces exerted on the urethra at leakage. Increases in abdominal pressure compress the urethra and result in reflex activation of the periurethral muscles, which are not assessed by resting urethral pressures.

CLINICAL RECOMMENDATIONS

- Urethral pressure measurements should be performed under the supervision of the urologist or urogynaecologist.
- The urologist or urogynaecologist should refer to the International Continence Society standardization report on urethral pressure measurements.
- An understanding of the limitations of the different urethral pressure measurements is required before embarking on research.
- Multidisciplinary collaboration is required when physical therapists perform research in this area with the urologist or urogynaecologist providing the urethral pressure measurements.
- Urethral pressure measurements, if performed correctly, are good valid measurements for assessing PFM strength.

REFERENCES

Abrams, P. (1997). *Urodynamics* (2nd ed.). London: Springer.

Abrams, P., Damaser, M., Niblett, P., et al. (2017). Air filled, including "air-charged," catheters in urodynamic studies: Does the evidence justify their use? *Neurourology and Urodynamics, 36*(5), 1234–1242.

Abrams, P. H., Martin, S., & Griffiths, D. J. (1978). The measurement and interpretation of urethral pressures obtained by the method of brown and wickham. *British Journal of Urology, 50*(1), 33–38.

Anderson, R. S., Shepherd, A. M., & Feneley, R. C. (1983). Micro-transducer urethral profile methodology: Variations caused by transducer orientation. *Journal of Urology, 130*(4), 727–728.

Awad, S. A., Bryniak, S. R., Lowe, P. J., et al. (1978). Urethral pressure profile in female stress incontinence. *Journal of Urology, 120*(4), 475–479.

Barnes, A. (1961). The method of evaluating the stress of urinary incontinence. *Obstetrics & Gynecology, 81*, 108.

Bhatia, N. N., & Ostergard, D. R. (1982). Urodynamics in women with stress urinary incontinence. *Obstetrics & Gynecology, 60*(5), 552–559.

Brown, M., & Wickham, J. E. (1969). The urethral pressure profile. *British Journal of Urology, 41*(2), 211–217.

Dorflinger, A., Gorton, E., Stanton, S., et al. (2002). Urethral pressure profile: Is it affected by position? *Neurourology and Urodynamics, 21*(6), 553–557.

Edwards, L., & Malvern, J. (1974). The urethral pressure profile: Theoretical considerations and clinical application. *British Journal of Urology, 46*(3), 325–335.

Fowler, C. J., Christmas, T. J., Chapple, C. R., et al. (1988). Abnormal electromyographic activity of the urethral sphincter, voiding dysfunction, and polycystic ovaries: A new syndrome? *British medical journal, 297*(6661), 1436–1438.

Griffiths, D. S. (1980). *Urodynamics*. Bristol: Adam Hilger.

Griffiths, D. (1985). The pressure within a collapsed tube, with special reference to urethral pressure. *Physics in Medicine and Biology, 30*(9), 951–963.

Hammerer, P., & Huland, H. (1997). Urodynamic evaluation of changes in urinary control after radical retropubic prostatectomy. *Journal of Urology, 157*(1), 233–236.

Harrison, N. W. (1976). The urethral pressure profile. *Urological Research, 4*(3), 95–100.

Harris, N., Swithinbank, L., Hayek, S. A., et al. (2011). Can maximum urethral closure pressure (MUCP) be used to predict outcome of surgical treatment of stress urinary incontinence. *Neurourology and Urodynamics, 39*(8), 1609–1612.

Henriksson, L., Andersson, K. E., & Ulmsten, U. (1979). The urethral pressure profiles in continent and stress-incontinent women. *Scandinavian Journal of Urology and Nephrology, 13*(1), 5–10.

Henriksson, L., Ulmsten, U., & Andersson, K. E. (1977). The effect of changes of posture on the urethral closure pressure in healthy women. *Scandinavian Journal of Urology and Nephrology, 11*(3), 201–206.

Hilton, P. (1982). Urethral pressure measurements at rest: An analysis of variance. *Neurourology and Urodynamics, 1*, 303.

Hilton, P. (1989). A clinical and urodynamic study comparing the Stamey bladder neck suspension and suburethral sling procedures in the treatment of genuine stress incontinence. *British Journal of Obstetrics and Gynaecology, 96*(2), 213–220.

Hilton, P., & Stanton, S. L. (1983a). Urethral pressure measurement by microtransducer: The results in symptom-free women and in those with genuine stress incontinence. *British Journal of Obstetrics and Gynaecology, 90*(10), 919–933.

Hilton, P., & Stanton, S. L. (1983b). A clinical and urodynamic assessment of the Burch colposuspension for genuine stress incontinence. *British Journal of Obstetrics and Gynaecology, 90*(10), 934–939.

Khayyami, Y., Klarskov, N., & Lose, G. (2016). The promise of urethral pressure reflectometry: An update. *Review International Urogynecology Journal, 27*(10), 1449–1458.

Klarskov, N., & Lose, G. (2007a). Urethral pressure reflectometry; a novel technique for simultaneous recording of pressure and cross-sectional area in the female urethra. *Neurourology and Urodynamics, 26*(2), 254–261.

Klarskov, N., & Lose, G. (2007b). Urethral pressure reflectometry vs urethral pressure profilometry in women: A comparative study of reproducibility and accuracy. *British Journal of Urology, 100*(2), 351–356.

Klünder, M., Amend, B., Sawodny, O., et al. (2017). Assessing the reproducibility of high definition urethral pressure profilometry and its correlation with an air-charged system. *Neurourology and Urodynamics, 36*(5), 1292–1300.

Klünder, M., Amend, B., Vaegler, M., et al. (2016). High definition urethral pressure profilometry: Evaluating a novel microtip catheter. *Neurourology and Urodynamics, 35*(8), 888–894.

Lose, G. (1992). Simultaneous recording of pressure and cross-sectional area in the female urethra: A study of urethral closure function in healthy and stress incontinent women. *Neurourology and Urodynamics, 11*, 55.

Lose, G., Griffiths, D., Hosker, G., et al. (2002). Standardisation of urethral pressure measurement: Report from the standardisation sub-committee of the international continence society. *Neurourology and Urodynamics, 21*(3), 258–260.

Pollak, J. T., Neimark, M., Connor, J. T., et al. (2004). Air-charged and microtransducer urodynamic catheters in the evaluation of urethral function. *International Urogynecology Journal and Pelvic Floor Dysfunction, 15*(2), 124–128.

Sand, P. K., Winkler, H., Blackhurst, D. W., et al. (2000). A prospective randomized study comparing modified Burch retropubic urethropexy and suburethral sling for treatment of genuine stress incontinence with low-pressure urethra. *American Journal of Obstetrics and Gynecology, 182*(1), 30–34.

Thind, P., Bagi, P., Lose, G., et al. (1994). Characterization of pressure changes in the lower urinary tract during coughing with special reference to the demands on the pressure recording equipment. *Neurourology and Urodynamics, 13*(3), 219–225.

Van Geelen, J. M., Doesburg, W. H., Thomas, C. M., et al. (1981). Urodynamic studies in the normal menstrual cycle: The relationship between hormonal changes during the menstrual cycle and the urethral pressure profile. *American Journal of Obstetrics and Gynecology, 141*(4), 384–392.

Versi, E. (1990). Discriminant analysis of urethral pressure profilometry data for the diagnosis of genuine stress incontinence. *British Journal of Obstetrics and Gynaecology, 97*(3), 251–259.

Wang, A. C., & Chen, M. C. (2002). A comparison of urethral pressure profilometry using microtip and double-lumen perfusion catheters in women with genuine stress incontinence. *British journal of obstetrics and gynaecology, 109*(3), 322–326.

5.7 Ultrasound in the Assessment of Pelvic Floor Muscle, Anal Canal and Pelvic Organ Descent

HP Dietz

INTRODUCTION

Ultrasound is increasingly used for the morphological and functional assessment of the muscles of the pelvic floor. Recent developments have greatly simplified the direct demonstration of the levator ani and anal canal by ultrasound. The advent of 3D ultrasound has given us access to the axial plane while using non-invasive techniques. A 4D ultrasound allows real-time imaging of the effect of manoeuvres such as cough, Valsalva and pelvic floor muscle contraction (PFMC) in any arbitrarily defined plane (Dietz, 2004b). Most recently, modern image processing techniques, both on- and offline, have enabled us to reach resolutions equivalent to magnetic resonance imaging (MRI) in all three dimensions for most of the structures in which we are interested while delivering temporal resolution far above anything possible on MRI today.

This discussion will be limited to translabial or transperineal ultrasound, which is the only sonographic imaging modality to allow direct assessment of both levator structure and function. When assessing the anal canal, the same modality is sometimes termed *exoanal* ultrasound (Dietz, 2018). Although transabdominal sonography has been used to describe levator activity (Thompson and O'Sullivan, 2003), such an assessment is necessarily indirect and quite limited. Endovaginal imaging can demonstrate static anatomy and biometric measures, but the presence of an instrument within the vagina severely limits the assessment of function via manoeuvres such as Valsalva and PFMC. The same holds for endoanal imaging, which has been the mainstay of sphincter assessment since the 1980s (Sultan, 2003).

Technique

Translabial or perineal ultrasound is performed by placing a transducer (usually a 3.5–5, 4–8 or 6–9 MHz curved array) on the perineum (Fig. 5.7.1), after covering the instrument with a glove or thin plastic wrap for hygienic reasons. Powdered gloves can markedly impair imaging quality due to reverberations and should be avoided. Imaging can be performed in dorsal lithotomy, with the hips flexed and slightly abducted, or in the standing position. Bladder filling should be specified; for some applications, prior voiding is preferable. The presence of a full rectum may impair diagnostic accuracy and sometimes requires repeat assessment after defecation. Parting of the labia can improve image quality. The transducer can generally be placed quite firmly against the symphysis pubis without causing significant discomfort, unless there is marked atrophy. The resulting image includes the symphysis anteriorly, the urethra and bladder neck, the vagina, cervix, rectum, and anal canal (see Fig. 5.7.1). Posterior to the anorectal junction a hyperechogenic area indicates the central portion of the levator plate (i.e., the puborectalis/pubococcygeus or pubovisceral muscle). The cul de sac may also be seen, filled with a small amount of fluid, echogenic fat or peristalsing small bowel. Parasagittal or transverse views may yield additional information, such as enabling assessment of the puborectalis muscle and its insertion on the arcus tendineus of the levator ani. For imaging of the anal canal, the transducer is rotated clockwise by 90 degrees and tilted from ventrocaudal to dorsocranial to obtain a cross-section of the anal canal (Fig. 5.7.2). The external anal sphincter (EAS) appears as a hyperechogenic

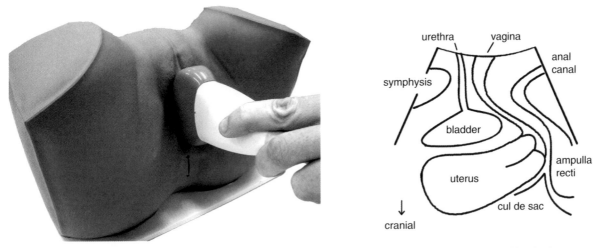

Fig. 5.7.1 Transducer placement (left) and field of vision (right) for translabial/perineal ultrasound, midsagittal plane. *(From Dietz [2010], with permission.)*

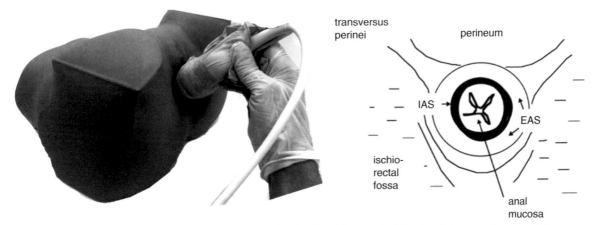

Fig. 5.7.2 Transducer placement (left) and field of vision (right) for translabial/perineal ultrasound, midsagittal plane. *EAS*, External anal sphincter; *IAS*, internal anal sphincter. *(Reproduced with permission from Dietz, H. P. Pelvic Floor Ultrasound In: Fleischer, A. C., Toy, E. C., FManning, F. A., et al (eds). Fleischer's Sonography in Obstetrics & Gynecology, Eighth Edition © 2018 McGraw Hill. All Rights Reserved. Figure 42-21.)*

(bright) ring structure, with the internal anal sphincter (IAS) seen as hypo- to anechoic (dark). Trauma to either structure is easily visible, with external sphincter tears appearing as hypoechoic defects in the ring. Likewise, internal sphincter defects are seen as isoechogenic defects in an anechoic ring structure.

Bladder Neck Position and Mobility

Bladder neck position and mobility can be assessed with a high degree of reliability (Dietz et al., 2005a; Tan et al., 2015). To obtain valid and reproducible results, it is essential, however, to ensure an adequate Valsalva manoeuvre which ought to be sustained for at least 5 seconds (Orejuela et al., 2012). The patient has to be coached to breathe

in, hold her breath, and 'push as if you had to push a baby out' or 'push as if you had to pass a hard bowel movement' to achieve adequate abdominal pressures. At the same time, one should ensure that the patient does not produce a concomitant levator contraction which will result in artificially low values for pelvic organ descent and hiatal dimensions. This is most common in young women with good pelvic floor muscle (PFM) function (Oerno and Dietz, 2007) and is evident as a reduction in the anteroposterior diameter of the levator hiatus, and as a posterior displacement of the prepubic fat pad, seen inferior or caudal to the inferior surface of the symphysis pubis, due to contraction of the superficial perineal muscles. Pressure on the transducer has to be reduced as much as possible

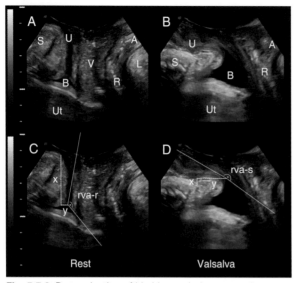

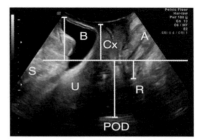

Fig. 5.7.4 Prolapse assessment by translabial ultrasound, mid-sagittal plane. There is a cystocele to about 3.5 cm and uterine prolapse to about 3 cm below the symphysis pubis. *A*, Anal canal; *B*, bladder; *Cx*, cervix; *POD*, pouch of Douglas; *R*, rectum; *S*, symphysis pubis; *U*, uterus.

Fig. 5.7.3 Determination of bladder neck descent and retrovesical angle. Ultrasound images show the midsagittal plane at rest (A, C) and on Valsalva (B, D). The lower images demonstrate the measurement of distances between the interior symphyseal margin and bladder neck (vertical, x; horizontal, y), and the retrovesical angle at rest (rva-r) and on Valsalva (rva-s). *A*, Anal canal; *B*, bladder; *L*, levator ani; *R*, rectal ampulla; *S*, symphysis pubis; *U*, urethra; *Ut*, uterus; *V*, vagina. *(From Dietz [2011a], with permission.)*

without losing contact during a Valsalva manoeuvre to allow full descent of pelvic organs.

Points of reference are the central axis of the symphysis pubis (Schaer, 1997) or its inferoposterior margin (Dietz, 2004c). Measurements of bladder neck position are generally performed at rest and on maximal Valsalva manoeuvre. The difference yields a numerical value for bladder neck descent (Fig. 5.7.3). On Valsalva, the proximal urethra is usually seen to rotate in a posteroinferior direction. The extent of rotation can be measured by comparing the angle of inclination between the proximal urethra and any other fixed axis. This is often accompanied by an opening of the retrovesical angle (see Fig. 5.7.3), although none of those changes in functional anatomy are diagnostic of urodynamic stress incontinence (Nazemian et al., 2013). Fig. 5.7.4 illustrates how pelvic floor ultrasound can be used to quantify descent not just of the bladder neck and urethra but also of the most dependent part of a cystocele, central and posterior compartment (Dietz et al., 2001a).

The aetiology of increased bladder neck descent is likely to be multifactorial. The wide range of values obtained in young nulliparous women suggests a

congenital component, and a twin study has confirmed a high degree of heritability for anterior vaginal wall mobility (Dietz et al., 2005a). Vaginal childbirth is probably the most significant environmental factor, with forceps being the strongest risk factor for future prolapse (Dietz et al., 2016). While the pelvic floor is undoubtedly affected by pregnancy and childbirth, labour and delivery are in turn affected by pelvic floor characteristics: anterior vaginal wall mobility on Valsalva has been found to be a potential predictor of delivery mode (Balmforth et al., 2003; Dietz et al., 2003), and this may also be true for hiatal distensibility (Lanzarone and Dietz, 2007).

Levator Activity

Perineal ultrasound has been used for the quantification of PFM activity, both in women with stress incontinence and continent controls (Wijma et al., 1991), as well as before and after childbirth (Dietz, 2004a; Peschers et al., 1997b). A cranioventral shift of pelvic organs imaged in a sagittal midline orientation is taken as evidence of a levator contraction (Dietz, 2011a). The resulting displacement of the internal urethral meatus is measured relative to the inferoposterior symphyseal margin (Fig. 5.7.5). Another means of quantifying levator activity is to measure reduction of the levator hiatus in the midsagittal plane, or the change in the main hiatal plane axis relative to the central symphyseal axis (see Fig. 5.7.5). Ultrasound can also be utilized for PFM exercise teaching by providing visual biofeedback (Dietz et al., 2001b). The technique has helped validate the concept of 'the knack'—that is, of a reflex levator contraction immediately prior to increases in intra-abdominal pressure such as those resulting from coughing (Miller et al., 1996). Correlations between cranioventral shift of the bladder neck on the one hand and palpation/perineometry on the other hand have been shown to be good (Dietz et al., 2002). However, it has to

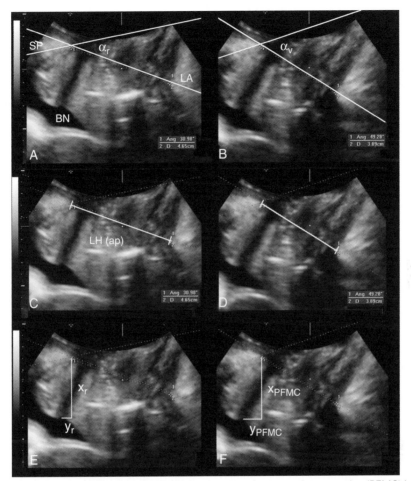

Fig. 5.7.5 Three methods of determining the effect of a pelvic floor muscle contraction (PFMC) in the midsagittal plane, using 2D translabial ultrasound. The left-hand images in each pair (A, C, E) represent the resting state, and the right-hand images (B, D, E) show findings on PFMC. The top pair illustrates measurement of the levator plate angle (the angle between the symphyseal axis and the levator hiatus in the midsagittal plane), the middle pair shows reduction of the anteroposterior diameter of the LH (ap) and the bottom pair illustrates bladder neck displacement on PFMC, analogous to the way bladder neck descent is measured on Valsalva. *BN*, Bladder neck; *LA*, levator ani; *LH (ap)*, levator hiatus; *SP*, symphysis pubis. *(From Dietz [2011a], with permission.)*

be recognized that measures of organ displacement have an obvious weakness when it comes to describing contractility. Whether a given force results in greater or lesser tissue displacement will depend on tissue stiffness or elasticity. Highly elastic tissues as in a patient with prolapse and marked hiatal ballooning may be displaced substantially by a relatively small force. Yet a much greater force may be required for a minor degree of displacement in women with less elastic tissues (Oversand et al., 2015).

Direct visualization of a levator contraction and shortening of fibres is possible on 2D ultrasound using an oblique parasagittal plane (Fig. 5.7.6), which can also be used to demonstrate levator trauma (Dietz and Shek, 2009).

In addition, it is possible to observe reflex activation of the levator ani and the bulbospongiosus/bulbocavernosus muscles, which is manifested as a reduction in the anteroposterior hiatal diameter and as a dorsal displacement of the clitoral area. Although childbirth seems to have some effect on such reflexes (Dietz et al., 2012a), clinical utility appears to be limited (Dietz et al., 2012b).

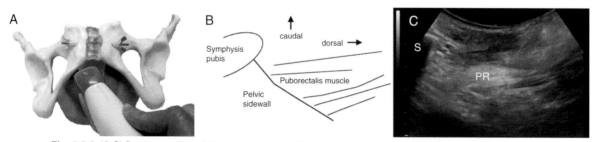

Fig. 5.7.6 (A-C) Demonstration of the pubococcygeus/puborectalis complex by oblique parasagittal imaging. This orientation can be used to directly observe shortening of the pubovisceral muscle complex on contraction. *PR*, Puborectalis muscle; *S*, symphysis pubis.

PROLAPSE QUANTIFICATION

Translabial ultrasound can diagnose uterovaginal prolapse (Dietz et al., 2001a). The inferior margin of the symphysis pubis serves as a line of reference against which maximal descent of the bladder, uterus, cul de sac and rectal ampulla on Valsalva manoeuvre can be measured (see Fig. 5.7.4). Findings have been validated against clinical staging and the results of POP-Q assessments, with the result that, in the opinion of the author, translabial ultrasound is now better defined as a methodology and validated against patient symptoms than clinical assessment (Shek and Dietz, 2016). An obvious advantage is the ability to differentiate different forms of posterior compartment descent that are indistinguishable clinically, such as rectocele, enterocele and rectal intussusception (Guzman Rojas et al., 2016).

Disadvantages of the method include incomplete imaging of bladder neck, cervix and vault with large rectoceles; the inability to reduce one compartment to assess another; and the potential underestimation of severe prolapse due to transducer pressure. Occasionally, apparent anterior vaginal wall prolapse will turn out to be due to a urethral diverticulum, a vaginal cyst such as a Gartner duct cyst (cystic remnant of the mesonephric or Wolffian ducts), or a cyst due to epithelial inversion after repair surgery or even a vaginal fibroma.

3D/4D PELVIC FLOOR IMAGING

Pelvic floor ultrasound in 3D and 4D is currently performed using systems that have evolved around transducers that allow motorized acquisition. The first such motorized probe was developed in 1974, and by 1987 transducers for clinical use were commercially available (Gritzky and Brandl, 1998). The first system platform, the Kretz Voluson, was developed around such a 'fan

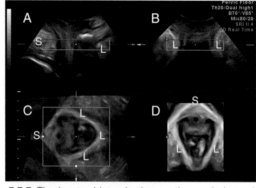

Fig. 5.7.7 The levator hiatus in three orthogonal planes (midsagittal on A, coronal on B, axial on C) and as a rendered volume (D). This case illustrates normal anatomy. *L*, Levator ani; *S*, symphysis pubis.

scan' probe. With such a transducer, automatic image acquisition is achieved by rapid oscillation of a group of piezoelectric elements. The widespread acceptance of 3D ultrasound in obstetrics and gynaecology was helped considerably by the development of such transducers as they do not require any movement relative to the investigated tissue during acquisition. 4D imaging implies the real-time acquisition of volume ultrasound data, which can be represented in orthogonal planes or rendered volumes. Modern systems allow the storing of cine loops of volumes, which is of major importance in pelvic floor imaging as it allows enhanced documentation of functional anatomy.

A single volume obtained at rest with an acquisition angle of 70 degrees or higher will include the entire levator hiatus with symphysis pubis, urethra, paravaginal tissues, the vagina, anorectum and levator ani muscle from the pelvic sidewall to the posterior aspect of the anorectal junction (Fig. 5.7.7). The levator hiatus as seen on translabial 3D/4D ultrasound or MRI is the plane of minimal dimensions between the symphysis pubis/pubic rami anteriorly and the pubovisceral or puborectalis muscle laterally and posteriorly. Hiatal dimensions can be measured both in the axial plane (Dietz et al., 2005b) and in a rendered volume (Dietz et al., 2011c). The latter method is easier and at least as reproducible and may be preferable, given the non-Euclidean (warped) nature of the plane of the hiatus (Kruger et al., 2010).

The main advantage of volume ultrasound for pelvic floor imaging is that the method gives access to the plane of the levator hiatus (i.e., the axial or transverse plane). Up until recently, pelvic floor ultrasound was limited to the midsagittal plane. Parasagittal (see Fig. 5.7.6) and coronal plane imaging (see Fig. 5.7.7, top right, for an example) may at times be helpful, although there are no obvious points of reference. Imaging planes on 3D ultrasound can be varied in a completely arbitrary fashion to enhance the visibility of a given anatomical structure, either at the time of acquisition or offline at a later time. The three orthogonal images (i.e., three planes at right angles to each other: sagittal, transverse and axial) are complemented by a 'rendered image' (i.e., a semitransparent representation of all voxels in an arbitrarily definable 'box'). The bottom right-hand image in Fig. 5.7.7 shows a standard surface-rendered image of the levator hiatus, with the rendering direction set from caudally to cranially, which is most convenient for imaging of the levator muscle. Midsagittal, axial and coronal views of the levator hiatus are given in the 'orthogonal' images in the top row and bottom left.

Over the past 15 years, a substantial body of research employing 3D/4D translabial ultrasound has been accumulated in the literature. We do know what a normal, healthy pelvic floor in a nulligravid young woman looks like and how it functions (Dietz et al., 2005b; Kruger et al., 2008; Yang et al., 2006) and that there is substantial variation between individuals (Svabik et al., 2009). There have been multiple studies examining the impact of pregnancy and childbirth, demonstrating that vaginal childbirth, particularly forceps delivery, is the most substantial environmental influence on pelvic floor anatomy and function (Dietz, 2015).

HIATAL AREA

Hiatal depth and area measurements (Fig. 5.7.8) seem highly reproducible (Dietz et al., 2005b; Hoff Braekken et al., 2008). Depth, width and area of the hiatus correlate strongly with pelvic organ descent, both at rest and on Valsalva (Dietz et al., 2008). Although this is not surprising for the correlation between the hiatal area on Valsalva and descent (as downward displacement of organs may push the levator laterally), it is much more

interesting that hiatal area at rest is associated with pelvic organ descent on Valsalva. This data constitutes the first real evidence for the hypothesis that the state of the levator ani is important for pelvic organ support (DeLancey, 2001), even in the absence of levator trauma. Excessive hiatal distension or 'ballooning' has been defined as a hiatal area of 25 cm^2 or more on maximal Valsalva, which seems to be the optimal cut-off on receiver operating characteristic statistics (Dietz et al., 2008) and, incidentally, represents the mean plus two standard deviations in young nulliparous women (Dietz et al., 2005b). This matters, as the levator hiatus is the largest potential hernial portal in the human body. Whether hernia (i.e., pelvic organ prolapse) ensues is largely dependent on the size or distensibility of this portal.

LEVATOR TRAUMA

The structure limiting and defining this hernial portal, the puborectalis component of the levator ani, is subjected to enormous distension in vaginal childbirth (Svabik et al., 2009). Not surprisingly, the puborectalis suffers macroscopic trauma in a substantial minority of women (Shek and Dietz, 2019).

The typical form of levator trauma, a unilateral avulsion of the levator ani muscle off the inferior ramus and body of the os pubis, is clearly related to childbirth (see Figs. 5.7.9, 5.7.10, 5.7.12, 5.7.13) and is palpable as an asymmetrical loss of substance in the anteromedial portion of the muscle. Digital evaluation for morphological abnormalities (Figs. 5.7.9 and 5.7.10) requires significant operator experience, but it is within the reach of every practitioner caring for women with pelvic floor disorders (Dietz and Shek, 2008b). It appears that those components of the levator ani which form the hiatus (i.e., those subdivisions that insert on the inferior pubic ramus) are most critical, as judged by the results of mathematical modelling on the basis of tomographic (multislice) imaging (Dietz, 2007; Dietz et al., 2011a) (as seen in Fig. 5.7.11). Hence, we rate an avulsion as present if we are unable to palpate contractile tissue attached to the inferior pubic ramus. Partial trauma is common in the form of generalized or irregular thinning or as slits or holes in the muscle insertion on the inferior pubic ramus, but this seems to be of less relevance than complete avulsion (Dietz et al., 2011a; Dietz et al., 2022).

In general, an avulsed muscle generates less force, resulting in reduced strength grading (Dietz and Shek, 2008a), but sometimes there is compensatory hypertrophy

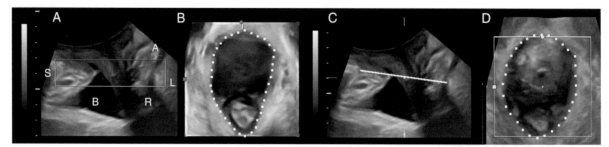

Fig. 5.7.8 Determination of the plane of minimal hiatal dimensions on Valsalva. The hiatus can be imaged in a rendered volume placed at the location of the minimal distance between the symphysis pubis (S) and the levator ani posterior to the anorectal angle (L) as shown in B (Dietz et al., 2011c). The original method described for measurement of hiatal dimensions is shown in C and D, which illustrate the location of the plane of minimal dimensions in the midsagittal plane (C) and its representation in the axial plane (D) (Dietz et al., 2005b). *A,* anal canal; *B,* bladder; *L,* levator ani; *R,* rectum; *S,* symphysis pubis. *(From Dietz [2011c], with permission.)*

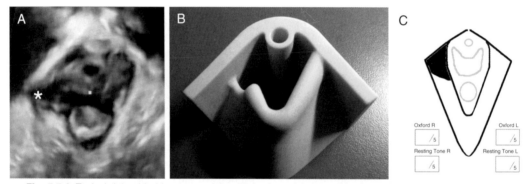

Fig. 5.7.9 Typical right-sided levator avulsion (*) in the axial plane (A), shown in a palpation model (B) and documented in a drawing. *(Panel C is modified from Dietz and Shek [2008b].)*

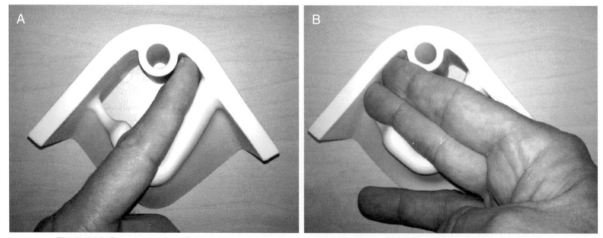

Fig. 5.7.10 Demonstration of the palpatory assessment of the levator ani for the diagnosis of avulsion. On the intact side (A), the vaginal formix, which is the space between the urethra medially, the inferior pubic ramus superiorly and the purobectalis muscle laterally, admits one finger only. On the abnormal side (B), there is much more room in that space, and no contractile tissue can be palpated on the inferior pubic ramus.

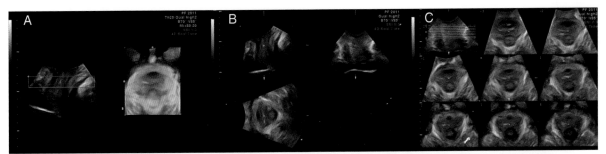

Fig. 5.7.11 The three main steps in producing a tomographic representation of the levator ani on translabial 4D ultrasound. (A) Recording of a pelvic floor contraction on volume imaging. (B) Identification of the axial plane of minimal hiatal dimensions (bottom panel) on sectional plane imaging. (C) Switch to tomographic mode in the axial plane with an interslice interval of 2.5 mm.

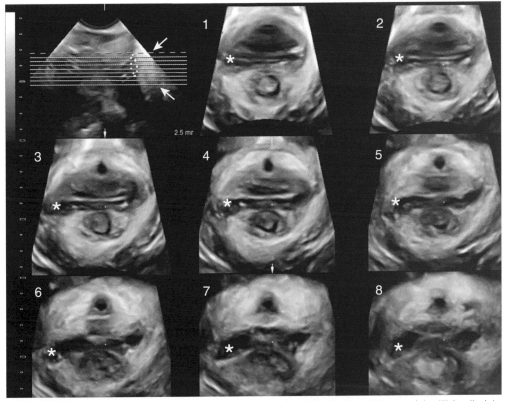

Fig. 5.7.12 Tomographic representation of a full right-sided avulsion indicated by asterisks (*) in all eight panels. The minimal criterion for the diagnosis of a full avulsion is a detachment of the puborectalis from the inferior pubic rami in slices 3 to 5, but, as in this case of a patient with above-average muscle mass, the damage is often much more extensive. The top left-hand corner shows the coronal reference plane in which the (largely) intact left puborectalis is indicated by an arrow. Minor partial trauma on this side is evident as an alteration of the normally smooth drop-shaped contour of the levator, outlined by dots. The right puborectalis muscle is entirely absent in this coronal plane view.

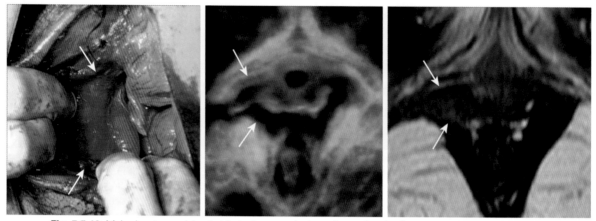

Fig. 5.7.13 Major levator avulsion behind a large vaginal tear immediately after a normal vaginal delivery at term (left panel). Despite attempts at repairing the defect, it is still evident 3 months later on ultrasound (middle) and magnetic resonance imaging (right). *(Modified from Dietz et al. [2007], with permission.)*

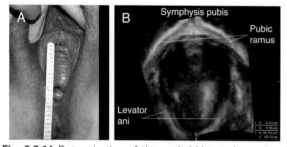

Fig. 5.7.14 Determination of the genital hiatus plus perineal body using the POPStix disposable wooden ruler (A) and measurement of hiatal dimensions on ultrasound (B). *(From Gerges et al. [2012], with permission.)*

of more cranial aspects of the levator ani. Avulsion also causes enlargement and asymmetry of the levator hiatus (Abdool et al., 2009; Dietz et al., 2011b), and both can sometimes be detected by simple observation during a Valsalva manoeuvre. Enlargement of the hiatus ('ballooning') is usually measured on axial plane imaging, but simple clinical measurement of the genital hiatus and perineal body is strongly correlated with the hiatal area, as well as symptoms and signs of prolapse (Fig. 5.7.14) (Gerges et al., 2013; Khunda et al., 2012). Measurements of 7 cm or more for the distance between external urethral meatus and anus (genital hiatus plus the perineal body) are defined as 'clinical ballooning' (Gerges et al., 2013).

Recent meta-analyses have clarified risk factors and clinical consequences of avulsion. It is likely that factors such as birth weight, length of second stage and size of the fetal head increase the probability of avulsion injury, but the use of forceps is by far the most major modifiable risk factor (Friedman et al., 2019). Forceps should

probably be regarded as obsolete, except in situations of imminent fetal demise. Unfortunately, many other 'predictors' of avulsion are of limited use since they are not available prior to the onset of labour. To prevent avulsion, we need risk factors that can be determined during pregnancy. The one useful predictor seems to be maternal age (Dietz and Kirby, 2010; Dietz and Simpson, 2007; Low et al., 2014; Speksnijder et al., 2019; Urbankova et al., 2019). Finally, one should point out that it is usually the first vaginal delivery that causes by far the most morphological and functional alteration, both in terms of actual tears as well as in terms of levator distensibility or pelvic organ support (Atan et al., 2018; Dickie et al., 2010; Dietz et al., 2020; Horak et al., 2014; Kamisan Atan et al., 2015).

Unsurprisingly, avulsion has substantial medium- and long-term consequences. The puborectalis muscle is the main determinant of intravaginal pressures (Jung et al., 2007) and has been termed the *love muscle* in the popular press. It is not surprising that women notice the effect of avulsion on PFM strength (Dietz et al., 2012d) and sexual function. The latter seems to primarily manifest as reduced tone and 'vaginal laxity' (Thibault-Gagnon et al., 2012).

In the long term, the most substantial consequence of levator trauma is pelvic organ prolapse (Deprest et al., 2022), especially of the anterior and central compartments (Dietz and Simpson, 2008). The larger a defect is, both in width and depth, the more likely are symptoms and/or signs of prolapse (Dietz, 2007). The effect of avulsion on prolapse is partly mediated through ballooning (Dietz et al., 2012c; Handa et al., 2019) or abnormal distensibility of the levator hiatus, which also is associated with prolapse (Dietz et al., 2008). One of the more intriguing findings is an association between rectal intussusception, an early form of rectal prolapse, and avulsion as well as ballooning (Rodrigo et al., 2011). The most important issue for the surgeon is that both avulsion and ballooning are the best-defined and most substantial risk factors for prolapse recurrence (Friedman et al., 2018). This implies that such findings are likely to become useful for surgical planning.

The effect of avulsion on urinary and fecal incontinence is much less clear. We often assume that urinary incontinence is a sign of a weak pelvic floor, which may be a misconception. There is some evidence that major levator avulsion defects may be *negatively* associated with stress urinary incontinence and urodynamic stress incontinence (Dietz et al., 2009; Morgan et al., 2010). How can this be explained in view of the fact that PFM training is a proven therapeutic intervention in women with stress urinary incontinence (Wilson et al., 2005)? If the puborectalis muscle is part of the urinary continence mechanism, should it not matter if this muscle is disconnected from the inferior pubic ramus?

The therapeutic success of PFM training does not prove a role of the levator ani muscle in stress urinary continence. The intervention trains not just the levator muscle but likely all muscle innervated by the pudendal nerve and associated pelvic nerves arising from S2 to S4. What is more, there are other mechanisms by which childbirth might affect urinary continence. Denervation is one (Allen et al., 1990), and damage to the urethral rhabdosphincter or the longitudinal smooth muscle of the urethra may be another. Finally, there is the issue of pressure transmission, likely mediated through the pubourethral ligaments and/or suburethral tissues. With regard to anal or faecal incontinence, some studies have identified no significant association with levator trauma (Chantarasorn et al., 2011; van de Geest and Steensma, 2010), whereas others found levator avulsion to be an independent risk factor for faecal incontinence after primary obstetric anal sphincter injury (OASI) repair (Shek et al., 2012). Such studies are complicated by the fact that obstetric anal sphincter tears and avulsion share many risk factors such as forceps, birth weight and maternal age. It is therefore not surprising that there is an increased incidence of OASI in women with avulsion, and vice versa (Heliker et al., 2021; Shek et al., 2016; Volloyhaug et al., 2019).

THE ANAL SPHINCTER

Anal sphincter imaging is more complex (and takes longer to teach and learn) than the imaging of levator trauma.

Avulsion is rarely diagnosed and never repaired, which means that findings on imaging are unaltered since the moment of trauma. Surgical repair of OASI can lead to substantial distortion and influence the association between trauma and subsequent symptoms. In addition, anal sphincter tears potentially affect two structures—the IAS and EAS—not just one. The association between imaging findings and symptoms is less clear than it is for levator trauma and weak to absent in postmenopausal women (Dietz and Shek, 2021); however, latency between trauma and symptoms is clearly less for OASI (Turel et al., 2019a).

The anal sphincters are usually imaged with endoanal ultrasound (Jha and Sultan, 2015) and MRI (Meriwether et al., 2019). Exoanal ultrasound of the sphincters was first described in 1997 (Peschers et al., 1997a) and is now widely used to image the anal sphincter. The use of 4D probes allows tomographic representation of the anal canal and can identify structures, such as the fascial plane between the EAS and levator ani, which have not been described before, and identify subdivisions of the EAS (Dietz, 2018; Turel et al., 2019b). Normal values for the IAS and EAS have been published (Magpoc Mendoza et al., 2019). There is fair to good agreement with endoanal ultrasound (Stuart et al., 2019; Taithongchai et al., 2019; Zhao et al., 2023). Abdominal probes may have advantages over vaginal transducers (Cattani et al., 2020).

The same transducers as for pelvic floor imaging can be used for the sphincters, by rotating them 90 degrees clockwise after performance of a standard pelvic floor ultrasound. Steep inclination from ventrocaudal to dorsocranial provides a coronal view of the anal canal (Fig. 5.7.15A). This results in a representation of orthogonal planes as in Fig. 5.7.15B, and tomographic imaging as shown in Figs. 5.7.15C, 5.7.16 and 5.7.17. Application of additional gel in the midline fills the labial fold; hirsute labia are parted. Imaging is preferably performed on PFMC, which seems to enhance the definition of muscular defects, but imaging at rest is also acceptable (Subramaniam et al., 2020). The interslice interval is adjusted individually, placing slice 1 above the external sphincter (see Fig. 5.7.15C) and slice 8 below the internal sphincter.

EAS defects as in Fig. 5.7.16 are associated with anal incontinence, both after primary repair (Shek et al., 2014; Turel et al., 2019a) and later in life (Guzman Rojas et al., 2015). To quantify the degree of trauma, the number of slices showing a defect of the EAS (see Figs. 5.7.16 and 5.7.17) is determined, with four to six abnormal slices defined as a 'residual defect'. The defect angle can be measured as in Fig. 5.7.17. As shown in this

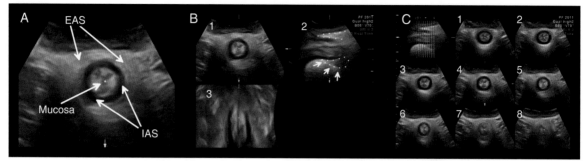

Fig. 5.7.15 The three main steps in producing a tomographic representation of the anal canal on translabial 4D ultrasound. (A) Identification of the external anal sphincter (EAS) and the internal anal sphincter (IAS) on volume imaging. (B) Identification of the fascial plane between the EAS (dots in panel 2) and the levator ani on sectional plane imaging during pelvic floor muscle contraction (arrows in panel 2). (C) Switch to tomographic mode in the coronal plane with an individually adjusted interslice interval, resulting in slice 1 being cranial to the EAS, whereas slice 8 is below the IAS.

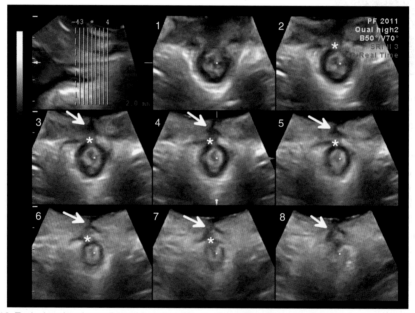

Fig. 5.7.16 Typical perineal tear (branching dark line in slices 3–8) in continuity with a suboptimally repaired 3B obstetric anal sphincter injury, with external anal sphincter defects remaining in slices 2 through 7. This appearance is rated as a 'residual defect' after obstetric anal sphincter injury repair.

figure, the adequacy of episiotomy can also be assessed, provided that one avoids compression of the perineum (Housmans et al., 2023; Subramaniam et al., 2022). Both the accuracy of clinical diagnosis (Gillor et al., 2020) as well as the quality of OASI repair (Shek et al., 2014; Turel et al., 2019a) can be monitored, which allows such measures to be documented as key performance indicators of obstetric services, together with levator trauma (Dietz et al., 2015). As with levator trauma, forceps are the main risk factor (Dietz et al., 2023).

CONCLUSION

Ultrasound imaging, and particularly translabial or transperineal ultrasound, has become an important clinical and research tool for assessing the pelvic floor. The methodology has been standardized by six international societies (AIUM/IUGA, 2019) and is taught online by the International Urogynecology Association (https://www.iuga.org/education/pfic/pfic-overview). Although much information on PFM morphology and

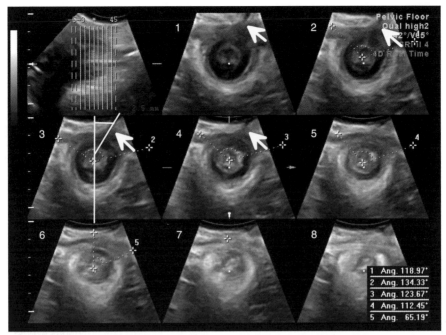

Fig. 5.7.17 Overlooked, unrepaired 3B obstetric anal sphincter injury with a well-repaired episiotomy. The angle measurements illustrate quantification of this tear which measures well over 30 degrees in slices 2 to 6. It is also evident that the episiotomy (arrow) was started 'contralaterally' (i.e., on the wrong side of the midline) and was cut too steep (i.e., towards the anal canal rather than away from it), as indicated by the lines in slice 3.

function can be gleaned easily and cheaply using 2D ultrasound systems, direct demonstration of the inferior aspects of the levator is much simplified by axial plane imaging (i.e., 3D/4D ultrasound). The availability of this technology is increasing rapidly, with hundreds of thousands of such systems installed worldwide. Physical therapists, urologists and gynaecologists are in the process of discovering the usefulness of such systems for their field. Undoubtedly, pelvic floor imaging by ultrasound provides a superior tool for research and clinical assessment. It will alter our perception of pelvic floor morbidity and hopefully enhance our means of treating the same.

There is currently no evidence to prove that modern imaging techniques improve patient outcomes, which is a limitation that is true for most diagnostic modalities in clinical medicine. Due to methodological issues, the situation is unlikely to improve soon. In the meantime, it has to be recognized that any diagnostic method is only as good as the operator behind the machine, and diagnostic ultrasound is well known for its operator-dependent nature. Teaching is therefore of paramount importance to ensure that imaging techniques are used appropriately and effectively.

RECOMMENDATIONS

Pelvic floor imaging is unlikely to become a routine intervention in the hands of each and every clinical practitioner providing pelvic floor re-education, but it already is a quite useful tool for research and the most convenient imaging method currently available. Next, a list is presented of recommendations for the clinical use of ultrasound equipment in assessing pelvic floor function via the translabial route.

Equipment

- Real-time B mode capable diagnostic ultrasound system
- Cine loop function
- 3.5- to 5- to 6-MHz curved array transducers with a footprint of at least 6 cm
- Black and white video printer
- Non-powdered gloves
- Ultrasound gel
- Alcoholic wipes for disinfection of probes between patients
- Optional: 3D/4D capability, tomographic/multislice imaging, speckle reduction

Examination

- Position the patient supine (lithotomy), with feet close to the buttocks, and the lower abdomen and legs covered with a sheet for privacy.
- Examine after voiding (and defaecation if possible).
  - Cover the contact surface of the transducer with gel, then with a glove/transducer cover while avoiding bubbles between the transducer and cover;
- Place the transducer in the midsagittal plane after parting the labia (if necessary).
- Ask the patient to cough to clear air bubbles/detritus.
  - Perform at least three manoeuvres (Valsalva, PFMC) each, and watch for incorrect manoeuvres such as levator activation with Valsalva and vice versa.
  - Observe the presence/absence of reflex muscle activation, in the sense of a dorsocaudal movement of the prepubic fat pad and ventral movement of the posterior aspect of the levator ani muscle on coughing.
  - Provide biofeedback teaching.
  - Compare images and measurements at rest and on manoeuvre.
  - Obtain hiatal dimensions (axial plane) at rest and on Valsalva.

Documentation for Assessment of Pelvic Floor Muscle Contraction

- Position of bladder neck or midsagittal hiatal diameter at rest and on PFMC
- Need for teaching/biofeedback and success of teaching
- Presence of reflex contraction on coughing
- Levator integrity assessment using axial plane tomographic imaging

REFERENCES

Abdool, Z., Shek, K., & Dietz, H. (2009). The effect of levator avulsion on hiatal dimensions and function. *American Journal of Obstetrics and Gynecology, 201*, 89.e1–89.e5.

AIUM/IUGA, 2019. AIUM/IUGA practice parameter for the performance of urogynecological ultrasound examinations: Developed in collaboration with the ACR, the AUGS, the AUA, and the SRU. *International Urogynecology Journal, 30*(9), 1389–1400.

Allen, R. E., Hosker, G. L., Smith, A. R., et al. (1990). Pelvic floor damage and childbirth: A neurophysiological study. *British Journal of Obstetrics and Gynaecology, 97*(9), 770–779.

Atan, I., Lin, S., Dietz, H., et al. (2018). It is the first birth that does the damage: A cross-sectional study 20 years after delivery. *International Urogynecology Journal, 29*, 1637–1643.

Balmforth, J., Toosz-Hobson, P., & Cardozo, L. (2003). Ask not what childbirth can do to your pelvic floor but what your pelvic floor can do in childbirth. *Neurourology and Urodynamics, 22*(5), 540–542.

Cattani, L., Van Schoubroeck, D., Housmans, S., et al. (2020). Exo-anal imaging of the anal sphincter: A comparison between introital and transperineal image acquisition. *International Urogynecology Journal, 31*, 1107–1113.

Chantarasorn, V., Shek, K., & Dietz, H. (2011). Sonographic detection of puborectalis muscle avulsion is not associated with anal incontinence. *The Australian and New Zealand Journal of Obstetrics and Gynaecology, 51*(2), 130–135.

DeLancey, J. O. (2001). Anatomy. In L. Cardozo, & D. Staskin (Eds.), *Textbook of female urology and urogynaecology* (pp. 112–124). London: Isis Medical Media.

Deprest, J. A., Cartwright, R., Dietz, H. P., et al. (2022). International Urogynecological Consultation (IUC): Pathophysiology of Pelvic Organ Prolapse (POP). *International Urogynecology Journal, 33*(7), 1699–1710.

Dickie, K., Shek, K., & Dietz, H. (2010). The relationship between urethral mobility and parity. *British Journal of Obstetrics and Gynaecology, 117*(10), 1220–1224.

Dietz, H. (2004a). Levator function before and after childbirth. *The Australian and New Zealand Journal of Obstetrics and Gynaecology, 44*(1), 19–23.

Dietz, H. (2004b). Ultrasound imaging of the pelvic floor: 3D aspects. *Ultrasound in Obstetrics and Gynecology, 23*(6), 615–625.

Dietz, H. P. (2004c). Ultrasound imaging of the pelvic floor. Part I: Two-dimensional aspects. *Ultrasound in Obstetrics and Gynecology, 23*(1), 80–92.

Dietz, H. (2007). Quantification of major morphological abnormalities of the levator ani. *Ultrasound in Obstetrics and Gynecology, 29*, 329–334.

Dietz, H. (2010). Pelvic floor ultrasound: A review. *American Journal of Obstetrics and Gynecology, 202*, 321–334.

Dietz, H. P. (2011a). Pelvic floor ultrasound in incontinence: what's in it for the surgeon? *International Urogynecology Journal, 22*(9), 1085–1097.

Dietz, H. P. (2011b). Pelvic floor ultrasound in prolapse: what's in it for the surgeon? *International Urogynecology Journal, 22*, 1221–1232.

Dietz, H. (2015). Forceps: Towards obsolescence or revival? *Acta Obstetricia et Gynecologica Scandinavica, 94*(4), 347–351.

Dietz, H. (2018). Exo-anal imaging of the anal sphincters: A pictorial introduction. *Journal of Ultrasound in Medicine, 2018*, 263–280.

Dietz, H., & Kirby, A. (2010). Modelling the likelihood of levator avulsion in a urogynaecological population. *The Australian and New Zealand Journal of Obstetrics and Gynaecology, 50*, 268–272.

Dietz, H. P., & Shek, C. (2008a). Levator avulsion and grading of pelvic floor muscle strength. *International Urogynecology Journal, 19*(5), 633–636.

Dietz, H. P., & Shek, K. L. (2008b). Validity and reproducibility of the digital detection of levator trauma. *International Urogynecology Journal, 19*, 1097–1101.

Dietz, H. P., & Shek, K. L. (2009). Levator trauma can be diagnosed by 2D translabial ultrasound. *International Urogynecology Journal, 20*, 807–811.

Dietz, H. P., & Shek, K. L. (2021). Confounders of the relationship between anal sphincter trauma and anal incontinence. *International Urogynecology Journal, 33*(S1), S40–S41.

Dietz, H. P., Shek, K. L., & Low, G. K. (2022). All or nothing? A second look at partial levator avulsion. *Ultrasound in Obstetrics and Gynecology, 60*(5), 693–697.

Dietz, H. P., Shek, K. L., & Low, G. (2023). Obstetric risk factors for anal sphincter trauma in a urogynecological population. *International Urogynecology Journal, 34*(2), 425–430.

Dietz, H., & Simpson, J. (2007). Does delayed childbearing increase the risk of levator injury in labour? *The Australian and New Zealand Journal of Obstetrics and Gynaecology, 47*, 491–495.

Dietz, H., & Simpson, J. (2008). Levator trauma is associated with pelvic organ prolapse. *British Journal of Obstetrics and Gynaecology, 115*, 979–984.

Dietz, H., Bernardo, M., Kirby, A., et al. (2011a). Minimal criteria for the diagnosis of avulsion of the puborectalis muscle by tomographic ultrasound. *International Urogynecology Journal, 22*(6), 699–704.

Dietz, H., Bhalla, R., Chantarasorn, V., et al. (2011b). Avulsion of the puborectalis muscle causes asymmetry of the levator hiatus. *Ultrasound in Obstetrics and Gynecology, 37*(6), 723–726.

Dietz, H., Bond, V., & Shek, K. (2012a). Does childbirth alter the reflex pelvic floor response to sudden increases in intra-abdominal pressure? *Ultrasound in Obstetrics and Gynecology, 39*, 569–573.

Dietz, H., De Leon, J., & Shek, K. (2008). Ballooning of the levator hiatus. *Ultrasound in Obstetrics and Gynecology, 31*, 676–680.

Dietz, H., Erdmann, M., & Shek, K. (2012b). Reflex contraction of the levator ani in women symptomatic for pelvic floor disorders. *Ultrasound in Obstetrics and Gynecology, 40*(2), 215–218.

Dietz, H., Franco, A., Shek, K., et al. (2012c). Avulsion injury and levator hiatal ballooning: Two independent risk factors for prolapse? An observational study. *Acta Obstetricia et Gynecologica Scandinavica, 91*(2), 211–214.

Dietz, H., Gillespie, A., & Phadke, P. (2007). Avulsion of the pubovisceral muscle associated with large vaginal tear after normal vaginal delivery at term. *The Australian and New Zealand Journal of Obstetrics and Gynaecology, 47*, 341–344.

Dietz, H., Hansell, N., Grace, M., et al. (2005a). Bladder neck mobility is a heritable trait. *British Journal of Obstetrics and Gynaecology, 112*, 334–339.

Dietz, H. P., Haylen, B. T., & Broome, J. (2001a). Ultrasound in the quantification of female pelvic organ prolapse. *Ultrasound in Obstetrics and Gynecology, 18*(5), 511–514.

Dietz, H. P., Jarvis, S. K., & Vancaillie, T. G. (2002). The assessment of levator muscle strength: A validation of three ultrasound techniques. *International Urogynecology Journal, 13*(3), 156–159.

Dietz, H., Kirby, A., Shek, K., et al. (2009). Does avulsion of the puborectalis muscle affect bladder function? *International Urogynecology Journal, 20*, 967–972.

Dietz, H. P., Moore, K. H., & Steensma, A. B. (2003). Antenatal pelvic organ mobility is associated with delivery mode. *The Australian and New Zealand Journal of Obstetrics and Gynaecology, 43*(1), 70–74.

Dietz, H., Pardey, J., & Murray, H. (2015). Pelvic floor and anal sphincter trauma should be key performance indicators of maternity services. *International Urogynecology Journal, 26*, 29–32.

Dietz, H., Shek, K., Chantarasorn, V., et al. (2012d). Do women notice the effect of childbirth-related pelvic floor trauma? *The Australian and New Zealand Journal of Obstetrics and Gynaecology, 52*(3), 277–281.

Dietz, H., Shek, K., & Clarke, B. (2005b). Biometry of the pubovisceral muscle and levator hiatus by three-dimensional pelvic floor ultrasound. *Ultrasound in Obstetrics and Gynecology, 25*, 580–585.

Dietz, H., Walsh, C., Friedman, T., et al. (2020). Levator avulsion and vaginal parity: Do subsequent vaginal births matter? *International Urogynecology Journal, 31*, 2311–2315.

Dietz, H., Wilson, P., & Milsom, I. (2016). Maternal birth trauma: Why should it matter to urogynaecologists? *Current Opinion in Obstetrics and Gynecology, 28*(5), 441–448.

Dietz, H. P., Wilson, P. D., & Clarke, B. (2001b). The use of perineal ultrasound to quantify levator activity and teach pelvic floor muscle exercises. *International Urogynecology Journal and Pelvic Floor Dysfunction, 12*(3), 166–168 discussion 168–169.

Dietz, H., Wong, V., & Shek, K. L. (2011c). A simplified method for determining hiatal biometry. *The Australian and New Zealand Journal of Obstetrics and Gynaecology, 51*, 540–543.

Friedman, T., Eslick, G., & Dietz, H. (2018). Risk factors for prolapse recurrence: Systematic review and meta-analysis. *International Urogynecology Journal, 29*(1), 13–21.

Friedman, T., Eslick, G., & Dietz, H. P. (2019). Delivery mode and the risk of levator muscle avulsion: A meta-analysis. *International Urogynecology Journal, 30*, 901–907.

Gerges, B., Kamisan Atan, I., Shek, K., et al. (2013). How to determine "ballooning" of the levator hiatus on clinical examination: A retrospective observational study. *International Urogynecology Journal, 24*(11), 1933–1937.

Gillor, M., Shek, K., & Dietz, H. (2020). How comparable is the clinical grading of obstetric anal sphincter injury with that determined by four-dimensional translabial ultrasound? *Ultrasound in Obstetrics and Gynecology, 56*(4), 618–623.

Gritzky, A., & Brandl, H. (1998). The Voluson (Kretz) technique. In E. Merz (Ed.), *3-D ultrasound in obstetrics and gynecology* (pp. 9–15). Philadelphia: Lippincott Williams & Wilkins Healthcare.

Guzman Rojas, R., Kamisan Atan, I., Shek, K., et al. (2015). Anal sphincter trauma and anal incontinence in urogynecological patients. *Ultrasound in Obstetrics and Gynecology, 46*, 363–366.

Guzman Rojas, R., Kamisan Atan, I., Shek, K., et al. (2016). The prevalence of abnormal posterior compartment anatomy and its association with obstructed defecation symptoms in urogynecological patients. *International Urogynecology Journal, 27*(6), 939–944.

Handa, V., Roem, J., Blomquist, J., et al. (2019). Pelvic organ prolapse as a function of levator ani avulsion, hiatus size, and strength. *American Journal of Obstetrics and Gynecology, 221*, 41.e1–41.e7.

Heliker, B., Kenton, K., Leader-Cramer, A., et al. (2021). Adding insult to injury: Levator ani avulsion in women with obstetric anal sphincter injuries. *Female Pelvic Medicine & Reconstructive Surgery, 27*(7), 462–467.

Hoff Braekken, I., Majida, M., Ellstrom Engh, M., et al. (2008). Test–retest and intra-observer repeatability of two-, three- and four-dimensional perineal ultrasound of pelvic floor muscle anatomy and function. *International Urogynecology Journal, 19*, 227–235.

Horak, A., Guzman Rojas, R., Shek, K., et al. (2014). Pelvic floor trauma: Does the second baby matter? *Ultrasound in Obstetrics and Gynecology, 44*(1), 90–94.

Housmans, S., Gillor, M., Shek, K. L., et al. (2023). Assessment of perineal scars on translabial pelvic floor ultrasound: A pilot study. *Journal of Ultrasound in Medicine, 42*(4), 881–888.

Jha, S., & Sultan, A. (2015). Obstetric anal sphincter injury: The changing landscape. *British Journal of Obstetrics and Gynaecology, 122*(7), 931.

Jung, S., Pretorius, D., Padda, B., et al. (2007). Vaginal high-pressure zone assessed by dynamic 3-dimensional ultrasound images of the pelvic floor. *American Journal of Obstetrics and Gynecology, 197*(1), 52.e1–52.e7.

Kamisan Atan, I., Gerges, B., Shek, K., et al. (2015). The association between vaginal childbirth and hiatal dimensions: A retrospective observational study in a tertiary urogynaecological centre. *British Journal of Obstetrics and Gynaecology, 122*(6), 867–872.

Khunda, A., Shek, K., & Dietz, H. (2012). Can ballooning of the levator hiatus be determined clinically? *American Journal of Obstetrics and Gynecology, 206*(3), 246.e1–246.e4.

Kruger, J., Heap, S., Murphy, B., et al. (2010). How best to measure the levator hiatus: Evidence for the non-euclidean nature of the 'plane of minimal dimensions. *Ultrasound in Obstetrics and Gynecology, 36*, 755–758.

Kruger, J., Heap, X., Murphy, B., et al. (2008). Pelvic floor function in nulliparous women using 3-dimensional ultrasound and magnetic resonance imaging. *Obstetrics & Gynecology, 111*, 631–638.

Lanzarone, V., & Dietz, H. (2007). Three-dimensional ultrasound imaging of the levator hiatus in late pregnancy and associations with delivery outcomes. *The Australian and New Zealand Journal of Obstetrics and Gynaecology, 47*(3), 176–180.

Low, L., Zielinski, R., Tao, Y., et al. (2014). Predicting birth-related levator ani tear severity in primiparous women: Evaluating Maternal Recovery from Labor and Delivery (EMRLD Study). *Open Journal of Obstetrics and Gynecology, 4*(6), 266–278.

Magpoc Mendoza, J., Turel Fatakia, F., Kamisan Atan, I., et al. (2019). Normal values of anal sphincter biometry by 4-dimensional translabial ultrasound. a retrospective study of pregnant women in their third trimester. *Journal of Ultrasound in Medicine, 38*(10), 2733–2738.

Meriwether, K., Lockhart, M., Meyer, I., et al. (2019). Anal sphincter anatomy prepregnancy to postdelivery among the same primiparous women on dynamic magnetic resonance imaging. *Female Pelvic Medicine & Reconstructive Surgery, 25*(1), 8–14.

Miller, J., Ashton-Miller, J., & DeLancey, J. O. (1996). The knack: Use of precisely timed pelvic floor muscle contraction can reduce leakage in SUI. *Neurourology and Urodynamics, 15*(4), 392–393.

Morgan, D., Cardoza, P., Guire, K., et al. (2010). Levator ani defect status and lower urinary tract symptoms in women with pelvic organ prolapse. *International Urogynecology Journal, 21*(1), 47–52.

Nazemian, K., Shek, K., Martin, A., et al. (2013). Can urodynamic stress incontinence be diagnosed by ultrasound? *International Urogynecology Journal, 24*, 1399–1403.

Oerno, A., & Dietz, H. (2007). Levator co-activation is a significant confounder of pelvic organ descent on Valsalva maneuver. *Ultrasound in Obstetrics and Gynecology, 30*, 346–350.

Orejuela, F., Shek, K., & Dietz, H. (2012). The time factor in the assessment of prolapse and levator ballooning. *International Urogynecology Journal, 23*, 175–178.

Oversand, S., Dietz, H., Kamisan Atan, I., et al. (2015). The association between different measures of pelvic floor muscle function and female pelvic organ prolapse. *International Urogynecology Journal, 26*(12), 1777–1781.

Peschers, U. M., DeLancey, J. O., Schaer, G. N., et al. (1997a). Exoanal ultrasound of the anal sphincter: Normal anatomy and sphincter defects. *British Journal of Obstetrics and Gynaecology, 104*(9), 999–1003.

Peschers, U. M., Schaer, G. N., DeLancey, J. O., et al. (1997b). Levator ani function before and after childbirth. *British Journal of Obstetrics and Gynaecology, 104*(9), 1004–1008.

Rodrigo, N., Shek, K., & Dietz, H. (2011). Rectal intussusception is associated with abnormal levator structure and morphometry. *Techniques in Coloproctology, 15*, 39–43.

Schaer, G. N. (1997). Ultrasonography of the lower urinary tract. *Current Opinion in Obstetrics and Gynecology, 9*, 313–316.

Shek, K., & Dietz, H. (2016). Assessment of pelvic organ prolapse: A review. *Ultrasound in Obstetrics and Gynecology, 48*, 681–692.

Shek, K., & Dietz, H. (2019). Vaginal birth and pelvic floor trauma. *Current Obstetrics Gynecology Reprod, 8*, 15–25.

Shek, K., Green, K., Hall, J., et al. (2016). Perineal and vaginal tears are clinical markers for occult levator ani trauma: A retrospective observational study. *Ultrasound in Obstetrics and Gynecology, 47*, 224–227.

Shek, K., Guzman Rojas, R., & Dietz, H. (2014). Residual defects of the external anal sphincter following primary repair: An observational study using transperineal ultrasound. *Ultrasound in Obstetrics and Gynecology, 44*, 704–709.

Shek, K., Guzman Rojas, R., & Dietz, H. P. (2012). Residual defects of the external anal sphincter are common after OASIS repair. *Neurourology and Urodynamics, 31*(6), 913–914.

Speksnijder, L., Oom, D., Van Bavel, J., et al. (2019). Association of levator injury and urogynecological complaints in women after their first vaginal birth with and without mediolateral episiotomy. *American Journal of Obstetrics and Gynecology, 220*(1), 93.e1–93.e9.

Stuart, A., Ignell, C., & Orno, A. (2019). Comparison of transperineal and endoanal ultrasound in detecting residual obstetric anal sphincter injury. *Acta Obstetricia et Gynecologica Scandinavica, 98*(12), 1624–1631.

Subramaniam, N., Robledo, K., & Dietz, H. (2020). Anal sphincter imaging: Better done at rest or on pelvic floor muscle contraction? *International Urogynecology Journal, 31*(6), 1191–1196.

Subramaniam, N., Shek, K. L., & Dietz, H. P. ((2022). Imaging characteristics of episiotomy scars on translabial ultrasound: An observational study. *Journal of Ultrasound in Medicine, 41*(9), 2287–2293.

Sultan, A. H. (2003). The role of anal endosonography in obstetrics. *Ultrasound in Obstetrics and Gynecology, 22*(6), 559–560.

Svabik, K., Shek, K., & Dietz, H. (2009). How much does the levator hiatus have to stretch during childbirth? *British Journal of Obstetrics and Gynaecology, 116*, 1657–1662.

Taithongchai, A., Van Gruting, I., Volloyhaug, I., et al. (2019). Comparing the diagnostic accuracy of 3 ultrasound modalities for diagnosing obstetric anal sphincter injuries. *American Journal of Obstetrics and Gynecology, 221*(2), 134.e1–134.e9.

Tan, L., Shek, K., Kamisan Atan, I., et al. (2015). The repeatability of sonographic measures of functional pelvic floor anatomy. *International Urogynecology Journal, 26*, 1667–1672.

Thibault-Gagnon, S., Yusuf, S., Langer, S., et al. (2012). Do women notice the impact of childbirth-related levator trauma on pelvic floor and sexual function? *International Urogynecology Journal, 23*(Suppl. 1), 183–185.

Thompson, J. A., & O'Sullivan, P. B. (2003). Levator plate movement during voluntary pelvic floor muscle contraction in subjects with incontinence and prolapse: A cross-sectional study and review. *International Urogynecology Journal, 14*(2), 84–88.

Turel, F., Langer, S., Shek, K., et al. (2019a). Long-term follow-up of obstetric anal sphincter injury. *Diseases of the Colon & Rectum, 62*(3), 348–356.

Turel, F., Subramaniam, N., Bienkiewicz, J., et al. (2019b). How repeatable is the assessment of external anal sphincter trauma by exoanal 4D ultrasound? *Ultrasound in Obstetrics and Gynecology, 53*, 836–840.

Urbankova, I., Grohregin, K., Hanacek, J., et al. (2019). The effect of the first vaginal birth on pelvic floor anatomy and dysfunction. *International Urogynecology Journal, 30*(10), 1689–1696.

Van de Geest, L., & Steensma, A. B. (2010). Three-dimensional transperineal ultrasound imaging of anal sphincter injuries after surgical primary repair. *Ultrasound in Obstetrics and Gynecology, 36*(Suppl. 1), 270.

Volloyhaug, I., Taithongchai, A., Van Gruting, I., et al. (2019). Levator ani muscle morphology and function in women with obstetric anal sphincter injury. *Ultrasound in Obstetrics and Gynecology, 53*(3), 410–416.

Wijma, J., Tinga, D. J., & Visser, G. H. (1991). Perineal ultrasonography in women with stress incontinence and controls: The role of the pelvic floor muscles. *Gynecologic and Obstetric Investigation, 32*(3), 176–179.

Wilson, P. D., Hay Smith, E. J., Nygaard, I. E., et al. (2005). Adult conservative management. In P. Abrams, L. Cardozo, S. Khoury, et al. (Eds.), *Incontinence: Third international consultation on incontinence, vol. 2* (pp. 855–964). Paris: Health Publications.

Yang, J., Yang, S., & Huang, W. (2006). Biometry of the pubovisceral muscle and levator hiatus in nulliparous Chinese women. *Ultrasound in Obstetrics and Gynecology, 26*, 710–716.

Zhao, B., Li, Y., Tang, Y., et al. (2023). Assessing obstetric anal sphincter injuries: A comparison of exoanal and endoanal ultrasound. *Journal of Ultrasound in Medicine, 42*(9), 2031–2038.

5.8 Magnetic Resonance Imaging of Intact and Injured Female Pelvic Floor Muscles

John OL DeLancey and James A Ashton-Miller

INTRODUCTION

Pelvic striated muscle activity is critical to normal continence and pelvic organ support. Three portions of the levator ani muscle support the pelvic organs, as described in Chapter 4. These muscles must constantly adjust to the widely varying stresses placed on the pelvic floor during daily activities that may range from sitting and reading to jumping on a trampoline to forcefully sneezing. This chapter will focus on the levator ani muscle damage seen after vaginal delivery and the implications of this damage for muscle rehabilitation.

Each muscle in the body has its own specific action. Knowing the functional loss that occurs when a muscle is injured is important to understanding the dysfunction that arises from muscle injury. When one of the levator ani muscle elements is damaged, knowing how pelvic muscle training is influenced by muscle injury type has relevance to clinical therapy. If one muscle in the shoulder, for example, is damaged, there is a characteristic impairment that results. Damage to the pectoral muscle, for example, would limit forward motion of the arm while not limiting its backward movement. Now that magnetic resonance imaging (MRI) can show us evidence of localized muscle injury in an individual, it will be possible to better understand the relationship between injury to a specific part of the muscle and specific female pelvic floor problems.

The mechanism of injury to a muscle may also influence its rehabilitation. If a muscle is weak, it can be strengthened. If a portion of the muscle is partially denervated, then the remaining muscle parts can be recruited to compensate for its muscle loss. However, if an entire muscle is lost through avulsion from its attachment and subsequent atrophy or is lost through complete denervation, then it may not be possible to improve the function of the missing muscle. In the past, knowing how a given type of pelvic floor muscle injury would respond to treatment has not been possible because it has not been possible to visualize and locate the injury. Now, with the advent of modern imaging, we can directly see the pelvic floor muscles and their injuries. There is the very real possibility that failure rates with muscle training will decline as patients are more appropriately selected for treatment based on each individual's specific situation.

MAGNETIC RESONANCE IMAGING ANATOMY OF THE NORMAL LEVATOR ANI MUSCLE STRUCTURE

The levator ani muscle consists of several parts. Each has its own origin and insertion. The suggested terms for these components, along with their origin/insertion and function, are listed in Table 5.8.1 based on a review of anatomical descriptions available in the literature (Kearney et al., 2004). These are shown in Figs. 5.8.1 and 5.8.2. Although these parts are simple and are described consistently by authors who have personally studied the muscle, a profusion of conflicting terms that have historically applied to this region makes it somewhat complicated to interpret the literature, as described in the work of Kearney et al. (2004).

The iliococcygeal muscle is a thin sheet of muscle that spans the pelvic canal from the tendinous arch of the levator ani to the midline iliococcygeal raphe where it interdigitates with the muscle of the other side and connects with the superior surface of the sacrum and coccyx.

Arising from the pubic bone and passing beside the pelvic organs is the pubovisceral muscle. This muscle has previously been called the *pubococcygeal muscle*, but we favour Lawson's term *pubovisceral* (Lawson, 1974) because it describes the origin and insertion accurately, whereas the older term is based on evolutionary considerations rather than human anatomy. Within the pubovisceral muscle are parts that attach to the perineal body (puboperinealis), and a part that inserts into the anal canal and skin (puboanal). The vaginal wall is attached to this mass of muscle, and those fibres to which the vaginal wall is attached belong to the pubovaginal portion of the pubovisceral muscle. Arising near the perineal membrane and coursing lateral to the remainder of the levator ani muscle is the puborectal muscle. It forms a sling behind the rectum and is distinct from the pubovisceral muscle. The puborectal muscle creates an angulation in the rectum, whereas the pubovisceral muscle elevates the anus, perineal body and vagina. (Lawson includes this muscle within the pubovisceral muscle complex, but we prefer a separate designation because, as Betschart et al. [2014] have shown, its line of action differs

TABLE 5.8.1 Overview of the Nomenclature and Functional Anatomy of the Levator Ani

Terminologia anatomica	Origin	Insertion	Function
Pubococcygeal (we favour 'pubovisceral')			
Puboperineal	Pubis	Perineal body	Tonic activity pulls perineal body ventrally toward pubis
Pubovaginal	Pubis	Vaginal wall at the level of the mid-urethra	Elevates vagina in region of mid-urethra
Puboanal	Pubis	Intersphineteric groove between internal and external anal sphincter to end in the anal skin	Inserts into the intersphineteric groove to elevate the anus and its attached anoderm
Puborectal	Pubis	Sling behind rectum	Forms sling behind the rectum forming the anorectal angle and closing the pelvic floor
Iliococcygeal	Tendinous arch of the levator ani	Two sides fuse in the iliococcygeal raphe	The two sides form a supportive diaphragm that spans the pelvic canal

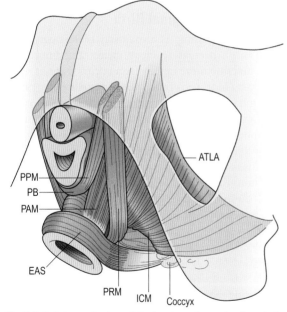

Fig. 5.8.1 Schematic view of the levator ani muscles from below after the vulvar structures and perineal membrane have been removed showing the arcus tendineus levator ani (ATLA), external anal sphincter (EAS), puboanal muscle (PAM), perineal body (PB) uniting the two ends of the puboperineal muscle (PPM), iliococcygeal muscle (ICM) and puborectal muscle (PRM). Note that the urethra and vagina have been transected just above the hymenal ring. *(From Kearney et al. (2004). © DeLancey.)*

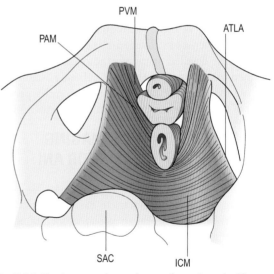

Fig. 5.8.2 The levator ani muscle seen from above looking over the sacral promontory (SAC) showing the pubovaginal muscle (PVM). The urethra, vagina and rectum have been transected just above the pelvic floor. (The internal obturator muscles have been removed to clarify levator muscle origins.) *ATLA*, Arcus tendineus levator ani; *ICM*, iliococcygeal muscle; *PAM*, puboanal muscle. *(From Kearney et al. (2004). © DeLancey.)*

by 60 degrees from that of the pubovisceral muscle.) Each of these different origin/insertion pairs has its unique mechanical action. Injury to one component may have different mechanical effects than damage to another. For example, loss of the pubovaginal muscle would prevent elevation of the anterior vaginal wall (and urethra), whereas loss of the puborectal muscle would prevent kinking of the rectum in the post-anal angle. Therefore knowing their subdivisions will make a difference to understanding how the pelvic floor works normally and what can change with a given injury.

MRI is an investigative tool that provides anatomical detail in the pelvic floor. It has allowed the detailed anatomy and integrity of the levator ani muscles to be examined with ever-improving spatial resolution and variety of radiofrequency pulse sequences and gradients. Not only has MRI revealed important insights about normal anatomy but it also allows investigators to study muscle damage while providing permanent records of muscle morphology that can be evaluated by researchers blinded to the subject's clinical status, minimizing potential observer bias. Systematic studies concerning repeatability of these techniques, their validity and their responsiveness to change are yet to be carried out. However, the detailed anatomical information that can be gained from these techniques has already established their use in research, and data concerning the performance of these measures are certain to be forthcoming.

MAGNETIC RESONANCE IMAGING APPEARANCE OF THE LEVATOR ANI MUSCLES

Damage to the levator ani muscle has been described in cadavers with pelvic organ prolapse for 100 years (Halban and Tandler, 1907). Matched cross-sections of a cadaver pelvis and MRI have clarified the anatomy of the levator ani muscles in cross-sectional imaging (Strohbehn et al., 1996). Recent advances in MRI and 3D ultrasound have allowed the muscles to be examined and demonstrated the anatomy of the muscles in serial 2D images (Fig. 5.8.3) and in 3D reconstructions (Fig. 5.8.4) (Margulies et al., 2006; Shobeiri et al., 2009). These scans show considerable variation in the normal thickness and configuration of the muscle from one individual to another (Tunn et al., 2003) (Fig. 5.8.5). As is true in other parts of the body, this variation in muscle bulk is likely attributable to a combination of genetic factors, daily demands and exercise. The amount of

muscle that an individual has should have implications for pelvic floor function and injury. A woman with a naturally bulky set of muscles may lose half of her muscle bulk due to injury or atrophy and still have the same amount of muscle as a woman with naturally delicate muscles. The consequences of these variations and damage remain to be determined.

BIRTH: A MAJOR EVENT CAUSING PELVIC FLOOR DYSFUNCTION

Vaginal birth increases the likelihood that a woman will have pelvic floor dysfunction (Mant et al., 1997; Rortveit et al., 2003), and vaginal birth has been identified as a cause of damage to the muscle (DeLancey et al., 2003). The levator ani muscle and pelvic floor undergo remarkable changes during the second stage of labour to dilate sufficiently for the fetal head to be delivered. Understanding how injury can occur and how recovery does or does not proceed are central to understanding the role of rehabilitation.

Recovery After Vaginal Birth

Pelvic muscle training is a mainstay of recovery after vaginal birth, decreasing incontinence and improving muscle function more rapidly than occurs without regular exercise (Mørkved et al., 2003; Sampselle et al., 1998). Imaging has allowed us to study the process of normal recovery and has given insight into changes the muscle must undergo to return to its normal healthy state.

Soon after delivery the pelvic floor sags and the urogenital hiatus is wider than normal (Fig. 5.8.6) (Krofta et al., 2009; Tunn et al., 1999). Muscle recovery results in resumption of the near-normal position in most women over the course of the first 6 months—the time when normal pelvic muscle strength also returns to normal (Sampselle et al., 1998). Chemical changes in the muscle where there is increased fluid from oedema in certain muscle parts early in the recovery reveal the changes in muscular tissue during the normal healing process (Fig. 5.8.7).

Injury From Vaginal Birth

Injury to the levator ani muscle has been reported in between 13% (Shek and Dietz, 2010) and 36% (Dietz and Lanzarone 2005) of women. These injuries involve the pubovisceral muscle and occasionally the iliococcygeal muscle (DeLancey et al., 2003) (Fig. 5.8.8). A recent review presents an overview of birth-related pelvic muscle injury (Dietz, 2021). Several factors indicating a

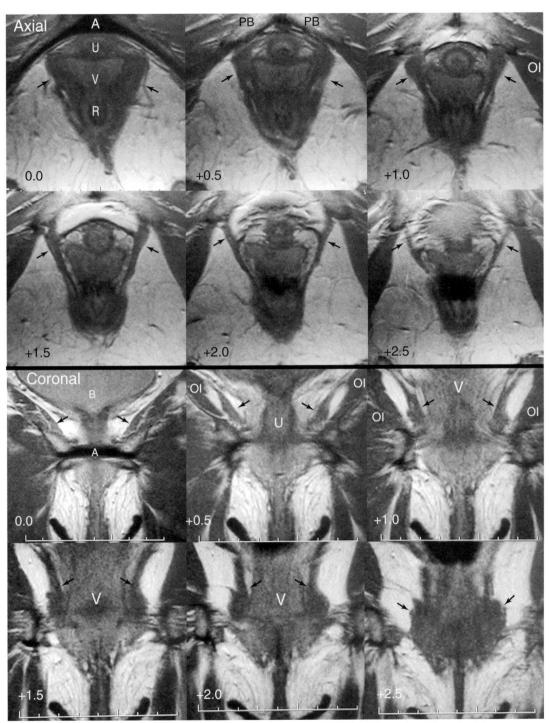

Fig. 5.8.3 Axial and coronal images from a 45-year-old nulliparous woman. The urethra (U), vagina (V), rectum (R), arcuate pubic ligament (A), pubic bones (PB) and bladder (B) are shown. Black arrows point to the levator ani muscles. The arcuate pubic ligament is designated as zero for reference, and the distance from this reference plane is indicated in the lower left corner. Note the attachment of the levator muscle to the pubic bone in axial 1.0, 1.5 and 2.0. Coronal images show the urethra, vagina and muscles of the levator ani and obturator internus (OI). *(From DeLancey et al. (2003). © DeLancey.)*

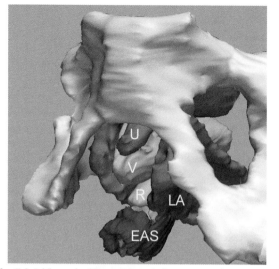

Fig. 5.8.4 View of a 3D model made from magnetic resonance imaging scans of a 34-year-old woman with normal anatomy showing the urethra (U), vagina (V), external anal sphincter (EAS), rectum (R) and levator ani (LA). *(Modified from Margulies (2006). © DeLancey.)*

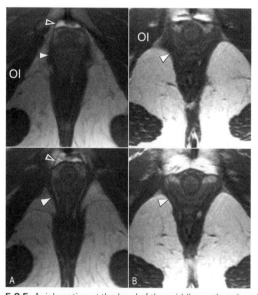

Fig. 5.8.5 Axial section at the level of the middle urethra showing the difference in levator ani muscle thickness and configuration. In this and subsequent illustrations, scans from two individuals are compared: scans from one individual are displayed on the left, and scans from the other individual are displayed on the right. (A) Thin muscle (31-year-old nulliparous woman). (B) Thicker muscle (36-year-old nulliparous woman). Note that the muscle is shaped more like a V in panel A and more like a U in panel B. The closed arrowhead points to the right levator ani muscle, and the open arrowhead points to the insertion of the arcus tendineus fasciae pelvis into the pubic bone in (B). *OI,* Obturator internus. *(From Tunn et al. (2003). © DeLancey.)*

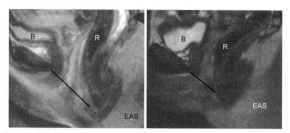

Fig. 5.8.6 T2-weighted sagittal sections of an 18-year-old woman, para 2, 1 day (left) and 6 months (right) after spontaneous vaginal delivery. The external anal sphincter (EAS) and perineal body that lies ventral to it are much lower on the first day after delivery compared with the anatomy 6 months later, and the urogenital hiatus is also larger (line). *B,* Bladder, *R,* rectum. *(From Tunn et al. (1999). © DeLancey.)*

difficult birth are associated with increased risk of injury, namely forceps, increased second stage length and larger head circumference. Forceps delivery is associated with an injury rate of 63% (Krofta et al., 2009), with an odds ratio of 3.8 for muscle avulsion, and increased second stage of labour length is associated with increased levator hiatus area (Shek and Dietz, 2010). The independent risk of forceps over and above a prolonged second stage is supported by the observation that women delivered with forceps for a prolonged second stage have a higher rate of levator injury (63%) compared to those delivered with forceps for fetal distress (42%) (Kearney et al., 2010). Head circumference greater than 35.5 cm was associated with an odds ratio of 3.3 (Valsky et al., 2009). Vacuum-assisted vaginal birth and epidural are not associated with increased risk.

Among the women with injury to the pubovisceral muscle, the amount of muscle injury varies from one individual to another. Some of these injuries involve complete bilateral loss of pubovisceral muscle bulk (see Fig. 5.8.8), whereas others have only unilateral loss (Fig. 5.8.9). There is also variation in the amount of architectural distortion that occurs. Some individuals show major changes in the overall architecture (Fig. 5.8.10), whereas others have intact spatial relationships (Fig. 5.8.11). Whether this represents the difference between a muscle rupture that distorts muscle appearance or denervation that simply results in loss of muscle without deformity remains to be determined.

What Are the Mechanisms of Levator Injury?

Several injury mechanisms have been hypothesized. Neuropathy, muscle tearing or stretch, and compression have all been suggested. The earliest studies of muscle

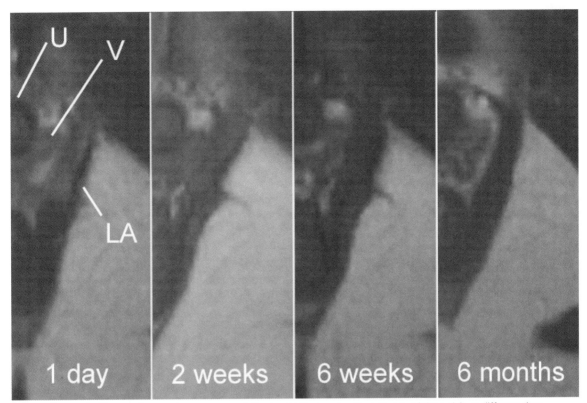

Fig. 5.8.7 Changes in muscle appearance following birth showing the left side of the pelvis at different time points after delivery. The urethra (U), vagina (V) and levator ani (LA) can be seen. Notice the increasing definition of the structures postpartum, especially the medial portion of the levator ani muscle adjacent to the vagina, which is quite pale 1 day after delivery but recovers its signal by 6 months. © *DeLancey.*)

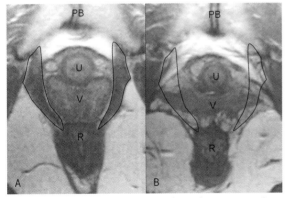

Fig. 5.8.8 (A) Axial proton density magnetic resonance imaging shows normal pubococcygeal muscle with the muscle outlined at the level of the mid-urethra. (B) A similar image from a woman with complete loss of the pubococcygeal muscle (expected location of the pubococcygeal muscle is shown by the outline). *PB*, Pubic bone; *R*, rectum; *U*, urethra, *V*, vagina. *(From DeLancey (2005). © DeLancey.)*

injury used electrodiagnostic techniques demonstrating that birth causes changes in mean motor unit duration after vaginal birth (Allen et al., 1990) as well as neuropathic changes outside the normal range in electromyographic examination turns/amplitude data in 29% of women at 6 months postpartum (Weidner et al., 2006). Abnormal tests have been seen in women with both prolapse and stress incontinence (Weidner et al., 2000). Although the pudendal nerve innervates the voluntary urethral and anal sphincters, it does not innervate the levator ani muscles, which receive their own nerve supply from the sacral plexus (Barber et al., 2002). These techniques, however, cannot distinguish between mechanisms for the visible abnormality seen in imaging.

Recently, techniques used in musculoskeletal MRI that allow injury mechanisms to be determined were applied to study the muscle in women at high risk for injury after vaginal birth (Miller et al., 2010). The injury

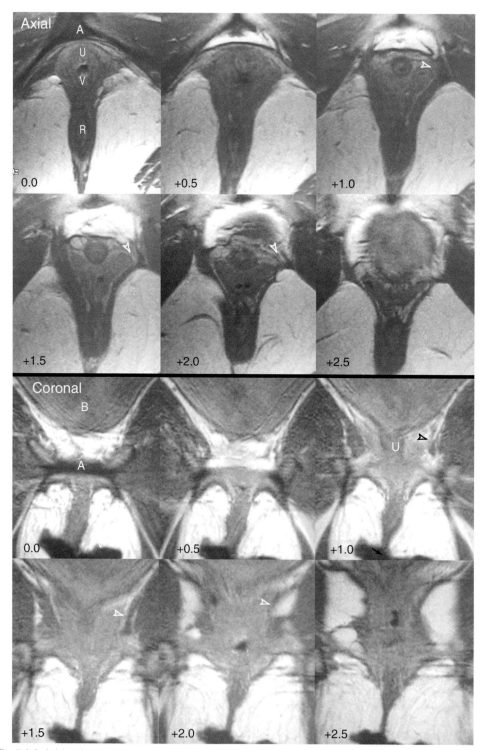

Fig. 5.8.9 Axial and coronal images from a 34-year-old incontinent primiparous woman showing a unilateral defect in the left pubovisceral portion of the levator ani muscle. The arcuate pubic ligament (A), urethra (U), vagina (V), rectum (R) and bladder (B) are shown. The location normally occupied by the pubovisceral muscle is indicated by the open arrowhead in axial and coronal images 1.0, 1.5 and 2.0. *(From DeLancey et al. (2003). © DeLancey.)*

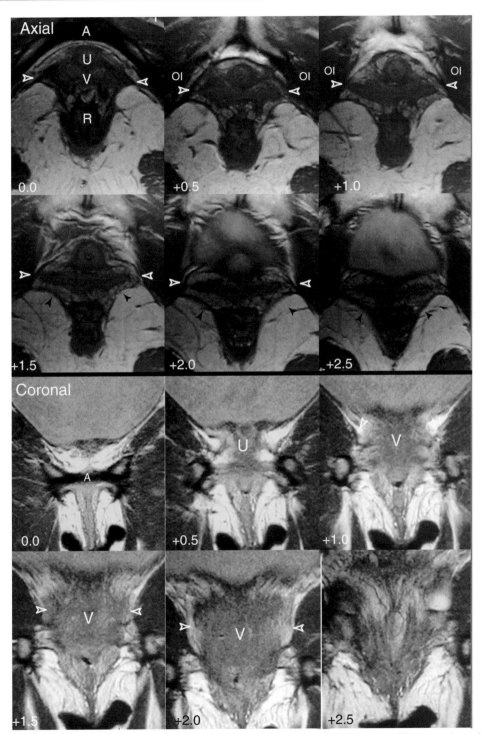

Fig. 5.8.10 Axial and coronal images of a 38-year-old incontinent primiparous woman. The area where the pubovisceral portion of the levator ani muscle is missing (open arrowhead) between the urethra (U), vagina (V), rectum (R) and obturator internus muscle (OI) is shown. The vagina protrudes laterally into the defects to lie close to the obturator internus muscle. *A,* Arcuate pubic ligament. *(From DeLancey et al. (2003). © DeLancey.)*

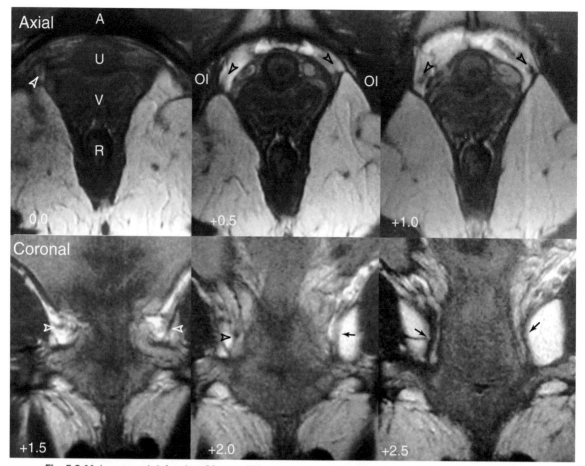

Fig. 5.8.11 Levator ani defect in a 30-year-old incontinent primiparous woman with loss of muscle bulk but preservation of pelvic architecture. The area where the levator is absent in this woman is shown (open arrowhead) in the axial images and coronal images 1.5 and 2.0. Note that in contrast to Fig. 5.8.3, where the vagina lies close to the obturator internus (OI), it has a normal shape. The normal appearance of the levator ani muscle is seen in coronal images 2.0 and 2.5 (arrows). *A,* Arcuate pubic ligament; *R,* rectum; *U,* urethra; *V,* vagina. *(From DeLancey et al. (2003). © DeLancey.)*

mechanisms were evaluated using fluid-sensitive and anatomical sequences made in the early (7 weeks) and late (7 months) postpartum period. Levator injuries were seen in 7 of 19 women. Focal tears at the muscle's insertion into the pubic bone were seen in all. Delayed atrophy, where the muscle is relatively normal early and shows loss of muscle bulk late, was not seen. Oedema could arise either from compression or muscle stretch. If it was compression, it would involve the internal obturator muscle that shares the space between the fetal head and pubic bone. Oedema was seen in all subjects in the levator ani muscle but never in the obturator, indicating that oedema was caused by muscle stretch rather than

compression. Subsequent studies in a larger sample have confirmed these findings and shown the associated bony injuries that occur as well (Miller et al., 2015).

Computer models have studied the stretching that occurs in the levator ani muscle. Those parts of the muscle that are stretched the most are those parts that are seen to be injured (Lien et al., 2004). Using a computer model of the levator ani muscle based on anatomy from a normal woman, the degree to which individual muscle bands are stretched could be studied (Fig. 5.8.12). This analysis revealed that the muscle injured most often, the pubovisceral (pubococcygeal) portion, was the portion of the muscle that underwent the greatest degree of stretch, and

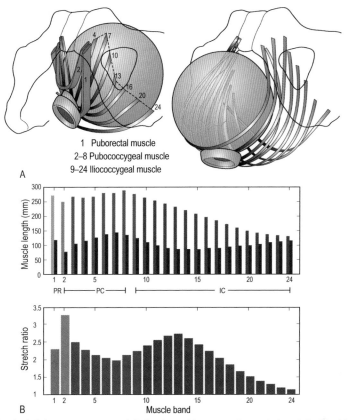

1 Puborectal muscle
2–8 Pubococcygeal muscle
9–24 Iliococcygeal muscle

Fig. 5.8.12 (A) On the left is a computer model of selected levator ani muscle bands before birth, with muscle fibres numbered and the muscle groups identified; the figure on the right demonstrates muscle band lengthening present at the end of the second stage of labour. (B) A graphic representation of the original and final muscle lengths (top) and the stretch ratio (bottom), indicating the degree to which each muscle band must lengthen to accommodate a normal-sized fetal head. Note that the pubococcygeal muscle fascicles labelled 'PC2' undergo the greatest degree of stretch and would be the most vulnerable to stretch-induced injury. *(From Lien et al. (2004), with permission. Biomechanics Research Laboratory.)*

the second area of observed injury, the iliococcygeal muscle, was the second most stretched muscle. Furthermore, when the portion of the muscle at risk was identified in cross-sections cut in the same orientation as axial MRI scans, the pattern of predicted injury matched the injury seen in MRI (Fig. 5.8.13). Further studies that include the viscoelastic properties of the muscle have revealed that the pubovisceral muscle enthesis and the muscle near the perineal body are the regions of greatest strain, thereby placing them at highest risk for stretch-related injury. Decreasing perineal body tissue stiffness significantly reduced tissue stress and strain, and therefore injury risk, in those regions (Jing et al., 2012).

Computer simulations indicating that the pubovisceral muscle is subject to the largest stretch are now confirmed clinically with information about oedema patterns within the muscle. Oedema in the levator that is a sign of muscle injury is localized and does not affect all parts of the muscle, and the location of these changes in the magnetic resonance signal can map areas of stretch-induced injury in the absence of muscle disruption (Pipitone et al., 2021). In a group of 78 women at high risk for levator ani muscle injury, 51% showed muscle oedema in the pubovisceral muscle, whereas 5% had involved the puborectal and 5% also involved the iliococcygeal. Therefore the pubovisceral muscle was seven times more likely than other muscles to show the oedema, adding further evidence that overstretching is an important mechanism of injury because it occurs in the parts of the muscle that are stretched the most.

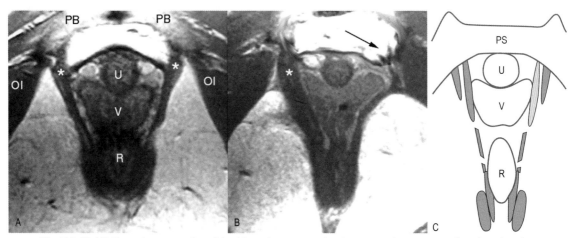

Fig. 5.8.13 (A) Normal anatomy in axial mid-urethra proton density magnetic resonance imaging showing the pubovisceral muscle (*) (see Fig. 5.8.1 for orientation). (B) A woman who has lost part of the left pubovisceral muscle (displayed on the right side of the image, according to standard medical imaging convention) with lateral displacement of the vagina into the area normally occupied by the muscle. The arrow points to the expected location of the missing muscle. The puborectalis is left intact bilaterally. (C) Axial, mid-urethral section of the model through the arch of the pubic bone (see the pubic symphysis [PS], top) and the model levator ani muscles corresponding to those from the patients shown in (A) and (B). Intact muscles are shown in dark shading. Simulated PC2 muscle atrophy is illustrated by the light shading of the left-side PC2 muscle. This location is shown to correspond with the location of muscle atrophy demonstrated in Fig. 5.8.6. *OI,* Obturator internus; *PB,* pubic bone; *R,* rectum; *U,* urethra; *V,* vagina. *(From Lien et al. (2004), with permission. Biomechanics Research Laboratory.)*

CLINICAL IMPLICATIONS OF LEVATOR ANI MUSCLE INJURY

Visible injury to the levator ani muscle is highly associated with pelvic organ prolapse. A more detailed discussion of this issue is presented in Chapter 7.5, which concerns pregnancy and pathophysiology of pelvic floor disorders. Highlights about the most important clinical implications will be covered here.

Levator injury is a major factor causing pelvic floor disorders, especially pelvic organ prolapse. In a case–control study comparing the occurrence of major levator ani muscle defects that involve loss of more than 50% of the pubovisceral portion of the levator ani muscle, major defects were found in 16% of women with normal support and 55% of women with prolapse (DeLancey et al., 2007). Among women attending a clinic for urogynaecologic problems, prolapse was seen in 150 of 181 (83%) women with avulsion and in 265 of 600 (44%) women without avulsion (Dietz and Simpson, 2008).

As is true with any muscle injury, the amount of muscle that is damaged and lost matters. Recent analysis has demonstrated the likelihood of having prolapse with varying degrees of pelvic floor injury (Berger et al., 2014) (Fig. 5.8.14). In a study comparing 284 cases (with prolapse) to 219 controls (normal support) defined by using Pelvic Organ Prolapse Quantification (POP-Q) examinations, levator ani defect scores were assessed on MRI, with scores from 0 (no defects) to 6 (complete, bilateral defects). In lesser degrees of pubovisceral injury, the remaining muscle can compensate for the lost fibers, but with increasing degrees of injury, essentially in those that involve more than half of the muscle, there is not enough residual for normal function to return.

There is also evidence that levator defects are associated with faecal incontinence. In a study of women with anal sphincter tears at birth, women who had a levator tear seen in association with the sphincter tear trended towards more faecal incontinence (35.3%) compared to women who had sphincter laceration but intact levator ani muscles (16.7%, p = 0.10) (Heilbrun et al., 2010).

Not all pelvic floor disorders, however, are similarly associated with levator ani muscle injury. As mentioned

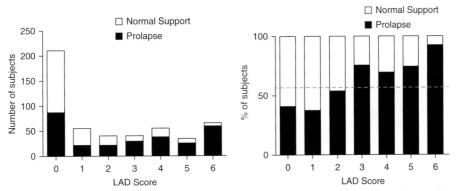

Fig. 5.8.14 The left panel shows the number of cases (black bars) and controls (white bars) at each levator ani defect (LAD) score. The right panel shows the proportion of cases (black bars) and controls (white bars) for each LAD score. The dashed line indicates the overall proportion of individuals with prolapse at least 1 cm beyond the hymen (56.5%). *(From Berger et al. (2014).)*

earlier in this chapter, visible injury is more common in women with stress incontinence 9 months after vaginal birth, but this is not true of women at mid-life who present for care with stress incontinence, in whom injury is seen in 13% compared with 18% seen in continent women (DeLancey et al., 2008).

Mechanism by Which Levator Injury Affects Pelvic Floor Dysfunction

Hiatal Closure

There are potentially both direct and indirect ways in which birth-induced levator injury may influence pelvic floor function. Pelvic organ support is provided by the combined action of the levator ani muscles and the endopelvic fascia. The levator ani closes the vagina by creating a high-pressure zone (Guaderrama et al., 2005) similar to the high-pressure zones created by the urethral and anal sphincter muscles. Women with levator defects have a lower vaginal closure force (2.0 Newtons) compared to women without defects (3.1 Newtons, p < 0.001) (DeLancey et al., 2007). There is also an increase in the levator hiatus area of 28% with injury compared to 6% in women without injury (Shek and Dietz, 2009). Women with an enlarged hiatus are also more likely in longitudinal follow-up to develop prolapse than those with a normal-sized hiatus (Handa et al., 2019, 2020).

The muscles and ligaments must resist the downward force applied on the pelvic floor by the superincumbent abdominal organs and the forces that arise from increases in abdominal pressure during cough, during sneeze or from inertial loads placed on them when landing from a jump, for example. This normal load sharing

between the adaptive action of the muscles and the energy efficient action of static connective tissues is part of the elegant load-bearing design of the pelvic floor. When injury to one of these two components occurs, the other must carry the increased demands placed on it. When the muscle is injured, the connective tissue is subjected to increased load. If this load exceeds the strength of the pelvic tissues, they may be stretched or broken and prolapse may result. This forms a causal chain of events by which pelvic muscle injury may influence pelvic organ prolapse or urinary incontinence. In addition, there is accumulating evidence that women operated on for pelvic organ prolapse or urinary incontinence have higher postoperative failure rates if they have levator ani muscle impairment assessed by biopsy (Hanzal et al., 1993), muscle function testing (Vakili et al., 2005) and ultrasound-detected levator damage (Dietz et al., 2010) than women who have normal muscles. There are early differences in pelvic organ support after surgery depending on whether a defect is present (Morgan et al., 2011). Muscle avulsion is seen more commonly in women with anatomical recurrence at 2 years compared to women with no avulsion (Weemhoff et al., 2012).

More recent studies have shown that as important as the levator ani muscle is, it is not the only factor in hiatal closure. For example, Nandikanti et al. (2018) have shown that less than 25% of variation in the hiatus size is attributable to the degree of muscle injury present on MRI). As well, control of the hiatus size is not simple. For example, only 4% of the hiatus size is explained by muscle contraction strength, and so many other factors must be considered (English et al., 2021). In addition,

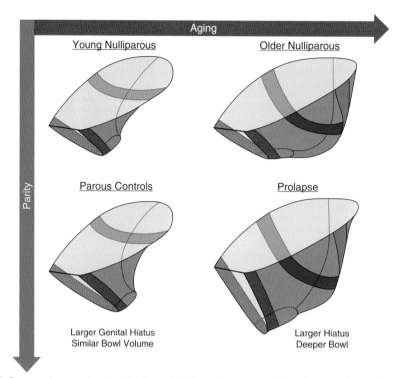

Fig. 5.8.15 Proposed conceptual model for pelvic floor changes resulting from ageing and vaginal parity showing birth-related increase in the hiatus surrounded by the pubovisceral muscle (red band) and age-related change in the region of the iliococcygeal muscle (blue band). *(From Swenson et al. (2020), © DeLancey.)*

although the iliococcygeal portion of the muscle has not received much attention, it is a site of specific age-related change where this region is much deeper in older nulliparas compared with young nulliparas, indicating an age effect separate from parity (Swenson et al., 2020). An overall conceptual model for evaluating the different effects of hiatal enlargement and iliococcygeal changes is shown in Fig. 5.8.15.

Birth-induced levator ani muscle injury may be accompanied by other types of injury that occurred during vaginal birth. A birth that was sufficiently difficult that it resulted in injury to the levator ani muscle may have also created injury to the connective tissue supports. This hypothesis is supported by observations made on the function of the urethral sphincter in women with injured levator ani muscle and those with intact muscles. Women with torn muscles had a 24% lower urethral closure pressure during a maximal pelvic muscle contraction than women without a tear (65.9 vs 86.8 cmH$_2$O, p = 0.004) (Sheng et al., 2020). This may be because individual women lose the ability to increase pressure. In an earlier study of 28 women with normal muscles and 17 women

TABLE 5.8.2   Urethral Closure Pressure Data in 28 Women With Intact Pubovisceral Muscles and 17 Women With Absent Pubovisceral Muscles

	Pubovisceral Muscle Intact	Pubovisceral Muscle Absent
Pressure increase >5 cmH$_2$O (%)	86	41
Mean MUCP (SD)	58 (21)	55 (19)
Mean volitional MUCP pressure increase (SD)	14 (11)	6 (9)

MUCP, Maximum urethral closure pressure.
Adapted from Miller et al., 2004.

with complete bilateral pubovisceral muscle loss, women with intact muscles generated a greater increase in urethral pressure during a maximal pelvic muscle contraction than those with absent pubovisceral muscles (14 ± 11 vs 6 ± 9 cmH$_2$O) (Table 5.8.2). This difference in the ability to increase pressure came from the fact that more of the women (86%) were able to elicit a measurable increase (>5 cmH$_2$O) in urethral closure than those with missing muscles (41%); among women who could increase urethral closure pressure the increase in urethral closure pressure was the same (Miller et al., 2004). Therefore women with complete levator muscle loss can volitionally elevate urethral pressure in the absence of the pubovisceral muscle (presumably using their still-intact striated urethral sphincter muscle), but fewer women are able to do this, suggesting the occurrence of sphincter injury as well in a subset of women in this group. This indicates that some women who are unable to contract their levator ani muscles due to muscle (or nerve) injury escape injury to the urethral sphincter (or pudendal nerve), whereas others do not, and this phenomenon occurs more often in women with muscle problems.

ISSUES IN REHABILITATION

According to the Committee on Trauma of the American College of Surgeons (1961), 'the injured patient is entitled to know at the outset, in general terms, what [her] injuries are, what the immediate treatment will be, and what may be the expected result' (p. 16). The committee also stated the following: 'The fate of the injured person depends to a large extent upon the initial care that [her] injuries receive. Skilled competent care may salvage function in seemingly hopeless situations; inept care for even a trivial injury may end in disaster' (p. 1).

This statement made more than 60 years ago articulates an enduring truth about injury management—that is, knowing the type of injury is an important guide to proper treatment. Imaging has now demonstrated specific evidence of localized muscle loss revealing a great variety of injury patterns in different women. At present, without specific testing, we do not know whether birth-induced muscle injury is caused by neurological injury or by muscle rupture. Whether there should be similar treatment of these two types of injury remains to be determined. Further research is needed to develop effective strategies to answer this question in individual women.

In addition, the nature of a woman's defect later in life may influence the type of therapy selected. Pelvic muscle training can have two effects. Firstly, it can improve a woman's skill in using her muscles, and secondly, it can improve the contractile force. Whether exercise changes resting urethral function is not known. If the ability to contract a normally innervated pelvic floor muscle during a cough is lost, for example, a woman can be taught to purposefully contract the muscle. As well, the muscles can be exercised to become stronger through hypertrophy. Therefore if the normally occurring muscle contraction occurs but is not strong enough, this muscle can be strengthened and continence improved. Most of a person's time is not spent coughing or jumping. Most of the time, there should be normal 'tone' in the muscle. This tonic activity is similar to the action of postural muscle in the back in that it automatically adjusts to the loads placed upon it. Whether this can be improved is unknown.

At present the success of muscle training in women with different types of levator ani muscle injury is not clear. If the pubovisceral muscle is missing, then the connections between the pubic bone and the vagina or perineal body are missing. Although the iliococcygeal and puborectal muscles remain, there are presently no data to know whether the success of pelvic muscle training is similar in women with and without muscle injury. This should be a fertile field for research as new imaging modalities make the detection of muscle injury routine.

ACKNOWLEDGEMENT

We gratefully acknowledge support of our research through NIH grants R01 DK 51405, R01 HD 38665 and P50 HD 44406.

REFERENCES

Allen, R. E., Hosker, G. L., Smith, A. R. B., et al. (1990). Pelvic floor damage and childbirth: A neurophysiological study. *British Journal of Obstetrics and Gynaecology, 97*, 770–779.

Barber, M. D., Bremer, R. E., Thor, K. B., et al. (2002). Innervation of the female levator ani muscles. *American Journal of Obstetrics and Gynecology, 187*, 64–71.

Berger, M. B., Morgan, D. M., & DeLancey, J. O. (2014). Levator ani defect scores and pelvic organ prolapse: Is there a threshold effect? *International Urogynecology Journal, 25*(10), 1375–1379.

Betschart, C., Kim, J., Miller, J. M., et al. (2014). Comparison of muscle fiber directions between different levator ani muscle subdivisions: In vivo MRI measurements in women. *International Urogynecology Journal, 25*(9), 1263–1268.

Committee on Trauma, American College of Surgeons. (1961). *Early care of acute soft tissue injuries* (2nd ed.). Philadelphia: W. B. Saunders.

DeLancey, J. O. (2005). The hidden epidemic of pelvic floor dysfunction: Achievable goals for improved prevention and treatment. *American Journal of Obstetrics and Gynecology, 192*, 1488–1495.

DeLancey, J. O., Kearney, R., Chou, Q., et al. (2003). The appearance of levator ani muscle abnormalities in magnetic resonance images after vaginal delivery. *Obstetrics & Gynecology, 101*, 46–53.

DeLancey, J. O., Morgan, D. M., Fenner, D. E., et al. (2007). Comparison of levator ani muscle defects and function in women with and without pelvic organ prolapse. *Obstetrics & Gynecology, 109*(2 Pt. 1), 295–302.

DeLancey, J. O., Trowbridge, E. R., Miller, J. M., et al. (2008). Stress urinary incontinence: Relative importance of urethral support and urethral closure pressure. *J. Urol., 179*(6), 2286–2290.

Dietz, H. P. (2021). Ultrasound imaging of maternal birth trauma. *International Urogynecology Journal, 32*(7), 1953–1962.

Dietz, H. P., Chantarasorn, V., & Shek, K. L. (2010). Levator avulsion is a risk factor for cystocele recurrence. *Ultrasound in Obstetrics and Gynecology, 36*, 76–80.

Dietz, H. P., & Lanzarone, V. (2005). Levator trauma after vaginal delivery. *Obstetrics & Gynecology, 106*(4), 707–712.

Dietz, H. P., & Simpson, J. M. (2008). Levator trauma is associated with pelvic organ prolapse. *British Journal of Obstetrics and Gynaecology, 115*(8), 979–984.

English, E. M., Chen, L., Sammarco, A. G., et al. (2021). Mechanisms of hiatus failure in prolapse: A multifaceted evaluation. *International Urogynecology Journal, 32*(6), 1545–1553.

Guaderrama, N. M., Nager, C. W., Uu, J., et al. (2005). The vaginal pressure profile. *Neurourology and Urodynamics, 24*, 243–247.

Halban, J., & Tandler, J. (1907). *Anatomie und Aetiologie der Genitalprolapse beim Weihe.* Vienna: Wilhelm Braumueller.

Handa, V. L., Blomquist, J. L., Carroll, M., et al. (2020). Genital hiatus size and the development of prolapse among parous women. *Female Pelvic Medicine & Reconstructive Surgery, 26*, 287–298.

Handa, V. L., Roem, J., Blomquist, J. L., et al. (2019). Pelvic organ prolapse as a function of levator ani avulsion, hiatus size, and strength. *American Journal of Obstetrics and Gynecology, 221*, 41.e1–41.e7.

Hanzal, E., Berger, E., & Koelbl, H. (1993). Levator ani muscle morphology and recurrent genuine stress incontinence. *Obstetrics & Gynecology, 81*, 426–429.

Heilbrun, M. E., Nygaard, I. E., Lockhart, M. E., et al. (2010). Correlation between levator ani muscle injuries on magnetic resonance imaging and fecal incontinence, pelvic organ prolapse, and urinary incontinence in primiparous women. *American Journal of Obstetrics and Gynecology, 202*(5), 488.e1–488.e6.

Jing, D., Ashton-Miller, J. A., & DeLancey, J. O. (2012). A subject-specific anisotropic visco-hyperelastic finite element model of female pelvic floor stress and strain during the second stage of labor. *Journal of Biomechanics, 45*(3), 455–460.

Kearney, R., Fitzpatrick, M., Brennan, S., et al. (2010). Levator ani injury in primiparous women with forceps delivery for fetal distress, forceps for second stage arrest, and spontaneous delivery. *International Journal of Gynaecology & Obstetrics, 111*(1), 19–22.

Kearney, R., Sawhney, R., & DeLancey, J. O. (2004). Levator ani muscle anatomy evaluated by origin-insertion pairs. *Obstetrics & Gynecology, 104*, 168–173.

Krofta, L., Otcenásek, M., Kasíková, E., et al. (2009). Pubococcygeus-puborectalis trauma after forceps delivery: Evaluation of the levator ani muscle with 3D/4D ultrasound. *International Urogynecology Journal and Pelvic Floor Dysfunction, 20*(10), 1175–1181.

Lawson, J. O. (1974). Pelvic anatomy. I. Pelvic floor muscles. *Annals of the Royal College of Surgeons of England, 54*, 244–252.

Lien, K. C., Mooney, B., DeLancey, J. O., et al. (2004). Levator ani muscle stretch induced by simulated vaginal birth. *Obstetrics & Gynecology, 103*, 31–40.

Mant, J., Painter, R., & Vessey, M. (1997). Epidemiology of genital prolapse: Observations from the oxford family planning association study. *British Journal of Obstetrics and Gynaecology, 104*, 579–585.

Margulies, R. U., Hsu, Y., Kearney, R., et al. (2006). Appearance of the levator ani muscle subdivisions in magnetic resonance images. *Obstetrics & Gynecology, 107*(5), 1064–1069.

Miller, J. M., Brandon, C., Jacobson, J. A., et al. (2010). MRI findings in patients considered high risk for pelvic floor injury studied serially after vaginal childbirth. *American Journal of Roentgenology, 195*(3), 786–791.

Miller, J. M., Low, L. K., Zielinski, R., et al. (2015). Evaluating maternal recovery from labor and delivery: Bone and levator ani injuries. *American Journal of Obstetrics and Gynecology, 213*(2) 188.e1–188.e11.

Miller, J. M., Umek, W. H., DeLancey, J. O., et al. (2004). Can women without visible pubococcygeal muscle in MR images still increase urethral closure pressures? *American Journal of Obstetrics and Gynecology, 191*, 171–175.

Morgan, D. M., Larson, K., Lewicky-Gaupp, C., et al. (2011). Vaginal support as determined by levator ani defect status 6 weeks after primary surgery for pelvic organ prolapse. *International Journal of Gynaecology & Obstetrics, 114*(2), 141–144.

Mørkved, S., Bø, K., Schei, B., et al. (2003). Pelvic floor muscle training during pregnancy to prevent urinary incontinence: A single-blind randomized controlled trial. *Obstetrics & Gynecology, 101*, 313–319.

Nandikanti, L., Sammarco, A. G., Kobernik, E. K., et al. (2018). Levator ani defect severity and its association with enlarged hiatus size, levator bowl depth, and prolapse size. *American Journal of Obstetrics and Gynecology, 218*(5), 537–539.

Pipitone, F., Miller, J. M., & DeLancey, J. O. L. (2021). Injury-associated levator ani muscle and anal sphincter oedema following vaginal birth: A secondary analysis of the EM-RLD study. *British Journal of Obstetrics and Gynaecology, 128*(12), 2046–2053.

Rortveit, G., Daltveit, A. K., Hannestad, Y. S., et al. (2003). Norwegian EPINCONT study. Urinary incontinence after vaginal delivery or cesarean section. *New England Journal of Medicine, 348*, 900–907.

Sampselle, C. M., Miller, J. M., Mims, B. L., et al. (1998). Effect of pelvic muscle exercise on transient incontinence during pregnancy and after birth. *Obstetrics & Gynecology, 91*, 406–412.

Shek, K. L., & Dietz, H. P. (2009). The effect of childbirth on hiatal dimensions. *Obstetrics & Gynecology, 113*(6), 1272–1278.

Shek, K. L., & Dietz, H. P. (2010). Intrapartum risk factors for levator trauma. *British Journal of Obstetrics and Gynaecology, 117*(12), 1485–1492.

Sheng, Y., Liu, X., Low, L. K., et al. (2020). Association of pu-bovisceral muscle tear with functional capacity of urethral closure: Evaluating maternal recovery from labor and delivery. *American Journal of Obstetrics and Gynecology, 222*(6), 598.e1–598.e7.

Shobeiri, S. A., Leclaire, E., Nihira, M. A., et al. (2009). Appearance of the levator ani muscle subdivisions in endovaginal three-dimensional ultrasonography. *Obstetrics & Gynecology, 114*(1), 66–72.

Strohbehn, K., Ellis, J. H., Strohbehn, I. A., et al. (1996). Magnetic resonance imaging of the levator ani with anatomic correlation. *Obstetrics & Gynecology, 87*, 277–285.

Swenson, C. W., Masteling, M., DeLancey, J. O., et al. (2020). Aging effects on pelvic floor support: A pilot study comparing young versus older nulliparous women. *International Urogynecology Journal, 31*(3), 535–543.

Tunn, R., DeLancey, J. O., Howard, D., et al. (1999). MR imaging of levator ani muscle recovery following vaginal delivery. *International Urogynecology Journal and Pelvic Floor Dysfunction, 10*, 300–307.

Tunn, R., DeLancey, J. O., Howard, D., et al. (2003). Anatomic variations in the levator ani muscle, endopelvic fascia and urethra in nulliparas evaluated by magnetic resonance imaging. *American Journal of Obstetrics and Gynecology, 188*, 116–121.

Vakili, B., Zheng, Y. T., Loesch, H., et al. (2005). Levator contraction strength and genital hiatus as risk factors for recurrent pelvic organ prolapse. *American Journal of Obstetrics and Gynecology, 194*, 1592–1598.

Valsky, D. V., Lipschuetz, M., Bord, A., et al. (2009). Fetal head circumference and length of second stage of labor are risk factors for levator ani muscle injury, diagnosed by 3-dimensional transperineal ultrasound in primiparous women. *American Journal of Obstetrics and Gynecology, 201*(1), 91.e1–91.e7.

Weemhoff, M., Vergeldt, T. F., Notten, K., et al. (2012). Avulsion of puborectalis muscle and other risk factors for cystocele recurrence: A 2-year follow-up study. *International Urogynecology Journal, 23*(1), 65–71.

Weidner, A. C., Barber, M. D., Visco, A. G., et al. (2000). Pelvic muscle electromyography of levator ani and external anal sphincter in nulliparous women and women with pelvic floor dysfunction. *American Journal of Obstetrics and Gynecology, 183*, 1390–1399.

Weidner, A. C., Jamison, M. G., Branham, V., et al. (2006). Neuropathic injury to the levator ani occurs in 1 in 4 primiparous women. *American Journal of Obstetrics and Gynecology, 195*(6), 1851–1856.

Pelvic Floor and Exercise Science

OUTLINE

6.1 Motor Learning

Kari Bø and Siv Mørkved

ABILITY TO CONTRACT THE PELVIC FLOOR MUSCLES

Before starting a training programme of the pelvic floor muscles (PFMs) one must ensure that the patients/clients are able to perform a correct PFM contraction. A correct PFM contraction has two components: squeeze around the pelvic openings and inward (cranial) lift (Kegel, 1952). Several research groups have shown that more than 30% of women are not able to voluntarily contract the PFMs at their first consultation even after thorough individual instruction (Benvenuti et al., 1987; Bø et al., 1988; Bump et al., 1991; Kegel, 1952). In a study of 343 Austrian women aged 18 to 79 years attending routine gynaecological visits, 44.9% were not able to contract the PFMs. It was reported that involuntary contraction was present before increase in intra-abdominal pressure (IAP) in only 26.5% (assessed by palpation) (Talasz et al., 2008). Freitas et al. (2018) studied knowledge of the pelvic floor, ability to contract and PFM function in a sample of 133 parous Brazilian women. They found that 23.4% were not able to contract the PFMs, whereas 35.3% had a grade 2 on the modified Oxford grading scale. The participants showed a low level of PFM knowledge, but no relationship between PFM knowledge and ability to contract or prevalence of urinary incontinence was observed. Uechi et al. (2019) studied 82 women with a mean age of 46.8 years (SD: 17.9). Most (98.8%) believed that they were able to voluntarily contract their PFMs, but only 33% correctly estimated their PFMs according to the examiner's assessment. Henderson et al. (2013) studied

779 women presenting to community-based primary care practices and compared the ability to contract the PFMs between women with and without pelvic floor dysfunction. Being able to contract on the first attempt were 85.5%, 83.4%, 68.6% and 85.8% of women with pelvic organ prolapse (POP), stress urinary incontinence (SUI), both POP and SUI, and neither POP nor SUI, respectively (p = 0.01 for a difference between POP and SUI vs neither POP nor SUI).

Correct contraction of the PFMs may be an extra challenge after childbirth. Vermandel et al. (2015) studied 958 women, mean age 30 years (± 4.9 years) using questionnaire and clinical assessment with visual observation within 1 week after childbirth. A total of 26% had no knowledge of the pelvic floor, 52.2% had trained the PFMs and 52.2% (n = 500) showed no inward perineal displacement during attempts to contract (29% showed no movement at all, and 24% showed some movement but no inward displacement). Interestingly, 45% of those who had trained the PFMs and were convinced they were doing it correctly were not. Hilde et al. (2013a) assessed 277 first-time pregnant women at gestational week 22 and 6 to 8 weeks postpartum. After vaginal delivery, vaginal resting pressure was reduced in 29% and PFM strength and endurance in 54% and 53%, respectively. Vaginal delivery had statistically significantly greater impact on vaginal resting pressure, PFM strength and endurance when compared with caesarean section (CS), with the CS group only showing a reduction of vaginal resting pressure (10%). PFM strength was also significantly reduced in women with instrumental vaginal delivery compared with non-instrumental deliveries, and continent women had significantly stronger and better PFM endurance than incontinent women. Stær-Jenssen et al. (2015) followed the same cohort of women from gestational weeks 21 to 37 and then 6 weeks, 6 and 12 months postpartum with ultrasound measurements of levator hiatus dimensions. After an increase from pregnancy to 6 weeks postpartum, there was an improvement in all measurements during the first 6 months postpartum (levator hiatus area: reduced with 3.5 cm^2). However, at 12 months postpartum, all measurements at rest were still increased compared to pregnancy. No negative changes were seen in the CS group. Hilde et al. (2013b) compared 55 primiparous women with and 120 without major PFM defects 6 weeks postpartum and found that only 4% of the total sample could not do a correct

PFM contraction, and with no difference between those with and without muscle defects. However, there was a statistically significant difference in strength and endurance of 47% in favour of those with no injuries but no difference in vaginal resting pressure. Most women with major defects were able to contract the PFMs correctly, which implies that PFM training (PFMT) might be worthwhile in this subgroup as well. Sheng et al. (2019) compared 21 women with puboviseral muscle tear confirmed by magnetic resonance imaging with 35 women without tears. They found no difference in urethral resting pressure but a statistically significant difference in urethral pressure during a voluntary PFM contraction, 65.9 versus 86.8 cmH$_2$O, in women with and without tears, respectively (p = 0.004). In contradiction to the latter study, Brincat et al. (2011) found no association between maximum urethral closure pressure and PFM contraction in 160 women with and without levator ani defects 9 to 12 months postpartum. The latter authors suggested that major tears of the PFMs may spare the urethral sphincter.

Common mistakes when trying to perform a PFM contraction are listed in Table 6.1.1. Bø et al. (1988, 1990a) found that many women contracted other muscles in addition to the PFMs, and 9 of 52 women were straining instead of lifting. Bump et al. (1991) found corresponding results in an American population, with as many as 25% of women straining instead of squeezing and lifting. These findings were later supported by Thompson and O'Sullivan (2003) in a population of Australian women.

There may be several explanations as to why a voluntary PFM contraction is difficult to perform:

- the PFMs have an invisible location inside the pelvis;
- neither men nor women have ever learned to contract the PFMs, and most people would be unaware of the automatic contractions of the muscles;
- the muscles are small and, from a neurophysiological point of view, therefore more difficult to contract voluntarily; and
- the common awareness of these pelvic and perineal areas of the body may be associated with voiding and defaecation, and straining at toilet is common.

Tries (1990) suggests that there may be a lack of sensory feedback during PFMT in some women, causing:

- problems with feedback from the correct muscles because other muscles are used instead of the PFMs;

TABLE 6.1.1 Common Errors in Attempts to Perform a Maximum Contraction of the Pelvic Floor Muscles

Error	Observation
Contraction of outer abdominal muscles instead of the PFMs	The person is either curving the back or starts the attempt to contract by 'hollowing'/tucking the stomach inwards (note that a small 'hollowing' can be seen in a correct contraction with the transverse abdominal muscle co-contracting)
Contraction of hip adductor muscles instead of the PFMs	A contraction of the muscles of the inner thigh can be seen
Contraction of gluteal muscles instead of the PFMs	The person is pressing the buttocks together, lifting up from the bench
Stop breathing	The person closes their mouth and holds their breath
Enhanced inhaling	The person takes a deep inspiration often accompanied by contraction of abdominal muscles and tries erroneously to 'lift up' the pelvic floor by the inspiration
Straining	The person presses downwards; when undressed, the perineum can be seen pressing in a caudal direction, and if the person has pelvic organ prolapse, the prolapse may protrude

PFM, Pelvic floor muscles.

- insufficient kinaesthetic feedback due to low-intensity contractions in weak PFMs; and
- lack of or reduced sensation, which may limit the sensory incentive that normally leads to a motor response or reflex preventing leakage.

Motor re-learning depends on sensory feedback (Tries, 1990). Following Gentile (1987), learning is generally facilitated by the use of feedback, and the physical therapist (PT) should give external feedback as 'knowledge of results' (KR) as a part of the intervention. KR

may compensate for a loss of normal sources for internal feedback in patients with central- or peripheral nerve injuries (Winstein, 1991). Although many women have reduced innervations in the pelvic floor (e.g., after injury related to pregnancy and delivery), the use of KR may be useful in learning correct PFM contraction.

Several trials have used the protocol by Bø et al. (1990a), where the women are specifically instructed to contract only the PFMs (Bø et al., 1999; Johannessen et al., 2017; Mørkved and Bø, 1997; Mørkved et al., 2002; Mørkved et al., 2003; Overgård et al., 2008; Stafne et al., 2012). Our reason for attempting to isolate the PFM contraction from outer pelvic muscles when training the muscles is not because we do not appreciate that many muscles in the body act together in a motor task and seldom work in isolation. However, such simultaneous contractions of outer and more commonly used larger muscle groups outside the pelvis may mask the awareness and strength of the PFM contraction. The person erroneously believes that he or she is performing a strong contraction, but the PFMs are not doing the job. Most importantly, to train and build up a muscle or muscle group's strength and volume, it is mandatory to work specifically with the targeted muscle. In an experimental study, Kruger et al. (2018) assessed simultaneous IAP and response from the PFMs on contraction of the PFMs and outer pelvic muscles. They found that pressure in the region of the pelvic floor was significantly higher during a targeted PFM contraction compared to that for all other exercises, except for cough and curl-ups, where the IAP was also quite high. They concluded that targeted PFM contractions develop higher pressures compared to IAP than any exercise tested in the study, and that exercising accessory muscles in an attempt to activate the pelvic floor sufficiently to illicit a training effect is not recommended.

More concerning than the contraction of outer pelvic muscles simultaneously with PFM contraction is straining. If patients are straining instead of performing a correct contraction the training may permanently stretch, weaken and harm the contractile ability of the PFMs. In addition, straining may stretch the connective tissue of fasciae and ligaments, thereby potentially increasing the risk of development of POP. Proper assessment of ability to contract the PFMs and feedback on performance is therefore mandatory before starting a training programme.

PRACTICAL TEACHING OF CORRECT PELVIC FLOOR MUSCLE CONTRACTION

The steps of learning a correct muscle contraction can be separated into five levels:

1. Understand: The patient needs to understand where the PFMs are located and how they work (cognitive function).
2. Search: The patient needs time to put this understanding into her or his body. Where is my pelvic floor?
3. Find: The patient must find where the PFMs are but often needs reassurance from the PT of the location.
4. Learn: After having found the PFMs, the patient needs to learn how to perform a correct contraction of the PFMs. Feedback from the PT is mandatory.
5. Control: After having learned to contract, most subjects still strive for a while to perform controlled and coordinated contractions, recruiting as many motor units as possible during each contraction. Most people are unable to hold the contraction, perform repetitive contractions, or conduct contractions of high velocity or strength during their first attempts of training.

Basically, four teaching tools can be used to facilitate skill acquisition (Gentile, 1972): the therapist can try to verbally indicate key aspects of the task or performance, supplementary visual input can be provided, direct physical contact with the learner might be employed and the therapist can structure the environmental conditions under which practice is to take place.

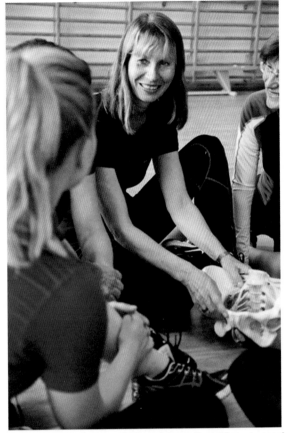

Fig. 6.1.1 Use of anatomical models or illustrations to teach anatomy and physiology of the pelvic floor. Place the anatomical model in front of the patient's pelvis so that she can see the correct position of the organs as they are located inside her.

Teaching Tools

To facilitate correct PFM contractions the PT can use different teaching tools.

Verbal instructions should be based on knowledge of the function of the PFMs, namely to form a structural support and to ensure less opening of the levator hiatus, maintaining a sufficient maximum urethral closure pressure, and less downward movement during abrupt increase in IAP. One example of a training command is 'squeeze and lift'.

To teach patients, the PT might use drawings and anatomical models of the pelvic floor to show the patient where the muscles are located anatomically (Fig. 6.1.1). We also recommend that the PT demonstrates a correct PFM contraction in the standing position, showing that there should be no movement of the pelvis or thighs visible from the outside. The patient can also palpate the PT's buttocks to feel the difference between gluteal muscle contraction and the relaxed position these muscles should hold during PFM contraction. Allow the patient to ask questions and practise a few contractions for herself or himself.

One way to help patients understand the action of the PFMs is to use imagery such as describing the contraction as a lift starting with closure of the doors (squeeze) and from there the elevator is moving upstairs (lift). Another way is to explain the action as eating spaghetti or the action of a vacuum cleaner. Many patients may have general low body awareness, and sometimes it is necessary first to focus on the pelvic area and make the patient move the pelvis in different directions by use of the outer pelvic muscles (Fig. 6.1.2). When the patient

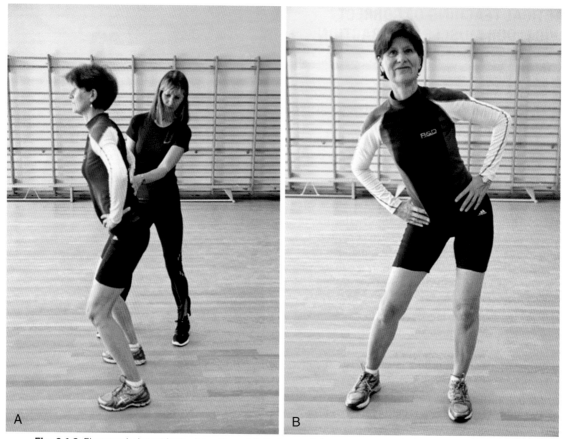

A   B

Fig. 6.1.2 First teach the patient where the pelvis is by practising movements of the pelvis in an anteroposterior direction (A) and sideways (B).

is familiar with the pelvic area, one can start to focus on the internal pelvic muscles (the PFMs).

One way of visualizing where the PFMs are located and how they work is to use a skeleton and place the patient's hand as if it was the pelvic floor inside the pelvis. Then the PT presses the hand towards the 'pelvic floor' to make the patient understand the role of the PFMs as a structural support for all pelvic organs and how it should resist increases in IAP (Fig. 6.1.3).

Direct physical contact may be used to enhance sensory stimulation and proprioceptive facilitation. An effective position to teach a correct PFM contraction is having the patient sit on an armrest or at the edge of a table with legs in abduction, feet on the floor, straight back and hip flexion. In this position the patient gets exteroceptive, and for some maybe proprioceptive, stimulus on the perineum/PFMs. The patient is then instructed to squeeze and lift away from the chair

without rising up, then relax again (Fig. 6.1.4). After this instruction, the patient is allowed to go to the toilet to empty the bladder. Observation and vaginal palpation then take place. Figure 6.1.5 shows the relationship between the PT and patient with vaginal palpation during attempts to contract the PFMs. Both the PT and patient give verbal feedback to each other during the contraction. In addition, proprioceptive facilitation may be used during vaginal palpation to enhance contraction of the PFMs. The palpation (rectal for men) is also important to give feedback of the strength of the contraction and to make the patient understand that although he or she is contracting correctly, it is possible to work much harder. Bump et al. (1991) found that in the group of women capable of doing a correct contraction, only 49% contracted hard enough to increase urethral pressure. Gentile (1987) claims that generally one of the most important roles of the instructor is to keep

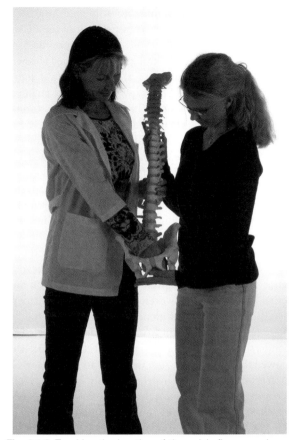

Fig. 6.1.3 Teaching the location of the pelvic floor muscles as a structural support for the internal organs and how they act to resist downward movement and increase in abdominal pressure by lifting upwards. The physical therapist presses downwards and the patient holds against the movement, mirroring the work of the pelvic floor muscles.

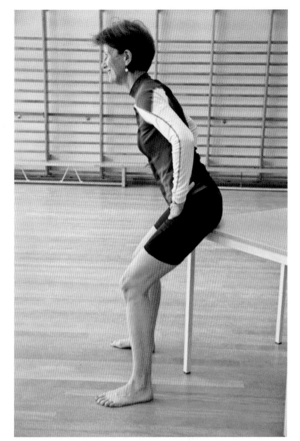

Fig. 6.1.4 The patient sits on an armrest (or edge of a table) with legs apart, feet on the floor, flexed hips and straight back with the perineum resting on the armrest. The instruction is to squeeze around the pelvic openings and lift the skin away from the armrest without rising up or putting any pressure on the feet.

the patient's motivation high because practice/training is a premise for learning. A distinction must be made between feedback aiming at giving information about performance or results, and verbal comments to motivate the patient to adherence.

It can be explained to men that if they perform a correct PFM contraction, they feel and see a lift of the scrotum. If appropriate, a mirror can be used for both men and women to see the inward lifting movement. However, some people feel uncomfortable observing their genitalia, and the PT must show tact before suggesting this method.

Another way of facilitating learning may be to structure the environmental conditions under which practice is to take place. We emphasize a situation during PFMT, both at home and in training groups, that allows thorough concentration. One consequence of this is that

during group training classes we do not use music when teaching the PFM contractions.

Although as many as 30% may not be able to conduct a correct PFM contraction at the first consultation, we have experienced that most women learn to contract if they are given advice to practise on their own at home for a week. It is important not to strain the patient at the first consultation if she is not able to contract. Ask the patient to exercise on an armrest at home and also ask her or him to try to stop the dribble at the end of voiding. However, stopping the urine stream is not recommended in a training protocol, as it may disturb the fine neurological balance between bladder and urethral pressures during voiding. There should be no PFM activity just before (opening of the urethra) and during voiding. Stopping the dribble at the very end of voiding

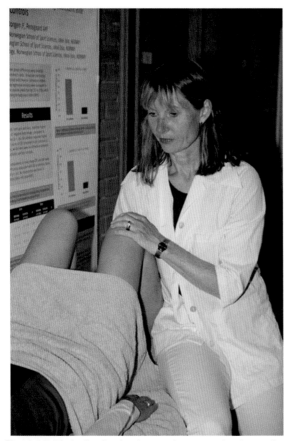

Fig. 6.1.5 Vaginal palpation is mandatory to give immediate feedback on correctness of the attempt to contract the pelvic floor muscles.

is therefore only recommended as a test of the ability to contract, and many patients have reported that they have learned to contract the PFMs with this method. Another way to improve the awareness of a correct PFM contraction is to contract other circular muscles (e.g., those surrounding the mouth; Liebergall-Wischnitzer et al., 2005). Two experimental studies evaluating the effect of contracting the circular muscles on the PFM contractions did not support that such contractions facilitated or augmented the effect of voluntary PFM contraction using surface electromyography (EMG) and ultrasound (Bø et al., 2011; Resende et al., 2011). However, it may give the patient an understanding of how a contraction around an opening may be perceived. The recommendation of all preceding methods to teach PFM contraction is based on clinical experience only.

If the patient is still unable to contract the PFMs after 1 week of rehearsal on her own, the PT may try general muscle facilitation techniques to stimulate awareness of the PFMs. Methods such as fast stretch of the PFMs, tapping on the perineum or muscles, pressure/massage techniques or electrical stimulation can be tried (Brown, 2001). Mateus-Vasconcelos et al. (2017) did a systematic review on physical therapy methods to facilitate voluntary PFM contraction. They found only six studies, including only two randomized controlled trials (RCTs), and no strict conclusions could be drawn. In a follow-up RCT, Mateus-Vasconcelos et al. (2018) randomized 132 women with 0 to 1 on the Oxford modified grading scale to 8 weeks of either PFMT with vaginal palpation, palpation during a pelvic tilt, intra-vaginal electrical stimulation or verbal instruction. They found that the number of women scoring 2 or higher on the Oxford scale was 63.6%, 69.7%, 33.3% and 18.2% in the preceding groups. The two palpation groups were statistically significantly better than the groups given electrical stimulation and verbal instruction. However, for reduction of urinary incontinence, palpation alone showed the best results. These results are different from the findings reported by Henderson et al. (2013) and Vermandel et al. (2015), who showed that more than 70% were able to learn a correct contraction after verbal instruction only. However, Henderson et al. (2013) found that women with POP were less likely to learn than women with neither POP nor SUI (54.3% vs 85.7%, p = 0.001). Studies using concentric needle EMG in the urethral sphincter and the PFMs have demonstrated that there is a co-contraction of the PFMs with the use of outer pelvic muscles (gluteal, hip adductor and rectus abdominis) in healthy volunteers (Bø and Stien, 1994). In addition, Sapsford and Hodges (2001) used surface EMG and found that there was a co-contraction of the PFM during transversus abdominus (TrA) contraction in healthy volunteers. Therefore many PTs recommend contractions of outer pelvic muscles and hope for a co-contraction of the PFMs if the patient is not able to perform a correct PFM contraction. However, we do not know whether there are such simultaneous co-contractions in persons with pelvic floor dysfunction, and we have only been able to find one RCT comparing contraction of other muscles (external and internal hip rotators) to PFM contractions (Jordre and Schweinle, 2014). They did not find any differences between groups, but this may be due to a small sample size (n = 27), no verification of ability to contract the PFMs, few visits with a PT and a short exercise period (6 weeks). If some of the outer pelvic muscles are to be used instead of the PFMs, we recommend hip adductor, gluteal and hip rotator muscle contractions and not TrA or other abdominal muscle training because contraction of all abdominal muscles may increase abdominal pressure (Hodges and Gandevia, 2000; Kruger et al., 2018). In addition, Bø et al. (2003) showed that when contracting the TrA, 30% of trained female PTs showed descent of the PFMs. In another study using perineal ultrasonography, it was shown that a PFM contraction was significantly more effective than a TrA contraction in reducing the levator hiatus area, and that in some women the levator hiatus opened up during TrA contraction (Bø et al., 2009). Therefore, if there is no co-contraction of the PFMs with the abdominal muscle contractions, this may strain and weaken the PFMs. So far, ultrasound and magnetic resonance imaging are not available in most clinical practices, and therefore physiotherapists cannot control for what happens inside the body (e.g., at the levator hiatus) by observing from the outside.

High-quality studies in the area of PFM awareness and motor learning of how to perform a correct and effective PFM contraction should be of high priority and are strongly encouraged in future research. However, it is important that PTs are aware that some subjects may never be able to perform a voluntary PFM contraction. In a study by Bø et al. (1990a), four of 52 patients were still unable to contract after 6 months of PFMT. Inability to contract the PFMs may be due to severe muscle, nerve and connective tissue damage or the inability to learn this specific task due to a general low body/muscle/movement awareness. These patients should not spend a lot of time and money with the PT, but should be referred back to their treating general practitioners, urologists or gynaecologists for other treatment options as soon as possible.

REFERENCES

Benvenuti, F., Caputo, G. M., Bandinelli, S., et al. (1987). Re-educative treatment of female genuine stress incontinence. *American Journal of Physical Medicine*, 66, 155–168.

Bø, K., Brækken, I. H., Majida, M., et al. (2009). Constriction of the levator hiatus during instruction of pelvic floor or transversus abdominis contraction: A 4D ultrasound study. *International Urogynecology Journal Pelvic Floor Dysfunct*, 20, 27–32.

Bø, K., Hagen, R. H., Kvarstein, B., et al. (1990a). Pelvic floor muscle exercise for the treatment of female stress urinary incontinence: III. Effects of two different degrees of pelvic floor muscle exercise. *Neurourology and Urodynamics*, 9, 489–502.

Bø, K., Hilde, G., Stær Jensen, J., et al. (2011). Can the Paula Method facilitate co-contraction of the pelvic floor muscles? A 4D ultrasound study. *International Urogynecology Journal and Pelvic Floor Dysfunction*, 22(6), 671–676.

Bø, K., Larsen, S., Oseid, S., et al. (1988). Knowledge about and ability to correct pelvic floor muscle exercises in women with urinary stress incontinence. *Neurourology and Urodynamics*, 7, 261–262.

Bø, K., Sherburn, M., & Allen, T. (2003). Transabdominal ultrasound measurement of pelvic floor muscle activity when activated directly or via a transversus abdominal muscle contraction. *Neurourology and Urodynamics*, 22(6), 582–588.

Bø, K., & Stien, R. (1994). Needle EMG registration of striated urethral wall and pelvic floor muscle activity patterns during cough, Valsalva, abdominal, hip adductor, and gluteal muscle contractions in nulliparous healthy females. *Neurourology and Urodynamics*, 13, 35–41.

Bø, K., Talseth, T., & Holme, I. (1999). Single blind, randomised controlled trial of pelvic floor exercises, electrical stimulation, vaginal cones, and no treatment in management of genuine stress incontinence in women. *British Medical Journal*, 318, 487–493.

Brincat, C. A., Delancey, J. O., & Miller, J. M. (2011). Urethral closure pressures among primiparous women with and without levator ani muscle defects. *International Urogynecology Journal*, 22(12), 1491–1495.

Brown, C. (2001). Pelvic floor reeducation: A practical approach. In J. Corcos, & E. Shick (Eds.), *The urinary sphincter* (pp. 459–473). New York: Marcel Dekker.

Bump, R., Hurt, W. G., Fantl, J. A., et al. (1991). Assessment of Kegel exercise performance after brief verbal instruction. *American Journal of Obstetrics and Gynecology*, 165, 322–329.

Freitas, L. M., Bø, K., Fernandes, A. C. N. L., et al. (2018). Pelvic floor muscle knowledge and relationship with muscle strength in Brazilian women: A cross-sectional study. *International Urogynecology Journal*, 30(11) 1930–1909.

Gentile, A. M. (1972). A working model of skill acquisition with applications to teaching. *Quest*, 17, 3–23.

Gentile, A. M. (1987). Skill acquisition: Action, movement, and neuromotor processes. In J. H. Carr, P. B. Shepherd, J. Gordon, et al. (Eds.), *Movement science: Foundations for physiotherapy in Rehabilitation* (pp. 93–154). London: Heinemann Physio Therapy.

Henderson, J. W., Wang, S., Egger, M. J., et al. (2013). Can women correctly contract their pelvic floor muscles without formal instruction? *Female Pelvic Medicine & Reconstructive Surgery*, 19(1), 8–12.

Hilde, G., Stær-Jensen, J., Brækken, I. H., et al. (2013a). Impact of childbirth and mode of delivery on vaginal resting pressure and on pelvic floor muscle strength and endurance. *American Journal of Obstetrics and Gynecology*, *208*, 5.e1–5.e7.

Hilde, G., Staer-Jensen, J., Siafarikas, F., et al. (2013b). How well can pelvic floor muscles with major defects contract? A cross-sectional comparative study 6 weeks after delivery using transperineal 3D/4D ultrasound and manometer. *An International Journal of Journal of Aging and Physical Activity*, *120*(11), 1423–1429.

Hodges, P. W., & Gandevia, S. C. (2000). Changes in intra-abdominal pressure during postal and respiratory activation of the human diaphragm. *Journal of Applied Physiology*, *89*, 967–976.

Johannessen, H. H., Wibe, A., Stordahl, A., et al. (2017). Do pelvic floor muscle exercises reduce postpartum anal incontinence? A randomised controlled trial. *An International Journal of Journal of Aging and Physical Activity*, *124*(4), 686–694.

Jordre, B., & Schweinle, W. (2014). Comparing resisted hip rotation with pelvic floor muscle training in women with stress urinary incontinence: A pilot study. *Journal Women's Health Physical Therapy*, *38*, 81–89.

Kegel, A. H. (1952). Stress incontinence and genital relaxation. *Clinical Symposia*, *4*(2), 35–51.

Kruger, J., Budgett, D., Goodman, J., et al. (2018). Can you train the pelvic floor muscles by contracting other related muscles? *Neurourology and Urodynamics*, *38*(2), 655–683.

Liebergall-Wischnitzer, M., Hochner-Celnikier, D., Lavy, Y., et al. (2005). Paula method of circular muscle exercises for urinary stress incontinence—a clinical trial. *International Urogynecology Journal and Pelvic Floor Dysfunction*, *16*, 345–351.

Mateus-Vasconcelos, E. C. L., Brito, L. G. O., Driusso, P., et al. (2018). Effects of three interventions in facilitating voluntary pelvic floor muscle contraction in women: A randomized controlled trial. *BJPT*, *22*, 391–399.

Mateus-Vasconcelos, E. C. L., Ribeiro, A. M., Antônio, F. I., et al. (2017). Physiotherapy methods to facilitate pelvic floor muscle contraction: A systematic review. *Physiotherapy Theory and Practice*, *34*(6), 420–432.

Mørkved, S., & Bø, K. (1997). The effect of postpartum pelvic floor muscle exercise in prevention and treatment of urinary incontinence. *International Urogynecology Journal and Pelvic Floor Dysfunction*, *8*, 217–222.

Mørkved, S., Bø, K., & Fjørtoft, T. (2002). Is there any effect of adding biofeedback to pelvic floor muscle training for stress urinary incontinence? A single blind randomized controlled trial. *Obstetrics & Gynecology*, *100*(4), 730–739.

Mørkved, S., Bø, K., Schei, B., et al. (2003). Pelvic floor muscle training during pregnancy to prevent urinary incontinence: A single-blind randomized controlled trial. *Obstetrics & Gynecology*, *101*(2), 313–319.

Overgård, M., Angelsen, A., Lydersen, S., et al. (2008). Does physiotherapist-guided pelvic floor muscle training reduce urinary incontinence after radical prostatectomy? A randomized controlled trial. *European Urology*, *54*(2), 438–448.

Resende, A. P., Zanetti, M. R. D., Petricelli, C. D., et al. (2011). Effects of the Paula method in electromyographic activity of the pelvic floor: A comparative study. *International Urogynecology Journal and Pelvic Floor Dysfunction*, *22*, 677–680.

Sapsford, R., & Hodges, P. (2001). Contraction of the pelvic floor muscles during abdominal maneuvers. *Archives of Physical Medicine and Rehabilitation*, *82*, 1081–1088.

Sheng, Y., Liu, X., Low, L. K., et al. (2019). Association of pubovisceral muscle tear with functional capacity of urethral closure: Evaluating maternal recovery from labor and delivery. *American Journal of Obstetrics and Gynecology*, *222*(6), 598.e1–598.e7.

Stafne, S. N., Salvesen, K. Å., Romundstad, P. R., et al. (2012). Does regular exercise including pelvic floor muscle training prevent urinary and anal incontinence during pregnancy? A randomized controlled trial. *British Journal of Obstetrics and Gynaecology*, *119*(10), 1270–1280.

Stær-Jensen, J., Siafarikas, F., Hilde, G., et al. (2015). Postpartum recovery of levator hiatus and bladder neck mobility in relation to pregnancy. *Obstetrics & Gynecology*, *125*(3), 531–539.

Talasz, H., Himmer-Perschak, G., Marth, E., et al. (2008). Evaluation of pelvic floor muscle function in a random group of adult women in Austria. *International Urogynecology Journal and Pelvic Floor Dysfunction*, *19*, 131–135.

Thompson, J. A., & O'Sullivan, P. B. (2003). Levator plate movement during voluntary pelvic floor muscle contraction in subjects with incontinence and prolapse: A cross-sectional study and review. *International Urogynecology Journal and Pelvic Floor Dysfunction*, *14*(2), 84–88.

Tries, J. (1990). Kegel exercises enhanced by biofeedback. . *Journal Enterostomal Therapeutics*, *17*, 67–76.

Uechi, N., Fernandes, A. C. N. L., Bø, K., et al. (2019). Do women have an accurate perception of their pelvic floor muscle contraction? A cross-sectional study. *Neurourology and Urodynamics*, *39*(1), 361–366.

Vermandel, A., De Wachter, S., Beyltjens, T., et al. (2015). Pelvic floor awareness and the positive effect of verbal instructions in 958 women early postdelivery. *International Urogynecology Journal*, *26*, 223–228.

Winstein, C. J. (1991). Knowledge of results and motor learning—implications for physiotherapy. In *Movement science* (pp. 181–189). Alexandria, VA: American Physiotherapy Association.

6.2 Strength Training

Kari Bø and Truls Raastad

INTRODUCTION TO THE CONCEPT OF STRENGTH TRAINING FOR PELVIC FLOOR MUSCLES

The pelvic floor muscles (PFMs) are regular skeletal muscles (Fig. 6.2.1) and will therefore adapt to strength training in the same way as other muscles as long as the basic principles for strength training are followed. The aim of a strength training regimen is to increase strength and function by changing muscle morphology such as increasing the cross-sectional area and optimizing muscle length (Franchi et al., 2017; Oranchuk et al., 2019), and by improving neurological factors such as activation level, timing of contraction and regulating muscle 'tone' or stiffness (DiNubile, 1991; Suchomel et al., 2018) (Fig. 6.2.2).

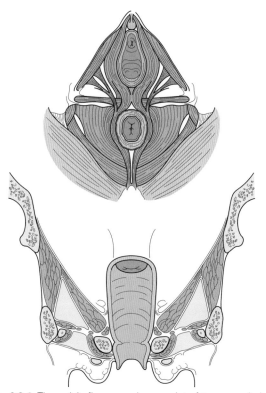

Fig. 6.2.1 The pelvic floor muscles consist of two muscle layers: the pelvic diaphragm (cranial location) and the urogenital diaphragm (caudal location, also named the *perineal muscles*).

Specific changes are dependent on the type of exercise and the training programme used, but response to a specific training programme also depends on genetics and hereditary factors (Haskel, 1994; Timmons, 2011), as well as the quality of contractions performed (Table 6.2.1). However, whenever starting to activate any muscle in the body, physiological changes will occur within the activated muscles. Table 6.2.2 presents a list of some of the physiological adaptations in the muscle fibre following regular strength training.

Connective tissue is abundant within and around all skeletal muscles including the epimysium, perimysium and endomysium. These connective tissue sheaths provide the tensile strength, contribute to viscoelastic properties ('stiffness') of muscle and provide support for the loading of muscle (Fleck and Kraemer, 2004; Roberts, 2016). There is evidence that strength training can increase connective tissue mass and change the mechanical properties, and that intensity of training and load bearing are major factors for effective training (Arampatzis et al., 2007). Magnusson et al. (2007) found in their study that the adaptability of tendon to loading differs in men and women. Tendons in women might have a lower rate of new tissue formation, respond less to mechanical loading and have a lower mechanical strength. Increased estradiol levels may slow down the rate of collagen synthesis. This may increase the risk of injury compared to men and could be important to take into consideration in training progression.

The theoretical rationale for intensive strength training of the PFMs is that strength training may build up the structural support of the pelvis by elevating the levator plate to a permanent higher location inside the pelvis and by enhancing hypertrophy and stiffness of the PFMs and connective tissue. This would facilitate a more effective co-contraction of the PFMs and prevent descent during increases in abdominal pressure. In an assessor-blinded randomized controlled trial (RCT) of 6 months of PFM training (PFMT) to prevent and treat pelvic organ prolapse, Brækken et al. (2010) found a significant increase in PFM thickness of 15.6%, a reduction in the levator hiatus area of 6.3%, reduction

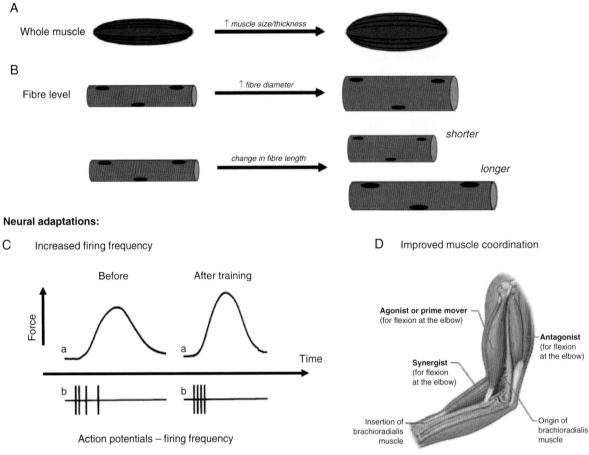

Fig. 6.2.2 Schematic overview of morphological and neural adaptations to strength training. Muscle adaptations include increase in muscle cross-sectional area (A), and increase in fibre cross-sectional area and optimization of muscle length (B). Neural adaptations include improved force (a) and rate of force development by increased firing frequency (b) (C), and improved coordination of involved agonists, synergists and antagonists (D).

TABLE 6.2.1	**Common Errors in Attempts to Contract the Pelvic Floor Muscles**
Error	**Observation**
Contraction of outer abdominal muscles instead of the PFMs	The person is either curving the back or starts the attempt to contract by 'hollowing'/tucking the stomach inwards (note that a small 'hollowing' can be seen in a correct contraction with the transverse abdominal muscle co-contracting)
Contraction of hip adductor muscles instead of the PFMs	A contraction of the muscles of the inner thigh can be seen
Contraction of gluteal muscles instead of the PFMs	The person is pressing the buttocks together, lifting up from the bench
Stop breathing	The person closes their mouth and holds their breath
Enhanced inhaling	The person takes a deep inspiration often accompanied by contraction of abdominal muscles and tries erroneously to 'lift up' the pelvic floor by the inspiration
Straining	The person presses downwards; when undressed, the perineum can be seen pressing in a caudal direction, and if the person has pelvic organ prolapse, the prolapse may protrude

PFMs, Pelvic floor muscles.

TABLE 6.2.2 Muscle Fibre Adaptation With Resistance Training

Variable	Muscle's Adaptational Response
Muscle fibre myofibrillar protein content	↑
Capillary density	↔ (↓↑) dependent on training status, number of repetitions per set and total volume
Mitochondrial volume density and content of mitochondrial (aerobic) enzymes	↔ (↓↑) dependent on training status, number of repetitions per set and total volume
Myoglobin	↓
Creatine phosphokinase	↑
Glycolytic enzymes	↔↑
Stored adenosine triphosphate	↑
Stored creatine phosphate	↑
Stored glycogen	↑ (dependent on diet)
Stored triglycerides	↑?
Myosin heavy chain composition	IIX to IIA

Modified from Kraemer and Fry (1995) and Groennebaek and Vissing (2017).

in muscle length of 4.2%, and a lift of the position of the bladder neck and rectal ampulla of 4.3 and 6.7 mm, respectively, compared to the control group. In addition, the levator hiatus area and muscle length were reduced during Valsalva, indicating increased PFM stiffness and improvement of automatic function. The pelvic floor can be considered as a trampoline with its position inside the pelvis. If the trampoline is stretched and sagging down, it is difficult to jump. However, a firm trampoline gives a quicker response and an effective 'push' upwards (Fig. 6.2.3). Increased stiffness in the connective tissue/tendons is probably important in all movements where we try to develop force as fast as possible. Arampatzis et al. (2007) found that to increase stiffness and cross-sectional area in the Achilles tendon, the loading/strain in the strength training regimen should be high (90% of maximum voluntary contraction). This is confirmed in later studies (Oranchuk et al., 2019).

As most individuals starting a PFMT regimen would be untrained, some improvements would probably occur regardless of the type of training programme applied (Kraemer and Ratamess, 2004). Because all PFMT studies have used different training dosages and different outcome measures, it is not possible to compare effects and conclude which training programme is the most effective. We will argue that proper strength training is needed to make a measurable change in muscle morphology and cure symptoms of pelvic floor dysfunction (Bræukken et al., 2010).

TERMINOLOGY AND DEFINITIONS

Muscle Strength

Muscle strength is 'the maximal amount of force or torque a muscle or muscle group can generate in a specific movement pattern at a specific velocity of movement' (Knuttgen and Komi, 2003; Knuttgen and Kraemer, 1987). To include different muscle actions, it has also been defined as the 'maximum force which can be exerted against an immovable object (static/isometric strength), the heaviest weight which can be lifted or lowered (concentric and eccentric dynamic strength), or the maximum torque which can be developed against a preset rate limiting device (isokinetic strength)' (Frontera and Meredith, 1989).

A *repetition* is one complete movement of an exercise (e.g., one contraction of the PFMs). It normally consists of two phases: the concentric muscle action and the eccentric muscle action (Fleck and Kraemer, 2004).

A *set* is a group of repetitions performed continuously without stopping or resting. In strength training, sets typically range from 1 to 15 repetitions (Fleck and Kramer, 2004).

Maximum Voluntary Contraction

Knuttgen and Kraemer (1987) described a *maximal voluntary contraction* as 'a condition in which a person attempts to recruit as many fibres in a muscle as possible for the purpose of developing force'. They focus on the importance of the word *voluntary* because inhibitory mechanisms in the central nervous system can limit the recruitment of motor units and thereby the total number of muscle fibres that will produce the force. An important part of strength training is to diminish the inhibitory mechanisms during maximal effort and allow the person to come as close as possible to full activation of the

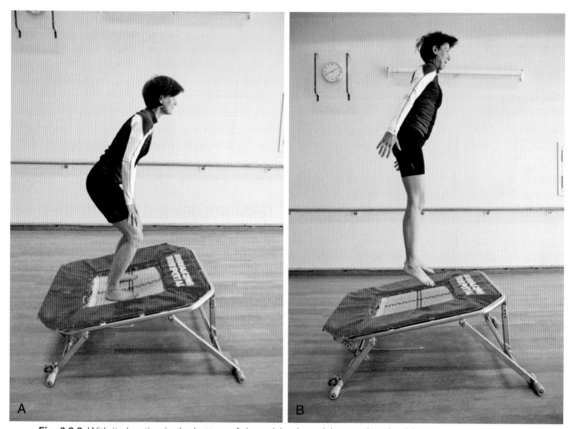

Fig. 6.2.3 With its location in the bottom of the pelvis, the pelvic muscles should act as a trampoline when abdominal pressure is increased. A stiff trampoline gives a quick response to load and pushes upwards.

muscle. The resistance at which the subject can perform only one lift of a free weight (dynamic contractions) and not be able to repeat it is termed the *one repetition maximum* (1RM) (Bompa and Carrera, 2005). For an isometric contraction, the max strength is often referred to as maximum voluntary contraction (Tan, 1999). The mass of the free weight that limits the person to 10 repetitions would be termed *10RM* (Knuttgen and Kraemer, 1987). Performing voluntary maximal muscular actions means that the muscles involved must contract against as much resistance as its present fatigue level will allow. This is often referred to as overloading the muscle.

Local Muscle Endurance

Local muscle endurance is usually defined as either the number of repetitions performed until failure with a specific load or duration of sustaining a submaximal isometric contraction. The number of repetitions until failure is inversely related to the percentage of 1RM, and

it varies with training status, sex and amount of muscle mass needed to perform the exercise (Hoeger et al., 1990). Training close to fatigue is a necessary component of local muscle endurance training (Kraemer and Ratamess, 2004). Importantly, increases in maximum strength usually increase local muscle endurance, especially at high intensities, whereas muscle endurance training does normally not improve maximum strength. Training to increase muscle endurance requires the performance of a high number of repetitions and minimizing recovery between sets. Adaptations to muscular endurance training is mostly related to increases in capillary density and mitochondrial proteins (Lim et al., 2019).

Muscle Power

Muscle power is the explosive aspect of strength, the product of force and speed of movement (force × distance)/time (Wilmore and Costill, 1999). Power is the functional application of both strength and speed, and it is the key component of most performances. Because force decreases with increasing velocity in a hyperbolic pattern, power production will be low at both low and very high velocities (Cormie et al., 2011a) (Fig. 6.2.4). Maximal power is therefore produced at a combination of submaximal force and velocity values. Maximal shortening velocity is higher in type II than in type I fibres, and the potential to produce power is therefore much higher in muscles with a large proportion of type II fibres. The proportion of type II fibres is, however, not easily changeable in skeletal muscle, so training strategies to improve power have to target other beneficial adaptations. In general, two different strategies can be used:

1. Training with moderate to high loads implies moderate to slow velocity contractions, but the expected increase in maximal strength will impact power production capacity.
2. Training with light to moderate loads performed at an explosive lifting velocity will not have the same effect on maximal strength, but the maximal effort in each contraction can increase the rate of force generation by improving the neural activation of the muscle (e.g., increased recruitment and rate coding). Rate coding is the rates at which motor units discharge action potentials.

These two strategies were used in the PFMT programme developed by Bø et al. (1990). The patient is asked to contract as close to maximum as possible, try to hold the contraction and then add three to four fast contractions on top of the holding period (Fig. 6.2.5). Notably, it might be possible to improve the neural activation to a similar extent with the heavy load strategy as long as the intent is to contract as fast as possible, but the combination of different strategies including specific exercise for the actual movement seems to give the best effect on power development (Cormie et al., 2011b).

DETERMINANTS OF MUSCLE STRENGTH

There are several determinants of muscle strength:

- Anatomical determinants: For skeletal muscle crossing a joint the lever arm is important. The longer the lever arm, the more torque the muscle can produce (torque = force × lever arm). For PFMs, there is, however, no real lever arm since there is no or little joint movement (the tail bone) (Bø et al., 2001). Nevertheless, a sagging pelvic floor may be more difficult to lift voluntarily, and the expected automatic co-contraction during increased abdominal pressure may be too slow to stop excessive downward movement. Furthermore, the total number of muscle fibres within a muscle, the cross-sectional area of the fibres, the distribution of type I and type II muscle fibres (especially in fast dynamic contractions), and the internal muscle architecture are determinants of muscle strength (Åstrand et al., 2003). All of these determinates differ between individuals.
- Length–tension: There is an optimal length at which muscle fibres generate maximal force. The total amount of force generated depends on the total number of myosin cross-bridges interacting with active sites on the actin. If a sarcomere or a muscle is stretched or shortened beyond the optimal length, less force can be developed (Fleck and Kraemer, 2004). This aspect might be of special importance for the strength in PFMs because the position of the pelvis floor will directly impact the length of the individual muscles.
- Force–velocity: As the velocity of a movement increases, the maximal force a muscle can produce concentrically decreases. Conversely, as the velocity of movement increases, the force that a muscle can develop eccentrically increases (Fleck and Kraemer, 2004).

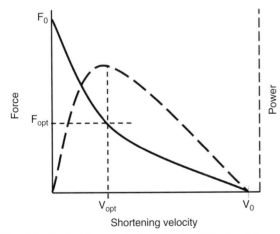

Fig. 6.2.4 Typical force–velocity curve (solid line) and the corresponding power–velocity (dashed line) relationship obtained from a hypothetical muscle or muscle group. F_{opt} corresponds to the muscle force (F) that overcomes the optimum external load that results in the optimum shortening velocity (V) for maximizing power.

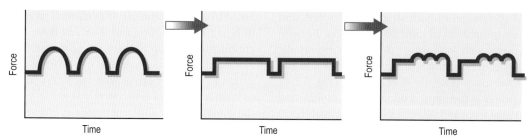

Fig. 6.2.5 Progression of pelvic floor muscle contraction. In the first stage the patient is instructed to contract as hard as possible; the second stage is to hold the contraction; and the third stage is to contract as hard as possible, hold the contraction and add three to four quick contractions on top of the holding period (third diagram).

- Muscle volume: There is a highly significant positive correlation between cross-sectional area and maximal strength, especially for experienced athletes (Brechue and Abe, 2002). The connection is less pronounced if untrained and in complex exercises because differences in technique can explain a bigger part of the result (Carroll et al., 2001). For the PFMs, the potential for maximal force production will also be proportional to the cross-sectional area of the individual muscles, but the individual strength will also be determined by the neural control.
- Neural control (motor unit recruitment, rate of firing and coordination of muscle activity) is an important component of muscle strength (Fleck and Kraemer, 2004). For most muscles, force is increased up to 80% of maximum by the gradual recruitment of more motor units, whereas the final 20% is mainly regulated by increasing the firing rate of each motor unit. The ability to obtain high firing rates in the beginning of a contraction is of special importance for the rate of force development. In more complex movements, the coordination of optimal activity and timing of activity in involved muscles is vital.

The two most important factors that can be influenced by strength training are neural adaptations and muscle cross-sectional area (hypertrophy) (Fleck and Kraemer, 2004), but muscle length can also be changed dependent on the muscle length at which the training is conducted (Oranchuk et al., 2019).

NEURAL ADAPTATIONS

Neural factors can be listed as neural drive (recruitment and rate of firing) to the muscle, increased synchronization of the motor units, increased activation of agonists,

decreased or more balanced activation of antagonists, coordination of all motor units and muscles involved in a movement, and inhibition of the protective mechanisms of the muscle (e.g., Golgi tendon organs) (Fleck and Kraemer, 2004). When a person attempts to produce a maximal contraction, all available motor units are activated. Force can be increased by recruiting more motor units and an increase in the motor unit firing rate. It has been suggested that untrained individuals are not able to voluntarily recruit the highest threshold motor units or maximally activate these motor units (Kraemer et al., 1996).

An important part of training adaptation is therefore developing the ability to recruit all motor units or the ability to fire all motor units at the rate needed for maximal force in a specific exercise. This seems to be especially important for PFMT because so few people are aware of the PFMs or have ever tried to contract the PFMs voluntarily. Another important neural adaptation to training is a reduction in antagonist activation. For the PFMs, it is difficult to say which muscles can be considered antagonists. However, abdominal contraction may be considered as an antagonist contraction because increased abdominal pressure will push the pelvic floor downwards. Consequently, an automatic co-contraction of the PFMs to counteract any increase in abdominal pressure or the increase from ground reaction force may be considered a goal for training.

The initial rapid gains in strength seen with strength training has been suggested to be due to neural adaptation (Sale, 1988), but this is probably most related to more complex movements where coordination of several muscle groups is central. A 50% increase in muscle strength within only weeks of training is common in such complex exercises, and this strength gain is much greater than can be explained by muscle hypertrophy (Fleck and Kraemer, 2004). In simpler movements, like elbow flexion, the strength gains are slower and more closely related to the increase in muscle cross-sectional area. After the initial period with neural adaptations, muscle hypertrophy becomes the predominant factor in strength increase.

Greater loading is needed to increase maximal strength as one progresses from intermediate to advanced levels of training, and loads greater than 80% to 85% of 1RM are needed to produce further neural adaptations during advanced resistance training with slow contractions (Kraemer and Ratamess, 2004), whereas neural adaptations with lighter loads require maximal effort and a more explosive contraction. This is important because maximizing strength, power and hypertrophy may be accomplished only when the maximal numbers of motor units are recruited. Another strategy to recruit all motor units with lighter loads is to perform sets until total failure. With this strategy, it is possible to achieve the same hypertrophy with 30RM loads as with heavy loads (Schoenfeld et al., 2017), but the increase in strength is less than with heavier loads and the training is less time efficient.

Some of the strength exercises are more difficult to coordinate than others and put the nervous system under greater demands. The potential for neural adaptations to influence the result are therefore higher during such exercises (e.g., squat vs arm curl) (Chilibeck et al., 1998). According to Shield and Zhou (2004), there is generally only small room for improvement in fully activating the muscles in simple movements in healthy people. The amount differs with the type of contraction (isometric, dynamic), muscle groups, injuries, degenerations and complexity of movements. But there are still disagreements in the amount of activation and the effect of strength training. Most studies imply that a full activation of most muscles is measured with early twitch interpolation techniques, whereas more sensitive techniques reveal that even healthy adults routinely fail to fully activate several different muscles despite maximal effort (Shield and Zhou, 2004). A typical activation deficit in untrained healthy people is 0% to 10%. Other factors that can only be explained by neural factors are the cross-education effect seen in unilateral training (Munn et al., 2004) and the effect where strength is increased after imagined contractions (Åstrand et al., 2003).

Hypertrophy

One of the most prominent adaptations to strength training is muscle enlargement. The growth in muscle size is primarily due to an increase in the size of the individual muscle fibre (Fleck and Kraemer, 2004). According to Fleck and Kraemer (2004), humans have a potential to hyperplasia, but it does not happen on a large scale and is far from the dominating cause of hypertrophy. An increase in the number of muscle fibres has been shown in birds and mammals, but there are limited data to prove this in humans.

The increase in cross-sectional area is attributed to increased size and number of the contractile structures (myofibrils) within existing muscle fibres. An increase in non-contractile proteins has also been suggested (Haun et al., 2019).

Activated satellite cells and centrally located myonuclei may indicate cellular repair after training, and the formation of new muscle cells, and the proportion of satellite cells that appear morphologically active, increase as a result of resistance training (Fleck and Kraemer, 2004). Another important function of the activated satellite cells is to fuse with the growing muscle fibres to ensure a constant nucleus to cytoplasmic ratio during hypertrophy.

Muscle fibre hypertrophy has been found in both type I and type II fibres after strength training. However, most studies show greater hypertrophy in type II and especially IIa fibres (Green et al., 1999; Kraemer et al., 1995). Genetic factors decide whether a person has predominantly type I or type II muscle fibres, and although transitions from type IIx to type IIa is normal in the first phase of strength training (Adams et al., 1993; Campos et al., 2002; Green et al., 1999), such changes only seem to happen within type II fibres (e.g., not from type II to type I; Fleck and Kraemer, 2004). Cessation of training leads to transitions back from IIa to IIx.

Different muscles have different distributions of fibre types, and the total number of muscle fibres varies between individuals. Because the number and distribution of muscle fibres does not seem to be the dominant factor for hypertrophy, and it is impossible to evaluate the number and distribution of muscle fibres in an individual without biopsies, types of muscle fibres should be disregarded as a factor when prescribing PFMT. The aim is to target as many motor units as possible in each contraction and thereby initiate a stimulus for hypertrophy in all fibres.

Greater hypertrophy has been associated with high-volume programmes compared to low-volume programmes (Kraemer and Ratamess, 2004). Short rest intervals have also been shown to be beneficial for hypertrophy and local muscle endurance (Kraemer and Ratamess, 2004). Some studies suggest that a fatigue stimulus with metabolic stress factors has an influence on optimal strength development and muscle growth, especially when exercising with lighter loads (Schoenfeld et al., 2017). Rooney et al. (1994) found that a 30-second rest between each lift gave a significant lower strength increase than the same amount of repetitions and loads with no rest between the lifts. Maximal hypertrophy may be best attained by a combination of strength and hypertrophy training.

With the initiation of a strength training regimen, changes in the types and amount of muscle proteins start to take place within a couple of workouts. This is caused by increased protein synthesis, a decrease in protein degradation or a combination of both. Protein synthesis is significantly elevated up to 48 hours after exercise (Fleck and Kraemer, 2004). However, to demonstrate significant muscle fibre hypertrophy, a longer training time is normally required (>8 weeks) (Fleck and Kraemer, 2004); however, with more sensitive measures, hypertrophy has been demonstrated after less than 4 weeks of training as well (DeFreitas et al., 2011). As studies are demonstrating an elevated muscle protein synthesis after an acute strength training bout (Biolo et al., 1995; MacDougall et al., 1995; Phillips et al., 1997), the discrepancy seen between increased strength and muscle growth early in a strength training regimen may be more due to methodological problems in measuring small changes in muscle cross-sectional area rather than the traditionally assumed effect of neural adaptation. Another contributing factor that can explain why the role of neural adaptation may be overestimated at the beginning of a strength training programme is an increase of muscle fibre girth at the expense of extracellular spaces (Åstrand et al., 2003). In most training studies, increase in muscle fibre cross-sectional area ranges from about 20% to 40% (Fleck and Kraemer, 2004). In an uncontrolled PFMT trial, Bernstein (1996) found an increase in levator ani thickness of 7.6% at rest and 9.3% during contraction,

whereas the increase in PFM thickness was 15.6% in the RCT by Brækken et al. (2010).

Normally, an isometric muscle action is considered as muscle activation without any joint movement, but in most cases, muscle fibres are shortening because the tendons are stretched. Is a voluntary PFM contraction a concentric or isometric muscle action? MRI studies (Bø et al., 2001) have shown that there is a movement of the coccyx during PFM contraction. Hence the contraction is concentric. However, this movement is small and therefore there must be an isometric component of PFMT. It has been suggested that 1 to 4 seconds is necessary to reach maximum contraction force in isometric muscle actions. However, holding times between 3 and 10 seconds are recommended for isometric contractions in training (Fleck and Kraemer, 2004). Daily isometric training is superior to less frequent training, but three training sessions per week will bring significant increases in maximal strength. Isometric training alone with no external weights has been shown to increase protein synthesis by 49% and muscular hypertrophy of both type I and II muscle fibres. Twelve weeks of training increased knee extensor cross-sectional area by 8% and muscle isometric strength by 41% (Fleck and Kraemer, 2004). Although PFM action is considered as isometric or concentric, eccentric actions do occur during rapid increases in intra-abdominal pressure.

DOSE–RESPONSE ISSUES

Dose–response issues deal with how much (or how little) exercise is needed to make a measurable training response (Bouchard, 2001; Bouchard et al., 1994). The dosage can be divided into mode of exercise, frequency, intensity, volume and duration of training. A training response is a progressive change in function or structure that results from performing repeated bouts of exercise.

Mode of Exercise

Mode of exercise refers to type of training (e.g., strength training, flexibility training, cardiovascular training and all types of specific exercises for different muscle groups). There is only one way to conduct a PFM contraction (squeeze around the pelvic openings and a lift inwards/forwards). However, the exercises can be conducted in different positions, and they can be performed as isometric, concentric and eccentric muscle actions (Fig. 6.2.6).

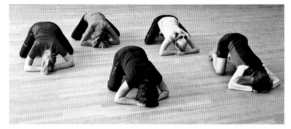

Fig. 6.2.6 Different positions can be used to vary pelvic floor muscle training.

Frequency

Frequency of exercise is usually defined as the number of training sessions per week in which a certain muscle group is being trained or a particular exercise is performed (Fleck and Kraemer, 2004). Training with heavy loads increases the recovery time needed before subsequent sessions. Most resistance training studies have used frequencies of 2 to 3 alternating days per week in previously untrained individuals. Power lifters typically train 4 to 6 days per week (Kraemer and Ratamess, 2004). The optimal training frequency is dependent on the stress put on the exercised muscles in each individual session and can be high (7 days/week) with less stressful training sessions and low (two to three sessions per week) with more normal strength training stress (Schoenfeld et al., 2016).

Intensity

Intensity of strength training is most often defined as the percentage of maximum (e.g., any given percentage of maximum or different repetition maximum resistances for the exercise; Fleck and Kraemer, 2004) but does also include the effort in each repetition. Intensity is by far the most important factor for an effective and quick response to a strength training programme (American College of Sports Medicine, 2009; Fatouros et al., 2005). Intensity is also one of the most important factors in maintaining the effects of resistance training (Fatouros et al., 2005).

Training intensity has traditionally been synonymous with training load, but it is the degree of activation and not the training resistance itself that determines the training intensity in strength training (Burd et al., 2012). Traditionally, the minimal intensity that was recommended to increase strength in young healthy individuals was 60% to 65% of 1RM. However, training with loads as low as 30% of 1RM has recently been shown

to increase muscle mass and strength as long as the training sets had been performed until failure (Schoenfeld et al., 2017). Although the hypertrophy was similar with the lighter loads, the increase in strength was lower compared to the effect with heavier loads. Furthermore, training with heavier loads is more time efficient and is more likely to induce positive adaptations in tendons and extracellular connective tissue. The following recommendations for intensity given by Garber et al. (2011) are therefore still valid:

Muscular endurance: 15 to 20 repetitions of less than 50% of 1RM

Power: 8 to 12 repetitions of 20% to 50% of 1RM and lighter for older people

Strength: 40% to 50% of 1RM (or 10–15 RM) for novice older adults and novice sedentary adults, 8 to 12 repetitions of 60% to 70% of 1RM for novice/intermediate exercisers and 80% or greater of 1RM for experienced strength trainers.

It is important to notice that all of these recommendations were based on studies on extremity muscles and not on the muscles of the abdomen, back or pelvic floor.

Single sets are recommended for novice and older adults to start with; two sets to improve strength and power, and two or more sets for muscular endurance. Breaks of 2 to 3 minutes are recommended between sets.

Performing many repetitions with very light resistance will result in no or minimal strength gain. This is quite contradictory to the recommendations for PFMT given by Kegel (1956). Although he emphasized to train against resistance, he advised performing at least 500 contractions per day, and for a long time this was the dominating recommendation for PFMT. Today, however, it is important to use modern evidence-based training principles to gain the best effect. Fewer contractions take less time and may therefore also be much more motivating. Hence exercise adherence and training efficiency may increase.

Duration

The *duration* of the training period (e.g., whether it is 3 weeks or 6 months) influences the results. The initial neural adaptations may manifest early in a training period, whereas other important adaptations such as hypertrophy increase linearly over several weeks and months (DeFreitas et al., 2011). Longer-duration training periods will therefore generally result in better effects on muscle strength, but the exact time course

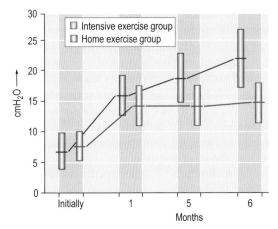

Fig. 6.2.7 Strength development during 6 months of two different training regimens for the pelvic floor muscles. There is 100% increase in muscle strength during the first month of exercise. After this first initial increase in strength, the group participating in supervised strenuous strength training in a class further develops muscle strength, whereas the other group exercising at home shows no further improvement.

differs between the individual adaptations and between individuals. Furthermore, training adaptations are not increasing linearly over longer periods, so periodical stagnation in strength gains should be expected.

In an RCT of PFM strength training to treat female stress urinary incontinence, Bø et al. (1990) demonstrated an increasing PFM strength in the intensive training group throughout the 6-month training period (Fig. 6.2.7). Short training periods may therefore not elicit the true effect of exercises. The American College of Sports Medicine (1998) recommends that to evaluate the efficacy of various intensities, frequencies and durations of exercise on fitness variables, a 15- to 20-week duration is an adequate minimum standard.

Training volume is a measure of the total amount of work (joules) performed in a training session, in a week of training, in a month of training or in some other period of time (Fleck and Kraemer, 2004). The simplest method to estimate training volume is to summate the number of repetitions performed in a specific time period or the total amount of weight lifted. More precisely, it can be determined by calculating the work performed (e.g., total work in a repetition is the resistance multiplied by the vertical distance a weight is lifted).

Periodization is the planned variation in the training volume and intensity (Fleck and Kraemer, 2004).

Variation is extremely important for continued gains in strength and other training outcomes. For improvements to occur, the programme used should be systematically altered so that the body is forced to adapt to changing stimuli. Variation can be achieved by altering muscle actions (isometric, concentric, eccentric), positions, repetitions, load, resting periods and types of exercises.

Adherence (often termed *compliance* in medical literature) is the extent to which the individual follows the exercise prescription. Adherence is the most important factor influencing outcome and should be reported in all exercise programmes.

HOW TO INCREASE MUSCLE STRENGTH AND UNDERLYING COMPONENTS

Four main principles are important in achieving measurable effects of strength training and underlying components: specificity, overload, progression and maintenance.

Specificity

The effect of exercise training is specific to the area of the body being trained (American College of Sports Medicine, 1998; Fleck and Kraemer, 2004). Strength training of the arms may therefore have little or no influence on the legs and vice versa. This principle is extremely important when it comes to the PFMs. There have been some suggestions that regular physical activity may enhance PFM strength (Bø, 2004). However, the prerequisite for this is that the load put on the pelvic floor by the increased intra-abdominal pressure or ground reaction force is counteracted by an adequate response from the PFMs. In an RCT, PFMT was compared with PFMT + running and jumping, and no effect was found from adding running and jumping to regular PFMT (Luginbuel et al., 2019). Obviously, in women with pelvic floor dysfunction the PFM are not co-contracting in adequate time or with enough strength to counteract the increased load. In such cases the PFMs are not trained but overloaded and stretched. There therefore needs to be a balance between the degree of loading and the counteraction of the PFMs. A gymnast may have adequate response from the PFMs during coughing and light activities. However, landing from a somersault on the balance beam may be too much load and cause urinary leakage. A small increase in abdominal pressure may therefore be an adequate stimulus for a co-contraction and thereby a 'training effect', whereas a huge increase may cause PFM descent and stretch and weaken the PFMs.

Although studies have shown that there are co-contractions of the PFMs with hip adductor, gluteal and different abdominal muscle contractions in healthy subjects (Bø and Stien, 1994; Neumann and Gill, 2002; Sapsford and Hodges, 2001), such contractions may not occur in persons with PFM dysfunction and may be weaker than a specific PFM contraction. Kruger et al. (2018) found that contraction of the PFMs was more effective and with only minimal increase in intra-abdominal pressure compared with abdominal contractions, for example. One should therefore focus on specific PFMT. In addition, Graves et al. (1988) have shown that resistance training should be conducted through a full range of motion for maximum benefit.

Overload

Muscular strength and endurance are developed by the progressive overload principle (e.g., by increasing more than normal the resistance to movement or frequency and duration of activity; American College of Sports Medicine, 2009). Muscular strength is best developed by using heavier weights/resistance (that require maximum or near-maximum tension development) with few repetitions, and muscular endurance is best developed by using lighter weights with a greater number of repetitions (American College of Sports Medicine, 2009). There are several ways to overload a muscle or muscle group:

- add weight or resistance;
- sustain the contraction;
- shorten resting periods between contractions;
- increase speed of the contraction;
- increase number of repetitions;
- increase frequency and duration of workouts;
- decrease recovery time between workouts;
- alternate forms of exercise; and
- alternate the range to which a muscle is being worked.

The physical therapist can manipulate all of the preceding factors when training the PFMs. However, certain important factors are difficult to apply for PFMT (e.g., to add weight and resistance). Plevnik (1985) invented vaginal weighted cones to make a progression of overload to the PFMs (Fig. 6.2.8). Vaginal cones come in different shapes and weights, and they are placed above the levator muscle. The patient is asked to start

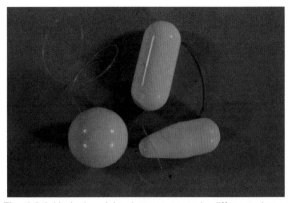

Fig. 6.2.8 Vaginal weighted cones come in different shapes and with different weights to make progression to pelvic floor muscle training. They were developed by Plevnik in 1985.

with a weight that she can hold for 1 minute in a standing position. The actual training is to try to stay in an upright position with the cone in place for 20 minutes. When the woman is able to walk around with a weight in place for 20 minutes, a heavier weight should replace the one used to make progression in workload. Although correct from a theoretical exercise science point of view, this method can be questioned from a practical point of view. In addition, holding a contraction for a long time may decrease blood supply, cause pain and reduce oxygen consumption (Bø, 1995). Many women report that they are unable to hold the cones in place, and adherence may be low (Bø et al., 1999; Cammu and Van Nylen, 1998).

Any magnitude of overload will result in strength development, but heavier resistance loads to maximal or near-maximal will elicit a significantly greater training effect (American College of Sports Medicine, 2009). Heavy resistance training may cause an acute increase in systolic and diastolic blood pressure, especially when a Valsalva manoeuvre is evoked (American College of Sports Medicine, 2011). This is of importance for PFMT because many women tend to erroneously perform a Valsalva manoeuvre when attempting to perform a PFM contraction. Ferreira et al. (2013) assessed heart rate during PFMT sessions and blood pressure before and after each training session in pregnant women. Heart rate significantly increased during training, but only for a limited time. Increase in blood pressure and heart rate during the training period was within normal ranges. Anecdotally, some women report slight headache, dizziness and discomfort during their first PFMT sessions, and this may be due to an increase in blood pressure or inadequate breathing. Normal breathing during attempts to perform maximal contractions is almost impossible. Therefore, an emphasis on normal breathing between each contraction is important.

Eccentric (lengthening) exercises are effective in increasing muscle strength (Fleck and Kraemer, 2004). However, the potential for skeletal muscle soreness and muscle injury is increased when compared to concentric (shortening) or isometric contractions, particularly in untrained individuals (American College of Sports Medicine, 2009; Fleck and Kraemer, 2004). Eccentric contractions are also more difficult to perform (require more motor skill and muscle awareness) than concentric or isometric contractions and are therefore not recommended at the beginning of a PFMT programme.

Progression

The three principles of progression are overload, variation and specificity.

Progressive overload is defined as 'continually increasing the stress placed on the muscle as it becomes capable of producing greater force or has more endurance' (Fleck and Kraemer, 2004, p. 7). One of the first reports of progression in strength training is from ancient Greece, where Milo, an Olympic 'wrestler', lifted a calf each day until it reached full growth (DiNubule, 1991).

The American College of Sport Medicine (2002, 2009) recommends that both concentric, eccentric and some isometric muscle actions are used in strength training programmes. For initial training, it is recommended that loads corresponding to 8 to 12 repetitions (60%–70% of repetition maximum) are used for novice training. For intermediate to advanced training, the recommendation is to use a wider range, from 1 to 12 repetitions (80%–100% of 1RM) in a periodized fashion, with eventually an emphasis on heavy loading (1–6 RM) with rest periods of at least 2 to 3 minutes between sets, and with a moderate to fast contraction velocity. Higher volume and emphasis on 6 to 12 RM is recommended for maximizing hypertrophy.

In practice, the principle of progressive overload is the most difficult factor to overcome in PFMT. It is difficult to put weight on the pelvic floor, and therefore other methods need to be used. In most cases the PT has tried to encourage the woman to contract the PFM

as close to maximum as possible. This can be done simultaneously with vaginal palpation (feedback) and with any measurement tool in situ (biofeedback). Using biofeedback to reach a maximum contraction can be important from an exercise science point of view. Strong verbal encouragement and motivation seem to be very important in reaching maximum effort. However, the physical therapist should always ensure that the patient is performing a correct contraction and not involving other muscles or increasing intra-abdominal pressure too much (to the extent that it is pressing the pelvic floor downwards). Leaving a patient to train alone is likely to result in loss of the overload and progression because only a few individuals can motivate themselves for maximal efforts.

Bø et al. (1990) have developed a method for progression in PFMT (see Fig. 6.2.5). The patient first learns to contract as hard as possible with no holding period, then the patient is encouraged to hold as long as possible, and the third step is to add three to four fast contractions on top of the sustained contraction. After this has been accomplished, the physical therapist encourages the patient to contract as hard as possible in each contraction.

One way to produce progression is to ask the patient to contract against progressively increasingly gravity going from a lying to a standing position (Fig. 6.2.9). Clinical experience has shown that most women find that PFM contractions are more difficult to conduct in the squatting position (Fig. 6.2.10). However, it is important that patients choose a position in which they can perceive the contraction, and also choose a position in which they feel a certain difficulty when training. In this way they stimulate the central nervous system and hopefully recruit an increasing number of motor units. In a group training setting the different positions are also used for variation in the training programme (Bø et al., 1990; Bø et al., 1999). So far, there are no studies comparing the effect of different positions on the development of PFM strength.

Another method to increase progression of the contraction is to use vaginal or rectal devices and ask the patient to hold back when the PT or the patient withdraws the device. This method implies eccentric muscle contraction and may be a quite effective method to increase strength. However, to date there are no studies comparing this training programme with no exercise

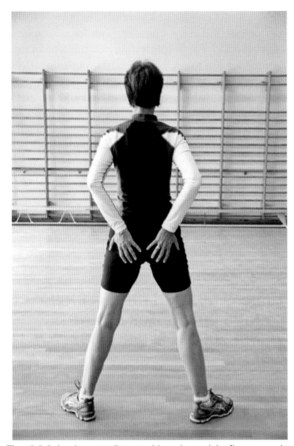

Fig. 6.2.9 In the standing position the pelvic floor muscles must contract against gravity, which is more difficult than in a supine or prone position.

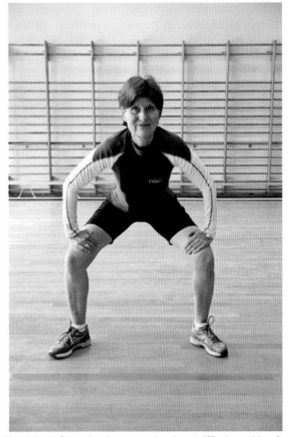

Fig. 6.2.10 Squatting is reported to be a difficult position for contracting the pelvic floor muscles and can therefore be used as a progression in loading.

or other exercise regimens, and one should be aware of the increased risk of injuries and development of muscle soreness in untrained individuals.

There is a need for more research evaluating different ways of adding progressive overload to PFMT.

Initial training status plays an important role in the rate of progression during strength training. Trained individuals have shown much slower rates of improvement than untrained individuals. Kraemer and Ratamess (2004) report that a literature review showed that muscular strength increased approximately 40% in 'untrained', 20% in 'moderately' trained, 16% in 'trained', 10% in 'advanced' and 2% in 'elite' individuals over periods of 4 weeks to 2 years. The only study looking at the development of PFM strength (see Fig. 6.2.7) showed a 100% increase after 1 month of exercise. This may be explained by

the PFMs being totally untrained and shows a huge potential for improvement. In a meta-analysis, Rea et al. (2003) confirmed statistically greater effect sizes in untrained compared to resistance-trained individuals with respect to training intensity, frequency and volume on progression. As the person approaches his or her genetic ceiling, small changes in strength require large amounts of training time.

Maintenance

Maintenance training is work to maintain the current level of muscular fitness. Cessation of exercise training is often referred to as detraining. Fleck and Kraemer (2004) described *detraining* as 'a deconditioning process that affects performance because of diminished physiological capacity'. Detraining from a muscle strengthening programme will reduce muscle girth, muscle fibre size, short-term endurance and strength/power, whereas capillary density, fat percentage, aerobic enzymes and mitochondrial density will increase (Fleck and Kraemer, 2004). However, following a shorter period of detraining, most individuals would still have higher values for these variables than untrained subjects, and physiological functions return quickly with retraining after the detraining period. Strength may be maintained for up to 2 weeks of detraining in power athletes, and in recreationally trained individuals, strength loss has been shown to take as long as 6 weeks. However, eccentric force and power seem to be more sensitive to detraining effects over a few weeks (Fleck and Kraemer, 2004).

In general, strength gains decline at a slower rate than strength increases due to training. There are few studies, however, investigating the minimal level of exercise necessary to maintain the training effect. A 5% to 10% loss of muscle strength per week has been shown after training cessation (Fleck and Kraemer, 2004). Greater loss has been shown in the elderly (65–75-year-olds) compared to younger people (20–30-year-olds); for both groups, most strength loss was from weeks 12 to 31 after cessation of training.

The rate of strength loss may depend on the duration of the training period before detraining, training intensity, type of strength test used and the specific muscle groups examined. Graves et al. (1988) showed that when strength training was reduced from 3 or 2 days a week to at least 1 day a week, strength was maintained for 12 weeks of reduced training. Reducing training frequency therefore does not seem to adversely affect muscular strength if intensity is maintained (Fatourus et al., 2005; Fleck and Kraemer, 2004). In one study, 24 weeks of heavy resistance training three times a week increased vertical jump ability by 13%. Twelve weeks of detraining decreased the ability, but it was still 2% above the pretraining value (Fleck and Kraemer, 2004). It is suggested that the ability to perform complex skills involving strength components may be lost if not included in the training programme (Fleck and Kraemer, 2004). Electromyography (EMG) studies have shown a change in motor unit firing rate and motor unit synchronization, and that this may cause the initial strength loss in the detraining period. Type II fibres may atrophy to a greater extent than type I fibres during short detraining periods in both men and women (Fleck and Kraemer, 2004).

Fleck and Kraemer (2004) concluded that research has not yet indicated the exact resistance, volume and frequency of strength training or the type of programme needed to maintain the training gains. However, studies indicate that to maintain strength gains or slow strength loss, the intensity should be maintained but the volume and frequency of training can be reduced: 1 to 2 days a week seems to be an effective maintenance frequency for those individuals already engaged in a resistance training programme (Kraemer and Ratamess, 2004).

Only one follow-up study measuring PFM strength after cessation of PFMT has been found. Bø and Talseth (1996) showed that there was no reduction in PFM muscle strength in the intensive training group 5 years after cessation of an RCT: 70% of the women in this group reported strength training of the PFMs at least once a week.

RECOMMENDATION FOR EFFECTIVE TRAINING DOSAGE FOR STRENGTH TRAINING OF THE PELVIC FLOOR MUSCLES

The American College of Sports Medicine has given the following recommendations for general strength training for (novice) adults (American College of Sports Medicine, 2009):

- Target major muscles.
- Perform 8 to 12 slow and moderate velocity, close-to-maximum contractions (even fewer repetitions are better to optimize strength and power).
- Perform one to three sets per exercise.
- Exercises should be conducted 2 to 3 days a week.
- It is difficult to improve at the same rate for long-term periods (e.g., >6 months) without manipulation of programme variables.

Although recommended for the use of external weights (resistance training), see the American College of Sports Medicine infographics in the work of Fiatarone et al. (2019).

Table 6.2.3 shows more specific recommendations for strength training regimens to effectively improve muscle strength, power and hypertrophy (Kraemer and Ratamess, 2004). Developing from untrained to intermediate and advanced, the progression is to get closer to maximum contraction and to add more training days per week.

TABLE 6.2.3   Recommendations for Progression of Training for Strength, Power and Hypertrophy in Novice Participants

	Strength	Power	Hypertrophy
Muscle Action	Eccentric and concentric	Eccentric and concentric	Eccentric and concentric
Exercise Selection	Single and multiple joint	Multiple joint	Single and multiple joint
Exercise Order	High before low intensity	High before low intensity	High before low intensity
Loading	60%–70% 1RM	60%–70% for strength 30%–60% for velocity/technique	60%–70% 1RM
Volume	1–3 sets × 8–12 repetitions	1–3 sets × 8–12 repetitions	1–3 sets × 8–12 repetitions
Rest Intervals	1–2 min	2–3 min for core 1–2 min for others	1–2 min
Velocity	Slow to moderate	Moderate	Slow to moderate
Frequency	2–3 days per week	2–3 days per week	2–3 days per week

1RM, One repetition maximum. *From Kraemer and Ratamess (2004).*

CLINICAL RECOMMENDATIONS

- Make sure the patient can perform a correct contraction.
- Ask the patient to contract as hard as possible.
- Progress with sustained contractions, and add contractions with higher velocity as a progression.
- Holding time should be 3 to 10 seconds.
- Recommend PFMT every day.
- Encourage and motivate patients to get as close to maximum contraction as possible. Use strong verbal encouragement.
- Advance to eccentric contractions if possible (no data are available on the effect of eccentric training for the PFMs).
- Inform the patient that strength training develops in steps and that the largest improvements come during the first training period. After that, the patient needs to work harder to achieve further improvement.

REFERENCES

Adams, G. R., Hather, B. M., Baldwin, K. M., et al. (1993). Skeletal muscle myosin heavy chain composition and resistance training. *Journal of Applied Physiology, 74*(2), 911–915.

American College of Sports Medicine. (1998). The recommended quantity and quality of exercise for developing and maintaining cardiorespiratory and muscular fitness, and flexibility in healthy adults. *Medicine & Science in Sports & Exercise, 30*, 975–991.

American College of Sports Medicine. (2002). Position stand. Progression models in resistance training for healthy adults. *Medicine & Science in Sports & Exercise, 34*, 364–380.

American College of Sports Medicine. (2009). Position stand. Progression models in resistance training for healthy adults. *Medicine & Science in Sports & Exercise, 41*(3), 687–708.

American College of Sports Medicine. (2011). Quantity and quality of exercise for developing and maintaining cardiorespiratory, musculoskeletal, and neuromotor fitness in apparently healthy adults: Guidance for prescribing exercise. *Medicine & Science in Sports & Exercise, 43*(7), 1334–1359.

Arampatzis, A., Karamanidis, K., & Albracht, K. (2007). Adaptational responses of the human Achilles tendon by modulation of the applied cyclic strain magnitude. *Journal of Experimental Biology, 210*, 2743–2753.

Åstrand, P. O., Rodahl, K., Dahl, H. A., et al. (2003). *Textbook of work physiology: Physiological basis of exercise.* Champaign, IL: Human Kinetics.

Bernstein, I. T. (1996). *The pelvic floor muscles. Doctoral thesis.* Hvidovre Hospital, Department of Urology, University of Copenhagen.

Biolo, G., Maggi, S. P., Williams, B. D., et al. (1995). Increased rates of muscle protein turnover and amino acid transport after resistance exercise in humans. *American Journal of Physiology, 268*(3 Pt. 1), E514–E520.

Bø, K. (1995). Vaginal weight cones. Theoretical framework, effect on pelvic floor muscle strength and female stress urinary incontinence. *Acta Obstetricia et Gynecologica Scandinavica, 74*, 87–92.

Bø, K. (2004). Urinary incontinence, pelvic floor dysfunction, exercise and sport. *Sports Medicine, 34*(7), 451–464.

Bø, K., Hagen, R. H., Kvarstein, B., et al. (1990). Pelvic floor muscle exercise for the treatment of female stress urinary incontinence: III. Effects of two different degrees of pelvic floor muscle exercise. *Neurourology and Urodynamics, 9*, 489–502.

Bø, K., Lilleås, F., Talseth, T., et al. (2001). Dynamic MRI of pelvic floor muscles in an upright sitting position. *Neurourology and Urodynamics, 20*, 167–174.

Bø, K., & Stien, R. (1994). Needle EMG registration of striated urethral wall and pelvic floor muscle activity patterns during cough, Valsalva, abdominal, hip adductor, and gluteal muscles contractions in nulliparous healthy females. *Neurourology and Urodynamics, 13*, 35–41.

Bø, K., & Talseth, T. (1996). Long-term effect of pelvic floor muscle exercise 5 years after cessation of organized training. *Obstetrics & Gynecology, 87*, 261–265.

Bø, K., Talseth, T., & Holme, I. (1999). Single blind, randomised controlled trial of pelvic floor exercises, electrical stimulation, vaginal cones, and no treatment in management of genuine stress incontinence in women. *British Medical Journal, 318*, 487–493.

Bompa, T. O., & Carrera, M. C. (2005). *Periodization training for sports* (2nd ed.). Champaign, IL: Human Kinetics.

Bouchard, C. (2001). Physical activity and health: Introduction to the dose–response symposium. *Medicine & Science in Sports & Exercise, 33*(Suppl. 6), 347–350.

Bouchard, C., Shephard, R. J., & Stephens, T. (1994). *Physical activity, fitness and health*. Champaign, IL: Consensus Statement. Human Kinetics.

Brækken, I. H., Majida, M., Engh, M. E., et al. (2010). Morphological changes after pelvic floor muscle training measured by 3D ultrasound. *Obstetrics & Gynecology, 115*(2 Pt. 1), 317–324.

Brechue, W. F., & Abe, T. (2002). The role of FFM accumulation and skeletal muscle architecture in powerlifting performance. *European Journal of Applied Physiology, 86*(4), 327–336.

Burd, N. A., Mitchell, C. J., Churchward-Venne, T. A., et al. (2012). Bigger weights may not beget bigger muscles: Evidence from acute muscle protein synthetic responses after resistance exercise. *Applied Physiology, Nutrition, and Metabolism, 37*, 551–554.

Cammu, H., & Van Nylen, M. (1998). Pelvic floor exercises versus vaginal weight cones in genuine stress incontinence. *European Journal of Obstetrics & Gynecology and Reproductive Biology, 77*, 89–93.

Campos, G. E., Luecke, T. J., Wendeln, H. K., et al. (2002). Muscular adaptations in response to three different resistance-training regimens: Specificity of repetition maximum training zones. *European Journal of Applied Physiology, 88*(1–2), 50–60.

Carroll, T. J., Riek, S., & Carson, R. G. (2001). Neural adaptations to resistance training: Implications for movement control. *Sports Medicine, 31*(12), 829–840.

Chilibeck, P. D., Calder, A. W., Sale, D. G., et al. (1998). A comparison of strength and muscle mass increases during resistance training in young women. *European Journal of Applied Physiology and Occupational Physiology, 77*(1–2), 70–175.

Cormie, P., McGuigan, M. R., & Newton, R. U. (2011a). Developing maximal neuromuscular power: Part 1—biological basis of maximal power production. *Sports Medicine, 41*(1), 17–38.

Cormie, P., McGuigan, M. R., & Newton, R. U. (2011b). Developing maximal neuromuscular power: Part 2—training considerations for improving maximal power production. *Sports Medicine, 41*(2), 125–146.

DeFreitas, J. M., Beck, T. W., Stock, M. S., et al. (2011). An examination of the time course of training-induced skeletal muscle hypertrophy. *European Journal of Applied Physiology, 111*(11), 2785–2790.

DiNubile, N. A. (1991). Strength training. *Clinics in Sports Medicine, 10*(1), 33–62.

Fatouros, I. G., Kambas, A., Katrabasas, I., et al. (2005). Strength training and detraining effects on muscular strength, anaerobic power, and mobility of inactive older men are intensity dependent. *British Journal of Sports Medicine, 39*, 776–780.

Ferreira, C. H., Naldoni, L. M., Ribeiro, Jdos. S., et al. (2014). Maternal blood pressure and heart rate response to pelvic floor muscle training during pregnancy. *Acta Obstetricia et Gynecologica Scandinavica, 93*(7), 678–683.

Fiataraone, M. S., Hackett, D., Schoenfeld, B., et al. (2019). *ACSM guidelines for strength training*. Featured Download [Online]. Available: https://www.acsm.org. [Accessed 07.31.19].

Fleck, S. J., & Kraemer, W. J. (2004). *Designing resistance training programs* (3rd ed.). Champaign, IL: Human Kinetics.

Franchi, M. V., Reeves, N. D., & Narici, M. V. (2017). Skeletal muscle remodeling in response to eccentric vs. concentric loading: Morphological, molecular, and metabolic adaptations. *Frontiers in Physiology, 8*, 447.

Frontera, W. R., & Meredith, C. N. (1989). Strength training in the elderly. In R. Harris, & S. Harris (Eds.), *Physical activity, aging and sports, 1: Scientific and medical research* (pp. 319–331). Albany, NY: Center for the Study of Aging.

Garber, C. E., Blissmer, B., Deschenes, M. R., et al. (2011). American College of Sports medicine position stand. Quantity and quality of exercise for developing and maintaining cardiorespiratory, musculoskeletal, and neuromotor fitness in apparently healthy adults: Guidance for prescribing exercise. *Medicine & Science in Sports & Exercise, 43*(7), 1334–1359.

Graves, J. E., Pollock, M. L., Leggett, S. H., et al. (1988). Effect of reduced frequency on muscular strength. *International Journal of Sports Medicine, 9*, 316–319.

Green, H., Goreham, C., Ouyang, J., et al. (1999). Regulation of fiber size, oxidative potential, and capillarization in human muscle by resistance exercise. *American Journal of Physiology, 276*(2 Pt. 2), 591–596.

Groennebaek, T., & Vissing, K. (2017). Impact of resistance training on skeletal muscle mitochondrial biogenesis, content, and function. *Frontiers in Physiology, 8*, 713.

Haskel, W. L. (1994). Dose–response issues from a biological perspective. In C. Bouchard, S. N. Blair, & W. L. Haskell (Eds.), *Physical activity, fitness and health* (pp. 1030–1039). Champaign, IL: Human Kinetics.

Haun, C. T., Vann, C. G., Roberts, B. M., et al. (2019). A critical evaluation of the biological construct skeletal muscle hypertrophy: Size matters but so does the measurement. *Frontiers in Physiology, 10,* 247.

Hoeger, W. W. K., Hopkins, D. R., Barette, S. L., et al. (1990). Relationship between repetitions and selected percentages of one repetition maximum: A comparison between untrained and trained males and females. *Journal of Strength and Conditioning Research, 4*(2), 47–54.

Kegel, A. H. (1956). Early genital relaxation. *Obstetrics & Gynecology, 8*(5), 545–550.

Knuttgen, H. G., & Komi, P. V. (2003). Basic considerations for exercise. In P. V. Komi (Ed.), *Strength and power in sport* (2nd ed.) (pp. 3–7). Oxford: Blackwell Scientific.

Knuttgen, H. G., & Kraemer, W. J. (1987). Terminology and measurement in exercise performance. *Journal of Applied Sport Science Research, 1,* 1–10.

Kraemer, W. J., Fleck, S. J., & Evans, W. J. (1996). Strength and power training: Physiological mechanisms of adaptation. *Exercise and Sport Sciences Reviews, 24,* 363–397.

Kraemer, W. J., & Fry, A. C. (1995). Strength testing: Development and evaluation of methodology. In P. J. Maud, & C. Foster (Eds.), *Physiological assessment of human fitness* (pp. 115–138). Champaign, IL: Human Kinetics.

Kraemer, W. J., Patton, J. F., Gordon, S. E., et al. (1995). Compatibility of high-intensity strength and endurance training on hormonal and skeletal muscle adaptations. *Journal of Applied Physiology, 78*(3), 976–989.

Kraemer, W. J., & Ratamess, N. A. (2004). Fundamentals of resistance training: Progression and exercise prescription. *Medicine & Science in Sports & Exercise, 36*(4), 674–688.

Kruger, J., Budgett, D., Goodman, J., Bø, K. (2018). Can you train the pelvic floor muscles by contracting other related muscles? https://doi.org/10.1002/nau.23890.

Koenig, I., Eichelberger, P., Luginbuehl, H., et al. (2021). Activation patterns of pelvic floor muscles in women with incontinence while running: A randomized controlled trial. *International Urogynecology Journal, 32*(2), 335–343.

Lim, C., Kim, H. J., Morton, R. W., et al. (2019). Resistance exercise-induced changes in muscle phenotype are load dependent. *Medicine & Science in Sports & Exercise, 51*(12), 2578–2585.

MacDougall, J. D., Gibala, M. J., Tarnopolsky, M. A., et al. (1995). The time course for elevated muscle protein synthesis following heavy resistance exercise. *Canadian Journal of Applied Physiology, 20*(4), 480–486.

Magnusson, S. P., Hansen, M., Langberg, H., et al. (2007). The adaptability of tendon to loading differs in men and women. *International Journal of Experimental Pathology, 88,* 237–240.

Munn, J., Herbert, R. D., & Gandevia, S. C. (2004). Contralateral effects of unilateral resistance training: A meta-analysis. *Journal of Applied Physiology, 96*(5), 1861–1866.

Neumann, P., & Gill, V. (2002). Pelvic floor and abdominal muscle interaction: EMG activity and intra-abdominal pressure. *International Urogynecology Journal and Pelvic Floor Dysfunction, 13,* 125–132.

Oranchuk, D. J., Storey, A. G., Nelson, A. R., et al. (2019). Isometric training and long-term adaptations: Effects of muscle length, intensity, and intent: A systematic review. *Scandinavian Journal of Medicine & Science in Sports, 29*(4), 484–503.

Phillips, S. M., Tipton, K. D., Aarsland, A., et al. (1997). Mixed muscle protein synthesis and breakdown after resistance exercise in humans. *American Journal of Physiology, 273*(1 Pt. 1), E99–E107.

Plevnik, S. (1985). A new method for testing and strengthening pelvic floor muscles. In *Proceedings of the 15th annual general meeting of the international continence society* (pp. 267–268). London: International Continence Society.

Rea, M. R., Alvar, B. A., Burkett, L. N., et al. (2003). A meta-analysis to determine the dose response for strength development. *Medicine & Science in Sports & Exercise, 35*(3), 456–464.

Roberts, T. J. (2016). Contribution of elastic tissues to the mechanics and energetics of muscle function during movement. *Journal of Experimental Biology, 219*(Pt. 2), 266–275.

Rooney, K. J., Herbert, R. D., & Balnave, R. J. (1994). Fatigue contributes to the strength training stimulus. *Medicine & Science in Sports & Exercise, 26*(9), 1160–1164.

Sale, D. (1988). Neural adaptation to resistance training. *Medicine & Science in Sports & Exercise, 20*(Suppl. 5), 135–145.

Sapsford, R., & Hodges, P. (2001). Contraction of the pelvic floor muscles during abdominal maneuvers. *Archives of Physical Medicine and Rehabilitation, 82,* 1081–1088.

Schoenfeld, B. J., Grgic, J., Ogborn, D., et al. (2017). Strength and hypertrophy adaptations between low- vs. high-load resistance training: A systematic review and meta-analysis. *Journal of Strength and Conditioning Research, 31*(12), 3508–3523.

Schoenfeld, B. J., Ogborn, D., & Krieger, J. W. (2016). Effects of resistance training frequency on measures of muscle hypertrophy: A systematic review and meta-analysis. *Sports Medicine, 46*(11), 1689–1697.

Shield, A., & Zhou, S. (2004). Assessing voluntary muscle activation with the twitch interpolation technique. *Sports Medicine, 34*(4), 253–267.

Suchomel, T. J., Nimphius, S., Bellon, C. R., et al. (2018). The importance of muscular strength: Training considerations. *Sports Medicine, 48*(4), 765–785.

Tan, B. (1999). Manipulating resistance training program variables to optimize maximum strength in men: A review. *Journal of Strength and Conditioning Research, 13*(3), 289–304.

Timmons, J. A. (2011). Variability in training-induced skeletal muscle adaptation. *Journal of Applied Physiology (1985), 110*(3), 846–853.

Wilmore, J. H., & Costill, D. L. (1999). *Physiology of Sport and exercise* (2nd ed.). Champaign, IL: Human Kinetics.

Female Pelvic Floor Dysfunction and Evidence-Based Physical Therapy

7.1 Female Stress Urinary Incontinence

Jacques Corcos

PREVALENCE, CAUSES AND PATHOPHYSIOLOGY

INTRODUCTION

The most fascinating aspect of medicine is its constant evolution over time. Its progression is based on new findings in our laboratories, new data from clinical research, new imaging techniques, and new views and theories. Looking back at 25 years of urology, it is not very apparent that major advances have been made in understanding the pathophysiology of most of the diseases seen in urology: stones, cancer, sexual and voiding dysfunction, infertility, benign prostate hyperplasia, and even hydrocele. Obvious changes have been introduced in the treatment of these diseases, with sophisticated techniques, such as shock wave lithotripsy, robotic surgery, advanced radiation therapy, precise sperm retrieval and utilization, lasers and mid-urethral slings, and new drugs. The overall result of new treatments (associated with better nutrition, prevention, hygiene, etc.) is that, according to the World Health Organization, life expectancy in the Western world has increased significantly over the past 25 years. In other words, we are improving patient care without really understanding our patient's diseases. Nevertheless, although we do not have a solid grasp of the pathophysiology of these diseases, we have at least eliminated some old concepts and beliefs that have served their time but were never really supported by high-level evidence from animal and human studies. This is particularly true in the field of female incontinence. We therefore propose to revisit the classical pathophysiology of female incontinence through the critical eyes of a long-standing researcher and clinician who has spent hours listening to others and who is trying today to synthesize what we presently know and do not know, and what we should focus on in research in the next decade.

PREVALENCE OF AND RISK FACTORS FOR STRESS URINARY INCONTINENCE

Prevalence of a condition is mainly important for health economics and to predict needs of a given population.

Most published surveys on the prevalence of incontinence have evaluated it as a whole. The reported prevalence of urinary incontinence (UI) among women varies widely in different studies due to the use of different definitions, heterogenicity of different study populations and population sampling procedures. In addition, different definitions of UI have been applied.

Prevalence

Two important studies in Europe and the United States defined UI as any leakage occurring in the past 30 days (Hunskaar et al., 2004; Kinchen et al., 2003). Their overall results were congruent, showing average UI prevalence of 35% and 37%, respectively. At 37% and 42%, respectively, stress urinary incontinence (SUI) seemed to be the most prevalent type in these studies, whereas mixed urinary incontinence (MUI) was found in 33% and 46%. Similar numbers were obtained in earlier surveys (Burgio et al., 1991; Hannestad et al., 2000; Yarnell et al., 1981). It is important to note that the number of symptomatic yet undiagnosed women remains substantial, suggesting significant under-reporting (Miller et al., 2009).

From a clinician point of view the most relevant prevalence should be the number of sufferers who seek treatment, although this number may vary according to the type of treatment offered and may also be a good argument for the development of awareness about treatment modalities. Incontinent patients likely will more readily accept a non-invasive approach, such as pelvic floor muscle training (PFMT) or injectables rather than a surgical procedure, and the number of sufferers seeking therapy may depend on the invasiveness of the intervention proffered. Future epidemiological studies should keep these important considerations in mind, as they explain why a large number of incontinent patients do not consult physicians.

Risk Factors

Among a multitude of risk factors, some need to be highlighted.

Age is an important parameter in prevalence, severity and 'bothersomeness'. Increased life expectancy translates in a similar increase of prevalence (Horbach and

Ostergard, 1994). In one study, it was noted that SUI occurred mainly in young and perimenopausal women (Hunskaar et al., 2004). The first peak in the prevalence curve occurs with postpartum incontinence, then the rate of incontinence drops and rises again beyond menopause. MUI has become the most ubiquitous type of incontinence in the seventh decade of life. Incident UI is relatively high after pregnancy (33%–40%) and remission rates are surprisingly low, depending on the UI definition used (MacArthur et al., 2016). It appears also that UI prevalence is double in the vaginal delivery group (31%; 95% CI: 30%–33%) compared to the caesarean section group (15%; 95% CI: 11%–18%) (Sangsawang, 2014; Thom and Rortveit, 2010).

Hysterectomy may also be associated with incident incontinence. The Swedish National Register for Gynecological Surgery noted that in more than 25,000 women without UI before hysterectomy, 8.5% developed de novo UI (Bohlin et al., 2017)

Type and level of sport activity also seems to be an important factor of incontinence with paradoxical effect. Veloso Teixeira et al. (2018) published an interesting meta-analysis on prevalence of incontinence in female athletes showing a 36% prevalence of UI in female athletes in different sports, and compared with sedentary women, the athletes had a 177% higher risk of presenting with UI. For more information about sports and the pelvic floor, see Chapter 7.1.

CAUSES AND PATHOPHYSIOLOGY OF STRESS URINARY INCONTINENCE

From a very simplistic viewpoint, UI occurs when bladder pressure rises higher than urethral pressure. Physiologically, this does not happen because bladder compliance on the one hand and adaptability of urethral pressure in response to increased bladder pressure on the other hand makes the equation impossible. Thus incontinence is always secondary to urethral incapacity to overcome bladder pressure either because there is a limit to what urethral pressure can resist physiologically or because it is weak.

UI is more frequent in women than in men (Hunskaar et al., 2004). Many reasons could account for this gender difference: dissimilarities in the anatomy of pelvic floor muscles and ligaments supporting the bladder and sphincter; the effect of childbirth and maternal injury on pelvic structures and the sphincter; and hormones that have receptors in the bladder, sphincter and vaginal area. Finally, genetic factors that are not yet well studied could explain racial and familial incontinence trends.

General Causes

The pathophysiology of secondary SUI is generally easy to understand. What seems the most frequently encountered is what is called *primary SUI*, which is most likely the result of many causes, such as pregnancy, delivery, ageing and hormonal changes, responsible for local anatomical changes. As already mentioned, the external urinary sphincter plays a central role in the pathophysiology of SUI. Any alteration of its function will lead to unbalance between bladder and sphincter normal functions and incontinence. Many SUI incontinence classifications still differentiate between changes in anatomical location of the urethra and external sphincter weakness (called *intrinsic sphincter deficiency* [ISD]). We always argued against such differentiation, being convinced that there is no incontinence without sphincter weakness. This viewpoint is shared by many authors, such as Chaikin et al. (1998) and Kayigil et al. (1999). However, the concepts of suburethral hammock (DeLancey, 1994) and 'fixed point' developed by Ulf Ulmsten and Peter Petros (Petros, 2015) brought a significant importance to the supportive structure needed for urethral function. Weakness of this supportive structure made of normal anatomical lie of the urethra, either at rest (urethral malposition) or during a rise in intra-abdominal pressure (urethral hypermobility), leads to a lack of compressive effect of the urethra and then to incontinence. More recent works have attempted to consolidate the anatomical and functional aetiologies into a unified approach listing the causes for an abnormal support of the urethra (Cundiff, 2004; Kalejaiye et al., 2015):

- Damage to the pubourethral ligament, causing posterior displacement of the urethra
- Impairment of the lateral supports, affecting the hammock normally provided by the vagina
- Deficiency in the endopelvic fascia, associated with descent of the proximal portion of the urethra, reducing the direct transmission of the intra-abdominal pressure enhancing urethral closure
- Damage or weakness to the pelvic floor muscles, especially the levator ani, allowing descent of the bladder base and outlet.

Specific Causes

Each of the causes developed hereafter are responsible for either sphincteric weakness or lack of urethral support responsible for a weak sphincteric action.

Congenital Anomalies

Congenital anomalies mainly involve the central nervous system (e.g., myelomeningocele, sacral agenesis, severe scoliosis). Most of these lesions produce neurogenic overactive bladder. However, the lowest lesions, involving the bottom segments of the spinal cord, may evoke cauda equina syndrome with pelvic floor weakness and/or areflexic bladder. Other congenital anomalies (e.g., bladder exstrophy) affect the bladder itself and its sphincter mechanism, which is often only partially developed (Koelbl et al., 2002).

Nervous System Injuries and Diseases

Nervous system injuries and diseases include, for example, multiple sclerosis, lipomas, and other benign or malignant tumors. In a similar line of thought, incontinence in these situations is mainly due to neurogenic overactive bladder, but lower lesions, such as disc compression, sacral tumors, sacral injuries and neuropathies (e.g., diabetes mellitus or toxins), are associated with pelvic floor weakness and hypofunctional bladder. With all of these lesions, incontinence is related to detrusor overactivity, leading to urgency incontinence, overflow in the case of detrusor hypocontractility or SUI if the pelvic floor is hypofunctional (Kessler, 2020; Kielb and Lia, 2020).

Detrusor Anomalies and Innervation

Connective tissue is not an important component of the normal detrusor because smooth muscle cells are arranged closely together (Gosling, 1997). Connective tissue is increased in obstructed bladders, indicating that some smooth muscle fibres convert from a contractile to a synthetic collagen phenotype. Bladder collagen transformation is not seen with ageing. Denervation is observed in both of these models but to a much lesser extent in ageing bladders. Except for the usual changes secondary to ageing, there are no structural bladder wall alterations in women with pure SUI (Camões et al., 2015).

Effect of Pregnancy and Delivery on the Lower Urinary Tract

Very little is known about the relationship between delivery, pelvic floor changes and SUI. It is widely recognized that SUI may be a consequence of pregnancy/delivery and that pregnancy usually worsens pre-existing SUI (Hojberg et al., 1999). Transient SUI is relatively common for a few weeks after normal vaginal delivery.

According to Koelbl et al. (2002), vaginal delivery might produce SUI via four major mechanisms:
1. Injury to connective tissue supports by the mechanical process of vaginal delivery
2. Vascular damage to pelvic structures as a result of compression by the presenting part of the fetus during labour
3. Wounds to pelvic nerves and/or muscles from trauma during parturition
4. Direct harm to the urinary tract during labour and delivery.

The physiological changes accompanying pregnancy may make women more susceptible to these pathophysiological processes.

Pelvic floor muscle strength decreases after delivery. According to some authors, it returns to the normal range a few weeks later (Peschers et al., 1997). To others, weakness is persistent (Dumoulin et al., 2004). For further references to studies in this area, see Chapter 7.1. Incontinence seems to be linked to several parameters (e.g., forceps use, labour duration, number of deliveries, preexisting bladder neck mobility). It also appears that a close relationship exists between epidural analgesia during labour and the severity of pelvic floor injuries (Cutner and Cardozo, 1992; Francis, 1960). Episiotomies are often reported to worsen postpartum pelvic floor dysfunction. However, evidence is seldom available, and its relationship to SUI is unproven (Hong et al., 1988; Lin et al., 2018).

Ageing

Incontinence at large is more frequent in the elderly. However, SUI prevalence is relatively decreased because of increased MUI. Ageing in women qualitatively modifies the pelvic floor muscles. Proportional numbers of slow- and fast-twitch muscle fibres change with age, as reported by Koelbl et al. (1989), who biopsied the pelvic floor of elderly, incontinent women. In addition, the response to electrical stimulation is decreased and electromyography modified by ageing (Smith et al., 1989). These findings are consistent with the two main classic causes of incontinence: bladder neck/urethral hypermobility and ISD (Nordling, 2002).

Bladder neck hypermobility. To be fully functional, the urethra must be supported by a 'non-elastic' structure, originally the urethral pelvic ligament, which provides a backboard against increasing abdominal forces compressing the urethra. This is the basis of the 'hammock theory' popularized by DeLancey (1994). Such loss of support results in what is classically called *urethral hypermobility* or rotational descent of the urethra around the pubic bone. For a long time, this defect was considered the main cause of SUI. It was also the basis behind the pressure transmission theory (Athanassopoulos et al., 1994; Enhorning, 1960) and the later development of 'slings' for the treatment of women with SUI. It is also the main background for explaining the effect of PFMT (Bø, 2004; Brækken et al., 2010). Lax urethral support could be ascribed to numerous factors, including childbirth, strenuous exercises, pelvic denervation after surgery or trauma, and probably genetic elements that remain to be proven.

The theory of urethral hypermobility is easy to understand and explains the success of surgery and PFMT in SUI repair. However, SUI can occur without urethral hypermobility, and failure of surgery is not always associated with recurrence of hypermobility, leaving plenty of room for ISD.

Intrinsic sphincter deficiency. The female urethra is a short but complex organ intimately connected to the bladder and pelvic floor structures. Anatomically, it can be isolated and described precisely (DeLancey et al., 2002), but its functionality cannot be studied separately (Corcos and Schick, 2001).

Besides its proximal smooth muscle sphincteric component and its mid-urethra rhabdosphincter, the urethral wall comprises an outer muscle coat and an inner epithelial membrane continuous with the bladder urothelium. The outer smooth muscle coat extends throughout the length of the urethra and is essentially made up of longitudinal fibres, whereas circular fibres are rare. Innervation of this coating is mainly parasympathetic, and its function appears to be to shorten and open the urethral lumen during micturition (Ek et al., 1977).

The urethral lamina propria covers the entire length of the urethra. It is lined by the urethral urothelium and lies on a rich layer of vascular plexus and mucous glands, which separates it from the smooth muscle layers. The vascular plexus is important for normal continence and has been shown to be highly sensitive to hormone levels in women (Dokita et al., 1991; Persson and Andersson,

1992). A defect in one of these entities elicits poor closure of the sphincteric urethra and SUI. Loss of sphincteric mass has been clearly demonstrated by different imaging modalities: electromyography, ultrasound and magnetic resonance imaging (Masata et al., 2000; Schaer et al., 1995; Yang et al., 1991).

However, it is hard to believe that urethral sphincter mechanisms, in continuous engagement during a lifetime, can spontaneously become anatomically incompetent. Ageing, through nerve and vascular 'injuries', can weaken the sphincter (Koelbl et al., 1989). Nerve and vascular injuries, provoked by declining hormone levels (menopause), pelvic surgery, radiation therapy and neuropathies (e.g., diabetes mellitus, toxins), are the most common causes of sphincteric weakness. Furthermore, a relationship probably exists between hypermobility and ISD. Repeated elongation of muscular fibres of the sphincter and surrounding tissues, including the nerves, may be responsible for sphincteric damage. A voluntary contraction of the pelvic floor muscles creates co-contractions of the intrinsic sphincter shown with concentric needle electromyography in women (Bø and Stien, 1994) and may explain how PFMT can also work for sphincteric weakness.

Mixed Urinary Incontinence

MUI is even more difficult to understand, and presently, only paper and pencil–based theories try to explain concomitance of the overactive bladder and defective sphincter. It is even difficult at times to understand a patient who gives hesitant answers to questions, which are supposed to help discriminate between stress and urgency incontinence (Bandukwala and Gousse, 2015).

We have already noted that PFMT can be successful in treating stress and urgency incontinence as well as MUI (Dumoulin et al., 2018). In addition, we know that two of three patients with MUI become free of symptoms after surgery directed solely against the stress component. If we add to this the epidemiological picture that stress incontinence is more common in younger women than MUI and urgency incontinence (Hannestad et al., 2000), and if we include the fact that the more pronounced stress incontinence they have, the more likely it is that they also have a component of urgency incontinence (Bump et al., 2003; Teleman et al., 2004), then the new, emerging picture seems easier to interpret but still does not give an answer about actual causes.

CONCLUSION

The prevalence of SUI is high, but not all women seek treatment because it is often not bothering them. Modern SUI pathophysiology proposes a model based mainly on sphincter weakness. Annualized incidence rates for UI in women vary between 1% and 10% (approximately 3% for each subtype) and are heavily influenced by the population surveyed and the survey tool used.

Bladder neck mobility, which is still often identified as a main cause, is only one of the multiple causes of this sphincteric weakness. However, it is an important factor, when present, because it is the main defect corrected by most SUI surgical treatments. Despite recent and quite effective new ways of SUI treatment, we have to admit that the real, intimate mechanism leading to external urinary sphincter weakness remains to be discovered and described.

REFERENCES

Athanassopoulos, A., Melekos, M. D., Speakman, M., et al. (1994). Endoscopic vesical neck suspension in female urinary stress incontinence: Results and changes in various urodynamic parameters. *International Urology and Nephrology, 26*(3), 293–299.

Bandukwala, N. Q., & Gousse, A. E. (2015). Mixed urinary incontinence: What first? *Current Urology Reports, 16*(3), 9.

Bø, K. (2004). Pelvic floor muscle training is effective in treatment of female stress urinary incontinence, but how does it work? *International Urogynecology Journal., 15*, 76–84.

Bø, K., & Stien, R. (1994). Needle EMG registration of striated urethral wall and pelvic floor muscle activity patterns during cough, Valsalva, abdominal, hip adductor and gluteal muscle contractions in nulliparous healthy females. *Neurourology and Urodynamics, 13*, 35–41.

Bohlin, K. S., Ankardal, M., Lindkvist, H., et al. (2017). Factors influencing the incidence and remission of urinary incontinence after hysterectomy. *American Journal of Obstetrics and Gynecology, 216* 53.e1–53.e9.

Brækken, I. H., Majida, M., Ellstrom-Engh, M., et al. (2010). Morphological changes after pelvic floor muscle training measured by 3-dimensional ultrasound: A randomized controlled trial. *Obstetrics & Gynecology, 115*(2), 317–324.

Bump, R. C., Norton, P. A., Zinner, N. R., et al. (2003). Mixed urinary incontinence symptoms: Urodynamic findings, incontinence severity, and treatment response. *Obstetrics & Gynecology, 102*(1), 76–83.

Burgio, K. L., Matthews, K. A., & Engel, B. T. (1991). Prevalence, incidence and correlates of urinary incontinence in healthy, middle-aged women. *Journal of Urology, 146*(5), 1255–1259.

Chaikin, D., Rosenthal, J., & Blaivas, J. (1998). Pubovaginal fascial sling for all types of stress urinary incontinence: Long-term analysis. *Journal of Urology, 160*(4), 1312–1316.

Camões, J., Coelho, A., Castro-Diaz, D., et al. (2015). Lower urinary tract symptoms and aging: The impact of chronic bladder ischemia on overactive bladder syndrome. *Urologia Internationalis, 95*(4), 373–379.

Corcos, J., & Schick, E. (Eds.). (2001). *The Urinary Sphincter.* New York: Marcel Dekker.

Cundiff, G. W. (2004). The pathophysiology of stress urinary incontinence: A historical perspective. *Reviews in Urology, 6*(Suppl. 3), 10–18.

Cutner, A., & Cardozo, L. D. (1992). The lower urinary tract in pregnancy and the puerperium. *International Urogynecology Journal and Pelvic Floor Dysfunction, 3*, 312–323.

DeLancey, J. O. (1994). Structural support of the urethra as it relates to stress urinary incontinence: The hammock hypothesis. *American Journal of Obstetrics and Gynecology, 170*(6), 1713–1720.

DeLancey, J. O., Gosling, J., Creed, K., et al. (2002). Gross anatomy and cell biology of the lower urinary tract. In P. Abrams, L. Cardozo, S. Khoury, et al. (Eds.), *Incontinence: second international consultation on incontinence* (pp. 17–82). Plymouth, UK: Health Publication/Plymbridge Distributors.

Dokita, S., Morgan, W. R., Wheeler, M. A., et al. (1991). NG-nitro-L-arginine inhibits non-adrenergic, non-cholinergic relaxation in rabbit urethral smooth muscle. *Life Sciences, 48*(25), 2429–2436.

Dumoulin, C., Cacciari, L. P., & Hay-Smith, E. J. C. (2018). Pelvic floor muscle training versus no treatment, or inactive control treatments, for urinary incontinence in women. *Cochrane Database of Systematic Reviews Issue, 10* Art. No. CD005654.

Dumoulin, C., Lemieux, M. C., Bourbonnais, D., et al. (2004). Physiotherapy for persistent postnatal stress urinary incontinence: A randomized controlled trial. *Obstetrics & Gynecology, 104*(3), 504–510.

Ek, A., Alm, P., Andersson, K. E., et al. (1977). Adrenergic and cholinergic nerves of the human urethra and urinary bladder. A histochemical study. *Acta Physiologica Scandinavica., 99*(3), 345–352.

Enhorning, G. (1960). Functional sphincterometry—a test for stress incontinence. *Urologia Internationalis, 10*, 129–136.

Francis, W. J. A. (1960). The onset of stress incontinence. *The Journal of Obstetrics and Gynaecology of the British Empire, 67*, 899–903.

Gosling, J. A. (1997). Modification of bladder structure in response to outflow obstruction and ageing. *European Urology, 32*(Suppl. 1), 9–14.

Hannestad, Y. S., Rortveit, G., Sandvik, H., et al. (2000). A community-based epidemiological survey of female urinary incontinence: The Norwegian EPINCONT study. Epidemiology of incontinence in the county of Nord-

Trondelag. *Journal of Clinical Epidemiology, 53*(11), 1150–1157.

Hojberg, K. E., Salvig, J. D., Winslow, N. A., et al. (1999). Urinary incontinence: Prevalence and risk factors at 16 weeks of gestation. *British Journal of Obstetrics and Gynaecology, 106*(8), 842–850.

Hong, P. L., Leong, M., & Selzer, V. (1988). Uroflowmetric observation in pregnancy. *Neurourology and Urodynamics, 7*, 61–70.

Horbach, N. S., & Ostergard, D. R. (1994). Predicting intrinsic urethral sphincter dysfunction in women with stress urinary incontinence Obstet. *Gynecol, 84*(2), 188–192.

Hunskaar, S., Lose, G., Sykes, D., et al. (2004). The prevalence of urinary incontinence in women in four European countries. *BJU International, 93*(3), 324–330.

Kalejaiye, O., Vij, M., & Drake, M. (2015). Classification of stress urinary incontinence World. *Journal of Urology, 33*, 1215–1220.

Kayigil, O., Iftekhar, A. S., & Metin, A. (1999). The coexistence of intrinsic sphincter deficiency with type II stress incontinence. *Journal of Urology, 162*(4), 1365–1366.

Kessler, T. (2020). Spinal cord injury and cerebral trauma. In J. Corcos, G. Karsenty, T. Kessler, et al. (Eds.), *Essentials of the adult neurogenic bladder* (pp. 113–118). Boca Raton, FL: CRC Press.

Kielb, S., & Lia, J. (2020). Systemic illnesses (diabetes mellitus, sarcoidosis, alcoholism, and porphyrias). In J. Corcos, G. Karsenty, T. Kessler, et al. (Eds.), *Essentials of the Adult Neurogenic Bladder* (pp. 44–49). Boca Raton, FL: CRC Press.

Kinchen, K. S., Burgio, K., Diokno, A. C., et al. (2003). Factors associated with women's decision to seek treatment for urinary incontinence. *Journal of Women's Health, 12*(7), 687–698.

Koelbl, H., Mostwin, J., Boiteux, J. P., et al. (2002). Pathophysiology. In P. Abrams, L. Cardozo, S. Khoury, et al. (Eds.), *Incontinence: second international consultation on incontinence* (pp. 203–242). Plymouth, UK: Health Publication/Plymbridge Distributors.

Koelbl, H., Strassegger, H., Riss, P. A., et al. (1989). Morphologic and functional aspects of pelvic floor muscles in patients with pelvic relaxation and genuine stress incontinence. *Obstetrics & Gynecology, 74*(5), 789–795.

Lin, Y. H., Chang, S. D., Hsieh, W. C., et al. (2018). Persistent stress urinary incontinence during pregnancy and one year after delivery; its prevalence, risk factors and impact on quality of life in Taiwanese women: An observational cohort study. *Taiwanese Journal of Obstetrics & Gynecology, 57*(3), 340–345.

MacArthur, C., Wilson, D., Herbison, P., et al. (2016). Urinary incontinence persisting after childbirth: Extent, delivery history, and effects in a 12–year longitudinal cohort study. *British Journal of Obstetrics and Gynaecology, 123*(6), 1022–1029.

Masata, J., Martan, A., Halaska, M., et al. (2000). [Ultrasonography of the funneling of the urethra]. *Ceská Gynekologie, 65*(2), 87–90.

Miller, D. C., Saigal, C. S., & Litwin, M. S. (2009). The demographic burden of urologic disease in America. *Urologic Clinics of North America, 36*, 11.

Nordling, J. (2002). The aging bladder—a significant but underestimated role in the development of lower urinary tract symptoms. *Experimental Gerontology, 37*(8–9), 991–999.

Persson, K., & Andersson, K. E. (1992). Nitric oxide and relaxation of pig lower urinary tract. *British Journal of Pharmacology, 106*(2), 416–422.

Peschers, U. M., Schaer, G. N., DeLancey, J. O., et al. (1997). Levator ani function before and after childbirth. *British Journal of Obstetrics and Gynaecology, 104*(9), 1004–1008.

Petros, P. (2015). Creating a gold standard surgical device: Scientific discoveries leading to TVT and beyond: Ulf Ulmsten Memorial Lecture 2014. *International Urogynecology Journal, 26*(4), 471–476.

Sangsawang, B. (2014). Risk factors for the development of stress urinary incontinence during pregnancy in primigravidae: A review of the literature. *European Journal of Obstetrics & Gynecology and Reproductive Biology, 178*, 27–34.

Schaer, G. N., Koechli, O. R., Schuessler, B., et al. (1995). Improvement of perineal sonographic bladder neck imaging with ultrasound contrast medium. *Obstetrics & Gynecology, 86*(6), 950–954.

Smith, A. R., Hosker, G. L., & Warrell, D. W. (1989). The role of partial denervation of the pelvic floor in the aetiology of genitourinary prolapse and stress incontinence of urine. A neurophysiological study. *British Journal of Obstetrics and Gynaecology, 96*(1), 24–28.

Teleman, P. M., Lidfeldt, J., Nerbrand, C., et al. (2004). Overactive bladder: Prevalence, risk factors and relation to stress incontinence in middle-aged women. *British Journal of Obstetrics and Gynaecology, 111*(6), 600–604.

Thom, D. H., & Rortveit, G. (2010). Prevalence of postpartum urinary incontinence: A systematic review. *Acta Obstetricia et Gynecologica Scandinavica, 89*(12), 1511–1522.

Veloso Teixeira, R., Colla, C., Sbruzzi, G., et al. (2018). Prevalence of urinary incontinence in female athletes: A systematic review with meta-analysis. *International Urogynecology Journal, 29*(12), 1717–1725.

Yang, A., Mostwin, J. L., Rosenshein, N. B., et al. (1991). Pelvic floor descent in women: Dynamic evaluation with fast MR imaging and cinematic display. *Radiology, 179*(1), 25–33.

Yarnell, J. W. G., Voyle, G. J., Richards, C. J., et al. (1981). The prevalence and severity of urinary incontinence in women. *Journal of Epidemiology & Community Health, 35*(1), 71–74.

Lifestyle Interventions

Pauline Chiarelli, Signe Nilssen Stafne and Siv Mørkved

MODIFIABLE FACTORS ASSOCIATED WITH URINARY INCONTINENCE

Epidemiological studies have shown lower urinary tract symptoms (LUTS) and urinary incontinence (UI) to be associated with several lifestyle factors or risk factors, some of which might be considered modifiable. Being modifiable, these factors should be of interest to health-care professionals when developing behavioural interventions aimed at reducing the symptoms of LUTS and UI. Available evidence most commonly refers to associations between lifestyle factors and urinary frequency, urgency, nocturia and incontinence. Regarding UI, the literature does not consequently subgroup into urgency urinary incontinence (UUI), stress urinary incontinence (SUI) or mixed urinary incontinence (MUI).

The literature is scarce regarding the association between modifiable lifestyle factors and other symptoms of pelvic floor dysfunction. This needs to be further addressed in future research.

Here we explore the strength of the association between selected modifiable lifestyle factors and LUTS/UI and the evidence currently available to support the inclusion of lifestyle changes within continence promotion interventions. The text also outlines some of the principles of behaviour change/health promotion and how these might best be incorporated within continence promotion interventions to help patients adopt relevant behaviours to maximize prescribed lifestyle changes.

Several epidemiological studies have shown a strong association between self-reports of LUTS/UI and lifestyle factors such as obesity (Chiarelli and Brown, 1999; Hunskaar, 2008; Litman et al., 2007; Townsend et al., 2008a; Wasserberg et al., 2009), physical activity (Bø and Borgen, 2001; Danforth et al., 2007; Litman et al., 2007; Maserejian et al., 2012; Morrisroe et al., 2014; Nygaard et al., 1994; Townsend et al., 2008b), smoking (Hannestad et al., 2003; Maserejian et al., 2012; Tahtinen et al., 2011; Tampakoudis et al., 1995) and dietary factors (Brown et al., 1999; Dallosso et al., 2004; Gleason et al., 2013; Jura et al., 2011; Kosilov et al., 2016; Tettamanti et al., 2011; Townsend et al., 2011; Townsend et al., 2012).

The fact that various peak bodies internationally recommended the inclusion of behavioural interventions aimed at modifying relevant lifestyle factors is a testament to the importance of their inclusion within continence promotion interventions (Abrams et al., 2009; Imamura et al., 2015; Landefeld et al., 2008; Myers, 2014; National Institute for Health and Care Excellence [NICE], 2006; NICE, 2019). Recent NICE guidelines highlight the need for a multidisciplinary approach and recommend lifestyle interventions (caffeine reduction, modifying fluid intake, and weight reduction in overweight and obese women) together with pelvic floor muscle training (PFMT) as first-line treatment of UI and pelvic organ prolapse (POP) (NICE, 2019).

EVIDENCE TO SUPPORT THE IMPACT OF LIFESTYLE CHANGES ON SYMPTOMS OF PELVIC FLOOR DYSFUNCTION

The Fourth International Consultation on Incontinence (ICI) (Abrams et al., 2009) examined the evidence relating to conservative treatment for UI in women, including lifestyle interventions (Hay-Smith et al., 2009). Systematic reviews of the literature pertaining to lifestyle interventions included lifestyle factors such as obesity, physical forces (exercise, work) and smoking, and dietary factors including caffeine, alcohol and fluid intake, as well as constipation. Strong evidence in favour of health behaviours or lifestyle changes to reduce pelvic floor muscle dysfunction was not available in most cases. The ICI updated the information in the Sixth International Consultation (Abrams et al., 2016). Committee 12 again reviewed the evidence related to lifestyle issues and UI (Dumoulin et al., 2016). Dumoulin et al. (2016) concluded that there was too little research to make any recommendations. The same conclusion remains relevant.

A summary of the findings of the ICI committee examining several lifestyle interventions and their impact on the management of UI are provided here (Dumoulin et al., 2016). Using the same search strategy, inclusion criteria and exclusion criteria as implemented by the initial reviewers (Hay-Smith et al., 2009), an update of the relevant literature examining lifestyle interventions from 2005 to the present has been added (Table 7.1.1).

In preparing the systematic review, levels of evidence and grades of recommendation were decided for each

(Continued on p. 185)

TABLE 7.1.1   Randomized Controlled Trials Assessing the Effect of Lifestyle Factors on Lower Urinary Tract Symptoms and Urinary Incontinence

Weight Loss	
Author and lifestyle factor	**Subak et al. (2009)**: intensive 6-month behavioural weight loss program intervention designed to produce an average loss of 7%–9% of initial body weight within the first 6 months of the program
Design	RCT with 2:1 ratio of assignment between intervention and control
Sample size and inclusion criteria	N = 338 overweight and obese women aged ≥30 years with BMI of 25–50 and able to walk unassisted 4 m to approximately 270 m without stopping, with ≥10 UI episodes/week as measured on a 7-day voiding diary
Response rate/ drop-out	226 assigned to weight loss intervention with 5 drop-outs; 112 assigned to control group with 15 drop-outs
Measures	BMI; 7-day voiding diary designed to identify incontinence episodes as predominantly SUI and UUI or 'other'
Results	At 6-month visit, compared with women in the control group, women in weight loss group had: Significant mean weight loss of 8% of body weight (p < 0.001) Mean decrease in total number of incontinence episodes/week of 47.4% vs 28.1% (p = 0.01) Reduction in stress incontinence episodes (p = 0.009) Reduction in urge incontinence episodes (p = 0.04)
Level of evidence provided	1
Author and lifestyle factor	**Gozukara et al. (2014)**: All participants received 1-h group education sessions in preceding month prior to randomization. Each session included about 20 women, and they consisted of information about beneficial effects of weight loss, physical activity and healthy eating on urinary complaints provided by an internist, dietitian and urogynecologists. Women randomized to intervention group received a 6-month structured weight loss program (calorie- and fat-restricted diet, monthly meetings in groups of 15–20 with nutrition, exercise and behavior change.
Design	RCT
Sample size and inclusion criteria	N = 378 overweight and obese women (BMI >25 kg/m²) with ≥5 episodes of any UI in a 3-day voiding diary
Response rate/ drop-out	46.5% response rate, 15% (31 in control group and 26 in study group) lost to follow-up; study completed by 158 women in control group and 163 women in weight loss group
Measures	Pelvic floor anatomy measured with POP-Q system, symptoms with the 20-item Pelvic Floor Distress Inventory (PFDI-20) and 3-day bladder diary
Results	Intervention group women had 9.4% weight loss, and control group women remained at same body weight. Intervention group women reported lower Pelvic Organ Prolapse Distress Inventory 6 (POPDI-6) and total PFDI scores compared to control group at follow-up. Intervention group reduced episodes of both SUI and UUI after intervention assessed with 3-day bladder diary. There was no change in leakage episodes in control group. Minimal anatomical changes were found with POP-Q system in intervention group but not in control group.
Level of evidence	1
Author and lifestyle factor	**Breyer et al. (2014)**: 6-month intensive lifestyle intervention (calorie restriction and moderate-intensity exercise 175 min/week with weekly/monthly meetings over 12 months) vs a diabetes support and educational control program (3 group sessions in 1 year) in overweight/obese men with type 2 diabetes

TABLE 7.1.1 **Randomized Controlled Trials Assessing the Effect of Lifestyle Factors on Lower Urinary Tract Symptoms and Urinary Incontinence—cont'd**

Design	RCT: secondary analysis
Sample size and inclusion criteria	N = 2049 men with diabetes type 2, aged 45–76 years with BMI ≥25 kg/m^2
Response rate/ drop-out	39% response rate, 6.8% lost to follow-up (59 in intervention group and 80 in control group), 1910 analysed
Measures	1-year outcome: self-reported any UI, SUI and UUI, nocturia and daytime voiding last 7 days
Results	Intervention group lost 9.4% of body weight, and control group lost 0.7%. Allocation to intervention group reduced odds of prevalent UI after adjusting for relevant comorbidities (OR: 0.62, 95% CI: 0.43-0.88, p < 0.01). Each 1 kg of weight loss reduced odds of weekly incontinence by 3% (OR: 0.97, 95% CI: 0.95-0.99, p = 0.04). Prevalence of UUI decreased from 6.9% to 4% in intervention group and increased from 5% to 7.3% in control group. Allocation to intervention group was associated with reduced incidence and increased resolution of UUI. Number of cases with SUI was too small to do group comparisons.
Level of evidence	1
Author and lifestyle factor	**De Oliveira et al. (2019)**: PFMT group + weight loss therapy (PFMT group + weight loss) vs PFMT group
Design	RCT: simple blinded PFMT group + weight loss: PFMT group + 3 meetings with nutritionist and individualized nutritional protocol targeting weight loss of 0.5–1 kg/week PFMT group: individualized PFMT twice weekly for 8 weeks (16 sessions)
Sample size and inclusion criteria	N = 22 women with MUI found by ICIQ-UI SF, 1-h pad test >1 g, aged 40–65 years, BMI 25–40 kg/m^2
Response rate/ drop-out	47% response rate, 0 losses to follow-up
Measures	ICIQ-UI SF, manometry (Peritron), quality of life (The Utian Quality of Life [UQOL] scale), 1-h pad test
Results	Neither intervention nor control group reduced weight. Both groups reduced MUI severity and improved pelvic floor muscle pressure. No between group differences.
Level of evidence	1
Author and lifestyle factor	**Hagovska et al. (2019)**: 2 different exercise intensities for weight reduction and effect on OAB symptoms; exercise protocols included both aerobic and strength training and lasted 12 weeks High-intensity group: supervised exercise training 3×/week for 60–90 min. Low-intensity group: supervised exercise training 1×/week for 60–90 min.
Design	RCT
Sample size and inclusion criteria	N = 93 women aged 18–35 years with BMI 25–29.9 kg/m^2, waist circumference >80 cm and OAB (urgency, urination frequency ≥8×/day and ≥2×/night)
Response rate/ drop-out	90% response rate, 16 (17%) dropped out; n = 77 included in final analysis
Measures	Body composition (bioelectric impedance analysis), voiding diary (total volume 24 h and separated by day and night, number of voids/24 h, nocturia, mean voided volume/24 h), Overactive Bladder Questionnaire–Short Form (OAB-q SF), Patient Perception of Intensity of Urgency Scale (PPIUS)
Results	High-intensity group but not low-intensity group reduced body weight >5% after 12-week intervention period. In high-intensity group 7.7% and in low-intensity group 89.5% still had persistent OAB symptoms.

Continued

TABLE 7.1.1   Randomized Controlled Trials Assessing the Effect of Lifestyle Factors on Lower Urinary Tract Symptoms and Urinary Incontinence—cont'd

Level of evidence	1
Physical Activity	
Author and lifestyle factor	**Talley et al. (2017)**: PFMT and behavioural incontinence strategies +/– 12-week physical activity program (150 min moderate-intensity walking [30 min/day, 5 days/week] and twice weekly 1-h group strength exercise sessions led by exercise instructor)
Design	Pilot RCT
Sample size and inclusion criteria	N = 42 women with any UI (≥1 on ICIQ), being frail (≥3 on Vulnerable Elders Survey), gait speed <0.8 m/s or using a walking assistive device
Response rate/dropout	68% response rate, 0 dropped out
Measures	3-day bladder diary, ICIQ and global self-ratings of satisfaction and perceptions of improvement with UI treatment
Results	Included women reported mixed UI (stress and urgency, 62%), urgency (22%), stress (14%) and functional (2%). Mean daily leakage episodes were reduced by 50% in intervention group and remained constant for control group. No other differences.
Level of evidence	1
Author and lifestyle factor	**Huang et al. (2014)**: All women received written, evidence-based information about behavioural incontinence self-management techniques (pelvic floor exercises, bladder training). Both groups consisted of supervised group exercise twice weekly (90 min) and once weekly at home (60 min) and lasted 3 months. Intervention program was a therapeutic yoga program aiming to maximize awareness and control of pelvic floor, reduce underlying stress and anxiety, and improve overall physical function. Control group received a non-specific muscle stretching and strengthening program.
Design	RCT: feasibility study
Sample size and inclusion criteria	N = 55 women >50 years, UI (SUI, UUI or MUI) last 3 months, ≥3 episodes of UI on screening 3-day voiding diary
Response rate/dropout	62% response rate, 6 (11%) dropped out
Measures	3-day voiding diary to register episodes of incontinence (frequency) and type of UI (urgency, stress or other), 28-item Incontinence Impact Questionnaire (IIQ), UDI-6, Patient Perception of Bladder Condition (PPBC)
Results	66% had UUI or urgency-predominant UI, and 34% had SUI or stress-predominant UI. Yoga group decreased UI episodes by 76% and non-specific strength and stretching group decreased UI episodes by 56% from baseline (p = 0.072). SUI frequency decreased by 61% in yoga group and 35% in control group (p = 0.45). UUI frequency decreased by 30% in yoga group and 17% in control group (p = 0.77).
Level of evidence	1
Author and lifestyle factor	**Wagg et al. (2019)** and **Haque et al. (2020)**: exercise including PFMT and education to promote healthy lifestyle (including continence)
Design	Cluster-randomized trial and 12-month follow-up study. Intervention groups received repeated individual education (on bladder health continence system and PFMT) using oral information and written/designated flash cards to promote healthy lifestyle (including continence). Physiotherapy-led 60 min exercise groups followed by 30 min brisk walking were held twice weekly for 12 weeks. A paramedic encouraged home exercises, organized group exercises and reinforced the education message for next 12 weeks. Control groups received education only at baseline and follow-up. Randomization by a random number generator.

TABLE 7.1.1 Randomized Controlled Trials Assessing the Effect of Lifestyle Factors on Lower Urinary Tract Symptoms and Urinary Incontinence—cont'd

Sample size and inclusion criteria	32 villages in Bangladesh, women aged 60–75 years, current UI (positive response on question 2, 3 or 4 on UDI-6 = SUI, UUI or drops of urine loss), independent in activities of daily living, able to understand and follow instructions
Response rate/ drop-out	62% response rate, 46 (7.4%) excluded from analysis (living too far from centre of village), 579 included in analysis 12-month follow-up included 9 villages (of original 16 exercise group villages), 130 of 150 (86.7%) women in original trial completed follow-up questionnaire and assessment
Measures	A 3-day continence record belt was used every fourth week. Primary outcome was change in number of leakage episodes from baseline to 24 weeks. Secondary outcomes were health-related quality of life (EuroQOL Health-Related Quality of Life [EQ-5D], depression (10-item Center of Epidemiologic Studies Depression Scale [CES-D-10]) and urinary samples.
Results	After 24-week intervention: significantly less leakage episodes (any UI) in exercise groups (1.7 ± 1) compared to control groups (8.2 ± 2.4) 12-months after intervention ended: 80/130 reported no leakage (continent); increase from 0.75 to 1.18 incontinence episodes (any UI) among incontinent; higher BMI at end of intervention weakly associated with incontinence after 12 months; continuing exercise post-trial strongly associated with continence 1 year later
Level of evidence	1
Caffeine Reduction	
Author and lifestyle factor	**Wells et al. (2014)**: effect of drinking caffeinated vs decaffeinated fluids on symptoms of OAB in women
Design	RCT: double-blind, crossover study; pilot study
Sample size and inclusion criteria	N = 15 women age ≥18 years, newly diagnosed with OAB symptoms and reported frequency of ≥7 voids/day and 2 at night (≥9 voided/24 h); self-rated urgency and/or UUI; consumption of ≥2 caffeinated drinks/day
Response rate/ drop-out	32% response rate, 4 (27%) dropped out; n = 11 analysed at follow-up
Measures	3-day bladder diary, ICIQ-OAB, ICIQ-OABqol, caffeine withdrawal visual analogue scale
Results	Reduction in urgency and frequency of urinary voids on day 3 of diary, total ICIQ-OAB score and non-significant directional change for total ICIQ-OABqol score in favour of period of decaffeinated drink intake
Level of evidence	1

BMI, Body mass index; *ICIQ,* International Consultation on Incontinence Questionnaire; *ICIQ–OAB,* International Consultation on Incontinence Questionnaire–Overactive Bladder; *ICIQ–OABqol,* International Consultation on Incontinence Questionnaire – Overactive Bladder Quality of Life; *ICIQ-UI SF,* International Consultation on Incontinence Questionnaire–Urinary Incontinence Short Form; *MUI,* mixed urinary incontinence; *OAB,* overactive bladder; *OR,* odds ratio; *PFMT,* pelvic floor muscle training; *POP-Q,* Pelvic Organ Prolapse Quantification; *RCT,* randomized controlled trial; *SUI,* stress urinary incontinence; *UDI-6,* six-item Urinary Distress Inventory; *UI,* urinary incontinence; *UUI,* urgency urinary incontinence.

We searched MEDLINE (languages English, Scandinavian, German) and the Cochrane Register of Controlled Trials from 2005 to 2020 using the following keywords linked to 'urinary incontinence' or 'urination disorders' or 'overactive bladder' or 'urinary urgency': *lifestyle interventions, weight, obesity, weight loss, exercise, work, physical activity, lifting, smoking, tobacco, coffee, caffeine, posture, constipation, bowel function, fluids, fluid restriction, pulmonary status, cough* and *diet.*

TABLE 7.1.2	Trials Included in the Review of Lifestyle Factors and Urinary Incontinence
Author and lifestyle factor	**Litman et al. (2007)**: relationship between LUTS and lifestyle and clinical factors
Design	Epidemiological survey—population-based, randomized stratified sample: cluster cells defined by age, gender and race
Sample size and inclusion criteria	5506 randomly selected community-dwelling adults, aged 30–79 years
Response rate/ drop-out	None reported
Measures	AUA LUTS Covariates: age, BMI, smoking status, physical activity, alcoholic drinks, depressive symptoms and other self-reported comorbidities
Results	LUTS increased significantly ($p < 0.001$) with age. Those aged 50–59 years had greatest odds for increased LUTS. In women, there was significant increase in odds of LUTS with BMI >30 kg/m^2 compared with <25 kg/m^2 in women ($p = 0.009$). BMI was not associated with LUTS in men. Increased physical activity was associated with significant decrease in odds of LUTS ($p = 0.003$). Depressive symptoms were only factor significantly associated with increase in odds of LUTS across gender and racial groups (OR: 2.4, 95% CI: 1.9–3.2).
Level of evidence	2
Author and lifestyle factor	**Auwad et al. (2008)**: weight loss
Design	Pilot study; prospective cohort design
Sample size and inclusion criteria	N = 64; BMI >30 kg/m^2; urodynamically proven UI
Response rate/ drop-out	65% response rate 42 women achieved weight loss >5%; 5 women did not lose required 5% body weight 17 women dropped out
Measures	BMI = weight loss ≥5%; waist circumference; body composition analysis; 24-h pad test; KHQ; 3-day FVC; incontinence severity; bladder neck mobility
Results	Mean weight loss = 8.8 kg (SD: 5.5) Median difference other parameters (CI): Body composition analysis 4.7 (4.05–5.55) Reduced waist circumference 4 cm (3–4.75) Pad weight 19 g (13–28) Bladder neck mobility: 2.44 cm (1.66–3.34) Other measures: KHQ: Significant change on all 9 parameters Incontinence severity: significant improvement Wilcoxon's signed-rank test ($p < 0.001$) 3-day FVC: nocturia significantly reduced but not frequency Significant correlation between pad test improvement and reduced waist circumference, as well as bladder neck mobility No correlation between reduced bladder neck mobility and waist circumference
Level of evidence provided	2

TABLE 7.1.2 Trials Included in the Review of Lifestyle Factors and Urinary Incontinence—cont'd

Author and lifestyle factor	**Wasserberg et al. (2009)**: surgically induced weight loss
Design	Prospective cohort study
Sample size and inclusion criteria	82 women who filled out pre-surgery questionnaire before undergoing bariatric surgery, consequently losing >50% of their excess body weight
Response rate/ drop-out	46 (56%) women agreed to repeat questionnaires
Measures	Pelvic Floor Distress Inventory (PFDI); Pelvic Floor Impact Questionnaire (PFIQ)
Results	Prevalence of any pelvic floor dysfunction (mainly urinary symptoms) was 87% before surgery and decreased to 65% after surgery (p = 0.02). The trend towards reductions in prevalence of pelvic organ prolapse and colorectal symptoms did not reach statistical significance.
Level of evidence provided	2
Author and lifestyle factor	**Townsend et al. (2008a)**: BMI and waist circumference
Design	Population-based longitudinal study
Sample size and inclusion criteria	Data from 1634 women were entered in the analysis: these were a random subset of 1939 women randomly chosen from among 6790 incontinent women from a sample of 35,754 women reported to be continent at baseline 2 years previously
Response rate/ drop-out	84.3% response rate
Measures	Continence and type, severity, and frequency of leaking; BMI; waist circumference
Results	Highly significant linear trends of increasing risk of any, frequent and severe UI with both increasing BMI and increasing waist circumference (p for trend $\leq$ 0.001) Reference group (women with BMI 21–22.9 kg/mg^2): risk of developing at least weekly UI reduced by 19% (CI: 4%–32%) Significant elevations in risk of 125% (CI: 83%–175%) in women with BMI $\geq$35 kg/m^2 Comparing extreme quintiles of waist circumference ($\geq$37.5 in. vs $\leq$ 29 in.): multivariable RR was 2% (CI: 1.65–2.44) for frequent UI and 2.09 (CI: 1.51–2.89) for severe UI
Levels of evidence	2
Author and lifestyle factor	**Subak et al. (2009)**: weight loss
Design	RCT with 2:1 ratio of assignment between intervention and control; intensive 6-month behavioural weight loss programme intervention designed to produce an average loss of 7%–9% of initial body weight within first 6 months of programme
Sample size and inclusion criteria	338 overweight and obese women aged $\geq$30 years with BMI of 25–50 and able to walk unassisted 4 m to approximately 270 m without stopping, with $\geq$10 UI episodes/week as measured on 7-day voiding diary
Response rate/ drop-out	226 assigned to weight loss intervention with 5 drop-outs; 112 assigned to control group with 15 drop-outs
Measures	BMI; 7-day voiding diary designed to identify incontinence episodes as predominantly stress and urge or 'other'
Results	At 6-month visit, compared with women in control group, women in weight loss group had: Significant mean weight loss of 8% of body weight (p < 0.001) Mean decrease in total number of incontinence episodes/week of 47.4% vs 28.1% (p = 0.01) Reduction in stress incontinence episodes (p = 0.009) Reduction in urge incontinence episodes (p = 0.04)

Continued

TABLE 7.1.2 Trials Included in the Review of Lifestyle Factors and Urinary Incontinence—cont'd

Level of evidence provided	1
Author and lifestyle factor	**Danforth et al. (2007)**: physical activity
Design	2-year longitudinal study
Sample size and inclusion criteria	2355 older (54–79 years) women who were continent at survey 1, then incontinent at survey 2
Response rate/drop-out	Additional UI information requested of 80% of incontinent women (n = 1193) and returned by 84% of these
Measures	Incontinence and its type; physical activity categorized as metabolic equivalent task hours
Results	After adjusting for potential confounding factors, increasing levels of total physical activity were associated with decreasing incidence of UI (test for trend p < 0.01). Women with highest levels of activity had 15%–20% lower risk of developing UI compared with women in lowest levels of activity.
Level of evidence provided	2
Author and lifestyle factor	**Townsend et al. (2008b)**: physical activity
Design	Longitudinal population-based study; sub-study of women developing frequent UI during study
Sample size and inclusion criteria	70,712 women aged 37–54 years who returned full-length versions of Nurses' Health Study (NHS II) questionnaire in 2001 and 2003
Response rate/drop-out	Supplementary questionnaire sent to 1058 women reporting incident frequent UI with 79.6% response rate
Measures	Calculation of long-term activity levels; UI and amount of leaking
Results	Mean age of women was 45.9 years. Median level of physical activities was 17 h/week of Motivational Enhancement Therapy, roughly equal to 5.7 h/week of walking at average pace. Among women in highest quintile of physical activity, RR for incident incontinence was 0.80 (95% CI: 0.7–0.89). Higher levels of physical activity are associated with 25%–30% reduction in risk of developing stress incontinence.
Level of evidence provided	2
Author and lifestyle factor	**Maserejian et al. (2012)**: physical activity, smoking and alcohol consumption
Design	Longitudinal observational study, with randomly selected participants interviewed face-to-face at baseline and 5 years later
Sample size and inclusion criteria	2301 men and 3201 women aged 30–79 years from 3 racial/ethnic groups
Response rate/drop-out	Completed follow-up interviews obtained for 1610 men and 2535 women; 80.5% response rate
Measures	The AUA Symptom Index (AUA-SI); BMI and waist circumference; physical activity for elderly; smoking status; alcohol consumption

TABLE 7.1.2 Trials Included in the Review of Lifestyle Factors and Urinary Incontinence—cont'd

Results	A total of 7.7% of men and 12.7% of women with no reported LUTS at baseline later reported LUTS at follow-up. Low level of physical activity was associated with 2–3 times greater likelihood of LUTS. There was no significant association between LUTS and physical activity in men.
	Storage symptoms were twice as likely to develop in women who were current smokers (OR: 2.15, 95% CI: 1.3–3.56, p = 0.003 compared to never-smokers). No association between smoking and LUTS in men.
	There was no significant association with alcohol consumption and LUTS in men or women.
Level of evidence provided	2
Author and lifestyle factor	**Tahtinen et al. (2011)**: smoking in women
Design	Postal survey, randomly selected participants from Finnish Population Register
Sample size and inclusion criteria	2002 women aged 18–79 years
Response rate/drop-out	67% response rate
Measures	Case definitions for SUI, urgency, and UUI were 'often' or 'always' based on reported occurrence (never, rarely, often, always). Case definitions for urinary frequency were based on reporting of longest voiding interval as <2 h and for nocturia reporting of ≥2 voids/night.
	Current smoking status was an additional measure.
Results	Frequency was reported by 7.1%, nocturia by 12.6%, SUI by 11.2%, urgency by 9.7% and UUI by 3.1%.
	Current smoking was significantly associated with:
	Urgency: OR 2.7 (95% CI: 1.7–4.24, current smokers) and OR 1.8 (CI 95% CI: 1.2–2.9, former smokers) when compared to never-smokers;
	Frequency: OR 3 (95% CI: 1.8–5, current smokers) and OR 1.7 (95% CI: 1–3.1, former smokers).
	There was no association found between smoking and nocturia. Current heavy smoking compared with light smoking was associated with an additional risk of urgency (OR: 2.1, 95% CI: 1.1–3.9) and frequency (OR: 2.2, 95% CI: 1.2–4.3).
	There was suggestion of a dose–response relationship.
Level of evidence provided	2
Author and lifestyle factor	**Tettamanti et al. (2011)**: coffee and tea consumption
Design	Population-based study using Swedish Twin Register and Web-based survey
Sample size and inclusion criteria	14,094 of 42,852 female twins born between 1959 and 1985 and with information related to 1 urinary symptom and coffee and tea consumption
Response rate/drop-out	66% response rate (n = 14,094)
Measures	Lower urinary tract conditions based on recommendations from International Continence Society; data on coffee and tea consumption categorized into 3 groups: 0 cups daily, 1 or 2 cups daily, and ≥3 cups daily
	Relevant covariates: age, smoking, parity, BMI

Continued

TABLE 7.1.2   Trials Included in the Review of Lifestyle Factors and Urinary Incontinence—cont'd

Results	Prevalence of overall SUI, UUI and mixed UI showed a near dose–response relationship with increasing age and with increasing BMI. All types of UI were more prevalent among women with largest consumption of coffee. There were significant associations between coffee intake and all incontinence subtypes except nocturia and OAB, and significant associations between highest daily tea intake and nocturia (p = 0.05) and OAB (p = 0.04). Smokers had lower rates of urinary tract dysfunction compared with non-smokers except for nocturia.
Level of evidence provided	2
Author and lifestyle factor	**Jura et al. (2011)**: caffeine intake **Townsend et al. (2011)**: fluid intake
Design	Prospective cohort study during 4 years of follow-up
Sample size and inclusion criteria	65,176 women aged 37–79 years without incontinence at baseline
Response rate/ drop-out	Of women who responded to UI questions at baseline, 93% provided UI information on ≥1 follow-up questionnaire.
Measures	UI and amount of urine lost; dietary information including intake of caffeinated beverages and fluid intake overall
Results	Daily caffeine intake and incidence rate of frequent UI was associated with significantly increased risk of incident, frequent UI in highest vs lowest category of caffeine intake (RR: 1.19, 95% CI: 1.06–1.34). Significant trend of steadily increasing risk with increasing caffeine intake (p for trend = 0.01). In women who consumed ≥450 mg of caffeine daily, frequent UI in 16% and UUI in 25% could be avoided by decreasing caffeine intake to between 0 and 149 mg of caffeine daily. No significant risk of incident UI was found with higher fluid intake in women.
Level of evidence provided	2
Author and lifestyle factor	**Townsend et al. (2012)**: caffeine intake over 1 year
Design	Retrospective analysis of data from population-based longitudinal study over 2 years
Sample size and inclusion criteria	21,564 women with moderate incontinence at baseline
Response rate/ drop-out	Not relevant
Measures	Frequency and amount and type of UI; increase of reported UI episodes from 1/month to 3/month; validated food frequency questionnaire including caffeinated beverages
Results	No association found between baseline level of caffeine intake and subsequent odds of progression of any type of UI over 2 years comparing women with highest caffeine intake against those with lowest caffeine intake
Level of evidence	3

AUA, American Urological Association; *BMI*, body mass index; *FVC*, frequency–volume chart; *KHQ*, King's Health Questionnaire; *LUTS*, lower urinary tract symptoms; *OAB*, overactive bladder; *OR*, odds ratio; *RCT*, randomized controlled trial; *RR*, risk ratio; *SD*, standard differentiation; *SUI*, stress urinary incontinence; *UI*, urinary incontinence; *UUI*, urgency urinary incontinence.

lifestyle factor reviewed. Abbreviated levels of evidence and grades of recommendations used within the ICI recommendations are as follows:

- Level 1: usually involves one well-designed randomized controlled trial (RCT)
- Level 2: includes at least one good-quality prospective cohort study
- Level 3: good-quality retrospective case–control study
- Level 4: includes good-quality case series.

Methodological quality of RCTs was further rated using the PEDro scale (Maher and Sherrington, 2003) (Table 7.1.3). Grades of recommendation are (Abrams, 2002):

- Grade A: consistent level 1 evidence, the recommendation being considered mandatory for placement within a clinical care pathway
- Grade B: based on consistent level 2 or 3 studies or 'majority' evidence from RCTs
- Grade C: based on level 4 studies or most evidence from level 2/3 studies
- Grade D: evidence is inconsistent/inconclusive or non-existent.

Obesity

Risk-Based Rationale for Including Obesity Within the Review

It seems reasonable to assume that an increased body mass index (BMI) might necessarily translate into increased abdominal forces acting upon the bladder itself, as well as the pelvic floor. However, increases in measured waist circumference rather than BMI show greater significant association with increased intravesical pressure, supporting the theory that improvements in UI after weight loss might be due more specifically to a reduction in the amount of abdominal fat rather than an overall decrease in BMI (Auwad et al., 2008). The urodynamic characteristics of incontinent, overweight or obese women also support this concept. Whereas increased waist circumference is significantly associated with both increased abdominal pressure and increased intravesical pressure, increased BMI has been shown to be significantly associated with increased abdominal pressure only (Richter et al., 2008).

A systematic review undertaken by Hunskaar (2008) found high-level evidence to support the view that moderate weight loss should be seen as an adequate first-line therapy for UI in women. This review highlighted the dose–response effect of increased BMI and increased waist–hip ratio that results predominantly in symptoms of SUI (including MUI) rather than symptoms of UUI or overactive bladder (OAB) (Hunskaar, 2008). Another review undertaken by Wesnes and Lose (2013) recommends aiming at normal weight before pregnancy and regaining pre-pregnancy weight postpartum to prevent UI in pregnancy and the postpartum period.

TABLE 7.1.3 PEDro Quality Score of Randomized Controlled Trials in Systematic Review of Lifestyle Factors and Urinary Incontinence

E – Eligibility criteria specified

1 – Subjects randomly allocated to groups

2 – Allocation concealed

3 – Groups similar at baseline

4 – Subjects blinded

5 – Therapist administering treatment blinded

6 – Assessors blinded

7 – Measures of key outcomes obtained from >85% of subjects

8 – Data analysed by intention to treat

9 – Statistical comparison between groups conducted

10 – Point measures and measures of variability provided

Study	E	1	2	3	4	5	6	7	8	9	10	Total Score
Subak et al. (2009)	+	+	+	+	–	–	+	+	–	+	+	7

+, Criterion is clearly satisfied; –, criterion is not satisfied; ?, not clear if the criterion was satisfied.
The total score is determined by counting the number of criteria that are satisfied, except the 'eligibility criteria specified' score is not used to generate the total score. Total scores are out of 10.

A systematic review that explored community-based prevalence studies using bivariate or multivariate analysis to explore the association of UI and increased BMI agreed that there was a clear dose–response effect of weight on UI and suggested that for each 5-unit increase of BMI there was an approximate 20% to 70% increase in UI risk (Subak et al., 2009a).

Increased BMI has also been implicated in the development of POP. Women with increased BMI are more likely to undergo surgery for prolapse than women with a normal BMI (Jelovsek et al., 2007).

International Consultation on Incontinence Summary and Recommendation

The Sixth International Consultation of the ICI determined obesity to be the most clearly established independent risk factor for UI (Abrams et al., 2016). Further, there is level 1 evidence to support that weight loss of 5% of initial body weight has an impact on the reduction of UI symptoms in women who are overweight and obese. Weight loss as a non-surgical intervention should be recommended to obese and overweight women with UI (grade of recommendation: A). Given the evidence of increasing obesity among women, recommendation was also made that weight loss advice should be included within continence promotion interventions. The prevention of weight gain was recommended as having a high research priority also including robust economic evaluation to determine the benefits of prevention strategies (Dumoulin et al., 2016).

Supporting Evidence: Obesity Reduction as a Management Strategy

In a study exploring the relationships between gender and lifestyle factors related to LUTS, a significant increase in such symptoms was found in women with a BMI of 30 kg/m^2 or greater when compared to women with a BMI less than 25 kg/m^2. However, BMI was not associated with any increase in the odds of LUTS among men (Litman et al., 2007) (level of evidence: 2).

Auwad et al. (2008) undertook a study in 64 obese women with urodynamically proven UI. The study was initially designed to be an RCT. However, when many of the women in the control group independently began dieting and lost weight, the study design, of necessity, became a longitudinal cohort study of the impact of weight loss on the incontinence symptoms of participant women. Participants' urine loss was measured by pad weight testing, and BMI as well as waist circumference were calculated. Forty-two women (65%) achieved a weight loss of at least 5% of initial body weight. A weak but statistically significant correlation was found between reductions in pad test weight, decreased waist circumference and bladder neck mobility. However, there was no correlation between reduction in BMI and reductions in UI measured by pad test weight (Auwad et al., 2008) (level of evidence: 2).

In a large longitudinal study of women in the United States aged between 54 and 79 years, study participants provided measures of height, weight and waist circumference in the baseline study. For the follow-up study 2 years later, women provided the same information along with information related to the onset of incontinence. Of the 35,754 women in this study, 34% were overweight and 17% were obese, and a multivariate analysis showed highly significant linear trends of increasing the risks of any, frequent and severe UI with both increasing BMI and increasing waist circumference. When BMI and waist circumference were included in the same model of analysis, only waist circumference remained a significant predictor of stress incontinence (Townsend et al., 2008a) (level of evidence: 2).

Wasserberg et al. (2009) explored the effect of surgically induced weight loss on pelvic floor disorders in morbidly obese women. A series of 178 women underwent bariatric surgery, 82 of whom achieved at least 50% reduction in excess body weight, and 46 (56%) of these women provided follow-up data showing a significant reduction in urinary symptoms. As well as this, there was a non-significant trend toward decreased prevalence of POP and measured colorectal symptoms in participant women (Wasserberg et al., 2009) (level of evidence: 2).

In a meta-analysis and systematic review, bariatric surgery was found to significantly improve UI in obese women at follow-up at 6 and 12 months (Zhang et al., 2020). Further, BMI was associated with poorer outcomes after incontinence surgery in both the short and long term (Bach et al., 2019; Laterza et al., 2018), suggesting that UI patients should be encouraged to change their BMI.

A search of the literature limited to RCTs studying weight loss to reduce UI symptoms retrieved five works. Four studies included women only (De Oliveira et al., 2019; Gozukara et al., 2014; Hagovska et al., 2019; Subak et al., 2009b), and one study included men only (Breyer et al., 2014). The intervention periods respectively lasted 8 weeks (De Oliveira et al., 2019), 12 weeks (Hagovska et al., 2019) and 6 months (Breyer et al., 2014; Gozukara et al., 2014; Subak et al., 2009b). No weight reduction was found in the study of de Oliveira et al. (2019), whereas a 5% to 9.4% weight reduction was found in the other studies. The inclusion criteria regarding UI phenotype differed as well as the outcome measure. However, all but one (De Oliveira et al., 2019) reported significant reduction in intervention groups regarding their outcome measure (UI, SUI, UUI, MUI or OAB) (Breyer et al., 2014; Gozukara et al., 2014; Hagovska et al., 2019; Subak et al., 2009b) (see Table 7.1.1).

Physical Activity

Risk-Based Rationale for Including Physical Activity Within the Review

Physical activity is one of the most important modifiable factors for promoting good health and in reducing premature death. The evidence is strong, and the current recommendation is a minimum of 150 minutes of weekly moderate-intensity exercise. However, it is questioned whether the increased intra-abdominal pressure during activity is good or bad for the pelvic floor. It might be reasonably assumed that increases in abdominal pressure inherent with some sporting or work activities might also contribute to pelvic floor dysfunction and UI. The topic is poorly investigated, and a recent narrative review by Bø and Nygaard (2020) identifies knowledge gaps and highlights the need for future research to understand the full effects of strenuous and non-strenuous activities on pelvic floor health. Studying the effect of physical activity and exercise in the prevention and treatment of UI is complex, as the effect might be mediated via an effect on weight. Further, women experiencing UI might refrain from physical activity due to fear of leaking.

An exploration of activity, sport and fitness levels among 82 UI women aged 28 to 80 years referred to a hospital gynaecology clinic for treatment of UI concluded that women seeking treatment for UI report similar levels of physical activity as continent women. Furthermore, the study reported that successful conservative or surgical cure of UI did not result in increases in activity levels in the women cured of incontinence in the longer term (Stach-Lempinen et al., 2004).

International Consultation on Incontinence Summary and Recommendation

Evaluating the association between physical activity and incontinence remains complex. Cross-sectional studies indicate that high-impact sports might be harmful, whereas low-impact sports might be protective (Abrams et al., 2016). The review undertaken in the Sixth International Consultation of the ICI reported no RCTs. However, the available literature suggests that moderate exercise decreases the incidence of UI (level of evidence: 3, grade of recommendation: C). Further, the evidence for strenuous physical activity and incontinence needs to be replicated using larger populations and more robust design before recommendations can be made (level of evidence: 3, grade of recommendation: C) (Dumoulin et al., 2016).

Supporting Evidence: Changes to Physical Activity as a Management Strategy

A longitudinal analysis of data available from the Nurses' Health Study (NHS) of women aged 54 to 79 years explored women's activity levels and their risk of developing UI and the type of UI (Danforth et al., 2007). Activity levels were averaged across all sequential questionnaires and calculated as 'metabolic equivalent task hours per week' which were divided into five groups (quintiles). The analysis revealed that total physical activity and walking were associated with significantly reduced odds of developing SUI but not symptoms of UUI (Danforth et al., 2007; Townsend et al., 2008b). It seems reasonable to assume that the role played by physical activity in maintaining a healthy body weight might make an important contribution to these findings (level of evidence: 2).

Similar results were found by Litman et al. (2007), who studied the association between physical activity and LUTS. The study involved 2301 men and 3205 women and showed that physical activity directly decreased the odds of LUTS, particularly in women when comparing study participants with high levels of physical activity against those with low levels of physical activity (Litman et al., 2007). The outcomes of this study are supported by other large prospective studies of the onset of UI and attributable factors (Townsend et al., 2008b) (level of evidence: 2).

Another large observational, US population-based longitudinal study among 3201 women and 2301 men again found low levels of physical activity to be associated with a two to three times greater likelihood of experiencing LUTS. Women were 68% less likely to experience LUTS if they reported high versus low levels of physical activity (Maserejian et al., 2012). In a secondary analysis of a the Caminemos trial, increasing time of walking in previously sedentary older (≥60 years) Latinos was associated with an increase in physical performance score and a 31% reduced risk of incident UI (Morrisroe et al., 2014) (level of evidence: 2). On the contrary, among young female athletes (mean age 19.9 years, all nulliparous) engaged in different sports, as many as 28% reported UI while participating in their respective sport activity. Prevalence varied from 0% to 67%, with high-impact sports reporting the highest prevalence (Nygaard et al., 1994). Bø and Borgen (2001) studied young athletes and found that 41% reported SUI and 16% reported UUI. There was no difference compared to controls (Bø & Borgen, 2001).

A search of the literature limited to RCTs studying the effect of increasing the level of physical activity on reducing UI symptoms retrieved three original studies and one follow-up study. All studies included women with UI. Talley et al. (2017) included frail women, whereas Huang et al. (2019) invited women older than 50 years and Wagg et al. (2019) invited women aged 60 to 75 years. The intervention programs differed from therapeutic yoga (Huang et al., 2019) to more general physical activity programs (Talley et al., 2017; Wagg et al., 2019), and the intervention period lasted from 12 to 24 weeks. The outcome measure was a 3-day bladder diary or 3-day incontinence record belt in all three studies, and all studies found a positive effect (Huang et al., 2019; Talley et al., 2017; Wagg et al., 2019). The positive effect was also seen after 12 months in the study by Wagg et al. (2019) (Haque et al., 2020).

All preceding trials included educative programs regarding bladder health and PFMT in the intervention program. Whether the positive effect is attributed to the physical activity intervention per se or the combination with PFMT is not to be concluded. However, the recent studies suggest that there is level 1 evidence to increase the level of physical activity in combination with PFMT to reduce UI.

No studies have examined the effect on UI of ceasing provocative activities, so the grade of recommendation remains at C.

Smoking

Risk-Based Rationale for Including Smoking Cessation Within the Review

It is commonly held that smokers are more likely than non-smokers to have a chronic cough. Because cough is related to increases in abdominal pressure, coughing might be likely to contribute to the lower urinary tract dysfunction usually associated with genuine SUI (Bump and McLish, 1994; Hannestad et al., 2003). However, the impact of nicotine on cholinergic detrusor pathways has also been implicated in animal studies (Koley et al., 1984), and several have associated past and current smokers with both SUI and symptoms of OAB (Danforth et al., 2006; Nuotio et al., 2001).

International Consultation on Incontinence Summary and Recommendation

The review of lifestyle interventions in relation to smoking concluded that although smoking might increase the chance of more severe UI (level of evidence: 3), no studies were found to show that smoking cessation resolves or reduces UI. The Sixth International Consultation of the ICI suggests the need for prospective studies to determine the impact of smoking cessation on both the onset and resolution of UI (Dumoulin et al., 2016) (grade of recommendation: C).

Supporting Evidence: Smoking Cessation as a Management Strategy

A well-conducted, prospective longitudinal analysis of the relationship between several lifestyle factors and the onset of SUI and OAB longitudinally over a 1-year period provides a higher level of evidence supporting the effect of smoking on the development of SUI and OAB. Exploration of data from a large longitudinal population study concluded that smoking might contribute to the development of UI in women but not in men (Maserejian et al., 2012) (level of evidence: 2).

Further exploration of the relationship between smoking status, smoking intensity and bladder symptoms among 3000 Finnish women revealed urinary urgency and frequency to be three times more common among current smokers than never-smokers. The association found between symptom severity and smoking intensity in study participants suggests a dose–response relationship. This study found no association between smoking and SUI (Tahtinen et al., 2011) (level of evidence: 2). In addition, a smaller study concluded that smokers are more likely to develop UI and that a dose relationship exists (Tampakoudis et al., 1995) (level of evidence: 2). A large cohort study including 27,936 women found that smoking status, and especially former heavy smoking, was independently associated with MUI (Hannestad et al., 2003) (level of evidence: 2).

No studies were found that examined the impact of smoking cessation on symptoms of UI. Therefore the grade of recommendation remains at C.

Dietary Factors

Risk-Based Rationale for Including Dietary Factors Within the Review

Several dietary factors are of interest regarding the management of UI. In the Sixth International Consultation of the ICI, dietary factors were divided into three groups: diet, fluid intake and caffeine. Each of these factors was reviewed individually by the Sixth International Consultation in relation to the conservative management of UI in women (Dumoulin et al., 2016). The association between alcohol and UI is far less studied, and only in men (Abrams et al., 2016).

Caffeine

Caffeine is the most widely consumed stimulant drug in the world and is well known for its diuretic and stimulant effects (Creighton and Stanton, 1990). The amount of caffeine in beverages varies considerably, and daily consumption of highly caffeinated beverages is on the rise (Arya et al., 2000).

The impact of caffeine ingestion in normal healthy people without LUTS was studied in a randomized, double-blind, placebo-controlled trial involving 80 healthy participants who received a twice-daily, standardized dose of caffeine (calculated equivalent to 200 mg in a person weighing 70 kg). Although the caffeine induced an initial diuresis in participants, there were no other significant or sustained effects on LUTS in the normal healthy study participants (Bird et al., 2005).

In exploring the impact of caffeine reduction on UI, an early RCT by Bryant et al. (2000) compared a bladder training protocol that included reduction of caffeine ingestion to 100 mg per day compared with a bladder training protocol without reduction of caffeine intake. Participants in this study experienced a significant reduction in the number of voids per 24 hours and reduced occasions of urgency per 24 hours, but the reduction in occasions of leakage per 24 hours did not reach significance (Bryant et al., 2000) (level of evidence: 2).

International Consultation on Incontinence Summary and Recommendation

Existing data suggests that caffeine consumption is likely to play a role in exacerbating UI and related symptoms such as urgency and frequency (level of evidence: 2). The committee recommended that caffeine reduction should be included as part of an intervention to reduce bladder symptoms (Dumoulin et al., 2016) (grade of recommendation: B).

Supporting Evidence: Caffeine Restriction as a Management Strategy

Population studies related to the impact of caffeine intake on LUTS provide conflicting results.

A population-based study of 14,031 Swedish twins explored the relationship between coffee and tea consumption and symptoms of UI. Women with high coffee intake were found to have lower risk of UI compared to women who did not drink coffee. Coffee intake was not found to be related to any specific subtypes of UI. However, significant associations were found between high levels of tea consumption and the risk of OAB symptoms and nocturia (Tettamanti et al., 2011) (level of evidence: 2).

A large prospective cohort study involving 65,176 female nurses aged 37 to 79 years was followed longitudinally over 4 years. Caffeine intake and symptoms of UI were measured, and findings suggest that high (but not low) coffee ingestion was associated with a modest but significantly increased risk of UI in women with the highest versus those with the lowest intake (>450 mg daily vs <150 mg daily). The attributable risk of UUI associated with high caffeine intake was calculated to be 25%. It was estimated that the onset of UI might be eliminated in 25% of the cases if the high caffeine intake were to be eliminated (Jura et al., 2011) (level of evidence: 2).

Longitudinal data from the same study mentioned earlier was also used to estimate the association between long-term caffeine intake and the progression of symptoms in 21,564 mildly incontinent women. Baseline caffeine intake and changes in caffeine intake over 4 years were measured, as were their symptoms of UI. The percentage of women with progressive symptoms of UI was similar across all categories based on the level of caffeine intake. It was therefore concluded that long-term caffeine intake over 2 years did not appear to be associated with the risk of the progression of UI symptoms in women (Townsend et al., 2012) (level of evidence: 2).

An observational study aimed to assess the association between caffeine intake and OAB in 1098 adults (>60 years of age) not previously diagnosed with OAB. The study found that a higher level of daily caffeine intake (≥300 mg/day) was associated with more episodes of urgency than a caffeine intake of 100 to 300 mg per day and <100 mg per day. No difference in leakage episodes were found (Kosilov et al., 2016) (level of evidence: 3).

Only one RCT was found (see Table 7.1.1). In a double-blinded, randomized, crossover pilot study, Wells et al. (2014) included 15 women newly diagnosed with OAB. Women were drinking caffeinated and decaffeinated fluids over 2 weeks with a 2-week wash-out period between. There was a reduction in urgency and frequency of urinary voids on the 3-day bladder diary, a reduction in the total International Consultation on Incontinence Questionnaire–Overactive Bladder (ICIQ-OAB) score, and a non-significant directional change for the total International Consultation on Incontinence Questionnaire–Overactive Bladder Quality of Life (ICIQ-OABqol) score in favour of the period of decaffeinated drink intake (Wells et al., 2014) (level of evidence: 1).

Although the level of evidence in support of caffeine reduction in the management of urgency, frequency and UUI is strengthening, the recommendation remains at level B.

Fluid Intake

The average fluid intake of healthy sedentary adults in temperate climates is estimated to be 1220 mL per person per day (Valtin, 2001). Incontinent people manipulate their fluid intake, reducing it in an attempt to prevent leakage episodes. Fluid intake is an important factor related not only to UI but also to bowel health, especially as an adjunct to the prevention of constipation.

International Consultation on Incontinence Summary and Recommendation

The review team concluded that fluid intake overall plays a minor role in the pathogenesis of UI, but since reduced fluid intake may lead to dehydration, urinary tract infections and constipation, fluid restriction as an intervention is recommended only in patients with abnormally high fluid intake (Dumoulin et al., 2016) (grade of recommendation: B).

Supporting Evidence: Manipulation of Fluid Intake as a Management Strategy

The prospective cohort study of 65,167 female nurses in the United States provided the opportunity to investigate associations between total fluid intake and incident UI (including symptoms of SUI, UUI and MUI) over 4 years. Comparing the group of women considered to have the highest fluid intake against women considered to have the lowest fluid intake, no significant risk of incident UI was found, with higher fluid intake in women suggesting that women should not be encouraged to restrict their fluid intake to prevent the onset of any type of UI (Townsend et al., 2011). The grade of recommendation remains at B.

Alcohol

International Consultation on Incontinence Summary and Recommendation

In the Sixth International Consultation of the ICI, only two surveys including Asian men were found indicating a significant association between alcohol consumption and UI (Abrams et al., 2016). In the face of these limited findings the ICI committee allocated no levels of evidence or grade of recommendation.

Supporting Evidence: Alcohol Reduction as a Management Strategy

A longitudinal study with follow-up over 4.8 years included 1610 men and 2535 women, exploring LUTS and several lifestyle factors, including alcohol intake, which was assessed by measuring both the type and amount of beverage consumed in the last 30 days. Women drinkers showed no association between alcohol intake and total LUTS other than nocturia (Maserejian et al., 2012) (level of evidence: 2). (By comparison, men reported as moderate drinkers, i.e., less than one alcoholic drink daily, were more than twice as likely to develop lower urinary tract storage symptoms when compared to men who did not drink alcohol. Men who drank more than moderately were not seen to be at any further increased risk for LUTS. The grade of recommendation related to men and lower urinary tract storage symptoms is B.)

Diet

Although diet might be seen to contribute to obesity and constipation, until now there has been scant evidence to support dietary manipulation in the management of UI.

A meta-analysis assessed studies related to the effectiveness of cranberry and blueberry products in preventing symptomatic urinary tract infections and concluded that there was some evidence from four scientifically robust RCTs that cranberry juice may decrease the number of symptomatic urinary tract infections over a 12-month period, particularly in women with recurrent urinary tract infections (Jepson and Craig, 2007) (level of evidence: 1).

International Consultation on Incontinence Summary and Recommendation

Dietary content may play a role in UI (level of evidence: 3). However, minimal evidence exists on the role of macronutrient intake and reduction of UI. The recommendations for dietary intake and fluid intake were unchanged in the Sixth International Consultation of the ICI (Dumoulin et al., 2016) (grade of recommendation: 3). RCTs on the role of diet in UI are warranted.

Supporting Evidence: Dietary Manipulation as a Management Strategy

No further evidence related to dietary manipulation as a management strategy for the prevention or management of LUTS was found.

Constipation

Epidemiological studies have shown associations between constipation and UI (Chiarelli et al., 2000), and some early studies showed a clear association between straining at stool and pelvic floor dysfunction (Lubowsi et al., 1988; Snooks et al., 1985). Medical relief of constipation has been shown to significantly improve LUTS in the elderly (Charach et al., 2001).

International Consultation on Incontinence Summary and Recommendation

Only small observational studies suggest that chronic straining may be a risk factor for UI (level of evidence: 3). There is too little research to make any recommendations (Dumoulin et al., 2016). The same conclusion remains relevant.

Supporting Evidence: Reducing Constipation as a Management Strategy

No studies were found to support the resolution of constipation as a management strategy to prevent or reduce LUTS.

Summary of Lifestyle Factors Associated With Urinary Incontinence

In light of the available evidence, it seems reasonable that interventions aimed at improving LUTS should include advice related to modifying relevant lifestyle risk factors. This might include advice about reducing waist circumference, constipation and caffeine consumption while encouraging increased physical activity levels in incontinent women. Advice about decreasing alcohol consumption would seem to be relevant only for incontinent men. Strategies for future research on lifestyle factors and UI should include a focus on better phenotyping and prevention.

MOTIVATING LIFESTYLE CHANGES

Just as there are models and theories used to predict and improve adherence to health behaviours, there are models and theories that address the processes of behaviour change. A commonly used definition of a theory is this: 'systematically organized knowledge applicable in a relatively wide variety of circumstances, devised to analyse, predict or otherwise explain the nature of behaviour of a specified set of phenomena that could be used as the basis for action' (Van Ryn and Heaney, 1992).

Knowing about a problem is insufficient to motivate change. Healthcare professionals commonly believe that simply by telling patients about their condition and likely contributing health behaviours is sufficient to motivate individuals towards changing their health behaviours.

Evidence to the contrary would appear to have had little effect on the way healthcare professionals go about inducing behaviour change in their patients. It is well known that knowledge relating to health risks is not sufficient to encourage people to adopt health behaviours. If knowledge itself were enough the rates of smoking in developed countries would be minimal, as would the health risks associated with an elevated BMI.

Individuals are bombarded with enormous amounts of information, which is interpreted through the filters of their past experiences, backgrounds, beliefs, values and attitudes. Human behaviour is complex, and understanding how to encourage behaviour change is even more complex. Many theories have been devised in an attempt to understand and promote changes in health behaviour. All such theories are based on the fact that health is mediated by some behaviour and that health behaviours have the potential for change.

Most behaviour change theories have emerged from the behavioural and social sciences, which in turn have borrowed from disciplines such as sociology, psychology, management and marketing. The theories derived from this variety of disciplines can be used to provide a framework or model that might be used to underpin the planning, adoption and evaluation of health behaviours.

Although some overlap of strategies might be observed, the models described in Table 7.1.4 are specifically related to health promotion—the adoption of specific health behaviours. In keeping with the evidence presented in relation to continence promotion, modifiable health behaviours that might be discussed with patients include restriction of caffeine, increasing physical activity, and maintenance or reduction of waist circumference. The attention to issues surrounding BMI and waist circumference must, of necessity, involve dietary manipulation and increased activity levels. However, simply telling the patient that weight loss is likely to improve their bladder symptoms is unlikely to have any impact unless behaviour modification strategies are implemented.

Behaviour modification strategies are based on a series of evolving theoretical models. Among the theoretical models that have been developed, some are intended to provide understanding, whereas others are

TABLE 7.1.4	**Theoretical Models of Behaviour Change and Their Implications for Practice**
Theory and authors	**Health Belief Model (HBM) (Becker, 1974)**
Description	The HBM is one of the earliest attempts to explain health behaviour.
	The HBM extends the use of psychosocial variables to explain preventive health behaviour by delineating people's subjective perceptions or beliefs about their health.
	Numerous studies of the HBM provide substantial empirical support for its usefulness in health education planning.
	Evidence supports the effectiveness of this model in developing continence promotion programmes.
Key concepts	The HBM is based on three essential factors: the readiness of the individual to consider behaviour changes to avoid disease or minimize health risks, the existence of forces in the individual's environment that urge change (cues to action) and make it possible, and the behaviours themselves.
	The HBM asserts that to undertake a preventive health action, individuals must believe that they are susceptible to the incontinence or that severity of present incontinence is likely to worsen, that incontinence and its sequelae are serious, that the action will be beneficial, and that the benefits will outweigh any costs or disadvantages.
	Barriers to action
	Cues to action
	Self-efficacy: confidence in performing the intervention
Implications for practice	The following concepts should be explored with the patient and relevant information supplied:
	Patients' perceptions of susceptibility, seriousness and progress of their condition should be assessed and corrected if unrealistic.
	Patients' understanding of the impact the health behaviour is likely to have on their condition should be assessed.
	There needs to be agreement that the health behaviour will be beneficial and worthwhile.
	Barriers to adoption of the health behaviour need to be explored, allowing the patient to suggest how perceived barriers might be overcome.
	Reminders need to be instigated to encourage the behaviour.
	Patients must demonstrate the required action.
	Patients must be able to practise repeatedly until proficient.
	Patients are encouraged to set initial, attainable goals related to the behaviour.

TABLE 7.1.4   Theoretical Models of Behaviour Change and Their Implications for Practice—cont'd

Theory and authors	**Theory of Reasoned Action and Planned Behaviour (Ajzen and Fishbein, 1980)**
Description	This theory was developed to explain behaviour that is able to be changed.
	It assumes that people make rational, predictable decisions in well-defined circumstances.
	The theory also assumes that the intention to act is the most important determinant of action and all factors relating to the particular action will need to be filtered through the initial intention.
	If personal beliefs and social pressures are strong enough, the intention is likely to translate into action.
	People's intentions are likely to be greater if they feel they have enough personal control over the behaviour.
Key concepts	Attitude towards behaviour
	Outcome expectations
	Value of outcome expectations
	Beliefs of others
	Motive to comply with others
	Perceived personal control over behaviour
Implications for practice	Explore:
	Patient's attitudes to required behaviour
	What patient believes outcome might be
	How important expected outcome is to patient
	What impact others might have on behaviour (e.g., a family attitude to eating more vegetables)
	What the patient believes others will think
	How much control patient feels in relation to behaviour
Theory and authors	**Transtheoretical Model (Stages of Change) (Prochaska and DiClemente, 1984)**
Description	This model integrates several principles and behaviours from other models.
	It is based on the assumption that an intention to act (or behave) immediately precedes that action or behaviour.
	The model looks closely at factors related to the intention to perform rather than the behaviour itself.
	Assessment of the stage a patient has reached can give an indication of the likelihood that the patient will comply with intervention requirements.
	Most patients seeking help have advanced through the initial stages of change and are in the contemplation or preparation stage.
Key concepts	Stages of change:
	Precontemplation: consciousness raising
	Contemplation: recognition of benefits of change
	Preparation: identification of barriers
	Action: programme or intervention
	Maintenance: recognition that relapse is a strong possibility
Implications for practice	Discuss the benefits of behaviour change.
	Discuss the consequences and progress likely if no changes are instigated.
	Allow the patient to identify barriers to behaviour change. Can the patient offer solutions to overcome the barriers?
	Work out tailored intervention.
	Allow the patient to repeat programme components in their own words to ensure understanding.
	Check self-efficacy.
	Monitor progress closely.
	Use patient-written records (e.g., diary) rather than self-reports for most variables.
	Discuss this with the patient, and put strategies into place in readiness.

Continued

TABLE 7.1.4	**Theoretical Models of Behaviour Change and Their Implications for Practice—cont'd**
Theory and authors	**Social Cognitive Theory (Bandura, 1977, 1982)**
Description	The model: Addresses underlying determinants of health behaviour as well as change methods Looks at continuous interplay among individual, environment and behaviour Adds cognitions to relationships Organizes cognitive and behavioural elements of behaviour change Recognizes behavioural reinforcement as external, internal, direct, observational or self-reinforcement Healthcare professionals are seen more as an agent of change than an interventionist by developing the patient's personal competencies.
Key concepts	Expectations: Self-control: goal-directed behaviour Observational learning: observing reward for a particular behaviour Self-efficacy: belief in ability to successfully perform behaviour
Implications for practice	What does the patient see as a likely outcome from behaviour change? Emphasize short-term, tangible benefits to begin with to booster the sense of self control. Explore the value placed on the outcome, especially by peers. The patient must feel confident of self-control regardless of the environment. Discuss coping strategies for situations when self-control might be less.

aimed more specifically at developing effective intervention protocols. Those models most used to develop strategies for use at an individual level include the Health Belief Model, Theory of Reasoned Action and Planned Behaviour, the Transtheoretical (or Stages of Change) Model and Social Cognitive Theory.

Table 7.1.4 sets out the health behaviour theories and how they might be implemented to optimize continence promotion/behaviour change/lifestyle interventions. From the table, it is clear that the theories presented overlap on several issues and generally have more in common than not (Nutbeam and Harris, 2004).

In summary, the main points emphasized by the collected theories are as follows:

- Regarding knowledge and beliefs about health while advocating health education, all theories emphasize the role of individualization—personalizing the information so that it is seen by individuals as relevant and pertinent.
- Regarding a patient's belief in their own ability to do what is asked, it is important to explore the patient's feelings of competency in relation to the behaviour and encouraging repeated, well-supervised practice to improve self-efficacy and self-esteem.

- It is important to perceive what is 'normal' by a patient in relation to the influences and values of their social group—the influence of the patient's social group as a role model, family and peer influences.
- Patients move forward and backwards along a continuum of change or readiness to change.
- It is important to be aware of the impact of socioeconomic and environmental factors on a patient's ability to adopt specific behaviours.
- It is important to encourage changing a patient's environment or perceptions of the environment when it impacts on their progress (Nutbeam and Harris, 2004).

HOW MIGHT LIFESTYLE CHANGES BE ENCOURAGED IN CLINICAL PRACTICE?

Much of healthcare today involves helping patients manage conditions whose outcomes can be greatly influenced by lifestyle or behaviour change. However, healthcare professionals tend to make inappropriate assumptions about patients and behaviour change. These are likely to have a negative impact on the outcome of consultation and include such assumptions as the patient 'should' and therefore 'wants' to change, that 'now' is the best time for the patient to change, and that the healthcare professional is the 'expert' and knows what is best for the patient (Emmons and Rollnick, 2001).

To improve the interactions of healthcare professionals with patients related to behaviour change, an excellent technique for negotiating behaviour change in a clinical setting has been developed by Rollnick and Heather (1992). On close examination, this patient-centred interviewing technique appears to be underpinned by several of the models described earlier. Originally developed to allow motivational interviewing (MI) related to substance abuse, the strategy is easily adaptable to suit any behavioural intervention related to lifestyle changes, and primary care clinicians have reported that the method is acceptable (Rollnick et al., 1997). This method of interviewing has been used successfully by various professions working in the fields of alcohol abuse, diabetes mellitus and tobacco smoking (Rollnick et al., 1999; Sellman et al., 2001), and a systematic review of the efficacy of the method shows it to be superior to other interviewing techniques (Dunn et al., 2001).

The technique is based on the concept of readiness to change and the fact that a patient's decision to change behaviour is apt to move forward and backwards along a continuum (Prochaska and DiClemente, 1984; see Table 7.1.4). This ambivalence is one of the main reasons advice giving has such limited effectiveness. Patients will only accept advice and act upon it when they are ready. They often experience feelings of ambivalence toward behaviour change, and using MI techniques provides the opportunity to build rapport with the patient and to explore the perceived importance of behaviour change through their eyes, to provide information if necessary, and also to explore their feelings of confidence (self-efficacy) related to the change in behaviour.

MI requires interviewing skills that are commonly used by healthcare professionals, such as active listening and empathizing. The use of open and closed questioning is also an important component of MI (Emmons and Rollnick, 2001).

The theoretical base of the interview strategy places importance on concepts such as readiness (related to the Stages of Change Model), the importance of the behaviour (related to the Health Belief Model), the patient's own concepts of beliefs and outcome expectations (related to the Theory of Planned Behaviour), and the patient's confidence in their ability to change (related to self-efficacy).

In general terms, MI has been shown to work better than 'usual' or 'traditional' care. Systematic reviews support MI as effective in fields as diverse as diet and exercise, diabetes, hypertension, asthma, and oral health (Knight et al., 2006; Martins and McNeil, 2009). Problems with bladder and bowel control are also considered chronic conditions, but to date no studies are available providing evidence of increased effectiveness specific to continence promotion when MI is incorporated into the intervention. It seems reasonable to assume that healthcare practitioners well trained in MI techniques might easily incorporate them into continence promotion programmes.

The study by Alewijnse et al. (2003) highlighted the fact that improved *implementation* of therapists' counselling skills significantly improved women's adherence to the pelvic floor muscle exercise programmes. This confirms the fact that when healthcare practitioners consciously implement specific counselling skills in which they have been trained, they are likely to optimize adherence to treatment programmes.

Although the techniques involved in MI may be appealing in their simplicity, practitioners tend to underestimate the complexity of MI and the need for adequate training (Mesters, 2009). Proficiency in effective utilization of MI techniques requires not only initial training but also ongoing feedback (Miller and Mount, 2001).

Although the focus of responsibility is changed when using MI, and the client is assigned more responsibility, this does not lessen the responsibility of the healthcare professional (Mesters, 2009). Using MI techniques can help both patients and practitioners talk about behaviour change in less confrontational ways that are likely to stimulate behaviour change.

Proficient, effective MI techniques need to be practised and well honed. Healthcare professionals willing to undertake training in MI techniques should realize that the training is just the beginning. As with any new skill, practice makes perfect.

IS THERE EVIDENCE OF THE USE OF BEHAVIOUR MODELS WITHIN CONTINENCE PROMOTION?

Healthcare practitioners use behavioural interventions daily without knowing it. Treatment protocols are regularly issued in a 'top-down' manner, with the health-care practitioners assuming that having been given the information, patients will know the importance of changing their behaviour and subsequently proceed to do so. Nothing could be further from the truth (Rollnick and Heather, 1992).

Many continence promotion programmes incorporate behavioural techniques within their programmes in an ad hoc fashion, but it is important to examine the available supporting evidence within continence promotion.

Chiarelli and Cockburn (1999) used the Health Belief Model as a framework to underpin the development of a successfully implemented postnatal continence promotion programme. The study by Chiarelli and Cockburn (1999) also employed social marketing strategies in the development of materials used within the programme. There was a significantly positive trend shown in the proportions of women adhering to pelvic floor exercise protocols at adequate levels in the intervention group when compared with those in the control group (p = 0.001, Mantel-Haenszel chi square).

There is little evidence, however, to show that other interventions have been based on any of the various models of behaviour change. When new continence promotion programmes are under development, whether individual treatment protocols for use in a physical therapy practice or continence promotion programmes for use in postnatal women or an aged care setting, it seems rational that they should be based on a proven framework such as that provided by the various models. In developing programmes aimed at behaviour change, further formative exploration is necessary to determine various beliefs and perceptions that underlie attitudes, motivation and behaviour. When this has been achieved, more effective health/continence promotion programmes might follow.

CLINICAL RECOMMENDATIONS

The following is the menu of strategies suggested as a framework for the interviewing technique that might easily be used within a continence promotion consultation (Rollnick and Heather, 1992; Emmons and Rollnick, 2001; Rollnick et al., 2008):
- Establishing rapport/introducing the subject: This provides an understanding of the client's concerns about the suggested change and allows deeper

understanding of the behaviour in the context of the person. The use of open-ended questions demonstrates to the patient that you are concerned about 'their story'. Explore what they know about the behaviour as it relates to them personally.
- Raising the subject: It is important here to check that the patient is happy to talk about the subject.
- Assessing the patient's readiness to change: Ask patients directly how they feel about changing the behaviour. By using phrases such as 'on a scale of 1 to 10, 1 being absolutely unwilling and 10 being ready, right now, to give it a go', the patient's readiness to change can easily be assessed.
- Provide feedback and raise awareness of the consequences of the behaviour: Objective data can be introduced at this point, the patient's need for more information can be explored and their concerns can be discussed, along with their feelings of self-efficacy. Offers of more support should be made at this point, especially if the patient feels little confidence in their ability to achieve the required change. If there is little readiness to change, this should be acknowledged, and questions such as 'What are the things about [the behaviour] that concern you?' should be asked.
- If the patient seems undecided: Describe how other patients have coped in the same situation, but be careful to emphasize that 'the patient knows best' and support them in whatever decision they make. In some instances, the subject is better postponed until the patient indicates more readiness to change.

The brief description is provided here to show how patients might be encouraged to become active collaborators in changing their health behaviours by using a method of empowerment that is underpinned by the most commonly used theories of behaviour change.

It is important that specialized healthcare providers realize the need for referral to other 'experts in the field'. For example, where weight loss is the desired outcome, brief MI within a continence promotion consultation might move the patient toward this behaviour, but referral to a dietician might be in the best interests of the patient.

MI has been used successfully in many fields of health promotion and is a powerful tool to enhance communication with patients and guide them in making choices to improve their health, from weight loss to exercise and smoking cessation to medication adherence.

REFERENCES

Abrams, P. (2002). Levels of evidence and grades of recommendation. In P. Abrams, L. Cardozo, S. Khoury, et al. (Eds.), *Incontinence: second international consultation on incontinence* (p. 8). Plymouth, UK: Health Publication/Plymbridge Distributors.

Abrams, P., Cardozo, L., Khoury, S., et al. (Eds.). (2009). *Incontinence: fourth international consultation on incontinence.* Paris: Health Publication/Editions 21.

Abrams, P., Cardozo, L., Wagg, A., et al. (Eds.). (2016). *Incontinence: sixth international consultation on incontinence.* Bristol, UK: ICUD.

Ajzen, I., & Fishbein, M. (1980). *Understanding Attitudes and Predicting Behaviour.* Englewood Cliffs, NJ: Prentice Hall.

Alewijnse, D., Metsemakers, J., Mesters, I. E. P. E., et al. (2003). Effectiveness of pelvic floor muscle exercise therapy supplemented with a health education program to promote long-term adherents among women with urinary incontinence. *Neurourology and Urodynamics, 22,* 284–295.

Arya, L. A., Myers, D. L., Jackson, N. D., et al. (2000). Dietary caffeine intake and the risk for detrusor instability: A case–control study. *Obstetrics & Gynecology, 96*(1), 85–89.

Auwad, W., Steggles, P., Bombieri, L., et al. (2008). Moderate weight loss in obese women with urinary incontinence: A prospective longitudinal study. *International Urogynecology Journal, 19*(9), 1251–1259.

Bach, F., Hill, S., & Toozs-Hobson, P. (2019). The effect of body mass index on retropubic midurethral slings. *American Journal of Obstetrics and Gynecology, 220*(4), 371 e1–371.e9.

Bandura, A. (1977). *Social learning theory.* Englewood Cliffs, NJ: Prentice Hall.

Bandura, A. (1982). Self-efficacy mechanism in human agency. *American Psychologist, 37*(2), 122–147.

Becker, M. (1974). The Health Belief Model and personal health behaviour. *Health Education Monographs, 2,* 324–508.

Bird, E. T., Parker, B. D., Kim, H. S., et al. (2005). Caffeine ingestion and lower urinary tract symptoms in healthy volunteers. *Neurourology and Urodynamics, 24*(7), 611–615.

Bø, K., & Borgen, J. (2001). Prevalence of stress and urge urinary incontinence in elite athletes and controls. *Medicine & Science in Sports & Exercise, 33*(11), 1797–1802.

Bø, K., & Nygaard, I. E. (2020). Is physical activity good or bad for the female pelvic floor? A narrative review. *Sports Medicine, 50*(3), 471–484.

Breyer, B. N., Phelan, S., Hogan, P. E., et al. (2014). Intensive lifestyle intervention reduces urinary incontinence in overweight/obese men with type 2 diabetes: Results from the Look AHEAD trial. *Journal of Urology, 192*(1), 144–149.

Brown, J., Grady, D., Ouslander, J. G., et al. (1999). Prevalence of urinary incontinence and associated risk factors in postmenopausal women. *Obstetrics & Gynecology, 94*(1), 66–70.

Bryant, C., Dowell, C., & Fairbrother, G. (2000). A randomised trial of the effects of caffeine upon frequency, urgency and urge incontinence. *Neurourology and Urodynamics, 19*(4) 96–96.

Bump, R., & McLish, D. (1994). Cigarette smoking and pure genuine stress incontinence of urine: A comparison of risk factors and determinants between smokers and non-smokers. *American Journal of Obstetrics and Gynecology, 170,* 579–582.

Charach, G., Greenstein, A., Rabinovich, P., et al. (2001). Alleviating constipation in the elderly improves lower urinary tract symptoms. *Gerontology, 47,* 72–76.

Chiarelli, P., & Brown, W. (1999). Urinary incontinence in Australian women: Prevalence and associated conditions. *Women & Health, 29*(1), 1–14.

Chiarelli, P., Brown, W., & McElduff, P. (2000). Constipation in Australian women: Prevalence and associated factors. *International Urogynecology Journal and Pelvic Floor Dysfunction, 11,* 71–78.

Chiarelli, P., & Cockburn, J. (1999). The development of a physiotherapy continence promotion program using a customer focus. *Australian Journal of Physiotherapy, 45*(2), 111–119.

Creighton, S., & Stanton, S. (1990). Caffeine: Does it affect your bladder? *British Journal of Urology, 66*(6), 613–614.

Dallosso, H., Matthews, R., McGrother, C., et al. (2004). Diet as a risk factor for the development of stress urinary incontinence: A longitudinal study in women. *European Journal of Clinical Nutrition, 58*(6), 920–926.

Danforth, K. N., Townsend, M. K., Lifford, K., et al. (2006). Risk factors for urinary incontinence among middle-aged women. *American Journal of Obstetrics and Gynecology, 194*(2), 339–345.

Danforth, K. N., Shah, A. D., Townsend, M. K., et al. (2007). Physical activity and urinary incontinence among healthy, older women. *Obstetrics & Gynecology, 109*(3), 721–727.

De Oliveira, M. C. E., de Oliveira de Lima, V. C., Pegado, R., et al. (2019). Comparison of pelvic floor muscle training isolated and associated with weight loss: A randomized controlled trial. *Archives of Gynecology and Obstetrics, 300*(5), 1343–1351.

Dumoulin, C., Adewuyi, T., Booth, J., et al. (2016). Committee 12: Adult conservative management. In P. Abrams, L. Cardozo, A. Wagg, et al. (Eds.), *Incontinence: sixth international consultation on incontinence* (pp. 1443–1628). Bristol, UK: ICUD.

Dunn, C., Deroo, L., & Rivara, F. P. (2001). The use of brief interventions adapted from motivational interviewing across behavioral domains: A systematic review. *Addiction, 96*(12), 1725–1742.

Emmons, K., & Rollnick, S. (2001). Motivational interviewing in health care settings: Opportunities and limitations. *American Journal of Preventive Medicine, 20*(1), 68–74.

Gleason, J. L., Richter, H. E., & Reddenm, D. T. (2013). Caffeine and urinary incontinence in US women. *International Urogynecology Journal and Pelvic Floor Dysfunction, 24*(2), 295–302.

Gozukara, Y. M., Akalan, G., Tok, E. C., et al. (2014). The improvement in pelvic floor symptoms with weight loss in obese women does not correlate with the changes in pelvic anatomy. *International Urogynecology Journal, 25*(9), 1219–1225.

Hagovska, M., Svihra, J., Bukova, A., et al. (2019). The impact of different intensities of exercise on body weight reduction and overactive bladder symptoms—randomised trial. *European Journal of Obstetrics & Gynecology and Reproductive Biology, 242*, 144–149.

Hannestad, Y., Rortveit, G., Daltveit, A. K., et al. (2003). Are smoking and other lifestyle factors associated with female urinary incontinence? The Norwegian EPINCONT study. *British Journal of Obstetrics and Gynaecology, 110*(3), 247–254.

Haque, R., Kabir, F., Naher, K., et al. (2020). Promoting and maintaining urinary continence: Follow-up from a cluster-randomized trial of elderly village women in Bangladesh. *Neurourology and Urodynamics, 39*(4), 1152–1161.

Hay-Smith, J., Berghmans, B., Burgio, K., et al. (2009). Committee 12: Adult conservative management. In P. Abrams (Ed.), *Health Publication/Editions 21. Incontinence: Fourth International Consultation on Incontinence* Paris: p. 1107.

Huang, A. J., Jenny, H. E., Chesney, M. A., et al. (2014). A group-based yoga therapy intervention for urinary incontinence in women: A pilot randomized trial. *Female Pelvic Medicine & Reconstructive Surgery, 20*(3), 147–154.

Hunskaar, S. (2008). A systematic review of overweight and obesity as risk factors and targets for clinical intervention for urinary incontinence in women. *Neurourology and Urodynamics, 27*(8), 749–757.

Imamura, M., Williams, K., Wells, M., et al. (2015). Lifestyle interventions for the treatment of urinary incontinence in adults. *Cochrane Database Systematic Reviews Issue, 12* Art. No. CD003505.

Jelovsek, J. E., Maher, C., & Barber, M. D. (2007). Pelvic organ prolapse. *Lancet, 369*, 1027–1038.

Jepson, R. G., & Craig, J. C. (2007). A systematic review of the evidence for cranberries and blueberries in UTI prevention. *Molecular Nutrition & Food Research., 51*(6), 738–745.

Jura, Y. H., Townsend, M. K., Curhan, G. C., et al. (2011). Caffeine intake, and the risk of stress, urgency and mixed urinary incontinence. *Journal of Urology, 185*(5), 1775–1780.

Knight, K. M., McGowan, L., Dickens, C., et al. (2006). A systematic review of motivational interviewing in physical health care settings. *British Journal of Health Psychology, 11*(2), 319–332.

Koley, B., Koley, J., & Saha, J. K. (1984). The effects of nicotine on spontaneous contractions of cat urinary bladder in situ. *British Journal of Pharmacology, 83*(2), 347–355.

Kosilov, K. V., Loparev, S. A., Ivanovskaya, M. A., et al. (2016). Caffeine as a probable factor for increased risk of OAB development in elderly people. *Current Urology, 9*(3), 124–131.

Landefeld, C. S., Bowers, B. J., Feld, A. D., et al. (2008). National Institutes of health State-of-the-Science Conference statement: Prevention of fecal and urinary incontinence in adults. *Annals of Internal Medicine, 148*(6), 449–458.

Laterza, R. M., Halpern, K., Ulrich, D., et al. (2018). Influence of age, BMI and parity on the success rate of midurethral slings for stress urinary incontinence. *PLoS One, 13*(8): Article e0201167.

Litman, H. J., Steers, W., Wei, J. T., et al. (2007). Relationship of lifestyle and clinical factors with lower urinary tract symptoms (LUTS): Results from the Boston Area community health (BACH) survey. *Urology, 70*(5), 916–921.

Lubowsi, D., Swash, M., Nicholls, R. J., et al. (1988). Increases in pudendal nerve terminal motor latency with defaecation straining. *British Journal of Surgery, 75*, 1095–1097.

Maher, C., & Sherrington, C. (2003). Reliability of the PEDro scale for rating quality of randomized controlled trials. *Physical Therapy, 83*, 713–721.

Martins, R. K., & McNeil, D. W. (2009). Review of motivational interviewing in promoting health behaviors. *Clinical Psychology Review, 29*(4), 283–293.

Maserejian, N. N., Kupelian, V., Miyasato, G., et al. (2012). Are physical activity, smoking and alcohol consumption associated with lower urinary tract symptoms in men or women? Results from a population based observational study. *Journal of Urology, 188*(2), 490–495.

Mesters, A. (2009). Motivational interviewing: Hype or hope? *Chronic Illn, 5*(3), 3–6.

Miller, W., & Mount, K. (2001). A small study of training in motivational interviewing: Does one workshop change clinician and client behaviour? *Behav. Cogn. Psychother., 29*, 457–471.

Morrisroe, S. N., Rodriguez, L. V., Wang, P. C., et al. (2014). Correlates of 1-year incidence of urinary incontinence in older Latino adults enrolled in a community-based physical activity trial. *Journal of the American Geriatrics Society, 62*(4), 740–746.

Myers, D. L. (2014). Female mixed urinary incontinence: A clinical review. *JAMA, 311*(19), 2007–2014.

National Institute for Health and Clinical Excellence (NICE). (2006). *Urinary incontinence: The Management of urinary incontinence in women. Guideline 40.* London: National Institute for Health and Clinical Excellence.

National Institute for Health and Clinical Excellence (NICE). (2019). *Urinary incontinence and pelvic organ prolapse in women: management.* Available: https://www.nice.org.uk/guidance/ng123/chapter/Recommendations (accessed 27.07.22).

Nuotio, M., Jylhä, M., Koivisto, A. M., et al. (2001). Association of smoking with urgency in older people. *European Urology, 40,* 206–212.

Nutbeam, D., & Harris, E. (2004). *Theory in a Nutshell.* Sydney: McGraw Hill.

Nygaard, I. E., Thompson, F. L., Svengalis, S. L., et al. (1994). Urinary incontinence in elite nulliparous athletes. *Obstetrics & Gynecology, 84*(2), 183–187.

Prochaska, J., & DiClemente, C. (1984). *The Transtheoretical Approach: Crossing Traditional Foundations of Change.* Homewood, IL: Don Jones/Irwin.

Richter, H. E., Creasman, J. M., Myers, D. L., et al. (2008). Urodynamic characterization of obese women with urinary incontinence undergoing a weight loss program: The program to reduce incontinence by diet and exercise (PRIDE) trial. *International Urogynecology Journal and Pelvic Floor Dysfunction, 19*(12), 1653–1658.

Rollnick, S., Butler, C., & Stott, N. (1997). Helping smokers make decisions: The enhancement of brief intervention for general medical practice. *Patient Education and Counseling, 31,* 191–203.

Rollnick, S., & Heather, N. (1992). Negotiating behaviour change in medical settings. *Journal of Mental Health, 1*(1), 25–38.

Rollnick, S., Mason, P., & Butler, C. (1999). *Health Behaviour Change: A Guide for Practitioners.* Edinburgh: Churchill Livingstone.

Rollnick, S., Miller, W., & Butler, C. (2008). *Motivational Interviewing in Health Care: Helping Patients Change Behavior. Applications of Motivational Interviewing.* New York: Guilford Press.

Sellman, J. D., Sullivan, P. F., Dore, G. M., et al. (2001). A randomized controlled trial of Motivational Enhancement Therapy (MET) for mild to moderate alcohol dependence. *Journal of Studies on Alcohol, 62*(3), 389–396.

Snooks, S. J., Barnes, P. R. H., Swash, M., et al. (1985). Damage to the innervation of the pelvic floor musculature in chronic constipation. *Gastroenterology, 89*(5), 977–981.

Stach-Lempinen, B., Nygard, C., Laippala, P., et al. (2004). Is physical activity influenced by urinary incontinence? *British Journal of Obstetrics and Gynaecology, 11,* 475–480.

Subak, L., Richter, H., & Hunskaar, S. (2009). Obesity and urinary incontinence: Epidemiology and clinical research update. *Journal of Urology, 182*(6 Suppl. l), 2–7.

Subak, L. L., Wing, R., West, D. S., et al. (2009). Weight loss to treat urinary incontinence in overweight and obese women. *New England Journal of Medicine, 360*(5), 481–490.

Tahtinen, R. M., Auvinen, A., Cartwright, R., et al. (2011). Smoking and bladder symptoms in women. *Obstetrics & Gynecology, 118*(3), 643–648.

Talley, K. M. C., Wyman, J. F., Bronas, U., et al. (2017). Defeating urinary incontinence with exercise training: Results of a pilot study in frail older women. *Journal of the American Geriatrics Society, 65*(6), 1321–1327.

Tampakoudis, P., Tantanassis, T., Grimbizis, G., et al. (1995). Cigarette smoking and urinary incontinence in women—a new calculative method of measuring exposure to smoke. *European Journal of Obstetrics & Gynecology and Reproductive Biology, 63,* 27–30.

Tettamanti, G., Altman, D., Pedersen, N. L., et al. (2011). Effects of coffee and tea consumption on urinary incontinence in female twins. *British Journal of Obstetrics and Gynaecology, 118*(7), 806–813.

Townsend, M. K., Curhan, G. C., Resnick, N. M., et al. (2008). BMI, waist circumference, and incident urinary incontinence in older women. *Obesity, 16*(4), 881–886.

Townsend, M. K., Danforth, K. N., Rosner, B., et al. (2008). Physical activity and incident urinary incontinence in middle-aged women. *Journal of Urology, 179*(3), 1012–1016 discussion 1016–1017.

Townsend, M. K., Jura, Y. H., Curhan, G. C., et al. (2011). Fluid intake and risk of stress, urgency, and mixed urinary incontinence. *American Journal of Obstetrics and Gynecology, 205*(1) 73.e1–73.e6.

Townsend, M. K., Resnick, N. M., & Grodstein, F. (2012). Caffeine intake and risk of urinary incontinence progression among women. *Obstetrics & Gynecology, 119*(5), 950–957.

Valtin, H. (2001). Drink at least eight glasses of water a day? Really? Is there scientific evidence for "8 × 8". *American Journal of Physiology - Regulatory, Integrative and Comparative Physiology, 283*(5), R993–R1004.

Van Ryn, M., & Heaney, C. (1992). What's the use of theory? *Health Education Quarterly, 19*(3), 315–330.

Wagg, A., Chowdhury, Z., Galarneau, J. M., et al. (2019). Exercise intervention in the management of urinary incontinence in older women in villages in Bangladesh: A cluster randomised trial. *Lancet Glob. Health, 7*(7), e923–e931.

Wasserberg, N., Petrone, P., Haney, M., et al. (2009). Effect of surgically induced weight loss on pelvic floor disorders in morbidly obese women. *Annals of Surgery, 249*(1), 72–76.

Wells, M. J., Jamieson, K., Markham, T. C., et al. (2014). The effect of caffeinated versus decaffeinated drinks on overactive bladder: A double-blind, randomized, crossover study. *Journal of Wound Ostomy & Continence Nursing, 41*(4), 371–378.

Wesnes, S. L., & Lose, G. (2013). Preventing urinary incontinence during pregnancy and postpartum: A review. *International Urogynecology Journal, 24*(6), 889–899.

Zhang, J., Gao, L., Liu, M., et al. (2020). Effect of bariatric surgery on urinary incontinence in obese women: A meta-analysis and systematic review. *Female Pelvic Medicine & Reconstructive Surgery, 26*(3), 207–211.

Pelvic Floor Muscle Training for Stress Urinary Incontinence

Kari Bø

INTRODUCTION

Kegel (1948) was the first to report pelvic floor muscle training (PFMT) to be effective in the treatment of female urinary incontinence. Despite his reports of cure rates greater than 84% (pre-/post-studies, no randomized controlled trials [RCTs]), surgery soon became the first choice of treatment, and not until the 1980s was there renewed interest in conservative treatment. This interest may have developed because of higher awareness among women regarding incontinence and health and fitness activities, cost of surgery and morbidity, complications and relapses reported after surgical procedures (Fantl et al., 1996).

Although several consensus statements based on systematic reviews have recommended conservative treatment and especially PFMT as the first choice of treatment for urinary incontinence (Dumoulin et al., 2017; Dumoulin et al., 2018; Hay-Smith et al., 2011; Herderschee et al., 2011; Imamura et al., 2010; National Institute for Health and Care Excellence (NICE), 2019), many surgeons seem to regard minimally invasive surgery as a better first-line option than PFMT. The skepticism against PFMT may be based on inappropriate knowledge of exercise science and physical therapy, beliefs that there is insufficient evidence for the effect of PFMT, that evidence for long-term effect is lacking or poor, and that women are not motivated to regularly perform PFMT. To date, we have only been able to find two RCTs comparing PFMT and surgery. In the RCT of Klarskov et al. (1986) the patients had different surgeries according to their problems. The PFMT program was described as group training with five or more sessions with a physical therapist (PT), and it is not clear whether the participants had vaginal palpation to make sure they were able to contract the pelvic floor muscles (PFMs) correctly. At 4 months the PFMT group was less likely to report cure compared to women who had surgery. However, there was no statistical difference in the proportions reporting cure/improvement. At 12 months, 10 of 24 women in the PFMT group reported satisfaction with the initial therapy versus 19 of 26 in the surgery group. Adverse effects were reported only in the surgery group, including new urgency incontinence, retropubic or pelvic pain, or dyspareunia.

Labrie et al. (2013) compared nine visits to physical therapy of PFMT + home exercise with mid-urethral sling surgery. The conclusion was that surgery was more effective in women with stress urinary incontinence (SUI) than PFMT. The results have been debated because of a possible selection bias (many women had tried PFMT earlier with no effect and the crossover design), no blinding of the assessors and the fact that 83 different PTs were conducting the training. The PTs could individually follow a guideline allowing for other interventions such as breathing and posture exercise, abdominal training, and change of general movement patterns, possibly lowering the actual dosage and time spent on actual strength training for the PFMs. In addition, adherence to the home PFMT program was not reported.

Recently, mid-urethral sling surgery has come under scrutiny following concerns raised regarding long-term complications. In some European countries, such as the UK, the use of synthetic mid-urethral slings has been paused following a parliamentary review published in July 2020 (Cumberledge, 2020). The review concluded the following: 'For many women mesh surgery is trouble-free and leads to improvements in their condition. However, this is not the case for all. There is no reliable information on the true number of women who have suffered complications. While they may be in the minority, that does not diminish the catastrophic nature of their suffering or the importance of providing support to them and learning from what has happened to them'. The NICE (2019) guideline concluded that PFMT is as effective as surgery for around half of women with SUI, and due to the risks following surgery and absence of adverse events of PFMT, they recommend 3 months of supervised PFMT as first-line treatment for SUI and mixed urinary incontinence (MUI).

The aim of this chapter is to report evidence-based knowledge about PFMT for SUI.

RATIONALE FOR PELVIC FLOOR MUSCLE TRAINING

To date, there are two main theories of mechanisms on how PFMT may be effective in the prevention and treatment of SUI (Bø, 2004):

1. Theory 1 states that women learn to consciously contract before and during an increase in intra-abdominal pressure and continue to perform such contractions as a behaviour modification to prevent descent of the pelvic floor.

2. Theory 2 states that women are taught to perform regular strength training over time to build up 'stiffness' and structural support of the pelvic floor. There is basic research, as well as case–control studies and RCTs, to support both hypotheses (Bø, 2004; Dumoulin et al., 2017).

In addition to these main theories, two other theories have been proposed:

1. Theory 3 is stated by Sapsford (2001, 2004), who claimed that the PFMs were effectively trained indirectly by contraction of the internal abdominal muscles, especially the transversus abdominus (TrA) muscle.

2. Theory 4, named *functional training*, has been claimed by many PTs.

'Functional training of the PFM' was described by Carriere (2002) in that women are asked to conduct a PFM contraction during different tasks of daily living. This was further defined by Bø et al. (2017) as follows: Functional training consists of training for tasks of daily living and self-care activities, such as squatting to train quadriceps and gluteal muscles. Functional PFMT includes training and exercises that incorporate a correct PFM contraction into activities of daily living such as lifting, transferring out of bed, or sneezing. A PFM contraction before a rise in intra-abdominal pressure, such as a cough ('the Knack'), is part of functional PFMT.

Evidence for Theory 1

By intentional contraction of the PFMs before and during an increase in abdominal pressure, there is a lift of the pelvic floor in a cranial and forward direction and a squeeze around the urethra, vagina and rectum (DeLancey, 1990, 1994a,b, 1997; Kegel, 1948). Ultrasonography and magnetic resonance imaging studies have verified a lift in a cranial direction and movement of the coccyx in a forward, anterior and cranial direction (Bø et al., 2001; Thompsen

and O'Sullivan, 2003). Miller et al. (1998) named this voluntary counterbracing-type contraction *the Knack* and in a single-blind RCT showed that the Knack performed during a medium and deep cough reduced urinary leakage by 98.2% and 73.3%, respectively. Cure rate in 'real life' was not reported. In addition, research on basic and functional anatomy research supports the Knack as an effective manoeuvre to stabilize the pelvic floor (Miller et al., 2001; Peschers et al., 2001c). A single voluntary contraction of the PFMs increases urethral closure pressure (Miller et al., 2018; Zubieta et al., 2016), causes simultaneous co-contraction of the urethral sphincter (Bø and Stien, 1994) and reduces the levator hiatus area by 25%, from a resting area of 20 cm^2 (95% CI: 17–23) to 15 cm^2 (95% CI: 13–17). The muscle length shortens 21%, from 12.5 cm (95% CI: 11.1–13.8) to 9.7 cm (95% CI: 8.7–10.7), and lifts the pelvic floor higher up in the pelvis (Brækken et al., 2009). In an RCT of 108 women with SUI and MUI, one group received a 15-minute slide show including a Knack tutorial on how to contract the PFMs to inhibit urgency and to contract before and during increase in intra-abdominal pressure. The other group saw a video containing good diet and exercise advice. Significant improvement was reported by 71% in the Knack tutorial group compared to 25% in the diet/exercise advice group (p < 0.001). Self-perceived improvement was 21% to 22% higher in the Knack tutorial group (p < 0.001) (Miller et al., 2018). However, many women did not leak on the paper towel test before the intervention, and we do not know whether they had urgency urinary incontinence (UUI). To date, there are no studies on how much strength is necessary to prevent descent during coughing and other physical exertions, and we do not know if regular counterbracing during daily activities is enough to increase muscle strength or cause morphological changes of the PFMs.

Evidence for Theory 2

Kegel (1948) originally described PFMT as physiological training or 'tightening up' of the pelvic floor. The theoretical rationale for intensive strength training (exercise) of the PFMs to treat SUI is that strength training may build up the structural support of the pelvis by elevating the levator plate to a permanent higher location inside the pelvis and by enhancing hypertrophy and stiffness of the PFMs and their connective tissue. This would facilitate a more effective automatic motor unit firing (neural adaptation), preventing descent during an increase in abdominal pressure. The pelvic openings and the levator hiatus may narrow and the pelvic organs are held in place during increases in abdominal pressure. In addition, a pelvic floor located at a higher level inside the pelvis may yield a much quicker and more coordinated response to an increase in abdominal pressure, closing the urethra by increasing the urethral pressure (Constantinou and Govan, 1981; Howard et al., 2000). The most likely theory is that a tight pelvic floor may prevent huge and uncontrolled downward movements and opening of the levator hiatus during increase in intra-abdominal pressure and ground reaction forces with no need for simultaneous PFM contractions.

Ultrasound studies have shown that parous women have a more caudal location of the pelvic floor than nulliparous women (Peschers et al., 1997). Difference in anatomical placement has also been shown between continent and incontinent women (Miller et al., 2001; Peschers et al., 2001a).

In an uncontrolled trial of PFMT for SUI, Balmforth et al. (2004) found that the position of the bladder neck was observed by ultrasound to be significantly elevated at rest, and during Valsalva manoeuvre and squeeze after 14 weeks of supervised PFMT and behavioural modifications. McLean et al. (2013) randomized 40 women with SUI to either 12 weekly physiotherapy sessions during which they learned how to properly contract their PFMs and a home exercise program or a control group with no treatment. Before and after the 12-week study period, ultrasound imaging was used to evaluate bladder neck position and mobility during coughing and Valsalva manoeuvre in supine and standing positions, as well as urethral morphology. The results showed that the women in the treatment group reduced bladder neck mobility during coughing and increased cross-sectional area of their urethra after as compared to before the training. There were no changes in the control group. No differences in the resting position of the bladder neck or in bladder neck excursion during Valsalva manoeuvre were noted in either group. Madill et al. (2015) reported in a pre-/post test study on women with SUI that the striated urethral sphincter increased significantly in thickness (21%, $p < 0.001$), cross-sectional area (20%, $p = 0.003$) and volume (12%, $p = 0.003$) following the intervention. The reported number of incontinence episodes and their bother also decreased significantly. In an assessor-blinded RCT of PFMT in women with pelvic organ prolapse where 102 participants had concomitant urinary incontinence (UI), Brækken et al. (2010) found statistically significant changes in PFM strength, thickness, muscle length, levator hiatus area and position of the rectal ampulla and bladder neck in favour of the PFMT group compared to the control group. The training group also had statistically significant reduction in SUI symptoms. As the results were found in women with pelvic organ prolapse, there is a need for a similar study in women with SUI only. However, since the results were consistent for all morphological changes in this more complicated group to treat, one may assume that even better results will be found in a group with SUI only.

Furthermore, in a pre-/post test study of 29 postmenopausal women, Mercier et al. (2020) found that PFMT significantly improved blood flow parameters in both arteries ($p < 0.05$) and significantly increased the speed of PFM relaxation after a contraction ($p = 0.003$). After the intervention, a marginally significant decrease in PFM tone was observed, as well as an increase in PFM strength ($p = 0.06$ and $p = 0.05$, respectively). In addition, improvements in skin elasticity and introitus width were observed as measured by the Vaginal Atrophy Index ($p < 0.007$). These findings are promising but need confirmation in future RCTs.

In some studies, the patients were tested both subjectively and objectively during physical activity, and had no leakage during strenuous tests after the training period (Bø et al., 1990a; Bø et al., 1999; Castro et al., 2008; Dumoulin et al., 2018; McLean et al., 2013; Mørkved et al., 2002; Pereira et al., 2011). Therefore the effect most likely was due to improved automatic muscle function and not only the ability to voluntarily contract before an increase in abdominal pressure. Brækken et al. (2010) found that there was less increase in the levator hiatus area during Valsalva in the PFMT group compared to the control group, and suggested that this may be due to increased automatic function of the PFMs.

Evidence for Theory 3

Sapsford (2001, 2004) suggested that the PFMs can be trained indirectly by training the TrA muscle. This is based on an understanding that the PFMs are part of the abdominal capsule surrounding the abdominal and pelvic organs. The structures included in this capsule (often referred to as the 'core') are the lumbar vertebrae and deeper layers of the multifidus muscle, the respiratory diaphragm, the TrA and the PFMs (Sapsford, 2001, 2004).

Several studies have shown that different abdominal muscles co-contract during PFM contraction (Bø and Stien, 1994; Bø et al., 1990b; Neumann and Gill, 2002; Peschers et al., 2001b; Sapsford et al., 2001). In addition, some studies have shown that there is a co-contraction of the PFMs during different abdominal muscle contractions in healthy volunteers. Bø and Stien (1994), using concentric needle electromyography (EMG), found that there was a co-contraction of the PFM during contractions of the rectus abdominis in continent women. Sapsford and Hodges (2001) found that PFM surface electromyography (EMG) increased with TrA contractions in six healthy females, and this was supported by a study of four continent women by Neumann and Gill (2002). In continent women, Sapsford et al. (1998) found that a sustained isometric abdominal contraction termed *hollowing* in which the TrA and internal obliques are contracted increased the urethral pressure as much as a maximal PFM contraction. However, they had also ensured that the women were simultaneously contracting the PFMs. Based on these findings, Sapsford (2001, 2004) recommends that incontinence training should begin by training the TrA rather than the PFMs specifically. However, it is important to note that all of these studies were in healthy women, in which such co-contractions are expected and a possible explanation of why they are continent.

To date, there are no RCTs comparing the effect of indirect training of the PFMs via the TrA on SUI with either untreated controls, conscious precontraction of the PFMs or PFM strength training. However, Dumoulin et al. (2004) compared PFMT with PFMT and TrA training and did not find any further benefit of adding TrA training to the protocol. In a systematic review, Bø and Herbert (2013) analysed the effect of alternative exercise regimens for the PFMs and found three RCTs for abdominal training with no additional effect of abdominal training for SUI. A new search in October 2020 revealed one new RCT. Ptak et al (2019) randomized women aged 45 to 60 years with SUI to either PFMT + TrA training or PFMT alone and found that women in the combined group had significantly better quality of life compared with the PFMT-only group. There was no information of control for the ability to contract the PFMs or any details on whether the program contained home training or visits with a PT, and adherence was not reported. There was no report of the effect of the program on

SUI variables. Hence there is still no evidence for the effect of combining PFMT with TrA training or for TrA training alone on SUI.

Evidence for Theory 4

In some physical therapy practices the PFMT protocol seems to include only teaching the patients to co-contract the PFMs with low load during all daily activities and movements (Carriere, 2002). No specific strength training protocol or follow-up training is undertaken. This can be considered using the same theory as use of conscious precontraction, or the Knack. However, unlike the use of a conscious contraction, the idea is that by learning to contract, over time this may become an automatic function and by itself be enough to prevent SUI. Therefore, in 'functional training' the conscious contraction is further developed to be performed in all daily activities where leakage may occur. This means that the woman is asked to contract while lifting, doing housework, playing tennis and so forth.

Because it is possible to learn to hold a hand over the mouth before and during coughing, it is perhaps possible to learn to precontract the PFMs before and during simple and single tasks such as coughing, lifting and performing abdominal exercises. However, multiple task activities and repetitive movements such as running, playing tennis, or participating in dance and aerobic activities most likely cannot be conducted with intentional co-contractions of the PFMs. The preceding study of Miller et al. (2018) found that such a program was effective compared to general diet and exercise advice.

METHODS

Only outcomes from RCTs and systematic reviews are included. Computerized search on PubMed, studies, data and conclusions from the Sixth International Consultation on Incontinence (ICI) (Dumoulin et al., 2017), as well as the Cochrane Library and other systematic reviews (Dumoulin et al., 2018; Hay-Smith et al., 2011; Herbison and Dean, 2013; Herderschee et al., 2011; Imamura et al., 2010), have been used as background sources. Physical therapy techniques to treat SUI include PFMT with or without biofeedback, electrical stimulation and use of vaginal cones (Bø et al., 2017). Because SUI and UUI are different conditions that may need different treatment approaches, only studies including female SUI are presented here. Methodological quality of RCTs reporting cure rates assessing the condition with pad tests are judged by use of the PEDro rating scale (Herbert and Gabriel, 2002).

Evidence for Pelvic Floor Muscle Training

Updated and comprehensive systematic reviews on PFMT in the treatment of SUI with detailed tables can be found in the Cochrane Library, the ICI book and the NICE guidelines (Dumoulin et al., 2017, Dumoulin et al., 2018, NICE, 2019), so we will not repeat the same detailed tables of each RCT here. We refer to the same studies and newer studies found in our updated search in the text and urge the reader to stay updated with new studies through the Cochrane Library and the PEDro database.

It is difficult to make meaningful comparisons between studies and groups of studies in this area because of heterogeneity between studies in inclusion criteria of the studies (several studies include women with SUI and urgency and mixed incontinence), different outcome measures and different exercise regimens with a huge variety of training dosage. In addition, many researchers have used combined interventions (e.g., electrical stimulation and strength training, bladder training and strength training).

In this textbook, in addition to looking at methodological quality (internal validity) we also try to address the interventional quality of the studies. A thorough discussion of the quality of the intervention is necessary to elaborate a correct cause–effect relationship found or not found in RCTs of PFMT (Herbert and Bø, 2005).

One important flaw in PFMT studies is not controlling for lack of ability to contract the PFMs. Several research groups have shown that more than 30% of women are unable to voluntarily contract the PFMs at their first consultation even after thorough individual instruction (Benvenuti et al., 1987; Bø et al., 1988; Bump et al. 1991; Kegel, 1952). Common mistakes are to contract other muscles such as abdominals, gluteals and hip adductor muscles instead of the PFMs (Bø et al., 1988; Bø et al., 1990b; Neels et al., 2018). In addition, Bump et al. (1991) showed that as many as 25% of women may strain instead of squeeze and lift. If women are straining instead of performing a correct contraction, the training may harm and not improve PFM function. Proper assessment of ability to contract the PFMs is therefore mandatory (Fig. 7.1.1).

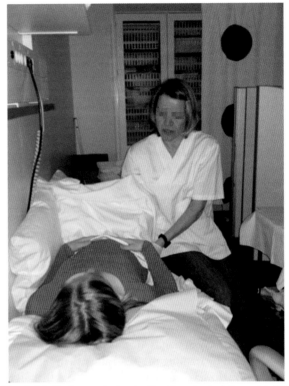

Fig. 7.1.1 During vaginal palpation the physical therapist (PT) instructs the patient about how to perform a contraction correctly ('Squeeze around my finger and try to lift the finger inwards') and tells her how well she is able to do it and also about coordination skills and strength. With encouragement, most patients are able to contract harder.

The numerous reports by Kegel, with a greater than 80% cure rate, comprised uncontrolled studies with the inclusion of a variety of incontinence types and no measurement of urinary leakage before and after treatment. However, since then, several RCTs have demonstrated that PFM exercise is more effective than no treatment to treat SUI (Dumoulin et al., 2018). In addition, several RCTs have compared PFMT alone with either the use of vaginal resistance devices, biofeedback or vaginal cones (Dumoulin et al., 2017; Hay-Smith et al., 2011; Herbison and Dean, 2013; Herderschee et al., 2011). Today there is level 1 evidence (recommendation A) that PFMT should be first-line treatment for UI in females (Dumoulin et al., 2017; Dumoulin et al., 2018; NICE, 2019). In the general population, women with SUI who do PFMT are eight times (95% CI: 4–19, 56% vs 6%) more likely to be cured than control groups with no or sham treatments (Dumoulin et al., 2018). PFMT reduced UI episodes among women with SUI (MD: 1.2 episodes per day, 95% CI: 0.7–1.8) and among women with any type of UI (MD: 1 episode per day, 95% CI: 0.6–1.4) (Dumoulin et al., 2018). On short pad tests, PFMT reduced the amount of urine lost by women with SUI (MD: 10 g, 95% CI: 1–19) and by women with any type of UI (MD: 4 g, 95% CI: 2–5) (Dumoulin et al., 2018). PFMT also caused women with any type of UI to report significantly better incontinence-related quality of life and reduced UI symptoms than those who did not receive the treatment. Because of substantial heterogeneity among the outcome measures used to assess quality of life, a meta-analysis of this variable was not conducted. PFMT has rare and minor adverse effects (Dumoulin et al., 2017; Dumoulin et al., 2018; Dumoulin et al., 2020).

The effects of PFMT are better if it is delivered with regular supervised training (e.g., once a week) (Dumoulin et al., 2017; Dumoulin et al., 2018; Hay-Smith et al., 2011). Supervised training is defined as a PFMT program taught and monitored by a health professional/clinician/instructor (Bø et al., 2017). This means that the PT teaches each PFM contraction either individually or in a group setting. Thus, if the PT only provides teaching and assessment at the first consultation, this would not be considered supervised training (Bø et al., 2017).

Combined Improvement and Cure Rates

As for surgery and pharmacology studies, a combination of cure and improvement measures is often reported. To date, there is no consensus on what outcome measure to choose as the gold standard for cure (urodynamic findings of SUI, number of leakage episodes, ≤2 g of leakage on pad test [tests with standardized bladder volume, 1-, 24- and 48 hour], women's report, etc.) (Hilton and Robinson, 2011). Subjective cure and improvement rates of PFMT reported in RCTs in studies including groups with SUI and mixed incontinence vary between 56% and 70% (Dumoulin et al., 2017).

Cure Rates

It is often reported that PFMT is more commonly associated with improvement of symptoms rather than a total cure. However, short-term cure rates of 20% to 75%, defined as 2 g or less of leakage on different pad tests, have been found after PFMT (Aksac et al., 2003; Bø et al., 1999; Castro et al., 2008; Dumoulin et al. 2004; Glavind et al., 1996; Henalla et al., 1989; Henalla et al.,

1990; Mørkved et al., 2002; Wong et al., 1997; Zanetti et al., 2007). Table 7.1.5 describes these studies, and Table 7.1.6 gives the methodological quality of the same studies. The highest cure rates were shown in two single-blind RCTs of high methodological quality. The participants had thorough individual instruction by a trained PT, combined training with biofeedback or electrical stimulation, and close follow-up once or every second week. Adherence was high, and drop-out was low (Dumoulin et al., 2004; Mørkved et al., 2002). Because biofeedback and electrical stimulation have not shown any additional effect on PFMT in RCTs and systematic reviews (biofeedback RCTs being flawed because of the difference in training dosage in favour of the biofeedback intervention) (Dumoulin et al. 2017; Herderschee et al., 2011), the conclusion is that the key factors for success are most likely close follow-up and more intensive training (Dumoulin et al., 2017; Dumoulin et al., 2018; Herderschee et al., 2011).

Quality of the Intervention: Dose–Response Issues

Because of use of different outcome measures and instruments to measure PFM function and strength, it is impossible to combine results between studies, and it is difficult to conclude which training regimen is more effective. In addition, the exercise dosage (type of exercise, frequency, duration and intensity) varies significantly between studies (Dumoulin et al., 2017). Looking into the studies on SUI patients included in the Cochrane systematic review, duration of the intervention varies between 6 weeks and 6 months, intensity (measured as holding time) varies between 3 and 40 seconds, and the number of repetitions per day between 36 and more than 200. Frequency of training is every day in all RCTs (Dumoulin et al., 2017).

Bø et al. (1990b) have shown that instructor followed-up training is significantly more effective than home exercise. In this study, individual assessment and teaching of correct contraction was combined with strength training in groups in a 6-month training program. The women were randomized to either an intensive training program consisting of seven individual sessions with a PT, combined with 45 minutes of weekly PFMT classes, and three sets of 8 to 12 contractions per day at home or the same program except for the weekly intensive exercise classes. The results showed a much better improvement in both muscle strength and

TABLE 7.1.5   Cure Rates Reported as Less Than 2 g of Leakage Measured With a Variety of Pad Tests in Randomized Controlled Trials of Pelvic Floor Muscle Training to Treat Stress Urinary Incontinence

Author	**Henalla et al. (1989)**
Design	Randomized to PFMT, interference therapy, oestrogen, or control
Sample size and age (years)	104 women; mean age with variance not reported
Diagnosis	Urodynamic stress incontinence
Training protocol	PFMT: vaginal palpation, contract PFMs 5×/h, hold 5 s; 10 sessions once a week with PT
	Interference: 10 sessions with PT, 0–100 Hz, 20 min
	Oestrogen: Premarin vaginal cream each night for 12 weeks (1.25 mg)
	Control: no treatment
Drop-out	4/104: not reported from which groups
Adherence	Not reported
Results	65% cured or >50% reduction
Author	**Henalla et al. (1990)**
Design	Randomized to PFMT, oestrogen, or control
Sample size and age (years)	26 postmenopausal women, mean age 54 (49–64)
Diagnosis	SUI on history
Training protocol	6-week intervention
	PFMT: protocol not explained
	Oestrogen: Premarin vaginal cream 2 g/night
Drop-out	Not reported
Adherence	Not reported
Results	PFMT: 50% cured or >50% reduction; oestrogen: 0; control: 0
Author	**Glavind et al. (1996)**
Design	Randomized to PFMT with PT or PFMT with BF
Sample size and age (years)	40 women age 40–48; mean age 45
Diagnosis	Urodynamic SUI
Training protocol	4-week intervention; vaginal palpation; both groups asked to perform PFMT at home at least 3×/day
	PFMT + PT: individual treatment with PT 3–4×/day
	PFMT + BF: individual treatment as above + 4 times with BF
Drop-out	PFMT + PT: 25%; PFMT + BF: 5%
Adherence	Not reported
Results	PFMT + PT: 20% cured; PFMT + BF: 58% cured
Author	**Wong et al. (1997)**
Design	Randomized to clinic-based PFMT or home-based PFMT
Sample size and age (years)	47 women, mean age 48.8 (SD: 9.4)
Diagnosis	Urodynamic SUI

TABLE 7.1.5   Cure Rates Reported as Less Than 2 g of Leakage Measured With a Variety of Pad Tests in Randomized Controlled Trials of Pelvic Floor Muscle Training to Treat Stress Urinary Incontinence—cont'd

Training protocol	4-week training period
	Clinic: 8 sessions + daily PFMT
	Home: daily PFMT at home
Drop-out	Not reported
Adherence	Not reported
Results	No difference between groups; 55% cured
Author	**Bø et al. (1999)**
Design	Randomized to PFMT, ES, cones, or control
Sample size and age (years)	107 women age 24–70; mean age 49.5
Diagnosis	Urodynamic SUI
Training protocol	6-month intervention; vaginal palpation
	PFMT: 3× 8–12 contractions/day at home; training diary; weekly 45-min exercise class; individual assessment of muscle strength and motivation for further training once a month
Drop-out	8%
Adherence	93%
Results	PFMT: 44% cured; control: 6.7% cured
Author	**Mørkved et al. (2002)**
Design	Randomized to PFMT or PFMT with BF
Sample size and age (years)	103 women age 30–70; mean age 46.6
Diagnosis	Urodynamic SUI
Training protocol	6-month intervention after vaginal palpation
	Both groups: same amount of exercise and meeting with PT once a week for the first 2 months, then once every second week; 3 sets of 10 contractions holding 6 s, add 3–4 fast contractions on top at each visit
	Home training: 3 sets of 10 contractions/day
	BF: same program with BF
Drop-out	8.7%
Adherence	PFMT: 85.3%; PFMT + BF: 88.9%
Results	PFMT: 69% cured; PFMT + BF: 67% cured
Author	**Aksac et al. (2003)**
Design	Randomized to PFMT, PFMT with BF, or control group on oestrogen
Sample size and age (years)	50 women, 20 in each training group and 10 in control group; mean age 52.9 (SD: 7.1)
Diagnosis	Urodynamic diagnosis of SUI
Training protocol	8 weeks
	PFMT: vaginal palpation, 10 contractions 3×/day, hold for 5 s, progressing to 10 after 2 weeks; weekly clinic sessions + 'regular' home training
	BF: weekly clinic sessions, use BF at home 3 ×/week, 20 min with 10-s hold and 20-s rest

Continued

TABLE 7.1.5   Cure Rates Reported as Less Than 2 g of Leakage Measured With a Variety of Pad Tests in Randomized Controlled Trials of Pelvic Floor Muscle Training to Treat Stress Urinary Incontinence—cont'd

Drop-out	None
Adherence	Not reported
Results	PFMT: 75% cure, 25% improvement; BF: 80% cured, 20% improvement; control: 0% cured, 20% improvement
Author	**Dumoulin et al. (2004)**
Design	Randomized to multimodal PFMT, multimodal PFMT + abdominal training, or control
Sample size and age (years)	64 women age 23.3–39; mean age 36.2
Diagnosis	Urodynamic SUI
Training protocol	8 weeks PFMT: supervised sessions once a week with PT, 15 min of ES, 25 min of PFMT, home exercise 5 days/week Same PFMT + 30 min of deep abdominal training Control: back and extremities massage
Drop-out	3.1%
Adherence	Not reported
Results	PFMT: 70% cured; PFMT + abdominals: 70% cured; control: 0% cured
Author	**Zanetti et al. (2007)**
Design	Parallel group RCT
Sample size	44 women with SUI
Diagnosis	Urodynamic assessment
Training protocol	12 weeks of individual 45-min PFMT twice a week including strength training and 'the Knack' with PT (n = 23) compared to unsupervised PFMT (n = 21) at home; both groups had monthly assessment (vaginal palpation) by PT
Drop-out	0
Adherence	Not reported
Results	11 (48%) in supervised PFMT vs 2 (9.8%) cured in control vs 11 (48%) in supervised PFMT
Author	**Castro et al. (2008)**
Design	4-group parallel group RCT using PFMT, ES, vaginal cones, or untreated control
Sample size	118 (PFMT 31, ES 30, vaginal cones 27, control 30)
Diagnosis	Urodynamic SUI
Training protocol	6 months of 45-min weekly group training after vaginal palpation of ability to contract
Drop-out	17.8%
Adherence	PFMT: 92%; ES: 91%; vaginal cones: 93%
Results	Negative pad test: PFMT 12 (46%); ES 13 (48%); vaginal cones 11 (46%); control 2 (8%)

BF, Biofeedback; *ES*, electrical stimulation; *PFM*, pelvic floor muscle; *PFMT*, pelvic floor muscle training; *PT*, physical therapist; *RCT*, randomized controlled trial; *SUI*, stress urinary incontinence.

TABLE 7.1.6   PEDro Quality Score of Randomized Controlled Trials in Systematic Review of Pelvic Floor Muscle Training to Treat Stress Urinary Incontinence

E – Eligibility criteria specified

1 – Subjects randomly allocated to groups

2 – Allocation concealed

3 – Groups similar at baseline

4 – Subjects blinded

5 – Therapist administering treatment blinded

6 – Assessors blinded

7 – Measures of key outcomes obtained from >85% of subjects

8 – Data analysed by intention to treat

9 – Statistical comparison between groups conducted

10 – Point measures and measures of variability provided

Study	E	1	2	3	4	5	6	7	8	9	10	Total Score
Henalla et al. (1989)	+	+	–	?	–	–	–	+	–	?	+	3
Henalla et al. (1990)	+	+	?	?	–	–	–	+	?	–	–	2
Glavind et al. (1996)	+	+	+	+	–	–	–	+	–	+	+	6
Wong et al. (1997)	–	+	?	+	–	–	–	?	?	–	–	2
Bø et al. (1999)	+	+	+	+	–	–	+	+	+	+	+	8
Mørkved et al. (2002)	+	+	+	+	–	–	+	+	+	+	+	8
Aksac et al. (2003)	+	+	+	+	–	–	–	+	+	+	+	7
Dumoulin et al. (2004)	+	+	?	+	–	+	+	+	+	+	+	8
Zanetti et al. (2007)	+	+	+	+	–	–	–	+	+	+	+	7
Castro et al. (2008)	+	+	–	+	–	–	+	+	–	+	+	6

+, Criterion is clearly satisfied; –, criterion is not satisfied; ?, not clear if the criterion was satisfied.
The total score is determined by counting the number of criteria that are satisfied, except the 'eligibility criteria specified' score is not used to generate the total score. Total scores are out of 10.

urinary leakage in the intensive exercise group: 60% were reported to be continent/almost continent in the intensive exercise group compared to 17% in the less intensive group. A significant reduction of urinary leakage, measured by a pad test with standardized bladder volume, was only demonstrated in the intensive exercise group (Fig. 7.1.2).

This study demonstrated that a huge difference in outcome can be expected according to the intensity and follow-up of the training program and very little effect can be expected after training without close follow-up. It is worth noting that the significantly less effective group in this study had seven visits with a skilled PT and that adherence to the home training program was high. Nevertheless, the effect was only 17%. That more intensive training (follow-up and training dosage) is more effective is now the conclusion of several systematic reviews (Dumoulin et al.,

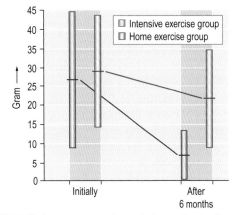

Fig. 7.1.2 Pad-test results showed that only the 'intensive' pelvic floor muscle training group had a statistically significant reduction in urinary leakage. (*From Bø, Hagen et al., 1990, with permission.*)

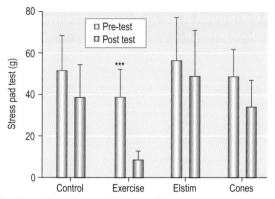

Fig. 7.1.3 The Norwegian Pelvic Floor Study demonstrated huge and statistically significant improvement pad-test results only for the training group. Elstim, electrical stimulation. (*From Bø et al., 1999, with permission.*)

2017; Dumoulin et al., 2018; Imamura et al., 2010; NICE, 2019). There is a dose–response issue in all sorts of training regimens. Therefore one reason for disappointing effects shown in some clinical practices or research studies may be due to insufficient training stimulus and low dosage. If low-dosage programs are chosen as one arm in a RCT comparing PFMT with other methods, PFMT is bound to be less effective (Herbert and Bø, 2005).

Pelvic Floor Muscle Training With Biofeedback

Biofeedback has been defined as 'a group of experimental procedures where an external sensor is used to give an indication on bodily processes, usually in the purpose of changing the measured quality' (Schwartz and Beatty, 1977). Biofeedback equipment has been developed within the area of psychology, mainly to measure sweating, heart rate and blood pressure during different forms of stress. Kegel (1948) always based his training protocol on thorough instruction of correct contraction using vaginal palpation and clinical observation. He combined PFMT with use of vaginal squeeze pressure measurement as biofeedback during exercise. Today, a variety of biofeedback apparatus is commonly used in clinical practice to assist with PFMT.

Unfortunately, the term *biofeedback* is often used to classify a method different from PFMT. However, biofeedback is not a treatment on its own. It is an adjunct to training, measuring the response from a single PFM contraction. In the area of PFMT, both vaginal and anal surface EMG, and urethral and vaginal squeeze pressure measurements, have been used to make patients more aware of muscle function, and to enhance and motivate patients' efforts during training (Herderschee et al., 2011). It is important to be aware that erroneous attempts at PFM contractions (e.g., by straining) may be registered by manometers and dynamometers, and contractions of muscles other than the PFMs may affect surface EMG activity. Therefore no biofeedback methods other than imaging methods such as ultrasound and magnetic resonance imaging that actually show the constriction and lift of the PFMs can be used to register a correct contraction.

Since Kegel first presented his results, several RCTs have shown that PFMT without biofeedback is more effective than no treatment for SUI (Dumoulin et al., 2017; Dumoulin et al., 2018; NICE, 2019). In a Cochrane review, Herderschee et al. (2011) found 24 RCTs or quasi-randomized trials comparing PFMT with and without biofeedback. They concluded that use of biofeedback *may* provide benefit in addition to PFMT.

None of the RCTs comparing PFMT with and without biofeedback have used the exact same training dosage in the two groups (Herderschee et al., 2011). For example, Pages et al. (2001) compared 60 minutes of group training 5 days a week with 15 minutes of individual biofeedback training 5 days a week, finding that the individualized biofeedback training protocol was more effectively assessed by the women's report and measurement of PFM strength. When the two groups under comparison receive different dosage of training in addition to biofeedback, it is impossible to conclude what is causing a possible effect. In addition, other factors flaw the results of studies comparing PFMT with and without biofeedback. Considering that PFMT is effective without biofeedback, a large sample size may be needed to show any beneficial effect of adding biofeedback to an effective training protocol. In most published studies comparing PFMT with PFMT combined with biofeedback, the sample sizes are small, and type II error may have been the reason for negative findings (Herderschee et al., 2011). In a recent study, Hagen et al. (2019) randomized 600 women with SUI and MUI to the same training dosage and attention of either PFMT with or without use of biofeedback (16 weeks of six individual visits + home training). They reported results after 6 months, 1 year and 2 years). No difference between groups were found in the International Consultation on Incontinence Questionnaire–Urinary Incontinence

Short Form (ICIQ-UI SF), participants' reported improvement or Oxford grading of PFM strength. A similar percentage had received surgery (12.3% biofeedback, 9.3% PFMT), and an adherence of about 50% to PFMT at 2-year follow-up was reported for both groups. The researchers concluded that use of biofeedback was therefore not cost effective.

Many women may not like to undress, go to a private room and insert a vaginal or rectal device to exercise (Prashar et al., 2000). However, some women find it motivating to use biofeedback to control and enhance the strength of the contractions when training. Any factor that may stimulate high adherence and intensive training should be recommended to enhance the effect of a training program. Therefore, when available, biofeedback should be given as an option for home training, and the PT should use any sensitive, reliable and valid tool to measure the contraction force at office follow-up.

Pelvic Floor Muscle Training With Vaginal Weighted Cones

Vaginal cones are weights that are put into the vagina above the levator plate (Herbison and Dean, 2013). The theory behind their use in strength training is that the PFMs are contracted reflexively or voluntarily when the cone is perceived to slip out. The weight of the cone is supposed to give a training stimulus and make women contract harder with progressive weight. In a Cochrane review, combining studies including 23 RCTs or quasi-randomized studies with 1806 women with both SUI and MUI (six trials published as abstracts only), it was concluded that training with vaginal cones is more effective than no treatment and can be offered as treatment option for women who find it acceptable (Cammu and van Nylen, 1998; Herbison and Dean, 2013). Cammu and van Nylen (1998) reported very low compliance and therefore did not recommend use of cones. In addition, in the study of Bø et al. (1999), women in the cone group had great motivational problems. Laycock et al. (2001) had a total drop-out rate in their study of 33%.

The use of cones can be questioned from an exercise science perspective. Holding the cone for the recommended time of 15 to 20 minutes may result in decreased blood supply, decreased oxygen consumption, muscle fatigue and pain, and recruit contraction of other muscles instead of the PFMs. In addition,

many women report that they dislike using cones (Bø et al., 1999; Cammu and van Nylen, 1998). However, the cones may add benefit to the training protocol if used in a different way: the subjects can be asked to contract around the cone and simultaneously try to pull it out in a lying or standing position, repeating this 8 to 12 times in three series per day, or they can use the cones during progressively graded activities of daily living. In this way, general strength training principles are followed, and progression can be added to the training protocol. Arvonen et al. (2001) used 'vaginal balls' and followed general strength training principles. They found that training with the balls was significantly more effective in reducing urinary leakage than regular PFMT.

Long-Term Effect of Pelvic Floor Muscle Training

Several studies have reported the long-term effect of PFMT (Bø and Hilde., 2013; Dumoulin et al., 2017; Dumoulin et al., 2018). However, usually women in the non-treatment or less effective intervention groups have gone on to receive treatment after cessation of the study period. Therefore, follow-up data are usually reported either for all women or for only the group with the best effect. As for surgery, there are only a few long-term studies including clinical examination (Bø and Herbert, 2013; Bø and Hilde, 2013). As for any exercise intervention, it is expected that the benefits gained from PFMT need maintenance training for continuing effects (Garber et al., 2011; Herbert et al., 2018). A systematic review on the long-term effects of PFMT included 19 studies with follow-up periods of 1 to 15 years; long-term adherence to PFMT varied between 10% and 70% (Bø and Hilde, 2013). Among participants who were treated with PFMT and whose UI resolved initially, five studies reported sustained success rates (i.e., percentage remaining free of UI at long-term follow-up) which were between 41% and 85%. Surgery rates in the long term varied between 5% and 58%. It was concluded that the short-term benefit of PFMT can be maintained at long-term follow-up without incentives for continued training, although there was high heterogeneity in both interventional and methodological quality in short- and long-term PFMT studies.

The general recommendations for maintaining muscle strength are one session per week of moderate-to-hard intensity exercises (Garber et al., 2011). The intensity of the contraction seems to be more important than frequency of training. So far, no studies have evaluated how many contractions patients must perform to maintain PFM strength after cessation of organized training. In a study by Bø and Talseth (1996), PFM strength was maintained 5 years after cessation of organized training with 70% exercising more than once a week. However, the number and intensity of exercises varied considerably between successful women (Bø, 1995). One series of 8 to 12 contractions could easily be instructed in aerobic dance classes or recommended as part of women's general strength training programs. However, we do not know how a voluntary precontraction before an increase in abdominal pressure will maintain or increase muscle strength. In the study of Cammu et al. (2000) the long-term effect of PFMT appeared to be attributed to the precontraction before sudden increases in intra-abdominal pressure and not so much to regular strength training. Muscle strength was not measured in their study. Although not taught in the original program, several women in the study of Bø et al. (2005) also had performed a voluntary contraction of the PFMs before and during a rise in intra-abdominal pressure (the Knack) during the long-term follow-up period.

Other Programs

Today, there is a lot of interest in PFMT in combination with so-called core training (stabilizing training for the lower spine including TrA and multifidus muscles). Yoga, Pilates, Feldenkrais and Mensendick classes are examples of exercise programs that may or may not include training of the PFMs. All of these programs except yoga (which is much longer established) were developed in the 1920s and 1930s, and as far as this author has ascertained, none originally included PFMT.

We refer to the systematic review of Bø and Herbert (2013) for an overview and discussion of the evidence for alternative methods to treat SUI, and to the article on when and how new therapies should become clinical practice from the same authors (Bø and Herbert, 2009). In the 2103 review, three RCTs on abdominal training, two RCTs for Pilates and two RCTs for the Paula method were found. Many of the studies were biased due to more attention and higher training dosage favouring the alternative methods. None of the alternative exercises proved to be better than or yielded additional

effect to PFMT. A new search on PubMed in September 2020 found one RCT on yoga but no RCTs on Tai Chi, the Paula method, balance training or respiratory exercise. The RCT on yoga compared twice weekly group yoga training with twice weekly group stretching exercises (Huang et al., 2019). Fifty-six women with a mean age of 65.4 (±8.1) years were randomized (28 to yoga, 28 to control). The mean baseline incontinence frequency was 3.5 (±2) episodes a day, and 37 women (66%) had urgency-predominant incontinence. A total of 50 women completed their assigned 3-month intervention program (89%), including 27 in the yoga and 23 in the control group (p = 0.19). Of those, 24 (89%) in the yoga and 20 (87%) in the control group attended at least 80% of group classes. Over 3 months, total incontinence frequency decreased by an average of 76% from baseline in the yoga and 56% in the control group (p = 0.07 for between-group difference). SUI frequency also decreased by an average of 61% in the yoga group and 35% in controls (p = 0.045 for between-group difference), but changes in UUI frequency did not differ significantly between groups. The yoga exercises included focus on the PFMs, whereas this was not the case for the stretching classes.

Luginbuehl et al. (2019) hypothesized that general physical activity, specifically running and jumping, would improve SUI and conducted an RCT including 96 women. The participants were randomized to PFMT or PFMT + running and jumping activities. No difference between groups were found between groups in SUI outcomes, EMG activity or quality of life.

HYPOPRESSIVE EXERCISE

Jose-Vaz et al. (2020) randomized 90 women with SUI to either 12 weeks of PFMT or hypopressive exercise. PFMT was superior to hypopressive exercise in UI leakage episodes in 7 days, with a mean difference of −1.27 (95% CI: −1.92 to −0.62), effect size 0.94 and total score of the International Consultation on Incontinence Questionnaire–Short Form (ICIQ-SF), with a mean difference between groups of −4.7 (95% CI: −6.90 to −2.50) and effect size 1.04 in favour of PFMT. PFM strength showed a mean difference between groups of 11 cm H_2O (95% CI: 6.33–15.67) and effect size 1.15 also in favour of PFMT.

In untrained individuals, all stimulus for regular training have the potential for improving function, and a focus on and incorporation of PFMT in any fitness program for women should therefore be welcomed. However, all studies that have shown effect include training of the PFMs. Hence it is not the training concepts as such (e.g., yoga or Pilates) that make the difference but the actual PFMT. One should be aware, however, that many women may not be able to perform correct contractions without proper individual instruction. Lack of effect of such general programs may therefore also be due to incorrect contractions. The effect of group training versus individual training of the PFMs has been elaborated on by Bø (2020), and in this chapter we will briefly summarize the findings.

Group Training

The first group training protocol in physical therapy for PFMT was developed by Bø et al. (1990a). In a systematic review comparing the effect of individual and group PFMT, 10 studies involving group training were included (Paiva et al., 2017). Five of six RCTs comparing group PFMT with individual PFMT were included in a meta-analysis. The authors found significant risk of bias in many of the studies: random sequence generation, allocation concealment and blinding of outcome assessment. The conclusion was that there was no significant difference in results between individual and group-based PFMT. There was a huge heterogeneity in outcome measures and exercise protocols between studies, but a more serious bias was the difference in supervision and content of the intervention between the individual and group training protocols within the same study.

In a well-designed, adequately powered, non-inferiority, multicenter randomized trial involving women with SUI and MUI, individual PFMT was compared to group training (Dumoulin et al., 2020). Both treatment arms contained the same dosage of training and the same contact and attention from the physiotherapist. Furthermore, both groups received the same individual information and underwent assessment and feedback of their ability to contract the PFMs before commencing the training period. At 1-year follow-up, the median reduction in the frequency of leakage episodes per week was similar: 70% (95% CI: 44–89) in the individual group and 74% (95% CI: 46–86) in the group training group. Furthermore, there were no important differences between the groups in any other outcome measures, and the researchers concluded that group PFMT is not inferior to individual training in the treatment of female UI.

Most group training regimens of PFMT include individual teaching of a correct contraction and assessment and feedback of ability to contract (Bø, 2020; Paiva et al., 2017). However, in a few studies, group training has been done without such confirmation of the participants' skills. Nevertheless, all of these studies found significant improvement in UI after the intervention and no difference between individual or group training. In a primary prevention study, 169 women in their first pregnancies were randomized to either an exercise group including PFMT three times a week or a control group without any intervention (Pelaez et al., 2014). The participants had no evaluation of their ability to perform a correct contraction. The results showed significant differences in incidence, frequency and amount of UI in favour of the exercise group, accompanied by a benefit on an incontinence-related quality of life score with an effect size of 0.8. The results were presented as per-protocol analyses only, but it shows that it is possible to do effective PFMT without individual teaching and control of ability to perform a correct contraction in a group of women with no symptoms and injuries to the PFMs. However, we do not know whether the effect would have been even higher with additional individual teaching and control of the women's ability to perform a correct contraction.

Motivation and Adherence

Several researchers have looked into factors affecting the outcome of PFMT on UI (Dumoulin et al., 2017). No single factor has been shown to predict outcome, and it has been concluded that many factors traditionally supposed to affect outcomes such as age and severity of incontinence may be less crucial than previously thought. Factors that appear to be most associated with a positive outcome are thorough teaching of correct contraction, motivation, adherence with the intervention and intensity of the program.

Some women may find the exercises hard to conduct on a regular basis (Alewijnse, 2002). However, when analysing results of RCTs, adherence to the exercise program is generally high and drop-out rate is low (Dumoulin et al., 2017). In a few studies, low adherence and high drop-out rates have been reported (Laycock et al., 2001; Ramsey and Thou, 1990). Knowledge about behavioural sciences such as pedagogy and health psychology, and

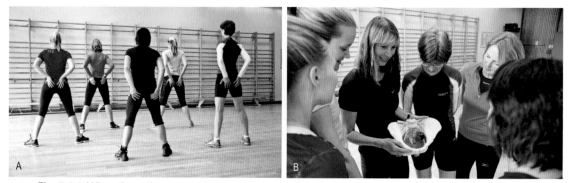

Fig. 7.1.4 When the patients are able to contract the pelvic floor muscles correctly it can be fun and motivating to conduct the strength training in a class. Group training classes for pelvic floor muscle training were developed by Bø in 1986 and the results of the first randomized controlled trial using group training for stress urinary incontinence were presented in the journal *Neurourology and Urodynamics* in 1990.

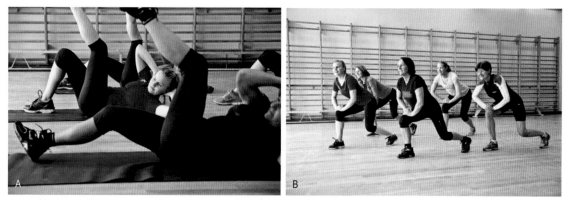

Fig. 7.1.5 In between the pelvic floor muscle strength training other exercises are performed to music. The original class emphasizes strength training of the abdominal (including transversus abdominis), back and thigh muscles in addition to body awareness and relaxation (breathing and stretching) exercises. The class is 60 minutes with 45 minutes of exercising and 15 minutes for information, conversation and motivation for home training.

the ability to explain and motivate patients, may be a crucial factor to enhance adherence and minimize drop-outs from training. In some studies, such strategies have been followed, and high adherence has been achieved (Alewijnse, 2002; Chiarelli and Cockburn, 2002). In other studies, specific strategies have not been reported, but emphasis has been put on creating a positive, enjoyable and supportive training environment. Group training after thorough individual instruction may be a good concept if led by a skilled and motivating person (Bø et al., 1990a; Bø et al., 1999) (Figs. 7.1.4 and 7.1.5).

PFMT concepts with no drop-outs (Berghmans et al., 1996) and adherence of greater than 90% (Bø et al., 1999) are possible. In a study of Alewijnse (2002), most women followed advice to train 4 to 6 times a week 1 year after cessation of the training program. The following factors predicted 50% adherence:
• positive intention to adhere,
• high short-term adherence levels,
• positive self-efficacy expectations, and
• frequent weekly episodes of leakage before and after initial therapy.

Patients do not comply with treatment for a wide variety of reasons: long-lasting and time-consuming treatments, requirement of lifestyle changes, poor client–patient interaction, cultural and health beliefs, poor social support, inconvenience, lack of time, motivational problems, and travel time to clinics have been listed (Paddison, 2002).

Sugaya et al. (2003) used a computerized pocket-size device giving a sound three times a day to remind the person to perform PFMT. To stop the sound the person needed to push a button, and by pushing the button for each contraction, adherence was registered: 46 women were randomly assigned to either instruction to contract the PFMs following a pamphlet or with the same pamphlet together with the sound device and instruction on how to use the device. The results showed a significant improvement in daily incontinence episodes and pad test only in the device group: 48% were satisfied in the device group compared to 15% in the control group. It was reported that patients in the device group felt obliged to perform PFMT when the chime sounded. Recently, apps have been developed to assist with PFMT. It is a strong belief that apps may solve the adherence problem for PFMT. However, the published articles show that many buy apps and do not use them, and adherence is not higher in apps compared to other regimens for PFMT (Nagib et al., 2020).

CONCLUSION

There is level 1 evidence (recommendation A) that PFMT is more effective than no treatment, sham or placebo treatment for SUI. PFMT is recommended as first-line treatment for SUI. There is no evidence to suggest that adding use of biofeedback, electrical stimulation or vaginal cones brings any additional effect over PFMT alone. Group training following individual instruction is not inferior to individual PFMT.

CLINICAL RECOMMENDATIONS

- Teach the patient about the PFMs and lower urinary tract function using diagrams, drawings and models.
- Explain a correct PFM contraction. Allow the patient to practice before checking the ability to contract.
- Assess PFM contraction.
- If the woman can contract, set up an individual training program to be conducted at home. Aim for close

to maximum PFM contractions, building up to three sets of 8 to 12 contractions per day. Ask the patient to suggest where and when exercises should be performed. Supply the patient with an exercise diary, apps or biofeedback with computerized adherence registration if the patient is motivated to use technology. If available, discuss whether the use of biofeedback motivates the patient to exercise.

- If the woman is unable to contract, try manual techniques such as touch, tapping, massage and fast stretch or electrical stimulation. Be aware that most patients learn to contract if they are given some time by themselves at home to practice.
- Follow up with weekly or more often supervised training. Supervised training can be conducted individually or in groups.
- Follow development in PFM function and strength closely, using responsive, reliable and valid assessment tools.
- In addition to a strength training regimen, ask the patient to precontract and hold the contraction before and during coughing, laughing, sneezing and lifting (conscious precontraction, the Knack).
- Suggested assessment of urinary leakage and quality of life before and after treatment:
  - ICIQ-SF (Avery et al., 2004),
  - 3-day leakage episodes (Lose et al., 1998),
  - leakage index (Bø, 1994),
  - pad test (48-, 24- and 1-hour short tests with standardized bladder volume) (Lose et al., 1998), and
  - general and disease-specific quality-of-life questionnaires (Short Form 37 Health Survey Questionnaire [SF-37], ICIQ-UI SF, King's College, B-FLUTS) (Corcos et al., 2002).
- For additional recommendations, refer to the ICI (Diaz et al., 2017).

REFERENCES

Aksac, B., Semih, A., Karan, A., et al. (2003). Biofeedback and pelvic floor exercises for the rehabilitation of urinary stress incontinence. *Gynecologic and Obstetric Investigation*, 56, 23–27.

Alewijnse, D. (2002). *Urinary incontinence in women. Long term outcome of pelvic floor muscle exercise therapy. Doctoral thesis*. Department of Health Education and Health Promotion, Maastricht Health Research Institute for Prevention and Care.

Arvonen, T., Fianu-Jonasson, A., & Tyni-Lenne, R. (2001). Effectiveness of two conservative modes of physiotherapy in women with urinary stress incontinence. *Neurourology and Urodynamics, 20,* 591–599.

Avery, K., Donovan, J., Peters, T. J., et al. (2004). ICIQ: A brief and robust measure for evaluating the symptoms and impact of urinary incontinence. *Neurourology and Urodynamics, 23*(4), 322–330.

Balmforth, J., Bidmead, J., Cardozo, L., et al. (2004). Raising the tone: A prospective observational study evaluating the effect of pelvic floor muscle training on bladder neck mobility and associated improvement in stress urinary incontinence. *Neurourology and Urodynamics, 23,* 553–554.

Benvenuti, F., Caputo, G. M., Bandinelli, S., et al. (1987). Re-educative treatment of female genuine stress incontinence. *American Journal of Physical Medicine, 66*(4), 155–168.

Berghmans, L. C. M., Frederiks, C. M. A., de Bie, R. A., et al. (1996). Efficacy of biofeedback, when included with pelvic floor muscle exercise treatment, for genuine stress incontinence. *Neurourology and Urodynamics, 15,* 37–52.

Bø, K. (1994). Reproducibility of instruments designed to measure subjective evaluation of female stress urinary incontinence. *Scandinavian Journal of Urology and Nephrology, 28,* 97–100.

Bø, K. (1995). Adherence to pelvic floor muscle exercise and long term effect on stress urinary incontinence. A five year follow up. *Scandinavian Journal of Medicine & Science in Sports, 5,* 36–39.

Bø, K. (2004). Pelvic floor muscle training is effective in treatment of stress urinary incontinence, but how does it work? *International Urogynecology Journal and Pelvic Floor Dysfunction, 15,* 76–84.

Bø, K. (2020). Physiotherapy management of female urinary incontinence. *Journal of Physiotherapy, 66*(3), 147–154.

Bø, K., Frawley, H. C., & Haylen, B. T. (2017). An International Urogynecological Association (IUGA)/International Continence Society (ICS) joint report on the terminology for the conservative and nonpharmacological management of female pelvic floor dysfunction. *Neurourology and Urodynamics, 36,* 221–244.

Bø, K., Hagen, R. H., Kvarstein, B., et al. (1990). Pelvic floor muscle exercise for the treatment of female stress urinary incontinence: III. Effects of two different degrees of pelvic floor muscle exercise. *Neurourology and Urodynamics, 9,* 489–502.

Bø, K., & Herbert, R. (2009). When and how should new therapies become routine clinical practice? *Physiotherapy, 95,* 51–57.

Bø, K., & Herbert, R. H. (2013). There is not yet strong evidence that exercise regimens other than pelvic floor muscle training can reduce stress urinary incontinence in women: A systematic review. *Journal of Physiotherapy, 59,* 159–168.

Bø, K., & Hilde, G. (2013). Does it work in the long term? A systematic review on pelvic floor muscle training for female stress urinary incontinence. *Neurourology and Urodynamics, 32,* 215–223.

Bø, K., Kvarstein, B., Hagen, R., et al. (1990). Pelvic floor muscle exercise for the treatment of female stress urinary incontinence: II. Validity of vaginal pressure measurements of pelvic floor muscle strength and the necessity of supplementary methods for control of correct contraction. *Neurourology and Urodynamics, 9,* 479–487.

Bø, K., Kvarstein, B., & Nygaard, I. (2005). Lower urinary tract symptoms and pelvic floor muscle exercise adherence after 15 years. *Obstetrics & Gynecology, 105*(5 Pt. 1), 999–1005.

Bø, K., Larsen, S., Oseid, S., et al. (1988). Knowledge about and ability to correct pelvic floor muscle exercises in women with urinary stress incontinence. *Neurourology and Urodynamics, 7*(3), 261–262.

Bø, K., Lilleås, F., Talseth, T., et al. (2001). Dynamic MRI of pelvic floor muscles in an upright sitting position. *Neurourology and Urodynamics, 20,* 167–174.

Bø, K., & Stien, R. (1994). Needle EMG registration of striated urethral wall and pelvic floor muscle activity patterns during cough, Valsalva, abdominal, hip adductor, and gluteal muscle contractions in nulliparous healthy females. *Neurourology and Urodynamics, 13,* 35–41.

Bø, K., & Talseth, T. (1996). Long term effect of pelvic floor muscle exercise five years after cessation of organized training. *Obstetrics & Gynecology, 87*(2), 261–265.

Bø, K., Talseth, T., & Holme, I. (1999). Single blind, randomised controlled trial of pelvic floor exercises, electrical stimulation, vaginal cones, and no treatment in management of genuine stress incontinence in women. *British Medical Journal, 318,* 487–493.

Brækken, I. H., Majida, M., Ellstrom-Engh, M., et al. (2010). Morphological changes after pelvic floor muscle training measured by 3-dimensional ultrasound: A randomized controlled trial. *Obstetrics & Gynecology, 115*(2), 317–324.

Brækken, I. H., Majida, M., Engh, M. E., et al. (2009). Test–retest reliability of pelvic floor muscle contraction measured by 4D ultrasound. *Neurourology and Urodynamics, 28,* 68–73.

Bump, R., Hurt, W. G., Fantl, J. A., et al. (1991). Assessment of Kegel exercise performance after brief verbal instruction. *American Journal of Obstetrics and Gynecology, 165,* 322–329.

Cammu, H., & Van Nylen, M. (1998). Pelvic floor exercises versus vaginal weight cones in genuine stress incontinence. *European Journal of Obstetrics & Gynecology and Reproductive Biology, 77,* 89–93.

Cammu, H., Van Nylen, M., & Amy, J. (2000). A ten-year follow-up after Kegel pelvic floor muscle exercises for genuine stress incontinence. *BJU International, 85*, 655–658.

Carriere, B. (2002). *Fitness for the pelvic floor*. Stuttgart: Georg Thieme Verlag.

Castro, R. A., Arruda, R. M., Zanetti, M. R. D., et al. (2008). Single-blind, randomized, controlled trial of pelvic floor muscle training, electrical stimulation, vaginal cones, and no active treatment in the management of stress urinary incontinence. *Clinics, 63*(4), 465–472.

Chiarelli, P., & Cockburn, J. (2002). Promoting urinary continence in women after delivery: Randomised controlled trial. *British Medical Journal, 324*, 1241.

Constantinou, C. E., & Govan, D. E. (1981). Contribution and timing of transmitted and generated pressure components in the female urethra. In *Female Incontinence* (pp. 113–120). New York: Allan R. Liss.

Corcos, J., Beaulieu, S., Donovan, J., et al. (2002). Quality of life assessment in men and women with urinary incontinence. *Journal of Urology, 168*, 896–905.

Cumberledge, J. (2020). *First Do No Harm*. Available: https://www.immdsreview.org.uk/downloads/IMMDSReview_Web.pdf (accessed 16.07.22).

DeLancey, J. (1990). Functional anatomy of the female lower urinary tract and pelvic floor. *Ciba Foundation Symposia, 151*, 57–76.

DeLancey, J. (1994). Structural support of the urethra as it relates to stress urinary incontinence: The hammock hypothesis. *American Journal of Obstetrics and Gynecology, 170*, 1713–1723.

DeLancey, J. (1994). The anatomy of the pelvic floor. *Current Opinion in Obstetrics and Gynecology, 6*, 313–316.

DeLancey, J. (1997). The pathophysiology of stress urinary incontinence in women and its applications for surgical treatment. *World Journal of Urology, 15*, 268–274.

Diaz, D. C., Robinson, D., & Bosch, R. (2017). Patient-reported outcome assessment. Committee 5b. In P. Abrams, L. Cardozo, & A. Wagg (Eds.), *Incontinence* (6th ed., vol 1) (pp. 541–598). Bristol, UK: ICUD.

Dudley, G. A., & Harris, R. T. (1992). Use of electrical stimulation in strength and power training. In P. V. Komi (Ed.), *Strength and power in sport* (pp. 329–337). Oxford: Blackwell Scientific.

Dumoulin, C., Adewuyi, T., Booth, J., et al. (2017). Adult conservative management. In P. Abrams, L. Cardozo, A. Wagg, et al. (Eds.), *Incontinence* (6th ed., vol. 2) (pp. 1443–1628). Bristol, UK: ICUD.

Dumoulin, C., Cacciari, L. P., & Hay-Smith, E. J. C. (2018). Pelvic floor muscle training versus no treatment, or inactive control treatments, for urinary incontinence in women. *Cochrane Database Systematic Reviews Issue, 10* Art. No. CD005654.

Dumoulin, C., Lemieux, M., Bourbonnais, D., et al. (2004). Physiotherapy for persistent postnatal stress urinary incontinence: A randomized controlled trial. *Obstetrics & Gynecology, 104*, 504–510.

Dumoulin, C., Morin, M., Danieli, C., et al. (2020). Group-based vs individual pelvic floor muscle training to treat urinary incontinence in older women: A randomized controlled trial. *JAMA Internal Medicine, 18*, 544. https://doi.org/10.1001/jamainternmed.2020.2993. Published online August 3.

Fantl, J. A., Newman, D. K., Colling, J., et al. (1996). *Urinary incontinence in adults: Acute and Chronic Management. Clinical Practice Guideline No. 2, update*. Rockville, MD: Department of Health and Human Services, Public Health Service, Agency for Health Care Policy and Research. [96–0682].

Ferguson, K. L., McKey, P. L., Bishop, K. R., et al. (1990). Stress urinary incontinence: Effect of pelvic muscle exercise. *Obstetrics & Gynecology, 75*, 671–675.

Garber, C. E., Blissmer, B., Deschenes, M. R., et al. (2011). Quantity and quality of exercise for developing and maintaining cardiorespiratory, musculoskeletal, and neuromotor fitness in apparently healthy adults: Guidance for prescribing exercise. *Medicine & Science in Sports & Exercise, 43*(7), 1334–1359.

Glavind, K., Nøhr, S., & Walter, S. (1996). Biofeedback and physiotherapy versus physiotherapy alone in the treatment of genuine stress urinary incontinence. *International Urogynecology Journal and Pelvic Floor Dysfunction, 7*, 339–343.

Hagen, S., Elders, A., Henderson, L., et al. (2019). Effectiveness and cost-effectiveness of biofeedback-assisted pelvic floor muscle training for female urinary incontinence: A multicenter randomised controlled trial. Available: https://www.ics.org/2019/abstract/489 (accessed 16.07.22).

Hay-Smith, E. J. C., Herderschee, R., Dumoulin, C., et al. (2011). Comparisons of approaches to pelvic floor muscle training for urinary incontinence in women. *Cochrane Database Systematic Reviews Issue, 12* Art. No. CD009508.

Henalla, S., Hutchins, C. J., Robinson, P., et al. (1989). Non-operative methods in the treatment of female genuine stress incontinence of urine. *Journal of Obstetrics and Gynaecology,, 9*, 222–225.

Henalla, S., Millar, D., & Wallace, K. (1990). Surgical versus conservative management for post-menopausal genuine stress incontinence of urine. *Neurourology and Urodynamics, 9*(4), 436–437.

Herbert, R., & Bø, K. (2005). Analysis of quality of interventions in systematic reviews. *British Medical Journal, 331*, 507–509.

Herbert, R., & Gabriel, M. (2002). Effects of stretching before and after exercising on muscle soreness and risk of injury: Systematic review. *British Medical Journal, 325*, 1–5.

Herbert, R. D., Kasza, J., & Bø, K. (2018). Analysis of randomised trials with long-term follow-up. *BMC Medical Research Methodology, 18*, 48.

Herbison, G. P., & Dean, N. (2013). Weighted vaginal cones for urinary incontinence. *Cochrane Database Syst Rev. Issue, 7*, CD002114.

Herderschee, R., Hay-Smith, E. J. C., Herbison, G. P., et al. (2011). Feedback or biofeedback to augment pelvic floor muscle training for urinary incontinence in women. *Cochrane Database Systematic Reviews Issue, 7* Art. No. CD009252.

Hilton, P., & Robinson, D. (2011). Defining cure. *Neurourology and Urodynamics, 30*, 741–745.

Howard, D., Miller, J., DeLancey, J., et al. (2000). Differential effects of cough, Valsalva, and continence status on vesical neck movement. *Obstetrics & Gynecology, 95*, 535–540.

Huang, A. J., Jenny, H. E., Chesney, M. A., et al. (2014). A group-based yoga therapy intervention for urinary incontinence in women: A pilot randomized trial. *Female Pelvic Medicine & Reconstructive Surgery, 20*(3), 147–154.

Huang, A. J., Chesney, M., Lisha, N., et al. (2019). A group-based yoga program for urinary incontinence in ambulatory women: Feasibility, tolerability, and change in incontinence frequency over 3 months in a single-center randomized trial. *American Journal of Obstetrics and Gynecology, 220*(1), 87 e1–87.e13.

Imamura, M., Abrams, P., Bain, C., et al. (2010). Systematic review and economic modelling of the effectiveness of non-surgical treatments for women with stress urinary incontinence. *Health Technology Assessment, 14*(40), 1–118 , iii–iv.

Kegel, A. H. (1948). Progressive resistance exercise in the functional restoration of the perineal muscles. *American Journal of Obstetrics and Gynecology, 56*, 238–249.

Kegel, A. H. (1952). Stress incontinence and genital relaxation. *Ciba Clinical Symposia, 2*, 35–51.

Klarskov, P., Belving, D., Bischoff, N., et al. (1986). Pelvic floor exercise versus surgery for female urinary stress incontinence. *Urologia Internationalis, 41*, 129–132.

Labrie, J., Berghmans, B. L. C. M., Fisher, K., et al. (2013). Surgery versus physiotherapy for stress urinary incontinence. *New England Journal of Medicine, 369*, 1124–1133.

Laycock, J., Brown, J., Cusack, C., et al. (2001). Pelvic floor re-education for stress incontinence: Comparing three methods. *British Journal of Community Nursing, 6*(5), 230–237.

Lose, G., Fantl, J. A., Victor, A., et al. (1998). Outcome measures for research in adult women with symptoms of lower urinary tract dysfunction. *Neurourology and Urodynamics, 17*(3), 255–262.

Luginbuehl, H., Lehmann, C., Koenig, I., et al. (2019). Involuntary reflexive pelvic floor muscle training in addition to standard training alone for women with stress urinary incontinence: A randomized controlled trial. *International Urogynecology Journal, 33*(3), 531–540.

Madill, S. J., Pontbriand-Drolet, S., Tang, A., et al. (2015). Changes in urethral sphincter size following rehabilitation in older women with stress urinary incontinence. *International Urogynecology Journal, 26*, 277–283.

McLean, L., Varette, K., & Gentilcore-Saulnier, E. (2013). Pelvic floor muscle training in women with stress urinary incontinence causes hypertrophy of the urethral sphincters and reduces bladder neck mobility during coughing. *Neurourology and Urodynamics, 32*(8), 1096–1102.

Mercier, J., Morin, M., Tang, A., et al. (2020). Pelvic floor muscle training: Mechanisms of action for the improvement of genitourinary syndrome of menopause. *Climacteric, 23*(5), 468–473.

Miller, J. M., Ashton-Miller, J. A., & DeLancey, J. (1998). A pelvic muscle precontraction can reduce cough-related urine loss in selected women with mild SUI. *Journal of the American Geriatrics Society, 46*, 870–874.

Miller, J. M., Hawthorne, K. M., Park, L., et al. (2018). Self-perceived improvement in bladder health after viewing a novel tutorial on Knack use: A randomized controlled trial pilot study. *Journal of Women's Health (Larchmt.), 29*(10), 1319–1327.

Miller, J. M., Perucchini, D., Carchidi, L., et al. (2001). Pelvic floor muscle contraction during a cough and decreased vesical neck mobility. *Obstetrics & Gynecology, 97*, 255–260.

Mørkved, S., Bø, K., & Fjørtoft, T. (2002). Is there any additional effect of adding biofeedback to pelvic floor muscle training? A single-blind randomized controlled trial. *Obstetrics & Gynecology, 100*(4), 730–739.

Nagib, A. B. L., Riccetto, C., & Martinho, N. M. (2020). Use of mobile apps for controlling of the urinary incontinence: A systematic review. *Neurourology and Urodynamics, 39*(4), 1036–1048.

National Institute for Health and Care Excellence (NICE). (2019). *Urinary incontinence and pelvic Organ Prolapse in women: Management.* London: NICE Guideline NG123. National Institute for Health and Care Excellence.

Neels, H., De Wachter, S., Wyndaele, J. J., et al. (2018). Common errors made in attempt to contract the pelvic floor muscles in women early after delivery: A prospective observational study. *European Journal of Obstetrics & Gynecology and Reproductive Biology, 220*, 113–117.

Neumann, P., & Gill, V. (2002). Pelvic floor and abdominal muscle interaction: EMG activity and intra-abdominal pressure. *International Urogynecology Journal and Pelvic Floor Dysfunction, 13*, 125–132.

Paddison, K. (2002). Complying with pelvic floor exercises: A literature review. *Nursing Standard, 16*(39), 33–38.

Pages, I., Schaufele, M., & Conradi, E. (2001). Comparative analysis of biofeedback and physiotherapy for treatment of urinary stress incontinence in women. *American Journal of Physical Medicine & Rehabilitation, 80*(7), 494–502.

Paiva, L. L., Ferla, L., Darski, C., et al. (2017). Pelvic floor muscle training in groups versus individual or home treatment of women with urinary incontinence: Systematic review and meta-analysis. *International Urogynecology Journal, 28*, 351–359.

Pelaez, M., Gonzalez-Cerron, S., Montejo, R., et al. (2014). Pelvic floor muscle training included in a pregnancy exercise program is effective in primary prevention of urinary incontinence: A randomized controlled trial. *Neurourology and Urodynamics, 33*, 67–71.

Pereira, V. S., Correia, G. N., & Driusso, P. (2011). Individual and group pelvic floor muscle training versus no treatment in female stress urinary incontinence: A randomized controlled pilot study. *European Journal of Obstetrics & Gynecology and Reproductive Biology, 159*(2), 465–471.

Peschers, U., Fanger, G., Schaer, G., et al. (2001). Bladder neck mobility in continent nulliparous women. *British Journal of Obstetrics and Gynaecology, 108*, 320–324.

Peschers, U., Gingelmaier, A., Jundt, K., et al. (2001). Evaluation of pelvic floor muscle strength using four different techniques. *International Urogynecology Journal and Pelvic Floor Dysfunction, 12*, 27–30.

Peschers, U., Schaer, G., DeLancey, J., et al. (1997). Levator ani function before and after childbirth. *British Journal of Obstetrics and Gynaecology, 104*, 1004–1008.

Peschers, U., Vodušek, D., Fanger, G., et al. (2001). Pelvic muscle activity in nulliparous volunteers. *Neurourology and Urodynamics, 20*, 269–275.

Prashar, S., Simons, A., Bryant, C., et al. (2000). Attitudes to vaginal/urethral touching and device placement in women with urinary incontinence. *International Urogynecology Journal and Pelvic Floor Dysfunction, 11*, 4–8.

Ptak, M., Ciećwież, S., Brodowska, A., et al. (2019). The effect of pelvic floor muscles exercise on quality of life in women with stress urinary incontinence and its relationship with vaginal deliveries: A randomized trial. *BioMed Research International, 2019*(6) Art. No. 5321864.

Ramsey, I. N., & Thou, M. (1990). A randomized, double blind, placebo controlled trial of pelvic floor exercise in the treatment of genuine stress incontinence. *Neurourology and Urodynamics, 9*(4), 398–399.

Jose-Vaz, L. A., Andrade, C. L., Cardoso, L. C., et al. (2020). Can abdominal hypropressive technique improve stress urinary incontinence? An assessor-blinded randomized controlled trial. *Neurourology and Urodynamics, 39*(8), 2314–2321.

Sapsford, R. (2001). The pelvic floor. A clinical model for function and rehabilitation. *Physiotherapy, 87*(12), 620–630.

Sapsford, R. (2004). Rehabilitation of pelvic floor muscles utilizing trunk stabilization. *Manual Therapy, 9*, 3–12.

Sapsford, R., & Hodges, P. (2001). Contraction of the pelvic floor muscles during abdominal maneuvers. *Archives of Physical Medicine and Rehabilitation, 82*, 1081–1088.

Sapsford, R., Hodges, P., Richardson, C., et al. (2001). Co-activation of the abdominal and pelvic floor muscles during voluntary exercises. *Neurourology and Urodynamics, 20*, 31–42.

Sapsford, R., Markwell, S., & Clarke, B. (1998). The relationship between urethral pressure and abdominal muscle activity. *Australian and New Zealand Continence Journal,, 4*, 102–110.

Schwartz, G., & Beatty, J. (1977). *Biofeedback: Theory and Research*. New York: Academic Press.

Sugaya, K., Owan, T., Hatano, T., et al. (2003). Device to promote pelvic floor muscle training for stress incontinence. *International Journal of Urology, 10*, 416–422.

Thompsen, J., & O'Sullivan, P. (2003). Levator plate movement during voluntary pelvic floor muscle contraction in subjects with incontinence and prolapse: A cross-sectional study. *International Urogynecology Journal and Pelvic Floor Dysfunction, 14*, 84–88.

Wong, K., Fung, B., Fung, L. C. W., et al. (1997). *Pelvic floor exercises in the treatment of stress urinary incontinence in Hong Kong Chinese women*. Yokohama, Japan: ICS 27th Annual Meeting, 62–63.

Zanetti, M. R. D., Castro, R. A., Rotta, A. L., et al. (2007). Impact of supervised physiotherapeutic pelvic floor exercises for treating female stress urinary incontinence. *Sao Paulo Medical Journal, 125*(5), 265–269.

Zubieta, M., Carr, R. L., Drake, M. J., et al. (2016). Influence of voluntary pelvic floor muscle contraction and pelvic floor muscle training on urethral closure pressures—a systematic review. *International Urogynecology Journal, 27*, 687–696.

Electrical Stimulation for Stress Urinary Incontinence

Bary Berghmans, Abdallahi N'Dongo and Georges Billard

INTRODUCTION

When a nerve is stimulated, signals travel both towards the periphery and towards the central nervous system. Electrical stimulation (ES) may elicit responses to these signals, which may come from the central nervous system or the tissues innervated by the nerve, or the central nervous system may be modified to re-interpret some signals (Chancellor and Leng, 2002; Fall and Lindström, 1994).

With respect to lower urinary tract dysfunction, ES is applied particularly to the pelvic floor muscles (PFMs), bladder and sacral nerve roots. ES of the pelvic floor aims at stimulating motor fibres of the pudendal nerve, which may elicit a direct contraction of the PFMs or the striated periurethral musculature, supporting the intrinsic part of the urethral sphincter closing mechanism (Fall and Lindström, 1991; Scheepens, 2003). As such, ES might contribute to the compensation of a weak intrinsic sphincter, but it is questionable whether or not ES in such cases would be the first choice treatment option or would have any additional value to a functional training (Ayeleke, 2015; Berghmans et al., 1998)

In patients with detrusor overactivity or symptoms of urgency and urgency urinary incontinence, ES can elicit direct contractions of the PFMs, which stimulate *afferent* fibres of the pudendal nerve going to the sacral spinal cord that reflexively decrease the feeling/sensation of urgency and inhibit parasympathetic activity at the level of the sacral micturition centre in the sacral cord, to reduce involuntary detrusor contractions and reflexively activate the striated periurethral musculature. ES may be used as stand-alone therapy or in combination with pelvic floor muscle training (PFMT) (Dumoulin et al., 2017). ES can be divided into two major forms: neurostimulation and neuromodulation. Neurostimulation of the pelvic floor aims at stimulating motor efferent fibres of the pudendal nerve, which may elicit a *direct* response from the effector organ, such as a contraction of the PFMs (Eriksen, 1989; Fall and Lindström, 1991; Scheepens, 2003). The object of neuromodulation is to remodel neuronal reflex loops, such as the detrusor inhibition reflex, by stimulating afferent nerve fibres of

the pudendal nerve that influence these reflex loops. Thus neuromodulation may elicit an *indirect* response from the effector organ, such as detrusor muscle inhibition (Berghmans et al., 2002; Fall and Lindström, 1994; Vodušek et al., 1986; Weil et al., 2000).

Even today, it is still quite difficult to clarify the potential value and benefits of ES in the treatment of urinary incontinence, which is the most prevalent form of lower urinary tract dysfunction (Dumoulin et al., 2017). There are several reasons for this.

Firstly, the nomenclature used to describe ES has been inconsistent. Stimulation has sometimes been described on the basis of the type of current being used (e.g., faradic stimulation, interferential therapy), but is also described on the basis of the structures being targeted (e.g., neuromuscular ES), the current intensity (e.g., low-intensity stimulation or maximal stimulation) and the proposed mechanism of action (e.g., neuromodulation). In the absence of a clear unequivocal classification of ES, the present authors will make no attempt to classify the interventions considered.

Secondly, although it has been suggested that ES as an intervention for urinary incontinence is using the natural neural pathways and micturition reflexes (Fall, 1998; Yamanishi and Yasuda, 1998) and the understanding of both neuroanatomy and neurophysiology of the central and peripheral nervous systems is increasing, there is still lack of a well-substantiated biological rationale supporting the use of ES (Dumoulin et al., 2017).

Thirdly, the lack of a clear biological rationale seems to hamper reasoned choices of ES parameters. Parameters, used in previous ES studies, such as the current source, pulse width and duration, current intensity (range), amplitudes, stimulus frequency, pulse shape, ramp-up and ramp-down (gradually changing the rate at which the current achieves maximal amplitude), time and total number of sessions and rest/work ratio, and electrode placements vary according to type of urinary incontinence and type of ES (Dumoulin et al., 2017; Stewart et al., 2017). Berghmans et al. (2002) reported that usually frequencies of 5 to 20 Hz are used for urgency urinary incontinence, 20 to 50 Hz for stress urinary incontinence (SUI) and for mixed urinary incontinence (around) 20 Hz or high/low alternately (Dumoulin et al., 2017). Pulse durations of 200 (Dumoulin et al., 2017), 300 (Yamanishi et al., 2010), 400 to 600 (Everaert et al., 1999) and 1000 µs (Moore et al., 1999) for SUI have been reported, and for detrusor overactivity 200 to 500 µs and for mixed urinary incontinence depending on the dominant factor of urinary incontinence (Berghmans et al., 2002). Pulse shape is generally rectangular, and biphasic pulses are preferred (Dumoulin et al., 2017).

Although a wide range of parameters has been claimed to be successful, the most optimal set of parameters for each type of urinary incontinence has not been determined (Dumoulin et al., 2017). Additional confusion is created by the relatively rapid developments in the area of ES. Even for the same health problem, a wide variety of stimulation devices, protocols and parameters have been used (Dumoulin et al., 2017) (see Table 7.1.7).

Parameters for Electrical Stimulation

Today, manufacturers of ES devices have programmed into their devices many protocols using parameters suitable for the different pelvic floor dysfunction. Unfortunately, stimulation protocols are not systematically documented in the literature, which limits the feasibility of meta-analysis and impedes the generalization of conclusions (Günter et al., 2019). To what extent the choice and selection of parameters are evidence based and proven to be effective remains largely unknown. Programming all parameters for preset protocols may lead to the undesirable situation that physical therapists just follow the instruction manuals of the devices and apply ES without adapting and adjusting parameters to the individual needs of patients suffering from a particular pelvic floor problem. In addition, so far, the relevant literature does not provide satisfactory evidence-based information and tools about when and how to select optimal parameters for each individual pelvic floor problem. This is certainly a complicated and maybe time-consuming endeavor—one of the reasons physical therapists continue to use the manufacturer's protocols.

To select adequate parameters themselves, first of all, physical therapists must apply to general rules for ES.

ES is applied via a probe through the vaginal walls and would be diffused over the entire pudendal plexus and nearby neuromuscular junctions. This stimulation would therefore provoke the recruitment of all PFMs in that area. As the current is applied directly on the vaginal mucosa or at the region of the vulva with superficial adhesive patches, it is important to eliminate any risk of electrolysis due to a unidirectional current which produces acid formation under the anode and base formation under the cathode (Tadej et al., 2010).

Safety limitations on pulse amplitude (and consequently, charge injection) are dependent on geometrical factors such as electrode placement, size and proximity to the stimulated fiber (Günter et al., 2019).

Since intra-cavitary ES is applied directly through the contact between vaginal/anal mucosa and probe electrodes, it has been suggested that the type of current used should always be symmetrical biphasic waveform (Günter et al., 2019).

Besides this, even using symmetrical biphasic waveform currents, the energy spent should be reasonable (Günter et al., 2019). Indeed, Joule's law of electricity ($W_J = R \times I^2 \times t$) reminds us that the heat produced is mainly due to the intensity of current (Hubert et al., 2019). With excessive intensity, physical burn by the Joule effect could occur from all current types. To ensure an excellent current flow between the probe and the mucosa, a glycerin-free aqueous conductive gel should be applied (Bolfe et al., 2009). Because of the risks associated with the Joule effect, medical devices that generate ES must comply with very high safety standards, and a current intensity greater than 50 mA should be avoided (La Norme Francaise, 2015). Therefore, if this critical threshold is reached without obtaining the expected effect, the pulse width should be enlarged to increase the amount of energy delivered without raising the intensity beyond 50 mA (Günter et al., 2019). Regarding pulse width and amplitude, short pulses require lower electric charges to elicit action potentials, and therefore short pulses should be preferred whenever the necessary higher current amplitudes are technically feasible (Günter et al., 2019). The application of ES with a constant current generator should never be uncomfortable or painful.

To improve the comfort of patients and the quality of electro-induced muscle recruitment, it has been suggested to apply ES through envelope curves that incorporate a rise, a plateau and a descent period (Fig. 7.1.6). However, a slowly rising stimulus slope may entail an elevation of the threshold (Wessale et al., 1992). Günter et al. (2019) stated that rectangular waveforms may be more effective in eliciting physiological responses. This statement seems to be supported by Wessale et al. (1992), who found that rectangular pulses require slightly lower currents to reach threshold.

TABLE 7.1.7 Randomized Controlled Trials on Electrical Stimulation to Treat Stress Urinary Incontinence

Author	Shepherd et al. (1984)
Design	2-arm RCT: ES; placebo ES
Sample size and age (years)	107 women (42 with SUI) age 26–72
Diagnosis	Urodynamic assessment with urethral profilometry and cystometry; cystoscopy under general anaesthesia; measurement of pelvic contraction
Training protocol	1 single session of maximum perineal stimulation while under anaesthesia ES group: vaginal and buttock ES; monophasic square wave pulses; I max 40 V, 10–50 Hz; 20 min Placebo ES: same but no current; assessment at 6 and 12 weeks post-treatment; questionnaires, pad test, diary, perineometry
Drop-out	12%
Adherence	Not applicable
Results	Only overall results available, but authors stated no difference between diagnostic groups No difference between groups regarding reduction frequency, severity, pads used, pelvic floor muscle strength, subjective improvement
Author	**Henalla et al. (1989)**
Design	4-arm RCT: PFMT; ES; oestrogens; no treatment
Sample size and age (years)	104 women; mean age not stated, age comparable between groups
Diagnosis	Urodynamically proven GSI
Training protocol	PFMT with digital feedback by patient + regular PFM exercises 5 s, 5×/h; PT 1×/week 10 ES sessions 20 min, 1×/week IFT 0–100 Hz, I max 2 g oestrogens + nightly applicator for 12 weeks No treatment
Drop-out	4%
Adherence	Not reported
Results	No in-between comparisons; pad test 50% reduction in 17/26 (65%) PFMT; in 8/25 (32%) ES; 3/24 (12%) after 3 months; pad weights reduction in PFMT and ES (p < 0.02); 3/17 PFMT and 1/8 ES recurrences of UI after 9 months; 3/3 immediate recurrence after discontinuing oestrogens
Author	**Olah et al. (1990)**
Design	2-arm RCT: VC; ES
Sample size and age (years)	69 women; mean age 43.2 ± 8.9 (VC), 47.9 ± 13 (ES)
Diagnosis	Continence-frequency chart 1 week pre-treatment, pelvic floor strength with VC, 1-h pad test
Training protocol	VC group 1×/week for 4 weeks, active PFMT with VC 2×/day for 15 min, increasing weight after 2 successful occasions; ES-IFT 3×/week for 4 weeks; 0–100 Hz, 4 vacuum electrodes, 2 abdominal, 2 thighs, I max, 15 min
Drop-out	15/69 (22%)
Adherence	Not reported
Results	Weekly leakages (g) mean ± SD: VC from 22 ± 31.4 to 8.2 ± 14.5 to 3.9 ± 9.4 (after 6 months); IFT 19.3 ± 22.6 to 7.7 ± 11.7 to 5.3 ± 9.2 (after 6 months) UI (g) mean ± SD: VC 27.7 ± 38.8 to 14 ± 36.7 to 2.8 ± 8.3; IFT from 32.2 ± 49.1 to 10.5 ± 17.3 to 9.7 ± 28.4 (after 6 months) No difference between groups Cured/improved: VC 4/15 of 24, 10/7 of 24 after 6 months; IFT 4/23 of 30, 12/15 of 30

TABLE 7.1.7 Randomized Controlled Trials on Electrical Stimulation to Treat Stress Urinary Incontinence—cont'd

Author	**Von Hofbauer et al. (1990)**
Design	4-arm RCT: ES + PFMT; PFMT; ES; sham treatment
Sample size and age (years)	43 women; mean age 57.5 ± 12
Diagnosis	Cystoscopy, cystometry, UPP, micturition diary
Training protocol	ES constant 3×/week for 10 min for 6 weeks perineal and lumbar electrodes, faradic, I variable until contraction; PFMT + abd/add 20 min 2×/week + home exercises; sham ES
Drop-out	Not reported
Adherence	Not reported
Results	Cured/improved/unchanged: ES + PFMT 3/4/4; PFMT 6/1/4; ES 1/2/8; sham ES 0/0/10 Maximal urethral closing pressure, functional urethral length and pressure transmission, no significant changes pre- and post-treatment
Author	**Blowman et al. (1991)**
Design	Double-blind 2-arm RCT: PFMT + ES; PFMT + sham ES
Sample size and age (years)	14 women age 33–68
Diagnosis	Urodynamics, filling cystometry, coughing-induced leakage while standing
Training protocol	PFMT + visual feedback with perineometer 4×/day; home (sham) surface ES 60 min/day; perineal and buttocks, ES 10 Hz, 4-s hold/relax, pulse width 80 µs, 2 weeks 35 Hz, 15 min/day; ES no contraction, minimal sensation, 4 weeks
Drop-out	1/14 (7%)
Adherence	Not reported
Results	No significant decrease median (range) IEF/week in sham ES from 12.5 (1–31) to 6 (0–21), significant decrease ES from 5 (0–14) to 0 (0–1) Max perineometer in sham ES median (range) pre-/post-treatment from 3.5 (1–5) to 5 (3–13), ES 1 (0–8) to 5 (2–16); no side effect of (sham) ES reported; IEF 0 in 6/7 ES, 1/6 in sham ES; questionnaire after 6 months ES no ES, 4 sham ES further treatment needed
Author	**Hahn et al. (1991)**
Design	2-arm RCT: PFMT; ES If not cured after 6 months, other arm offered
Sample size and age (years)	20 women; mean age 47.2 (range 24–64) 13 women had both arms
Diagnosis	Urodynamics, cystometry, pad test, cystourethroscopy
Training protocol	PFMT fast Pmax 5-s hold and relax and slow-twitch P submax 2-s hold and relax in various positions, 5–10 times, 6–8×/day, endurance 30–40 s; IFT vaginal probe, alternating pulses 10/20/50 Hz, home device (Contelle) 6–8 h/night
Drop-out	2 IFT after unsuccessful PFMT/13
Adherence	Not reported
Results	Pad test: 5/20 cured in 1 treatment course (1 PFMT, 4 IFT); PFMT, IFT significant improvement, in-between NS; 13 in second course had significant improvement; subjective improvement 2 cured/11 improved Pad test after 4 years: 4/14 further improvement, 8/14 unchanged, 2/14 deterioration; subjective improvement: 1/14 improved, 8/14 unchanged, 5 deteriorated
Author	**Laycock and Jerwood (1993)** (study 1)
Design	2-arm RCT: ES; PFMT + interferential therapy VC
Sample size and age (years)	46 women age 28–59

Continued

TABLE 7.1.7 Randomized Controlled Trials on Electrical Stimulation to Treat Stress Urinary Incontinence—cont'd

Diagnosis	Urodynamically proven GSI; digital palpation (Oxford scale grading)
Training protocol	Mean 10 ES-IFT sessions, bipolar, perineal and symphysis pubis, 30 min, I max, 1/10–40/40 Hz 10 min each; 6 weeks PFMT, 5 maximal voluntary contractions every hour, from second visit VC 10 min, 2×/day
Drop-out	ES: no drop-outs PFMT: 6/23 (26%)
Adherence	After therapy in ES group, 1 subject (7%) home maintenance PFMT every day, 6 (40%) nearly every day, 8 (53%) 1×/week
Results	Pad test: significant decrease (p < 0.003) in both groups PFM strength: ES significant improvement (p = 0.0035), PFMT NS Micturition diary: IEF significant decrease in both groups Subjective assessment: IEF in both groups equally effective Review questionnaire: after 2 years, >30% ES maintained improvement
Author	**Laycock and Jerwood (1993)** (study 2)
Design	2-arm RCT: ES; sham ES
Sample size and age (years)	30 women age 16–66
Diagnosis	See study 1 of Laycock and Jerwood (1993)
Training protocol	IFT: see study 1 of Laycock and Jerwood (1993) Sham IFT: no current, rest similar IFT
Drop-out	IFT no drop-outs; sham IFT 4/15 (27%)
Adherence	After therapy in ES group, 2 subjects (15.4%) home maintenance PFMT every day, 5 (38.5%) nearly every day, 4 (30.8%) 1×/week, 2 (15.4%) <1×/week
Results	Pad test: IFT mean 56.8% decrease weight pre-/post-treatment, sham IFT 21.4%; in between significant difference Perineometer: PFMC significant increase in strength only in IFT Micturition chart: IEF reduction only in IFT, severity reduction idem Review questionnaire after mean 16 months: 20% IFT maintained improvement
Author	**Sand et al. (1995)**
Design	Multicentre 2-arm RCT: ES; sham ES
Sample size and age (years)	52 women age mean ± SD 53.2 ± 11.4
Diagnosis	Urodynamically proven GSI, urethral closing pressure >20 cmH$_2$O, leak point pressure >60 cmH$_2$O at max cyst. capacity
Training protocol	Vaginal electrode, ES pulse duration 0.3 ms, I max, first 2 weeks 5/10 s, later 5/5-s hold/relax; sham ES 1 mA max, 15–30 min 2×/day for 12 weeks
Drop-out	8/52 (15%)
Adherence	61% used ES >50 out of planned 70 h (80%) vs 89% sham ES
Results	ES vs sham ES after 12 weeks IEF/24 h, IEF/week, UI during pad test, PFM strength on perineometry significantly better in ES; no irreversible adverse events, vaginal irritation/infection/urinary tract infection/pain 14%/11%/3%/9% ES and 12%/12%/12%/6% sham ES
Author	**Smith (1996)**
Design	2-arm RCT: ES; PFMT
Sample size and age (years)	Subgroup GSI (type II): 18 women age 26–72
Diagnosis	Cystoscopy only when indicated, complex video urodynamic study (i.e., uroflow, UPP, cystometrography, Valsalva leak point pressure)

TABLE 7.1.7 Randomized Controlled Trials on Electrical Stimulation to Treat Stress Urinary Incontinence—cont'd

Training protocol	ES: 5-s contractions (range: 3–15), duty circle 1:2, treatment time 15–60 min 2×/day for 4 months, I 5–80 mA PFMT: 60 contractions/day, fast and slow twitch
Drop-out	None
Adherence	80%
Results	IEF, pads >50% improved, objective improvement 44% PFMT, 1/4/5 cured/improved/unchanged; 66% ES, 2/4/3; in between NS
Author	**Brubaker et al. (1997)**
Design	2-arm RCT: ES; sham ES
Sample size and age (years)	148 women, subgroup with GSI 60 women; mean age 57 (SD: 12)
Diagnosis	Urodynamics, micturition diary
Training protocol	ES: transvaginal, 20 Hz, 2/4-s work/rest, pulse width 0.1 μs, bipolar square wave, I 0–100 mA Sham ES: same parameters, no I Both groups: 8-week treatment
Drop-out	18%
Adherence	ES vs sham ES mean compliance 87% vs 81% at 4 and 8 treatment weeks
Results	ES vs sham ES, 6 weeks 24-h frequency NS; 6 weeks, number of accidents/24 h (average) NS; adequate subjective improvement p = 0.027; QoL NS; no analysis diaries because of incomplete data
Author	**Luber and Wolde-Tsadik (1997)**
Design	2-arm double-blind RCT: ES; sham ES
Sample size and age (years)	45 women with GSI; mean age 53.8
Diagnosis	Urodynamics, micturition diary, questionnaire, cotton swab test: hypermobility urethra
Training protocol	ES: 15-min sessions 2×/day for 12 weeks, home device, pulse width 2 ms, 2/4-s work/rest, frequency 50 Hz, I 10–100 mA Sham ES: same parameters, I no sensation
Drop-out	1/45 (2.2%)
Adherence	Measured by internal memory home device
Results	Difference NS between groups (ES 20 women, sham ES 24 women in subjective cure/improvement, objective cure (diaries, incontinence questionnaire, urodynamics); no adverse events
Author	**Knight et al. (1998)**
Design	3-arm RCT: clinic ES + PFMT/BF; home ES + PFMT/BF; PFMT/BF
Sample size and age (years)	70 women with GSI age 24–68
Diagnosis	Urodynamics, micturition diary, pad test, perineometry
Training protocol	Baseline treatment: home PFMT after instruction with PT, 10/4-s hold/relax (max 10), repetitions recorded, max 10 fast-twitch contractions, 6×/day Baseline treatment nightly low I home ES, vaginal probe, trains of 10 Hz, 35 Hz occasionally, pulse width 200 μs, duty circle 5/5 s Baseline treatment + 30-min clinic ES (16 sessions), I max, 35 Hz, pulse width 250 ms, together with voluntary contraction
Drop-out	13/70 (18.6%); 24% in home ES (NS), ITT analysis of all
Adherence	Median percentage compliance home ES (72.5%); PFMT/BF (90%); difference between groups NS

Continued

TABLE 7.1.7   Randomized Controlled Trials on Electrical Stimulation to Treat Stress Urinary Incontinence—cont'd

Results	Pad test after 6 months: significant reduction in urine loss in all 3 groups, clinic ES best, after 12 > reduction; objective improvement/cured after 6 months of clinic ES (n = 20) vs home ES (n = 19) vs controls (n = 18) 80%/52.8%/72.3% Micturition diaries data incomplete, not analysed; PFM strength significant increase in all groups, biggest in clinic ES (NS)
Author	**Bø et al. (1999)**
Design	4-arm RCT: PFMT; ES; VC; no treatment
Sample size and age (years)	122 women with GSI; mean age (range) 49.5 (24–70)
Diagnosis	Urodynamics, uroflowmetry, cystometry, pad test with standard bladder volume
Training protocol	PFMT: 8–12 voluntary PFM contractions 3×/day at home % 1×/week in office ES: vaginal intermittent stimulation, 50 Hz 30 min/day VC: 20 min/day
Drop-out	15/122 (12%) primary analysis and ITT analysis of all
Adherence	Mean (SE) adherence PFMT 93% (1.5%), ES 75% (2.8%), VC 78% (4.4%); PFMT vs ES or VC significantly better, ES vs VC NS
Results	Significant improvement pre-/post-treatment in all treatment groups: PFMT vs no treatment significant difference (p < 0.01); PFMT 44% cured, no treatment 6.7%; change in PFM strength significantly greater in PFMT (p = 0.03), not in ES or VC; ITT analysis same results; PFMT vs no treatment significant change in pad test after 6 months, IEF (p < 0.01), Social Activity Index (p < 0.01) and Leakage Index (p < 0.01); no urodynamic parameters changed in any group pre-/post-treatment
Author	**Jeyaseelan et al. (2000)**
Design	2-arm RCT: ES; sham ES
Sample size and age (years)	27 women with GSI, age not reported
Diagnosis	Urodynamics, 7-day micturition diary, 20-min pad test
Training protocol	ES: background low frequency (target slow-twitch fibres) and intermediate frequency with an initial doublet (target fast-twitch fibres), vaginal probe, 1 h/day, 8 weeks Sham ES: 250 µs/min for 1 h (1 session) I no effect
Drop-out	3/27 (11%)
Adherence	ES 71%–98%; sham ES 64%–100%
Results	Perineometry: PFM strength between and within groups no significant changes pre-/post-treatment (p = 0.86) Digital assessment: significant within changes pre-/post-treatment Endurance PFM by perineometry: ES 73% ± 116% improved, sham ES reduction −6% ± 24%, difference between groups NS Pad test, micturition diary, Incontinence Impact Questionnaire (IIQ): no significant changes between groups UDI: ES > reduction than sham ES (p = 0.03)
Author	**Goode et al. (2003)**
Design	3-arm RCT: ES + PFMT/BF; PFMT/BF; controls (self-administered PFMT)
Sample size and age (years)	200 women age 40–78
Diagnosis	Urodynamics, cystometry, micturition diary, QoL questionnaires
Training protocol	PFMT: 1×/2 weeks for 8 weeks, anorectal BF for awareness PFM, hold/relax 20 min, verbal and written instructions for 3×/day PFMT at home, duration hold/relax max 10 s each ES: vaginal probe, biphasic, 20 Hz, pulse width 1 ms, hold/relax 1:1, I max up to 100 mA 15 min/2 days Controls: written instructions, booklet

TABLE 7.1.7 Randomized Controlled Trials on Electrical Stimulation to Treat Stress Urinary Incontinence—cont'd

Drop-out	18.2% in PFMT, 11.9% in ES, 37.3% in controls, ITT analysis
Adherence	Not reported
Results	Mean reduction 68.6% PFMT/BF, 71.9% ES + PFMT/BF, 52.5% controls condition
	In comparison with controls, both interventions significantly more effective but not significantly different from each other (p = 0.60)
	ES + PFMT/BF significantly better patient self-perception of outcome (p < 0.001) and satisfaction with progress (p = 0.02)
Author	**Castro et al. (2008)**
Design	4-arm RCT: ES; VC; PFMT; no treatment (controls)
Sample size and age (years)	118 women with urodynamically proven (predominant) SUI; mean age (range) 54.2 (41–69)
Diagnosis	Urodynamically proven SUI
Training protocol	PFMT: 10× 5-s contractions, 5-s rest, then 20× 2/2, 20× 1/1, 5× 10/10, followed by 5× strong contractions with stimulated cough/1-min rest; general warming-up and stretching exercises at end
	ES: transvaginal 20 min, 3×/week, 50 Hz, biphasic, pulse width 500 μs, I 0–100 mA, duty cycle 5/10 s
	VC: 1 session with PT 3 days/week supervised physical therapy; 45 min holding heaviest weight
	Duration training period 6 months
Drop-out	17 (14%) of which 9 (7.6%) lack of success (2 PFMT, 1 ES, 4 VC, 2 controls); 8 (7.4%) other reasons (1 PFMT, 2 ES, 2 VC, 3 controls)
Adherence	Mean compliance PFMT 92%, ES 91%, VC 93% after 6 months of treatment
Results	Cure objective (pad test): 12 (46%) PFMT, 13 (48%) ES, 11 (46%) VC, 2 (8%) controls; active treatment significantly better than controls (p = 0.003); difference between active groups NS
	QoL: active treatment significantly better than controls (p = 0.002); increase QoL, PFMT 28.4%, 32.4% ES, 30.3% VC, −3.6% controls; difference between active groups NS
Author	**Eyjólfsdóttir et al. (2009)**
Design	2-arm RCT: PFMT + ES; PFMT
Sample size and age (years)	24 women age 27–73
Diagnosis	SUI
Training protocol	PFMT both groups: 15 min/twice a day for 9 weeks
	ES: intermittent ES
Drop-out	Not reported
Adherence	Not reported
Results	UI episode frequency and quantity questionnaire and visual analogue scale: subjective cure/improvement in 70% of all women, no report on rates cured/improved or group differences
	Oxford scale, vaginal palpation, electromyography: both groups significant increase in PFM strength (PFMT, p = 0.007; PFMT + ES, p = 0.005; difference between groups NS)

Abd/add; Abduction/adduction; *BF,* biofeedback; *cyst.,* cystometry; *ES,* electrical stimulation; *GSI,* genuine stress incontinence; *IEF,* incontinence episode frequency; *IFT,* inferential therapy; *ITT,* intention to treat; *NS,* not statistically significant; *PFM,* pelvic floor muscle; *PFMC,* pelvic floor muscle contraction; *PFMT,* pelvic floor muscle training; *PT,* physical therapist; *QoL,* quality of life; *RCT,* randomized controlled trial; *SUI,* stress urinary incontinence; *UI,* urinary incontinence; *UDI,* Urogenital Distress Index; *UPP,* urethral pressure profile; *VC,* vaginal cone.

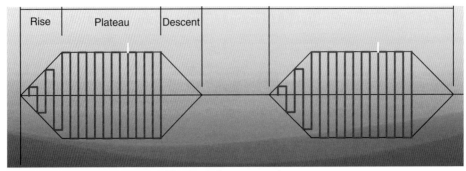

Fig. 7.1.6 Current envelope.

The choice for an optimal set of parameters depends on the particular device being used, the type of electrical current, the type of urinary incontinence, and the individual patient's needs and circumstances (Bø et al., 2017).

A standard list of parameters to be selected consists of (Belanger, 2010; Bø et al., 2017):
- *current amplitude* or intensity, ranging from micro- to milliamps;
- *pulse width* (i.e., time from the beginning to the end of one pulse cycle, usually expressed in microseconds or milliseconds pulse shape);
- *pulse shape* (rectangular, envelope, Gaussian, triangle, biphasic, sinusoidal, etc.);
- *type of current*, (direct [continuous, unidirectional flow], alternating [continuous, bidirectional flow] and pulsed [the non-continuous, interrupted and periodic flow of direct or alternating currents]);
- *pulse frequency*, or rate, in hertz (Hz);
- *train*, which is the continuous series of pulse cycles over time, usually lasting seconds;
- *train ramp-up time and ramp-down time*, where ramp-up time is the time elapsed from the onset (or baseline) to the plateau and ramp-down is the time elapsed from end plateau to end stimulus);
- *duty cycle* (D), the ratio of ON time to the summation of ON time + OFF time, expressed as a percentage (duty cycle = [ON]/[ON + OFF time] × 100, e.g., a duty cycle of 20% is calculated when the ON and OFF times equal 10 and 40 seconds, respectively);
- *impedance*, electric resistance of each tissue under influence of the ES, in ohms and designated as Z; and
- *time of each session*.

It has been suggested that ES restores continence by:
- strengthening the structural support of the urethra and the bladder neck (Plevnic et al., 1991);
- securing the resting and active closure of the proximal urethra (Erlandson and Fall, 1977);
- strengthening the PFMs (Sand et al., 1995);
- inhibiting reflex bladder contractions (Berghmans et al., 2002; Fall and Lindström, 1994);
- modifying the vascularity of the urethral and bladder neck tissues (Fall and Lindström, 1991, 1994; Plevnic et al., 1991); and
- improvement in electric activation, improving the proprioception and coordination of the pelvic floor during situations that cause SUI (Correia et al., 2014; Monga et al., 2012).

In the context of conservative or non-surgical, non-medical therapy, ES can be applied using surface electrodes (Brubaker, 2000; Goldberg and Sand, 2000; Govier et al., 2001; Jabs and Stanton, 2001).

Surface electrodes include *transcutaneous ES* (Berghmans et al., 2002; Brubaker, 2000; Jabs and Stanton, 2001) or transcutaneous electrical nerve stimulation (TENS), via suprapubic, sacral or penile/clitoral attachment of electrodes (Yamanishi et al., 2000), vaginal/anal plug electrodes (Dumoulin et al., 2017), plantar/thigh and similar stimulation (Walsh et al., 1999), and other surface placement of electrodes such as for interferential or maximum ES, and *percutaneous ES* (Amarenco et al., 2003; Govier et al., 2001), such as posterior tibial nerve stimulation, percutaneous nerve evaluation and electroacupuncture.

There are two main types of ES:
1. Long-term or chronic ES is delivered below the sensory threshold aiming at detrusor inhibition by afferent pudendal nerve stimulation. The electrically

evoked activity is suggested to result in reflex activation of hypogastric efferents and central inhibition of pelvic efferent mechanisms sensitive to low-frequency stimulation (Fall and Lindström, 1994). The device is used 6 to 12 hours a day for several months (Eriksen, 1989).

2. Maximal ES uses a high-intensity stimulus (just below the pain threshold). It aims to improve urethral closure. Fall and Lindström (1991) suggested a direct and reflexogenic contraction of striated periurethral musculature. In addition, detrusor inhibition by afferent pudendal nerve stimulation has been suggested (Berghmans et al., 2002). Maximal ES is applied with short duration (15–30 minutes) and is used several times a week (1–2 times daily, also using portable devices at home) (Yamanishi and Yasuda, 1998; Yamanishi et al., 1997; Yamanishi et al., 2000).

In addition to clinic-based mains-powered ES, portable ES devices for self-care by patients themselves at home have been developed (Berghmans et al., 2002). In the literature, some authors suggest that intermittent, short-term stimulation (maximal ES) by means of a portable, home-use device should usually be employed.

ES has been used for patients with SUI, symptoms of urgency, frequency and/or urge urinary incontinence, nocturia, detrusor overactivity and mixed urinary incontinence (Dumoulin et al., 2017).

In the rest of this chapter we will address the question about the most appropriate ES protocol for female patients with SUI, whether ES is better than no treatment, placebo or control treatment; whether ES is better than any other single treatment; and whether or not (additional) ES to other (additional) treatments adds any benefit. Finally we will address the results of ES on PFM strength and adverse events reported in the included studies. Information about male patients with SUI can be found in Chapter 11.

METHODS

The following qualitative summary of the evidence regarding ES in adult patients with SUI is based on RCTs included in five systematic reviews (Berghmans et al., 1998; Berghmans et al., 2000; Dumoulin et al., 2017; Schreiner et al., 2013; Stewart et al., 2017), with addition of trials performed after publication of the reviews and/or located through additional electronic searching on PubMed from 1998 to 2020 and the Cochrane Library.

Additionally, we searched the literature used in the most recent (Sixth) International Consultation on Incontinence (Dumoulin et al., 2017). Published abstracts were excluded.

EVIDENCE FOR ELECTRICAL STIMULATION TO TREAT STRESS URINARY INCONTINENCE SYMPTOMS

Table 7.1.7 provides details of results of all included studies (n = 19); one study consisted of two separate randomized controlled trials (RCTs) (Laycock and Jerwood, 1993). The PEDro rating scale was used to classify the methodological quality of the included studies (Table 7.1.8). PEDro scores were between 1 and 9, meaning that the studies had low to high methodological quality. It appeared that there was considerable variation in ES protocols with no consistent pattern emerging.

Interferential therapy was used in four trials (Alves et al., 2011; Henalla et al., 1989; Laycock and Jerwood, 1993; Olah et al., 1990). Few trials clearly stated whether direct or alternating currents were being used.

The most commonly used descriptors were frequency and pulse duration. Ten trials used a single frequency, ranging from 20 Hz (Brubaker et al., 1997; Goode et al., 2003) to 50 Hz (Alves et al., 2011; Bø et al., 1999; Castro et al., 2008; Correia et al., 2014; Dmochowski et al., 2019; Hahn et al., 1991; Luber and Wolde-Tsadik, 1997; Smith, 1996). Two trials included stimulation at both 10 and 35 Hz (Blowman et al., 1991; Knight et al., 1998), although the protocols were different, one at combined low and intermediate frequency (Jeyaseelan et al., 2000). Other protocols included stimulation at 12.5 and 50 Hz (Sand et al., 1995), 10 to 50 Hz (Shepherd et al., 1984), 0 to 100 Hz (Henalla et al., 1989; Olah et al., 1990), and finally a 30-minute treatment including 10 minutes at 1 Hz, 10 minutes 10 to 40 Hz and 10 minutes at 40 Hz (Laycock and Jerwood, 1993). Pulse durations ranged from 0.08 ms (Blowman et al., 1991) up to 100 ms (Alves et al., 2011; Brubaker et al., 1997). Twelve trials also detailed the duty cycle used during stimulation. The ratios ranged from 1:3 (Bø et al., 1999) and 1:2 (Alves et al., 2011; Brubaker et al., 1997; Castro et al., 2008; Correia et al., 2014; Luber and Wolde-Tsadik, 1997) to 1:1 (Blowman et al., 1991; Dmochowski et al., 2019; Goode et al., 2003; Knight et al., 1998), and two trials alternated between a ratio of 1:1 and 1:2 (Sand et al., 1995; Smith, 1996).

TABLE 7.1.8   **PEDro Quality Score of Randomized Controlled Trials in Systematic Review of Electrical Stimulation to Treat Stress Urinary Incontinence**

E – Eligibility criteria specified

1 – Subjects randomly allocated to groups

2 – Allocation concealed

3 – Groups similar at baseline

4 – Subjects blinded

5 – Therapist administering treatment blinded

6 – Assessors blinded

7 – Measures of key outcomes obtained from >85% of subjects

8 – Data analysed by intention to treat

9 – Statistical comparison between groups conducted

10 – Point measures and measures of variability provided

Study	E	1	2	3	4	5	6	7	8	9	10	Total Score
Shepherd et al. (1984)	+	+	+	+	+	−	+	+	−	−	−	6
Henalla et al. (1989)	+	+	−	?	−	−	−	+	−	?	+	3
Olah et al. (1990)	+	+	−	+	−	−	−	+	+	+	+	6
Von Hofbauer et al. (1990)	+	+	−	+	−	−	−	+	−	−	−	3
Blowman et al. (1991)	+	+	−	+	+	+	+	+	−	−	+	7
Hahn et al. (1991)	+	+	−	+	−	−	−	+	−	+	−	4
Laycock and Jerwood (1993) (Study 1)	+	+	−	+	−	−	−	+	−	+	+	5
Laycock and Jerwood (1993) (Study 2)	+	+	−	+	+	−	−	+	−	+	+	6
Sand et al. (1995)	+	+	+	+	+	+	+	−	+	+	+	9
Smith (1996)	+	+	−	−	−	−	−	+	−	+	+	4
Brubaker et al. (1997)	+	+	+	+	+	−	+	−	−	+	+	7
Luber and Wolde-Tsadik (1997)	+	+	+	+	+	+	+	−	−	+	+	8
Knight et al. (1998)	+	+	+	+	−	−	−	−	+	+	+	6
Bø et al. (1999)	+	+	+	+	−	−	+	+	+	+	+	8
Jeyaseelan et al. (2000)	+	+	+	+	−	−	+	+	+	+	+	8
Goode et al. (2003)	+	+	+	+	−	−	−	−	+	+	+	6
Castro et al. (2008)	+	+	+	−	−	+	+	−	+	+	+	7
Eyjólfsdóttir et al. (2009)	+	+	?	−	−	−	?	?	?	−	−	1

+, Criterion is clearly satisfied; −, criterion is not satisfied; ?, not clear if the criterion was satisfied.
The total score is determined by counting the number of criteria that are satisfied, except the 'eligibility criteria specified' score is not used to generate the total score. Total scores are out of 10.

Nine trials asked women to use the maximum tolerable intensity of stimulation (Alves et al., 2011; Bø et al., 1999; Brubaker et al., 1997; Castro et al., 2008; Correia et al., 2014; Goode et al., 2003; Laycock and Jerwood, 1993; Olah et al., 1990; Sand et al., 1995), and one trial increased output until there was a noticeable muscle contraction (Von Hofbauer et al., 1990). The trial compared 'low intensity' and 'maximal intensity' protocols. The trials by Von Hofbauer et al. (1990), Knight et al. (1998) and Goode et al. (2003) also asked women to add a voluntary PFM contraction to the stimulated contraction, although in the trial of Knight et al. (1998) this was only for the maximal stimulation group.

Current was most commonly delivered via a single vaginal electrode (Alves et al., 2011; Bø et al., 1999; Brubaker et al., 1997; Castro et al., 2008; Goode et al., 2003; Hahn et al., 1991; Luber and Wolde-Tsadik, 1997; Sand et al., 1995; Smith, 1996). One trial used both vaginal and buttock electrodes (Shepherd et al., 1995). In five trials external electrodes were used: abdomen and inside thighs (Olah et al., 1990), perineal body and symphysis pubis (Correia et al., 2014; Laycock and Jerwood, 1993), perineal and buttock (Blowman et al., 1991), and buttocks and thighs (Dmochowski et al., 2019), and in two studies the electrode placement was not clearly described (Henalla et al., 1989; Von Hofbauer et al., 1990).

The length and number of treatments was also highly variable. The longest treatment periods included daily treatment at home for 6 months (Bø et al., 1999; Hahn et al., 1991; Knight et al., 1998) and 20 minutes of clinic-based treatment three times a week for 6 months (Castro et al., 2008). Medium-length treatment periods were based on once-daily treatment at home for 8 weeks every other day (Goode et al., 2003) and twice-daily treatment for 6 weeks (Correia et al., 2014) and at home for 8 weeks (Brubaker et al., 1997) to 12 weeks (Dmochowski et al., 2019; Luber and Wolde-Tsadik, 1997; Sand et al., 1995). The shortest treatment periods were all for clinic-based stimulation, ranging from 10 (Henalla et al., 1989; Laycock and Jerwood, 1993) to 12 (Olah et al., 1990) to 16 (Knight et al., 1998) and 18 sessions in total (Von Hofbauer et al., 1990).

Comparing two protocols with different intensity of ES, Knight et al. (1998) found a trend, across a range of outcomes including self-report of cure or improvement, pad test and PFM strength measurement, measured by vaginal squeeze pressure, for women who received clinic-based maximal stimulation to benefit more women in the low-intensity stimulation group, although most differences were not significant.

Also comparing two protocols but now with low- and medium-frequency current, Alves et al. (2011) found that the two ES protocols applied were equally effective in the treatment of SUI, based on a 1-hour pad test as an objective outcome measure of urinary incontinence, a visual analogue scale to evaluate subjective severity of urinary incontinence and perineal pressure performed with a perineometer to test PFM maximum voluntary contraction.

Effects of surface ES were compared with intravaginal electrical stimulation (IVES). The authors found that both surface ES and IVES improved SUI, quality of life, strength and pressure of PFM contraction (Correia et al., 2014).

Dmochowski et al. (2019) compared in a multicenter study, conducted at 12 urology clinics in the United States over 12 weeks, an external neuromuscular electrostimulation (NMES) with a comparator device (IVES) and found that both devices provided broadly similar, clinically meaningful improvements in a range of subjective and objective measures of SUI.

Is Electrical Stimulation Better Than No Treatment, Control or Placebo Treatment?

Henalla et al. (1989) compared ES with no treatment in women with SUI. Eight of the 25 women receiving ES were 'objectively' cured or improved (negative pad test or >50% reduction in the pad test) at 3 months versus none of the 25 women in the no treatment group. One trial compared ES with control intervention (women were offered use of the Continence Guard [Coloplast, Minneapolis, MN], used infrequently by 14 of 30 controls) in women with SUI (Bø et al., 1999). Bø et al. (1999) found that ES was better than control intervention for change in leakage episodes over 3 days, using the Social Activity Index and Leakage Index. However, only one of these measures (change in leakage episodes over 3 days) remained significant (p = 0.047) with intention-to-treat analysis. PFM activity was significantly improved in the ES group after treatment, but the change in activity was not significant when compared with controls. There was no difference in the primary outcome measure (i.e., pad test with standardized bladder volume). Two of 30 controls were cured (<2 g leakage) on the pad test compared to 7 of 25 in the ES group. One of 30 women in the control group reported that the condition was 'unproblematic' after treatment versus 3 of 25 in the ES group, but 28 of 30 and 19 of 25 wanted further treatment, respectively.

Six trials compared ES with placebo ES in women with urodynamic stress incontinence (Blowman et al., 1991; Jeyaseelan et al., 2000; Laycock and Jerwood, 1993; Luber and Wolde-Tsadik, 1997; Sand et al., 1995; Von Hofbauer et al., 1990). Blowman et al. (1991) compared ES/PFMT versus placebo ES/PFMT in women with urodynamic stress incontinence, and for the purposes of analysis this trial was considered to be a comparison of

ES with placebo ES. Von Hofbauer et al. (1990) provided minimal detail of participants, methods and stimulation parameters. Laycock and Jerwood (1993) used clinic-based, short-term (10 treatments) maximal stimulation with an interferential current applied with external surface electrodes. The ES treatment regimen of Jeyaseelan et al. (2000) consisted of a new stimulation pattern, such as background low frequency (to target the slow-twitch fibres) and intermediate frequency with an initial doublet (to target the fast-twitch fibres) applied with a vaginal probe. Four trials were based on daily home stimulation for 6 (Blowman et al., 1991), 8 (Jeyaseelan et al., 2000) or 12 weeks (Luber and Wolde-Tsadik, 1997; Sand et al., 1995).

The two most comparable trials in terms of stimulation parameters reported contrasting findings. Sand et al. (1995) found that the ES group has significantly greater changes in the number of leakage episodes in 24 hours, number of pads used, amount of leakage on the pad test and PFM activity (PFM strength measurement, measured by vaginal squeeze pressure) than the placebo stimulation group. In addition, the ES group had significantly improved subjective measures (e.g., visual analogue measure of severity) than the placebo group. Neither group demonstrated significant change in the quality-of-life measure (Short Form 36 Health Survey Questionnaire [SF-36]). In contrast, Luber and Wolde-Tsadik (1997) did not find any statistically significant differences between ES and placebo ES groups for rates of self-reported cure or improvement, objective cure (negative stress test during urodynamics), number of incontinence episodes in 24 hours or Valsalva leak point pressure.

The other trials generally favoured ES over placebo ES. Laycock and Jerwood (1993) generally found significantly greater improvements in the ES group (pad test, PFM activity, self-reported severity), although the decrease in incontinence episodes was not significantly different between the groups post-treatment. Blowman et al. (1991) found a significant decrease in the number of leakage episodes in the ES group only. Von Hofbauer et al. (1990) reported that 3 of 11 women in the ES group were cured/improved (not defined) versus 0 of 11 in the placebo ES group.

Jeyaseelan et al. (2000) did not find statistically significant differences between the two study groups when PFM strength was measured by a device

measuring vaginal squeeze pressure, but in contrast, when strength was assessed using digital assessment a statistical significant difference was found. When endurance was assessed, an improvement in favour of ES was found over time in the ES group, but not in the sham ES group. The authors suggested that between-group differences may not be significant as a result of the high degree of variance combined with a small sample size. No changes were reported using a pad test or diaries, but a significant change in favour of the ES group using the Urogenital Distress Index (UDI) score (Jeyaseelan et al., 2000).

Is Electrical Stimulation Better Than Any Other Single Treatment?

Henalla et al. (1989) compared ES (interferential) with vaginal oestrogens (Premarin). Eight of 25 women in the stimulation group reported that they were cured or improved versus 3 of 24 in the oestrogen therapy group. There was a significant reduction in leakage on the pad test in the stimulation group but not in the oestrogen group. In contrast, the maximum urethral closure pressure was significantly increased in the oestrogen group but not in the stimulation group. Long-term follow-up (9 months) found that subjectively, 1 of the 8 women in the ES group who had reported cure/improvement post-treatment had recurrent symptoms, as did all 3 women in the oestrogen group once oestrogen therapy ceased.

Comparing ES with PFMT, using a pad test as mentioned before, only Bø et al. (1999) found a statistically significant difference in favour of PFMT. It was not clear if the cure data reported by Von Hofbauer et al. (1990) were derived from a symptom scale or voiding diary; these data were therefore excluded. Only Bø et al. (1999) measured leakage episodes and quality of life (Social Activity Index) in SUI women. There was no statistically significant difference between the groups for either outcome. At 9 months post-treatment, Henalla et al. (1989) found that 3 of 17 PFMT women and 1 of 8 in the ES group reported recurrent symptoms.

In both the trials of Olah et al. (1990) and of Bø et al. (1999) there was no statistically significant difference between vaginal cone (VC) and ES groups for self-reported cure, self-reported cure/improvement or leakage episodes in 24 hours. Bø et al. (1999) did not find any statistically significant difference between the groups in quality of life (Social Activity Index). Olah et al. (1990) had to exclude some women from their trial prior to randomization because they could not use cones in the vagina (e.g., wedging of cones).

One study (Castro et al., 2008) in a four-arm RCT compared women with urodynamically proven SUI with ES, PFMT, VC and a control group with no treatment. Only data of those women (101 of 118) who completed the study were analysed for final results. Based on a pad test with standardized bladder volume, 48% of ES, 46% of PFMT, 46% of VC and only 8% of controls were cured, defined as <2 g in pad weight. All active groups were effective but superior to no treatment, with no significant difference between the active groups (Castro et al., 2008). The increase of quality of life was 32.4% in the ES group, 28.4% in the PFMT group and 30.3% in the VC group, whereas there was a decrease in the no treatment group of 3.6%. There was no significant difference in quality of life between groups.

Is (Additional) ES Better Than Other (Additional) Treatments?

For comparisons of ES with biofeedback-assisted PFMT versus biofeedback-assisted PFMT alone versus a control condition, reporting was limited to a single trial. In the study of Goode et al. (2003), intention-to-treat analysis showed that incontinence was reduced by a mean of 68.6% with biofeedback-assisted PFMT, 71.9% with ES with biofeedback-assisted PFMT and 52.5% with the control condition. In comparison with the control group, both interventions were significantly more effective, but they were not significantly different from each other (p = 0.60). The ES with biofeedback-assisted PFMT had significantly better patient self-perception of outcome (p < 0.001) and satisfaction with progress (p = 0.02).

Two trials compared ES in combination with PFMT versus PFMT alone in women with stress incontinence (Von Hofbauer et al., 1990; Luber and Wolde-Tsadik, 1997). As both arms in these trials received the same PFMT, the trials are essentially investigating the effect of ES. Von Hofbauer et al. (1990) gave minimal detail of participants, methods and stimulation parameters. In a three-arm RCT, Knight et al. (1998) compared PFMT versus PFMT with home-based low-intensity

ES versus PFMT with clinic-based maximal-intensity stimulation. Ten of 21 women in the PFMT group, 9 of 25 women in the low-intensity stimulation group and 16 of 24 in the maximum-intensity stimulation group reported cure or great improvement. All three groups had significant improvements in the pad test after treatment, with no significant differences in the percentage reduction between the groups. Similarly, all three groups had improvements in vaginal squeeze pressure, but there were no significant differences in improvement.

Overall, Knight et al. (1998) did not find any clear benefits of ES in addition to PFMT. This finding is similar to that of Von Hofbauer et al. (1990), who found no significant differences between the groups receiving combined ES/PFMT and PFMT alone.

Muscle Strength

Several studies reported on PFM strength as an outcome measure (Alves et al., 2011; Blowman et al., 1991; Bø et al., 1999; Jeyaseelan et al., 2000; Knight et al., 1998; Laycock and Jerwood, 1993; Sand et al., 1995; Shepherd et al., 1984). In all but study 1 in the trial of Laycock and Jerwood (1993), a (kind of) device, measuring PFM strength by vaginal squeeze pressure, was used with contrasting results between the studies. Laycock and Jerwood (1993) did use digital assessment in that trial.

Shepherd et al. (1984) did not find any difference in PFM strength between groups, although no statistical tests were performed to confirm this.

An improvement of PFM strength in both groups (PFMT + ES vs PFMT + sham ES) was noted, with more improvement in the PFMT + ES group reported in the study of Blowman et al. (1991). However, no statistical tests were performed to test statistical significance.

When digitally tested, Laycock and Jerwood (1993) found a pre-/post-treatment statistically significant improvement (p = 0.0035) only in the ES group (PFMT vs ES [interferential therapy]). In this trial they did not report the in-between results. In the second trial they used PFM strength measurement, measured by vaginal squeeze pressure to measure PFM strength at PFM maximal contraction and found a significant increase only in the ES group.

Sand et al. (1995) performed PFM strength measurements using a device measuring vaginal squeeze pressure in 35 patients and 17 controls who used identical sham devices before and after a 15-week treatment period. The active group had a significant improvement in vaginal muscle strength when compared to the controls. In the active group mean (± standard error), change of vaginal muscle strength (mmHg) before and after treatment was 4.6 ± 1.4, and in the control group it was 1.1 ± 1.5 (p = 0.02).

Knight et al. (1998) found a significant increase of PFM strength in all groups, the biggest in the ES group in a clinical setting. However, there was no significant difference between groups. In contrast with the ES group, Bø et al. (1999) reported significant improvement of PFM strength only in the PFMT group (compared with no treatment). As indicated before, Jeyaseelan et al. (2000) did not detect any statistically significant differences between ES and sham ES when PFM strength was measured using a device measuring vaginal squeeze pressure. However, if strength was assessed using digital assessment, a statistical significant difference in favour of ES was found.

The difference between included studies with respect to outcome of PFM strength, using a device measuring PFM strength by vaginal squeeze pressure, can be explained by the huge variation in measurement protocols, devices used and assessment differences. For instance, in the studies of Shepherd et al. (1984) and Blowman et al. (1991), no statistical tests were performed. Knight et al. (1998) and Laycock and Jerwood (1993) did not blind the outcome measurement assessors, whereas Sand et al. (1995), Bø et al. (1999) and Jeyaseelan et al. (2000) did.

Adverse Events

Four trials (Bø et al., 1999; Hahn et al., 1991; Sand et al., 1995; Smith, 1996;) reported side effects related to ES, including vaginal irritation or infection, urinary tract infection, pain, and/or vaginal bleeding. Sand et al. (1995) reported that all adverse events were reversible. Besides the ES group, the VC group also reported adverse events in the trial by Bø et al. (1999). Dmochowski et al. (2019) reported that there were similar, not treatment-related, proportions of mild to moderate adverse events in both groups, with 9% of NMES users and 8.8% of comparator users, and serious adverse events in 2 of 89 NMES users and 5 of 91 comparator users.

CONCLUSION

- There is a marked lack of consistency in the ES protocols; this implies a lack of understanding of the physiological principles of rehabilitating urinary incontinence through ES used in clinical practice to treat women with SUI.
- There is insufficient evidence to judge whether ES is better than no treatment or placebo treatment for women with SUI.
- Although conclusive evidence is lacking, PFMT seems to be better than ES in women with SUI.
- There is insufficient evidence to determine whether ES is better than vaginal oestrogens or VCs in women with SUI.
- At present, it seems that there is no extra benefit in adding ES to PFMT.
- There is need for more basic research to explore the working mechanism of ES in women with SUI, and to determine the best ES protocol(s) and outcome measures for this kind of patient.

CLINICAL RECOMMENDATIONS

- As yet, there is no convincing evidence from RCTs that ES is a useful treatment in women with SUI. So far, it is impossible to recommend the most optimal ES regimen and protocol.
- A protocol based on the hypothesis that ES might help patients who are unaware of how to contract the PFMs and are not capable of doing so voluntarily to regain awareness of the PFMs should be considered for testing in a high-quality RCT.

REFERENCES

Alves, P. G., Nunues, F. R., & Guirro, E. C. (2011). Comparison between two different neuromuscular electrical stimulation protocols for the treatment of female stress urinary incontinence: A randomized controlled trial. *Revista Brasileira de Fisioterapia, 15*(5), 393–398.

Amarenco, G., Ismael, S. S., Even-Schneider, A., et al. (2003). Urodynamic effect of acute transcutaneous posterior tibial nerve stimulation in overactive bladder. *Journal of Urology, 169,* 2210–2215.

Ayeleke, R. O., Hay-Smith, E. J., & Omar, M. I. (2015). Pelvic floor muscle training added to another active treatment versus the same active treatment alone for urinary incontinence in women. *Cochrane Database of Systematic Reviews, 11* CD010551.

Berghmans, L. C. M., Hendriks, H. J., Bø, K., et al. (1998). Conservative treatment of genuine stress incontinence in women: A systematic review of randomized clinical trials. *British Journal of Urology, 82*(2), 181–191.

Berghmans, L. C. M., Waalwijk van Doorn, E. S. C., van Nieman, F., et al. (2000). Efficacy of extramural physical therapy modalities in women with proven bladder over-activity: A randomised clinical trial. *Neurourology and Urodynamics, 19*(4), 496–497.

Berghmans, L. C. M., Waalwijk van Doorn, E. S. C., van Nieman, F. H., et al. (2002). Efficacy of physical therapeutic modalities in women with proven bladder overactivity. *European Urology, 41*, 581–588.

Blowman, C., Pickles, C., Emery, S., et al. (1991). Prospective double blind controlled trial of intensive physiotherapy with and without stimulation of the pelvic floor in the treatment of genuine stress incontinence. *Physiotherapy, 77*, 661–664.

Bø, K., Frawley, H. C., Haylen, B. T., et al. (2017). An International Urogynecological Association (IUGA)/International Continence Society (ICS) joint report on the terminology for the conservative and nonpharmacological management of female pelvic floor dysfunction. *International Urogynecology Journal, 28*(2), 191–213.

Bø, K., Talseth, T., & Holme, I. (1999). Single blind, randomised controlled trial of pelvic floor exercises, electrical stimulation, vaginal cones, and no treatment in management of genuine stress incontinence in women. *British Medical Journal, 318*, 487–493.

Brubaker, L. (2000). Electrical stimulation in overactive bladder. *Urology, 55*(Suppl. 5A), 17–23.

Brubaker, L., Benson, T., Bent, A., et al. (1997). Transvaginal electrical stimulation for female urinary incontinence. *American Journal of Obstetrics and Gynecology, 177*, 536–540.

Castro, R. A., Arruda, R. M., Zanetti, M. R., et al. (2008). Single-blind, randomized, controlled trial of pelvic floor muscle training, electrical stimulation, vaginal cones, and no active treatment in the management of stress urinary incontinence. *Clinics, 63*, 465–472.

Chancellor, M. B., & Leng, W. (2002). The mechanism of action of sacral nerve stimulation in the treatment of detrusor overactivity and urinary retention. In U. Jonas, & V. Grünewald (Eds.), *New Perspectives in Sacral Nerve Stimulation*. London: Martin Dunitz. Chapter 3.

Correia, G. N., Pereira, V. S., Hirakawa, H. S., et al. (2014). Effects of surface and intravaginal electrical stimulation in the treatment of women with stress urinary incontinence: randomized controlled trial. *European Journal of Obstetrics & Gynecology and Reproductive Biology, 173*, 113–118.

Dmochowski, R., Lynch, C. M., Efros, M., et al. (2019). External electrical stimulation compared with intra-vaginal electrical stimulation for the treatment of stress urinary incontinence in women: A randomized controlled noninferiority trial. *Neurourology and Urodynamics, 38*(7), 1834–1843.

Dumoulin, C., Adewuyi, T., & Booth, J. (2017). Adult conservative management. In P. Abrams, L. Cardozo, A. Wagg, & A. Wein (Eds.), *Incontinence*. Tokyo: 6th International Consultation on Incontinence. September 2016. ICS-ICUD 2017.

Eriksen, B. C. (1989). *Electrostimulation of the pelvic floor in female urinary incontinence*. Norway: Doctoral thesis. University of Trondheim.

Erlandson, B. E., & Fall, M. (1977). Intravaginal electrical stimulation in urinary incontinence. An experimental and clinical study. *Scandinavian Journal of Urology and Nephrology, 44*, 1.

Everaert, K., Lefevere, F., Hagens, P., et al. (1999). *Influence of FES parameters on urethral pressure (Abstract)*. Denver, Colorado: Proceedings of the International Continence Society 29th Annual Meeting.

Eyjólfsdóttir, H., Ragnarsdóttir, M., & Geirsson, G. (2009). [Pelvic floor muscle training with and without functional electrical stimulation as treatment for stress urinary incontinence]. *Laeknabladid, 95*(9), 575–580 quiz 581.

Fall, M. (1998). Advantages and pitfalls of functional electrical stimulation. *Acta Obstetricia et Gynecologica Scandinavica, 77*(Suppl. 168), 16–21.

Fall, M., & Lindström, S. (1991). Electrical stimulation: A physiologic approach to the treatment of urinary incontinence. *Urologic Clinics of North America, 18*, 393–407.

Fall, M., & Lindström, S. (1994). Functional electrical stimulation: Physiological basis and clinical principles. *International Urogynecology Journal, 5*, 296–304.

Goldberg, R. P., & Sand, P. K. (2000). Electromagnetic pelvic floor stimulation: Applications for the gynecologist. *Obstetrical and Gynecological Survey, 55*(11), 715–720.

Goode, P. S., Burgio, K. I., Locher, J. L., et al. (2003). Effect of behavioral training with and without pelvic floor electrical stimulation on stress incontinence in women. A randomized controlled trial. *JAMA, 290*, 345–352.

Govier, F. E., Litwiller, S., Nitti, V., et al. (2001). Percutaneous afferent neuromodulation for the refractory overactive bladder: Results of a multicenter study. *Journal of Urology, 165*, 1193–1198.

Günter, C., Delbeke, J., & Ortiz-Catalan, M. (2019). Safety of long-term electrical peripheral nerve stimulation: review of the state of the art. *Journal of NeuroEngineering and Rehabilitation, 16*, 13.

Hahn, H. N., Sommar, S., & Fall, M. (1991). A comparative study of pelvic floor training and electrical stimulation for the treatment of genuine female urinary incontinence. *Neurourology and Urodynamics, 10*(6), 545–554.

Hay-Smith, J., Berghmans, B., Burgio, K., et al. (2009). Committee 12: Adult conservative management. In P. Abrams, L. Cardozo, S. Khoury, et al. (Eds.), *Incontinence: fourth international consultation on incontinence* (pp. 1025–1120). Paris: Health Publication/Editions 21.

Hay-Smith, E. J., Bø, K., Berghmans, L. C., et al. (2001). Pelvic floor muscle training for urinary incontinence in women. *Cochrane Database Systematic Reviews Issue, 1* Art. No. CD001407.

Henalla, S. M., Hutchins, C. J., Robinson, P., et al. (1989). Non-operative methods in the treatment of female genuine stress incontinence of urine. *Journal of Obstetrics and Gynaecology,, 9*(3), 222–225.

Hubert, C., Andre, D., Dubar, L., et al. (2019). *Stimulation of continuum electrical stimulation conduction and Joule heating using DEM domain.* https://hal.archives-ouvertes.fr/hal-02354556.

Jabs, C. F. I., & Stanton, S. L. (2001). Urge incontinence and detrusor instability. *International Urogynecology Journal, 12*, 58–68.

Jeyaseelan, S. M., Haslam, E. J., Winstanley, J., et al. (2000). An evaluation of a new pattern of electrical stimulation as a treatment for urinary stress incontinence: A randomized, double-blind, controlled trial. *Clinical Rehabilitation, 14*, 631–640.

Knight, S., Laycock, J., & Naylor, D. (1998). Evaluation of neuromuscular electrical stimulation in the treatment of genuine stress incontinence. *Physiotherapy, 84*(2), 61–71.

La Norme Française (NF), la Norme Européenne (EN) Appareils électromédicaux: 60601-2-10, C 74-313, ICS: 11.040.60, Septembre 2015.

Laycock, J., & Jerwood, D. (1993). Does pre-modulated interferential therapy cure genuine stress incontinence? *Physiotherapy, 79*, 553–560.

Luber, K. M., & Wolde-Tsadik, G. (1997). Efficacy of functional electrical stimulation in treating genuine stress incontinence: A randomized clinical trial. *Neurourology and Urodynamics, 16*, 543–551.

Monga, A. K., Tracey, M. R., & Subbaroyan, J. (2012). A systematic review of clinical studies of electrical stimulation for treatment of lower urinary tract dysfunction. *International Urogynecology Journal, 23*, 993–1005.

Moore, K. N., Griffiths, D., & Hughton, A. (1999). Urinary incontinence after radical prostatectomy: A randomized controlled trial comparing pelvic muscle exercises with or without electrical stimulation. *BJU International, 83*, 57–65.

Olah, K. S., Bridges, N., Denning, J., et al. (1990). The conservative management of patients with symptoms of stress incontinence: A randomized, prospective study comparing weighted vaginal cones and interferential therapy. *American Journal of Obstetrics and Gynecology, 162*(1), 87–92.

Plevnic, S., Janez, J., & Vodušek, D. B. (1991). Electrical stimulation. In K. J. Krane, & M. B. Siroky (Eds.), *Clinical Neuro-Urology*. Boston, MA: Little Brown.

Sand, P. K., Richardson, D. A., Staskin, D. R., et al. (1995). Pelvic floor electrical stimulation in the treatment of genuine stress incontinence: A multicenter placebo-controlled trial. *American Journal of Obstetrics and Gynecology, 173*, 72–79.

Scheepens, W. A. (2003). *Progress in sacral neuromodulation of the lower urinary tract*. Maastricht, The Netherlands: Doctoral thesis. University of Maastricht.

Shepherd, A. M., Tribe, E., & Bainton, D. (1984). Maximum perineal stimulation: A controlled study. *British Journal of Urology, 56*, 644–646.

Smith, J. J. (1996). Intravaginal stimulation randomized trial. *Journal of Urology, 155*, 127.

Stewart, F., Gameiro, L. F., El Dib, R., Gameiro, M. O., Kapoor, A., & Amaro, J. L. (2016). Electrical stimulation with non-implanted electrodes for overactive bladder in adults. *Cochrane Database of Systematic Reviews, 12* CD010098.

Tadej, B. A., & Marko, M. U. (2010). Basic functional electrical stimulation (FES) of extremites - an Engineer's view, Technology and health care. *Journal of the European society for engineering and Medicine*. https://doi.org/10.3233/THC-2010-0588

Van Balkan, M. R., Vandoninck, V., Gisolf, K. W. H., et al. (2001). Posterior tibial nerve stimulation as neuromodulative treatment of lower urinary tract dysfunction. *Journal of Urology, 166*, 914–918.

Vodušek, D. B., Light, J. K., & Libby, J. M. (1986). Detrusor inhibition induced by stimulation of pudendal nerve afferents. *Neurourology and Urodynamics, 5*, 2381–2389.

Von Hofbauer, J., Preisinger, F., & Nurnberger, N. (1990). [The value of physical therapy in genuine female stress incontinence]. *Zeitschrift für Urologie und Nephrologie, 83*, 249.

Walsh, I. K., Johnston, R. S., & Keane, P. F. (1999). Transcutaneous sacral neurostimulation for irritative voiding dysfunction. *European Urology, 35*, 192–196.

Weil, E. H., Ruiz Cerda, J. L., & Eerdmans, P. H. (2000). Sacral root neuromodulation in the treatment of refractory urinary urge incontinence: A prospective randomized clinical trial. *European Urology, 37*(2), 161–171.

Wessale, J. L., Geddes, L. A., Ayers, G. M., et al. (1992). Comparison of rectangular and exponential current pulses for evoking sensation. *Annals of Biomedical Engineering, 20*, 237–244.

Yamanishi, T., Mizuno, T., Watanabe, M., et al. (2010). Randomized, placebo controlled study of electrical stimulation with pelvic floor muscle training for severe urinary incontinence after radical prostatectomy. *Journal of Urology, 184*, 2007–2012.

Yamanishi, T., Sakakibara, R., Uchiyama, T., et al. (2000). Comparative study of the effects of magnetic versus electrical stimulation on inhibition of detrusor overactivity. *Urology, 56*, 777–781.

Yamanishi, T., & Yasuda, K. (1998). Electrical stimulation for stress incontinence. *International Urogynecology Journal, 9*, 281–290.

Yamanishi, T., Yasuda, K., Sakakibara, R., et al. (1997). Pelvic floor electrical stimulation in the treatment of stress incontinence: An investigational study and a placebo controlled double-blind trial. *Journal of Urology, 158*(6), 2127–2131.

7.2 Overactive Bladder

Bary Berghmans, Gommert Van Koeveringe and Nol Bernards

PREVALENCE, CAUSES AND PATHOPHYSIOLOGY OF OVERACTIVE BLADDER AND URGENCY

Overactive bladder (OAB) is defined by the International Continence Society (ICS) as a symptom complex of urinary urgency, usually with urinary frequency and nocturia, with or without urinary incontinence, in the absence of urinary tract infection or other obvious pathology (Haylen et al., 2010). Urgency is defined as a complaint of a sudden, compelling desire to pass urine which is difficult to defer (Haylen et al., 2010). When urgency is accompanied by urinary incontinence, this is called *urgency urinary incontinence*.

Urgency is a symptom that fits a quite heterogeneous patient group, making it difficult to identify clear comorbid conditions or even causes for urgency within a classification of problem areas.

PREVALENCE OF OVERACTIVE BLADDER AND URGENCY URINARY INCONTINENCE

OAB is bothersome (Coyne et al., 2009; Irwin et al., 2008; Vaughan et al., 2011) and associated with a decrease of physical health, comorbidity such as skin infections in the genital area, lower urinary tract infections, sleep disorders (Castro Díaz et al., 2009), significantly higher body mass index, thyroid dysfunction (Robles-Mejía et al., 2019), impaired quality of life (Vaughan et al., 2011), anxiety, depression and sick leave from work (Coyne et al., 2008). OAB is likely to be associated with increased risk of falls and fractures (Moon et al., 2011).

In both women and men, a large number of OAB cases cannot be attributed to any comorbid condition and are therefore referred to as idiopathic.

Prevalence estimates from as low as 2% up to 53% have been reported (Milsom et al., 2016). Many studies on OAB have reported prevalence estimates between 10% and 20% (Irwin et al., 2011). However, many of these studies have not measured bothersomeness, which limits their impact. Overall, in the latest recommendations of the International Consultation on Incontinence (ICI), the median OAB prevalence estimate based on the included studies was 16.5% (range: 2%–35% in men and 3%–41% in women) (Milsom et al., 2016). In more recent studies, however, prevalence numbers are lower compared to earlier estimates (Milsom et al., 2016).

Overall, approximately 9% to 13% of women are bothered by urgency urinary incontinence (UUI) (Coyne et al., 2009; Irwin et al., 2008; Stewart et al., 2003). UUI increases linearly with age, with only 2% of women aged 18 to 24 years affected compared to 19% of women aged 65 to 74 years (Coyne et al., 2009; Dumoulin et al., 2018; Irwin et al., 2008; Stewart et al., 2003). Common risk factors for UUI in women include age, parity, obesity, neurological disease and chronic constipation (Gamble et al., 2010). UUI in women imposes an immense cost burden on the healthcare system and society, and it is associated with a significantly poorer quality of life and increased psychosomatic comorbidity such as depression (Stewart et al., 2003).

In men, global risk factors for UUI include bladder outlet obstruction, ageing, neurological conditions, various inflammatory processes of the bladder and psychosocial stressors (Smith and Wein, 2011).

To provide insight into the biological rationale for urgency, the normal physiological mechanism of bladder filling will first be explained, supplemented with the working mechanisms at the level of the bladder and at the level of the processing and interpretation of signals in the central nervous system that underlie the development of the perception of urgency.

NATURE OF THE BLADDER FILLING SENSATION

Current views on bladder sensation are derived largely from urodynamic studies (De Wachter et al., 2011). Relevant literature has shown that authors disagreed on the character of the sensation: episodic or continuous. Chapple et al. (2005) have described the pattern in which normal sensations of bladder filling are episodic in nature; the individual sensations gradually increase in intensity. As the bladder fills, the sensations appear in a standard order. The first sensation appears first, then declines and is followed by further episodic sensations with increasing intensity, namely the first desire to void and the normal desire to void. Eventually, the final, strong desire to void, also called *urge*, triggers the subject to find a toilet to void (Chapple et al., 2005).

Another way in which normal bladder sensations can develop is a continuous sensation model (Gillespie et al., 2009). This model states that signals are continuously generated within the bladder. This means that there are no episodic, waxing and waning sensations but that, as the bladder fills, continuous signalling increases in intensity and possibly changes in character. Modulated by different aspects, these afferent signals can be suppressed, probed or sampled by the mind if desired and finally may be transformed into a sensation of urge that consequently leads to finding a toilet (Heeringa, 2012).

Nathan (1956) pointed out that different sensations might be originating from different anatomical locations. But is there any conclusive anatomical evidence for different sensations of bladder filling? Gillespie et al. (2009) suggested that the perception of the degree of filling is determined by, among other things, the effect of the afferent signal coming from the bladder and/or the urethra, by supraspinal control (attention, concentration) both in a facilitating and inhibiting sense. De Wachter et al. (2011) stated, reviewing relevant and often-cited studies, that there is no real evidence to support the view that different filling sensations are conducted through different peripheral nerves. These authors concluded that an anatomical basis for perceiving different sensations is therefore wide open.

To date, the nature and thus the development of urgency (urinary incontinence) is also unclear. The following questions still arise in the literature: Is the sensation of filling in patients with 'urgency' the same and only stronger compared to that in 'normal people' who have the urge to go to the toilet (intensification of the normal urge)? Is the sensation of filling completely different and may it be generated by a different mechanism (Blaivas et al., 2009; Gillespie et al., 2009)?

Heeringa (2012) stated that urgency is seen as a pathological, all-or-none sensation that can clearly be differentiated from a sensation of bladder fullness (Chapple et al., 2005; Morrison et al., 2002). Urgency is experienced in different pathological conditions, such as OAB, but also in, for example, urolithiasis, in urinary tract infection and after bladder/pelvic radiotherapy (Dutz et al., 2019). Consequently, different causes of urgency, such as caused by involuntary detrusor contractions, exist. (Hyman et al., 2001). But urgency may not always be pathological. During cystometry, both patients with the sensation of urgency but no detrusor overactivity (e.g., no detrusor overactivity during bladder filling) (Oliver et al., 2003) and healthy persons without lower urinary tract symptoms with detrusor overactivity report to have urgency (Robertson et al., 1994). Urgency can also be caused by spontaneous relaxations of the urethra (Kulseng-Hanssen and Kristoffersen, 1988). These relaxations have been described as urethral instability or overactivity. The location of the urgency sensation can be different for different subjects (FitzGerald et al., 2005). For example, more than half of the patients with painful bladder syndrome and a minority of patients with OAB localized their urgency to both suprapubic and vulvar/urethral locations, whereas most OAB patients located the sensation only perineally. Healthy subjects and patients with stress urinary incontinence, however, locate the sensation of urge in the suprapubic region (FitzGerald et al., 2005). Urgency might be a sensation that can be graded. At the same time, as described before, it can be questioned whether urgency is in fact a different sensation than the normal urge to void or, alternatively, it is the same sensation but more pronounced (Blaivas et al., 2009; de Wachter and Hanno, 2010). Blaivas et al. (2009) showed by means of questionnaires that there are two types of urgency. One is an intensification of the normal urge to void, and the other is a different sensation. These different types of urgency might represent different etiology and respond differently to treatment options. This indicates that a comprehensive classification of these possible different types of urgency can be of great importance.

AFFERENT INPUT TO THE CENTRAL NERVOUS SYSTEM

Afferent information originates from different areas, such as the bladder wall, bladder neck, trigone, proximal urethra and sphincters. From there, bladder afferent output is transmitted by different functional subsets of afferent nerve fibres, and depending on the situation and/or intensity of the transmission of the stimulus, it can be perceived or not.

Thus the central nervous system receives information from different sources and of different nature. It is still unclear how and when the central nervous system uses this information to perceive filling, and how and when this is followed by a micturition reflex. It seems that only part of the afferent information contributes to conscious perception (sensibility).

It remains unclear which subsets of nerve fibers have which properties (Gillespie et al., 2009; Janssen et al., 2017). Gillespie et al. (2009) distinguished five functional subsets in afferent nerve fibres classified according to the nature of the stimuli to which they are sensitive:
1. sensitive to noxious stimuli;
2. sensitive to mechanical stimuli (stretch, pressure);
3. sensitive to various substances released from the urothelium in response to stretch, such as prostaglandins, adenosine triphosphate, nitrogen oxide and acetylcholine ('chemical response');
4. sensitive to myofibroblast contraction; and
5. sensitive to events taking place in the bladder wall: rapid stretching of the bladder wall induces local contractions, and this phasic motor activity then produces a phasic afferent stimulus.

With an increase in filling, the afferent signal will become stronger, and in this continuum of bladder filling, indications such as 'sensation', 'need', 'strong need', 'urge' and possibly 'pain' can be placed. Gillespie et al. (2009) suggested other terminology, originating from urodynamic investigation, such as 'first sensation to void', 'second sensation to void' and 'urge'. The fact that a urodynamic investigation is based on artificial filling makes it questionable whether these sensation markers can be compared with the normal filling sensations.

Similar diagrams have been drawn to describe the situation in patients with 'urgency'. In such patients the first sensations occur at low bladder volumes, and strong sensations, now called *urgency*, are experienced at low volume. Urgency is followed shortly after by voiding, the interval being described as the 'warning time'. Thus, in the case of OAB, urgency is associated with a small bladder volume and results in a decreased voiding volume and a reduction in the intervoid interval, which could explain the frequency and nocturia (Gillespie et al., 2009).

The location, character and duration of the urgency still need to be considered. In the study by Digesu et al. (2009), according to urodynamic diagnosis, women with detrusor overactivity and with mixed urinary incontinence experienced the bladder sensations mainly in the perineal and vaginal area. Women with urodynamic stress urinary incontinence described the bladder sensations usually at a suprapubic location. Digesu et al. (2009) reported that women's description of the *nature* of the bladder sensations was not significantly different between the diagnostic groups and the intensity increased with larger bladder volume. The duration that voiding could be delayed by women was significantly different between different urodynamic groups. The Digesu study results showed that the *location* of the sensation of needing to micturate is felt in different places with different pathologies.

In men the urgency also seems to be felt more peripherally (in the glans penis) as a kind of 'referred sensation' (Salvatore et al., 2017). It seems quite likely that these referred sensations are elicited by stimulation and/or dilatation of the proximal urethra (Mattiasson and Teleman, 2006; Peyronnet et al., 2019).

NORMAL PHYSIOLOGICAL MECHANISM IN BLADDER FILLING AND VOIDING

The initial volume increase of the bladder, during natural filling by urine entering via the ureters from the kidneys, gives relatively little increase in the tension in the bladder wall, indicating that the filling of the bladder is a more or less isotonic process.

During the storage phase, bladder filling activates mechanosensitive myelinated Aδ-afferent nerve fibres in the bladder wall. Action potentials are conducted by axons and transmitted at axonal terminals to connecting neurons to enter the dorsal root ganglia at S2–S4 segmental levels. Within the spinal cord, ascending tracts transmit the information towards the pontine micturition center, well known as a central coordination center for the micturition/storage process. This center, in a complex interplay, sends and receives signals from centers under conscious and unconscious control throughout the central nerve system such as the periaquaductal grey, prefrontal cortex, right insular cortex, cerebellum, limbic system and others (Fowler et al., 2008).

This afferent input results in stimulation of sympathetic efferent activity (via the hypogastric nerve TH10–L2), leading to increase in tone of smooth muscles in the bladder base and proximal urethra (via activation of α-adrenergic receptors) and relaxation of the detrusor (via activation of β-adrenergic receptors in the bladder body). Somatic efferent activity (via the pudendal nerve S1–S3) also increases, resulting in increased tone of the striated external urethral sphincter. These responses occur through spinal reflex pathways organized in the lumbosacral region of the spinal cord and represent 'guarding reflexes', which promote continence (Clemens, 2010).

The voiding phase of micturition is initiated voluntarily by signals from the cerebral cortex. The initial event, coordinated by the pons, is relaxation of the striated external urethral sphincter, caused by reflex inhibition of somatic efferent activity based on the stretching stimulus in the bladder wall. At the same time, there is inhibition of sympathetic efferent activity, with concomitant activation of parasympathetic outflow to the bladder and urethra. Bladder contraction is mediated via muscarinic receptors in the bladder body, and urethral smooth muscle relaxation is mediated through the release of nitric oxide (Clemens, 2010).

CAUSES OF URGENCY

Urgency is not a normal perception of bladder filling but the result of sensitization in the regulatory systems involved (Yamaguchi, 2007).

In the case of OAB, the following pattern can be observed. The sensation of urgency arises with a relatively small bladder volume. In normal urine production, this leads to frequency and nocturia and an increased chance of a micturition that can no longer be consciously controlled. This may often also lead to urine leakage related to urgency.

What causes an afferent signal with such a relatively small bladder volume often without significant activity of the detrusor? When connective tissue is elongated, fibroblasts become longer and flatter, and this change in shape is accompanied by a decrease in the tension in the connective tissue (Langevin et al., 2013). Suburothelial myofibroblasts, when challenged with their capacity to contract, can inhibit this extension of the suburothelial connective tissue, simultaneously increasing tension and generating an afferent signal at a relatively small bladder volume (Gillespie et al., 2009; Sui et al., 2008).

This mechanism may explain the feeling of incomplete emptying that patients with a high Overactive Bladder Symptom Score report despite a low post-void residual volume (Lee and Koo, 2020). The function of the suburothelial myofibroblasts is sometimes compared to intrafusal muscle fibres in a muscle spindle, which form a syncitium that causes a link between cells like in skeletal muscle cells or in the Auerbach plexus in the gastrointestinal tract that causes coordinated peristalsis. The contraction state of the myofibroblast determines the sensitivity of the afferent nerve endings located in the connective tissue. Several indications exist for an efferent influence on these myofibroblasts. A relationship between an increase in tissue tension and an increase in the sensitivity of mechanoreceptors under the influence of the sympathetic nervous system has been demonstrated previously (Roberts and Elardo, 1985). The vascularization of connective tissue is innervated by sympathetic nerve fibres that release noradrenaline.

Interestingly, 'cold stress' by cooling the skin induces urgency and detrusor overactivity, both of which can be reduced under the influence of α-adrenergic receptor antagonists (Chen et al., 2009). Imamura et al. (2013) showed that cold stress through a rapid change in room temperature from 27°C to 2°C resulted in a detrusor overactivity including increased basal pressure and decreased voiding interval, micturition volume and bladder capacity. The sympathetic nervous system is associated with transient hypertension and decreases of skin surface temperature that are closely correlated with detrusor overactivity. They showed that α1-adrenergic receptor antagonists have the potential to treat cold stress–exacerbated lower urinary tract symptoms (Imamura et al., 2013). In addition, adrenoceptors in the urothelium have been shown to facilitate mechano-sensitive bladder afferent nerve activity and reflex voiding under the influence of efferent sympathetic activity (Ishihama et al., 2006).

The cold stress involves a centrally mediated stress response. It is therefore plausible that the same mechanism applies to stress responses based on other stressors.

Many people will be aware, from their own experience, of the non-pathological relationship between moments of emotional tension and stress and the urge to urinate. It is also true that urgency and frequency are troublesome lower urinary tract symptoms which are found in 20% of women aged between 20 and 65 years. In a study of psychological aspects in women undergoing urodynamics, Macaulay et al. (1987) found that patients with urodynamic stress urinary incontinence showed changes comparable to other patients with longstanding physical complaints. Patients with sensory urgency lacked self-esteem and were more anxious than those with urodynamic stress urinary incontinence. Patients with detrusor overactivity were as anxious and lacking in self-esteem as patients with sensory urgency and additionally had morbid thoughts and worries and higher scores on the hysteria subscale of the Crown Crisp Experiential Index. Roughly a quarter of all patients reported that their urinary symptoms rendered life intolerable and were as anxious, depressed and phobic as psychiatric inpatients (Macaulay et al., 1987; Vrijens et al., 2015). Urgency of micturition is even a symptom of somatic anxiety that may cause significant stress and disability in public spaces (Frías et al., 2014). In this form of urgency, there is not only sensitization at the level of the bladder but also the centers involved in the control of storage and voiding of urine in the spinal cord and brainstem, and there is overactivity in the insular cortex—the cerebral alarm center of body perception (Leue et al., 2017; Peyronnet et al., 2019, Tadic et al., 2012).

This mechanism probably plays a role in other stress-related health problems such as obesity, metabolic syndrome, oxidative stress, systemic inflammation and insulin resistance (Peyronnet et al., 2019). Obstructive sleep apnea syndrome has similar association with urgency (Kemmer et al., 2009).

Different examples of the association of urgency with other comorbidities and anatomical and functional disorders that have been studied are mentioned next:

- Inflammation of the urothelium in the lower urinary tract causes urgency with a strong association with pain. This pain in the association with urgency is a red flag. Urgency in this association can refer to serious pathology, other than OAB. Urgency is also a key symptom of lower urinary tract tumors (Lunney et al., 2019), inflammation, kidney stones and bladder stones (Zamecnik et al., 2021).
- Chronic stress can lead to a sensitization of the dorsal horn in the spinal cord. Noxious stimulation from sacral innervated structures can cause urgency and pelvic pain. Noxious stimulation from other sacral structures than the bladder can cause irritation of the urothelium through dorsal root reflexes and create a picture of interstitial cystitis and prostatitis (Sluka et al., 1995; Wesselmann, 2001; Westlund and Zhang, 2013).
- Neurogenic etiology has been proposed by de Groat (1997) suggesting that subclinical neurological changes (either sensitization of afferents to the bladder or diminished central inhibition) produce detrusor overactivity including urgency.
- Cystocele/pelvic organ prolapse: Traction on the bladder with change in position and/or activity can stimulate urgency in women (Potts and Payne, 2018). In this case, urgency will not occur at rest and is relieved when the prolapse is corrected with a pessary or surgery (Potts and Payne, 2018).
- Next to causes of neurogenic or psychological origin, there are myogenic causes. Bladder muscle dysfunction may cause OAB (Miller and Hoffman, 2006b; Mills et al., 2000). Specific structural changes of a myogenic nature in the bladder wall could include infiltration of smooth muscle by elastin and collagen and patchy denervation in addition to changes in the cell-to-cell junctions resulting in increased excitation and electrical coupling between muscle cells (Brading, 1997). Such changes in intercellular electrical coupling could induce uncontrolled spread of the muscle contraction over the bladder, leading to sensations of urgency and even UUI (Brading, 1997; Elbadawi et al., 1993) The sensation of urgency has also been linked to the stretching of small portions of the bladder wall due to the localized contraction of smooth muscle, leading to activation of a set of

stretch-sensitive neurons that mediate the sensation of urgency (Elbadawi et al., 1993).

- Bladder outlet obstruction results in an increase in bladder pressure, a hypertrophy of the detrusor muscle, which can cause partial neurological denervation of bladder smooth muscle cells and may cause detrusor activity through cholinergic denervation of the detrusor and subsequent supersensitivity to acetylcholine. This increases the number of spontaneous action potentials and the ability of these action potentials to spread from cell to cell (myogenic theory) (Appukuttan et al., 2018). Rather than a normal detrusor contraction that would empty the bladder, this denervation causes 'micro-movements' of the bladder smooth muscle, increasing pressure in the bladder and triggering sensors in the smooth muscle. The afferent signal from these sensors leads to the development of urgency and is associated with OAB (Wein and Rackley, 2006). It seems that (partial) denervation of the detrusor is the cause of the changes in both bladder outlet obstruction and detrusor overactivity.

- In some cases of chronic stress, an overload of stimulation of the β2-adrenoceptors by the hormone adrenaline can lead to a shortage of β2-adrenoceptors (downregulation) (Miller and Chen, 2006a). As a result, the smooth muscle of the detrusor is no longer inhibited by adrenaline and the smooth muscle tissue becomes quite sensitive/irritable (Buckner et al., 2002). Due to the increased sensitivity of the smooth muscle cells, detrusor contractions can occur independent of parasympathetic activity and could stimulate the mechanosensitive neural elements in the suburothelial connective tissue. Thus there is smooth muscle cell activity without control from the sacral spinal cord (Buckner et al., 2002).

- In addition, disorders that can influence the continence mechanism are more common in the older population, such as diabetes, neurological diseases and cognitive impairments (Milsom et al., 2016).

A special form of urgency associated with detrusor overactivity is in old age, the result of reduced supraspinal inhibitory control on the micturition reflex. This can be caused by the loss of frontal inhibition of the pontine micturition center or by loss of the descending inhibitory tracts from the pontine micturition center (Peyronnet et al., 2019). It was demonstrated that older age and a greater burden of white matter damage in patients with detrusor overactivity are associated with more severe functional urinary impairment (Tadic et al., 2012).

This 'white matter disease' could be the anatomical substrate for the brain etiology of OAB associated with detrusor overactivity, maybe through frontal hypoperfusion. Other white matter disease such as multiple sclerosis could lead to symptoms of OAB due to impairment of myelinated pathways in the nervous system (Milsom et al., 2016; Peyronnet et al., 2019).

- In old age, there is also a decrease in the number of motor neurons and a decrease in the number of striated muscle fibres. This will reduce the strength of the external sphincter and decrease the pressure in the urethra. This does not necessarily lead to incontinence. With the decreased ability to close the urethra, when the abdominal pressure increases, such as during physical effort, urethral instability (sudden loss of urethral pressure during filling) and/or loss of the tonic inhibitory effect of the urethral sphincter leads to urgency (Potts and Payne, 2018). This feeling of urgency is called *stress-induced urgency*. This combination of urgency and physical effort related factors may explain the frequent occurrence of mixed urinary incontinence in the elderly (Mattiasson, 2007; Potts and Payne, 2018).

- In patients with a spinal cord injury between the brainstem and the sacral center, a reflex bladder function will occur. This spinal cord lesion interrupts the descending inhibition which leads to an uninhibited reflex arc which on its turn provokes overactive efferent fibres to fire leading to overactive detrusor contraction with or without urgency depending on the completeness of the spinal cord lesion. The reflex pathways at the sacral level are still intact, and the bladder is emptied via a disinhibited (sacral) micturition reflex (Taweel and Seyam, 2015). A reflex bladder should not be confused with the existence of an autonomic bladder as a consequence of a lesion of the S2–S4 efferents. Lesion of the S2–S4 segments causes the bladder to function without control, as an autonomic bladder as a result of parasympathetic denervation of the bladder and denervation of the sphincter. In cases of complete lesion, conscious awareness of bladder filling is lost, and the micturition reflex is absent. The findings are a competent but non-relaxing smooth sphincter and a striated sphincter that retains some fixed tone but is not under voluntary control (Taweel and Seyam, 2015).

As indicated before, urgency and OAB can occur in nervous system disorders. There is a pathological substrate (cerebral and/or spinal). The health problem has been identified and diagnosed, such as spinal cord injury, cerebral infarction/cerebral haemorrhage, Parkinson's disease, multiple sclerosis, spinal cord injury or amyotrophic lateral sclerosis. These neurogenic syndromes almost always involve a disinhibited micturition reflex and not necessarily urgency.

Research shows that in cases of neurogenic detrusor overactivity in patients with multiple sclerosis and in cases of OAB in Parkinson's disease, transcutaneous tibial nerve stimulation could be useful (Araujo et al., 2021). Some evidence suggests that posterior tibial nerve stimulation could also trigger plastic reorganization of the cortical network involved in micturition control (Finazzi-Agrò et al., 2010).

INDICATION FOR PHYSICAL THERAPY

The research and clinical evidence mentioned earlier show that the development of the symptom urgency is complex and fits a heterogeneous patient group. This makes it difficult to classify causes of urgency and UUI indicated for physical therapy.

Based on the biological rationale, there would be an indication for physical therapy for those patients in which anatomical abnormalities or pathologies have been ruled out by the referrer. This implies that physical therapy is especially indicated in a group of patients who suffer from urgency, frequency, nocturia and UUI that cannot be explained from a pathological substrate. This involves a disorder in which an increased sensitivity of parts of the micturition reflex is the result. With a smaller bladder volume, an afferent signal is created which enters a spinal cord that is in a facilitated state.

The physical therapist may encounter patients with detrusor overactivity due to sensitization within the afferent system, detrusor overactivity as a result of downregulation of the β2-adrenoceptors or non-relaxation of the pelvic floor muscles.

Detrusor Overactivity Due to Sensitization within the Afferent System

The two types of sensitization are central and peripheral:
- Central sensitization: This type of sensitization can arise from fatigue of the descending pathways, causing the inhibition to disappear. This occurs more often in the central nervous system, such as a result of a long-term stress response (including chronic fatigue and fibromyalgia). The inhibition of, for example, nocisensory stimulation (stress-induced analgesia) associated with the stress response fails, resulting in an increased sensitivity of the dorsal horn of the spinal cord (Leue et al., 2017). Dorsal root reflexes may then develop in this sensitized dorsal horn (Puopolo and Mendell, 2017; Westlund and Zhang, 2013). By retrograde activation of afferent nerve fibres that have their endings in this dorsal horn, neurogenic inflammatory reactions can occur in the peripheral innervation area (Sluka et al., 1995). Under the influence of the tachykinins released in this process, the free nerve fibres in the peripheral receptive field of these afferents also become more sensitive (peripheral sensitization) and there is an association with hyperalgesia (Sluka et al., 1995; Wesselmann, 2001; Westlund and Zhang, 2013).
- Peripheral sensitization: Acetylcholine can be released during the bladder filling phase from a non-neuronal source (probably the urothelium), or from postganglionic cholinergic neurons that can be activated by increased activity of the afferents via reflex pathways. The release of acetylcholine can increase detrusor contraction activity, as explained in the myogenic hypothesis (Mostwin et al., 2005; Wein and Rackley, 2006). In addition, sensors in the urothelium may be more sensitive to the released acetylcholine. Subsequently, the increased activation of the central nervous system gives the feeling of urgency (Wein and Rackley, 2006). Finally, as a result of a neurogenic inflammatory reaction, tachykinins can be released, resulting in sensitization of the sensors and producing local hyperalgesia of mechanosensitive receptors (mechanical pain).

Urgency means that, during the bladder filling phase, the continuous and intense afferent flow of stimuli from the periphery will be perceived by nuclei in the central nervous system, which are not (adequately) able to suppress this sensation. The delicate physiological process of bladder filling is disturbed.

Because OAB and urgency are associated with tension and emotions, it is obvious to strive for behavioural change and emotional stability and resilience in addition to physical therapeutic modalities, whereby local and general relaxation and stress reduction should be the therapeutic goal. Wyman et al. (2009) suggested that relevant healthcare providers should be familiar with the practical details of promoting healthy bladder habits, lifestyle modifications and training techniques not only to optimize treatment outcomes but also as the foundation for patient education and counselling to promote bladder health as part of routine healthcare. Fluid intake may play a minor role in the pathogenesis of urinary incontinence (level of evidence: 2) (Dumoulin et al., 2016). Caffeine (cola, coffee) consumption is likely to play a role in exacerbating urinary incontinence and related symptoms such as urgency and frequency. Small clinical trials suggest that decreasing caffeine intake improves continence (level of evidence: 2) (Dumoulin et al., 2016).

The aim of physical therapy in this group of patients is to suppress the urgency and to inhibit the unwanted micturition reflex (reflex inhibition of the motor neurons in the sacral spinal cord which are responsible for the contraction of the detrusor and desensitize or block the disrupted reflex circles). Physical therapy aims to influence this pathophysiological transmission and perception of afferent stimuli, using several strategies and therapy modalities.

Therapy modalities which activate large, myelinated fibres within the sacral segments include low thoracic/high lumbar (interferential) electrostimulation (Kaur and Narkeesh, 2014), intracavity electrostimulation (Berghmans et al., 2002), percutaneous tibial nerve stimulation (a kind of neuromodulation) (Finazzi-Agrò et al., 2010) and pelvic floor muscle training (Shafik & Shafik, 2003a, 2003b) have been used. For pelvic floor muscle training for OAB and UUI, the reader is also referred to the earlier sections of the chapter, for electrical stimulation also to Chapter 7.1. All of these modalities aim to introduce an effect of *neuromodulation*, which is defined as 'the alteration of nerve activity through targeted delivery of a stimulus, such as electrical stimulation, to specific neurological sites in the body' (in this case the pudendal nerves or the tibial posterior nerve) (La Rosa et al., 2019).

Detrusor Overactivity as a Result of Downregulation of the β2-Adrenoceptors

Due to the downregulation of the β2-adrenoceptors, the smooth muscle cells are disinhibited and detrusor overactivity arises more or less independently of the parasympathetic control (Moro et al., 2013). It then resembles an autonomic bladder, as seen after bladder denervation (in lesions of the sacral roots/sacral spinal nerves or sacral spinal cord). It seems plausible that reflex inhibition of the detrusor is no longer possible in

this situation. Physical therapy applying effective relaxation techniques may contribute to the reduction of the chronic stress factor responsible for the downregulation of the β2-adrenoceptors. Wyman et al. (2009) suggested that urgency can be controlled by performing general relaxation techniques, including slow deep breathing exercises to relax the bladder, decrease the intensity of the urgency and allow the patient to delay voiding, and distraction techniques in which patients get involved in tasks that involve mental concentration. However, up to now there is no RCT evidence to support relaxation therapy for OAB and urgency.

Non-Relaxation of Pelvic Floor Muscles

In a small proportion of patients, the OAB syndrome (of which UUI is a part) has been postulated to be associated with non-relaxation of the pelvic floor muscles, which is often accompanied by constipation and dyspareunia (Lagro-Janssen et al., 2006). Timely assessment of non-relaxation of the pelvic floor muscles allows earlier tailored intervention for patients. Down-training physical therapy is an emerging concept for the management of non-relaxation of the pelvic floor muscles, with emphasis on pelvic floor muscle awareness, relaxation exercises, pain point release techniques and/or manual stretches (Lukban et al., 2001). For patients undergoing surgery for stress incontinence, the identification of concomitant non-relaxation of the pelvic floor muscles and early physical therapy may reduce risks of postoperative voiding difficulties. Long-term follow-up of these patients is needed to assess their responses to down-training physical therapy (Aw et al., 2017). When non-relaxation of the pelvic floor muscles and detrusor overactivity coexist, non-relaxation of the pelvic floor muscles may be the driving factor (Aw et al., 2017). As such, combination therapy with pelvic floor relaxation and pharmaceuticals (anticholinergics/Botox injections) may yield better results than medications alone (Aw et al., 2017).

Aw et al. (2017) concluded that targeted intervention with pelvic floor physical therapy is central in the multimodal approach of non-relaxation pelvic floor muscles associated with urgency.

In the challenging field of diagnostic and therapeutic management of urgency, different physical therapy modalities are attractive first-line interventions, on one hand because of only a few side effects and the possibility to combine them with other interventions, and on the other hand because, in the case of insufficient effect, all more invasive surgical and pharmaceutica options will be left open. To validate and increase the level of evidence for physical therapy in patients with urgency and UUI, more high-quality research remains warranted.

REFERENCES

Appukuttan, S., Padmakumar, M., Young, J. S., et al. (2018). Investigation of the syncytial nature of detrusor smooth muscle as a determinant of action potential shape. *Frontiers in Physiology*, 9, 1–13.

Araujo, T. G., Schmidt, A. P., Sanches, P. R. S., Silva Junior, D. P., Rieder, C. R. M., & Ramos, J. G. L. (2021). Transcutaneous tibial nerve home stimulation for overactive bladder in women with Parkinson's disease: A randomized clinical trial. *Neurourology and Urodynamics*, 40(1), 538–548.

Aw, H. C., Ranasinhe, W., Tan, P. H. M., et al. (2017). Overactive pelvic floor muscles (OPFM): Improving diagnostic accuracy with clinical examination and functional studies. *Translational Andrology and Urology*, 6(Suppl. 2), 64–67.

Berghmans, L. C. M., van Waalwijk van Doorn, E. S. C., Nieman, F., et al. (2002). Efficacy of physical therapeutic modalities in women with proven bladder overactivity. *European Urology*, 41, 581–587.

Blaivas, J. G., Panagopoulos, G., Weiss, J. P., et al. (2009). Two types of urgency. *Neurourology and Urodynamics*, 28, 188–190.

Brading, A. (1997). A myogenic basis for the overactive bladder. *Urology*, 50, 57.

Buckner, S. A., Milicic, I., Daza, A. V., et al. (2002). Spontaneous phasic activity of the pig urinary bladder smooth muscle: Characteristics and sensitivity to potassium channel modulators. *British Journal of Pharmacology*, 135, 639–648.

Castro Díaz, D., Rebollo, P., & González-Segura Alsina, D. (2009). Comorbilidad asociada al síndrome de vejiga hiperactiva. *Espanola Urology*, 62(8), 639–645.

Chapple, C. R., Artibani, W., Cardozo, L. D., et al. (2005). The role of urinary urgency and its measurement in the overactive bladder symptom syndrome: Current concepts and future prospects. *BJU International*, 95, 335.

Chen, Z., Ishizuka, O., Imamura, T., et al. (2009). Role of α1-adrenergic receptors in detrusor overactivity induced by cold stress in conscious rats. *Neurourology and Urodynamics*, 28(3), 251–256.

Clemens, J. Q. (2010). Basic bladder neurophysiology. *Urology Clinical North American*, 37(4), 487–494.

Coyne, K. S., Sexton, C. C., Irwin, D. E., et al. (2008). The impact of overactive bladder, incontinence and other lower urinary tract symptoms on quality of life, work productivity, sexuality and emotional well-being in men and women: Results from the EPIC study. *BJU International*, 101(11), 1388–1395.

Coyne, K. S., Sexton, C. C., Thompson, C. L., et al. (2009). The prevalence of lower urinary tract symptoms (LUTS) in the USA, the UK and Sweden: Results from the Epidemiology of LUTS (EpiLUTS) study. *BJU International*, 104(3), 352–360.

De Groat, W. C. (1997). A neurologic basis for the overactive bladder. *Urology*, 50, 36–52.

De Wachter, S., & Hanno, P. (2010). Urgency: All or none phenomenon? *Neurourology and Urodynamics*, 29, 616.

De Wachter, S. G. G., Heeringa, R., van Koeveringe, G. A., et al. (2011). On the nature of bladder sensation: The concept of sensory modulation. *Neurourology and Urodynamics*, 30(7), 1220–1226.

Digesu, G. A., Basra, R., Khullar, V., et al. (2009). Bladder sensations during filling cystometry are different according to urodynamic diagnosis. *Neurourology and Urodynamics*, 28, 191–196.

Dumoulin, C., Adewuyi, T., Booth, J., et al. (2016). Adult conservative management. In P. Abrams, L. Cardozo, A. Wagg, et al. (Eds.), *Incontinence: Sixth international consultation on incontinence* (pp. 1443–1628). Bristol, UK: ICUD.

Dumoulin, C., Cacciari, L. P., & Hay-Smith, E. J. (2018). Pelvic floor muscle training versus no treatment, or inactive control treatments, for urinary incontinence in women. *Cochrane Database of Systematic Reviews* Issue 10, Art. No. CD005654.

Dutz, A., Agolli, L., Baumann, M., et al. (2019). Early and late side effects, dosimetric parameters and quality of life after proton beam therapy and IMRT for prostate cancer: A matched-pair analysis. *Acta Oncologica*, 58(6), 916–925.

Elbadawi, A., Yalla, S. V., & Resnick, N. M. (1993). Structural basis of geriatric voiding dysfunction. III. Detrusor overactivity. *Journal Urology*, 150, 1668.

Finazzi-Agrò, E., Petta, F., Sciobica, F., et al. (2010). Percutaneous tibial nerve stimulation effects on detrusor overactivity incontinence are not due to a placebo effect: A randomized, double-blind, placebo controlled trial. *Journal Urology*, 184(5), 2001–2006.

FitzGerald, M. P., Kenton, K. S., & Brubaker, L. (2005). Localization of the urge to void in patients with painful bladder syndrome. *Neurourology and Urodynamics*, 24, 7.

Fowler, C. J., Griffiths, D., & Groat, W. C. (2008). The neural control of micturition. *Nature Reviews Neuroscience*, 9(6), 453–466.

Frías, A., Palma, C., & Farriols, N. (2014). Frequent urgency of micturition in public spaces: A possible subtype of agoraphobia. *Minerva Psichiatrica*, 55(4), 226–229.

Gamble, T. L., Du, H., Sand, P. K., et al. (2010). Urge incontinence: Estimating environmental and obstetrical risk factors using an identical twin study. *International Urogynecology Journal and Pelvic Floor Dysfunction*, 21, 939–946.

Gillespie, J. I., van Koeveringe, G. A., de Wachter, S. G., et al. (2009). On the origins of the sensory output from the bladder: The concept of afferent noise. *BJU International*, *103*, 1324–1333.

Haylen, B. T., de Ridder, D., Freeman, R. M., et al. (2010). An International Urogynecological Association (IUGA)/International Continence Society (ICS) joint report on the terminology for female pelvic floor dysfunction. *International Urogynecology Journal and Pelvic Floor Dysfunction*, *21*(1), 5–26.

Heeringa, R. (2012). *The evaluation of normal and pathological bladder sensations*. Maastricht, Netherlands: Doctoral thesis. Maastricht University.

Hyman, M. J., Groutz, A., & Blaivas, J. G. (2001). Detrusor instability in men: Correlation of lower urinary tract symptoms with urodynamic findings. *Journal Urology*, *166*, 550.

Imamura, M., Sugino, Y., Long, X., et al. (2013). Myocardin and microRNA-1 modulate bladder activity through connexin 43 expression during post-natal development. *Journal of Cellular Physiology*, *228*(9), 1819–1826.

Irwin, D. E., Kopp, Z. S., Agatep, B., et al. (2011). Worldwide prevalence estimates of lower urinary tract symptoms, overactive bladder, urinary incontinence and bladder outlet obstruction. *BJU International*, *108*(7), 1132–1138.

Irwin, D. E., Milsom, I., Kopp, Z., et al. (2008). Symptom bother and health care seeking behavior among individuals with overactive bladder. *European Urology*, *53*(5), 1029–1037.

Ishihama, H., Momota, Y., Yanase, H., et al. (2006). Activation of alpha1D adrenerg receptors in the rat urothelium facilitates the micturition reflex. *Journal Urology*, *175*(1), 358–364.

Janssen, D. A. W., Schalken, J. A., & Heesakkers, J. P. F. A. (2017). Urothelium update: How the bladder mucosa measures bladder filling. *Acta Physiologica*, *220*(2), 201–217.

Kaur, B., & Narkeesh, A. (2014). Review study on the effect surface spinal stimulation on autonomic nervous system in spinal cord injury patient. *Journal of Exercise Science & Physiotherapy*, *10*(1), 46.

Kemmer, H., Mathes, A. M., Dilk, O., et al. (2009). Obstructive sleep apnea syndrome is associated with overactive bladder and urgency incontinence in men. *Sleep*, *32*(2), 271–275.

Kulseng-Hanssen, S., & Kristoffersen, M. (1988). Urethral pressure variations in females with and without neurorological symptoms. *Scandinavian Journal of Urology & Nephrology - Supplementum*, *114*, 48–52.

Lagro-Janssen, A. L. M., Breedveldt Boer, H. P., van Dongen, J. J. A. M., et al. (2006). NHG-Standaard incontinentie voor urine. *Huisards Wet*, *49*(10), 501–510.

Langevin, H. M., Nedergaard, M., & Howe, A. (2013). Cellular control of connective matrix tension. *Journal of Cellular Biochemistry*, *114*(8), 1714–1719.

La Rosa, V. L., Platania, A., Ciebiera, M., et al. (2019). A comparison of sacral neuromodulation vs. transvaginal electrostimulation for the treatment of refractory overactive bladder: The impact on quality of life, body image, sexual function, and emotional well-being. *Prz. Menopauzalny*, *18*(2), 89–93.

Lee, K. S., & Koo, K. C. (2020). Clinical factors associated with the feeling of incomplete bladder emptying in women with little postvoided residue. *International Neurourology Journal*, *24*(2), 172–179.

Leue, C., Kruimel, J., Vrijens, D., et al. (2017). Functional urological disorders: A sensitized defence response in the bladder-gut-brain axis. *Nature Reviews Urology*, *14*(3), 153–163.

Lukban, J., Whitmore, K., Kellogg-Spadt, S., et al. (2001). The effect of manual physical therapy in patients diagnosed with interstitial cystitis, high-tone pelvic floor dysfunction, and sacroiliac dysfunction. *Urology*, *57*, 121–122.

Lunney, A., Haynes, A., & Sharma, P. (2019). Moderate or severe LUTS is associated with increased recurrence of non-muscle-invasive urothelial carcinoma of the bladder. *International Braz J Urol*, *45*(2), 306–314.

Macaulay, A. J., Stern, R. S., & Holmes, D. M. (1987). Micturition and the mind: Psychological factors in the aetiology and treatment of urinary symptoms in women. *Brtish Medicine Journal (Clinical Research Education)*, *294*(6571), 540–543.

Mattiason, A. (2007). Overactive bladder. In K. Bø, B. Berghmans, S. Mørkved, et al. (Eds.), *Evidence-based physical therapy for the pelvic floor: Bridging science and clinical practice* (pp. 201–208). Edinburgh: Butterworth Heinemann Elsevier.

Mattiason, A., & Teleman, P. (2006). Abnormal urethral motor function is common in female stress, mixed, and urge incontinence. *Neurourology and Urodynamics*, *25*, 703–708.

Miller, G. E., & Chen, E. (2006). Life stress and diminished expression of genes encoding glucocorticoid receptor and β2-adrenergic receptor in children with asthma. *Proceedings of the National Academy Science U S A.*, *103*(14), 5496–5501.

Miller, J., & Hoffman, E. (2006). The causes and consequences of overactive bladder. *Journal Womens Health (Larchmt.)*, *15*(3), 251–260.

Mills, I. W., Greenland, J. E., McMurray, G., et al. (2000). Studies of the pathophysiology of idiopathic detrusor instability: The physiological properties of the detrusor smooth muscle and its pattern of innervation. *Journal Urology*, *163*, 646–651.

Milsom, I., Altman, D., Cartwright, R., et al. (2016). Epidemiology of urinary incontinence (UI) and other lower urinary tract symptoms (LUTS), pelvic organ prolapse (POP) and anal incontinence (AI). In P. Abrams, L. Cardozo, A. Wagg, et al. (Eds.), *Incontinence: Sixth international consultation on incontinence* (pp. 49–61). Bristol, UK: ICUD.

Moon, S. J., Kim, Y. T., Lee, T. Y., et al. (2011). The influence of an overactive bladder on falling: A study of females aged 40 and older in the community. *International Neurourology Journal, 15*(1), 41–47.

Moro, C., Tajouri, L., & Chess-Williams, R. (2013). Adrenoceptor function and expression in bladder urothelium and lamina propria. *Urology, 81*(1), 211.e1–211.e7.

Morrison, J. F. B., Steers, W. D., Brading, A., et al. (2002). Neurophysiology and neuropharmacology. In P. Abrams, L. Cardozo, S. Khoury, et al. (Eds.), *Incontinence: Second international consultation on incontinence* (pp. 83–163). Plymouth, UK: Health Publication.

Mostwin, J., Bourcier, A., Haab, F., et al. (2005). Pathophysiology of urinary incontinence, fecal incontinence and pelvic organ prolapse. In P. Abrams, L. Cardozo, R. Khoury, et al. (Eds.), *Incontinence: Third international consultation on incontinence* (pp. 255–312). Plymouth, UK: Health Publication.

Nathan, P. W. (1956). Sensations associated with micturition. *British Journal of Urology, 28*, 126.

Oliver, S., Fowler, C., Mundy, A., et al. (2003). Measuring the sensations of urge and bladder filling during cystometry in urge incontinence and the effects of neuromodulation. *Neurourology and Urodynamics, 22*, 7.

Peyronnet, B., Krupp, L. B., Reynolds, W. S., et al. (2019). Nocturia in patients with multiple sclerosis. *Reviews in Urology, 21*(2–3), 63–73.

Potts, J. M., & Payne, C. K. (2018). Urinary urgency in the elderly. *Gerontology, 64*, 541–550.

Puopolo, M., & Mendell, L. M. (2017). *Nociceptors: The gateway to pain. Neuroscience and biobehavioral psychology.* Elsevier Reference Collection.

Roberts, W. J., & Elardo, S. M. (1985). Sympathetic activation of A-delta nociceptors. *Somatosensory Research, 3*(1), 33–44.

Robertson, A. S., Griffiths, C. J., Ramsden, P. D., et al. (1994). Bladder function in healthy volunteers: Ambulatory monitoring and conventional urodynamic studies. *British Journal of Urology, 73*, 242.

Robles-Mejía, M., Rodríguez-Ayala, C., & González-Aldeco, P. M. (2019). Prevalence of overactive bladder syndrome and associated comorbidities in patients from a climacteric clinic. *Review Sanidad Military Mexico, 73*(2), 120–125.

Salvatore, S., DeLancey, J., & Igawa, Y. (2017). Pathophysiology of urinary incontinence, faecal incontinence and pelvic organ prolapse. In P. Abrams, L. Cardozo, A. Wagg, et al. (Eds.), *Incontinence: Sixth international consultation on incontinence* (pp. 361–497). Bristol, UK: ICS-ICUD.

Shafik, A., & Shafik, I. A. (2003). Overactive bladder inhibition in response to pelvic floor muscle exercises. *World Journal of Urology, 20*(6), 374–377.

Sluka, K. A., Willis, W. D., & Westlund, K. N. (1995). The role of dorsal root reflexes in neurogenic inflammation. *Pain Forum, 4*(3), 141–149.

Smith, A., & Wein, A. (2011). Urinary incontinence: Pharmacotherapy options. *Annals of Medicine, 43*(6), 461–476.

Stewart, W. F., Van Rooyen, J. B., Cundiff, G. W., et al. (2003). Prevalence and burden of overactive bladder in the United States. *World Journal of Urology, 20*, 327–336.

Sui, G. P., Wu, C., Roosen, A., et al. (2008). Modulation of bladder myofibroblast activity: Implications for bladder function. *American Journal Physiology Renal Physiology, 295*(3), F688–F697.

Tadic, S. D., Griffiths, D., Schaefer, W., et al. (2012). Brain activity underlying impaired continence control in older women with overactive bladder. *Neurourology and Urodynamics, 31*, 652–658.

Taweel, W. A., & Seyam, R. (2015). Neurogenic bladder in spinal cord injury patients. *Research and Reports in Urology, 7*, 85–89.

Vaughan, C. P., Johnson, T. M. 2nd, Ala-Lipasti, M. A., et al. (2011). The prevalence of clinically meaningful overactive bladder: Bother and quality of life results from the population-based FINNO study. *European Urology, 59*(4), 629–636.

Vrijens, D., Drossaerts, J., van Koeveringe, G., et al. (2015). Affective symptoms and the overactive bladder—a systematic review. *Journal of Psychosomatic Research, 78*(2), 95–108.

Wein, A. J., & Rackley, R. R. (2006). Overactive bladder: A better understanding of pathophysiology, diagnosis and management. *Journal Urology, 175*, S5–S10.

Wesselmann, U., et al. (2001). Neurogenic inflammation and chronic pelvic pain. *World Journal of Urology, 19*(3), 180–185.

Westlund, K., & Zhang, L. (2013). Detection of sensitized nerve responses: Dorsal root reflexes, live cell calcium and ROS imaging. *NeuroMethods, 78*, 261–273.

Wyman, J. F., Burgio, K. L., & Newman, D. K. (2009). Practical aspects of lifestyle modifications and behavioural interventions in the treatment of overactive bladder and urgency urinary incontinence. *International Journal of Clinical Practice, 63*(8), 1177–1191.

Yamaguchi, O., Honda, K., Nomiya, M., et al. (2007). Defining overactive bladder as hypersensitivity. *Neurourology and Urodynamics*, 904–907.

Zamecnik, L., Martan, A., Svabik, K., et al. (2021). Laparoscopic removal of intravesically inserted transobturator tape. *International Urogynecology Journal, 32*(12), 3309–3312.

Bladder Training

Jean F. Wyman

INTRODUCTION

Bladder training has been advocated for treatment for overactive bladder (OAB) symptoms (e.g., urgency, frequency, urgency incontinence and nocturia) since the late 1960s (Jeffcoate and Francis, 1966). It has also been recommended as a treatment for mixed urinary incontinence and stress urinary incontinence in women (Fantl et al., 1996; Moore et al., 2013). Bladder training is used for highly motivated adult patients without cognitive or physical impairments (Hadley, 1986; Wallace et al., 2009). The goal of bladder training is to restore normal bladder function through a process of patient education along with a mandatory or self-adjustable voiding regimen that gradually increases the time interval between voiding. How bladder training achieves its effects on improving lower urinary tract symptoms is unclear. One hypothesis is that it strengthens the brain's control over bladder sensations and urethral closure (Fantl et al., 1981; Fantl et al., 1991). An alternative hypothesis is that individuals change their behaviour in ways that increase the 'reserve capacity' of the lower urinary tract system as they become more knowledgeable of circumstances that cause bladder leakage (Fantl et al., 1991; Wyman et al., 1998).

Bladder training offers the advantages of being simple, relatively inexpensive and free from unpleasant side effects (Wyman and Fantl, 1991). This makes it particularly attractive for use in older adults, particularly those with high comorbidity who are already on multiple drug regimens and for whom OAB drug therapy, because of its anticholinergic properties, would place them at higher risk for adverse drug effects (Rovner et al., 2019). Bladder training can be used alone or in combination with drug therapy or with types of non-surgical treatments such as pelvic floor muscle training (PFMT).

Bladder training has now been recommended as a first-line treatment for urinary incontinence in men and women, including frail older adults, by several national and international professional societies and groups (Burkhard et al., 2018; Corcos et al., 2017; Dumoulin et al., 2017; Gormley et al., 2019; Gravas et al., 2020; National Clinical Guideline Centre, 2015, 2019; Wagg

et al., 2017). Although primarily used for treatment of urgency incontinence and OAB in women, some guidelines also recommend it for treatment of mixed urinary incontinence (Wagg et al., 2017).

This chapter will describe the evidence base for the use of bladder training in the prevention and treatment of urinary incontinence and OAB in adults. Systematic reviews and meta-analyses that included bladder training will be summarized, along with the methodological quality of individual studies. Clinical recommendations on the use of bladder training in adults with urinary incontinence will be provided.

PROTOCOLS

Bladder training typically consists of three main components: (1) patient education about the bladder, how continence is maintained, and urgency suppression strategies; (2) a scheduled voiding regimen that gradually extends the intervoiding intervals; and (3) positive reinforcement techniques provided by a healthcare professional (Wyman and Fantl, 1991). How these components are delivered varies considerably in practice. In early bladder training protocols, bladder training (also referred to as bladder discipline, bladder drill, bladder re-education and bladder retraining) was conducted through 5 to 13 days of hospitalization to ensure mandatory adherence to a strict voiding schedule; voiding off schedule was not permitted even if incontinence resulted (Jeffcoate and Francis, 1966; Ramsey et al., 1996). Patients were given anticholinergic drug therapy or sedatives to help cope with severe urgency. In a modification of this approach, Frewen (1979, 1980) found that patients with less severe symptoms could be treated in a 3-month outpatient programme.

Several variations became incorporated in bladder training programmes as they evolved over the decades. Outpatient protocols became the norm, and they differed in duration from 6 to 12 weeks. Although most protocols involved individual training, recent protocols have tested bladder training in a small group session (Hulbæk et al., 2016; Sherburn et al., 2011). The initial voiding interval is established based on the individual's voiding pattern from their baseline voiding diary and typically is set at 1 hour. Self-adjustable schedules permitted patients to void off schedule with severe urgency if they perceived that an incontinent episode was imminent (Wyman and Fantl, 1991). Education on urgency suppression strategies such as distraction and relaxation techniques and/or use of pelvic floor muscle contraction provides patients with specific methods to control urgency episodes. Self-monitoring of voiding behaviour using voiding diaries or logs is used frequently. Fluid and caffeine modifications might be recommended (Bryant et al., 2002; Ramsey et al., 1996); however, in clinical trials this generally has been avoided to test the effect of bladder training as a sole intervention. Advice on constipation prevention (Dougherty et al., 2002), high-fibre diets or weight loss reduction diets if appropriate (Ramsey et al., 1996) might also be provided. Alternative delivery strategies have been incorporated into clinical practice or trials such as a facsimile machine submission of voiding diaries with weekly telephone feedback (Visco et al., 1999), a simplification of the teaching method using a brief written instruction sheet (Mattiasson et al., 2003), use of a programmable electronic voiding timing device (Davila and Promozich, 1998) and group-based teaching methods (Hulbæk et al., 2016; Sampselle et al., 2005).

Systematic Literature Reviews

Four systematic reviews have been published that provide qualitative synthesis with evidence grading on bladder training in the treatment of urinary incontinence or urgency urinary incontinence (Dumoulin et al., 2017; Moore et al., 2013; PEDro, 2020; Wallace et al., 2009). The International Consultation on Incontinence (ICI) has also updated its previous reviews (Dumoulin et al., 2017; Moore et al., 2013). The Cochrane Collaboration (Wallace et al., 2009) and the Agency for Healthcare Quality and Research (AHRQ) (Balk et al., 2018; Shamilyan et al., 2007; 2012) published quantitative analyses of randomized controlled trial (RCT) data. Each systematic review varies in its objectives, its methodology, and the number and type of studies included. These variations contribute to differences in the number of studies reviewed and the conclusions regarding the effect of bladder training.

Berghmans et al. (2000) focused their review on RCTs that assessed physical therapies including bladder training as well as other forms of conservative therapies used in the treatment of urgency urinary incontinence. Of the nine bladder training trials they located that met inclusion criteria, they concluded that there was only weak evidence to suggest that bladder training is more effective than no treatment, and that bladder training is better than drug therapy.

The Cochrane Collaboration (Wallace et al., 2009) published an edited review updated from their 2004 review that included quantitative analyses of 12 RCTs (n = 1473 participants) on five prespecified primary outcomes: (1) the participant's perception of cure of urinary incontinence, (2) the participant's perception of improvement of urinary incontinence, (3) the number of incontinent episodes, (4) the number of micturitions and (5) quality of life. Adverse events were also noted. Their review is limited to RCTs with participants who had urinary incontinence; OAB studies in which it could not be determined that participants had urinary incontinence were excluded. However, subanalyses did examine urgency urinary incontinence as a variable. The Cochrane Group concluded that there was inconclusive evidence to judge the effects of bladder training in both the short and long term. The results of the trials reviewed tended to favour bladder training in the treatment of urinary incontinence; however, the trials were of variable quality and small size. They found no evidence of adverse effects. They also found no evidence to determine whether first-line therapy should be bladder training or anticholinergic drug therapy or whether bladder training was useful as a supplement to another therapy.

The ICI (Dumoulin et al., 2017) updated its previous systematic reviews that addressed a broader set of questions than the Cochrane review:

- What is the most appropriate bladder training protocol?
- Is bladder training better than no treatment, placebo or control treatments?
- Is bladder training better than other treatments?
- Does the addition of bladder training to other treatments add benefit?
- What is the effect of bladder training on other lower urinary tract symptoms?
- What factors might affect the outcome of bladder training?

In contrast to the Cochrane review, the updated ICI review included 17 RCTs with 3194 women who had urinary incontinence (urgency, stress and mixed incontinence) as well as those who had OAB without urinary incontinence. The ICI concluded that there was still no trial evidence to suggest the most effective method or specific parameters of bladder training. For those undertaking bladder training, having more health professional contact will be better than less, based on the developing evidence for PFMT, which, like bladder training, requires behavioural change. They recommended that clinicians should provide the most intensive bladder training supervision possible within service constraints. The ICI also concluded from the few available trials in women that bladder training may be effective for women with urgency urinary incontinence, stress urinary incontinence and mixed urinary incontinence, and they recommended bladder training as a first-line therapy for urinary incontinence in women. They also found unclear evidence on whether bladder training or drug therapy is more effective for women with detrusor overactivity or urgency urinary incontinence, or whether augmenting bladder training with drug therapy was effective. The ICI did recommend that bladder training may be preferred by clinicians and women because it does not produce the adverse effects associated with drug therapy. The ICI concluded that there was evidence from one trial combining bladder training with PFMT that led to improved short-term outcomes when compared to PFMT alone, but the added benefit did not persist 3 months later. They also found no evidence for an added benefit of combining written bladder training instructions with antimuscarinic drug therapy for women with OAB.

The AHRQ published two systematic reviews on urinary incontinence that included a meta-analysis on the effect of bladder training (Shamilyan, et al., 2007; 2012) and a third review using network meta-analysis (Balk et al., 2018). The first review examined the evidence to support specific clinical interventions (e.g., bladder training) in reducing the risk of urinary incontinence in adults residing in community and long-term care settings (Shamilyan et al., 2007). No prevention studies were located for bladder training alone, and there was limited evidence on the effectiveness of bladder training in community-dwelling adults. The second review focused on non-surgical treatments for urinary incontinence in women and addressed several questions on non-pharmacological treatments that were relevant to bladder training (Shamilyan et al., 2012). These included how the non-pharmacological treatments affected incontinence, incontinence severity and frequency, and quality of life either alone or combined with drugs; what their effectiveness was in comparison to other treatments; what their harms were when compared to other treatments; and what patient characteristics modified the effects of treatment outcomes and harms. Outcomes used in this meta-analysis included urinary continence and improvement (≥50% reduction of urinary incontinent episodes on a 3–7-day diary; 70% improvement on a quality-of-life scale or 60% improvement on a global improvement scale). This review concluded that there was a low level of evidence indicating that bladder training improved urinary incontinence when compared to usual care for urgency incontinence. When bladder training is combined with PFMT for mixed urinary incontinence, a high level of evidence was found that indicates significant benefits on continence and improvement in urinary incontinence. However, the evidence was low for reducing the bother of urinary incontinence, and it was insufficient for improving quality of life. In comparing bladder training to other forms of treatment, the review found that continence did not differ between bladder training alone versus bladder training combined with PFMT for continence or improvement (Shamilyan et al., 2012). Continence did not differ between bladder training and PFMT, nor did satisfaction with current urinary incontinence and feelings of no impact from urinary incontinence on quality-of-life measures. Adverse effects were uncommon. The specific characteristics of women associated with better benefits and compliance to bladder training were unclear.

In the third AHRQ review (Balk et al., 2018) that involved a network analysis which combined data from direct (head-to-head) and indirect comparisons through a common comparator, urinary incontinence outcomes (e.g., cure, improvement, satisfaction and quality of life) were analysed with comparison of first-line (behavioural therapies) and second-line (pharmacological) interventions and summarized by incontinence type (stress, urgency incontinence). Behavioural therapies (e.g., bladder training, PFMT, biofeedback and other non-pharmacological therapies) were grouped together, making it difficult to identify outcomes associated with bladder training alone.

EVIDENCE BASE

Overview

This section describes the evidence base for bladder training in the prevention of and treatment for urinary incontinence and other OAB symptoms in adults. Bladder training has been (1) compared as a sole treatment to no treatment; (2) compared as a sole treatment to another treatment (non-surgical or pharmacological) and (3) compared as a sole treatment to its use in combination with a non-surgical or pharmacological treatment. Comment will be made on the search strategy and selection criteria used in selecting studies included in the evidence base, the systematic literature reviews on bladder training and the methodological qualities of the included studies as they relate to the type of comparison being made using the PEDro Quality Scale (PEDro, 2020).

The following criteria were used to distinguish levels of evidence based on a modification of criteria proposed by Berghmans et al. (2000):

- To conclude that there was *strong evidence for or against bladder training* for OAB patients, at least three high-quality studies with a PEDro score of 6 or greater were needed.
- The conclusion of *weak evidence for bladder training* required at least three high-quality studies with inconsistent results (e.g., 25%–75% considered positive) or at least three low-quality studies with PEDro scores less than 6 with consistent results in favour of bladder treatment.
- To conclude that there is *weak evidence against bladder training*, there needed to be at least three low-quality studies with consistent results with regard to bladder training on at least one outcome measure (e.g., urgency, urinary frequency, nocturia or urgency incontinence).
- The conclusion of *insufficient evidence* was based on low-quality studies with inconsistent results or with fewer than three studies of whatever quality.

The OVID MEDLINE, CINAHL, PSYCHInfo and Cochrane Collaboration databases were searched (1980–2020) using the following keywords: *urinary incontinence, overactive bladder, detrusor overactivity, detrusor hyperactivity, detrusor instability, urgency, frequency, nocturia, bladder training, bladder retraining, behavioral therapy, behavioral techniques, adult, aged, randomized controlled trial, clinical trial* and *systematic review.*

Studies were included if they were RCTs and met the following criteria: bladder training in at least one treatment arm alone; comparison of bladder training with another treatment in one arm versus a comparison of the other treatment alone; included results for community-residing adult participants with urgency incontinence, urodynamic detrusor overactivity (previously diagnosed as detrusor instability), OAB with or without urinary incontinence reported exclusively or separately from those for participants with mixed urinary incontinence, or stress urinary incontinence; published full-length report and trial report published in English. Studies were excluded that focused on participants with neurological conditions such as stroke, Parkinson's disease or spinal cord injury, or provided bladder training techniques as part of a multicomponent behavioural intervention without details regarding the specific bladder training protocol.

PREVENTION

There are no studies testing bladder training as a sole intervention in the prevention of OAB in adults. Therefore, there is no evidence to base clinical practice decisions in the use of bladder training to prevent or delay urinary incontinence and other OAB symptoms.

TREATMENT

Trial Comparisons

Fifteen RCTs on bladder training involving 1933 adults (predominantly female) met the inclusion criteria. A summary of these trials is presented in Table 7.2.1 with a rating of their quality using the PEDro scale in Table 7.2.2. Overall, the PEDro rating of these studies ranged from 2 to 9; 10 studies (Dougherty et al., 2002; Fantl et al., 1991; Hulbæk et al., 2016; Kaya et al., 2013; Mattiasson et al., 2003; Sherburn et al., 2011; Szonyi et al., 1995; Wiseman et al., 1991; Wyman et al., 1998; Yoon et al., 2003) had good methodological quality (PEDRro = 6–8), 1 study (Kafri et al., 2015) had excellent quality (PEDro = 9–10) and 4 studies (Hadley, 1986; Jarvis, 1981; Jarvis and Millar, 1980; Bryant et al., 2002) had fair quality (PEDro = 4–5). With the exception of four trials (Dougherty et al., 2002; Fantl et al., 1991; Mattiasson et al., 2003; Wyman et al., 1998), most trials included sample sizes with groups of less than 50 participants. Mean age of the participants ranged from 46.5 to 82.2 years.

TABLE 7.2.1   Randomized Controlled Trials on Bladder Training to Treat Overactive Bladder and Urinary Incontinence in Community-Residing Women

Author	**Bryant et al. (2002)**
Design	2-arm RCT: BT; BT and caffeine reduction
Sample size and age (years)	95 women and men with urinary symptoms; mean age 57 (SD: 17)
Diagnosis	Clinical assessment time/volume/caffeine charts indicating urinary urgency, frequency, with or without urgency incontinence and ingested ≥100 mg of caffeine/24 h
Training protocol	4 weekly visits; increase voiding intervals, maintain or increase fluid intake to 2 L/24 h, urgency suppression techniques, cease 'just in case' voiding
Drop-out	Not assessed
Adherence	Not reported
Results	No difference between groups on reduction in incontinent episodes/24 h (p = 0.219) Caffeine reduction with BT led to significantly greater decreases than BT alone in urgency (p < 0.002) and urinary frequency (p = 0.037)
Author	**Columbo et al. (1995)**
Design	2-arm RCT: BT; oxybutynin
Sample size and age (years)	81 women age <65 with UUI age 24–65; mean age 48.5
Diagnosis	Clinical assessment, cystometry, cystoscopy, post-void residual determination, voiding diary
Training protocol	6-week outpatient programme, initial interval based on maximal voiding interval, encouraged to hold urine 30 min beyond initial voiding interval, progressively increase interval every 4–5 days to reach goal of 3–4 h voiding interval; at appointments every 2 weeks, encouragement and BT advice provided
Drop-out	BT arm: 2/39 (5.1%); drug arm: 4/42 (9.5%)
Adherence	Not reported
Results	In BT arm, 27/37 (73%) were clinically cured (e.g., no UUI or pad use) vs drug arm 28/38 (74%) at 6 weeks At 6 months, fewer relapses with BT (1/27) vs drug arm (12/28) BT clinically cured 8/13 (62%) with detrusor overactivity, 6/8 (75%) with low-compliance bladder and 13/16 (81%) with OAB without detrusor overactivity vs drug arm 13/14 (93%), 6/9 (67%) and 9/15 (60%), respectively Significant increase in first desire to void BT resolved diurnal frequency in 20/29 (69%) and nocturia in 11/18 (61%) In BT arm, 17/27 (63%) clinically cured with detrusor overactivity returned to stable bladders vs drug arm 16/28 (57%)
Author	**Dougherty et al. (2002)**
Design	2-arm RCT conducted in 3 phases, BT; no treatment
Sample size and age (years)	218 women age ≥55; mean age 67.7 (SD: 8.3)
Diagnosis	Clinical assessment, urinalysis, voiding diary
Training protocol	6–8-week programme according to Fantl et al. (1991); gradually increasing voiding interval with no times given, constipation prevention education, fluid and caffeine advice if problem noted, positive reinforcement and continence goals decided at onset
Drop-out	BT arm: 21%; control arm: 15%
Adherence	Not reported
Results	In 89 women who underwent BT, 48% reduction in grams of urine lost on 24-h pad test and 57% reduction in incontinent episodes; unable to determine results compared to control group

TABLE 7.2.1 **Randomized Controlled Trials on Bladder Training to Treat Overactive Bladder and Urinary Incontinence in Community-Residing Women—cont'd**

Author	**Fantl et al. (1991)**
Design	2-arm RCT: BT; 6-week delayed treatment
Sample size and age (years)	131 women age ≥55 with detrusor overactivity with or without genuine stress incontinence or stress incontinence alone; mean age 67 (SD: 8.5)
Diagnosis	Clinical assessment, urodynamics, voiding diary ≥1 incontinent episode/week
Training protocol	6-week outpatient programme, initial voiding schedule based on voiding diary, typically set at 1-h intervals during waking hours only; increased by 30 min depending on schedule tolerance; instructed in urgency control strategies; encouraged to avoid voiding off schedule but not prohibited; instructed to maintain usual fluid intake pattern and keep treatment log; at weekly appointments, positive reinforcement, support and optimism in successful outcome provided
Drop-out	8/131 (6%) at 6 weeks; 20/131 (15.3%) at 6 months
Adherence	Not reported
Results	At 6-week follow-up, 12% were continent and 75% reduced their incontinence 50% or better on voiding diary with results maintained at 6 months In OAB group, frequency was improved for those with ≥57 micturitions/week, nocturia was unchanged and IIQ scores were improved at 6 weeks and maintained at 6 months
Author	**Hulbæk et al. (2016)**
Design	2-arm, 6-site RCT: individual BT; small group BT
Sample size and age (years)	91 women with OAB; individual BT: mean age 57.4 (SD: 13.8); group BT: mean age 57.7 (SD: 15.1)
Diagnosis	Gynaecologist diagnosis of OAB, clinical assessment, urine dipstick, pregnancy test
Training protocol	8-week programme with 3 training sessions and progressive voiding intervals of 15–30 min/week, urgency suppression techniques; education covered fluid intake, obstipation, lifestyle modification and helping aids
Drop-out	Individual BT: 5/43 (11.6%); group BT: 7/48 (14.6%)
Adherence	At least 75% adherence to reporting BT in voiding diary; median of 14 days between first 2 sessions to median of 28 days between third visit and follow-up; similar in both groups
Results	No differences between individual and group BT in urgency episodes, UUI episodes, voiding frequencies, VAS or global improvement scores VAS scores unchanged in both groups Non-significant 50% median reduction in daily UUI episodes in both groups; no difference in treatment satisfaction, although higher in individual BT (88%) vs group BT (74%)
Author	**Jarvis (1981)**
Design	2-arm RCT: inpatient BT; outpatient drug therapy (flavoxate and imipramine)
Sample size and age (years)	50 women age 17–78 with detrusor overactivity; mean age 46.5 (SD: 13.6)
Diagnosis	Clinical assessment, cystometry, cystoscopy
Training protocol	Inpatient BT programme (details not provided)
Drop-out	5/25 (20%) drug therapy group only
Adherence	Not reported
Results	Greater improvement in BT group: 84% became continent and 76% symptom free vs 56% continent and 48% symptom free in drug therapy group BT improvements: frequency 78%, nocturia 81%, urgency 84%, UUI 84%

Continued

TABLE 7.2.1 **Randomized Controlled Trials on Bladder Training to Treat Overactive Bladder and Urinary Incontinence in Community-Residing Women—cont'd**

Author	**Jarvis and Millar (1980)**
Design	2-arm RCT: inpatient BT; control (e.g., advised that they should be able to hold urine 4 h, be continent and allowed home)
Sample size and age (years)	60 women age 27–79 with detrusor overactivity
Diagnosis	Clinical assessment, cystoscopy, urethral dilatation
Training protocol	Inpatient BT programme; initial voiding schedule typically set at 1.5 h during waking hours only; schedule increases by 30 min daily until 4-h interval reached; instructed to wait to assigned time or be incontinent; encouraged to maintain usual fluid intake and keep fluid intake record; introduced to patient successfully treated by BT
Drop-out	None reported
Adherence	Not reported
Results	27/30 (90%) became continent and 25/30 (83.3%) symptom free Improvements noted with frequency (83.3%), nocturia (88.8%), urgency (86.7%) and urgency incontinence (80%), which were significantly better than control group (p < 0.01)
Author	**Kafri et al. (2015)**
Design	Multicenter, 4-arm RCT: BT; PFMT; combined pelvic floor rehabilitation (BT + PFMT + lifestyle advice); drug therapy (tolterodine)
Sample size and age (years)	164 women age 45–75 with UUI; mean age 56.7 (SD: 8)
Diagnosis	Diagnosed by health professional with UUI, clinical assessment, bladder ultrasound, voiding diary
Training protocol	12-week programme (4 visits every 3 weeks) using predetermined or self-adjusted voiding schedule to achieve voiding interval of 3–4 h
Drop-out	BT: 2/41 (4.9%); PFMT: 6/40 (15%); combined pelvic floor rehabilitation: 4/41 (9.8%); drug therapy: 15/42 (35.7%)
Adherence	BT: 85%; PFMT: 90%; combined pelvic floor rehabilitation: 95%; drug therapy: 64%
Results	All groups had significant improvements in 24-h voiding frequency, voided volume, UUI episodes, QoL (I-QOL) and pad use at 3 months and 1-year; slight advantage for combined pelvic floor rehabilitation group in decreasing voiding frequency and improving self-reported function Significant decrease in symptoms (ISI) in BT compared to drug therapy and significant improvement in overall disability limitations
Author	**Kaya et al. (2013)**
Design	2-arm RCT: BT; BT + PFMT
Sample size and age (years)	108 women age ≥18 with SUI, UUI or MUI; BT: mean age 50.9 (SD: 8.4); BT + PFMT: mean age 48.7 (SD: 10.1)
Diagnosis	Clinical evaluation, urinalysis, voiding diary, and QUID (stress scores ≥3 for SUI; urge scores ≥6 for UUI)
Training protocol	6-week programme over 4 visits with progressive increases of voiding interval by 15 min/week if tolerated, urgency suppression techniques, no fluid adjustments; brief instruction sheet provided along with voiding diary
Drop-out	BT arm: 13/65 (20%); BT + PFMT arm: 11/67 (16.4%)
Adherence	No significant differences in compliance with BT regimen between groups; details not reported

TABLE 7.2.1 Randomized Controlled Trials on Bladder Training to Treat Overactive Bladder and Urinary Incontinence in Community-Residing Women—cont'd

Results	Significantly more patients in BT + PFMT group reported cured or improved symptoms than in BT group (100% vs 82.7%) (p = 0.001) BT + PFMT group had significantly lower ISI scores (p = 0.001), improved symptom distress scores (p = 0.001) and lower QoL impact scores (p = 0.005) Significant differences in more patients reporting cured or improved symptoms for BT + PFMT who had SUI (p = 0.001) and MUI (p = 0.038) but not for UUI (p = 0.352); similarly improved ISI scores for those with SUI (p = 0.001) and MUI (p = 0.039) but not with UUI (p = 0.098); those with SUI in the BT + PFMT group had significantly greater improvement in symptom distress (UDI-6, p = 0.001) and QoL impact (IIQ-7, p = 0.040) than those in BT group; no differences between changes in symptom distress (UDI-6, p = 0.108) or QoL impact (IIQ-7, p = 0.283) scores for patients with MUI PFMT + BT group and those with SUI in BT + PFMT had fewer UI episodes (p = 0.025 and p = 0.047, respectively); no differences between treatments for patients with UUI or MUI and no difference between groups in micturition frequency
Author	**Mattiasson et al. (2003)**
Design	2-arm multicentre RCT: BT and tolterodine; tolterodine alone
Sample size and age (years)	501 women and men (75% women) age ≥18 with OAB with and without UI; median age 63
Diagnosis	Clinical assessment, voiding diary
Training protocol	Brief written instruction sheet on BT, emphasize bladder stretching through delaying urination with goal to reduce urinary frequency to 5–7×/24 h, urgency suppression techniques, keep voiding diary every other week to chart progress, no other training or follow-up by study personnel
Drop-out	391/505 (23%)
Adherence	Subsample of BT group (n = 95): 68% kept voiding diary for 1 day, 72% at 11 weeks, not reported at 23 weeks; 60% kept diary for 7 days at 1 week, 62% at 11 weeks and 46/56 (82%) at 23 weeks
Results	BT yielded greater reductions in number of voids/24 h (p < 0.001) and volume voided (p < 0.0001) No difference in BT + tolterodine compared to tolterodine alone in number of urgency episodes/24 h, incontinent episodes/24 h and patient perceptions of symptoms
Author	**Sherburn et al. (2011)**
Design	2-arm, 2-site RCT: group BT; group PFMT
Sample size and age (years)	83 women age >65 with SUI; mean age 71.8 (SD: 5.3)
Diagnosis	Clinical assessment, urodynamics voiding diary
Training protocol	4 weekly group sessions, individually set and progressed voiding intervals, and use of cognitive strategies for urgency suppression; also included stretching exercises as control for PFMT
Drop-out	BT: 35/40 (12.5%); PFMT: 2/43 (4.7%)
Adherence	BT: 93.1% mean completion of 3-day diaries PFMT: 96.8% mean completion of daily exercises
Results	PFMT group had significantly lower median grams of urine lost on cough stress test (p = 0.006), improved overall symptom change (ICIQ-UI SF), improved bother scores (VAS) and greater perception of change than BT group (p = 0.002) No difference between groups in mean voided volume and generic health-related QoL
Author	**Szonyi et al. (1995)**
Design	2-arm double-blinded RCT: oxybutynin and BT; placebo
Sample size and age (years)	60 adults age ≥70 with OAB; mean age 82.2

Continued

TABLE 7.2.1   Randomized Controlled Trials on Bladder Training to Treat Overactive Bladder and Urinary Incontinence in Community-Residing Women—cont'd

Diagnosis	Clinical assessment, cystometry, laboratory studies, urine culture, voiding diary
Training protocol	Not specified
Drop-out	8/30 (26.7%) BT and drug group; 5/30 (16.7%) placebo group
Adherence	Not specified for BT; 80% for drug and 80% in placebo group
Results	Greater reduction in diurnal frequency (p = 0.003) and superior subjective benefit (86% vs 55%, p = 0.02) in BT and drug therapy group; no difference in nocturia or incontinent episodes
Author	**Wiseman et al. (1991)**
Design	2-arm double-blinded RCT: terodiline and BT; placebo and BT
Sample size and age (years)	37 adults age ≥70 with OAB due to detrusor overactivity; mean age 80.4
Diagnosis	Clinical assessment, cystometry, laboratory studies, urine culture, voiding diary
Training protocol	Asked to delay bladder emptying for as long as possible whenever they experienced the need to void
Drop-out	BT and drug group: 1/19 (5.2%); BT and placebo group: 2/18 (11.1%)
Adherence	Not reported
Results	Both groups improved slightly, but no difference between groups in micturition frequency and incontinence episodes
Author	**Wyman et al. (1998)**
Design	3-arm, 2-site RCT: BT; PFMT; BT and PFMT
Sample size and age (years)	204 women age ≥55 with detrusor overactivity with or without genuine stress incontinence or stress incontinence alone; mean age 61 (SD: 9.7)
Diagnosis	Clinical assessment, urodynamics, voiding diary ≥1 UI episode/week
Training protocol	12-week outpatient BT programme: 6 weekly visits (first 6 weeks), 6 mailed-in logs (second 6 weeks) Same training protocol as Fantl et al. (1991) presented earlier
Drop-out	11/204 (5.4%) at 12 weeks, 16/204 (7.8%) at 24 weeks
Adherence	57% of office visits, 85% to voiding schedule during treatment and 44% to voiding schedule at 24 weeks
Results	At 12 weeks, BT + PFMT had less incontinent episodes than BT alone (p = 0.004), but by 24 weeks, no difference noted between groups No differences noted in treatment response by urodynamic diagnosis Women with detrusor overactivity had less symptom distress (UDI, p = 0.054) and greater improvement in life impact (IIQ, p = 0.03) than those with stress incontinence alone at 12 weeks; no differences at 24 weeks
Author	**Yoon et al. (2003)**
Design	3-arm RCT: BT; PFMT; control
Sample size and age (years)	50 women with urinary incontinence age 35–55
Diagnosis	Clinical assessment, pad test ≥1 g, urinalysis and urine culture, voiding diary
Training protocol	8-week programme with progressive increases in voiding interval
Drop-out	BT: 2/21 (9.5%); PFMT: 2/14 (14.3%); control: 2/15 (13.3%)
Adherence	Not reported
Results	BT group significantly reduced urinary frequency (p < 0.01) and nocturia (p <0.01) and increased voided volume (p < 0.01) when compared to PFMT and control groups; no differences among groups in pad test amounts

BT, Bladder training; *ICIQ-UI SF*, International Consultation on Incontinence Questionnaire-Urinary Incontinence, Short Form; *IIQ*, Incontinence Impact Questionnaire; *I-QOL*, Incontinence Quality of Life; *ISI*, Incontinence Severity Index; *MUI*, mixed urinary incontinence; *OAB*, overactive bladder; *PFMT*, pelvic floor muscle training; *QoL*, quality of life; *QUID*, Questionnaire for Urinary Incontinence Diagnosis; *RCT*, randomized controlled trial; *SUI*, stress urinary incontinence; *UDI*, Urogenital Distress Index; *UI*, urinary incontinence; *UUI*, urgency urinary incontinence; *VAS*, visual analogue scale.

TABLE 7.2.2   PEDro Quality Scores of Randomized Controlled Trials of Bladder Training

E – Eligibility criteria specified
1 – Subjects randomly allocated to groups
2 – Allocation concealed
3 – Groups similar at baseline
4 – Subjects blinded
5 – Therapist administering treatment blinded
6 – Assessors blinded[b]
7 – Measures of key outcomes obtained from >85% of subjects
8 – Data analysed by intention to treat
9 – Comparison between groups conducted
10 – Point measures and measures of variability provided[b]

Study	E	1	2	3[a]	4	5	6[b]	7	8	9	10[b]	Total Score
Bryant et al. (2002)	+	+	−	+	−	−	−	−	−	−	+	4
Columbo et al. (1995)	+	+	?	?	−	−	−	+	−	−	−	2
Dougherty et al. (2002)	+	+	?	+	−	−	−	+	+	+	+	7
Fantl et al. (1991)	+	+	?	+	−	−	−	+	−	+	+	6
Hulbæk et al. (2016)	+	?	+	+	−	−	−	+	+	+	+	7
Jarvis and Millar (1980)	−	+	−	−	+	−	−	+	?	+	−	4
Jarvis (1981)	−	+	−	+	−	−	−	+	?	+	+	5
Kafri et al. (2015)	+	+	+	+	−	−	+	+	+	+	+	9
Kaya et al. (2013)	+	+	+	+	−	−	−	+	?	+	+	7
Mattiasson et al. (2003)	+	+	?	+	−	−	−	−	+	+	+	6
Sherburn et al. (2011)	+	+	+	+	−	−	+	+	+	+	+	9
Szonyi et al. (1995)	+	+	+	−	+	−	−	−	−	+	+	6
Wiseman et al. (1991)	+	+	−	?	+	+	+	+	+	+	−	8
Wyman et al. (1998)	+	+	+	+	−	−	−	+	−	+	+	7
Yoon et al. (2003)	+	+	?	+	−	−	+	+	−	+	+	6

[a]Based on overactive bladder symptoms (e.g., urinary frequency, nocturia, urinary incontinent episodes).
[b]Blinded to active versus placebo drug; no studies were able to blind for use of bladder training in protocol.
+, Criterion is clearly satisfied; −, criterion is not satisfied; ?, not clear if the criterion was satisfied.
The total score is determined by counting the number of criteria that are satisfied, except scale item 1 (eligibility criteria specified) is not used to generate the total score. Total scores are out of 10.

Bladder Training Versus No Treatment or Control

Three RCTs of good methodological quality (Dougherty et al., 2002; Fantl et al., 1991; Yoon et al., 2003) and one trial of poor quality (Jarvis and Millar, 1980) compared the effect of a 6- to 8-week outpatient programme of bladder training to no treatment or a control in 441 women with detrusor overactivity with or without stress incontinence or women with urinary incontinence. The results in two trials (Fantl et al., 1991; Yoon et al., 2003) favoured bladder training in improving incontinent episodes and the symptoms of urgency incontinence as well as urinary frequency, urgency and nocturia. In one study (Yoon et al., 2003), bladder training also led to increased voided volumes. One trial (Dougherty et al., 2002) did not clearly report outcomes to judge the evidence. Overall, there was weak evidence that bladder training is more effective than no treatment (control) in reducing urinary incontinence and OAB symptoms.

Bladder Training Versus Other Treatments

Six trials were located in which bladder training was compared to other treatments: PFMT in four studies of good to excellent quality (Kafri et al., 2015; Sherburn et al., 2011; Wyman et al., 1998; Yoon et al., 2003), and antimuscarinic drug therapy in one study of excellent quality (Kafri et al., 2015) and two studies of fair quality (Jarvis, 1981). In trials comparing bladder training to PFMT involving 239 women, there were inconsistent results regarding its comparative efficacy. Group bladder training was found to be inferior to group PFMT in women with stress urinary incontinence on improving symptoms, bother and perception of change, but there were no differences in mean voided volume and generic quality of life (Sherburn et al., 2011). In one trial in women with urgency urinary incontinence (Kafri et al., 2015), bladder training had similar efficacy as PFMT in improving 24-hour voiding frequency, voided volume, urgency urinary incontinent episodes, quality of life and pad use at 2 months and 1 year, and in another trial (Wyman et al., 1998), PFMT had greater efficacy at 12 weeks in reducing incontinent episodes in women with detrusor overactivity with and without stress incontinence or stress incontinence alone; however, by 24 weeks, bladder training and PFMT had similar efficacy. In a smaller trial in women with urinary incontinence (Yoon et al., 2003), bladder training resulted in significantly reduced urinary frequency and nocturia and increased voided volume when compared to PFMT, and similar results in pad test amounts.

There were inconsistent findings in the three trials involving 214 women with urgency urinary incontinence or detrusor overactivity that compared bladder training alone or with placebo to antimuscarinic drug therapy (Columbo et al., 1995; Jarvis, 1981; Kafri et al., 2015;). In one study of excellent quality (Kafri et al., 2015), bladder training had similar efficacy as sustained-release tolterodine 4 mg daily on 24-hour voiding frequency, incontinent episodes and quality of life but better efficacy on decreasing symptoms and improving overall disability limitations. In a fair-quality trial (Jarvis, 1981), an inpatient bladder training programme was superior to an outpatient programme of flavoxate and imipramine (now rarely used for urinary incontinence) in reducing urinary frequency and improving symptom-free continence status in women with detrusor overactivity. A third poor quality trial (Columbo et al., 1995) found that a 6-week course of immediate-release 5-mg

oxybutynin chloride three times a day had a similar clinical cure rate (e.g., self-reported total disappearance of urgency incontinence, no protective pads or further treatment) as bladder training. The relapse rate at 6 months was higher for the drug group, whereas those in the bladder training group showed better maintenance of their results. Although there were higher clinical cure rates (e.g., no urgency urinary incontinence episodes or pad use) in the drug group for women with urgency urinary incontinence, bladder training resulted in higher clinical cure rates for those with OAB without detrusor overactivity. Women in the bladder training group also had a significant increase in the first desire to void and higher reductions in diurnal frequency and nocturia. There have been no published trials comparing bladder training to electrical stimulation, incontinence devices or surgical management. Overall, there is insufficient evidence for or against bladder training in comparison to PFMT or drug therapy in women with OAB, urgency urinary incontinence or stress urinary incontinence.

Bladder Training Versus Bladder Training and Other Treatments

Four trials involving 352 women were located in which bladder training was compared to an intervention combining bladder training with other treatments. These included three studies of good to excellent quality (Kafri et al., 2015; Kaya et al., 2013; Wyman et al., 1998) that compared bladder training to bladder training combined with PFMT and lifestyle advice, and one study of low quality (Bryant et al., 2002) that included a comparison to bladder training with caffeine reduction.

There are inconsistent results in studies comparing bladder training to bladder training with PFMT. In one trial of good quality involving a 12-week intervention with more than 50 participants in each treatment arm (Wyman et al., 1998), slightly less than half of the participants had OAB symptoms (48.5%), whereas the number of women who actually had detrusor overactivity was less than a quarter of the sample (24.5%). Although more women reported that they were much or somewhat better with PFMT than bladder training, the difference did not reach statistical significance at 3 or 6 months. Similarly, although women in the PFMT group had fewer incontinent episodes per day than those in the bladder training group, the difference was not statistically significant at 3 or 6 months post-treatment (Wyman et al., 1998). An excellent-quality RCT (Kafri et al., 2015) involving women with urgency urinary incontinence found no differences between a 12-week programme of bladder training and combined pelvic floor rehabilitation (bladder training, PFMT and lifestyle advice) compared to bladder training alone with respect to 24-hour voiding frequency, voided volume, incontinent episodes, quality of life and pad use at 3 months and 1 year. There was a slight advantage for the combined pelvic floor rehabilitation group to decrease voiding frequency and improve self-reported function. The results in a small RCT (Yoon et al., 2003) in women with urinary incontinence that compared an 8-week outpatient bladder training programme to biofeedback-assisted PFMT are difficult to interpret because of low power and unclear reporting of incontinent episodes and between group changes. No significant differences at post-treatment were found between groups on volume of urine leaked on a clinic pad test. The bladder training group was found to have a significant decrease in micturition and nocturia, and a significant increase in voided volume when compared to the combined group. With only four trials, small sample sizes and a limited number of OAB participants, there is insufficient evidence for an improved effect of combining bladder training with PFMT versus bladder training alone in the treatment for urgency incontinence and OAB.

A small RCT (Bryant et al., 2002) that compared bladder training alone to bladder training with caffeine reduction in adults with OAB found that the combination intervention was more successful than bladder training in reducing urgency episodes. Although the combination therapy group also had a greater reduction in incontinent episodes, this was not statistically significant and could have been affected by lower power. Overall, there was insufficient evidence to determine whether bladder training and caffeine reduction for individuals who consume more than 100 mg of caffeine daily is superior to bladder training alone.

Bladder Training and Drug Therapy Versus Drug Therapy or Placebo

Three trials of good quality were located involving 602 adults that combined bladder training with drug therapy or placebo (Mattiasson et al., 2003; Szonyi et al., 1995; Wiseman et al., 1991). One study (Szonyi et al., 1995) conducted with older adults found that bladder training and oxybutynin (2.5 mg immediate release twice daily) was superior to a placebo group in reducing daytime frequency and producing subjective benefit. However, there were no differences between groups in reducing incontinent episodes or nocturia. One large RCT (Mattiasson et al., 2003) compared bladder training and tolterodine (2 mg twice daily) to drug alone in adults with OAB with and without urgency incontinence. In this trial, bladder training significantly augmented drug therapy, resulting in reduced voiding frequency and increased volume per void compared to drug alone. However, there was no difference between groups in their reduction of incontinence episodes and urgency episodes. A small trial (Wiseman et al., 1991) conducted in older adults with OAB due to detrusor overactivity found that there was no difference between terodiline (now withdrawn from the market) and bladder training as compared to a placebo and bladder training in micturition frequency and incontinent episodes. Overall, there is weak evidence that favours augmenting OAB drug therapy with bladder training for OAB. The results tend to favour that bladder training does improve urinary frequency; it is inconclusive, however, that it benefits urgency incontinence or nocturia.

CONCLUSION

In summary, the evidence base on bladder training comprises relatively few good- to excellent-quality trials, with most having small sample sizes. There is no evidence to judge the benefit of bladder training as a sole intervention in the prevention of OAB and only weak evidence to judge its effectiveness in treatment as a sole intervention. Bladder training may be helpful in the short-term treatment of OAB in women, but evidence regarding its long-term effects is inconclusive. There is insufficient evidence comparing bladder training to other non-surgical treatments and current drug therapies. The additional benefits of combining bladder training with other treatments were inconsistent, although it may be beneficial to add caffeine reduction and PFMT to bladder training for patients with OAB. There may be a benefit of augmenting drug therapy with bladder training, but these benefits were not consistently noted on all OAB symptoms.

CLINICAL RECOMMENDATIONS

Bladder training has no known adverse effects and can be used safely as a first-line treatment for OAB in women. Although it may be helpful for men as well, there is insufficient evidence regarding its use. Its effects might be augmented by caffeine reduction for individuals who have difficulty with urinary urgency and who drink more than 100 mg of caffeine daily. Bladder training may also further improve urinary symptoms in those on drug therapies for OAB and urinary incontinence.

Bladder training programmes can be successfully implemented in outpatient settings. Some evidence suggests that individual and small group bladder training programmes are equally effective in improving OAB symptoms (Hulbæk et al., 2016). The ICI has recommended that bladder training be initiated by assigning an initial voiding interval based on the baseline voiding frequency (Dumoulin et al., 2017; Wallace et al., 2009). Typically, this is set at a 1-hour interval during waking hours, although a shorter interval (e.g., ≤30 minutes) may be necessary. The schedule is increased by 15 to 30 minutes per week depending on tolerance to the schedule (i.e., fewer incontinent episodes than the previous week, minimal interruptions to the schedule and the individual's control over urgency). Ideally the healthcare provider should monitor a patient's progress on a weekly basis during the training period. More intensive supervision is preferable to less intensive supervision.

Patient education should be provided about normal bladder control and methods to control urgency such as distraction and relaxation techniques including pelvic floor muscle contraction. Self-monitoring of voiding behaviour using voiding diaries is a useful adjunct to treatment and can help the patient and clinician evaluate adherence to the schedule, evaluate progress and determine whether the voiding schedule should be changed.

Clinicians should monitor progress, determine adjustments to the voiding interval and provide positive reinforcement during the training period. If there is no improvement after 3 weeks of bladder training, the patient should be re-evaluated with consideration given to other treatment options.

REFERENCES

Balk, E., Adam, G. P., Kimmel, H., et al. (2018). *Nonsurgical treatments for urinary incontinence in women: A systematic review update. Comparative effectiveness review No. 212. AHRQ publication No. 18-EHCO016-EF. PCORI publication No. 2018-SR-03*. Rockville, MD: Agency for Healthcare Research and Quality.

Berghmans, K. C. M., Hendriks, H. J. M., de Bie, R. A., et al. (2000). Conservative treatment of urge urinary incontinence in women: A systematic review of randomized clinical trials. *BJU International, 85*, 254–263.

Bryant, C., Dowell, C. J., & Fairbrother, G. (2002). Caffeine reduction education to improve urinary symptoms. *British Journal of Nursing, 11*, 560–565.

Burkhard, F. C., Bosch, J. L. H. R., Cruz, F., et al. (2018). *Urinary incontinence guidelines, European association of Urology [online]*. Available https://uroweb.org/guideline/urinary-incontinence (accessed 14.07.22).

Columbo, M., Zanetta, G., Scalambrino, S., et al. (1995). Oxybutynin and bladder training in the management of female urinary urge incontinence: A randomized study. *International Urogynecology Journal and Pelvic Floor Dysfunction, 6*(1), 63–67.

Corcos, J., Przydacz, M., Campeau, L., et al. (2017). CUA guideline on adult overactive bladder. *Cancer Urology Associate Journal, 11*(5), E142–E143.

Davila, G. W., & Promozich, J. (1998). Prospective randomized trial of bladder retraining using an electronic voiding device versus self-administered bladder drills in women with detrusor instability. *Neurourology and Urodynamics, 17*(4), 324–325.

Dougherty, M. C., Dwyer, J. W., Pendergast, J. F., et al. (2002). A randomized trial of behavioral management for continence with older rural women. *Research in Nursing and Health, 25*, 3–13.

Dumoulin, C., Adequyi, T., Booth, J., et al. (2017). Committee 12: Adult conservative management. In P. Abrams, L. Cardozo, A. Wagg, et al. (Eds.), *Incontinence: Sixth international consultation on incontinence* (pp. 1443–1628). Bristol, UK: ICUD.

Fantl, J. A., Hurt, W. G., & Dunn, L. J. (1981). Detrusor instability syndrome: The use of bladder retraining drills with and without anticholinergics. *American Journal of Obstetrics and Gynecology, 140*(8), 885–890.

Fantl, J. A., Newman, D. K., Colling, J., et al. (1996). *Urinary incontinence in adults: Acute and chronic management. Clinical practice guideline, No. 2. 1996 update*. Rockville, MD: Agency for Health Care Policy and Research.

Fantl, J. A., Wyman, J. F., McClish, D. K., et al. (1991). Efficacy of bladder training in older women with urinary incontinence. *JAMA, 265*(5), 609–613.

Frewen, W. K. (1979). Role of bladder training in the treatment of the unstable bladder in the female. *Urology Clinical North America, 6*(1), 273–277.

Frewen, W. K. (1980). The management of urgency and frequency of micturition. *British Journal of Urology, 52*, 367–369.

Gormley, E. A., Lightner, D. J., Burgio, K. L., et al. (2019). *Diagnosis and treatment of non-neurogenic overactive bladder*

(OAB) in adults: An AUA/SUFU guideline (2019) [online]. Available: https://www.auanet.org/guidelines/overactive-bladder-(oab)-guideline (accessed 14.07.22).

Gravas, S., Cornu, J. N., Gacci, M., et al. (2020). *Management of non-neurogenic Male LUTS guidelines, European Association of Urology [online]*. Available: https://uroweb.org/guideline/treatment-of-non-neurogenic-male-luts (accessed 14.07.22).

Hadley, E. D. (1986). Bladder training and related therapies for urinary incontinence in older people. *JAMA, 256*(3), 372–379.

Hulbæk, M., Kayse, K., & Kesmodel, U. S. (2016). Group training for overactive bladder in female patients: A clinical, randomized, non-blinded study. *International Journal Urology Nursing, 10*(2), 88–96.

Jarvis, G. J. (1981). A controlled trial of bladder drill and drug therapy in the management of detrusor instability. *British Journal of Urology, 53*(6), 565–566.

Jarvis, G. J., & Millar, D. R. (1980). Controlled trial of bladder drill for detrusor instability. *BMJ, 281*(6251), 1322–1323.

Jeffcoate, T. N. A., & Francis, W. J. (1966). Urgency incontinence in the female. *American Journal of Obstetrics and Gynecology, 94*, 604–618.

Kafri, S., Akbayrak, T., Gursen, C., et al. (2015). Short-term effect of adding pelvic floor muscle training to bladder training for female urinary incontinence: A randomized controlled trial. *International Urogynecology Journal, 26*, 285–293.

Kaya, R., Deutscher, D., Shames, J., et al. (2013). Randomized trial of a comparison of rehabilitation or drug therapy for urgency urinary incontinence: 1-year follow-up. *International Urogynecology Journal, 24*, 1181–1189.

Mattiasson, A., Blaakaer, J., Hoye, K., et al. (2003). Simplified bladder training augments the effectiveness of tolterodine in patients with an overactive bladder. *BJU International, 91*(1), 54–60.

Moore, K., Dumoulin, C., Bradley, C., et al. (2013). Adult conservative management. In P. Abrams, L. Cardozo, S. Khoury, et al. (Eds.), *Incontinence* (5th ed.) (pp. 1101–1227). Paris: Health Communications Press.

National Clinical Guideline Centre (NICE). (2015). *Lower urinary tract symptoms in men: Management (clinical guideline CG97) [online]*. Available: https://www.nice.org.uk/guidance/cg97 (accessed 14.07.22).

National Clinical Guideline Centre (NICE). (2019). *Urinary incontinence and pelvic organ prolapse in women: Management (clinical guideline NG123) [online]*. Available: https://www.nice.org.uk/guidance/ng123 (accessed 14.07.22).

PEDro. (2020). *Physiotherapy evidence database*. Available: https://pedro.org.au (accessed 14.07.22).

Ramsey, I. N., Ali, H. M., Hunger, M., et al. (1996). A prospective randomized controlled trial of inpatient versus outpatient continence programs in the treatment of urinary incontinence in the female. *International Urogynecology Journal, 7*, 260–263.

Rovner, E. S., Wyman, J., & Lam, S. (2019). Urinary incontinence. In J. T. DiPiro, G. C. Yee, L. M. Posey, et al. (Eds.), *Pharmacotherapy: A pathophysiologic approach* (11th ed.) (pp. 1431–1450). New York: McGraw Hill.

Sampselle, C. M., Messer, K. L., Seng, J. S., et al. (2005). Learning outcomes of a group behavioral modification program to prevent urinary incontinence. *International Urogynecology Journal, 16*, 441–446.

Shamilyan, T., Wyman, J., Bliss, D. Z., et al. (2007). *Prevention of urinary and fecal incontinence. Publication No. 08-E003*. Rockville, MD: Agency for Healthcare Policy and Research.

Shamilyan, T., Wyman, J., Sainfort, F., et al. (2012). *Nonsurgical treatments for urinary incontinence in adult women: Diagnosis and comparative effectiveness*. Rockville, MD: Agency for Healthcare Research and Quality.

Sherburn, M., Bird, M., Carey, M., et al. (2011). Incontinence improves in older women after intensive pelvic floor muscle training: An assessor-blinded randomized controlled trial. *Neurourology and Urodynamics, 30*, 317–324.

Szonyi, G., Collas, D. M., Ding, Y. Y., et al. (1995). Oxybutynin with bladder retraining for detrusor instability in elderly people: A randomized controlled trial. *Age and Ageing, 24*(4), 287–291.

Visco, A. G., Weidner, A. C., Cuniff, G. W., et al. (1999). Observed patient compliance with a structured outpatient bladder retraining program. *American Journal of Obstetrics and Gynecology, 181*(6), 1392–1394.

Wagg, A., Chen, L. K., Johnson, T., II., et al. (2017). Committee 11: Incontinence in frail older persons. In P. Abrams, L. Cardozo, A. Wagg, et al. (Eds.), *Incontinence: Sixth International Consultation on Incontinence* (pp. 1311–1441). Bristol, UK: ICUD.

Wallace, S. A., Roe, B., Williams, K., et al. (2009). Bladder training for urinary incontinence in adults. *Cochrane Database of Systematic Reviews* Issue 1, Art. No. CD001308.

Wiseman, P. A., Malone-Lee, J., & Rai, G. S. (1991). Terodiline with bladder training for treating detrusor instability in elderly people. *BMJ, 302*(6783), 994–996.

Wyman, J. F., & Fantl, J. A. (1991). Bladder training in ambulatory care management of urinary incontinence. *Urologic Nursing, 11*(3), 11–17.

Wyman, J. F., Fantl, J. A., McClish, D. K., et al. (1998). Comparative efficacy of behavioral interventions in the management of female urinary incontinence. *American Journal of Obstetrics and Gynecology, 179*(4), 999–1007.

Yoon, J. S., Song, J. J., & Ro, Y. J. (2003). A comparison of effectiveness of bladder training and pelvic muscle exercise on female urinary incontinence. *International Journal of Nursing Studies, 40*, 45–50.

Pelvic Floor Muscle Training

Kari Bø and Cristine Homsi Jorge

INTRODUCTION

In clinical practice, many patients with overactive bladder (OAB) symptoms are treated with lifestyle interventions, pelvic floor muscle training (PFMT) with and without biofeedback, electrical stimulation, bladder training or medication, and often many of the interventions are combined. When different methods are combined, it is not possible to analyse the cause–effect of the different interventions. In most systematic reviews on efficacy of PFMT to prevent and treat urinary incontinence, studies including patients with symptoms or urodynamic diagnosis of stress urinary incontinence (SUI), urgency urinary incontinence (UUI) and mixed urinary incontinence are combined (Dumoulin et al., 2018; Hay-Smith et al., 2011; Herderschee et al., 2011). This makes it impossible to understand the real effect of the individual interventions on each condition.

Although there are theories suggesting pelvic floor muscle (PFM) dysfunction as a common cause of the two main diagnoses (SUI and UUI) (Artibani, 1997; Mattiasson, 1997), the mechanisms behind the PFM dysfunction in each of these diagnoses are not yet thoroughly understood, and pathophysiological factors may be quite different (rupture of the pelvic floor and connective tissue during childbirth for SUI, caffeine-induced UUI in an elderly woman). Optimally, the physical therapy intervention should relate to the underlying pathophysiological condition. PFMT may have different cure and improvement rates for SUI and UUI, and the combination of heterogeneous patient groups in systematic reviews and meta-analyses may disseminate the real cure rate for each of the diagnoses. In addition, and most important, an optimal PFMT protocol may be different for the two conditions due to a different theoretical rationale. In this chapter we will therefore cover studies including only female patients with symptoms and diagnosis of OAB and studies where PFMT with or without biofeedback or vaginal cones was the only intervention.

RATIONALE FOR THE EFFECT OF PELVIC FLOOR MUSCLE TRAINING

The rationale behind the use of PFMT to treat symptoms of OAB is based on observations from electrical stimulation and urodynamic assessment during PFM contraction. Godec et al. (1975) studied 40 patients with cystometrograms, taken during and after 3 minutes of 20-Hz functional electrical stimulation. The results showed that during such stimulation, hyperactivity of the bladder was diminished or completely abolished in 31 of 40 patients. One minute after stimulation cessation, the inhibition was still present. Mean bladder capacity also increased significantly, from 151 ± 126 mL to 206 ± 131 mL (p < 0.05).

De Groat (1997) noted that during the storage of urine, distension of the bladder produces low-level vesical afferent firing. This stimulates the sympathetic outflow to the bladder outlet (base and urethra) and the pudendal outflow to the external urethral sphincter. He stated that these responses occur by spinal reflex pathways, representing 'guarding reflexes' that promote continence. Sympathetic firing also inhibits the detrusor muscle and bladder ganglia. Morrison (1993) claimed that the excitatory loop through Barrington's micturition centre is switched on at bladder pressures between 5 and 25 mmHg, whereas the inhibitory loop through the raphe nucleus is active predominantly above 25 mmHg. The inhibition is at the automatic level, with the person not being conscious of the increasing tone in the PFMs and urethral wall striated muscles.

Shafik and Shafik (2003) investigated the effect of a voluntary PFM contraction on detrusor and urethral pressures in 28 patients with OAB (mean age 48.8 ± 10.2 years, 18 men and 10 women) and 17 healthy volunteers (mean age 42.6 ± 9.8 years, 12 men and 5 women). They found that during PFM contraction the urethral pressure significantly increased and vesical pressure significantly decreased in both patients and healthy subjects. The change during PFM contraction was significantly larger in the healthy participants. The authors concluded that PFM contractions led to a decline of detrusor pressure, an increase of urethral pressures and suppression of the micturition reflex, and that the results encourage PFM contractions in treatment of OAB.

Clinical experience suggests that patients can successfully inhibit urgency, detrusor contraction and urinary leakage also by walking, bending forwards, crossing their legs, using hip adductor muscles with or without conscious co-contraction of the PFMs, or by conscious contraction of the PFMs alone. After inhibition of the urgency to void and detrusor contraction, the patients may gain time to reach the toilet and thereby prevent leakage. The reciprocal inhibition reflex runs via cerebral control, recruiting ventral horn motor neurons for voluntary PFM contraction and inhibiting the parasympathetic excitatory pathway for the micturition reflex via Onuf's ganglion. This mechanism has been exploited as part of bladder training regimens (Burgio et al., 1998). There may therefore be two main hypotheses for the mechanism of PFMT to treat urgency incontinence:

- intentional contraction of the PFMs during urgency and holding of the contraction until the urge to void disappears, and
- strength training of the PFMs with the aim of long-lasting changes in muscle morphology, which may stabilize neurogenic activity.

None of the studies in this field (neither uncontrolled studies nor randomized controlled trials [RCTs]) have evaluated whether changes in the inhibitory mechanisms really occur after PFMT. In addition, research in this area is relatively new, and there does not seem to be any consensus on the optimal exercise protocol to prevent or treat OAB (Bø et al., 2020; Monteiro et al., 2018). The theoretical basis of how PFMT may work in the treatment of OAB therefore remains unclear.

METHODS

This systematic review is based on a Cochrane review (Rai et al., 2012) and three published systematic reviews (Bø et al., 2020; Greer et al., 2012; Monteiro et al., 2018). In addition we conducted an electronic search on PubMed limited to the past 5 years on 1 April 2020. No additional RCTs were found. Only fully published RCTs including female patients with OAB symptoms (frequency, urgency, nocturia and UUI) alone with PFMT as the only treatment were included. RCTs in women during pregnancy and in neurological patients

and children were excluded. Methodological quality is classified according to the PEDro rating scale, which has been found to have high reliability (Maher et al., 2003).

EVIDENCE FOR PELVIC FLOOR MUSCLE TRAINING TO TREAT OVERACTIVE BLADDER SYMPTOMS

Twelve RCTs were identified using PFMT alone to treat symptoms of OAB. One of the RCTs was a 4-year follow-up of another RCT (Azuri et al., 2017). The outcome measures, content of the intervention and results of the studies are presented in Table 7.2.3. The heterogeneity of outcome measures and interventions was too huge to justify a statistical meta-analysis of the results. PFMT provided a significant reduction of OAB symptoms compared to the control interventions in only four of 11 studies (Alves et al., 2015; Firra et al., 2013; Kim et al., 2011a; Wang et al., 2004). Breathing exercises are believed to be effective in treatment of pelvic floor dysfunction by some physical therapists. Huang et al. (2019) randomized 161 women with OAB to either 12 weeks of respiration exercise with biofeedback (n = 82) or a control group using an identical-appearing control device reprogrammed to play music without guiding breathing (n = 79). The breathing exercise group was not superior to the music-listening control in reducing urinary symptoms or changing autonomic function.

Methodological quality is presented in Table 7.2.4. The studies had moderate to high methodological quality with total scores on PEDro between 4 and 7.

Quality of the Intervention: Dose–Response Issues

Quality of the interventions is difficult to judge because there are no direct recommendations on how PFMT should be conducted to inhibit urgency and detrusor contraction. The published studies have all used different exercise protocols. Table 7.2.3 shows that frequency of supervised training varied between 4 and 24 sessions and the duration of the exercise period lasted between 6 and 12 weeks. The number of slow PFM contractions per day varied from 8 to 50, and the contractions were sustained for 6 to 12 seconds. The number of fast contractions per day varied from 10 to 40. Intensity of this contraction varied between submaximal to maximum contractions or different combinations of the two, but

TABLE 7.2.3   Randomized Controlled Trials of Pelvic Floor Muscle Training Alone to Treat Overactive Bladder Symptoms in Women

Author	Yoon et al. (2003)
Design	3-arm RCT: bladder training vs PFMT vs inactive control
Sample size and age (years)	N = 50; age 35–45
Outcome	Bladder diary
PFMT protocol	8-week intervention; 30 PFM contractions sustained for 6 s in the first week and extending with 1 s each week until reaching 12 s, performed every day at home + 20-min weekly supervised session with biofeedback
Drop-out	12%
Adherence	Not reported
Results	Non-significant
Author	**Wang et al. (2004)**
Design	3-arm RCT: PFMT; PFMT + biofeedback; ES
Sample size and age (years)	N = 120; mean age 52.7 (SD: 13.7)
Outcome	Symptoms of OBA >6 months, frequency ≥8 ×/day, urge incontinence ≥1×/day
PFMT protocol	12 weeks Home exercise: based on individual PFM strength 3×/day Same home training + in-clinic biofeedback twice a week
Drop-out	14%
Adherence	PFMT: 83% PFMT + biofeedback: 75% ES: 79% Home exercise PFMT: 14.5 days PFMT + biofeedback: 8.5 days
Results	PFMT mean number of leakages/day 0.73 (SD: 1.82) vs PFMT + biofeedback 0.70 (SD: 1.80) vs ES 1.95 (SD: 2.84) (significant difference between both PFMT groups and ES at post-test); with PFMT, UUI resolved in 30%, modified 6%, unchanged 64% PFMT + biofeedback: UUI resolved in 38%, modified 12%, unchanged 40%; no change in urodynamic parameters Improvement/cured: PFMT 38%; PFMT + biofeedback 50% PFM strength with vaginal palpation (0–5 scale: significant difference at post-test in PFMT + biofeedback –2.5 (–5.1) vs ES 0 (–2.2) Times of fast contraction: PFMT + biofeedback –6.21 (SD: 4.56) vs ES –3.03 (SD: 4.98) vs PFMT –2 (–5) vs ES 0 (2.2) Number of fast contraction: PFMT 5.82 (SD: 5.05) vs ES 3.03 (SD: 4.98) Manometry at post-test: significant difference in PFM strength in PFMT + biofeedback –38.35 (SD: 29.62) vs ES –8.91 (SD: 12.83); PFMT 36.03 (SD: 21.79) vs ES 8.91 (SD: 12.83)
Author	**Arruda et al. (2008)**
Design	3-arm RCT: oxybutynin (5 mg) vs functional electrostimulation vs PFMT
Sample size and age (years)	N = 64; age 35–80
Outcome	7-day bladder diary: women's self-report of urgency
PFMT protocol	Supervised PFMT twice a week for 12 weeks: 40 fast (2- and 5-s) and 20 sustained (10-s) PFM contractions + home training
Drop-out	16.8%
Adherence	Not reported
Results	Non-significant

TABLE 7.2.3 Randomized Controlled Trials of Pelvic Floor Muscle Training Alone to Treat Overactive Bladder Symptoms in Women—cont'd

Author	**Kim et al. (2011a)**
Design	2-arm RCT: PFMT + fitness exercise, 24 sessions, twice a week for 12 weeks vs general education classes once a month for 3 months not including PFMT information
Sample size and age (years)	N = 127; age 75.9
Outcome	ICIQ-UI SF
PFMT protocol	10 fast contractions (3 s), 5-s interval, 10 sustained contractions (8–10 s), 10-s interval performed in different positions
Drop-out	5.5%
Adherence	70.3%
Results	Mean urinary leakage score at post-test, significant difference between groups; PFMT T0 5 (SD: 1), T1 3 (SD: 2), T2 3.6 (SD: 2.2) vs control group T0 5.1 (SD: 1), T1 4.4 (SD: 1.6), T2 4.8 (1.6) ANOVA group × time F = 7.64
Author	**Kim et al. (2011b)**
Design	4-arm RCT: supervised PFMT + general strength and stretching exercises vs heat and steam generating vs supervised PFMT + general strength and stretching exercises + heat and steam generating for 3 months vs general education group once a month for a total of 3 times
Sample size and age (years)	N = 147; mean age 76
Outcome	ICIQ-UI SF
PFMT protocol	10 fast contractions (3 s), 5-s interval, 10 sustained contractions (8–10 s), 10-s interval performed in different positions, 24 sessions, twice a week for 12 weeks
Drop out	2.7%
Adherence	Not reported
Results	Non-significant
Author	**Kafri et al. (2013)**
Design	4-arm RCT: tolterodine SR 4 mg vs bladder training vs PFMT vs combined pelvic floor rehabilitation (bladder training + PFMT + bowel education)
Sample size and age (years)	N = 164; mean age 56.7
Outcome	Bladder diary: women's report of urinary frequency, 3 episodes of UUI over 4 weeks
PFMT protocol	4 sessions, once every 3 weeks for 3 months: 3 sets of 8–12 slow maximal contractions sustained for 6–8 s, progressing from lying to standing + home with repeated contractions to diminish urgency
Drop-out	17.6%
Adherence	Not reported
Results	Non-significant
Author	**Firra et al. (2013)**
Design	3-arm RCT: control group (inactive) vs PFMT vs PFMT + ES
Sample size and age (years)	N = 64; mean age 58.01
Outcome	Urodynamic testing or the MESA self-report questionnaire
Training protocol	8 weeks, twice a week (16 sessions): 6 different PFM exercises including transverse abdominals and multifidus, 10 contractions sustained for 10 s, 20-s rests between contractions, 5 times per day + biofeedback
Drop-out	25%

Continued

TABLE 7.2.3   Randomized Controlled Trials of Pelvic Floor Muscle Training Alone to Treat Overactive Bladder Symptoms in Women—cont'd

Adherence	Not reported
Results	Urinary frequency post-treatment: control group mean 24.2 (SD: 10.4) vs PFMT mean 23.5 (SD: 5.9), p < 0.05
	Manometry, significant at post-test: control group mean 34.3 cmH$_2$O (SD: 25.5) vs PFMT mean 47.2 (SD: 22.7)
Author	**Alves et al. (2015)**
Design	2-arm RCT: supervised PFMT + fitness programme vs information of PFMT
Sample size and age (years)	N = 30; mean age 65.93
Outcome	ICIQ-UI SF and ICIQ-OAB: urgency with or without UI, urinary frequency >8 voids/day and nocturia
PFMT protocol	12 sessions of supervised PFMT + fitness programme twice a week for 6 weeks vs only instructions about PFM function and how to contract; protocol included 4 series of ten fast contractions together with 4 series of ten 8-s contractions, 16-s relaxation period, different positions
Drop-out	28.57%
Adherence	Not reported
Results	ICIQ-OAB: a significant reduced score of UI found only in PFMT group (at post-test); effect size: 0.47 ICIQ-UI SF
	Palpation of PFM strength (0–5 scale)
	Significant difference at post-test PFMT: mean 3.16 (SD: 1.09) vs control mean 2.58 (SD: 0.99)
	sEMG at post-test, significant difference:
	PFMT mean 28.12 µV (SD: 16.80) vs control group mean 27.80 (SD: 13.96)
Author	**Azuri et al. (2017)**
Design	4-arm RCT: tolterodine SR 4 mg vs bladder training vs PFMT vs combined pelvic floor (bladder training + PFMT + bowel education)
Sample size and age (years)	N = 120; mean age 59.5
Outcome	Bladder diary: women's report of urinary frequency, 3 episodes of UUI over 4 weeks
PFMT protocol	4 sessions, once every 3 weeks for 3 months: three sets of 8–12 slow maximal contractions sustained for 6–8 s, progressing from lying to standing + PFMT home with repeated contractions to diminish urgency
Drop-out	26.8%
Adherence	Not reported
Results	Non-significant
Author	**Rizvi et al. (2018)**
Design	3-arm RCT: bladder training vs PFMT vs PFMT + biofeedback
Sample size and age (years)	N = 150; age 22–65
Outcome	UDI-SF6
PFMT protocol	Submaximal to maximal PFM contractions for 6 s, 5 times and 10 fast contractions per session; all patients were instructed to practice this protocol at home at least 3 times daily in different positions; PFMT + biofeedback group performed supervised sessions twice a week + PFMT following audiovisual signals
Drop-out	2%
Adherence	Not reported

TABLE 7.2.3 Randomized Controlled Trials of Pelvic Floor Muscle Training Alone to Treat Overactive Bladder Symptoms in Women—cont'd

Results	Non-significant
Author	**Bykoviene et al. (2018)**
Design	3-arm RCT: control group (behavioural treatment + PFMT orientation) vs PFMT group vs PFMT + electrical stimulation of tibial nerve
Sample size and age (years)	N = 67; mean age 62.4
Outcome	3-day bladder diary
PFMT protocol	Protocols were determined according to PERFECT scheme, 5 times daily in different positions + participants taught to contract PFMs during an urge to void
Drop-out	8.9%
Adherence	Not reported
Results	Non-significant
Author	**Furtado-Albanezi et al. (2019)**
Design	2-arm RCT: electrical stimulation vs PFMT
Sample size and age (years)	N = 48; mean age 57.5
Outcome	Self-report of ≤1 episode of nocturia/night
PFMT protocol	Supervised 12 sessions 30 min once a week: 8–12 maximal contractions sustained for 6 to 8 s, 6-s rest interval performed in different static and dynamic positions
Drop-out	16.6%
Adherence	Not reported
Results	Non-significant

ES, Electrical stimulation; *ICIQ-OAB,* International Consultation on Incontinence Questionnaire–Overactive Bladder; *ICIQ-UI SF,* International Consultation on Incontinence Questionnaire–Urinary Incontinence Short Form; *MESA,* Medical, Epidemiologic, and Social aspects of Aging; *OAB,* overactive bladder; *PFM,* pelvic floor muscle; *PFMT,* pelvic floor muscle training; *RCT,* randomized controlled trial; *sEMG,* surface electromyography; *SR,* sustained release; *UDI-SF6,* Urinary Distress Inventory, Short Form; *UI,* urinary incontinence; *UUI,* urgency urinary incontinence.

some studies did not report this information (see Table 7.2.4). Building on the research from Shafik and Shafik (2003) showing that a PFM contraction can inhibit detrusor contraction and urinary leakage, it seems reasonable to put more emphasis on the immediate effect of a voluntary PFM contraction. However, only 2 of the 11 original RCTs included contractions during urge to void in the training programme (Bykoviene et al., 2018; Kafri et al., 2013), and these exercise programmes did not show any effect on OAB symptoms. The other studies included only regular strength training of the PFMs like protocols used for SUI. Six of the 11 studies assessed PFM function before and after treatment (Alves et al., 2015; Arruda et al., 2008; Firra et al., 2013; Kim et al., 2011a; Wang et al., 2004; Yoon et al., 2003), and they used three different assessment tools (vaginal palpation, surface electromyography and vaginal manometry).

Three of the six studies (Alves et al., 2015; Firra et al., 2013; Wang et al., 2004) found significant improvement in PFM variables in the groups receiving PFMT compared to other groups, and these results are shown in Table 7.2.3 All three studies reporting significant improvement in PFM variables also found significant improvement in OAB symptoms.

CONCLUSION

Eleven original RCTs and one follow-up study were found on PFMT to treat OAB symptoms in women. The studies had moderate to high methodological quality, but the heterogeneity of outcome measures and exercise protocols was too huge to justify a meta-analysis. Because the pathophysiological background for OAB is not clear, it is difficult to plan an optimal training

TABLE 7.2.4   PEDro Quality Score of Randomized Controlled Trials in Systematic Review of Pelvic Floor Muscle Training to Treat Overactive Bladder Symptoms

E – Eligibility criteria specified
1 – Subjects randomly allocated to groups
2 – Allocation concealed
3 – Groups similar at baseline
4 – Subjects blinded
5 – Therapist administering treatment blinded
6 – Assessors blinded
7 – Measures of key outcomes obtained from >85% of subjects
8 – Data analysed by intention to treat
9 – Statistical comparison between groups conducted
10 – Point measures and measures of variability provided

Study	E	1	2	3	4	5	6	7	8	9	10	Total Score
Yoon et al. (2003)	+	+	-	+	-	-	+	+	-	+	+	6
Wang et al. (2004)	+	+	+	-	-	-	+	+	-	+	-	5
Arruda et al. (2008)	+	+	-	+	-	-	-	-	-	+	+	4
Kim et al. (2011a)	+	+	-	+	-	-	+	+	-	+	+	6
Kim et al. (2011b)	+	+	-	+	-	-	-	+	-	+	+	5
Kafri et al. (2013)	+	+	+	+	-	-	-	-	+	+	+	6
Firra et al. (2013)	+	+	-	+	-	-	-	-	-	+	+	4
Alves et al. (2015)	+	+	+	+	-	-	+	-	-	+	+	6
Azuri et al. (2017)	+	+	+	+	-	-	-	-	-	+	+	5
Rizvi et al. (2018)	+	+	+	-	-	-	+	-	-	-	+	4
Bykoviene et al. (2018)	+	+	-	+	-	-	-	+	-	+	+	5
Furtado-Albanezi et al. (2019)	-	+	+	+	-	-	+	-	+	+	+	7

+, Criterion is clearly satisfied; –, criterion is not satisfied.
The total score is determined by counting the number of criteria that are satisfied, except the 'eligibility criteria specified' score is not used to generate the total score. Total scores are out of 10.

protocol. Based on the theoretical knowledge and symptoms of bladder overactivity, it seems reasonable to put more emphasis on the inhibition mechanisms of the PFM contraction and teaching and follow-up of patients trying to contract the PFMs when there is an urge to void. There is a need for more basic research to understand the role of a voluntary PFM contraction in inhibition of the micturition reflex and how this contraction should be performed (e.g., a long maximal contraction or repeated submaximal contractions?). Future RCTs with high interventional and methodological quality are recommended.

CLINICAL RECOMMENDATIONS

- Although four RCTs have shown some effect of PFMT in treatment of OAB, there are no convincing training protocols to recommend over others.
- Clinical experience and basic research show that it may be possible to learn to inhibit detrusor contraction by intentionally contracting the PFMs and holding the contraction to stop the urge to void. More basic knowledge on this mechanism is needed.
- Training protocols based on patients' and clinicians' experiences need to be tested in a high-quality RCT.

REFERENCES

Alves, F. K., Riccetto, C., Adami, D. B., et al. (2015). A pelvic floor muscle training program in postmenopausal women: A randomized controlled trial. *Maturitas, 81*(2), 300–305.

Arruda, R. M., Castro, R. A., Sousa, G. C., et al. (2008). Prospective randomized comparison of oxybutynin, functional electrostimulation, and pelvic floor training for treatment of detrusor overactivity in women. *International Urogynecology Journal and Pelvic Floor Dysfunction, 19*(8), 1055–1061.

Artibani, W. (1997). Diagnosis and significance of idiopathic overactive bladder. *Urology, 50*(Suppl. 6A), 25–32.

Azuri, J., Kafri, R., Ziv–Baran, T., et al. (2017). Outcomes of different protocols of pelvic floor physical therapy and anti–cholinergics in women with wet over–active bladder: A 4–year follow up. *Neurourology and Urodynamics, 36*(3), 755–758.

Bø, K., Fernandes, A. C. N. L., Duarte, T. B., et al. (2020). Is pelvic floor muscle training effective for symptoms of overactive bladder in women? A systematic review. *Physiotherapy, 106*, 65–76.

Burgio, K. L., Locher, J. L., Goode, P. S., et al. (1998). Behavioral vs drug treatment for urge urinary incontinence in older women: A randomized controlled trial. *JAMA, 280*(23), 1995–2000.

Bykoviene, L., Kubilius, R., Aniuliene, R., et al. (2018). Pelvic floor muscle training with or without tibial nerve stimulation and lifestyle changes have comparable effects on the overactive bladder. A randomized clinical trial. *Urology Journal, 15*(4), 186–192.

De Groat, W. (1997). A neurologic basis for the overactive bladder. *Urology, 50*(Suppl. 6A), 36–52.

Dumoulin, C., Cacciari, L. P., & Hay-Smith, E. J. C. (2018). Pelvic floor muscle training versus no treatment, or inactive control treatments, for urinary incontinence in women. *Cochrane Database of Systematic Reviews* Issue 10, Art. No. CD005654.

Firra, J., Thompson, M., & Smith, S. S. (2013). Paradoxical findings in the treatment of predominant stress and urge incontinence: A pilot study with exercise and electrical stimulation. *Journal Womens Health Physics Therapy, 37*(3), 113–123.

Furtado-Albanezi, D., Jürgensen, S. P., Avila, M. A., et al. (2019). Effects of two nonpharmacological treatments on the sleep quality of women with nocturia: A randomized controlled clinical trial. *International Urogynecology Journal, 30*(2), 279–286.

Godec, C., Cass, A., & Ayala, G. (1975). Bladder inhibition with functional electrical stimulation. *Urology, 6*(6), 663–666.

Greer, J. A., Smith, A. L., & Arya, L. A. (2012). Pelvic floor muscle training for urgency urinary incontinence in women: A systematic review. *International Urogynecology Journal, 23*, 687–697.

Hay-Smith, E. J. C., Herderschee, R., Dumoulin, C., et al. (2011). Comparisons of approaches to pelvic floor muscle training for urinary incontinence in women. *Cochrane Database of Systematic Reviews* Issue 12, Art. No. CD009508.

Herderschee, R., Hay-Smith, E. J. C., Herbison, G. P., et al. (2011). Feedback or biofeedback to augment pelvic floor muscle training for urinary incontinence in women. *Cochrane Database of Systematic Reviews* Issue 7, Art. No. CD009252.

Huang, A. J., Grady, D., & Mendes, W. B. (2019). A randomized controlled trial of device-guided slow-paced respiration in women with overactive bladder syndrome. *J Urol, 202*(4), 787–794.

Kafri, R., Deutscher, D., Shames, J., et al. (2013). Randomized trial of a comparison of rehabilitation or drug therapy for urgency urinary incontinence: 1-year follow-up. *International Urogynecology Journal, 24*(7), 1181–1189.

Kim, H., Yoshida, H., & Suzuki, T. (2011). The effects of multidimensional exercise treatment on community-dwelling elderly Japanese women with stress, urge, and mixed urinary incontinence: A randomized controlled trial. *International Journal of Nursing Studies, 48*(10), 1165–1172.

Kim, H., Yoshida, H., & Suzuki, T. (2011). Effects of exercise treatment with or without heat and steam generating sheet on urine loss in community–dwelling Japanese elderly women with urinary incontinence. *Geriatrics and Gerontology International, 11*(4), 452–459.

Maher, C., Sherrington, C., Herbert, R. D., et al. (2003). Reliability of the PEDro scale for rating quality of RCTs. *Physiotherapy, 83*(8), 713–721.

Mattiasson, A. (1997). Management of overactive bladder—looking to the future. *Urology, 50*(Suppl. 6A), 111–113.

Monteiro, S., Riccetto, C., Araújo, A., et al. (2018). Efficacy of pelvic floor muscle training in women with overactive bladder syndrome: A systematic review. *International Urogynecology Journal, 29*(11), 1565–1573.

Morrison, J. (1993). The excitability of the micturition reflex. *Scandinavian Journal of Urology and Nephrology, 29*(Suppl. 175), 21–25.

Rai, B. P., Cody, J. D., Alhasso, A., et al. (2012). Anticholinergic drugs versus non-drug active therapies for non-neurogenic overactive bladder syndrome in adults. *Cochrane Database of Systematic Reviews* Issue 12, Art No. CD003193.

Rizvi, R. M., Chughtai, N. G., & Kapadia, N. (2018). Effects of bladder training and pelvic floor muscle training in female patients with overactive bladder syndrome: A randomized controlled trial. *Urologia Internationalis, 100*(4), 420–427.

Shafik, A., & Shafik, I. A. (2003). Overactive bladder inhibition in response to pelvic floor muscle exercises. *World Journal of Urology, 20*, 374–377.

Wang, A., Wang, Y., & Chen, M. (2004). Single-blind, randomized trial of pelvic floor muscle training, biofeedback-assisted pelvic floor muscle training, and electrical stimulation in the management of overactive bladder. *Urology, 63*(1), 61–66.

Yoon, H. S., Song, H. H., & Ro, Y. J. (2003). A comparison of effectiveness of bladder training and pelvic muscle exercise on female urinary incontinence. *International Journal of Nursing Studies, 40*(1), 45–50.

Electrical Stimulation

Bary Berghmans

INTRODUCTION

Clinical experience has shown that overactive bladder (OAB) function with associated urgency urinary incontinence (UUI) is not amenable to surgical correction (Millard and Oldenburg, 1983; Ulmsten, 1999). Based on poor studies that did not compare sacral neuromodulation with other treatment methods, a Cochrane review concluded that sacral neuromodulation can be of benefit in selected patients with OAB symptoms in which other methods of treatment have failed (Dmochowski et al., 2017; Herbison and Arnold, 2009). Therefore it is important first to find another satisfactory treatment modality for patients with this problem. Pharmaceutical agents generally lead to disappointing results, with success rates of 60% to 70% in all adults and 25% to 75% in adults older than 65 years (Andersson et al., 2017) for the most effective single agents. But all of these agents show side effects to a greater or lesser extent in most of the patients, limiting their usefulness (Andersson et al., 2017). They are frequently not continued indefinitely (Andersson et al., 2017) and lead to poor tolerability in about 15% of patients (Sussman and Garely, 2002). The short duration of most clinical trials and the lack of long-term follow-up give little information about the short- and long-term efficacy and acceptability of drugs (Hsu et al., 2019; Madhuvrata et al., 2012). Although combination therapy is claimed to be more successful, the use of drugs produces many side effects, inevitably leading to non-compliance and the recurrence of incontinence (Hsu et al., 2019). A systematic review concluded that persistence rates regardless of relevant drug was generally poor, with median rates of 12% to 39.4% at 12 months and 6% to 12% at 24 months (Veenboer and Bosch, 2014). Risk factors for discontinuation included younger age groups (Veenboer and Bosch, 2014).

Besides bladder (re)-training and pelvic floor muscle training (PFMT) with or without biofeedback, electrical stimulation (ES) is one of the physical therapy treatment modalities used for management of women with OAB.

The theoretical basis of how ES for the treatment of OAB actually works remains unclear. Is it the *change* in pelvic floor muscle (PFM) activity during nervous excitation that automatically should inhibit or better prevent detrusor overactivity (Messelink, 1999; Lewis and Cheng, 2007)? Is it a *learning process* that should make the patient aware of contracting the PFMs during urgency to inhibit involuntary detrusor contraction (reciprocal inhibition) (Messelink, 1999) or a *cortical inhibition* (Pannek et al., 2010)? Is it that increase in *strength* of the PFMs could provide more inhibition of the overactivity of the bladder (Messelink, 1999)? The different physical therapy treatment modalities are therefore still based on hypotheses for the underlying pathologies causing OAB. However, clinical experience has shown that different physical therapy treatment modalities generally will provide some progress in most individuals with OAB. Improved bladder control can occur even in the cognitively impaired individual (Colling et al., 1992; Engel et al., 1990; McCormick et al., 1990; Schnelle et al., 1990).

RATIONALE FOR ELECTRICAL STIMULATION

The literature concerning ES in the management of OAB and UUI is quite difficult to interpret, due to the lack of a well-substantiated biological rationale underpinning the use of ES. The mechanisms of action may vary depending on the cause(s) of OAB and the structure(s) being targeted by ES, such as PFMs or detrusor muscle, or the peripheral or central nervous system (Dumoulin et al., 2017). Eriksen (1989), Eriksen and Eik-Nes (1989) and Fall (2000) claimed that ES theoretically stimulates the detrusor inhibition reflex and pacifies the micturition reflex, resulting in a decrease of OAB dysfunction. Schmidt (1988) hypothesized that the electrical stimulus was thought to activate the pudendal nerve, contracting the pelvic floor musculature and external urinary sphincter.

Elabbady et al. (1994) and Weil (2000) suggested that ES of PFMs induces a reflex contraction of the striated paraurethral and periurethral muscles, accompanied by a simultaneous reflex inhibition of the detrusor muscle. This reciprocal response depends on a preserved reflex arc through the sacral micturition reflex centre (Janssen et al., 2017). To obtain a therapeutic effect of pelvic floor stimulation in women with OAB, peripheral innervation of the PFMs must at least partially be intact (Eriksen, 1989; Janssen et al., 2017).

This means that when increasing stimulation is applied on the nerve, improved contraction of the muscles is obtained, resulting in more efficient detrusor inhibition (Elabbady et al., 1994; Hoebeke et al., 2001; Schmidt, 1988).

However, according to Weil (2000), detrusor inhibition is not the result of activating somatosensory efferents of the pudendal nerve (Schultz-Lampel, 1997). Schultz-Lampel (1997) holds the β-fibres of the sacral nerve afferents responsible for the electrically induced inhibition of detrusor contraction. Pudendal afferent β-fibres from the urinary sphincter and/or pelvic floor induce electrical inhibition of detrusor contractions (Schultz-Lampel, 1997). As these fibres are large in diameter, these nerve cells can be depolarized with minimal amounts of energy. Therefore ES should not be applied through muscle contraction, nor should excess energy be applied to produce depolarization of the smaller nerve fibres, like B- and unmyelinated C-fibres, which result in a painful sensation (Weil, 2000).

ES therapy alone, both external or internal, is suggested to inhibit the parasympathetic motor neurons to the bladder and to enable an effective reduction or inhibition of detrusor activity by stimulation of (large diameter) afferents of the pudendal nerve (Elabbady et al., 1994; Eriksen, 1989; Eriksen and Eik-Nes, 1989; Fall, 2000; Fall and Lindström, 1994; Hoebeke et al., 2001; Weil, 2000).

EVIDENCE FOR ELECTRICAL STIMULATION TO TREAT OVERACTIVE BLADDER SYMPTOMS

At present, few studies are performed regarding the efficacy of ES for OAB (Dumoulin et al., 2017). Systematic reviews revealed only weak evidence on the efficacy of ES alone or in combination with PFMT for women with UUI (Berghmans et al., 2000; Dumoulin et al., 2013).

However, these findings did not prove the noneffectivity of ES as a treatment modality for OAB as a whole. It was our assumption that the lack of efficacy is most likely caused by methodological flaws like heterogeneity of study groups and suboptimal research designs.

ES for OAB is provided by clinic-based mainspowered machines or portable battery-powered stimulators (Fig. 7.2.1). Also in this area, ES offers a seemingly infinite combination of current types, waveforms, frequencies, intensities, electrode placements, ES probes and so forth (Fig. 7.2.2). Without that clear biological rationale, mentioned earlier, it is difficult to make reasoned choices of ES parameters. Hence, as in ES studies for stress urinary incontinence, we see a wide variety of stimulation devices and protocols being used for OAB.

This section reviews the evidence in women comparing non-surgical ES with no treatment, placebo ES and comparisons of different ES protocols. It also includes trials comparing non-surgical ES with any other single intervention (e.g., magnetic stimulation, PFMT,

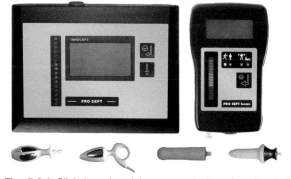

Fig. 7.2.1 Clinic-based and home-use devices for electrical stimulation.

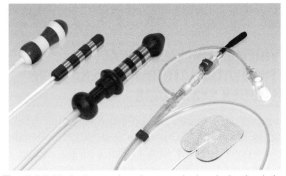

Fig. 7.2.2 Vaginal, rectal and external electrical stimulation probes.

weighted vaginal cones, surgery, medication) and trials comparing ES with any other combined intervention versus that other combined intervention alone.

Methods

Five systematic reviews (Berghmans et al., 1998; Berghmans et al., 2000; Dumoulin et al., 2017; Hay-Smith et al., 2001; Stewart et al., 2016) have been published that include trials relevant to this chapter. The following qualitative summary of the evidence regarding ES is based on the trials included in all of the previous systematic reviews with addition of trials performed after publication of the reviews and/or located through additional searching. This search was conducted in the same fashion as described earlier in the section of this chapter on ES in women with stress urinary incontinence.

To be included here, a trial needed to (1) be a randomized controlled trial (RCT), (2) include women with OAB or UUI symptoms, and (3) compare different ES protocols or investigate the effect of ES versus no treatment, placebo treatment or any other single treatment with any other combined intervention versus that other combined intervention. Published abstracts and reports of trials in progress were excluded.

Quality of Data

The two trials by Yamanishi and co-workers (Yamanishi et al., 2000a; Yamanishi et al., 2000b), the trial by Soomro et al. (2001) and that of Walsh et al. (2001) included both men and women with OAB and urinary incontinence. It is possible that the effects of stimulation might be different between genders (e.g., due to difference in electrode placement). Thus, although some of these studies included a large number of women with OAB and/or UUI symptoms and reported significant objective and/or subjective results in favour of ES in comparison to no or placebo treatment, for reasons of heterogeneity of inclusion criteria, such as differences in gender, we decided not to use these studies for the analysis of results where they did not perform subgroup analysis or did not differentiate the effects of treatment in women versus men. Only the study of Yamanishi et al. (2000b) could partly be used, where the authors did report results from subgroups according to gender. Table 7.2.5 provides details of results of all included studies (n = 16).

Again, the PEDro rating scale was used to classify the methodological quality of the included studies (Table 7.2.6). The PEDro scores were between 3 and 8 points out of 10, meaning that the studies had low (n = 2), moderate (n = 2) to high (n = 12) methodological quality.

Quality of the Intervention: Dose–Response Issues

Some ES protocols were poorly reported, lacking detail of stimulation parameters, devices and methods of delivery. However, on the basis of the details that have been reported, it appeared that there was considerable variation in ES protocols. In addition, the ES dosage (type of current, frequency, duration and intensity) varies significantly between studies (Dumoulin et al., 2017; Hay-Smith et al., 2001; Stewart et al., 2016). Looking into the studies on OAB patients included in the Cochrane systematic review reveals that length of the intervention varies between 4 months of daily stimulation (Smith, 1996) and a single episode of stimulation (Bower et al., 1998), intensity varies between 5 mA and maximal tolerable intensity, and length of each session varies between 20 minutes and several hours. Frequency of stimulation is once or twice every day in all RCTs except in studies by Abdelbary et al. (2015), Dumoulin et al. (2017), Franzen et al. (2010), Jacomo et al. (2020), Ozdedeli et al. (2010), Smith (1996), and Wang et al. (2006, 2017).

Despite the many clinical series that have been reported, the common issues of patient selection, dose–response issues and electrical parameters remain unsolved.

TABLE 7.2.5 Randomized Controlled Trials on Electrical Stimulation to Treat Overactive Bladder and/or Urgency Urinary Incontinence Symptoms

Author	Arruda et al. (2008)
Design	3-arm RCT: ES; oxybutynin; PFMT
Sample size and age (years)	64 women; age 35–80
Diagnosis	DO subjective response, voiding diary, urodynamics; UUI dominant in all MUI; SUI factor in 28.6% ES, 31.8 oxybutynin, 28.6% PFMT
Training protocol	12 weeks; 2×/week 20-min clinic ES: vaginal electrode, 10 Hz, pulse with 1 ms, intermittent biphasic, I max (range: 10–100 mA) Oxybutynin: immediate release 5 mg 2×/day PFMT: 2×/week 45-min clinic sessions: in supine, sitting and orthostatic positions forty fast (2 and 5 s) and twenty 10-s sustained contractions, 10-s relaxation, same home regimen
Drop-out	13/77 women: 4 unable to comply with ES, 4 oxybutynin, 5 PFMT, 1 no show at post-treatment urodynamics
Adherence	1 no show at post-treatment urodynamics
Results	Subjective symptomatic improvement: ES 52%, oxybutynin 77%, PFMT 76% Urgency resolved: ES 52%, oxybutynin 64%, PFMT 57% Urodynamic evaluation normal: ES 57%, oxybutynin 36%, PFMT 52% Maximum detrusor involuntary contraction pressure decreased in all groups ($p < 0.05$); all treatments equally effective Oxybutynin: high percentage of dry mouth Side effects (only reported for oxybutynin): 72.7% dry mouth, micturition difficulty 9.1% Follow-up 1 year: ES 36.4%; oxybutynin 58.8%, PFMT 56.2% persistent improvement
Author	**Berghmans et al. (2002)**
Design	4-arm RCT: LUTEs; ES; ES + LUTEs; no treatment
Sample size and age (years)	68 women; mean age 55.2 (SD: 14.4)
Diagnosis	Ambulatory urodynamics + micturition diary (DAI score ≥0.5 included)
Training protocol	9 treatments once a week daily home programme LUTEs: bladder retraining; selective contraction of the PFM to inhibit detrusor contraction; 20-s hold; toilet behaviour
Drop-out	10/68 (15%) ITT analysis of all
Adherence	92% (reported for all groups together)
Results	Dunnett's t-test: ES compared to no treatment significant difference in decrease in DAI score (0.23, $p > 0.039$), other treatment groups no difference compared with no treatment
Author	**Bower et al. (1998)**
Design	3-arm RCT: LF ES; HF ES; sham ES
Sample size and age (years)	80 women (49 OAB, 31 sensory urge); mean age 56.5 (SD: 16.9)
Diagnosis	Urodynamics (cystometry)
Training protocol	LF ES: transcutaneous, 10 Hz, pulse width 200 μs, sacral placement, I max HF ES: 150 Hz, 200 μs, suprapubic placement, I max Sham ES (placement at random): 1 session during filling cystometry
Drop-out	None
Adherence	Not applicable
Results	OAB: sham ES no sign change in first desire to void ($p = 0.69$), max cystometric capacity and detrusor pressure idem; both active ES groups reduction max detrusor pressure, significant increase in first desire to void, no change max cystometric capacity; no change in detrusor pressure at first desire to void; 44% in both active ES groups stable Sensory urgency: significant increase in first desire to void only in 150-Hz active ES; max cystometric capacity increase only in sham ES!

Continued

TABLE 7.2.5 **Randomized Controlled Trials on Electrical Stimulation to Treat Overactive Bladder and/or Urgency Urinary Incontinence Symptoms—cont'd**

Author	**Brubaker et al. (1997)**
Design	2-arm RCT: ES; sham ES
Sample size and age (years)	148 women, subgroup OAB 28 women; age mean 57 (SD: 12)
Diagnosis	Urodynamics, micturition diary
Training protocol	ES: transvaginal, 20 Hz, 2/4 s work/rest, pulse width 0.1 ms, bipolar square wave, I 0–100 mA
	Sham ES: same parameters, no I, both groups 8-week treatment
Drop-out	18%
Adherence	ES vs sham ES mean compliance 87% vs 81% at 4 and 8 treatment weeks
Results	ES vs sham ES
	54% (n = 33) OAB pre-treatment reduced to 27% (n = 16) post-treatment (p = 0.0004) vs sham ES 47% (n = 28) to 42% (p = 0.22)
	24-h frequency NS; 6-week number of accidents/24 h (average) NS; adequate subjective improvement p = 0.027; QoL NS difference; no analysis diaries because of incomplete data
Author	**Franzen et al. (2010)**
Design	2-arm RCT: ES; tolterodine 4 mg 1×/day
Sample size and age (years)	72 women with urgency/UUI (predominant)
	ES: n = 37; mean age 55 (SD: 11); range 37–79
	Tolterodine: n = 35; age 61 (SD: 12); range 37–83
Diagnosis	History taking, physical examination; optional urodynamics, cystoscopy
Training protocol	ES: Ten 20-min sessions 1–2x/week, vaginally and/or transanally, 5–10 Hz, I max tolerable
	Tolterodine SR: 6 months 4 mg orally 1×/day, with dose reduction allowed to 2 mg if intolerable side effects
Drop-out	15%: ES 6/37; tolterodine 5/35
Adherence	Tolterodine: 2/32 stopped at 6 weeks, 8/31 at 6 months, 1/32 ES switched to tolterodine
Results	Micturitions/24 h no significant difference between groups; mean voided volume idem
	Within groups: both groups had significant decrease in micturitions/24 h and increase in mean voided volume
	Subjective: at 6 months, ES 73%, tolterodine 71% lesser degree of bother from bladder symptoms; tolterodine 6% higher bother, ES equal
	Cured/improved no significant difference between groups
Author	**Ozdedeli et al. (2010)**
Design	2-arm RCT: ES; trospium hydrochloride 30 mg
Sample size and age (years)	35 women with UUI (OAB symptoms predominantly); age, median (range) ES (n = 18) 57.5 (36–78); trospium hydrochloride (n = 17) 60.0 (37–78)
Diagnosis	History taking, physical examination; urodynamics
Training protocol	ES: Eighteen 20-min sessions 3×/week, vaginal probe, 5 Hz, biphasic, symmetrical rectangular pulse, I max tolerable total duration 100 μs
	Trospium hydrochloride (Spasmex 30 mg tablet): 6 weeks, dose 45 mg/day
Drop-out	11.4%: ES 2/18; trospium hydrochloride: 2/17
Adherence	Compliance measured in trospium hydrochloride group but results not given

TABLE 7.2.5 Randomized Controlled Trials on Electrical Stimulation to Treat Overactive Bladder and/or Urgency Urinary Incontinence Symptoms—cont'd

Results	Urodynamic parameters: no significant differences between groups during all controls (after 6 [end treatment], 10 and 18 weeks); both groups equal progress
	Voiding diary: no significant differences between groups during all controls (after 6 [end treatment], 10 and 18 weeks); ES better progress
	Subjective: VAS urgency severity; IIQ-7 significant decrease in both groups; no significant difference between groups
	Treatment satisfaction: 87.6% ES and 93.3% trospium hydrochloride
	Side effects significantly less in ES (5/18, 27.7%) than in trospium hydrochloride (8/17, 47%)
Author	**Smith (1996)**
Design	2-arm RCT: ES; propantheline bromide
Sample size and age (years)	Subgroup detrusor instability, 38 women; age 44–73
Diagnosis	Cystoscopy only when indicated, complex video urodynamic study (i.e., uroflow, UPP, cystometrography, Vasalva LPP)
Training protocol	Study group: ES 5-s contractions (range: 3–15), duty circle 1:2, treatment time 15–60 min 2×/day for 4 months, I 5-max 25 mA
	Control group: propantheline bromide 7.5–45 mg 2–3×/day; written/verbal instructions timed voiding and bladder retraining
Drop-out	None
Adherence	>80%
Results	Control group: IEF 50% improved; Study group ES: IEF 72% improved, including 4 patients cured, greater bladder capacity trend in both groups; no improvement in urodynamic variables; in between NS
Author	**Soomro et al. (2001)[b]**
Design	2-arm RCT: ES; oxybutynin
Sample size and age (years)	43 patients: 30 women, 13 men; mean age 50 (SD: 15)
Diagnosis	OAB symptoms, SF-36 QoL, Bristol urinary symptom questionnaire; clinical assessment urodynamics, uroanalysis, urine cytology
Training protocol	ES: transcutaneous, 2 self-adhesive pads bilateral perianal region (S2/3 dermatome), I variable tickling sensation, 20 Hz, 200 μs, continuous, 6 h daily
	Oxybutynin: 2.5 mg orally 2×/day, titrated to 5 mg, orally 3×/day by day 7
Drop-out	Not reported
Adherence	Not reported
Results	Overall no differences between groups in symptoms, urodynamic data or SF-36 QoL, side effects
Author	**Walsh et al. (2001)[b]**
Design	2-arm RCT: ES; sham ES
Sample size and age (years)	146 patients: 111 women, 35 men with urgency incontinence age 17-79; mean age 47
Diagnosis	Clinical assessment: history and examination, uroanalysis, pelvic ultrasonography, cystourethroscopy, urodynamics
	ES: n = 74, DI/DH/SU 28/18/28
	Sham ES: n = 72, 27/17/28
Training protocol	Both groups: transcutaneous neurostimulator, bilateral S3 dermatomes; ES antidromic S3 neurostimulation, 10 Hz, 200 μs, continuous mode, I max
	Sham ES: no current
	Comparison first and second cystometry fill, and between groups

Continued

TABLE 7.2.5   Randomized Controlled Trials on Electrical Stimulation to Treat Overactive Bladder and/or Urgency Urinary Incontinence Symptoms—cont'd

Drop-out	None
Adherence	Not applicable
Results	ES: pre-/post-stimulation significantly greater mean volumes in bladder capacity at first desire to void (+57.3), strong desire to void (+68.4), urge (+55.2) and max capacity (+59.5) (p = 0.0002) Sham ES: no changes
Author	**Wang et al. (2004)**
Design	3-arm RCT: PFMT; PFMT + BF; ES
Sample size and age (years)	120 women; mean age 52.7 (SD: 13.7)
Diagnosis	Symptoms of OAB >6 months, frequency ≥8×/day, urge incontinence ≥1×/day
Training protocol	12 weeks Home exercise based on individual PFM strength 3×/day Same home training in addition to clinic BF twice a week
Drop-out	17/120 (14%)
Adherence	PFMT: 83%; PFMT + BF: 75%; ES: 79% Home exercise: PFMT 14.5 days; PFMT + BF 8.5 days
Results	PFMT: urge incontinence resolved 30%, modified 6%, unchanged 64% PFMT + BF: resolved 38%, modified 12%, unchanged 50% ES: resolved 40%, modified 11.5%, unchanged 48.5% Improvement/cured: PFMT 38%; PFMT + BF 50%; ES 51.5% PFM strength: no significant differences between exercise groups, but between both exercise groups and ES in favour of exercise groups; no change in urodynamic parameters; significant change in several QoL measures for different groups Between ES and PFMT + BF, no significant differences in improvement/reduction rate; between ES and PFMT, yes
Author	**Yamanishi et al. (2000a)[a]**
Design	2-arm RCT: ES; sham ES
Sample size and age (years)	68 patients: 39 women, 29 men; mean age 70 (SD: 11.2)
Diagnosis	Uroanalysis, urine cytologic examination, clinical assessment, neurological, anatomical, urodynamics (cystometrogram, cystometry)
Training protocol	ES: alternating 10-Hz pulses, 1-ms pulse duration, I max tolerable; in women, vaginal plug; 15 min 2×/day for 4 weeks
Drop-out	12%
Adherence	Not reported
Results	N IEF significance less in ES, not in sham ES, significant intergroup difference in favour of ES, favouring ES significant intergroup change in nocturia (p = 0.03), same for QoL (p = 0.045), significantly greater maximum cystometric capacity and first desire to void in ES vs sham ES; trend favouring ES daily frequency of pad changes (p = 0.06) Subgroup analysis of self-report of cure/improvement according to sex: in women, significant difference in favour of ES (p = 0.0091) in number of cured/improved
Author	**Yamanishi et al. (2000b)[b]**
Design	2-arm RCT: ES; MS
Sample size and age (years)	32 patients: 17 women, 15 men; mean age 62.3 (SD: 16.6)

TABLE 7.2.5 Randomized Controlled Trials on Electrical Stimulation to Treat Overactive Bladder and/or Urgency Urinary Incontinence Symptoms—cont'd

Diagnosis	Urodynamics (cystometrogram, cystometry)
Training protocol	ES: home- and clinic-bound device; alternating 10-Hz pulses, 1-ms pulse duration, I max tolerable; in women, vaginal plug- 15 min 2×/day for 4 weeks MS: continuous, low-impedance coil, armchair type seat, perineum centre of coil, I max, 10 Hz, maximum output 100% setting ≥270
Drop-out	None
Adherence	Not reported
Results	No significant intergroup differences between groups for max cystometric capacity and bladder capacity at first desire to void; OAB cured in 3/15 (20%) in MS and 0/17 in ES; >50-mL increase in max cystometric capacity in 13/15 patients in MS and 6/17 in ES; no adverse events in either group
Author	**Abdelbary et al. (2015)**
Design	3-arm RCT: A: vaginal ES B: local vaginal oestrogen C: ES + local vaginal oestrogen
Sample size and age (years)	N: 315 randomised, 300 analysed Mean age: A, 49.7 (SD: 6); B, 47.7 (SD: 6); C, 48 (SD: 6)
Diagnosis	Voiding diary, urine analysis, urodynamics
Training protocol	A: pelvic floor stimulator (Mod. MS-106 Twin; Vitacon AS, Trondheim, Norway) utilizing a vaginal probe was used in the study; treatment sessions twice weekly (12 sessions, 30 min each); stimulation pulses of 20 Hz for 320 ms; pulse intensity most tolerable intensity (with pulse intensity of 30–60 mA and mean of 43 mA) B: local vaginal estrogen cream 0.625 mg/g (Premarin; Wyeth, Dallas, TX) 2 g once daily C: combination of A and B
Drop-out	A, 5 patients; B, 7; C, 3 lost to follow-up after 3 months
Adherence	Not reported
Results	Significant difference between groups in all parameters: C > B in all parameters except DO (p = 0.7); C > A in all parameters except voiding frequency/day (p = 0.88), incontinence episodes (p = 0.81) and QoL (p = 0.94); A > B in all parameters except DOA (p = 0.68) All 3 groups showed deterioration in all parameters during 6 months follow-up except for incontinence episodes in group C (p = 0.158) Urgency episodes (n = 105): End of treatment: A, mean 2 (SD: 0.7); B, mean 4 (SD: 1.3); C, mean 1.4 (SD: 0.7) 3 months: A, mean 2.7 (SD: 1.0); B, mean 4.5 (SD: 1.5); C, mean 1.6 (SD: 0.9) 6 months: A, mean 4.7 (SD: 1.3); B, mean 4 (SD: 1.3); C, mean 2 (SD: 0.8)
Author	**Wang et al. (2006)**
Design	3-arm RCT: ES; oxybutynin; placebo
Sample size and age (years)	N: 82 eligible; 74 randomised, 68 analysed; mean age (SD) not reported ES: n = 25; oxybutynin: n = 26; placebo, n = 23
Diagnosis	Voiding diary, urodynamics (uroflowmetry, cystometry)

Continued

TABLE 7.2.5   Randomized Controlled Trials on Electrical Stimulation to Treat Overactive Bladder and/or Urgency Urinary Incontinence Symptoms—cont'd

Training protocol	ES: clinic-based ES group, intravaginal electrode (Periform; Neen Health-Care, Oldham, United Kingdom); biphasic, symmetric, pulsed current with a frequency of 10 Hz, pulse width of 400 μs, duty cycle 10 s on and 5 s off, and intensity varying with patient tolerance (minimum 20–63 mA and maximum 40–72 mA); 20 min/session, twice/week for 12 weeks
	Oxybutynin: starting dose 2.5 mg, 3×/day (TDS) without dose titration for 12 weeks
	Placebo: tablet looking exactly the same as oxybutynin (2.5 mg/tablet) containing microcrystalline cellulose powder, TDS for 12 weeks
Drop-out	ES, 1 patient; oxybutynin, 3; placebo, 3
Adherence	Not reported
Results	No improvement in urgency: ES 10/24; oxybutynin 14/23; placebo 19/21
	Urgency episodes/24 h (median, range, N):
	ES 1 (0–12.3), 24; oxybutynin 6 (0.5–13), 23; placebo 7.4 (3.9–13.4), 21
	Frequency/24 h (median, range, N): ES 7.8 (1.8–13), 24; oxybutynin 7.4 (2–14), 23; placebo 10 (6.6–16.3), 21
	Nocturia episodes per night (median, range, N): ES 0 (0–3), 24; oxybutynin 0 (0–2), 23; placebo 1 (0–3.6), 21
	Urgency incontinence episodes/24 h (median, range, N): ES 0.5 (0–2), 24; oxybutynin 0 (0–2), 23; placebo 1 (0–2), 21
	Change in urgency episodes/24 h (median, range, N): ES –3 (–14 to 0.5), 24; oxybutynin –3 (–12 to –0.1), 23; placebo –1.3 (–10.5 to 2)
	Change in frequency/24 h (median, range, N): ES –3.0 (–14 to 0.5), 24; oxybutynin –2.15 (–12.8 to 2.3), 23; placebo –0.75 (–6.5 to 2.3)
	Change in nocturia episodes/night (median, range, N): ES –0.8 (–6.5 to 0.4), 24; oxybutynin 0 (–2 to 1), 23; placebo 0 (–1.5 to 2)
	Change in urgency incontinence episodes/24 h (median, range, N): ES 0 (–2 to 2), 24; oxybutynin 0 (–1 to 1), 23; placebo 0 (–2 to 1), 21
Author	**Wang et al. (2017)**
Design	2-arm RCT: EPNS; TES
Sample size and age (years)	N: 120 randomised
	Mean age: EPNS 65.8 (±13.6); TES: 62.2 (±11.9)
Diagnosis	7-day voiding diary, urodynamics
Training protocol	EPNS: 4 sacrococcygeal points were selected for deep insertion of long acupuncture needles (Suzhou Shenlong Medical Apparatus Factory, Suzhou, China)
	TES: Device PHENIX USB 4 neuromuscular stimulation therapy system (Electronic Concept Lignon Innovation, Montpellier, France); current intensity <60 mA and frequency 12.5–30 Hz for 45 min 3×/week for 4 weeks; current intensity applied in 5% increments from 0 mA to intensity sensed without obvious discomfort
	Total treatment time was same in both arms: 540 min TES and 540 min EPNS.
Drop-out	EPNS: 5 patients; TES: ?
Adherence	Not reported

TABLE 7.2.5   Randomized Controlled Trials on Electrical Stimulation to Treat Overactive Bladder and/or Urgency Urinary Incontinence Symptoms—cont'd

Results	In EPNS, post-treatment complete symptom resolution occurred in 34 (42.5%) with a 50% or greater improvement rate in 70.1%; in TES, complete symptom resolution in 1 (2.5%) with a ≥50% improvement rate in 45% of patients Post-treatment UUI total, urgency incontinence index and QoL index scores with EPNS lower than TES and therapeutic effect in EPNS higher than TES
Author	**Jacomo et al. (2020)**
Design	2-arm RCT: A: n = 29 TTNS B: n = 29 TPS
Sample size and age (years)	N = 58 randomized; mean age 68.62 (±5.9)
Diagnosis	Clinical diagnosis of OAB, defined by presence of urgency, with or without UUI, nocturia, frequency
Training protocol	Biphasic current and surface electrodes; both groups underwent 8 sessions of 30 min of ES 2×/week using a DUALPEX 961s (Quark, Piracicaba, Sao Paulo, Brasil) ES device TTNS: 1 surface electrode below left medial malleolus, and other 5 cm cephalad to distal electrode; frequency 10 Hz; intensity just less than motor response TPS: symmetrically in parasacral region under posterior superior iliac spines to stimulate nerve roots S2 and S3; frequency 10 Hz; pulse width 700 µs; intensity maximal tolerance
Drop-out	4 in each group
Adherence	Not reported
Results	Post-treatment: both groups had significant improvements in the signs and symptoms of OAB, but TTNS showed a significant decrease in urgency episodes and UUI episodes, whereas TPS showed no significant differences in these assessments; no significant difference between groups

[a]Partly included in results for subgroup analysis according to gender.
[b]Not included in analysis of results because of inclusion of both women and men.
BF, Biofeedback; *DAI,* Detrusor Overactivity Index; *DO,* detrusor overactivity; *EPNS,* electrical pudendal nerve stimulation; *ES,* electrical stimulation; *HF,* high frequency; *IEF,* incontinence episode frequency; *IIQ-7,* Incontinence Impact Questionnaire; *ITT,* intention to treat; *LF,* low frequency; *LPP,* leak point pressure; *LUTEs,* lower urinary tract exercises; *MS,* magnetic stimulation; *MUI,* mixed urinary incontinence; *NS,* not statistically significant; *OAB,* overactive bladder; *PFM,* pelvic floor muscle; *PMFT,* pelvic muscle floor training; *QoL,* quality of life; *RCT,* randomized controlled trial; *SF-36,* Short Form 36 Health Survey Questionnaire; *SR,* sustained release; *SUI,* stress urinary incontinence; *TDS,* three times per day; *TES,* transvaginal electrical stimulation; *TPS,* transcutaneous parasacral stimulation; *TTNS,* transcutaneous tibial nerve stimulation; *UPP,* urethral pressure profile; *UUI,* urgency urinary incontinence; *VAS,* visual analogue scale.

Patient selection criteria should most likely have to include neurophysiological sacral arc testing and assessment of detrusor muscle status, because some forms of muscle dysfunction respond less to neural inhibitory effects (Brubaker, 2000). In addition, there is still no consensus on how much stimulation is required for an optimal effect (Dumoulin et al., 2017). Currently, most RCTs stimulate patients to use such an intensity of current that a maximally tolerable motor response of the pelvic floor is achieved (Dumoulin et al., 2017). But it remains unknown whether or not a contraction of the pelvic floor is really necessary to achieve detrusor inhibition or whether just excitation of the pudendal afferents is sufficiently effective for this kind of inhibition.

TABLE 7.2.6   PEDro Quality Score of Randomized Controlled Trials in Systematic Review of Electrical Stimulation to Treat Overactive Bladder and/or Urgency Urinary Incontinence Symptoms

E – Eligibility criteria specified
1 – Subjects randomly allocated to groups
2 – Allocation concealed
3 – Groups similar at baseline
4 – Subjects blinded
5 – Therapist administering treatment blinded
6 – Assessors blinded
7 – Measures of key outcomes obtained from >85% of subjects
8 – Data analysed by intention to treat
9 – Statistical comparison between groups conducted
10 – Point measures and measures of variability provided

Study	E	1	2	3	4	5	6	7	8	9	10	Total Score
Arruda et al. (2008)	+	+	+	+	−	−	−	−	−	+	+	5
Berghmans et al. (2002)	+	+	+	+	−	−	+	+	+	+	+	8
Bower et al. (1998)	+	+	−	+	+	?	+	+	+	+	+	8
Brubaker et al. (1997)	+	+	+	+	+	−	+	−	−	+	+	7
Franzen et al. (2010)	+	+	+	+	−	−	−	+	+	+	+	7
Ozdedeli et al. (2010)	+	+	+	+	−	−	+	+	−	+	+	7
Smith (1996)	+	+	−	+	−	−	−	+	−	+	+	5
Soomro et al. (2001)[a]	+	+	−	−	−	−	−	+	−	−	+	3
Walsh et al. (2001)[a]	+	+	−	+	−	−	−	+	+	+	+	6
Wang et al. (2004)	−	+	+	−	−	−	+	+	−	+	+	6
Yamanishi et al. (2000a)[b]	+	+	−	+	−	−	−	+	−	+	+	5
Yamanishi et al. (2000b)[a]	+	+	−	+	+	+	−	+	−	+	+	7
Abdelbary et al. (2015)	+	+	?	+	−	?	?	+	−	+	+	5
Wang et al. (2006)	+	+	+	+	−	−	−	+	−	+	+	6
Wang et al. (2017)	+	+	+	+	−	−	−	+	+	+	+	7
Jacomo et al. (2020)	+	+	+	+	−	+	+	+	−	+	+	8

[a]Partly included in results for subgroup analysis according to gender.
[b]Not included in analysis of results because of inclusion of both women and men.
+, Criterion is clearly satisfied; −, criterion is not satisfied; ?, not clear if the criterion was satisfied.
The total score is determined by counting the number of criteria that are satisfied, except the 'eligibility criteria specified' score is not used to generate the total score. Total scores are out of 10.

Electrical Parameters

Current

Although it appeared that all the ES trials reviewed here used alternating current, only nine trials specifically stated this to be biphasic (Berghmans et al., 2002; Jacomo et al., 2020; Ozdedeli et al., 2010; Wang et al., 2017), bipolar (Brubaker et al., 1997) and biphasic pulsed current (Arruda et al., 2008; Smith, 1996; Wang et al., 2004; Wang et al., 2006).

Pulse Shape

Six trials and the trials of Yamanishi and co-workers (Yamanishi et al., 2000a; Yamanishi et al., 2000b) were the only ones to detail the pulse shape: rectangular

(Berghmans et al., 2002; Ozdedeli et al., 2010); square (Brubaker et al., 1997; Yamanishi et al., 2000a; Yamanishi et al., 2000b); symmetric (Wang et al., 2004; Wang et al., 2017); asymmetric (Smith, 1996); and balanced with 2-second ramp up and 1-second ramp down.

(Pulse Repetition) Frequency

Seventeen trials gave details of the frequencies used, and these ranged from 5 Hz (Ozdedeli et al., 2010), 5 to 10 Hz (Franzen et al., 2010), 10 Hz (Arruda et al., 2008; Bower et al., 1998; Jacomo et al., 2020; Walsh et al., 2001; Wang et al., 2004; Wang et al., 2006; Yamanishi et al., 2000a; Yamanishi et al., 2000b) to 20 Hz (Abdelbary et al., 2015; Brubaker et al., 1997; Soomro et al., 2001), a combination of 12.5 to 30 Hz (Wang et al., 2017) and 12.5 and 50 Hz (Smith, 1996), 150 Hz (Bower et al., 1998), and a random frequency of 4 to 10 Hz (Berghmans et al., 2002).

Pulse Duration or Pulse Width

Pulse durations were also reported in 15 trials, and these were 0.1 ms (Brubaker et al., 1997; Ozdedeli et al., 2010), 0.2 ms (Berghmans et al., 2002; Bower et al., 1998; Jacomo et al., 2020; Soomro et al., 2001; Walsh et al., 2001), 0.3 ms (Smith, 1996), 0.4 ms (Wang et al., 2004; Wang et al., 2006), 1 ms (Arruda et al., 2008; Yamanishi et al., 2000a; Yamanishi et al., 2000b), 2 ms (Wang et al., 2017) and 320 ms (Abdelbary et al., 2015).

Duty Circle

Two trials used a duty cycle ratio of 1:2 (Brubaker et al., 1997; Smith, 1996), and in two trials this was 2:1 (Wang et al., 2004; Wang et al., 2006).

Intensity of Stimulation

Intensity of stimulation progressed from 5 to 25 mA in the trial by Smith (1996). Thirteen trials used the maximum tolerable intensity (Abdelbary et al., 2015; Arruda et al., 2008; Berghmans et al., 2002; Bower et al., 1998; Brubaker et al., 1997; Franzen et al., 2010; Jacomo et al., 2020; Ozdedeli et al., 2010; Walsh et al., 2001; Wang et al., 2004; Wang et al., 2006; Yamanishi et al., 2000a; Yamanishi et al., 2000b). In the trial of Soomro et al. (2001), patients were asked to control the amplitude of intensity to produce a tickling sensation. Wang et al. (2017) described a current intensity less than 60 mA applied in 5% increments from 0 mA to the intensity that was sensed without obvious discomfort.

Mode of Delivery of Current

Current was most commonly delivered by vaginal electrode (Abdelbary et al., 2015; Arruda et al., 2008; Berghmans et al., 2002; Brubaker et al., 1997; Franzen et al., 2010; Ozdedeli et al., 2010; Smith, 1996; Wang et al., 2004; Wang et al., 2006; Wang et al., 2017; Yamanishi et al., 2000a; Yamanishi et al., 2000b), transcutaneous parasacral (Jacomo et al., 2020) and over S3 sacral dermatomes (Walsh et al., 2001), although one trial used external surface electrode placements with two electrodes over S2–S3 sacral foramina or two electrodes just above the symphysis pubis (Bower et al., 1998). Transcutaneous ES was applied bilaterally over the perianal region using two self-adhesive electrodes (Soomro et al., 2001).

Length and Number of Treatments

The length and number of treatments was also highly variable. The longest treatment period was 4 months of daily stimulation (Smith, 1996). Medium-length treatment periods were based on two-weekly stimulations for 4 weeks (Jacomo et al., 2020); three-weekly stimulations for 4 weeks (Wang et al., 2017); and twice-daily stimulations for 4 (Yamanishi et al., 2000a), 8 (Brubaker et al., 1997), 6 (Abdelbary et al., 2015), 9 (Berghmans et al., 2002) or 12 weeks (Arruda et al., 2008; Wang et al., 2004; Wang et al., 2006). In the crossover trial of Soomro et al. (2001), after randomization, patients received 6 weeks of ES for 6 hours daily or oxybutynin. After a washout period of 2 weeks, they started in the second arm of treatment for another 6 weeks. The shortest treatment period consisted of a single episode of stimulation after the voiding phase of cystometry before filling was repeated (Bower et al., 1998).

Is Electrical Stimulation Better Than No Treatment, Control or Placebo Treatment?

In a four-arm RCT that included 83 women with detrusor overactivity, Berghmans et al. (2002) investigated the effect of no treatment, ES alone, a combination of PFMT and bladder training alone (which in this study was defined as lower urinary tract exercises), and ES in combination with lower urinary tract exercises. An important fact in this study was that women in the ES group received not only weekly clinic-based ES but also a twice-daily ES programme with a home device, which also measured the patient's compliance of use of ES. The main outcome measures were change in the Detrusor Overactivity Index (Berghmans et al., 2002), the Incontinence Impact

Questionnaire (Berghmans et al., 2001) and the adapted Dutch Incontinence Quality of Life questionnaire. The no treatment group showed no significant change at all pre- to post-treatment. In comparison with no treatment, there was a significant improvement in the ES alone group for the Destrusor Overactivity Index (Berghmans et al., 2002). The ES alone group turned out to have statistically significant lower self-professed impact of incontinence on daily life activities (Berghmans et al., 2001). Using the Dutch Incontinence Quality of Life questionnaire, ES alone improved self-professed incontinence control in daily life activities.

Yamanishi et al. (2000b) investigated maximum-intensity stimulation delivered daily for 4 weeks in 29 men and 39 women with detrusor overactivity. There was significantly more improvement in several outcomes in the ES group compared with the placebo ES group post-treatment (i.e., nocturia, number of leakage episodes, number of pad changes, quality-of-life score [using a questionnaire chart recording '0 = delighted', '1 = mostly satisfied', '2 = dissatisfied' and '3 = mostly dissatisfied or unhappy'], urodynamic evidence of improvement in detrusor overactivity, self-report of cure or improvement). For a single outcome, self-report of cure/improvement, subgroup analysis on the basis of sex was reported. Women in the active ES group were much more likely to report cure/improvement than women in the placebo ES group.

Bower et al. (1998) used a single stimulation episode given after the voiding phase of cystometry and before bladder filling was repeated. The results were reported separately for women with detrusor overactivity and those with urgency. For women with detrusor overactivity, both stimulation groups (10-Hz sacral electrodes and 150-Hz symphysis pubis electrodes) showed significant improvements in urodynamic measures when compared with the placebo stimulation group (i.e., reduction in maximum detrusor pressure, increase in first desire to void, proportion of women with a stable bladder). However, there were no significant differences between stimulation and placebo groups for change in maximum cystometric capacity or detrusor pressure at first desire to void. Fewer measures were reported for women with urgency. The only significant findings were a significant increase in first desire to void in the 150-Hz group and a significant increase in the maximum cystometric capacity in the placebo ES group.

One further trial (Brubaker et al., 1997) that compared ES with placebo ES in a group of women with urodynamic stress incontinence, detrusor overactivity or both conducted a subgroup analysis on the basis of diagnosis and found that women with pre-treatment detrusor overactivity who received active stimulation were significantly less likely to have urodynamic evidence of detrusor overactivity post-treatment.

Due to availability of only a single study in women comparing ES with no treatment and the variation in stimulation protocols comparing ES with placebo stimulation, it is difficult to interpret the findings of trials. However, for women with detrusor overactivity, there is an absolute trend in favour of active stimulation over no treatment or placebo stimulation.

Is Electrical Stimulation Better Than Any Other Single Treatment?

In a three-arm RCT including 103 women with OAB, Wang et al. (2004) compared the effects of ES with PFMT and with biofeedback-assisted PFMT (BAPFMT). Assessment was performed pre- and post-treatment using the King's Health Questionnaire for subjective cure/improvement, and urinary symptoms like urgency, diurnal frequency, urgency incontinence, dysuria and nocturia for more objective outcomes. As secondary outcomes, PFM strengthening and urodynamic data were used. More study details can be found in Table 7.2.5.

Wang et al. (2004) did not find any statistically significant difference between the groups for self-reported cure or cure/improvement. PFMT women had statistically significantly fewer leakage episodes per day. Although there were no statistically significant differences in the general health perception, incontinence impact, role limitation, physical limitation, social limitation, sleep/energy and personal relationships—domains of the quality-of-life measure (King's Health Questionnaire)—the ES group had statistically significantly better scores post-treatment for emotions and severity measures compared to the exercise regimens and in total score compared to PFMT only. Some women using ES reported discomfort during treatment.

Wang et al. (2017) compared in a two-arm RCT, at a ratio of 2:1 in 120 women with drug refractory idiopathic UUI, whether electrical pudendal nerve stimulation (EPNS) (group 1, n = 80) or transvaginal ES (group 2, n = 40) was more effective. Outcome measures were the 24-hour pad test and a questionnaire to measure the severity of symptoms and quality of life. The median severity of symptoms and quality-of-life score on the

UUI questionnaire (UUI total score) was 13 (range: 7–18.75) in group 1 and 11 (range: 8–16) in group 2 before treatment, which decreased to 2 (range: 0–6.75) in group 1 and 6.5 (range: 3.25–10.75) in group 2 (both p < 0.01) after the completion of treatment. At the end of treatment, in group 1, complete symptom resolution was noted in 34 patients (42.5%), with a 50% or greater symptom improvement rate in 70.1%. In group 2, complete symptom resolution was noted in 1 patient (2.5%) with a 50% or greater symptom improvement rate in 45%. The post-treatment UUI total score was lower and the therapeutic effect was better in group 1 than in group 2 (both p < 0.01). The authors concluded that electrical pudendal nerve stimulation is more effective than transvaginal ES in treating drug refractory idiopathic UUI.

In a two-arm RCT, Jacomo et al. (2020) randomized 50 female volunteers, mean age 68.62 (±5.9) years into two groups: those receiving transcutaneous tibial nerve stimulation (group 1, n = 25) and those receiving transcutaneous parasacral stimulation (group 2, n = 25). The primary outcome was the International Consultation on Incontinence Questionnaire–Overactive Bladder score, and secondary outcomes were the International Consultation on Incontinence Questionnaire—Short Form score and 3-day bladder diary measurements.

Both groups' symptoms improved statistically significantly as measured by the International Consultation on Incontinence Questionnaire–Overactive Bladder and International Consultation on Incontinence Questionnaire—Short Form. In the 3-day bladder diary assessments after treatment, group 1 showed a statistically significant reduced number of nocturia, urgency and urge urinary incontinence episodes, whereas group 2 showed only a reduced number of nocturia episodes. No difference between groups was found.

The conclusion was that both groups' symptoms of OAB improved but that transcutaneous tibial nerve stimulation had better, but not significant, results measured by the 3-day bladder diary.

The trial of Smith (1996) compared ES and medication (propantheline bromide) in women with detrusor overactivity with or without urodynamic stress incontinence. He did not find any statistically significant differences in outcome (self-reported improvement and urodynamic parameters) between the two groups.

Arruda et al. (2008) compared, in a three-arm study, intermittent ES with medication (oxybutynin immediate-release 5 mg) in women with detrusor overactivity and mixed urinary incontinence (UUI dominant on urodynamics) and with PFMT. No significant differences between groups were found in outcome of effects (based on self-reported cure/improvement and on urodynamics, equally effective directly after treatment and after 12-month follow-up). No side effects were reported for ES, only for oxybutynin.

Franzen et al. (2010) showed no significant differences comparing ES with tolterodine sustained-release 4 mg orally once per day for 6 months in women with (predominant) urgency and UUI symptoms. Both therapies were effective without any statistical difference in cured or improved patients between groups.

Wang et al. (2006) conducted a 3-arm RCT for 68 patients with OAB, placing emphasis on urinary urgency, comparing during a 12-week treatment period a vaginal ES programme (group 1, n = 24) using biphasic symmetric pulsed current with a 10-Hz frequency, 400-second pulse width, 10/5 duty cycle and varying intensity with oxybutynin (2.5 mg) (group 2, n = 23) or placebo (group 3, n = 21) three times per day. Outcome measures were warning time, urodynamics, voiding diaries and King's Health Questionnaire.

Between-group comparison showed statistically significant improvements in daily voided volume, pad count, number of urgency and nocturia episodes, and the King's Health Questionnaire domain 2 score and total score between the ES and the other groups. The reduction rate of OAB was 58.4% for the ES, 39.1% for the oxybutynin and 9.5% for the placebo groups. The conclusion was that ES had the greatest subjective outcome for OAB and was the most effective of the three treatments.

Abdelbary et al. (2015) carried out a three-arm RCT on 315 perimenopausal women with OAB. Group 1 underwent pelvic floor ES using vaginal probes twice weekly for 12 sessions. Group 2 received local vaginal estrogen, whereas group 3 received both pelvic floor ES and local estrogen. All patients were evaluated by a voiding diary, quality-of-life questionnaire, vaginal examination, urine analysis, blood sugar, ultrasonography and urodynamic study before and after therapy. Patients were followed up 1 week, 3 months and 6 months post-therapy. The analysed variables included day and nighttime frequency, incontinence episodes, urgency, quality of life, detrusor overactivity and functional bladder capacity. The outcome measure was urge incontinence. Urgency was statistically significantly improved in group 3 compared to groups 1 and 2. Incontinence improved statistically significantly more in groups 1 and 3 than in group 2.

Follow-up showed worsening of symptoms within 6 months in all groups, except incontinence in group 3. The authors concluded that that vaginal pelvic floor ES and estrogen are effective in treating OAB symptoms in perimenopausal females. In a trial comparing ES with trospium hydrochloride 45 mg daily in women with (predominant) UUI, no statistically significant differences were found between groups using both objective (urodynamic parameters, voiding diary) and subjective (visual analogue scale urgency severity, Incontinence Impact Questionnaire 7, treatment satisfaction) outcome measures. Side effects were statistically significantly higher in the medication group.

With only a few single trials comparing ES with PFMT, BAPFMT or medication, there is insufficient evidence to determine if ES is better than PFMT, BAPFMT, propantheline bromide, and anticholinergic or antimuscarinic therapy in women with detrusor overactivity. From the studies comparing ES with medication, it seems that ES is equally as effective as medication. However, one has to be quite cautious about such statements because different kinds of ES (protocols) were compared to different kinds of medication.

In summary, because of sparse availability of trials, there is insufficient evidence to determine if ES is better than PFMT, BAPFMT or medication for women with detrusor overactivity.

Is (Additional) Electrical Stimulation Better Than Other (Additional) Treatments?

In this section, no studies were found, so no conclusion can be drawn as to whether or not there is any benefit of adding ES to another treatment modality in women with OAB.

CONCLUSION

- ES protocols and designs in studies for women with OAB and/or UUI symptoms are largely inconsistent. One reason for this is insufficient understanding of the physiological rationale of the working mechanism and basic principles of ES used in clinical practice to treat these women.
- There is some evidence to judge that an intensive programme of clinic-based *and* home ES is better than no or placebo treatment for women with OAB and/or UUI symptoms. Unfortunately, some of the relevant studies in this area included both women and men, making interpretation of results in women only quite difficult.

- There is insufficient evidence to determine whether ES is better than PFMT, BAPFMT or medication in women with OAB and/or UUI symptoms.
- At present, no studies have investigated the extra benefit of adding ES to other treatment (modalities).
- There is need for more basic research to find out the working mechanism of ES in women with OAB and/or UUI symptoms, and to determine the best ES protocol(s) for this kind of patient.

CLINICAL RECOMMENDATIONS

- If available, ES should be applied both in clinical practice and at the patient's home, maybe as the treatment of first choice in this diagnostic group. So far, it is impossible to recommend the most optimal ES regimen and protocol. However, if ES is applied, do use an intensive (parameters, number of sessions, duration of therapy) ES regimen with both clinic-based and home devices. A protocol that has proven to be effective (Fall and Madersbacher, 1994; Berghmans et al., 2002) consisted of the following parameters:
- F0A1 Stochastic frequency: 4 to 10 Hz; frequency modulation 0.1 second
- F0A1 Intensity: I max
- F0A1 Pulse duration: 200 to 500 μs
- F0A1 Biphasic, duty circle 13 seconds 5/8
- F0A1 Shape of current: rectangular
- F0A1 Number and time schedule of sessions: daily at home 2 × 20 minutes per day; clinic 1 × 30 minutes per week
- F0A1 Duration of treatment period: 3 to 6 months
- Use intravaginal probes for ES therapy only after inspection and digital intra-vaginal examination to assess integrity of vaginal tissue and to avoid adverse events of ES use.
- Follow up with weekly or more often supervised training. Supervised training must be conducted individually.
- At follow-up, get as much as possible feedback from the patient about compliance, performance, potential side effects and adverse events. Micturition diaries are quite useful and should be filled out regularly to provide feedback to the patient and to monitor progress.
- As much as possible, try to use ES devices that digitally measure compliance of use. During clinic-based sessions, use these data to provide feedback to the patient and to support motivation to continue ES at home.

REFERENCES

Abdelbary, A. M., El-Dessoukey, A. A., Massoud, A. M., et al. (2015). Combined vaginal Pelvic Floor Electrical Stimulation (PFS) and local vaginal estrogen for treatment of Overactive Bladder (OAB) in perimenopausal females. Randomized controlled trial (RCT). *Urology, 86*, 482–486.

Andersson, K. E., Cardozo, L., Cruz, F., et al. (2017). Committee 8: Pharmacological treatment of urinary incontinence. In P. Abrams, L. Cardozo, A. Wagg, et al. (Eds.), *Incontinence: Sixth international consultation on incontinence* Tokyo, September 2016, ICUD-ICS 2017, pp. 805–959.

Arruda, R. M., Castro, R. A., Sousa, G. C., et al. (2008). Prospective randomized comparison of oxybutynin, functional electrostimulation, and pelvic floor training for treatment of detrusor activity in women. *International Urogynecology Journal, 19*, 1055–1061.

Berghmans, L. C. M., Hendriks, H. J., Bø, K., et al. (1998). Conservative treatment of genuine stress incontinence in women: A systematic review of randomized clinical trials. *British Journal of Urology, 82*(2), 181–191.

Berghmans, L. C. M., Nieman, F., Van Waalwijk van Doorn, E. S. C., et al. (2001). Effects of physiotherapy, using the adapted Dutch I-QOL in women with Urge Urinary Incontinence (UUI). Abstract 62 IUGA 2001 *International Urogynecology Journal, 12*(Suppl. 3), S40.

Berghmans, L. C. M., van Waalwijk van Doorn, E. S. C., Nieman, F., et al. (2002). Efficacy of physical therapeutic modalities in women with proven bladder overactivity. *European Urology, 41*, 581–587.

Berghmans, L. C. M., van Waalwijk van Doorn, E. S. C., Nieman, F., et al. (2000). Efficacy of extramural physical therapy modalities in women with proven bladder overactivity: A randomised clinical trial. *Neurourology and Urodynamics, 19*(4), 496–497.

Bower, W. F., Moore, K. H., Adams, R. D., et al. (1998). A urodynamic study of surface neuromodulation versus sham in detrusor instability and sensory urgency. *The Journal of Urology, 160*(6 pt.1), 2133–2136.

Brubaker, L. (2000). Electrical stimulation in overactive bladder. *BJU International, 85*(Suppl. 3), 17–24.

Brubaker, L., Benson, T., Bent, A., et al. (1997). Transvaginal electrical stimulation for female urinary incontinence. *American Journal of Obstetrics and Gynecology, 177*, 536–540.

Colling, J. C., Ouslander, J., Hadley, B. J., et al. (1992). *Patterned urge–response toileting for incontinence*. Research funded by NIH, National Center for Nursing Research under Grant No. NR01554 to Oregon Health Sciences University, Portland. (Eds.), New Perspectives in Sacral Nerve Stimulation. Martin Dunitz, London, ch 3.

Dumoulin, C., Adewuyi, T., & Booth, J. (2017). Adult conservative management. In P. Abrams, L. Cardozo, A. Wagg, & A. Wein (Eds.), *Incontinence. 6th international consultation on incontinence* Tokyo, September 2016. ICS-ICUD 2017.

Elabbady, A. A., Hassouna, M. M., & Elhilali, M. M. (1994). Neural stimulation for chronic voiding dysfunctions. *The Journal of Urology, 152*(6 Pt 1), 2076–2080.

Engel, B. T., Burgio, L. D., McCormick, K. A., et al. (1990). Behavioral treatment of incontinence in the long-term care setting. *Journal of the American Geriatrics Society, 38*(3), 361–363.

Eriksen, B. C. (1989). *Electrostimulation of the pelvic floor in female urinary incontinence*. Norway: Thesis University of Trondheim.

Eriksen, B. C., & Eik-Nes, S. H. (1989). Long-term electrical stimulation of the pelvic floor: Primary therapy in female stress incontinence? *Urologia Internationalis, 44*, 90.

Fall, M. (2000). Reactivation of bladder inhibitory reflexes – an underestimated asset in the treatment of overactive bladder. *Urology, 55*(5a), 29–30.

Fall, M., & Lindström, S. (1994). Functional electrical stimulation: Physiological basis and clinical principles. *International Urogynecology Journal, 5*, 296–304.

Fall, M., & Madersbacher, H. (1994). Peripheral electrical stimulation. In A. R. Mundy, T. P. Stephenson, & A. J. Wein (Eds.), *Urodynamics – principles, practice and application* (2nd ed.) (pp. 495–520). Edinburgh: Churchill Livingstone.

Franzen, K., Jahansson, J. E., Lauridse, I., et al. (2010). Electrical stimulation compared with tolterodine for treatment of urge/urge incontinence amongst women – a randomized clinical trial. *International Urogynecology Journal, 21*, 1517–1524.

Hay-Smith, E. J., Herbison, P., & Mørkved, S. (2001). *Physical therapies for prevention of incontinence in adults (Cochrane Protocol)*. Oxford: Update Software.

Herbison, G. P., & Arnold, E. P. (2009). Sacral neuromodulation with implanted devices for urinary storage and voiding dysfunction in adults. *Cochrane Database of Systematic Reviews* (Issue 2), Art. No. CD004202.

Hoebeke, P., Van Laecke, E., Everaert, K., et al. (2001). Transcutaneous neuromodulation for the urge syndrome in children: A pilot study. *The Journal of Urology, 166*(6), 2416–2419.

Hsu, F. C., Weeks, C., Shelley, S., et al. (2019). Updating the evidence on drugs to treat overactive bladder. A systematic review. *International Urogynecology Journal, 30*(10), 1603–1617.

Jacomo, R. H., Alves, A. T., Lucio, A., et al. (2020). Transcutaneous tibial nerve stimulation versu parasacral stimulation in the treatment of overactive bladder in elderly people: A triple-blinded randomized controlled trial. *Clinics, 75*, e1477.

Janssen, D. W., Martens, F. M., & de Wall, L. L. (2017). Clinical utility of neurostimulation devices in the treatment of overactive bladder: Current perspectives. *Medical Devices: Evidence and Research, 10*, 109–122.

Lewis, J. M., & Cheng, E. Y. (2007). Non-traditional management of the neurogenic bladder: Tissue engineering and neuromodulation. *The Scientific World Journal, 7*, 1230–1241.

Madhuvrata, P., Cody, J. D., Ellis, G., et al. (2012). Which anticholinergic drug for overactive bladder symptoms in adults. *Cochrane Database of Systematic Reviews* (Issue 1), Art. No. CD005429.

McCormick, K. A., Celia, M., Scheve, A., et al. (1990). Cost-effectiveness of treating incontinence in severely mobility-impaired long-term care residents. *QRB Quality Review Bulletin, 16*(12), 439–443.

Messelink, E. J. (1999). The overactive bladder and the role of the pelvic floor muscles. *British Journal of Urology, 83*, 31–35.

Millard, R. J., & Oldenburg, B. F. (1983). The symptomatic, urodynamic and psychodynamic results of bladder re-education programs. *The Journal of Urology, 130*, 715–719.

Ozdedeli, S., Karapolat, H., & Akkoc, Y. (2010). Comparison of intravaginal electrical stimulation and trospium hydrochloride in women with overactive bladder syndrome: A randomized controlled study. *Clinical Rehabilitation, 24*, 342–351.

Pannek, J., Janek, S., & Noldus, J. (2010). Neurogene oder idiopathische Detrusorüberaktivität nach erfolgloser antimuskarinerger Therapie. *Urologe A, Der, 49*, 530–535.

Rovner, Athanasiou, S., Choo, M., et al. (2017). Surgery for urinary incontinence in women. In P. Abrams, L. Cardozo, A. Wagg, et al. (Eds.), *Incontinence: Sixth international consultation on incontinence* ICUD-ICS 2016, Tokyo, pp. 1741–1854.

Schmidt, R. (1988). Applications of neurostimulation in urology. *Neurourology and Urodynamics, 7*, 585–592.

Schnelle, J. F. (1990). Treatment of urinary incontinence in nursing home patients by prompted voiding. *Journal of the American Geriatrics Society, 38*(3), 356–360.

Schultz-Lampel, D. (1997). *Neurophysiologische Grundlagen und klinische Anwendungen der sacralen Neuromodulation zur Therapie von Blasenfunktionsstörungen (Habilitationsschrift).* Wuppertal: Fakultätsklinik Witten/Herdecke.

Smith, J. J. (1996). Intravaginal stimulation randomized trial. *The Journal of Urology, 155*, 127.

Soomro, N. A., Khadra, M. H., Robson, W., et al. (2001). A crossover randomized trial of transcutaneous electrical nerve stimulation and oxybutynin in patients with detrusor instability. *The Journal of Urology, 166*, 146–149.

Stewart, F., Gameiro, L. F., El Dib, R., Gameiro, M. O., Kapoor, A., & Amaro, J. L. (2016). Electrical stimulation with non-implanted electrodes for overactive bladder in adults. *Cochrane Database of Systematic Reviews* (Issue 12). https://doi.org/10.1002/14651858.CD010098.pub4. Art. No.: CD010098.

Sussman, D., & Garely, A. (2002). Treatment of overactive bladder with once-daily extended release tolterodine or oxybutynin: The Antimuscarinic Clinical Effectiveness Trial (ACET). *Current Medical Research and Opinion, 18*(4), 177.

Ulmsten, U. I. (1999). *The role of surgery in womenAbstract presented at the symposium 'freedom' at the 14th Annual Meeting of EAU.* Stockholm, Sweden, April 7–11.

Veenboer, P. W., & Bosch, J. L. (2014). Long-term adherence to antimuscarinic therapy in everyday practice: A systematic review. *The Journal of Urology, 191*(4), 1003–1008.

Walsh, I. K., Thompson, T., Loughridge, W. G., et al. (2001). Non-invasive antidromic neurostimulation: A simple effective method for improving bladder storage. *Neurourology and Urodynamics, 20*(1), 73–84.

Wang, A. C., Wang, Y. Y., & Chen, M. C. (2004). Single-blind, randomized trial of pelvic floor muscle training, biofeedback-assisted pelvic floor muscle training, and electrical stimulation in the management of overactive bladder. *Urology, 63*(1), 61–66.

Wang, A. C., Chih, S. Y., & Chen, M. C. (2006). Comparison of electric stimulation and oxybutynin chloride in management of overactive bladder with special reference to urinary urgency: A randomized placebo-controlled trial. *Urology, 68*(5), 999–1004.

Wang, S., Lv, J., Feng, X., et al. (2017). Efficacy of electrical pudendal nerve stimulation versus transvaginal electrical stimulation in treating female idiopathic urgency urinary incontinence. *The Journal of Urology, 197*(6), 1496–1501.

Weil, E. H. J. (2000). *Clinical and experimental aspects of sacral nerve neuromodulation in lower urinary tract dysfunction.* Maastricht, The Netherlands: Thesis, University of Maastricht.

Yamanishi, T., Sakakibara, R., Uchiyama, T., et al. (2000a). Comparative study of the effects of magnetic versus electrical stimulation on inhibition of detrusor overactivity. *Urology, 56*, 777–781.

Yamanishi, T., Yasuka, K., Sakakibara, R., et al. (2000b). Randomized double-blind study of electrical stimulation for urinary incontinence due to detrusor overactivity. *Urology, 55*, 353–357.

Pudendal Neuralgia and Other Intrapelvic Nerve Entrapments

Nucelio Lemos and Jessica Nargi

INTRODUCTION

Pudendal neuralgia (PNA) was first described by Amarenco et al. (1987) and, since then, PNA and Alcock's canal syndrome have been used almost interchangeably in the literature. However, PNA can be caused by entrapments of the pudendal nerve or the sacral nerve roots in the intrapelvic spaces, with Alcock's canal being just one of those. In fact, in our case series, entrapments at the level of Alcock's canal correspond to only 8% of the cases, whereas most entrapments happen to more proximal portions of the plexus (Lemos et al., 2021). These more proximal entrapments are probably underdiagnosed due to lack of awareness and understanding of the intrapelvic portions of the lumbosacral plexus.

Intrapelvic nerve entrapments (IPNEs) are also a cause of extraspinal sciatica, a condition that is among some of the most challenging diagnoses in medicine. Low awareness and lack of a systematic approach to the intrapelvic portions of the lumbosacral plexus probably also play a role in underdiagnosis and mismanagement of these patients. For example, about 7% of patients undergoing a vaginal hysterectomy and uterosacral suspension for treating uterine prolapse develop sciatica and/or PNA postoperatively (Montoya et al., 2012); although the lithotomy position and spinal blocks often take the blame for these de novo neuropathic symptoms, IPNE by the reconstructive sutures/grafts are the most likely cause (Possover and Lemos, 2011).

The preceding examples illustrate how, even though more than five centuries have passed since described a large portion of the lumbosacral plexus located intra-abdominally Huard (1968), most of the clinical knowledge on this plexus refers to its extra-abdominal parts, whereas its intrapelvic portions, as well as the fact that these portions are subject to entrapments, are often neglected (Possover et al., 2011).

Possover et al. (2007) described the laparoscopic neuronavigation technique, opening the doors to accessing the retroperitoneal portion of the lumbosacral plexus through a safe, minimally invasive and objective way. Since then, multiple causes of IPNEs have been described and a new field in medicine—named *neuropelveology*—was created (Possover et al., 2015).

In this chapter, we will introduce the concept of IPNE and its diagnosis, and treatment rationale, highlighting the role of physiotherapy in treating this condition.

INTRAPELVIC NERVE ENTRAPMENT SYNDROME

Definition and Symptoms

Nerve entrapment syndrome, or compression neuropathy, is a clinical condition caused by compression on a single nerve or nerve root. Its symptoms include pain, tingling, numbness and muscle weakness on the affected nerve's dermatome (Bouche, 2013). IIPNEs are entrapment neuropathies of the intrapelvic portions of the lumbosacral plexus and will, as such, produce symptoms related to the lumabosacral dermatomes and myotomes.

The preceding definition refers to the entrapment of somatic nerves. Considering that many intrapelvic nerves contain both somatic and autonomic fibres, when IPNE occurs, their autonomic component will also produce visceral symptoms, such as urinary frequency or urgency, dysuria, rectal pain, suprapubic and/or abdominal cramps, and chills.

Symptoms and signs related to IPNEs are primarily centred on these nerves' dermatomes and myotomes; thus, knowledge of intrapelvic neuroanatomy and innervation territories (discussed later in this chapter) are essential during anamnesis, allowing for the formulation of a plausible diagnostic hypothesis.

In a concise manner, the main symptoms of IPNEs include the following (Lemos and Possover, 2015):
- Sciatica associated with urinary symptoms (urgency, frequency, dysuria) and without any clear orthopedic cause;
- Gluteal pain associated with perineal, vaginal or penile pain;
- Dysuria and/or painful ejaculation;
- Refractory lower urinary tract symptoms;
- Refractory pelvic and perineal pain.

It is important to emphasize that, due to the distance between both plexuses, IPNEs will usually cause unilateral symptoms. The most common presentations will be discussed later.

Diagnostic Workup

Once the hypothesis of an intrapelvic entrapment is raised, it is mandatory to perform the topographic diagnosis, which is the determination of the exact point of entrapment. So far, careful neuropelveological evaluation, with detailed anamnesis and neurological examination, is the most reliable method for this (Lemos and Possover, 2015).

To increase objectivity and accuracy of the diagnosis, we have been examining the use of high-definition pelvic magnetic resonance imaging (MRI) and sacral plexus tractography, which is a technique for functional MRI of peripheral nerves (Van der Jagt et al., 2012). In a case series of 13 patients, magnetic resonance tractography was able to identify asymmetries of signal on 11 of 13 patients, corresponding to IPNEs found in subsequent surgery (Lemos et al., 2021) (Fig. 7.2.3).

Our results so far are quite promising, but the accuracy of this method still needs to be investigated. Therefore, for further assurance, our next step is a diagnostic block, guided by ultrasound or fluoroscopy and performed by an intervention pain therapist or interventional radiologist; the exact point where a signal gap was identified at the tractography is infiltrated with 1 to 3 mL of bupivacaine 0.5%. If complete resolution of neuropathic pain is observed for at least 2 to 3 hours, the test is considered positive (Fig. 7.2.4).

Treatment Rationale

As a general rule, once a nerve entrapment has been diagnosed, decompression (usually surgical) is essential, as chronic ischemia can lead to endoneurial degeneration (Rempel et al., 1999). Therefore, the longer the time between the beginning of symptoms and detrapment, the lower the chance of success.

Surgical decompression tends to solve the problem in about 40% of patients; another 40% of patients will experience 50% or more reduction in pain and about 20% will not improve or, in some cases, experience worsening of their pain (Lemos et al., 2017). Approximately 56% of patients will present post-decompression neuropathic pain and 23% will present neuropraxia (muscle power loss on the decompressed nerve myotome), both of which tend to be transient; the former will last an average of 6 months and the latter about 4 months Lemos et al., 2021.

Some conservative methods for mechanical detrapment can be attempted, depending on the aetiology of the entrapment, and will be discussed more specifically in the next session of this chapter. Multiprofessional/multidisciplinary care plays a crucial role on preoperative and postoperative care of these patients; they are essential for post-decompression pain management, re-establishment of muscle power and recurrence prevention.

Perioperative Care

Medical management. Medical pain management plays a substantial role in postoperative pain control. However, this topic is an extensive and complex one and would constitute a chapter on its own; it is also not the topic of this book and will therefore not be approached in this chapter. As a general rule, prescribers should agree to institutional/regional guidelines for managing neuropathic pain.

Physiotherapy. Considering that pelvic floor muscle dysfunction will almost invariably be present, either as a consequence or a cause of IPNE, pelvic physical therapists are a fundamental part of the multiprofessional team and essential for treating this population of patients. With the exception of cases of neoplastic entrapment, where there is risk of disease progression and progressive irreversible nerve damage, pelvic floor physiotherapy is the first-line treatment for PNA (Khoder and Hale, 2014) and can provide effective treatment modalities for non-emergent cases of sciatica (Lewis et al., 2015).

Although nerve entrapments directly cause focal symptoms on the specific dermatomes and myotomes of the affected nerve(s), antalgic attitude will generate a global biomechanical imbalance; thus, the physical therapist must look beyond the pelvic floor, using a whole-person approach. The pelvic floor works synergistically with the deep abdominal muscles in healthy controls (Ferla et al., 2016). When pelvic floor dysfunction is present, mechanical changes may occur in the lumbopelvic region and thoracic spine (Pool-Goudzwaard et al., 2004; Hodges et al., 2007). When looking at the whole person, the therapist gains a better understanding of the individuals' learned protective postures, respiratory patterns, altered gait, movement strategies and overall functional limitations.

Notwithstanding, when treating this population, a biopsychosocial framework is imperative due to the complex nature of pelvic pain, especially in females with sexual pain. The frequency and intimacy of encounters puts the pelvic physiotherapist in an apposite position to utilize strategies such as cognitive behavioral therapy, mindfulness-based stress reduction, yoga and graded imagery for implementing and/or facilitating the biopsychosocial interventions (Vandyken and Hilton, 2017).

A thorough history must be taken to diagnose the functional limitations and psychosocial impact of

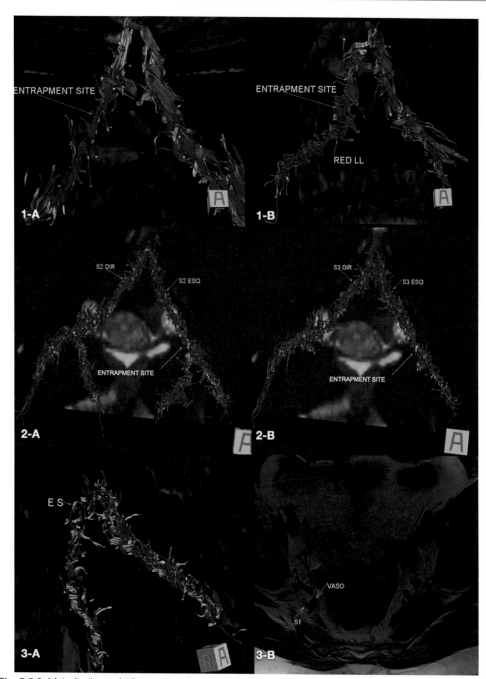

Fig. 7.2.3 Main findings of 3D tractography reconstruction. On case 1, at the entrapment site (ES), a reduction on the multitude of colours can be observed on S2 (1-A) and S3 (1-B) and narrowing of the tract bundle can be observed on S2 (1-A). Still in this case, the tracts proximally to the ES are deviated (more colours), in comparison with the contralateral side. On case 2, a narrowing of the tract bundle can be seen at the level of the ES both in S2 (2-A) and S3 (2-B). On case 3, a signal gap can be noticed at the ES (3-A), which correlates with the crossing of a dilated vein over S1 on the anatomical image (3-B).

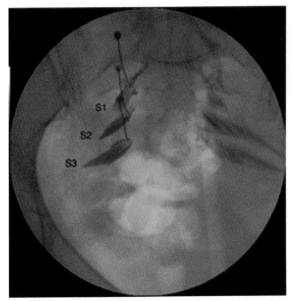

Fig. 7.2.4 Fluoroscopy guided block of S1, S2 and S3. (*Courtesy Dr. Alexadra Raffaini.*)

symptoms on the patient's daily life, to better understand the patient's goals and manage expectations for physical therapy and the overall treatment. For that, the physical therapist must act in an integrated manner with the medical team and have a thorough understanding of the aetiopathophysiology and natural history of IPNEs, as well as the different management strategies available. Integrated care is key to the success of IPNE treatment at improving symptoms, function and quality of life.

In addition, reliable and validated outcome measures help construct the assessment and treatment. Among those, the Pain Catastrophizing Scale is a quite useful tool, as pain catastrophizing has been associated with outcomes related to pain including increased pain severity, changes in central nervous system pain processing, postsurgical pain outcomes and disability (Quartana et al., 2009). Kinesiophobia is another factor that the physical therapist must consider when designing a successful treatment plan. Using a simple questionnaire such as the Tampa Kinesiophobia Scale can help quantify avoidance behaviors in this population (Lundberg et al., 2006).

The Depression Anxiety Stress Scale is a self-reported questionnaire that can be used as a screening tool to help identify those in need for additional and more specialized mental healthcare support. Specifically, this scale helps measure hopelessness, autonomic arousal, skeletal muscle effects, difficulties relaxing, nervous arousal and irritability

(Lovibond and Lovibond, 1995). Moreover, it can help frame the treatment strategies used by the physical therapist—for instance, those scoring high in depression may benefit from yoga-based approaches (De Manincor et al., 2016; Schmid et al., 2019), whereas those who score high on depression, anxiety and stress may benefit from mindfulness-based approaches (Khoury et al., 2013).

The Central Sensitization Inventory is a self-reported screening instrument to help identify patients with central sensitivity. When the patient scores higher than 40, it may suggest the presence of central sensitization (Neblett et al., 2013). Considering the visceral symptoms that occur with IPNEs, such as urinary frequency/urgency and rectal pain, using a urolog and bowel diary to measure micturition and bowel patterns is also necessary to help identify the need for re-training and/or other behavioral modifications.

A thorough mechanical assessment must be completed for all three layers of the pelvic floor through external and internal vaginal and/or rectal examination. Sacral nerves innervate the pelvic floor muscles; IPNEs can therefore cause over/underactivity of these muscles. Musculoskeletal dysfunction findings are more frequent in women with chronic pelvic pain than in healthy controls (Neville et al., 2012). Similarly, this population of patients has a higher pelvic floor resting tone, decreased maximal pelvic floor strength and relaxation capacity when compared to pain-free controls (Loving et al., 2014).

The therapist will also assess for both superficial and deep allodynia, hyperalgesia and pudendal nerve sensitivity using Tinnel's test. The internal examination also allows the physical therapist to evaluate the obturator internus and piriformis muscles, which are especially important if a piriformis entrapment is suspected. Pelvic floor muscle overactivity, tenderness and/or trigger points often cause/result from/contribute to chronic pelvic pain (Faubion et al., 2012; Neville et al., 2012; Loving et al., 2014), dyspareunia, dysfunctional voiding (urgency, frequency, hesitation, retention, dysuria, bladder pain, incontinence) (Faubion et al., 2012; Neville et al., 2012), constipation (difficulties with evacuation, a sensation of incomplete bowel emptying) (Faubion et al., 2012) and low back pain (Faubion et al., 2012; Dufour et al., 2018; Keizer et al., 2019).

Even though about two-thirds of patients with IPNE will need surgical management, there are many additional potential mediators that can drive pelvic floor dysfunction in this population. Therefore, working with the physical therapist preoperatively can help identify potential drivers, help triage appropriate surgical candidates, and aid in the development and effective implementation of a patient-centred, team-based approach (Berghmans, 2018).

Postoperative Care

Immediate postoperative care. Analgesic techniques including electrotherapy (Thakral et al., 2013) and low-level laser (Fallah et al., 2017) can help control the painful symptoms, without significant side effects. Another important aspect of postoperative care is plexular mobilization exercises. The mobilization strategy can be used to break fibrotic bands in formation and prevent recurrence of symptoms due to fibrotic entrapment. Hip mobilization should be performed for 10 to 15 minutes, two to three times daily, to avoid recurrent entrapment by postoperative fibrosis (Fig. 7.2.5).

Physical therapy management. Reassessment from the pelvic physical therapist is recommended at 6 weeks postoperatively, when an intracavitary myofascial assessment and treatment techniques can be administered safely. If performed earlier than the sixth postoperative

week, it can cause severe retroperitoneal bleeding. The physical therapist will administer the same outcome measures that were completed preoperatively to subjectively evaluate surgical outcomes and help construct a new treatment plan. A mechanical assessment will be completed to identify global and local contributors driving functional limitations. Neuropraxia is expected in the postoperative course and must always be considered when assessing functional strength, flexibility and sensory changes.

Treatment is tailored specifically to the patient, as every patient is unique. That being said, therapeutic neuroscience pain education is a modality used for all patients. There is fascinating evidence demonstrating the value of taking the time to educate the patient on the neurophysiological and neurobiological changes that occur with chronic pain. Doing so can help reduce pain ratings, increase physical performance, decrease catastrophizing and decrease perceived disability (Louw et al., 2011).

A properly trained physical therapist can detect evidence of neuroplastic changes in the central nervous

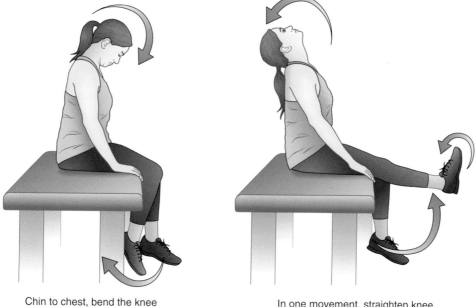

Chin to chest, bend the knee
and point the toe

In one movement, straighten knee
and look up

Fig. 7.2.5 Lumbar nerve flossing exercises are used postoperatively to break perineurial adhesions by making the lumbar nerve roots and sciatic nerve glide back-and-forth through the space that's allowing it to move more freely. This is accomplished by pulling on one end of the plexus while simultaneously providing slack on the other end. Next, the movements are reversed, making the nerves slide back and forth through their path. In this example, the nerves are pulled towards the spine by flexing the head ventrally (chin to chest), while simultaneously bending the nee and pointing the toes down. Sequentially, the nerves are pulled away from the spine doing a dorsal flexion of the head while simultaneously extending the knee and pointing the toes up. Although nerve flossing techniques are considered standard of care by many centers performing nerve detrapment procedures, based on the theory that it would break fibrotic bands while these are lose in the scarring process, there are, at the time of writing, no RCTs confirming or quantifying that effect. Therefore, these exercises are based only on specialist recommendations (Recommendation grade D).

system and of processing errors of the sensorimotor cortex, and use treatment strategies such as cognitive behavioral approaches, mindfulness meditation, graded exposure therapy, imagery, qi gong and manual therapy that is non-threatening to help desensitize allodynic tissues (Moseley and Flor, 2012; Vandyken and Hilton, 2017).

Manual therapy can be effective to address the mechanical changes in the lumbopelvic region, thoracic spine and hips, and help facilitate healthy movement patterns and restore function.

Interventional pain management. Interventional pain procedures are a valuable tool for postoperative pain management, usually providing targeted pain control with a low incidence of side effects. Currently, however, there is no good-quality evidence on interventional management for post-decompression pain specifically related to IPNEs. The information that follows corresponds to our group's experience and extrapolation of evidence from other kinds of peripheral entrapment; as such, it should be regarded as grade E evidence.

Caudal blocks are especially useful in the management of post-decompression pain. They consist of 'flushing' the sacral nerve roots with local anesthetics +/– a corticosteroid (Fig. 7.2.6). This procedure usually breaks the pain cycle and perineurial inflammation, producing prolonged symptom relief that usually lasts weeks or months. They are technically easier to perform than selective blocks and tend to provide better symptom relief than their more technically challenging counterparts.

Pulsed radiofrequency of the dorsal root ganglion may also be an option for targeted therapy, but evidence is still lacking. Its efficacy on lumbosacral neuropathies at a spinal level (Chang, 2018) make it a promising technique for post-decompression pain related to IPNEs.

When all of the preceding have failed, targeted therapy delivery with local anesthetics (ropivacaine or bupivacaine) has been showing promising results (Lemos et al., 2019b).

Surgical neuromodulation is also an option in refractory cases. It can be delivered epidurally (Hou et al., 2016) or specifically to the affected nerve (Possover et al., 2009; Possover et al., 2011).

THE MOST COMMON INTRAPELVIC NERVE ENTRAPMENT PRESENTATIONS

Topographic Diagnosis

The medical diagnostic sequence starts with a syndromic diagnosis, which is the collection of symptoms and signs reported by the patient (in this case, peripheral nerve

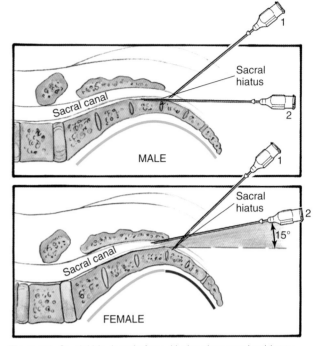

Fig. 7.2.6 Caudal block technique. Under ultrasound guidance, a needle is passed through the sacrococcygeal ligament and sacral hiatus into the sacral canal, and the sacral nerve roots are epidurally 'flushed' with local anesthetics +/– corticosteroids, breaking the chronic pain cycle. (From Mounir-Soliman, L., Farag, E., Brown, D. L. (2021). Brown's Atlas of Regional Anesthesia, Sixth Edition. Elsevier Inc.)

entrapment syndrome), followed by the topographic diagnosis, which is figuring out which organ or tissue is dysfunctional and generating those symptoms, and finally an aetiological diagnosis, which is finding what is causing that given organ or tissue to be dysfunctional.

For the topographic diagnosis, understanding this distribution and correlating the dermatomes (Fig. 7.2.7) with the potential nerve entrapment is crucial. Fig. 7.2.8 depicts the sites of IPNE in our series (Lemos et al., 2021).

The most frequent entrapment location is on the proximal aspect of S2, S3 and S4 nerve roots, in 35% of the cases. Entrapments at this level will produce pudendal, gluteal and medial sciatic pain, associated with urinary and faecal urgency, with or without incontinence, and voiding and defaecatory dysfunction. Urodynamics will show detrusor overactivity, due to irritation of the pelvic splanchnic nerves (parasympathetic) and detrusor-sphincter incoordination (due to pudendal activation). These entrapments are usually associated with piriformis entrapment, parametrial endometriosis, neurovascular conflict or primary nerve sheath tumors, from the most to least frequent aetiologies.

One-quarter of the cases affect the lumbosacral trunk and lateral sciatic fibers. Most of these cases are caused by abnormal variants of the superior gluteal vein (Lemos et al., 2019a), therefore following the cyclic pattern typical of neurovascular conflict, described later in this chapter.

Eighteen percent of the cases involve the distal aspect of S2, S3 and S4 nerve roots, which cause similar dermatomeric distribution to their proximal counterparts, as well as urinary urgency, with anorectal symptoms being less intense; urodynamics will show sensory-type urgency, without detrusor overactivity, since the pelvic splanchnic nerves are not affected—this is a key feature during diagnostic workup. Entrapments at this level are usually caused by parametrial endometriosis or scarring from reconstructive surgery, such as sacrospinous ligament fixation. These are also the most common causes of entrapments at the level of the pudendal (Alcock's) canal, which account for 8% of the cases and follow the pattern of the Nantes criteria (Labat et al., 2008).

In 12% of cases, entrapment was found on the proximal aspect of S1 and S2 nerve roots, mainly producing sciatica restricted to the posterior aspect of the thigh and leg and sole of the foot. These patients also complain of anterior perineal pain, not configuring the full pudendal dermatome. Such cases are usually caused by abnormal piriformis fibers (see the following) or by ovarian endometriomas that attach and infiltrate the pelvic sidewall.

The remaining 2% of the cases involve the obturator nerve and are usually caused by pelvic reconstructive procedures, causing pain on the medial thigh.

Etiological Diagnosis
Endometriosis
The first report of IPNE was made by Denton and Sherill (1955), who described a case of cyclic sciatica due to endometriosis in 1955. After that, some other case reports and small series were published, until 2011, when Possover et al. (2011) described the largest series to that date, with 175 patients, all treated laparoscopically.

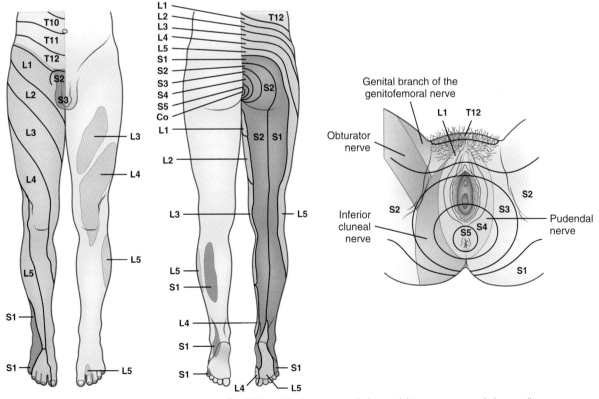

Fig. 7.2.7 Lumbosacral dermatomes. Familiarity with dermatomes in intrapelvic neuroanatomy is key to diagnosing intrapelvic nerve entrapment.

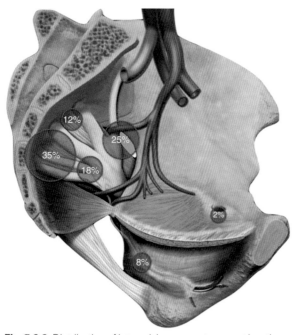

Fig. 7.2.8 Distribution of intrapelvic nerve entrapment locations: 35% on the proximal S2, S3 and S4 nerve roots; 25% on the lateral sciatic/lumbosacral trunk; 18% on the proximal pudendal/medial sciatic nerve; 12% on the S1 and S2 nerve roots; 8% at Alcock's canal level; and 2% on the obturator nerve.

Endometriotic entrapments present with cyclic symptoms, worsening in the periovulatory and peri-menstrual days, and ameliorating or even disappearing in the postmenstrual period (Lemos et al., 2011; Possover et al., 2011; Lemos et al., 2015).

Treatment consists of preoperatively identifying the symptoms and determining the topography of the lesions (by means, mainly, of anamnesis and neurological examination and, sometimes, by MRI) and laparoscopically exploring all suspect segments of the plexus, with radical removal of all endometriotic foci and fibrosis (Lemos et al. 2011; Possover et al., 2011; Lemos et al 2015) (Fig. 7.2.9).

Considering that no medical treatment has been shown to halt the progression of endometriosis, the risk of nerve infiltration, destruction of nerve fibers and its consequent permanent functional loss make surgical treatment mandatory in patients with IPNEs secondary to endometriosis (Lemos and Possover, 2015).

The true incidence of endometriosis involving the sacral plexus is unknown, as this presentation of the disease is often neglected. On average, patients undergo four surgical procedures seeking to treat the pain before

getting the right diagnosis (Possover, 2013). Moreover, about 40% of women with endometriosis have unilateral lower limb pain (Missmer and Bove, 2011), and in 30% of patients with endometriosis, leg pain was demonstrated to be neuropathic (Pacchiarotti et al., 2013), which leads to the conclusion that endometriotic involvement of the lumbosacral plexus is probably underdiagnosed and much more frequent than reported.

Physical therapy management. Endometriosis can adversely affect women's physical, mental and social well-being (Moradi et al., 2014). Loss in both work and household productivity are not uncommon due to the severe symptoms of endometriosis (Soliman et al., 2017). Women often complain of dysmenorrhoea, dyschezia, chronic pelvic pain (Ferrero et al., 2005) and deep dyspareunia (Bourdel et al., 2015; Lukic et al., 2016).

Physical therapy pre- and/or postoperatively can help improve penetrative sexual function and chronic pain management. Independent of the endometrial lesions, deep dyspareunia has been shown to be strongly related to pelvic floor tenderness and painful bladder syndrome; thus, the physical therapist can assess for the potential myofascial drivers and potential central mechanisms (Orr et al., 2018). Intravaginal manual techniques, digital biofeedback, electrotherapy and supervised pelvic floor exercises can be useful modalities (Ghaderi et al., 2019). Furthermore, vaginal re-mapping strategies with graded exposure can help the patient learn how to experience vaginal input without associated pain. Visceral mobilizations are especially effective postoperatively to prevent formation of adhesions (Bove and Chapelle, 2012). In addition, a bladder and bowel diary may be provided to assess fluid and fibre intake. Modification of defaecatory/voiding habits and postural/positional changes while toileting may be encouraged; abdominal massages to assist with bowel function can also be effective (Lämås et al., 2009). Low-intensity exercises, including yoga and stretching, as well as heat therapy, can also be effective to help manage dysmenorrhoea (Armour et al., 2019). Lastly, addressing functional limitations to help improve work and household productivity and ultimately quality of life will be ongoing in treatment.

Fibrosis

Fibrosis is one of the most frequent causes of IPNEs and possibly the most well-known etiology since Amarenco et al. (1987) first described PNA in cyclists, in whom the pain is a consequence of fibrotic entrapment due to continued trauma.

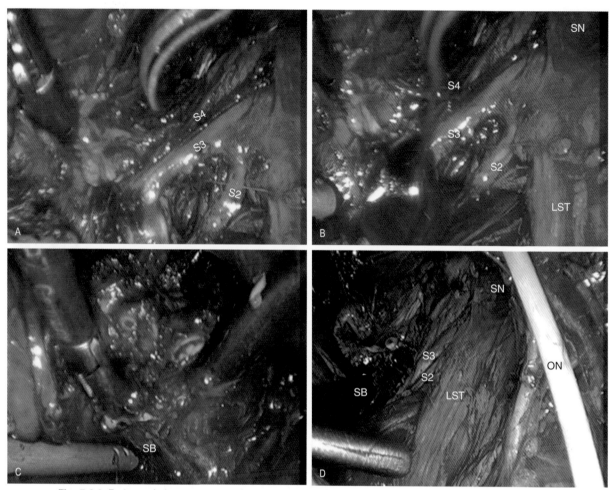

Fig. 7.2.9 Endometriotic entrapment of the right sacral plexus. (A) After partial detachment of the nodule, allowing for visualization of S2, S3 and S4 nerve roots, S3 was found to be dilated on its proximal part. (B) Opening of the S3 nerve root sheath revealed an endometrioma inside the nerve. (C) The nodule was detached from the sacral bone (SB). (D) The final aspect of the right pelvic sidewall. *LST,* Lumbosacral trunk; *ON,* obturator nerve; *SN,* sciatic nerve. (From Lemos et al. (2011).)

Despite the historical aspect, however, surgical manipulation seems to be the most frequent cause of fibrosis over the sacral plexus (Fig. 7.2.10). Among the surgeries with higher risks of inducing such kinds of entrapments are pelvic reconstructive procedures (Possover and Lemos, 2011); as mentioned previously, about 7% of women undergoing a vaginal hysterectomy for treatment of uterovaginal prolapse develop postoperative neuropathic pain on lumbosacral dermatomes (Montoya et al., 2012).

Considering that fibrosis is not a progressive condition, therapeutic blocks with high volumes of diluted local anesthetics, in an attempt to cause some hydrodissection,

and a dose of corticosteroids, to reduce inflammation and soften the fibrotic tissue, can be attempted before surgical detrapment (Khoder and Hale, 2014). Osteopathic and physiotherapy manipulation has also been suggested (Origo and Tarantino, 2019) and should be attempted in an effort to avoid more invasive approaches.

Physical therapy management. Although there is limited research, specifically looking at pelvic physical therapy effectiveness in treating IPNEs due to fibrosis, empirical observations suggest that pelvic physical therapy can successfully help this population avert surgery. The therapist will address overactive pelvic floor tissues through manual techniques (intravaginally or

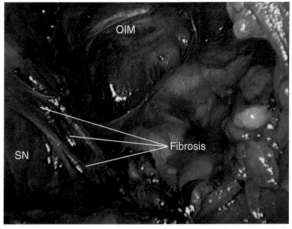

Fig. 7.2.10 Fibrotic entrapment of the left sciatic nerve (SN). *OIM*, Obturator Internus Muscle.

rectally) and use external connective tissue manipulation to help resolve any motion restrictions and to improve blood flow. Nerve mobilizations and flossing can also be effective. Often these patients need to modify sport or recreational activity to help manage symptoms. Depending on the sport or activity, the therapist must consider all moving parts; looking at global contributors is necessary to help resolve reported symptoms and, most importantly, to work towards returning to the preferred activity safely, whenever possible. Specifically, when working with a cyclist, much time is spent looking at bike fit and saddle shape—broader and conventionally shaped saddles cause fewer pelvic floor and genitourinary issues when compared to cut-out saddle designs (Trofaier et al., 2016). Reducing the rate of recurrence is salient to help these patients forestall surgery.

Neurovascular Conflict

Pelvic congestion syndrome is a well-known cause of cyclic pelvic pain. Patients commonly present with a cyclic, visceral type of pelvic pain, without evidence of inflammatory disease. The pain is worse during the premenstrual period and pregnancy, and is exacerbated by fatigue and prolonged standing (Ganeshan et al., 2007).

However, what is much less known is the fact that dilated or malformed branches of the internal or external iliac vessels can entrap the nerves of the sacral plexus against the pelvic sidewalls, producing symptoms such as sciatica, or refractory urinary and anorectal dysfunction (Possover, 2011; Lemos et al., 2016b; Lemos et al., 2019a) (Fig. 7.2.11).

Similarly to pelvic congestion syndrome, IPNEs secondary to neurovascular conflict are also cyclic in women. Patients are usually asymptomatic in the first half of the

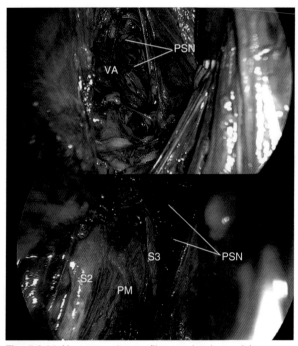

Fig. 7.2.11 Neurovascular conflict causing intrapelvic entrapment of S2 and S3. Varicose tributary (VA) of the left internal iliac vein entrapping the S2 and S3 nerve roots against the left piriformis muscle (PM). *PSN*, Pelvic Splancnic Nerves. (*From Lemos et al., 2015.*)

menstrual cycle; in most women, symptoms begin with ovulation and progressively become more intense, with the worst period being 2 days preceding menses. In both men and women, there is also a circadian pattern—patients present mild or no symptoms in the morning and then symptoms progressively worsen throughout the day, as gravity causes the pelvic varicosities to engorge/dilate, increasing the pressure over the nerves (Lemos et al., 2019a).

In these cases, conservative approaches can also be attempted before surgical management. Therapeutic nerve blocks associated with pelvic physiotherapy may be enough to mitigate symptoms. Embolization is associated with very high symptom recurrence in patient with lower urinary tract, pudendal and/or sciatic symptoms (Nasser et al., 2014), and should not be attempted in cases of neurovascular conflict, as it will make surgical detrapment more challenging and riskier.

Pelvic physical therapy management. The literature is lacking when it comes to examining the role of pelvic physical therapy in pelvic congestion syndrome. Notwithstanding this, considering these patients will often complain of dyspareunia, abdominal and pelvic tenderness, dysmenorrhoea, rectal discomfort and urinary frequency

(Ignacio et al., 2008), and when considering the proximity of the pelvic floor, it is no surprise that many patients report benefits from pelvic physical therapy. The therapist will often work with the patient in developing pacing strategies, considering their pain is often worsened at the end of the day or with prolonged standing. Having the patient get their legs up on the wall and/or elevated can help with increasing circulation to the pelvic floor, decrease pressure on the perineum and reduce pelvic tension. Lastly, ensuring the pelvic floor muscles are working efficiently for optimal bladder, bowel and sexual function is paramount.

Piriformis Syndrome

Numerous malformations of the piriformis muscle have been described in the deep gluteal space that can entrap branches of the sciatic nerve (Beaton & Anson, 1938): The laparoscopic approach has revealed that the intrapelvic fibers of this muscle can also entrap the sacral nerve roots (Sermer et al., 2021). Typically, these fibers originate laterally to the sacral foramina on the sacral bone; piriformis fibers originating medially to the sacral foramina can entrap the sacral nerve roots against the typical piriformis fibers (Fig. 7.2.12).

The prevalence of this anatomical variant is, however, quite high (Russell et al., 2008). A piriformis slip originating medially to the sacral foramina and, hence, with potential to entrap the underlying sacral nerve roots, can be found in about one-quarter of the population (cadaver study data is not yet published). Therefore, thorough clinical assessment is key to determining if the entrapment is caused by the variant piriformis bundle or if it is merely an incidental imaging finding.

One of the key features of the examination is a piriformis stretch test, which needs to be performed by two examiners. With the patient in the lateral decubitus position, an initial neurological examination is performed on the sacral dermatomes. The second examiner then performs a piriformis stretch manoeuvre by flexing the hip to 90 degrees, adducting the hip past the midline and performing an internal hip rotation. This manoeuvre should trigger/exacerbate the patient's symptoms and/or exacerbate the asymmetry in sensation on the affected sacral dermatomes (Fig. 7.2.13).

Differentiating intrapelvic from extrapelvic piriformis syndrome can also be quite challenging. Bowel and urinary symptoms are a good indication that the entrapment is intrapelvic, but these are not always present.

After imaging is complete, a transforaminal diagnostic nerve block is the next step. As mentioned previously, the block should resolve 100% of the radicular symptoms for the duration of the local anesthetic and render the piriformis stretch test negative.

Conservative management yields a higher success rate in piriformis syndrome than it does in other aetiologies of IPNE. Physiotherapy should focus on piriformis stretching and relaxation, ultimately aiming at reducing the pressure over the sacral nerve roots. Botulinum toxin can also be used at the abnormal muscle slip in an attempt to reduce its tonus.

If conservative treatment fails to control the symptoms, a laparoscopic approach is performed, aiming at transecting the abnormal bundle and resecting all of its intrapelvic segment (Li et al., 2018).

Pelvic physical therapy management. When assessing this population, it is important to rule out lumbopelvic dysfunction and other spinal pathologies (Hicks et al., 2020). There are various causes of compression, including, but not limited to, acute trauma, overuse trauma (from activity or prolonged sitting) or muscle hypertrophy (Chang et al., 2020) that are important for the therapist to understand to help them construct their assessment and treatment plan. The therapist will look at range of motion of the lumbar spine, thoracic spine and hips. General lower-extremity strength testing will be completed, with special attention to the gluteus maximus and gluteus medius muscles. Palpating the piriformis intrarectally will allow the therapist to understand the integrity, sensitivity and strength of the muscle. If needed, provocative testing can be completed to help with clinical reasoning. The assessment should also include a functional component, looking at gait, transitional movements, squats and/or movements that reproduce their pain. Treatment focus is to reduce any overactivity/spasm over the piriformis using manual techniques and active stretches to help reduce pressure over the sacral nerve roots. The gluteus maximus and medius often require strengthening, as weakness may be the cause or the result of piriformis irritability. Modifying functional activities such as sitting duration and frequency and/or sport may be necessary until the patient successfully completes a graded exposure program tailored to their limitations.

Neoplasms

Tumors can also entrap the nerves or nerve roots. Tumors can be primary neural tumors, such as schwannomas, or metastatic tumors entrapping the nerves, such as pelvic lymph nodes, in pelvic malignancies (Fig. 7.2.14).

Treatment in this case is primarily surgical, and the role of conservative treatment is restricted to the general perioperative care described previously.

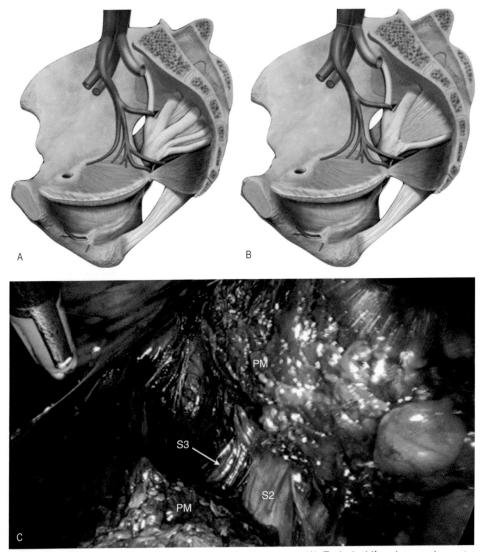

Fig. 7.2.12 Piriformis bundle entrapping the sacral nerve roots. (A) Typical piriformis muscle anatomy. Observe the sacral nerve roots overlying the muscle on its ventromedial aspect, as all muscle fibers are originating laterally to the sacral foramina. (B) Variant piriformis anatomy. Note that a muscle bundle originates medially to the sacral foramina and can potentially entrap the sacral nerve roots against the typical piriformis belly. (C) Muscular entrapment of the right S2 and S3 nerve roots (laparoscopic view). Observe the transected piriformis muscle bundle (PM) originating from the sacral bone medially from the sacral nerve roots and therefore crushing the nerves every time the muscle contracts.

CONCLUSION

Laparoscopy provides minimally invasive access with optimal visualization to virtually all abdominal portions of the lumbosacral plexus, which are also subject to entrapment neuropathies. Therefore. when facing sciatica, gluteal or perineal pain without any obvious spinal or deep gluteal causes, the examiner should always remember that the entrapment could be in the intrapelvic portions, especially when urinary or anorectal symptoms are present.

The laparoscopic approach to the intrapelvic bundles of the lumbosacral nerves has opened myriad possibilities to assess and treat this neglected portion of the plexus, and has allowed for better understanding of IPNEs, which will ultimately result in the development of better surgical/conservative strategies.

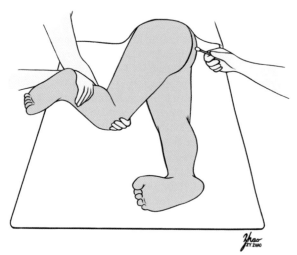

Fig. 7.2.13 Piriformis stretch test. With the patient in the lateral decubitus position, an initial neurological examination is performed on the sacral dermatomes. The second examiner then performs a piriformis stretch manoeuvre by flexing the hip to 90 degrees, adducting the hip past the midline and performing an internal hip rotation. This manoeuvre should trigger/exacerbate the patient's symptoms and/or exacerbate the asymmetry in sensation on the affected sacral dermatomes.

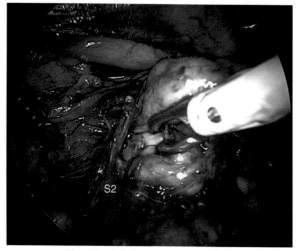

Fig. 7.2.14 Schwannoma in S2 (left).

REFERENCES

Amarenco, G., Lanoe, Y., Perrigot, M., et al. (1987). [A new canal syndrome: Compression of the pudendal nerve in Alcock's canal or perinal paralysis of cyclists]. *Presse Medicine, 16*(8), 399.

Armour, M., Smith, C. A., Steel, K. A., et al. (2019). The effectiveness of self-care and lifestyle interventions in primary dysmenorrhea: A systematic review and meta-analysis. *BMC Complement. Alternative Medicine, 19*(1), 22.

Barber, M. D., Bremer, R. E., Thor, K. B., et al. (2002). Innervation of the female levator ani muscles. *American Journal of Obstetrics and Gynecology, 187*(1), 64–71.

Beaton, L., Anson, B. (1938). The sciatic nerve and the piriformis muscle: their interrelation and possible cause of coccygodynia. *J Bone Joint Surg [Am], 20*, 686–688.

Berghmans, B. (2018). Physiotherapy for pelvic pain and female sexual dysfunction: An untapped resource. *International Urogynecology Journal, 29*(5), 631–638.

Bouche, P. (2013). Compression and entrapment neuropathies. *Handbook of Clinical Neurology, 115*, 311–366.

Bourdel, N., Alves, J., Pickering, G., et al. (2015). *Human Reproduction Update, 21*(1), 136–152.

Bove, G. M., & Chapelle, S. L. (2012). Visceral mobilization can lyse and prevent peritoneal adhesions in a rat model. *Journal of Bodywork and Movement Therapies, 16*(1), 76–82.

Chang, A., Ly, N., & Varacallo, M. (2020). *Piriformis injection [online]*. Available: https://www.ncbi.nlm.nih.gov/books/NBK448193/ (accessed 09.30.22).

Chang, M. C. (2018). Efficacy of pulsed radiofrequency stimulation in patients with peripheral neuropathic pain: A narrative review. *Pain Physician, 21*(3), e225–e234.

De Manincor, M., Bensoussan, A., Smith, C. A., et al. (2016). Individualized yoga for reducing depression and anxiety, and improving well-being: A randomized controlled trial. *Depression and Anxiety, 33*(9), 816–828.

DeGroat, W. C., & Yoshimura, N. (2015). Anatomy and physiology of the lower urinary tract. In *Handbook of clinical Neurology (3rd series)* (pp. 61–108). Oxford, UK: Elsevier.

Denton, R. O., & Sherrill, J. D. (1955). Sciatic syndrome due to endometriosis of sciatic nerve. *Southern Medical Journal, 48*(10), 1027–1031.

Dufour, S., Vandyken, B., Forget, M. J., et al. (2018). Association between lumbopelvic pain and pelvic floor dysfunction in women: A cross sectional study. *Musculoskelet Science Practice, 34*, 47–53.

Fallah, A., Mirzaei, A., Gutknecht, N., et al. (2017). Clinical effectiveness of low-level laser treatment on peripheral somatosensory neuropathy. *Lasers Medicine Science, 32*(3), 721–728.

Faubion, S. S., Shuster, L. T., & Bharucha, A. E. (2012). Recognition and management of nonrelaxing pelvic floor dysfunction. *Mayo Clinic Proceedings, 87*(2), 187–193.

Ferla, L., Darski, C., Paiva, L. L., et al. (2016). Synergism between abdominal and pelvic floor muscles in healthy women: A systematic review of observational studies. *Fisioterapia em Movimento, 29*(2), 399.

Ferrero, S., Esposito, F., & Abbamonte, L. H. (2005). Quality of sex life in women with endometriosis and deep dyspareunia. *Fertility and Sterility, 83*, 573–579.

Ganeshan, A., Upponi, S., Hon, L. Q., et al. (2007). Chronic pelvic pain due to pelvic congestion syndrome: The role of diagnostic and interventional radiology. *CardioVascular and Interventional Radiology, 30*(6), 1105–1111.

Ghaderi, F., Bastani, P., Hajebrahimi, S., et al. (2019). Pelvic floor rehabilitation in the treatment of women with dyspareunia: A randomized controlled clinical trial. *International Urogynecology Journal*, 30(11), 1849–1855.

Grigorescu, B. A., Lazarou, G., Olson, T. R., et al. (2008). Innervation of the levator ani muscles: Description of the nerve branches to the pubococcygeus, iliococcygeus, and puborectalis muscles. *International Urogynecology Journal and Pelvic Floor Dysfunction*, 19(1), 107–116.

Hicks, B. L., Lam, J. C., & Varacallo, M. (2020). *Piriformis syndrome. [Online].* Available: https://www.ncbi.nlm.nih.gov/books/NBK448172/ (accessed 09.30.22).

Hodges, P. W., Sapsford, R., & Pengel, L. H. (2007). Postural and respiratory functions of the pelvic floor muscles. *Neurourology and Urodynamics*, 26(3), 362–371.

Huard, P. (1968). Esboços do nervo isquiático. Windsor Collection-Na.B.f.18/ Clark1903 5 r/c. Windsor Collection—Q IV f. 9 r/Clark 1911 4 r/c.1495-1499. In *Léonard de Vinci, Dessins Anatomiques.* Paris: Dacosta pp. XX–XX.

Ignacio, E. A., Dua, R., Sarin, S., et al. (2008). Pelvic congestion syndrome: Diagnosis and treatment. *Seminars in Interventional Radiology*, 25(4), 361–368.

Keizer, A., Vandyken, B., Vandyken, C., et al. (2019). Predictors of pelvic floor muscle dysfunction among women with lumbopelvic pain. *Physical Therapy*, 99(12), 1703–1711.

Khoder, W., & Hale, D. (2014). Pudendal neuralgia. *Obstetrics Gynecology Clinical North American*, 41(3), 443–452.

Khoury, B., Lecomte, T., Fortin, G., et al. (2013). Mindfulness-based therapy: A comprehensive meta-analysis. *Clinical Psychology Review*, 33(6), 763–771.

Labat, J. J., Riant, T., Robert, R., et al. (2008). Diagnostic criteria for pudendal neuralgia by pudendal nerve entrapment (Nantes criteria). *Neurourology and Urodynamics*, 27(4), 306–310.

Lämås, K., Lindholm, L., Stenlund, H., et al. (2009). Effects of abdominal massage in management of constipation—a randomized controlled trial. *International Journal of Nursing Studies*, 46(6), 759–767.

Lemos, N., Cancelliere, L., Li, A. K., et al. (2019). Superior gluteal vein syndrome: An intrapelvic cause of sciatica. *Journal Hip Preserv Surgery.*, 6(2), 104–108.

Lemos, N., D'Amico, N., Marques, R., et al. (2016). Recognition and treatment of endometriosis involving the sacral nerve roots. *International Urogynecology Journal*, 27(1), 147–150.

Lemos, N., Fernandes, G. L., Qiao, L., et al. (2019). Laparoscopic catheter implantation for targeted therapy delivery in the treatment of pudendal neuralgia and other intrapelvic causes of neuropathic pain. *Journal of Minimally Invasive Gynecology*, 26(7), S80.

Lemos, N., Kamergorodsky, G., Ploger, C., et al. (2012). Sacral nerve infiltrative endometriosis presenting as perimenstrual right-sided sciatica and bladder atonia: Case report and description of surgical technique. *Journal of Minimally Invasive Gynecology*, 19(3), 396–400.

Lemos, N., Marques, R. M., Kamergorodsky, G., et al. (2016). Vascular entrapment of the sciatic plexus causing

catamenial sciatica and urinary symptoms. *International Urogynecology Journal*, 27(2), 317–319.

Lemos, N., Possover, M. (2015). Laparoscopic approach to intrapelvic nerve entrapments. *J Hip Preserv Surg*, 2(2), 92–98.

Lemos, N., Sermer, C., Fernandes, G., et al. (2021). Laparoscopic approach to refractory extraspinal sciatica and pudendal pain caused by intrapelvic nerve entrapment: report of a 10-year experience. *Nature Scientific Reports*, 11(1), 10820. DOI: 10.1038/s41598-021-90319-y.

Lewis, R. A., Williams, N. H., Sutton, A. J., et al. (2015). Comparative clinical effectiveness of management strategies for sciatica: Systematic review and network meta-analyses. *The Spine Journal*, 15(6), 1461–1477.

Li, A. L. K., Polesello, G., Tokechi, D., et al. (2018). Prize award: Best video abstract. Laparoscopic treatment of intrapelvic entrapment of sacral nerve roots by abnormal piriformis bundles causing sciatica, pudendal neuralgia, pelvic floor dysfunction, and lower urinary tract symptoms. *Neurourology and Urodynamics*, 37(Suppl. 5), 239–240.

Louw, A., Diener, I., Butler, D. S., et al. (2011). The effect of neuroscience education on pain, disability, anxiety, and stress in chronic musculoskeletal pain. *Archives of Physical Medicine and Rehabilitation*, 92(12), 2041–2056.

Lovibond, S. H., & Lovibond, P. F. (1995). *Manual for the depression anxiety stress scales* (2nd ed.). Sydney: Psychology Foundation.

Loving, S., Thomsen, T., Jaszczak, P., et al. (2014). Pelvic floor muscle dysfunctions are prevalent in female chronic pelvic pain: A cross-sectional population-based study. *European Journal of Pain*, 18(9), 1259–1270.

Lukic, A., Di Properzio, M., & De Carlo, S. (2016). Quality of sex life in endometriosis patients with deep dyspareunia before and after laparoscopic treatment. *Archives of Gynecology and Obstetrics*, 293, 583–590.

Lundberg, M., Larsson, M., Ostlund, H., et al. (2006). Kinesiophobia among patients with musculoskeletal pain in primary healthcare. *Journal of Rehabilitation Medicine*, 38(1), 37–43.

Missmer, S. A., & Bove, G. M. (2011). A pilot study of the prevalence of leg pain among women with endometriosis. *Journal Body Movement Therapy*, 15(3), 304–308.

Montoya, T. I., Luebbehusen, H. I., Schaffer, J. I., et al. (2012). Sensory neuropathy following suspension of the vaginal apex to the proximal uterosacral ligaments. *International Urogynecology Journal*, 23(12), 1735–1740.

Moradi, M., Parker, M., Sneddon, A., et al. (2014). Impact of endometriosis on women's lives: A qualitative study. *BMC Women's Health*, 14(1), 123.

Moseley, G. L., & Flor, H. (2012). Targeting cortical representations in the treatment of chronic pain: A review. *Neurorehabil. Neural Repair*, 26(6), 646–652.

Nasser, F., Cavalcante, R. N., Affonso, B. B., et al. (2014). Safety, efficacy, and prognostic factors in endovascular treatment of pelvic congestion syndrome. *International Journal of Gynaecology & Obstetrics, 125*(1), 65–68.

Neblett, R., Cohen, H., Choi, Y., et al. (2013). The central sensitization Inventory (CSI): Establishing clinically significant values for identifying central sensitivity syndromes in an outpatient chronic pain sample. *The Journal of Pain, 14*(5), 438–445.

Neville, C. E., Fitzgerald, C. M., Mallinson, T., et al. (2012). A preliminary report of MSK dysfunction in female pelvic pain: A blinded study of examination findings. *Journal of Bodywork and Movement Therapies, 6*(1), 50–56.

Origo, D., & Tarantino, A. G. (2019). Osteopathic manipulative treatment in pudendal neuralgia: A case report. *Journal of Bodywork and Movement Therapies, 23*(2), 247–250.

Orr, N. L., Noga, H., Williams, C., et al. (2018). Deep dyspareunia in endometriosis: Role of the bladder and pelvic floor. *The Journal of Sexual Medicine, 15*(8), 1158–1166.

Pacchiarotti, A., Milazzo, G. N., Biasiotta, A., et al. (2013). Pain in the upper anterior-lateral part of the thigh in women affected by endometriosis: Study of sensitive neuropathy. *Fertility and Sterility, 100*(1), 122–126.

Pool-Goudzwaard, A., van Dijke, G. H., van Gurp, M., et al. (2004). Contribution of pelvic floor muscles to stiffness of the pelvic ring. *Clinical biomechanics, 19*(6), 564–571.

Possover, M. (2009). Laparoscopic management of endopelvic etiologies of pudendal pain in 134 consecutive patients. *Journal Urology, 181*(4), 1732–1736.

Possover, M. (2009). The sacral LION procedure for recovery of bladder/rectum/sexual functions in paraplegic patients after explantation of a previous Finetech-Brindley controller. *Journal of Minimally Invasive Gynecology, 16*(1), 98–101.

Possover, M. (2013). Use of the LION procedure on the sensitive branches of the lumbar plexus for the treatment of intractable postherniorrhaphy neuropathic inguinodynia. *Hernia, 17*(3), 333–337.

Possover, M. (2014). Recovery of sensory and supraspinal control of leg movement in people with chronic paraplegia: A case series. *Archives of Physical Medicine and Rehabilitation, 95*(4), 610–614.

Possover, M., Chiantera, V., & Baekelandt, J. (2007). Anatomy of the sacral roots and the pelvic splanchnic nerves in women using the LANN technique. *Surgery Laparoscopy Endoscopy Percutaneous Technology, 17*(6), 508–510.

Possover, M., Forman, A., Rabischong, B., et al. (2015). Neuropelveology: New groundbreaking discipline in medicine. *Journal of Minimally Invasive Gynecology, 22*(7), 1140–1141.

Possover, M., & Lemos, N. (2011). Risks, symptoms, and management of pelvic nerve damage secondary to surgery

for pelvic organ prolapse: A report of 95 cases. *International Urogynecology Journal, 22*(12), 1485–1490.

Possover, M., Schneider, T., & Henle, K. P. (2011). Laparoscopic therapy for endometriosis and vascular entrapment of sacral plexus. *Fertility and Sterility, 95*(2), 756–758.

Possover, M., Schurch, B., & Henle, K. (2010). New strategies of pelvic nerves stimulation for recovery of pelvic visceral functions and locomotion in paraplegics. *Neurourology and Urodynamics, 29*, 1433–1438.

Quartana, P. J., Campbell, C. M., & Edwards, R. R. (2009). Pain catastrophizing: A critical review. *Expert Review Neurother., 9*(5), 745–758.

Rempel, D., Dahlin, L., & Lundborg, G. (1999). Pathophysiology of nerve compression syndromes: Response of peripheral nerves to loading. *Journal Bone Joint Surgery American, 81*(11), 1600–1610.

Russell, J. M., Kransdorf, M. J., Bancroft, L. W., et al. (2008). Magnetic resonance imaging of the sacral plexus and piriformis muscles. *Skeletal Radiology, 37*(8), 709–713.

Schmid, A. A., Van Puymbroeck, M., Fruhauf, C. A., et al. (2019). Yoga improves occupational performance, depression, and daily activities for people with chronic pain. *Work, 63*(2), 181–189.

Sermer, C., Adrienne L. K. Li, Fernandes, G. L., et al. (2021). Intrapelvic entrapment of sacral nerve roots by abnormal bundles of the piriformis muscle: description of an extra-spinal cause of sciatica and pudendal neuralgia. *Journal of Hip Preservation Surgery, 8*(1), 132–138.

Soliman, A. M., Coyne, K. S., Gries, K. S., et al. (2017). The effect of endometriosis symptoms on absenteeism and presenteeism in the workplace and at home. *Journal Management Care Specialist Pharmaceutical, 23*(7), 745–754.

Thakral, G., Kim, P. J., LaFontaine, J., et al. (2013). Electrical stimulation as an adjunctive treatment of painful and sensory diabetic neuropathy. *Journal Diabetes Science Technology, 7*(5), 1202–1209.

Trofaier, M. L., Schneidinger, C., Marschalek, J., et al. (2016). Pelvic floor symptoms in female cyclists and possible remedies: A narrative review. *International Urogynecology Journal, 27*(4), 513–519.

Van der Jagt, P. K., Dik, P., Froeling, M., et al. (2012). Architectural configuration and microstructural properties of the sacral plexus: A diffusion tensor MRI and fiber tractography study. *NeuroImage, 62*(3), 1792–1799.

Vandyken, C., & Hilton, S. (2017). Physical therapy in the treatment of central pain mechanisms for female sexual pain. *Sex Medicine Review, 5*(1), 20–30.

Wallner, C., van Wissen, J., Maas, C. P., et al. (2008). The contribution of the levator ani nerve and the pudendal nerve to the innervation of the levator ani muscles; a study in human fetuses. *European Urology, 54*(5), 1136–1142.

7.3 Pelvic Organ Prolapse

Douglas Luchristt and Matthew D. Barber

PREVALENCE AND INCIDENCE

Pelvic organ prolapse (POP) is the downward descent of the female pelvic organs (vagina, uterus, bladder and/or rectum) into or through the vagina. POP is a clinical condition encountered frequently by physical therapists specializing in the care of women with pelvic floor disorders. Loss of vaginal or uterine support is common, with rates observed on examination among women presenting for routine gynaecology care ranging from 43% to 92% (Ellerkmann et al., 2001; Swift, 2000). Among postmenopausal women, observed rates are higher, ranging from 86% to 98% (Nygaard et al., 2004; Swift et al., 2005). However, many women with loss of pelvic support are asymptomatic and do not require treatment, particularly among women with prolapse that does not extend beyond the hymen. Indeed, the hymen seems to be an important cut-off point for symptom development. Approximately 3% to 10% of women have descent of the uterus or vagina beyond the hymen, and approximately 3% to 8% of women report symptomatic vaginal bulging across diverse practice settings and populations (Cooper et al., 2015; Nygaard, Barber, Burgio, & et al., 2008a, 2008b; Trowbridge et al., 2008; Walker and Gunasekera, 2011).

Although increasing prevalence of POP is seen among older women, individual progression of disease is dynamic. One prospective longitudinal study of 270 postmenopausal women over a 4-year period found an estimated annual incidence of 26% and spontaneous resolution rate of 21%. Over 3 years, the incidence of POP was estimated to be 40% and resolution 19% without any intervention. The level and direction of change appears to be related to the baseline stage of disease, with women more likely to have a reduction in the descent of their prolapse when baseline measures were above the level of the hymen (Bradley et al., 2007).

RISK FACTORS

There are several well-established risk factors for POP. On average, each decade of increasing age is associated with a 40% increase in the relative rate of POP with a 12.6% lifetime risk of surgery for POP by age 80 years among all women (Swift et al., 2005; Wu et al., 2014). Among younger women, childbirth appears to be an important risk factor for symptomatic POP. An observational study from the UK found a direct linear relationship between the number of deliveries and risk of POP, with an 11-fold increased rate observed among women with four or more deliveries when compared to their nulliparous counterparts (Mant et al., 1997). The route of delivery also appears to independently influence risk of POP, with one cross-sectional study of more than 3000 women in a large healthcare system showing that vaginal delivery accounts for 46% of the attributable risk of symptomatic POP (Lukacz et al., 2006).

Obesity is another important risk factor for development of POP across all age ranges. Among women presenting for routine gynaecological care, overweight and obese individuals had a greater than threefold increase in odds of POP compared to normal-weight women (Swift et al., 2005). Moreover, when assessing the progression of disease, overweight and obese women had more than a twofold increased risk of worsening prolapse over a 3-year period (Bradley et al., 2007).

PATHOPHYSIOLOGY

When considering the prevalence of different forms of POP, prolapse of the anterior vaginal wall, or cystocele, is the most common form, detected twice as often as posterior vaginal prolapse (i.e., rectocele) and three times more often than apical prolapse (i.e., uterine and/or post-hysterectomy vaginal vault prolapse). However, although different organs may represent the leading edge of prolapse observed on physical examination, isolated defects in the anterior, apical or posterior compartments are rarely seen. In a functional magnetic resonance imaging study of 153 women presenting to a urogynaecology clinic, Summers et al. (2006) demonstrated a strong correlation between anterior and apical compartment descent, regardless of the stage of prolapse or symptoms reported by the patient. They estimated 53% of bladder, 67% of urethral and 71% of paravaginal descent was explained by loss of apical support. As a result, women presenting for evaluation of POP may present with a variety of symptoms (Box 7.3.1). Ellerkmann et al. (2001) found that in 237 women evaluated for POP, 73% reported urinary incontinence, 86% reported urinary urgency and/or frequency, 34% to 62% reported voiding dysfunction, and 31% complained of faecal incontinence.

The underlying mechanisms driving the development and progression of POP remain unclear, but function of the levator ani muscle complex appears to play an important role. Computational models based on functional magnetic resonance imaging has suggested that the levator complex stretches up to 350% of its resting length to accommodate crowning at vaginal delivery, with the greatest stretch forces experienced by the pubococcygeus (Lien et al., 2004). These forces are well beyond the typical forces tolerated by striated muscle and can lead to dysfunction related to stretch injury, rupture or avulsion. In a 10-year observational cohort study of parous women, risk of POP was directly related to levator strength and hiatus size, with the effects of injury or avulsion mediated through these key variables (Handa et al., 2019). In turn, opening of the genital and levator hiatus related to injury or weakness is thought to apply additional pressure to the apical compartment, leading to lengthening and weakening of the cardinal and uterosacral ligaments which provide the primary support (Kieserman-Shmokler et al., 2020).

CLINICAL ASSESSMENT OF PELVIC ORGAN PROLAPSE

POP, as with other pelvic floor disorders, rarely results in severe morbidity or mortality; rather, it causes symptoms that can impact a woman's daily activities and negatively affect her quality of life. As such, it is essential to understand not only the symptoms a particular patient experiences, but the degree of bother caused by these symptoms and how it impacts her quality of life. This understanding is essential for determining what treatment to offer and when. Current management options for women with symptomatic POP include observation, pessary use, pelvic floor muscle training and surgery. Women with advanced POP may have minimal symptoms and report little or no bother as a result of their POP. In these cases, observation or 'watchful waiting' is perfectly appropriate; in theory, this would be an appropriate time to consider starting a program of pelvic floor muscle training, but evidence is limited. To date, there is only one randomized controlled trial assessing the role of physical therapy for the prevention of worsening prolapse in women with symptomatic POP, and no studies in asymptomatic women (primary prevention). Women with advanced POP who choose observation should be evaluated periodically to identify the development of new symptoms or conditions that might prompt treatment.

> ### BOX 7.3.1 Common Symptoms in Women With Pelvic Organ Prolapse
>
> **Vaginal**
> Sensation of a bulge or protrusion
> Seeing or feeling a bulge from the vagina
> Pressure
> Heaviness
>
> **Urinary**
> Incontinence (stress, urge or mixed)
> Frequency
> Urgency
> Weak or prolonged urinary stream
> Hesitancy
> Feeling of incomplete emptying
> Manual reduction of prolapse to start or complete voiding (splinting)
> Position change to start or complete voiding
>
> **Bowel**
> Incontinence of flatus or liquid/solid stool
> Feeling of incomplete emptying
> Straining during defaecation
> Urgency to defaecate
> Digital evacuation to complete defaecation
> Splinting, or pushing on or around the vagina or perineum, to start or complete defaecation
> Feeling of blockage or obstruction during defaecation
>
> **Sexual**
> Dyspareunia

Reprinted with permission from Elsevier (Jelovsek et al. (2007). *The Lancet* 369(9566), 1027–1038).

HISTORY

As women with POP can present with multiple pelvic floor symptoms, a comprehensive clinical assessment is critical. This requires a complete history including an assessment for vaginal bulge symptoms and associated lower urinary and gastrointestinal symptoms and symptoms of sexual dysfunction (see Box 7.3.1). The symptom that most strongly correlates with advanced POP is the presence of a vaginal bulge that can be seen or felt (Bradley and Nygaard, 2005; Swift et al., 2003; Tan et al., 2005). The specificity of a vaginal bulge symptoms for predicting the presence of prolapse beyond the hymen on a straining examination is 99% to 100% (Barber et al., 2006; Bradley and Nygaard, 2005). Less specific symptoms such as pressure, heaviness and fullness have a much weaker relation to loss of vaginal support (Burrows et al., 2004; Ellerkmann et al., 2001; Samuelsson et al., 1999; Swift et al., 2005). Symptoms of POP, particularly bulging and pressure, are generally worse after long periods of standing or exercise and are often improved when the patient is lying supine. Complaints of vaginal bleeding, discharge or infection may result from vaginal ulcerations sometimes seen with advanced prolapse. Unexplained vaginal bleeding should prompt a workup for other causes of bleeding, particularly in postmenopausal women without hysterectomy, where an evaluation of the endometrium via biopsy or ultrasound is typically warranted.

Lower urinary tract complaints frequently coexist with symptoms of POP (Ellerkmann et al., 2001; Nygaard et al., 2008a, 2008b). In some circumstances, loss of vaginal support directly affects bladder or urethral function. In other cases the relationship between prolapse and lower urinary tract dysfunction, particularly irritative bladder symptoms, is less clear. Descent of the apical compartment is highly correlated with descent of the bladder and urethra. The underlying dysfunction and weakness in the pelvic floor musculature and connective tissues along the anterior vaginal wall are thought to contribute to development of stress urinary incontinence (Delancey and Ashton-Miller, 2004). Therefore, the fact that POP and stress urinary incontinence sometimes coexist is not surprising, particularly when prolapse is mild. In contrast, women with POP that extends beyond the hymen are less likely to report stress incontinence and more likely to have obstructed voiding symptoms such as urinary hesitancy, intermittent flow, weak or prolonged stream, feeling of incomplete emptying, the need to manually reduce (splint) the prolapse to initiate or complete urination and, in rare cases, urinary retention (Barber, 2005; Burrows et al., 2004; Ellerkmann et al., 2001; Samuelsson et al., 1999). The mechanism for this appears to be mechanical obstruction resulting from urethral kinking that occurs with progressively worsening anterior vaginal prolapse (Figure 7.3.1). As many as 30% of women with stage 3 or 4 POP have elevated post-void residuals (>100 mL),

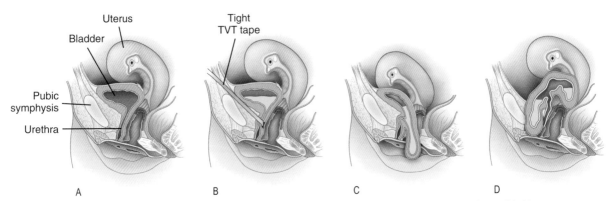

Fig. 7.3.1 (a) Normal anatomy. (b) Urethral obstruction. (c) Large prolapse, kinking urethra. (d) Flaccid, floppy bladder.

and development of de novo stress urinary incontinence after surgical correction of POP is seen in up to 43% of women (Coates et al., 1997; Wei et al., 2012).

QUESTIONNAIRES

Pelvic floor symptoms can be assessed in several ways. Obviously, taking a thorough clinical history is an important method of assessing the patient's symptoms and their effect on the patient's life. However, in situations where a standardized, reproducible assessment is desired, clinical histories can be problematic, as they typically take on a different form for each clinician and patient encounter. The most valid way of measuring the presence, severity and impact of pelvic floor symptoms on a patient's activities and well-being is through the use of psychometrically robust self-administered questionnaires (Barber et al., 2005). Several valid, reliable and responsive questionnaires are available and have been widely used in women with POP, including symptom questionnaires, measures of health-related quality of life and sexual function questionnaires (Box 7.3.2).

BOX 7.3.2 Recommended Questionnaires for Women With Pelvic Organ Prolapse

Symptom Questionnaires

Pelvic Floor Distress Inventory (PFDI) (Barber et al., 2001)

Pelvic Floor Distress Inventory–Short Form (PFDI-20) (Barber et al., 2005)

ICIQ Vaginal Symptoms Questionnaire (ICIQ-VS) (Price et al., 2006)

Quality-of-Life Questionnaires

Pelvic Floor Impact Questionnaire (PFIQ) (Barber et al., 2001)

Pelvic Floor Impact Questionnaire–Short Form (PFIQ-7) (Barber et al., 2005)

Prolapse Quality of Life Questionnaire (P-QOL) (Digesu et al., 2005)

Sexual Function Questionnaires

Prolapse and Incontinence Sexual Function Questionnaire (PISQ) (Rogers et al., 2001)

Prolapse and Incontinence Sexual Function Questionnaire–Short Form (PISQ-12) (Rogers et al., 2003)

Prolapse and Incontinence Sexual Function Questionnaire–IUGA Revised (PISQ-IR) (Rogers et al., 2013)

PHYSICAL EXAMINATION

Patients presenting with symptoms suggestive of POP should undergo a pelvic examination. The pelvic examination should be performed with the patient resting and straining while supine and standing to define the extent of the prolapse and determine the compartments involved (anterior, posterior and/or apical) (Bump et al., 1996). To start, a bivalve speculum is inserted into the cervix or, in women who have had a hysterectomy, the vaginal cuff is identified to evaluate apical vaginal support. While the patient strains, the speculum is slowly withdrawn and the descent of the vaginal apex is noted. The extent of prolapse of the anterior vaginal wall can be evaluated by placing a vaginal speculum or the posterior blade of a bivalve speculum in the vagina to retract the posterior vaginal wall. The patient is asked to strain, and the extent of anterior vaginal prolapse is noted. The blade is then placed to retract the anterior vaginal wall and the patient strains to reveal any posterior prolapse. As noted previously, there is strong correlation between apical and anterior and posterior descent on Valsalva; therefore, caution must be taken during examination to ensure that positioning of or pressure applied to the speculum does not reduce the prolapse and bias examination findings. A rectovaginal examination can be useful to identify the presence of a rectocele and determine the integrity of the perineal body.

In women with prolapse that protrudes beyond the hymen for a long duration, the vagina and/or cervix can become hypertrophied and develop erosions. A bimanual examination is performed to rule out coexistent gynaecologic pathology and pelvic muscle strength is assessed as described in the previous sections.

Although numerous prolapse grading systems have been described, the most widely used and accepted is the Pelvic Organ Prolapse Quantification (POP-Q) system. The POP-Q system was introduced in 1996 jointly by the Society of Gynecologic Surgeons, the American Urogynecologic Society and the International Continence Society as the accepted method for describing pelvic support and comparing examinations over time and after interventions (Bump et al., 1996). This system has since been similarly adopted by the National Institutes of Health, the International Urogynecological Association and the World Health Organization's International Consultation on Incontinence (Haylen et al., 2016). This prolapse grading system has been shown to have good

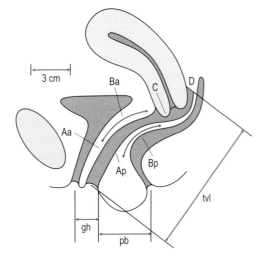

Fig. 7.3.2 The six vaginal segments (Aa, Ba, C, D, Ap and Bp), genital hiatus (gh), perineal body (pb) and total vaginal length (tvl) measured to complete the Pelvic Organ Prolapse Quantification (POP-Q) profile.

Stage	Definition
	TABLE 7.3.1 Staging system for pelvic organ prolapse, based on the POP-Q system
0	No prolapse is demonstrated. Points Aa, Ap, Ba and Bp are all at −3 and C and D are both <0 and the absolute value of either point is ≥[tvl −2] cm
I	Criteria for stage 0 are not met, but the most distal portion of the prolapse is >1 cm above the hymen (its value is <−1 cm)
II	The most distal portion of the prolapse is ≤1 cm proximal to or distal to the hymen (its value is ≤+1 but ≥−1 cm)
III	The most distal portion of the prolapse is >1 cm below the plane of the hymen but protrudes no further than 2 cm less than tvl (its value is >+1 but <[tvl −2] cm)
IV	Essentially, complete eversion of the total length of the vagina is demonstrated. The distal portion of the prolapse protrudes to at least [tvl −2] cm (its value is ≥[tvl −2] cm)

For description of measurement points see Fig. 7.3.2 and Bump et al., 1996. *tvl*, Total vaginal length.

inter- and intra-examiner reproducibility in multiple studies, and although other prolapse grading systems are still used by some, POP-Q has become the most commonly used system in the peer-review literature (Hall et al., 1996; Kobak et al., 1996; Muir et al., 2003). Specifically, inter-rater reliability has been assessed among physical therapy and gynaecologic providers, with substantial agreement noted (weighted kappa = 0.63) (Stark et al., 2010). The POP-Q system is an appropriate tool for use among physiotherapists.

The POP-Q examination systematically defines the degree of prolapse during a pelvic examination by measuring anterior, posterior and apical segments of the vaginal wall in centimeters relative to a fixed anatomical structure, the vaginal hymen (not the introitus). Six points (two on the anterior vaginal wall, two in the superior vagina and two on the posterior vaginal wall) are identified (Fig. 7.3.2), and the examiner then measures and records their anatomical position with the patient performing maximal strain. Measurements should be captured as centimeters above or proximal to the hymen (negative number) or centimeters below or distal to the hymen (positive number), with the plane of the hymen being defined as zero. For example, a cervix that protrudes 3 cm distal to the hymen should be described as +3 cm. In addition, three other measurements are made in centimeters: the length of the perineal body (from the posterior forchette to mid-anus), the length of the genital hiatus (from the external urethral meatus to posterior forchette) and the total vaginal length (measured from the hymen to the apex/posterior fornix, non-straining). In addition to these site-specific measurements, the POP-Q system provides a highly reliable and reproducible staging system (Table 7.3.1) to describe the overall extent of pelvic organ descent. Stages are assigned according to the most severe portion of the prolapse when the full extent of protrusion has been demonstrated.

In addition to its widespread adoption and proven reproducibility, another advantage of the POP-Q system is its relative precision (nine site-specific measurements in 1-cm increments), which has allowed an improved understanding of the relationship between the anatomical characteristics of POP and the development of specific pelvic floor symptoms. When evaluating pelvic organ support in a study, investigators should perform a standardized evaluation including POP-Q before and after the intervention. Details of this evaluation should be reported, including the position in which the examination was performed, the fullness of the bladder, the type of vaginal specula, retractors and measuring devices used, and the method used to ensure that the maximal extent of prolapse is seen. It is critical that the examiner asks the patient to confirm that the examination has captured the maximum protrusion noted by the individual during her daily activities. Disadvantages of the system include its relative complexity and the exclusion of some anatomical findings that some investigators believe to be essential for complete patient description, such as vaginal caliber, status of paravaginal support, pelvic floor descent and urethral mobility.

CONCLUSION

POP is a common condition encountered by physical therapists specializing in the care of women with pelvic floor disorders. Key risk factors for POP are advancing age, obesity and increasing parity. The presentation of POP varies, and the type, number and severity of symptoms do not necessarily correlate with physical examination findings. The clinical evaluation of a patient with POP requires a comprehensive review of the full spectrum of pelvic floor symptoms, an assessment of how these symptoms affect their quality of life, and a pelvic examination to evaluate and measure pelvic organ descent. Ancillary testing will largely depend upon the symptoms that the patient presents with but may include cystoscopy, urodynamics, dynamic magnetic resonance imaging and/or pelvic floor ultrasound. Several valid, reliable questionnaires exist to measure the presence and severity of pelvic floor symptoms and their impact on a patient's activities and quality of life, which complement the information gained from the clinical history. Pelvic examination using the POP-Q system to quantitatively assess the degree of anterior, posterior and apical pelvic organ support is essential. The POP-Q system is a valid and reliable system that provides a comprehensive description of pelvic organ support and overall stage of prolapse that is easy to learn and clinically useful as both the baseline assessment and outcome measure after treatment.

REFERENCES

Barber, M. D. (2005). Symptoms and outcome measures of pelvic organ prolapse. *Clinical Obstetrics and Gynecology*, *48*, 648–661.

Barber, M. D., Kuchibhatla, M. N., Pieper, C. F., et al. (2001). Psychometric evaluation of 2 comprehensive condition-specific quality of life instruments for women with pelvic floor disorders. *American Journal of Obstetrics and Gynecology*, *185*, 1388–1395.

Barber, M. D., Walters, M. D., & Bump, R. C. (2005). Short forms of two condition-specific quality-of-life questionnaires for women with pelvic floor disorders (PFDI-20 and PFIQ-7). *American Journal of Obstetrics and Gynecology*, *193*, 103–113.

Barber, M. D., Neubauer, N. L., & Klein-Olarte, V. (2006). Can we screen for pelvic organ prolapse without a physical examination in epidemiologic studies? *American Journal of Obstetrics and Gynecology*, *195*(4), 942–948.

Bradley, C. S., & Nygaard, I. E. (2005). Vaginal wall descensus and pelvic floor symptoms in older women. *Obstetrics & Gynecology*, *106*, 759–766.

Bradley, C. S., Zimmerman, M. B., Qi, Y., et al. (2007). Natural history of pelvic organ prolapse in postmenopausal women. *Obstetrics & Gynecology*, *109*, 848–854.

Bump, R. C., Mattiasson, A., Bø, K., et al. (1996). The standardization of terminology of female pelvic organ prolapse and pelvic floor dysfunction. *American Journal of Obstetrics and Gynecology*, *175*, 10–17.

Burrows, L. J., Meyn, L. A., Walters, M. D., et al. (2004). Pelvic symptoms in women with pelvic organ prolapse. *Obstetrics & Gynecology*, *104*, 982–988.

Coates, K. W., Harris, R. L., Cundiff, G. W., et al. (1997). Uroflowmetry in women with urinary incontinence and pelvic organ prolapse. *British Journal of Urology*, *80*, 217–221.

Cooper, J., Annappa, M., Dracocardos, D., et al. (2015). Prevalence of genital prolapse symptoms in primary care: A cross-sectional survey. *International Urogynecology Journal*, *26*, 505–510.

Delancey, J. O., & Ashton-Miller, J. A. (2004). Pathophysiology of adult urinary incontinence. *Gastroenterology*, *126*, S23–S32.

Digesu, G. A., Khullar, V., Cardozon, L., et al. (2005). P-QOL: A validated questionnaire to assess the symptoms and quality of life of women with urogenital prolapse. *International Urogynecology Journal and Pelvic Floor Dysfunction*, *16*, 176–181 discussion 181.

Ellerkmann, R. M., Cundiff, G. W., Melick, C., et al. (2001). Correlation of symptoms with location and severity of pelvic organ prolapse. *American Journal of Obstetrics and Gynecology*, *185*, 1332–1337 discussion 1337–1338.

Hall, A. F., Theofrastous, J. P., Cundiff, G. W., et al. (1996). Interobserver and intraobserver reliability of the proposed international continence Society, Society of Gynecologic Surgeons, and American Urogynecologic Society pelvic organ prolapse classification system. *American Journal of Obstetrics and Gynecology*, *175*, 1467–1470 discussion 1470–1471.

Handa, V. L., Roem, J., Blomquist, J. L., et al. (2019). Pelvic organ prolapse as a function of levator ani avulsion, hiatus size, and strength. *American Journal of Obstetrics and Gynecology*, 221, 41.e1–41.e7.

Haylen, B. T., Maher, C. F., Barber, M. D., et al. (2016). An International Urogynecological Association (IUGA)/International Continence Society (ICS) joint report on the terminology for female pelvic organ prolapse (POP). *International Urogynecology Journal*, 27, 165–194.

Jelovsek, J. E., Maher, C., & Barber, M. D. (2007). Pelvic organ prolapse. *Lancet*, 369, 1027–1038.

Kieserman-Shmokler, C., Swenson, C. W., Chen, L., et al. (2020). From molecular to macro: The key role of the apical ligaments in uterovaginal support. *American Journal of Obstetrics and Gynecology*, 222, 427–436.

Kobak, W. H., Rosenberger, K., & Walters, M. D. (1996). Interobserver variation in the assessment of pelvic organ prolapse. *International Urogynecology Journal and Pelvic Floor Dysfunction*, 7, 121–124.

Lien, K. C., Mooney, B., Delancey, J. O., et al. (2004). Levator ani muscle stretch induced by simulated vaginal birth. *Obstetrics & Gynecology*, 103, 31–40.

Lukacz, E. S., Lawrence, J. M., Contreras, R., et al. (2006). Parity, mode of delivery, and pelvic floor disorders. *Obstetrics & Gynecology*, 107, 1253–1260.

Mant, J., Painter, R., & Vessey, M. (1997). Epidemiology of genital prolapse: Observations from the Oxford Family Planning Association study. *British Journal of Obstetrics and Gynaecology*, 104, 579–585.

Muir, T. W., Stepp, K. J., & Barber, M. D. (2003). Adoption of the pelvic organ prolapse quantification system in peer-reviewed literature. *American Journal of Obstetrics and Gynecology*, 189, 1632–1635 discussion 1635–1636.

Nygaard, I., Barber, M. D., Burgio, K. L., et al. (2008). Prevalence of symptomatic pelvic floor disorders in US women. *JAMA*, 300, 1311–1316.

Nygaard, I., Bradley, C., Brandt, D., et al. (2004). Pelvic organ prolapse in older women: Prevalence and risk factors. *Obstetrics & Gynecology*, 104, 489–497.

Price, N., Jackson, S. R., Avery, K., et al. (2006). Development and psychometric evaluation of the ICIQ vaginal symptoms questionnaire: The ICIQ-VS. *BJOG*, 113, 700–712.

Rogers, R. G., Coates, K. W., Kammerer-Doak, D., et al. (2003). A short form of the pelvic organ prolapse/urinary incontinence sexual questionnaire (PISQ-12). *International Urogynecology Journal and Pelvic Floor Dysfunction*, 14, 164–168 discussion 168.

Rogers, R. G., Kammerer-Doak, D., Villarreal, A., et al. (2001). A new instrument to measure sexual function in women with urinary incontinence or pelvic organ prolapse. *American Journal of Obstetrics and Gynecology*, 184, 552–558.

Rogers, R. G., Rockwood, T. H., Constantine, M. L., et al. (2013). A new measure of sexual function in women with pelvic floor disorders (PFD): The pelvic organ prolapse/incontinence sexual questionnaire, IUGA-revised (PISQ-IR). *International Urogynecology Journal*, 24, 1091–1103.

Samuelsson, E. C., Victor, F. T., Tibblin, G., et al. (1999). Signs of genital prolapse in a Swedish population of women 20 to 59 years of age and possible related factors. *American Journal of Obstetrics and Gynecology*, 180, 299–305.

Stark, D., Dall, P., Abdel-Fattah, M., et al. (2010). Feasibility, inter- and intra-rater reliability of physiotherapists measuring prolapse using the pelvic organ prolapse quantification system. *International Urogynecology Journal*, 21(6), 651–656.

Summers, A., Winkel, L. A., Hussain, H. K., et al. (2006). The relationship between anterior and apical compartment support. *American Journal of Obstetrics and Gynecology*, 194, 1438–1443.

Swift, S. E. (2000). The distribution of pelvic organ support in a population of female subjects seen for routine gynecologic health care. *American Journal of Obstetrics and Gynecology*, 183, 277–285.

Swift, S. E., Tate, S. B., & Nicholas, J. (2003). Correlation of symptoms with degree of pelvic organ support in a general population of women: What is pelvic organ prolapse? *American Journal of Obstetrics and Gynecology*, 189, 372–377 discussion 377–379.

Swift, S., Woodman, P., O'Boyle, A., et al. (2005). Pelvic organ support study (POSST): The distribution, clinical definition, and epidemiologic condition of pelvic organ support defects. *American Journal of Obstetrics and Gynecology*, 192, 795–806.

Tan, J. S., Lukacz, E. S., Menefee, S. A., et al. (2005). Predictive value of prolapse symptoms: A large database study. *International Urogynecology Journal and Pelvic Floor Dysfunction*, 16, 203–209 discussion 209.

Trowbridge, E. R., Fultz, N. H., Patel, D. A., et al. (2008). Distribution of pelvic organ support measures in a population-based sample of middle-aged, community-dwelling African American and white women in southeastern Michigan. *American Journal of Obstetrics and Gynecology*, 198, 548.e1–548.e6.

Walker, G. J., & Gunasekera, P. (2011). Pelvic organ prolapse and incontinence in developing countries: Review of prevalence and risk factors. *International Urogynecology Journal*, 22, 127–135.

Wei, J. T., Nygaard, I., Richter, H. E., et al. (2012). A midurethral sling to reduce incontinence after vaginal prolapse repair. *New England Journal of Medicine*, 366, 2358–2367.

Wu, J. M., Matthews, C. A., Conover, M. M., et al. (2014). Lifetime risk of stress urinary incontinence or pelvic organ prolapse surgery. *Obstetrics & Gynecology*, 123, 1201–1206.

Pessaries

Patricia Neumann and Rebekah Das

INTRODUCTION

A pessary is an intravaginal device designed to provide support to the vaginal walls in women with pelvic organ prolapse (POP), which is recognized as a huge global health issue (De Albuquerque et al., 2020). Pessaries are a conservative management option recommended as first-line treatment for POP by the International Consultation on Incontinence (Adewuyi et al., 2017). Modern pessaries are made of medical-grade silicon which is flexible and hypoallergenic (De Albuquerque et al., 2016). Different shapes and sizes are available (Fig. 7.3.3). A clinical practice survey in the UK revealed that pessaries were most commonly prescribed for older women who were unsuitable for, or unwilling to undergo, surgery (Bugge et al., 2013). Pessaries were also prescribed by most clinicians for pregnant and postpartum women, but there is little published evidence on the role pessaries may have in the childbearing years and their potential to prevent or delay the progression of POP. Pessaries are not well known to women as a management option (Brown et al., 2016) and not necessarily promoted by the medical profession (Vasconcelos et al., 2020), but they can be a life-changing treatment for women with POP, as it allows re-engagement in activities of daily living, physical activities and sport, with psychological and physical benefits (Storey et al., 2009).

Economic Considerations

Pessaries are widely advocated as an inexpensive way to manage POP. However, there are no data evaluating the economic benefits of pessaries compared with surgery (Adewuyi et al., 2017) and only scant data suggesting that pessary treatment may have fewer direct costs than pelvic floor muscle training (PFMT) (Panman et al., 2016). Research is urgently needed to determine the benefits of pessaries from a health economics perspective.

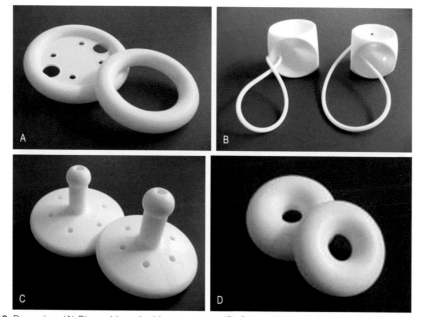

Fig. 7.3.3 Pessaries. (A) Ring with and without support. (B) Cube with and without holes. (C) Gellhorn, short and long stem. (D) Donut.

Physical Therapists' Role in Pessary Management

Pessaries have traditionally been managed by gynaecologists, urogynaecologists or specialist nurses, but in the past decade there has been increasing interest in pessaries by pelvic and women's health physical therapists to complement PFMT and lifestyle advice (Brown et al., 2020).

A clinical practice guideline (CPG) and management pathway produced by the University of South Australia (2012) clearly outlines the roles and responsibilities of a physical therapist providing pessary management in a shared-care model with the patient's medical practitioner, which will be mandated in most countries due to limitations of physical therapy scope of practice. The medical officer will have responsibility for the diagnosis of POP, prescribing of medication, and diagnosis and management of medical complications. The physical therapist will make clinical decisions, as outlined in the management pathway, and interact with the patient's responsible medical officer to remain within the physical therapy scope of practice. This scope will be mandated by local laws and regulations.

Training

There are currently no international training standards for physical therapists to guide the development of competence in pessary management (Brown et al., 2020; Dwyer et al., 2019). In their recent review, Dwyer et al. (2019, p. S23) cautioned that 'the current lack of policy or guidance related to pessary practitioner training is a concern for both health professionals and service users'. However, a UK clinical guideline for best practice in the use of vaginal pessaries, including training standards, was released in March 2021 (UK Pessary Guidelines 2021).

Although pessary management is considered by gynaecologists to be a simple way to treat POP, there are no studies on the efficacy or safety of pessaries managed by physical therapists, despite the documented pessary-related side effects and complications, which may be life threatening in rare cases (Abdulaziz et al., 2015). This potential for complications associated with pessary use has raised concerns about possible harm from the lack of physical therapy training standards. Parallels have been drawn with the situation with surgical mesh, which have evolved since the first edition. Dwyer et al. (2019) recommend that lessons should be learned from mesh and that health professionals, including physical therapists, should protect themselves as practitioners, to protect the availability of pessaries as a treatment option, and, most importantly, to protect patients' (p. S23).

In most countries, physical therapists' undergraduate training does not include competence in pelvic health management. Thus in consideration of the complexity of this area of practice, a case has been made for postgraduate competency-based training for physical therapists managing prolapse and other pelvic health conditions (Frawley et al., 2018). One-day pessary training workshops, where competence was not assessed, have been found to be insufficient for all participants to develop the confidence required to adopt pessary management into their clinical practice (Neumann et al., 2015). This would suggest that more rigorous training is needed to become competent and confident in pessary management.

Using e-Delphi methodology with an international, multidisciplinary panel of experts, a recent study has developed a framework of competency standards to guide standards to guide physiotherapy managment for the Australian health care setting (Neumann 2021). There was consensus that pessary management was advanced physical therapy practice and that physical therapists seeking to use pessaries in their clinical practice should be experienced and have competency-based training in pelvic health before commencing pessary training, in line with previous recommendations (Frawley et al., 2018). The e-Delphi expert panel also agreed on the competencies needed for physical therapists to manage pessaries in a shared-care model. Complex pessary cases, such as women unable to perform self-care, should be reserved for environments with on-site medical support. Recommendations for training in pessary management covered a range of physical therapy roles, in line with advanced practice models in other areas of physical therapy (Fennelly et al., 2020). These competency standards should assist practitioners to self-assess their level of competence and seek further training where they identify gaps. The competence framework should also provide guidance for training institutions to develop curricula in pessary management.

EVIDENCE FOR PESSARY USE IN PELVIC ORGAN PROLAPSE MANAGEMENT

Five randomized controlled trials (RCTs) have compared pessary types (Cundiff et al., 2007), pessaries versus PFMT (Panman et al., 2016) and in combination with PFMT, testing whether combined therapy is more effective than either strategy alone (Bugge et al., 2013; Cheung et al., 2016; Manonai et al., 2012) (Table 7.3.2). The PEDro rating scale was used to classify the methodological quality of the included studies, with a range of scores from 6 to 8, indicating medium to high methodological quality (Table 7.3.3). The PESSRI crossover trial of rings versus Gellhorns, worn 3 months each (average stage 3 POP), found the two types equally effective (Cundiff et al., 2007), with 60% patients successfully fitted with a pessary. Panman et al. (2016) had a similar fitting success rate and found that pessaries had a small advantage over PFMT, both in improving POP symptoms and economically. There is a persuasive rationale for using a pessary together with PFMT to elevate the pelvic organs above the levator plate and then train the muscles. However, a study designed to test whether PFMT would add benefit to wearing a pessary did not progress after difficulties encountered in a feasibility trial (Bugge et al., 2013). Two other studies have assessed whether adding pessaries to PFMT would add benefit, concluding no difference (Cheung et al., 2016; Manonai et al., 2012). More research is needed to determine if combining PFMT and pessaries is more effective and/or economical than either treatment alone.

Comparing pessaries with surgery via RCTs is ethically problematic, so relevant studies have investigated whether outcomes differ when the treatment approach is directed by patient choice. In studies with at least 1-year follow-up, surgery has demonstrated either no benefit over pessaries (Abdool et al., 2011; Lone et al., 2015) or a benefit in some outcomes (Coolen et al., 2018; Sung et al., 2016). However, surgery has higher complication rates and more severe complications (Miceli & Dueñas-Diez, 2019), whereas treatment satisfaction with pessaries is high, with Coolen et al. (2018) reporting that 72% of pessary users opted not to have surgery after their pessary trial. Given that prior reconstructive pelvic surgery predicts pessary fitting failure, it has been suggested that a pessary trial should be offered prior to surgery, as it will not always be possible to offer a pessary after surgery (Nemeth et al., 2017).

Apart from comparison with other treatment methods, effectiveness of pessaries has been explored in single-arm clinical trials assessing symptom changes, quality of life (QoL), treatment satisfaction and continuation rates. A 2016 systematic review of RCTs, observational cross-sectional and cohort studies, found that all seven studies reported improved QoL and treatment satisfaction, with more than 50% of women continuing with pessary use (De Albuquerque et al., 2016). They specifically reported on improved body perception and sexual function with pessary use. Other studies have investigated POP symptom change, with vaginal bulge symptoms improving the most (Clemons et al., 2004; Deng et al., 2017; Dueñas and Miceli, 2018; Fernando et al., 2006; Manchana and Bunyavejchevin, 2012; Mao et al., 2018b; Mao et al., 2019; Nemeth et al., 2013; Radnia et al., 2019). Resolution of urinary symptoms associated with POP tended to be lower (e.g., Clemons et al., 2004; Ding et al., 2015; Nemeth et al., 2013), although overactive bladder symptoms appeared to improve more than other lower urinary tract symptoms (Mao et al., 2018b; Zacharakis et al., 2018) and bowel symptoms changed the least (Brazell et al., 2014; Mao et al., 2019).

Apart from symptom change, there is some evidence that pessaries may also have a therapeutic effect, improving POP stage (Handa and Jones, 2002; Lukban et al., 2006) or reducing genital hiatus (GH) size measured on Valsalva (Jones et al., 2008; Lukban et al. 2006). There have also been published case series/studies reporting complete resolution of POP after pessary use (Matsubara and Ohki, 2010; Nemeth and Ott, 2011).

COMPLICATIONS

A systematic review of complications associated with pessaries identified reports of all Clavien-Dindo grades of severity and found no pessary design that has been complication free, with three reported deaths from complications of poorly managed pessaries (Abdulaziz et al., 2015). Since 2015, numerous studies of pessaries have reported complications. A recent prospective study (Miceli and Dueñas-Diez, 2019) compared complication rates and severity between ring pessary and surgery. A total of 31% of pessary users experienced grade 1 Clavien-Dindo complications (which included pessary expulsions) compared with 39% post-surgery, with severity grades 1 to 3. The highest complication rate was

TABLE 7.3.2   Studies Assessing the Effect of Pessaries in Randomized Controlled Trials

Author	Cundiff et al. (2007)
Design	Randomized crossover trial; ring (n = 125) vs Gellhorn pessary (n = 117)
Study population	N = 134 women with POP-Q stage ≥2 POP (median = POP-Q stage 3); mean age 61 years (range: 30–89) Multicentre: 6 tertiary sites in United States
Protocol	3 months with each pessary; initial pessary randomly assigned
Drop-out	31/125 (24.8%) from ring pessary; 18/117 (15.4%) from Gellhorn pessary
Outcomes	Initial successful fit of ring: 119/125 (95.2%) Initial successful fit of Gellhorn: 107/117 (91.5%) PFDI and PFIQ: Statistically significant improvement in pre-/post-intervention for both pessaries on all subscales except NS for stress subscale for ring Differences NS between pessaries at 3 months in symptom improvement on POPDI and POPIQ subscales
Adverse events	Not reported
Author	**Manonai et al. (2012)**
Design	2-arm RCT: Control: (n = 46) PFM exercise Intervention: (n = 45) Colpexin sphere + PFM exercise 16 weeks
Study population	N = 91 women with POP-Q stage 1 (49.5%) and 2 (50.5%). Mean age 44 + 8.9 years Single centre: Thailand, recruited from urogynaecology department and advertising
Protocol	Both groups: taught PFM exercise by nurse with visual perineal inspection Home PFM exercise: all received booklet; 10 repetitions with 10-s contraction/10-s relaxation 3×/day Intervention: taught to insert/remove Colpexin sphere, worn vaginally all day
Drop-out	6/91 (intervention: 3; control: 3)
Adherence	85/91 (93.4%) completed the study with >80% adherence to daily PFM exercise and use of Colpexin sphere (n = 2 <80% adherence)
Outcomes	Both groups: statistically significant improvement in PFM strength, ICIQ–VS subscale, Colpexin pull test, manual muscle test (Brink digital test), ICIQ (Thai version): differences NS between groups; n = 2 improvement in POP-Q stage from 2 to 1 in both arms
Adverse events	Intervention: heavy vaginal discharge, discomfort (n = 4)
Author	**Panman et al. (2016)**
Design	2-arm RCT: pessary (n = 82); PFMT (n = 80)
Study population	N = 162 women ≥55 years of age with symptomatic POP (POP-Q advanced stage 2 [at or beyond the hymen] or stage 3) Multicentre 20 primary care practices: Netherlands
Protocol	PFMT by physiotherapist, with confirmation of correct action, with BF or ES if unable to contract Individualized programs, based on digital assessment for strength and function ("knack"); lifestyle and toileting advice HEXP: Training 3×/day, 3–5×/week over median 15.9 weeks (IQR: 12–29.5 weeks) Pessary fitted, managed by physician with up to 3 attempts (starting with ring, ring with support, Shaatz or Gellhorn) Successful fit = retained comfortably for 2 weeks Follow-up: 3, 6, 12, 24 months

TABLE 7.3.2	Studies Assessing the Effect of Pessaries in Randomized Controlled Trials—cont'd
Drop-out	At 24 months: PFMT19/80 (23.75%); pessary 47/82 (57.3%)
Adherence	PFMT: not reported
Outcomes	47/82 (57%) successful initial pessary fit; 62/80 (77.5%) completed PFMT PFDI: difference between groups NS, ITT analysis: p = 0.43; PP analysis: p = 0.35 Significant difference in PFDI (subgroup POPDI-6) in favour of pessary group over 24 months (−3.2; 95% CI: −6.3 to −0.0; p = 0.047); difference NS in other secondary measures, including POP-Q stage Direct medical costs per person over 2 years: pessary, $309; PFMT, $437
Adverse events	Pessary group: 21/35 women (60%) had ≥1 side effect PFMT group: nil
Author	**Cheung et al. (2016)**
Design	2-arm RCT: Control: (n = 137) PF exercise Intervention: (n = 139) PF exercise + pessary
Study population	N = 276 women with POP-Q stage 1–3; mean age 62.6 (SD: 9.6) on 12-month wait list for surgery Tertiary centre: Hong Kong
Protocol	Intervention: ring pessary fitted by gynaecologist, up to 3 trials; successful fit = retained comfortably for 2 weeks Both groups: PF exercise in standardized program by nurse continence advisors, 4 individual sessions at 0–2, 4, 8, 16 weeks; HEXP: ≥2 sets of 8–12 preset exercise repetitions per day Follow-up: 6 and 12 months
Drop-out	At 12 months: control 6.6%; intervention 5%
Adherence	Adherence performing PF exercise at least twice a day, 3 days/week Intervention: 39.2% and 53.3% at 6 and 12 months, respectively Control: 49.3% and 43.1% at 6 and 12 months; difference NS at 6 and 12 months
Outcomes	Intervention: 92/139 (66%) successfully fitted with pessary; 87/139 (63%) continued at 6 months and 83/139 (60%) at 12 months Control: 129/137 (94%) continued PF exercise at 6 months and 120/137 (88%) at 12 months PFDI (POPDI subscale): control: within-group difference at 6 and 12 months NS; intervention: significant within-group difference at 6 months (p = 0.02) and 12 months (p = 0.04) PFIQ (POPIQ subscale): in control group, within-group difference at 6 and 12 months NS; in intervention group, significant within-group differences at 12 months (p = 0.02) PFDI and PPIQ at 12 months: significant difference in favour of intervention group (p < 0.01 and p < 0.01, respectively)
Adverse events	Abnormal bleeding, discharge: difference NS in both groups De novo SUI: intervention 48%; control 22.4% (p = 0.01)

BF, Biofeedback; *ES,* electrical stimulation; *HEXP,* home exercise program; *ICIQ,* International Classification on Incontinence Questionnaire; *ICIQ-VS,* International Classification on Incontinence–Vaginal Symptoms; *IQR,* interquartile range; *ITT,* intention to treat; *NS,* not statistically significant; *PF,* pelvic floor; *PFDI,* Pelvic Floor Distress Inventory; *PFIQ,* Pelvic Floor Impact Questionnaire; *PFM,* pelvic floor muscle; *PFMT,* pelvic floor muscle training; *POPDI,* Pelvic Organ Prolapse Distress Inventory; *POPIQ,* Pelvic Organ Prolapse Impact Questionnaire; *POP-Q,* Pelvic Organ Prolapse Quantification; *PP,* per protocol; *RCT,* randomized controlled trial; *SUI,* stress urinary incontinence.

TABLE 7.3.3 **PEDro Quality Score of Randomized Controlled Trials Assessing the Effect of Pessaries and Pessaries With Pelvic Floor Muscle Exercise**

E – Eligibility criteria specified
1 – Subjects randomly allocated to groups
2 – Allocation concealed
3 – Groups similar at baseline
4 – Subjects blinded
5 – Therapist administering treatment blinded
6 – Assessors blinded
7 – Measures of key outcomes obtained from >85% of subjects
8 – Data analysed by intention to treat
9 – Statistical comparison between groups conducted
10 – Point measures and measures of variability provided

Study[a]	E	1	2	3	4	5	6	7	8	9	10	Total Score
Cundiff et al. (2007)	+	+	+	+	–	–	+	–	–	+	+	6
Manonai et al. (2012)	+	+	+	+	–	–	+	+	+	+	+	7
Panman et al. (2016)	+	+	+	?	–	–	+	–	+	+	+	7
Cheung et al. (2016)	+	+	+	+	–	–	+	+	+	+	+	8

[a]Only full text studies included
+, Criterion is clearly satisfied; –, criterion is not satisfied; ?, not clear if the criterion was satisfied.
The total score is determined by counting the number of criteria that are satisfied, except the 'eligibility criteria specified' score is not used to generate the total score. Total scores are out of 10.

just over 50% minor complications (Deng et al., 2017). Reports of changing vaginal flora with pessary use vary, from no change (Coelho et al., 2017), inflammatory change rather than flora change (Collins et al., 2015) or finding that the presence of vaginal lactobacillus prior to pessary use protects against flora disturbance (Yoshimura et al., 2016). Although complications have often been associated with neglected pessaries, there have also been reports of vaginal evisceration during pessary fitting (Yoshimura et al., 2016) and fistula development 8 months after pessary removal (Penrose et al., 2014). More research is required on complication prevention. Although teaching patient self-management has been attributed to decreasing complication rates in clinical practice (Te West and Moore, 2014), others

have suggested that leaving pessaries in place, for as long as 2 years without removal, may reduce tissue trauma (Dueñas and Miceli, 2018; Miceli et al., 2020).

PRACTICE POINTS: CHOOSING PESSARY TYPES, SIZES AND FITTING EXPECTATIONS

With little evidence-based guidance, pessary choice requires clinicians' judgement on the type, size and number of trials that could be justified before deciding that a pessary is not an appropriate option. CPGs (Guidelines, 2012; UK clinical guidelines, 2021) recommend starting with a ring as the easiest type to use and trialling other types, if unsuccessful. Most research published since 2012 has followed this pattern (De Albuquerque et al., 2020), and ring pessaries have been shown to have high success rates, even in advanced POP (Cheung et al., 2018; Dueñas and Miceli, 2018; Mao et al., 2018b; Miceli and Dueñas-Diez, 2019; Miceli et al., 2020; Radnia et al. 2019). However, Nemeth et al. (2013) reported successful use of cubes as the first and only option in 97% of women, whereas Ding et al. (2016) demonstrated that women with shorter total vaginal length (TVL) (including previous hysterectomy) and wider vaginal introitus predicted success with a Gellhorn rather than a ring. Some studies have also described double pessary use (Myers et al., 1998; Singh and Reid, 2001). Many studies have had patients self-managing their pessaries (De Albuquerque et al., 2020), and although rings are considered the easiest to self-manage, cubes and Gellhorns have also been successfully self-managed (Deng et al., 2017; Nemeth et al., 2013).

Fitting success rates vary between 58% and 97% (Mao et al., 2018a). Data on repeated fittings are scarce but relatively consistent with approximately 30% to 40% of patients requiring up to three trials of different pessary sizes or types (Komesu et al., 2007; Maito et al., 2006; Mao et al., 2019; Wolff et al., 2017). A good fit has been described as a pessary that allows a finger between the pessary and vaginal wall, reduces POP above the hymen, involves no discomfort or dysuria, and is retained on Valsalva, coughing and walking (Yang et al., 2018). A pessary in situ does not significantly affect assessment of pelvic floor muscle strength in women with stage 2 to 4 POP (Bø et al., 2012).

According to a recent systematic review, pessary fitting failure (defined as the inability to achieve a comfortable fit with up to three trials in 3 weeks) is predicted by higher body mass index, advanced prolapse and previous reconstructive pelvic surgery (De Alburquerque et al., 2020). Advanced prolapse was the most important factor, with a fourfold risk of pessary expulsion (but note the preceding success achieved in recent trials). Previous hysterectomy, age, GH and TVL measurements were not found to be predictors of fitting failure, which is in contrast to recent, large prospective and retrospective studies, which found that vaginal dimensions (shorter TVL, larger GH, smaller GH/TVL ratio and larger vaginal introitus) predict failure (Lone and Palmer, 2019; Ma et al., 2020). Based on patients who could not be fitted either with a ring or a Gellhorn, it has been recommended that a TVL shorter than 7.3 cm will not allow pessary use (Deng et al., 2017). Levator ani muscle avulsion has also been associated with fitting failure of a ring pessary (Cheung et al., 2017). For rings specifically, posterior compartment POP predicts failure (Ma et al., 2020). Interestingly, two studies have also identified that significant posterior compartment prolapse predicts pessary discontinuation (Maito et al., 2006; Yang et al., 2018). Discontinuation, as compared with initial fitting failure, is additionally predicted by a patient's desire for surgery, pessary expulsion or vaginal discomfort (De Albuquerque et al., 2020). The initial month of pessary trials seems to be most important. Patients who continue with pessary use at this point are highly likely to continue in the longer term (Lone et al., 2011; Miceli et al., 2020).

CONCLUSION

Pessaries are an effective conservative management option for POP and may complement other forms of management offered by physical therapists (PFMT, lifestyle management). As such, pessary management could fit within the physical therapy scope of practice. There is no research to date describing the efficacy and safety of physical therapy–led pessary management, but adequate training is recommended to protect patients and the profession, as serious complications can result from poorly managed pessaries. Research is also needed to determine the possible economic benefit for both healthcare systems and consumers from physical therapists managing pessaries and to evaluate the consumers' perspectives.

CLINICAL RECOMMENDATIONS

- Competence in pelvic and women's health physical therapy is advised prior to managing pessaries.
- Training in pessary management is needed to achieve competence and provide safe practice.
- Physical therapists should understand pessary management within the wider context of conservative management of prolapse.
- Physical therapists should follow CPGs and work in a shared-care medical model.
- The ring pessary is generally the first choice unless complete avulsion is present, then a space-occupying pessary may be more successful. Several pessary trials may be needed, but not all women can be fitted successfully.
- Recording of patient attendance and regular monitoring is needed to mitigate risk and avoid complications.

REFERENCES

Abdool, Z., Thakar, R., Sultan, A. H., et al. (2011). Prospective evaluation of outcome of vaginal pessaries versus surgery in women with symptomatic pelvic organ prolapse. *International Urogynecology Journal, 22*(3), 273–278.

Abdulaziz, M., Stothers, L., Lazare, D., et al. (2015). An integrative review and severity classification of complications related to pessary use in the treatment of female pelvic organ prolapse. *Cancer Urology Associate Journal., 9*(5–6), E400–E406.

Adewuyi, T., Booth, J., Bradley, C., et al. (2017). Adult conservative management. In *Incontinence* (pp. 1443–1628). Bristol, UK: International Continence Society.

Bø, K., Majida, M., & Engh, M. E. (2012). Does a ring pessary in situ influence the pelvic floor muscle function of women with pelvic organ prolapse when tested in supine? *International Urogynecology Journal, 23,* 573–577.

Brazell, H. D., Patel, M., O'Sullivan, D. M., et al. (2014). The impact of pessary use on bowel symptoms: One-year outcomes. *Female Pelvic Medicine & Reconstructive Surgery, 20*(2), 95–98.

Brown, C. A., Pradhan, A., & Pandeva, I. (2020). Current trends in pessary management of vaginal prolapse: A multidisciplinary survey of UK practice. *International Urogynecology Journal, 32*(4), 1015–1022.

Brown, L. K., Fenner, D. E., DeLancey, J. O., et al. (2016). Defining patient knowledge and perceptions of vaginal pessaries for prolapse and incontinence. *Female Pelvic Medicine & Reconstructive Surgery, 22*(2), 93–97.

Bugge, C., Hagen, S., & Thakar, R. (2013). Vaginal pessaries for pelvic organ prolapse and urinary incontinence: A multiprofessional survey of practice. *International Urogynecology Journal*, 24(6), 1017–1024.

Bugge, C., Williams, B., Hagen, S., et al. (2013). A process for decision-making after pilot and feasibility trials (ADePT): Development following a feasibility study of a complex intervention for pelvic organ prolapse. *Trials, 14* 353–353.

Cheung, R. Y., Lee, J. H., Lee, L. L., et al. (2016). Vaginal pessary in women with symptomatic pelvic organ prolapse: A randomized controlled trial. *Obstetrics & Gynecology*, 128(1), 73–80.

Cheung, R. Y. K., Lee, J. H. S., Lee, L. L., et al. (2017). Levator ani muscle avulsion is a risk factor for expulsion within 1 year of vaginal pessary placed for pelvic organ prolapse. *Ultrasound in Obstetrics and Gynecology*, 50(6), 776–780.

Cheung, R. Y. K., Lee, L. L. L., Chung, T. K. H., et al. (2018). Predictors for dislodgment of vaginal pessary within one year in women with pelvic organ prolapse. *Maturitas*, 108, 3–57.

Clemons, L., Aguilar, V. C., Tillinghast, T. A., et al. (2004). Patient satisfaction and changes in prolapse and urinary symptoms in women who were fitted successfully with a pessary for pelvic organ prolapse. *American Journal of Obstetrics and Gynecology*, 190(4), 1025–1029.

Coelho, S., Paulo, G., Florentino, J., et al. (2017). Can the pessary use modify the vaginal microbiological flora? A cross-sectional study. *Revista Brasileira de Ginecologia e Obstetrícia*, 39(4), 169–174.

Collins, S., Beigi, R., Mellen, C., et al. (2015). The effect of pessaries on the vaginal microenvironment. *American Journal of Obstetrics and Gynecology*, 212(1), 60.e1–60.e6.

Coolen, A. W. M., Troost, S., Mol, B. W. J., et al. (2018). Primary treatment of pelvic organ prolapse: Pessary use versus prolapse surgery. *International.Urogynecology Journal*, 29(1), 99–107.

Cundiff, G. W., Amundsen, C. L., Bent, A. E., et al. (2007). The PESSRI study: Symptom relief outcomes of a randomized crossover trial of the ring and Gellhorn pessaries. *American Journal of Obstetrics and Gynecology*, 196(4), 405.e1–405.e8.

De Albuquerque Coelho, S. C., Brito, L. G. O., de Araujo, C. C., et al. (2020). Factors associated with unsuccessful pessary fitting in women with symptomatic pelvic organ prolapse: Systematic review and metanalysis. *Neurourology and Urodynamics*, 39(7), 912–921.

De Albuquerque Coelho, S. C., de Castro, E. B., & Juliato, R. (2016). Female pelvic organ prolapse using pessaries: Systematic review. *International Urogynecology Journal*, 27(12), 1797–1803.

Deng, M., Ding, J., Ai, F., et al. (2017). Successful use of the Gellhorn pessary as a second-line pessary in women with advanced pelvic organ prolapse. *Menopause, 24*(11), 1277–1281.

Ding, J., Chen, C., Song, X. C., et al. (2015). Successful use of ring pessary with support for advanced pelvic organ prolapse. *International Urogynecology Journal*, 26(10), 1517–1523.

Ding, J., Song, X. C., Deng, M., et al. (2016). Which factors should be considered in choosing pessary type and size for pelvic organ prolapse patients in a fitting trial? *International Urogynecology Journal*, 27(12), 1867–1871.

Dueñas, J., & Miceli, A. (2018). Effectiveness of a continuous-use ring-shaped vaginal pessary without support for advanced pelvic organ prolapse in postmenopausal women. *International Urogynecology Journal*, 29(11), 1629–1636.

Dwyer, L., Kearney, R., & Lavender, T. (2019). A review of pessary for prolapse practitioner training. *British Journal of Nursing*, 28(9), S18–S24.

Fennelly, O., Desmeules, F., O'Sullivan, C., et al. (2020). Advanced musculoskeletal physiotherapy practice: Informing education curricula. *Musculoskelet Science Practice*, 48, 1–10.

Fernando, R. J., Thakar, R., & Sultan, A. H. (2006). Effect of vaginal pessaries on symptoms associated with pelvic organ prolapse. *Obstetrics & Gynecology*, 108(1), 93–99.

Frawley, H. C., Neumann, P., & Delany, C. (2018). An argument for competency-based training in pelvic floor physiotherapy practice. *Physiotherapy Theory and Practice*, 35(12), 1117–1130.

Guideline for the use of support pessaries in the management of pelvic organ prolapse. (2012). https://unisa.edu.au/site-assets/episerver-6 files/global/health/sansom/documents/icahe/the-pessary-guideline_18-7-2012.pdf. accessed 11.01.21.

Handa, V. L., & Jones, M. (2002). Do pessaries prevent the progression of pelvic organ prolapse? *International Urogynecology Journal and Pelvic Floor Dysfunction*, 13(6), 349–352.

Jones, K., Yang, L., Lowder, J. L., et al. (2008). Effect of pessary use on genital hiatus measurements in women with pelvic organ prolapse. *Obstetrics & Gynecology*, 112(3), 630–636.

Komesu, Y. M., Rogers, R. G., Rode, M. A., et al. (2007). Pelvic floor symptom changes in pessary users. *American Journal of Obstetrics and Gynecology*, 197(6), 620.e1–620.e20.

Lone, F., Thakar, R., & Sultan, A. H. (2015). One-year prospective comparison of vaginal pessaries and surgery for pelvic organ prolapse using the validated ICIQ-VS and ICIQ-UI (SF) questionnaires. *International Urogynecology Journal*, 26(9), 1305–1312.

Lone, F., Thakar, R., Sultan, A. H., et al. (2011). A 5-year prospective study of vaginal pessary use for pelvic organ prolapse. *International Journal of Gynaecology & Obstetrics*, *114*(1), 56–59.

Lone, W., & Palmer, J. (2019). Predictors of successful fitting of vaginal pessary for female pelvic organ prolapse. *Journal Gynecology Research Obstetric*, *5*(1), 17–21.

Lukban, J. C., Aguirre, O. A., Davila, G. W., et al. (2006). Safety and effectiveness of Colpexin Sphere in the treatment of pelvic organ prolapse. *International Urogynecology Journal and Pelvic Floor Dysfunction*, *17*(5), 449–454.

Ma, C., Xu, T., Kang, J., et al. (2020). Factors associated with pessary fitting in women with symptomatic pelvic organ prolapse: A large prospective cohort study. *Neurourology and Urodynamics*, *39*(8), 2238–2245.

Maito, J. M., Quam, Z. A., Craig, E., et al. (2006). Predictors of successful pessary fitting and continued use in a nurse-midwifery pessary clinic. *J Midwifery Womens Health*, *51*(2), 78–84.

Manchana, T., & Bunyavejchevin, S. (2012). Impact on quality of life after ring pessary use for pelvic organ prolapse. *International Urogynecology Journal*, *23*, 873–877.

Manonai, J., Harnsomboon, T., Sarit-Apirak, S., et al. (2012). Effect of Colpexin Sphere on pelvic floor muscle strength and quality of life in women with pelvic organ prolapse stage I/II: A randomized controlled trial. *International Urogynecology Journal*, *23*, 307–312.

Mao, M., Ai, F., Kang, J., et al. (2019). Successful long-term use of Gellhorn pessary and the effect on symptoms and quality of life in women with symptomatic pelvic organ prolapse. *Menopause*, *26*(2), 145–151.

Mao, M., Ai, F., Zhang, Y., et al. (2018a). Predictors for unsuccessful pessary fitting in women with symptomatic pelvic organ prolapse: A prospective study. *BJOG*, *125*(11), 1434–1440.

Mao, M., Ai, F., Zhang, Y., et al. (2018b). Changes in the symptoms and quality of life of women with symptomatic pelvic organ prolapse fitted with a ring with support pessary. *Maturitas*, *117*, 51–56.

Matsubara, S., & Ohki, Y. (2010). Can a ring pessary have a lasting effect to reverse uterine prolapse even after its removal? *Journal of Obstetrics and Gynaecology Research*, *6*(2), 459–461.

Miceli, A., & Dueñas-Diez, J.-L. (2019). Effectiveness of ring pessaries versus vaginal hysterectomy for advanced pelvic organ prolapse. A cohort study. *International Urogynecology Journal*, *30*(12), 2161–2169.

Miceli, A., Fernández-Sánchez, M., Polo-Padillo, J., et al. (2020). Is it safe and effective to maintain the vaginal pessary without removing it for 2 consecutive years? *International Urogynecology Journal*, *31*, 2521–2528.

Myers, D. L., LaSala, C. A., & Murphy, J. A. (1998). Double pessary use in grade 4 uterine and vaginal prolapse. *Obstetrics & Gynecology*, *91*(6), 1019–1020.

Nemeth, Z., Farkas, N., & Farkas, B. (2017). Is hysterectomy or prior reconstructive surgery associated with unsuccessful initial trial of pessary fitting in women with symptomatic pelvic organ prolapse? *International Urogynecology Journal*, *28*(5), 757–761.

Nemeth, Z., Nagy, S., & Ott, J. (2013). The cube pessary: An underestimated treatment option for pelvic organ prolapse? Subjective 1-year outcomes. *International Urogynecology Journal*, *24*(10), 1695–1701.

Nemeth, Z., & Ott, J. (2011). Complete recovery of severe postpartum genital prolapse after conservative treatment—a case report. *International Urogynecology Journal*, *22*(11), 1467–1469.

Neumann, P. B., Scammell, A. E., Burnett, A. M., et al. (2015). Training of Australian health care providers in pessary management for women with pelvic organ prolapse: Outcomes of a novel program. *ANZCJ*, *21*(1), 6–12.

Neumann, P., Radi, N., Gerdis, T., Tonkin, C., Wright, C., Chalmers, K. & Nurkic, I. (2021). Development of a multinational, multidisciplinary competency framework for physiotherapy training in pessary management: an E-Delphi study. *International Urogynecology Journal*, *33*(2), 253–265.

Panman, C. M., Wiegersma, M., Kollen, B. J., et al. (2016). Effectiveness and cost-effectiveness of pessary treatment compared with pelvic floor muscle training in older women with pelvic organ prolapse: 2-year follow-up of a randomized controlled trial in primary care. *Menopause*, *23*(12), 1307–1318.

Penrose, K. J., Ma Yin, J., & Tsokos, N. (2014). Delayed vesicovaginal fistula after ring pessary usage. *International Urogynecology Journal*, *25*(2), 291–293.

Radnia, N., Hajhashemi, M., Eftekhar, T., et al. (2019). Patient satisfaction and symptoms improvement in women using a vaginal pessary for the treatment of pelvic organ prolapse. *Journal Medicine Life*, *12*(3), 271–275.

Rubin, R., Jones, K. A., & Harmanli, O. H. (2010). Vaginal evisceration during pessary fitting and treatment with immediate colpocleisis. *Obstetrics & Gynecology*, *116*(Suppl. 2), 496–498.

Singh, K., & Reid, W. M. N. (2001). Non-surgical treatment of uterovaginal prolapse using double vaginal rings. *BJOG*, *108*, 112–113.

Storey, S., Aston, M., Price, S., et al. (2009). Women's experiences with vaginal pessary use. *Journal of Advanced Nursing*, *65*(11), 2350–2357.

Sung, V. W., Wohlrab, K. J., Madsen, A., et al. (2016). Patient-reported goal attainment and comprehensive functioning outcomes after surgery compared with pessary for pelvic organ prolapse. *American Journal of Obstetrics and Gynecology*, *215*(5), 659.e1–659.e9.

Te West, N. I. D., & Moore, K. H. (2014). Recent developments in the non-surgical management of pelvic organ prolapse. *Current Obstetric Gynecology Report.*, 3(3), 172–179.

UK Clinical Guidelines for Best Practice in the use of Vaginal Pessaries for Pelvic Organ prolapse. (2021). https://www.ukcs.uk.net/UK-Pessary-Guideline-2021. accessed 30.3.21.

Vasconcelos, C. T. M., Silva Gomes, M. L., Ribeiro, G. L., et al. (2020). Women and healthcare providers' knowledge, attitudes and practice related to pessaries for pelvic organ prolapse: A systematic review. *European Journal of Obstetrics & Gynecology and Reproductive Biology*, 247, 132–142.

Wolff, B., Williams, K., Winkler, A., et al. (2017). Pessary types and discontinuation rates in patients with advanced pelvic organ prolapse. *International Urogynecology Journal*, 28(7), 993–997.

Yang, J., Han, J., Zhu, F., et al. (2018). Ring and Gellhorn pessaries used in patients with pelvic organ prolapse: A retrospective study of 8 years. *Archives of Gynecology and Obstetrics*, 298(3), 623–629.

Yoshimura, K., Morotomi, N., & Fukuda, K. (2016). Effects of pelvic organ prolapse ring pessary therapy on intravaginal microbial flora. *International Urogynecology Journal*, 27(2), 219–227.

Zacharakis, D., Grigoriadis, T., Pitsouni, E., et al. (2018). Assessment of overactive bladder symptoms among women with successful pessary placement. *International Urogynecology Journal*, 29(4), 571–577.

Pelvic Floor Muscle Training in Prevention and Treatment of Pelvic Organ Prolapse

Kari Bø and Helena Frawley

INTRODUCTION

The prevalence of symptomatic pelvic organ prolapse (POP) is reported to be 3% to 28% (Lawrence et al., 2008; Milsom et al., 2017; Nygaard et al., 2008a, 2008b; Slieker-Ten Hove et al., 2009; Tegerstedt et al., 2005). Mechanical symptoms such as vaginal bulging and perception of pelvic heaviness are the most prevalent and specific symptoms of POP (Mouritsen, 2005; Srikrishna et al., 2010), and these symptoms may greatly impair quality of life and result in restriction of participation in, for example, physical activity (Srikrishna et al., 2008).

It is estimated that approximately 50% of all women lose some of the supportive mechanisms of the pelvic floor due to childbirth, leading to different degrees of POP (Thakar and Stanton, 2002). In the UK, POP accounts for 20% of women on waiting lists for major gynaecological surgery (Thakar and Stanton, 2002). The prevalence of surgery for POP is considerable: up to 19% of women in Australia (Smith et al., 2010) and 20% in the Netherlands (De Boer et al., 2011). Prolapse recurs in up to 70% of women after surgery (Iglesia et al., 2010), and about one-third of operated women undergo at least one further surgical procedure for prolapse (Olsen et al., 1997). Potential risk factors for POP have been listed as constipation, pelvic surgery, genetic factors, familial transmission, Caucasian ethnicity, pregnancy and vaginal delivery (especially instrumental vaginal delivery), generalized connective tissue disorders (Ehlers–Danlos disease and Marfan's syndrome), chronic anaemia, chronic obstructive pulmonary disorders, low educational level/low income and hard work/exercise (Milsom et al., 2017). In a one-to-one age- and parity-matched case–control study, Brækken et al. (2009) compared 49 women with Pelvic Organ Prolapse Quantification (POP-Q) stage 2 or above with 49 controls with stage 0 and 1 and found no difference in postmenopausal status, current smoking, current low-intensity exercise, type of birth, birth weight, presence of striae, diastasis recti abdominis and joint hypermobility. However, body mass index, socioeconomic status, heavy occupational work, anal sphincter lacerations, pelvic floor muscle (PFM) strength and endurance were independently related to POP. The combination of weak PFMs and low vaginal resting pressure gave the highest odds ratio for POP (Brækken et al., 2009). The high prevalence and its increase with age highlight the need for preventative measures that could reduce both the incidence and the impact of POP.

Prolapse may be asymptomatic until the descending organ reaches the introitus, and therefore POP may not be recognized until an advanced stage is present (Handa et al., 2004; Milsom et al., 2017). In some women the prolapse advances rapidly, whereas others remain stable for many years. Traditional belief has been that POP does not regress. However, Handa et al. (2004) found that spontaneous regression is common, especially for minor prolapse. In addition, in a 5-year follow-up of 160 women with symptomatic POP and 120 women without symptomatic POP, Miedel et al. (2011) found that 47% had an unchanged POP-Q stage, 40% showed regression and only 13% showed progression. A total of 30% had no change in 'feeling of a vaginal bulge', and 2% of control women developed symptomatic POP. The authors concluded that only a small proportion of women with symptomatic POP worsen within 5 years.

Treatment of POP can be conservative (lifestyle interventions and/or pelvic floor muscle training [PFMT]), mechanical (use of a pessary) or surgical (Hagen and Stark, 2011). A survey of UK women's health physical therapists (PTs) showed that many women attending physical therapy sessions presented with a mixture of pelvic floor dysfunctions such as stress urinary incontinence (SUI) and prolapse, and that 92% of the PTs assessed and treated women with POP (Hagen et al., 2004). The most commonly used treatment was PFMT with and without biofeedback. In a systematic review, Dumoulin et al. (2017) found level 1A evidence/recommendation for PFMT to treat POP. Based on this, the International Consensus on Incontinence recommends that PFMT should be first-line treatment for POP together with lifestyle interventions (Dumoulin et al., 2017). The National Institute for Health and Care Excellence (2019) supports this recommendation.

RATIONALE FOR PELVIC FLOOR MUSCLE TRAINING

There are two main hypotheses of mechanisms of how PFMT may be effective in prevention and treatment of SUI (Bø, 2004), and the same theories may apply for the effect of PFMT to prevent and treat POP. The two hypotheses are as follows: hypothesis 1, in which women learn to consciously contract before and during increases in abdominal pressure (also termed *bracing* or *performing the Knack*), and continue to perform such voluntary contractions as a behaviour modification to prevent descent of the pelvic floor, and hypothesis 2, in which women are taught to perform regular strength training to build up 'stiffness' and structural support of the pelvic floor over time (Bø, 2004). These two hypotheses coexist,

as they both build on an anatomical and biomechanical understanding of the function of the PFMs—that is, a voluntary contraction of the PFMs constricts the levator hiatus and elevates the pelvic floor into a higher position. This results in an immediate effect during the PFM contraction—the Knack (Miller et al., 2001)—or may have an effect over time where long-term strength training changes the morphology and underlying causes of POP.

Conscious Contraction (Bracing or 'Performing the Knack') to Prevent and Treat Pelvic Organ Prolapse

Research on basic and functional anatomy supports conscious contraction of the PFMs as an effective manoeuvre to stabilize the pelvic floor (Miller et al., 2001; Peschers et al., 2001). However, to date, there are no studies on how much strength or what neuromotor control strategies are necessary to prevent descent during cough and other rises in intra-abdominal pressure, nor how to prevent gradual descent due to activities of daily living or over time. In a randomized controlled trial (RCT) comparing PFMT plus lifestyle advice plus the Knack to lifestyle advice plus the Knack, Brækken et al. (2010a) found no effect of lifestyle advice plus the Knack on vaginal resting pressure, PFM strength and endurance, whereas the PFMT group significantly increased PFM strength by 13 cmH$_2$O, an effect size of 1.2, and the effect size in change of muscle endurance in favour of the PFMT group was 0.9. There was no assessment of adherence to the Knack protocol, so it is unknown whether the women actually performed this manoeuvre during the 6-month training period. An interesting but difficult research question to test is whether women at risk for POP can prevent development of prolapse by performing the Knack during increases in intra-abdominal pressure. Since it is possible to learn to cough into the elbow, it is perhaps possible to learn to voluntarily precontract the PFMs before and during simple and single tasks such as coughing and lifting, and isolated exercises such as performing abdominal exercises. However, it is unlikely that multiple-task activities and repetitive movements such as running, playing tennis, aerobics and dance activities can be conducted simultaneously with intentional co-contractions of the PFMs. There is no knowledge whether this voluntary precontraction can become an automatic contraction (Box 7.3.3).

BOX 7.3.3 How to Tell if You Are Contracting the Pelvic Floor Muscles Correctly

- Sit on the arm of a chair or the edge of a table. Lift the pelvic floor up from the surface you are sitting on by pulling up and contracting around the urethra, vagina and rectum. Squeeze so hard that you feel a slight trembling in your vagina. When you squeeze hard enough, you can feel the lower part of the stomach being pulled in slightly at the same time. Release the contraction without pressing downward. Try to feel the difference between relaxing and tightening the pelvic floor.
- Try to stop the flow when you are urinating. If these muscles are weak, it may be difficult to stop the flow when it is strongest. You can then test yourself towards the end of urination, which is much easier. This is only a test to see whether you are using the muscles correctly. Do not use 'stop the flow' as part of training, as this can interfere with the ability to empty your bladder completely.
- If you are not sure about whether you are contracting correctly, contact your doctor and ask for a referral to a physical therapist with special training in women's health.

Training Programme

Lift upwards and inwards around your urethra, vagina and rectum. Squeeze as hard as you can during each contraction and try to hold it for 6 to 8 seconds before you gently relax. Relax and breathe with a slow, regular and gentle rhythm out and in both during and between the muscle contractions. Do 8 to 12 repetitions in three sets. If this seems too difficult, start with fewer repetitions. Choose one or more of these starting positions:

1. Sit with your legs apart and your back straight. Lift upwards and inwards around the openings in the pelvic floor.
2. Stand with your legs apart, and check that the buttock muscles are relaxed while you squeeze the pelvic floor muscles.
3. Kneel on all fours with your knees out to the side and feet together. Lift the pelvic floor upwards and inwards.

Strength Training

The theoretical rationale for intensive strength training (exercise) of the PFMs to treat POP is that strength training may build up the structural support of the pelvic floor by elevating the levator plate to a permanently higher location inside the pelvis, narrowing the levator hiatus and enhancing hypertrophy and stiffness of the PFMs and connective tissue. This would prevent or decrease descent during increases in intra-abdominal pressure (Bø, 2004). Brækken et al. (2010a) showed that the PFMT group had a statistically significant increased thickness of the PFMs, elevation of the bladder neck and rectal ampulla, and decrease of the levator hiatus area and length of the PFMs compared to the control group.

The aim of this section is to provide an updated systematic review of RCTs of PFMT to prevent and treat POP.

EVIDENCE FOR PELVIC FLOOR MUSCLE TRAINING

Research Methods

The basis for this review included searches on Cochrane, PubMed and PEDro databases and the abstract books from International Continence Society and International Urogynecology Association annual meetings from 2000 to March 2020 for RCTs of PFMT to prevent or treat POP. Methodological quality of the studies is classified according to the PEDro scoring system (Maher et al., 2003).

Results

Prevention

No RCTs or studies using other designs have been found to evaluate the effect of PFMT on POP in primary prevention—that is, to stop prolapse from developing (Dumoulin et al., 2017). Hagen et al. (2017) recruited 407 women (mean age 46.6 years [SD: 4.6], median parity 2 [1–11]) with POP-Q stage 1 to 3 who had not previously sought treatment for POP, in a 2-year follow-up study. POP symptoms were assessed by the Pelvic Organ Prolapse Symptom Score (POP-SS: 0–28). The women were randomized to either a lifestyle advice leaflet or five appointments with a PT over 16 weeks + two 6-week blocks of once weekly Pilates classes including specific PFMT. They reported a statistically significant, but small, reduction in POP symptoms in the exercise group compared with the control group. The mean POP-SS score at 2 years was 3.2 (SD: 3.4) in the intervention group versus 4.2 (SD: 4.4) in the control group (adjusted mean difference −1.01, 95% CI: −1.70 to −0.33; p = 0.004).

Treatment

Table 7.3.4 shows the 12 RCTs assessing PFMT to treat anatomical POP or POP symptoms. Three studies compared PFMT with no treatment (Alves et al., 2015;

TABLE 7.3.4 **Randomized Controlled Trials on Pelvic Floor Muscle Training to Treat Pelvic Organ Prolapse**

Author	**Piya-Anant et al. (2003)**
Design	RCT
Study population	654 women >60 years in Thailand; anterior vaginal wall POP
Intervention	PFMT: 2 years of 30 contractions/day + eat more fruit and vegetables and drink 2 L of water/day Control: no intervention, same follow-up
Drop-out/Adherence	Drop-out: not reported Adherence: not reported No report of changes in water and vegetable intake
Outcome measures	No, mild or severe prolapse assessed by Valsalva on vaginal examination
Results	PFMT: 27% worsening; control: 72% worsening; p = 0.005; effect only seen in severe prolapse
Author	**Ghroubi et al. (2008)**
Design	RCT
Study population	47 women from Tunisia, mean age 53.4 years (SD: 11), stage 1 and 2 anterior vaginal wall POP
Intervention	12 weeks PFMT: 2×/week for 5 weeks with individual PFMT + advice on healthy living by PT; home training 20 contractions/day for 7 weeks Control: no treatment
Drop-out/Adherence	Drop-out: 0 Adherence: not reported
Outcome measures	Clinical examination; MUH; urodynamic tests; Ditrovie QoL scale; patient satisfaction (VAS)
Results	PFMT: heaviness, 18.5%; control: heaviness, 70%; significantly better report on urinary handicap in PFMT Pelvic heaviness: 18.5% in PFMT and 70% in control after treatment, p < 0.001 Uroflowmetry showed significant improvement in maximum flow rate
Author	**Hagen et al. (2009)**
Design	Assessor-blinded RCT
Study population	47 women, mean age 56 years (SD: 9) with symptomatic stage 1 and 2 POP in UK, all kinds of POP
Intervention	1: PFMT for 16 weeks, 5 visits with PT; home exercise: 6 sets of max 10 contractions/day, use of diary + lifestyle advice sheet 2: Lifestyle advice sheet only
Drop-out/Adherence	Drop-out not reported; POP-Q data missing for 27/47 91% attended ≥3 physical therapy sessions, 65% attended 5 visits; 61% rated as good/moderate compliers
Outcome measures	POP-Q; prolapse symptoms; QoL/interference of daily living; self-report of change in POP; Oxford grading for PFM strength only in exercise group
Results	PFMT significantly more likely to have improved POP stage (45% vs 0%, p = 0.04), significantly greater decrease in POP symptoms (3.5 vs 0.1, p = 0.021), significantly more likely to say their POP was better (63% vs 24%) No difference in urinary, bowel or vaginal symptoms Oxford grading (n = 15): significant improvement in exercise group: mean 0.5 (95% CI: 02–0.8)
Author	**Brækken et al. (2010a, 2010b)**
Design	Assessor-blinded RCT

Continued

TABLE 7.3.4   Randomized Controlled Trials on Pelvic Floor Muscle Training to Treat Pelvic Organ Prolapse—cont'd

Study population	109 women, mean age 48.8 years (SD: 11.8), mean body mass index 25.6 (SD: 4.5), mean parity 2.4 (0.7) with POP-Q stage 1–3; all compartments of POP
Intervention	6 months PFMT: information on not to strain on toilet + 'the Knack'; 3 sets of 8–12 contractions/day, diary; weekly visits with PT for 3 months, every second week for 3 months Control: information on not to strain on toilet; 'the Knack'
Drop-out/Adherence	1 drop-out in each group; 79% adhered to ≥80% of exercise sessions
Outcome measures	POP-Q; ultrasound of bladder and rectal position at rest; symptoms and bother (Mouritsen and Larsen, 2003); ICIQ-UI SF; muscle strength
Results	POP-Q stage: 11 (19%) in the PFMT vs 4 (8%) controls improved 1 stage (p = 0.04) Elevation of the bladder neck: 12.3 mm vs ↓0.6 mm; diff. 3 mm (95% CI: 1.5–4.4), p < 0.001 Elevation of rectal ampulla: 14.4 mm vs ↓1.1 mm, diff. 5.5 mm (95% CI: 1.4–7.3), p = 0.02 Symptoms: Vaginal bulging/heaviness: ↓ frequency 32/43 vs 8/26, p < 0.01; ↓ bother 29/43 vs 11/26, p < 0.01 ICIQ-UI SF: effect size 0.66 in favour of PFMT, diff. 2.63 (95% CI: 0.95–4.30), p < 0.01 Bowel symptoms: no effect on emptying or solid FI Flatus: frequency diff. 31.2% (95% CI: 0.7–55) p < 0.01, bother diff. 25.3% (95% CI: 1.5–49.1) p < 0.01; loose FI: frequency diff. 68.6% (95% CI: 40.2–97) p < 0.01, bother diff. 64.3% (95% CI: 39.2–89.4) p < 0.01 Strength (p < 0.01): PFMT: ↑13.1 cmH$_2$O (95% CI: 10.6–15.5); control: 11.1 cmH$_2$O (95% CI: 0.4–2.7); effect size: 1.21 Endurance (p < 0.01): PFMT: ↑107 cmH$_2$O/s (95% CI: 77–136.4); control: ↑8 cmH$_2$O/s (95% CI: −7.4 to 24.1); effect size: 0.96
Author	**Hagen et al. (2014)**
Design	Assessor-blinded multicentre RCT
Study population	447 women, mean age 56.8 years (SD: 11.5); symptomatic POP-Q stage 1–3; 72% had stage 2
Intervention	PFMT (n = 224): 5 appointments with PT over 16 weeks + home exercise (see Hagen et al. [2009]) and lifestyle advice Control (n = 222): lifestyle advice
Drop-out/Adherence	Drop-out at 6 months: PFMT, 16%; control, 14% Adherence: 80% attended 4 or 5 physical therapy sessions
Outcome measures	Primary: POP symptom severity (POP-SS) Secondary: POP-Q, perceived change of POP, uptake of further treatment, cost-effectiveness
Results	Bulging at 6 months: PFMT, 13.8% reduction in n; control, 3.4% reduction in n Bulging at 12 months: PFMT, 20.5% reduction in n; control, 17% reduction in n POP stage: PFMT, 20% improved; control, 12% improved; p = 0.052 Uptake of further treatment: PFMT, 30%; control, 55%; p < 0.001 Net cost for effective treatment: £127 per woman
Authors	**Stupp et al. (2011), Bernardes et al. (2012), Rensende et al. (2012)**
Design	Assessor-blinded RCT
Study population	37 women, mean age 55 years (SD: 8) with stage 2 POP; 56.7% had anterior vaginal wall POP, 10.8% posterior and 32.4% a combination

TABLE 7.3.4 Randomized Controlled Trials on Pelvic Floor Muscle Training to Treat Pelvic Organ Prolapse—cont'd

Intervention	Group 1 (n = 21): PFMT 7 visits with PT; 14-week training period; use of quick pull of a vaginal cone and stretch reflex followed by active PFM contraction; use of Knack during different tasks; home exercise: 3 sets of 8–12 maximum voluntary contractions held for 6–10 s; PTs called patients every fortnight; global stretching and lifestyle: weight loss, fluid intake, constipation, avoidance of heavy lifting
	Group 2 (n = 16): control group taught how to perform PFM contractions with no protocol; same lifestyle and global stretching as PFMT group
Drop-out/Adherence	Drop out: 0%
	Adherence: 100% in intervention and 76.2% in control; 91% adherence to home training programme
Outcome measures	Primary: POP-Q
	Secondary: PFM function (Oxford grading, PERFECT, sEMG, P-QoL, QoL including symptoms)
Results	POP-Q stage: significantly greater improvement in training group (anterior vaginal wall: p < 0.001, posterior vaginal wall: p = 0.025)
	PFM function: significant difference in favour of PFMT
	QoL: significant difference in favour of PFMT
	Symptoms: significant difference in favour of PFMT
Author	**Frawley et al. (2012)**
Design	Assessor-blinded multicentre RCT
Study population	168 women, mean age 55.9 years (SD: 9.9) with symptomatic POP-Q stage 1–3; 80% had stage 2 POP, 73% had anterior POP
Intervention	PFMT: 5 appointments with PT over 16 weeks, home exercise (see Hagen et al. [2009]) + lifestyle advice
	Control: lifestyle advice
Drop-out/Adherence	Drop-out at 6 months: PFMT, 14.3%; control, 10.7%
	Drop-out at 12 months: PFMT, 5.6%; control, 21.3%
	Adherence: 82.1% attended 4 or 5 physical therapy sessions
Outcome measures	Primary: prolapse symptom severity (POP-SS), manometric strength and endurance
	Secondary: POP-Q stage
Results	Significant difference in symptoms in favour of PFMT at 6 and 12 months
	Manometry: borderline significant better endurance in PFMT group at 6 months; no difference in other manometry variables
	No difference between groups in POP-Q stage
	Significant difference in points Ap and Bp at 6 months and Ap and Bp relative to hymen in favour of PFMT
Author	**Kashyap et al. (2013)**
Design	RCT, not blinded
Study population	140 women, mean age 47 years (SD: 12) with POP-Q stage 1–3; 63.5% had POP-Q stage 1
Intervention	6 months; all had vaginal palpation
	Group A: 1-to-1 PFMT instruction + SIM; 6 follow-up visits at weeks 1, 3, 6, 12, 24; home exercise: 1 set of 10 contractions held for 10 s 3×/day; diary
	Group B: SIM + home training programme; 3 follow-up visits at weeks 6, 18, 24
Drop-out/Adherence	Loss to follow-up week 6: group A, 27.1%; group B, 12.9%
	Week 18: group A, 22.9%; group B, 31.4% Week 24: group A, 7.1%; group B, 21.4% Adherence not reported

Continued

TABLE 7.3.4   Randomized Controlled Trials on Pelvic Floor Muscle Training to Treat Pelvic Organ Prolapse—cont'd

Outcome measures	POP-Q stage POP symptom scale, VAS, QoL (PFIQ-7)
Results	Significant improvement in POP-Q stage 1 and 2 and bulging at weeks 6, 18 and 24 in favour of PFMT; significant difference between groups in favour of PFMT in VAS at weeks 18 and 24 Complete relief of symptoms in 24.5% in the PFMT group compared to 0 in the SIM group
Author	**Wiegersma et al. (2014)**
Design	RCT, not blinded
Study population	287 women, mean age 62.2 years (SD: 6.6) with POP-Q stage 1 and 2
Intervention	3 months of 'watchful waiting' or PFMT PFMT: individualized, not standardized following vaginal palpation, weekly visit to start with + home exercise
Drop-out/Adherence	Drop out: 26 in PFMT, 10 in watchful waiting Adherence: not reported
Outcome measures	PFDI-20, PFIQ-7, PISQ-12, vaginal palpation
Results	Significant improvement in PFDI-20 in PFMT vs control; 57% in PFMT vs 13% in control reported overall improvement in symptoms; No difference in POP-Q or PFM function
Author	**Alves et al. (2015)**
Design	Assessor-blinded RCT
Study population	46 postmenopausal women, mean age 65.9 years
Intervention	12 group sessions, 30 min, twice a week compared to control
Drop-out/Adherence	Drop out: 34.8% Adherence: not reported
Outcome measures	Digital palpation, sEMG, POP-Q, ICIQ
Results	sEMG ($p = 0.003$), digital palpation ($p = 0.001$), decrease in urinary incontinence symptoms ($p < 0.001$ for ICIQ-OAB scores, $p = 0.036$ for ICIQ-UI SF, anterior POP ($p = 0.03$) in favor of PFMT
Author	**Due et al. (2016a, 2016b)**
Design	Assessor-blinded RCT
Study population	109 women with symptomatic POP-Q ≥ stage 2
Intervention	3 months of PFMT, 1 individual session with PT to learn PFM contraction, 6 group visits with PT, Knack + lifestyle + home exercise 3 sets of 10 contractions/day compared to lifestyle information 6 group sessions
Drop-out/Adherence	Drop out: 18% at 3 months, 22% at 6 months Adherence: not reported
Outcome measures	Global improvement scale, POP symptoms, POP-Q
Results	Significantly better results in global improvement scale and POP symptoms in PFMT; no difference in POP-Q stage
Author	**Resende et al. (2019)**
Design	Assessor-blinded RCT
Study population	70 women, mean age 55.7 years (SD: 5.2) with symptomatic POP-Q stage 2
Intervention	All participants had 3 sessions with PT to learn how to do PFMT/hypopressive, then 3 months of either PFMT or hypopressive exercise at home with biweekly appointments with PT; exercise diary
Drop-out/Adherence	Drop-out: 4 in hypopressive, 5 in PFMT Adherence: 89% in hypopressive, 84% in PFMT

TABLE 7.3.4 Randomized Controlled Trials on Pelvic Floor Muscle Training to Treat Pelvic Organ Prolapse—cont'd

Outcome measures	Primary: P-QoL, POP-Q Secondary: Modified Oxford grading, sEMG
Results	All measures significantly better in PFMT Symptoms: effect size, 1.01 (95% CI: 1.002–1.021); 19 (67%) of anterior prolapse lifted 1 stage, 4 (45%) of posterior prolapse lifted 1 stage after PFMT; significant difference in favor of PFMT vs hypopressive in anatomic POP

FI, Faecal incontinence; *ICIQ,* International Consultation on Incontinence Questionnaire; *ICIQ-OAB,* International Consultation on Incontinence Questionnaire-Overactive Bladder; *ICIQ-UI SF,* International Consultation on Incontinence Questionnaire-Urinary Incontinence, Short Form; *MUH,* Measurement of Urinary Handicap scale; *n,* number; *PERFECT,* P represents power (or pressure, a measure of strength using a manometric perineometer), E = endurance, R = repetitions, F = fast contractions, and finally ECT = every contraction timed; *PFDI-20,* Pelvic Floor Distress Inventory-Short Form; *PFIQ-7,* Pelvic Floor Impact Questionnaire-Short Form; *PFM,* pelvic floor muscle; *PFMT,* pelvic floor muscle training; *PISQ-12,* Prolapse and Incontinence Sexual Function Questionnaire-Short Form; *POP,* pelvic organ prolapse; *POP-Q,* Pelvic Organ Prolapse Quantification; *POP-SS,* Pelvic Organ Prolapse Symptom Score; *P-QoL,* Prolapse Quality of Life Questionnaire; *PT,* physical therapist; *QoL,* quality of life; *RCT,* randomized controlled trial; *sEMG,* surface electromyography; *SIM,* self-instruction manual; *VAS,* visual analogue scale.

Ghroubi et al., 2008; Wiegersma et al., 2014), whereas Piya-Anant et al. (2003) compared a combination of PFMT and advice to drink water and eat vegetables to reduce constipation and straining at stool and compared this with no treatment. Three studies (two reporting data from the same study) compared PFMT with hypopressive exercise (Resende et al., 2012; Resende et al., 2019; Stupp et al., 2011). Typically, most RCTs compared PFMT plus lifestyle intervention against lifestyle interventions alone. Lifestyle intervention included use of precontraction of the PFMs before and during increase in intra-abdominal pressure (the Knack) and advice to avoid pushing down during defaecation (Brækken et al., 2010a, 2010b) or general lifestyle advice (Due et al., 2016a and 2016b; Frawley et al., 2012; Hagen et al., 2009; Hagen and Stark 2011). None has compared the effect of these lifestyle interventions with untreated controls, and there is no report of adherence to these protocols. Hence, the effect of lifestyle interventions alone on POP is still unknown. Brækken et al. (2010a) did not find any effect of advice to use the Knack on muscle morphology.

The RCTs are all in favour of PFMT to be effective in treating POP, demonstrating statistically significant improvement in POP symptoms (Alves et al., 2015; Brækken et al., 2010b; Due et al., 2016a and 2016b; Frawley et al., 2012; Ghroubi et al., 2008; Hagen et al., 2009; Hagen and Stark, 2011; Kashyap et al., 2013; Resende et al., 2012; Resende et al., 2019; Stupp et al., 2011; Wiegersma et al., 2014) and/or POP stage (anatomical POP) (Alves et al., 2015; Brækken et al., 2010b;

Hagen et al., 2009; Kashyap et al., 2013; Piya-Anant et al., 2003; Resende et al., 2019; Stupp et al., 2011). Frawley et al. (2012) did not find a significant change in stage of POP, but significant improvements were found in some of the individual POP-Q measurements. Wiegersma et al. (2014) and Due et al. (2016a and 2016b) did not find statistically significant difference between the PFMT group and control in stage of POP. The studies with no effect on POP stage had a lower training dosage compared with studies finding statistically significant improvement in anatomical POP. The methodological score on PEDro ranged from 4 to 8, with five of the studies scoring 7 to 8 (Table 7.3.5).

Pelvic Floor Muscle Training to Treat Pelvic Organ Prolapse in the Peripartum Period

As pregnancy and childbirth may cause damage to the pelvic floor, early intervention to prevent and treat POP should optimally start in the peripartum period. We have only been able to find one RCT evaluating the effect of PFMT in this period. In an assessor-blinded RCT including 175 primiparous women, no effect was found on symptoms of bulging, bladder neck position or POP stage after 4 months of group PFMT starting at 6 weeks postpartum (Bø et al., 2015). The study included women with and without POP, and the women presenting with POP had POP-Q stage 1 and 2. The primary outcome of this RCT was urinary incontinence, and since the study included women with and without POP, the sample size may have been too small to detect differences in POP

TABLE 7.3.5 PEDro Quality Score of Randomized Controlled Trials in Systematic Review of Pelvic Floor Muscle Training to Treat Pelvic Organ Prolapse

E – Eligibility criteria specified
1 – Subjects randomly allocated to groups
2 – Allocation concealed
3 – Groups similar at baseline
4 – Subjects blinded
5 – Therapist administering treatment blinded
6 – Assessors blinded
7 – Measures of key outcomes obtained from >85% of subjects
8 – Data analysed by intention to treat
9 – Statistical comparison between groups conducted
10 – Point measures and measures of variability provided

Study	E	1	2	3	4	5	6	7	8	9	10	Total Score
Piya-Anant et al. (2003)	+	+	?	+	–	–	+	–	–	+	–	4
Ghroubi et al. (2008)	+	+	–	+	–	–	–	+	+	+	+	6
Hagen et al. (2009)	+	+	+	+	–	–	+	–	–	+	+	6
Brækken et al. (2010a, 2010b)	+	+	+	+	–	–	+	+	+	+	+	8
Stupp et al. (2011)	+	+	?	+	–	–	+	+	+	+	+	7
Hagen et al. (2014)	+	+	+	+	–	–	+	+	+	+	+	8
Frawley et al. (2012)	+	+	+	+	–	–	+	–	+	+	+	7
Kashyap et al. (2013)	+	+	+	+	–	–	–	–	+	+	+	6
Wiegersma et al. (2014)	+	+	–	+	–	–	–	–	+	+	+	5
Alves et al. (2015)	+	+	+	+	–	–	+	–	–	+	+	6
Due et al. (2016a and 2016b)	+	+	+	+	–	–	+	–	+	+	+	7
Resende et al. (2019)	–	+	–	+	–	–	+	+	–	+	+	6

+, Criterion is clearly satisfied; –, criterion is not satisfied; ?, not clear if the criterion was satisfied.
The total score is determined by counting the number of criteria that are satisfied, except the 'eligibility criteria specified' score is not used to generate the total score. Total scores are out of 10.

symptoms. Further RCTs are warranted to test early prevention and treatment of POP in the peripartum period.

Quality of the Intervention for Randomized Controlled Trials Across All Populations: Dose–Response Issues

There was some variation in the content of the interventions. The study from Ghroubi et al. (2008) was published in the French language and only provided the abstract in English. All studies instructed in strength training of the PFMs except Wiegersma et al. (2014), where the exercise was up to the PT with no standardization of the training protocol. All research groups included digital palpation to determine correctness of PFM contractions. The training period varied between 12 weeks and 2 years, and the number of visits with the PT varied between 4 and 18 times. PFMT was taught individually in all but one trial (Due et al., 2016a and 2016b) and was combined with a home training programme. Drop-outs were low and adherence high in most studies. The highest number of visits with the PT was in the study of Brækken et al. (2010a, 2010b), which included 18 visits over 6 months. This study had high adherence and only two drop-outs, and showed the best overall results in change in POP stage and symptom reduction. An RCT from India compared 6 visits over 6 months' training using a self-instruction manual only with the instruction manual plus one-to-one

PFMT for the patients as well, and showed the same overall beneficial results in symptoms and POP-Q stage (Kashyap et al., 2013) as Brækken et al. (2010). Because of the use of different outcome measures in POP symptoms, it is difficult to compare results based on dose–response outcomes. No studies compared different training dosages.

Long-Term Effect

There are few studies on the long-term effect of PFMT for POP. Due et al. (2016b) performed a 12-month follow-up study. Thirty-four of the women had not sought further treatment, which included 13 (30%) of the 43 women in the control group (lifestyle) and 21 (52%) of the 40 women in the lifestyle plus PFMT group (p = 0.05). Based on all other outcomes, the authors concluded that at 12-month follow-up, the effects of adding PFMT to a structured lifestyle advice program were limited. Panman et al. (2016) did a 2-year follow up of a trial comparing 'watchful waiting' and PFMT. They found that PFMT resulted in greater pelvic floor symptom improvement and more often led to women's perceived improvement of symptoms and lower absorbent pads costs, and was more effective in women experiencing higher pelvic floor symptom distress. McClurg et al. (2019) did an 8- to 10-year follow-up of 11 of 23 centers, including 293 out of 447 original women participating in the original RCT (Hagen et al., 2014). They linked the participants to hospital data relating to activity between the date of randomization to the original study and the end of the follow-up period. A lower proportion of the intervention group (43.6%) received follow-up treatment than the control group (52.8%). The median time to first treatment was 3008 days (interquartile range: 589–3396) and 2242 days (interquartile range: 628.5–3279) in the intervention and control groups, respectively. However, there was no significant difference between groups in use of pessary, neurostimulation or undergoing any type of POP-related surgery during the follow-up period.

Hypopressive Technique

The 'hypopressive technique' is a technique developed by Caufriez (1997) and involves a combination of a breathing technique and contraction of the abdominal muscles. Resende et al. (2012) assessed 36 nulliparous patients with vaginal surface electromyography (sEMG) during PFM contraction, hypopressive technique and a combination of the two. They found that PFM

contraction was more effective than the hypopressive technique to increase sEMG activation of the PFMs and that there were no additional effects from adding the hypopressive technique. In this study, the hypopressive technique was significantly more effective than PFM contraction in activation of the transverse abdominal muscle (Resende et al. (2012). In an RCT, Stupp et al. (2011) found that both PFMT and PFMT plus the hypopressive technique were significantly more effective than lifestyle advice in increasing PFM strength (Oxford grading) and PFM activation (sEMG), but there was no additional effect of adding the hypopressive technique to PFMT. Ultrasound assessment of the cross-sectional area (CSA) of the levator ani muscle showed increased CSA in the PFMT and the PFMT plus the hypopressive technique groups compared to the lifestyle group, but there was no additional effect of the hypopressive technique on CSA (Bernardes et al., 2012). Resende et al. (2019) found that PFMT was superior to the hypopressive technique in treatment of POP, assessed both by symptoms and stage of POP.

Should Pelvic Floor Muscle Training Be an Adjunct to Prolapse Surgery?

As POP surgery is prevalent and results not always satisfactory, it is reasonable to investigate the effect of adding PFMT to surgery in order to test if PFMT benefits surgical outcomes. Refer to Fig. 7.3.4 to understand pelvic floor muscles' location.

Jarvis et al. (2005) studied the effect of PFMT and bladder/bowel training in an RCT on 60 women undergoing surgery for POP/urinary incontinence. The number of women undergoing POP-only surgery was not specified. The intervention consisted of PFMT, functional bracing of PFMs prior to rises in abdominal pressure, bladder/bowel training, and advice to reduce straining during voiding and defecation. There was a significant benefit in favour of the intervention group in bladder-related quality of life, urinary symptom-specific scores and PFM function. In a feasibility RCT, McClurg et al. (2014) found benefits in the intervention group (n = 28) over the control group (n = 29) in terms of fewer POP symptoms at 12 months (mean difference 3.94; 95% CI: 1.35–6.75; t=3.24; p=0.006) but concluded that the results must be viewed with caution due to possible selection bias.

In contrast, several studies have not found any additional effect of adding PFMT before and after surgery. In

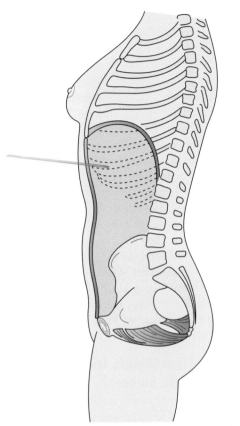

Fig. 7.3.4 The pelvic floor muscles are located inside the pelvis and form a structural support for internal organs.

an assessor-blinded RCT comparing the effect of POP surgery with and without a structured physical therapy programme, no significant effect of PFMT on de novo onset or relapse of comorbidities such as SUI was identified at 1-year follow-up; further, there were no objective measures of POP stage reported pre- or postoperatively (Frawley et al. 2010). The physical therapy intervention included a PFM strength training protocol, supplemented by bladder and bowel advice. This was provided over eight sessions: one preoperative and seven postoperative sessions; day 3 postoperatively, weeks 6, 7, 8, 10 and 12, and a final appointment at 9 months postoperatively. Neither Pauls et al. (2014), Barber et al. (2014), Duarte et al. (2020) nor Nyhus et al. (2020) found any additional effect of adding PFMT to prolapse surgery. Given the demonstrated effect of PFMT to treat POP, these results are somewhat counterintuitive. However, for women in whom POP surgery is effective, it may be difficult to show further improvement by PFMT, at

least in the short term. In a 5-year follow-up study of uterosacral ligament suspension or sacrospinous ligament fixation with perioperative behavioral therapy and PFMT compared with usual care for women undergoing vaginal prolapse surgery, Jelovsek et al. (2018) found that failure rates for vaginal prolapse surgery are high despite maintenance of improved prolapse symptoms, with an estimated probability of surgical failure of 61.5% with uterosacral ligament suspension versus 70.3% with sacrospinous ligament fixation. Anatomical failure was 48% with perioperative behavioral therapy and PFMT and 49.5% with usual care (the difference was not significant). However, adherence to PFMT was not reported in the 5-year follow-up period. If long-term effects are expected from adding PFMT to surgery, this must be evaluated in future RCTs with diligent follow-up and ensuring high adherence to the training protocol for many years. Such studies may be quite difficult to perform.

CONCLUSION

There is level 1, grade A evidence that PFMT is effective in treatment of POP. PFMT can typically reduce the prolapse by one stage, improves symptoms and has beneficial effects on pelvic floor comorbidities. There are no severe complications/side effects reported after PFMT. There are no studies in primary prevention or lifestyle intervention; there is a need for further RCTs to investigate the effect of such interventions. Morphological changes have been found after PFMT, which may indicate a possible preventive effect. There are few long-term studies on the effectiveness of PFMT for POP, and where these exist, the results should be interpreted with caution as only a subset of the original study population have participated in the follow-up study. Long-term studies are difficult to perform, as women are frequently offered other treatments, such as surgery, after cessation of the PFMT intervention or PFMT if they have been in the control group (Herbert et al., 2018). It is reasonable to assume that PFMT must be continued to maintain short-term results.

CLINICAL RECOMMENDATIONS

- Watchful waiting is recommended for POP stage 1 to 3 if symptom bother is absent or low, as POP stage and symptoms can both regress.

- There are convincing results from 12 RCTs that PFMT is effective in reducing symptoms and stage of POP in women who have not had previous POP surgery; therefore, PFMT should be first-line treatment for women presenting with symptoms of POP.
- PFMT for POP patients requires proper teaching, assessment and feedback of correct contraction (vaginal palpation).
- PFMT must be supervised in addition to a home training programme.
- There are not yet convincing results that PFMT yields additional benefit in conjunction with POP surgery.

REFERENCES

Alves, F. K., Riccetto, C., Adami, D. B., et al. (2015). A pelvic floor muscle training program in postmenopausal women: A randomized controlled trial. *Maturitas, 81*(2), 300–305.

Barber, M. D., Brubakery, L., Burgio, K. L., et al. (2014). Comparison of 2 transvaginal surgical approaches and perioperative behavioral therapy for apical vaginal prolapse: The OPTIMAL randomized trial. *JAMA, 311*(10), 1023–1034.

Bernardes, B. T., Resende, A. P. M., Stupp, L., et al. (2012). Efficacy of pelvic floor muscle training and hypopressive exercises for treating pelvic organ prolapse in women: Randomized controlled trial. *Sao Paulo Medical Journal, 130*(1), 5–9.

Bø, K. (2004). Pelvic floor muscle training is effective in treatment of female stress urinary incontinence, but how does it work? *International Urogynecology Journal and Pelvic Floor Dysfunction, 15*(2), 76–84.

Bø, K., Hilde, G., Stær-Jensen, J., et al. (2015). Postpartum pelvic floor muscle training and pelvic organ prolapse—a randomized trial of primiparous women. *American Journal of Obstetrics and Gynecology, 212*(1), 38.e1–38.e7.

Braekken, I. H., Majida, M., Engh, M. E., et al. (2009). Pelvic floor function is independently associated with pelvic organ prolapse. *BJOG, 116*(13), 1706–1714.

Bräkken, I. H., Majida, M., Engh, M. E., et al. (2010). Morphological changes after pelvic floor muscle training measured by 3D ultrasound. *Obstetrics & Gynecology, 115*(2 Pt. 1), 317–324.

Bräkken, I. H., Majida, M., Engh, M. E., et al. (2010). Can pelvic floor muscle training reverse pelvic organ prolapse and reduce prolapse symptoms? *American Journal of Obstetrics and Gynecology, 203*(2), 170e.1–170.e7.

Caufriez, M. (1997). In *Gymnastique abdominale hypopressive* (pp. 8–10). Brussels: MC Editions.

De Boer, T. A., Slieker-Ten Hove, M. C. P., Burger, C. W., et al. (2011). The prevalence and factors associated with previous surgery for pelvic organ prolapse and/or urinary incontinence in a cross-sectional study in The Netherlands. *European Journal of Obstetrics & Gynecology and Reproductive Biology, 158*(2), 343–349.

Duarte, T. B., Bø, K., Brito, L. G. O., et al. (2020). Perioperative pelvic floor muscle training did not improve outcomes in women undergoing pelvic organ prolapse surgery: A randomised trial. *Journal of Physiotherapy, 66*(1), 27–32.

Due, U., Brostrøm, S., & Lose, G. (2016). Lifestyle advice with or without pelvic floor muscle training for pelvic organ prolapse: A randomized controlled trial. *International Urogynecology Journal, 27*, 555–563.

Due, U., Brostrøm, S., & Lose, G. (2016). The 12-month effects of structured lifestyle advice and pelvic floor muscle training for pelvic organ prolapse. *Acta Obstetricia et Gynecologica Scandinavica, 95*(7), 811–819.

Dumoulin, C., Adewuyi, T., Booth, J., et al. (2017). Adult conservative management. In P. H. Abrams, L. Cardoza, A. E. Khoury, et al. (Eds.), *Incontinence: Sixth international consultation on urinary incontinence* (pp. 1443–1628). Plymouth, UK: Health Publication/Plymbridge Distributors.

Frawley, H., Hagen, S., Sherburn, M., et al. (2012). Changes in prolapse following pelvic floor muscle training: A randomised controlled trial. *Neurourology and Urodynamics, 31*(6), 938–939.

Frawley, H. C., Phillips, B. A., Bø, K., et al. (2010). Physiotherapy as an adjunct to prolapse surgery: An assessor-blinded randomized controlled trial. *Neurourology and Urodynamics, 29*, 719–725.

Ghroubi, S., Kharrat, O., Chaari, M., et al. (2008). Effect of conservative treatment in the management of low-degree urogenital prolapse. *Annales de Readaptation et de Medecine Physique, 51*, 96–102.

Hagen, S., Glazener, C., McClurg, D., et al. (2017). Pelvic floor muscle training for secondary prevention of pelvic organ prolapse (PREVPROL): A multicentre randomised controlled trial. *Lancet, 389*(10067), 393–402.

Hagen, S., & Stark, D. (2011). Conservative prevention and management of pelvic organ prolapse in women. *Cochrane Database of Systematic Reviews* Issue 12, Art. No. CD003882.

Hagen, S., Stark, D., & Cattermole, D. (2004). A United Kingdom-wide survey of physiotherapy practice in the treatment of pelvic organ prolapse. *Physiotherapy, 90*, 19–26.

Hagen, S., Stark, D., Glazener, C., et al. (2009). A randomized controlled trial of pelvic floor muscle training for stages I and II pelvic organ prolapse. *International Urogynecology Journal and Pelvic Floor Dysfunction, 20*, 45–51.

Hagen, S., Stark, D., Glazener, C., et al. (2014). Individualised pelvic floor muscle training in women with pelvic organ prolapse (POPPY): A multicentre randomised controlled trial. *Lancet, 383*(9919), 796–806.

Handa, V. L., Garrett, E., Hendrix, S., et al. (2004). Progression and remission of pelvic organ prolapse: A longitudinal study of menopausal women. *American Journal of Obstetrics and Gynecology, 190*, 27–32.

Herbert, R. D., Kasza, J., & Bø, K. (2018). Analysis of randomised trials with long-term follow-up. *BMC Medical Research Methodology, 18*(1), 48.

Iglesia, C. B., Sokol, A. I., Sokol, E. R., et al. (2010). Vaginal mesh for prolapse: A randomized controlled trial. *Obstetrics & Gynecology, 116*(2 Pt. 1), 293–303.

Jarvis, S. K., Hallam, T. K., Lujic, S., et al. (2005). Perioperative physiotherapy improves outcomes for women undergoing incontinence and or prolapse surgery: Results of a randomised controlled trial. *The Australian and New Zealand Journal of Obstetrics and Gynaecology, 45*(4), 300–303.

Jelovsek, J. E., Barber, M. D., & Brubaker, L. (2018). Effect of uterosacral ligament suspension vs sacrospinous ligament fixation with or without perioperative behavioral therapy for pelvic organ vaginal prolapse on surgical outcomes and prolapse symptoms at 5 years in the OPTIMAL randomized clinical trial. *JAMA, 319*(15), 1554–1565.

Kashyap, R., Jain, V., & Singh, A. (2013). Comparative effect of 2 packages of pelvic floor muscle training on the clinical course of stage I–III pelvic organ prolapse. *International Journal of Gynecology & Obstetrics, 121*(1), 69–73.

Lawrence, J. M., Lukacz, E. S., Nager, C. W., et al. (2008). Prevalence and co-occurrence of pelvic floor disorders in community-dwelling women. *Obstetrics & Gynecology, 111*, 678–685.

Maher, C. G., Sherrington, C., Herbert, R. D., et al. (2003). Reliability of the PEDro scale for rating quality of randomized controlled trials. *Physical Therapy, 8*, 713–721.

McClurg, D., Hagen, S., Berry, K., et al. (2019). A 10 year data-linkage follow-up study of a trial of pelvic floor muscle training for prolapse. *Neurourology and Urodynamics, 38*, S368–S369.

McClurg, D., Hilton, P., Dolan, L., et al. (2014). Pelvic floor muscle training as an adjunct to prolapse surgery: A randomised feasibility study. *International Urogynecology Journal, 25*(7), 883–891.

Miedel, A., Ek, M., Tegerstedt, G., et al. (2011). Short-term natural history in women with symptoms indicative of pelvic organ prolapse. *International Urogynecology Journal and Pelvic Floor Dysfunction, 22*, 461–468.

Miller, J. M., Perucchini, D., Carchidi, L. T., et al. (2001). Pelvic floor muscle contraction during a cough and decreased vesical neck mobility. *Obstetrics & Gynecology, 97*(2), 255–260.

Milsom, I., Altman, D., Lapitan, M. C., et al. (2009). Committee 1: Epidemiology of urinary (UI) and faecal (FI) incontinence and pelvic organ prolapse (POP). In P. Abrams, L. Cardozo, S. Khoury, et al. (Eds.), *Incontinence: Fourth international consultation on incontinence* (pp. 35–111). Paris: Health Publication/Editions 21.

Milsom, I., et al., (2017). Committee 1. Epidemiology of Urinary Incontinence (UI) and other Lower Urinary Tract Symptoms (LUTS), Pelvic Organ Prolapse (POP) and Anal (AI) Incontinence, In: INCONTINENCE, 6th Ed, Tokyo, Japan: International Consultation on Incontinence (ICI), 1–141.

Mouritsen, L. (2005). Classification and evaluation of prolapse. *Best Practice & Research Clinical Obstetrics & Gynaecology, 19*(6), 895–911.

Mouritsen, L., & Larsen, J. P. (2003). Symptoms, bother and POPQ in women referred with pelvic organ prolapse. *International Urogynecology Journal and Pelvic Floor Dysfunction, 14*, 122–127.

National Institute for Health and Care Excellence. (2019). *Urinary incontinence and pelvic organ prolapse in women: Management [online]*. Available: https://www.nice.org.uk/guidance/ng123 (accessed 07.10.20).

Nygaard, I., Barber, M. D., Burgio, K. L., et al. (2008). Prevalence of symptomatic pelvic floor disorders in US women. *JAMA, 300*, 1311–1316.

Nyhus, M., Mathew, S., Salvesen, Ø., et al. (2020). Effect of preoperative pelvic floor muscle training on pelvic floor contraction and symptomatic and anatomical pelvic organ prolapse after surgery: A randomized controlled trial. *Ultrasound in Obstetrics and Gynecology, 56*(1), 28–36.

Olsen, A. L., Smith, V. J., Bergstrom, J. O., et al. (1997). Epidemiology of surgically managed pelvic organ prolapse and urinary incontinence. *Obstetrics & Gynecology, 89*, 501–506.

Panman, C., Wiegersma, M., Kollen, B. J., et al. (2016). Two-year effects and cost-effectiveness of pelvic floor muscle training in mild pelvic organ prolapse: A randomised controlled trial in primary care. *BJOG, 124*(3), 511–520.

Pauls, R. N., Crisp, C. C., Novicki, K., et al. (2014). Pelvic floor physical therapy: Impact on quality of life 6 months after vaginal reconstructive surgery. *Female Pelvic Medicine & Reconstructive Surgery, 20*(6), 334–341.

Peschers, U. M., Fanger, G., Schaer, G. N., et al. (2001). Bladder neck mobility in continent nulliparous women. *BJOG, 108*(3), 320–324.

Piya-Anant, M., Therasakvichya, S., Leelaphatanadit, C., et al. (2003). Integrated health research program for the Thai elderly: Prevalence of genital prolapse and effectiveness of pelvic floor exercise to prevent worsening of genital prolapse in elderly women. *Medical Journal of the Medical Association of Thailand, 86*, 509–515.

Resende, A. P. M., Bernardes, B. T., Stüpp, L., et al. (2019). Pelvic floor muscle training is better than hypopressive exercises in pelvic organ prolapse treatment: An assessor-blinded randomized controlled trial. *Neurourology and Urodynamics, 38*(1), 171–179.

Resende, A. P. M., Stupp, L., Bernardes, B. T., et al. (2012). Can hypopressive exercises provide additional benefits to pelvic floor muscle training in women with pelvic organ prolapse? *Neurourology and Urodynamics, 31*, 121–125.

Slieker-Ten Hove, M. C., Pool-Goudzwaard, A. L., Eijkemans, M. J., et al. (2009). Symptomatic pelvic organ prolapse and possible risk factors in a general population. *American Journal of Obstetrics and Gynecology, 200*, 184–187.

Smith, F. J., Holman, C. D. J., Moorin, R. E., et al. (2010). Lifetime risk of undergoing surgery for pelvic organ prolapse. *Obstetrics & Gynecology, 116*(5), 1096–1100.

Srikrishna, S., Robinson, D., Cardozo, L., et al. (2008). Experiences and expectations of women with urogenital prolapse: A quantitative and qualitative exploration. *BJOG, 115*(11), 1362–1368.

Srikrishna, S., Robinson, D., & Cardozo, L. (2010). Validation of the patient global impression of improvement (PGI-I) for urogenital prolapse. *International Urogynecology Journal and Pelvic Floor Dysfunction, 21*(5), 523.

Stupp, L., Resende, A. P. M., Oliveira, E., et al. (2011). Pelvic floor muscle training for treatment of pelvic organ prolapse: An assessor-blinded randomized controlled trial. *International Urogynecology Journal and Pelvic Floor Dysfunction, 22*, 1233–1239.

Tegerstedt, G., Maehle-Schmidt, M., & Nyren, O. (2005). Prevalence of symptomatic pelvic organ prolapse in a Swedish population. *International Urogynecology Journal and Pelvic Floor Dysfunction, 16*, 497–503.

Thakar, R., & Stanton, S. (2002). Management of genital prolapse. *BMJ, 324*(7348), 1258–1262.

Wiegersma, M., Panman, C. M. C. R., Kollen, B. J., et al. (2014). Effect of pelvic floor muscle training compared with watchful waiting in older women with symptomatic mild pelvic organ prolapse: Randomized controlled trial in primary care. *BMJ, 349*, g7378.

7.4 Female Sexual Dysfunction

Sohier Elneil

PREVALENCE

Sexual dysfunction is a serious medical and social symptom that occurs in 10% to 52% of men and 25% to 63% of women (Dalpiaz et al., 2008; Levin, 2002). Sexuality is a crucial component of general health and well-being in both men and women. Female sexual dysfunction (FSD) is often a cause of pelvic floor dysfunction, commonly caused by childbirth in younger women and by menopause in older women (Addis et al., 2006; Baessler et al., 2004; Srivastava et al., 2008). It is multifactorial and multidimensional, and may be described as having biological, psychological, medical, interpersonal, and social components. Consequently, it impacts on relational quality of life. Numerous central and peripheral neural circuits control sexual activity. Impairment of one or more of these functional circuits may have a significant impact one or all of the preceding factors. Although several aspects of sexual motivation and performance are known, a complete picture of the various factors that control human sexual activity remain unknown. Sexual dysfunction may be classified as hypoactive sexual desire, or disorders of sexual aversion/desire, sexual arousal, sexual orgasms or sexual pain (Marthol and Hilz, 2004).

FSD has not been as extensively studied as erectile dysfunction (ED) in men nor adequately quantified within the wider community. In the published literature, FSD is often quoted as being a problem of the postpartum period, menopause, following radical surgery for various types of malignancies or a consequence of ED in the woman's partner. What is now known is that FSD is common and increases with age and pelvic floor disorders, such as urinary incontinence and pelvic organ prolapse, female genital mutilation (FGM), and neurological disorders such as multiple sclerosis. Surgical treatment of pelvic floor disorders has been poorly studied but has the potential to improve sexual satisfaction or cause sexual difficulties. There is now recognition of this fact, and new instruments such as condition-specific sexual questionnaires have recently been developed that will help to better evaluate the results of incontinence and prolapse surgery on sexual function.

PHYSIOLOGY OF SEXUAL FUNCTION AND ITS NEUROLOGICAL CONTROL

The neurological complexity of human sexual function is immense: higher centres determine the cognitive and emotional aspects of sexuality, hormonal levels drive libido and desire through the hypothalamus, and the ability to affect a sexual response depends on spinal autonomic reflexes. Malfunction of some aspect of this highly distributed system is therefore common in neurological disease.

Functional imaging techniques have been applied to examine brain responses on sexual arousal, using erotic visual stimulation compared with erotically neutral viewing in healthy subjects of both genders (Arnow et al., 2002; Hamann et al., 2004; Mouras et al., 2003; Park et al., 2001). Activation of the prefrontal cortex, the anterior cingulate, occipitotemporal cortex, thalamus, amygdala, hypothalamus, insula and claustrum is seen, with those regions being part of the limbic and paralimbic system long known to be important in mediating sexual motivation. The hypothalamus has been linked to most aspects of sexual behaviour, and animal experiments have shown that stimulation of medial preoptic nucleus of the hypothalamus results in erection in the rat (Andersson, 2001).

Comparison of brain activation between the genders is interesting since greater activation of the amygdala was seen in men than women (Hamann et al., 2004; Karama et al., 2002). A study of brain activation during penile stimulation by the subjects' females partners showed strong activation predominantly on the right side of the insula and secondary somatosensory cortex and deactivation of the amygdala but no activation of the hypothalamus (Georgiadis and Holstege, 2005). The same group reported brain activation during male ejaculation, and Holstege et al. (2003) showed prominent activity in the dopamine-rich mesodiencephalic junction/ventral tegmental area, an area which is also activated with the 'rush' experienced by heroin and cocaine addicts, who describe an orgasmic-like sensation with heroin use.

Animal and clinical studies of men following spinal cord injury (Bors and Comarr, 1960) pointed to the existence of two independent pathways for the male erectile response: a psychogenic pathway mediated by the thoracolumbar sympathetic outflow from T12 to L2 and a spinal reflex pathway which exists at the level of the sacral spinal cord, whereby genital stimulation results in a short-lived erection. It is thought that in neurological health, these two responses fuse to produce an erection adequate for intercourse. Comparable pathways mediate vaginal lubrication, the female sexual response analogous to penile erection, and have been identified by studies in women following spinal cord injury (Sipski et al., 2001).

In women the cavernous nerve runs along with the cavernous artery as it enters the corporal bodies of the clitoris. Large deep dorsal nerves perforate the glans of the clitoris on the dorsal aspect of its junction with the corporal bodies (O'Connell et al., 1998). Sexual arousal leads to increased vaginal blood flow, erection of the cavernous tissue of the clitoris and the outer part of the vagina. As in men, the erectile response of these tissues is nitric oxide (NO) dependent and neuronal NO synthetase has been detected in both the body and glans of the clitoris. Nerve fibres containing vasoactive intestinal polypeptide, calcitonin gene-related peptide and substance P have also been described in human clitoral tissue (Hauser-Kronberger et al., 1999). Vaginal lubrication is also NO mediated. Sexual arousal, either through direct stimulation of the genital region or through cerebral mechanisms, can result in quite rapid vaginal lubrication (i.e., within 30 seconds). Normal lubrication is dependent both on intact innervation and on normal oestrogen levels.

During female orgasm, there may be a series of synchronous contractions of the sphincter and vaginal muscles, and as many as 20 consecutive contractions have been registered lasting for 10 to 50 seconds. The sensory changes are generally described as being an intensely pleasurable pelvic event.

CLASSIFICATION

Various classifications of sexual dysfunction have been proposed, the most recent being one which included hypoactive sexual desire, or disorders of sexual desire, sexual arousal, orgasms or sexual pain. Many of these disorders are common among the general population: the Male Massachusetts study showed an increasing prevalence of ED with age, in which of a group of men aged 60 to 70 years, almost 60% had ED to a greater or lesser extent (Feldman et al., 1994)—data that has been confirmed by other studies worldwide. The prevalence of FSD has been estimated to be between 25% and 63%, the figure depending on the definition used and population studies. Among groups of patients with neurological disease, the prevalence of all types of disorder is even higher, although precise figures are not known.

PATHOPHYSIOLOGY AND CAUSES OF FEMALE SEXUAL DYSFUNCTION

The causes of FSD can be divided into neurological and non-neurological causes.

Neurological Causes of Sexual Dysfunction

Patients with neurological disease have a higher prevalence of all types of sexual function disorder (Borello-France et al., 2004; Burina and Sinanovic, 2006), although precise figures are not known. As they are a complex set of disorders, the different manifestations of each condition are outlined in Table 7.4.1.

Non-Neurological Causes of Sexual Dysfunction

Most women do not have a neurological cause for their sexual dysfunction, but their symptoms can originate from physical, hormonal, psychological or social factors (Table 7.4.2). Perhaps one condition which encapsulates all four groups is FGM, and this is discussed in further detail next.

TABLE 7.4.1 **Neurological Causes of Female Sexual Dysfunction**	
CORTICAL DISEASE Definition: Cortical disease affects the temporal or frontal regions which may result in sexual disturbances. The impact can differ on the extent and complexity of the condition.	
Head Injury	• Cognitive damage: Typically women present with a hypoactive sexual desire (Sandel et al., 1996). Both the amount of brain tissue and the location determine the outcome. • Prefrontal areas: Typically, women present with either erotic apathy or disinhibition with inappropriate sexually demanding behaviour (Miller et al., 1986). Similar problems can be seeing following encephalitis. • Brain injury: Partner dissatisfaction plays an important part in influencing sexual activity in women affected (Hibbard et al., 2000; O'Carroll et al., 1991). • Hypothalamic and pituitary damage, following head injury, can result in partner dissatisfaction and also in hypopituitarism (Bondanelli et al., 2004) requiring a full endocrine evaluation some months after a significant brain injury (Aimaretti et al., 2004).
Stroke	• Impact: This depends on pre-existing sexual dysfunction due to diseases such as hypertension, diabetes and myocardial infarction, which may mean that there is less impact of stroke on sexual behaviour (Sjogren and Fugl-Meyer, 1981). • Frequency and spectrum of sexual problems: This can be comparable to those problems seen following head injury (Korpelainen et al., 1999).
Epilepsy	• Temporal lobe disease causing epilepsy: This is associated with sexual manifestations including sexual auras which can occur as part of complex partial seizures and genital automatisms (observed in 11% of patients undergoing diagnostic video-telemetry [Dobesberger et al., 2004]). Temporal lobe epilepsy is also associated with hypersexuality (Blumer, 1970). • Other epileptic conditions: Although various sexual perversions can occur, the picture most commonly seen is that of a profound failure of arousal (Remillard et al., 1983; Scott and Prior, 1984; Spark et al., 1984).

Continued

TABLE 7.4.1 Neurological Causes of Female Sexual Dysfunction—cont'd

Parkinson's Disease	• Main presentation: Genital dysfunction usually is considered a feature of Parkinson's disease, but this situation is not entirely resolved. • Using questionnaire surveys, several studies have shown that dissatisfaction with the quality of sexual experiences in men (mainly erectile dysfunction [Jacobs et al., 2000]) and women (mainly hypoactive disorders [Oertel et al., 2003; Welsh et al., 1997; Wermuth and Stenager, 1995]) with Parkinson's disease is more likely than in control subjects.
Multiple System Atrophy	• In men, the main symptom is dysfunction of ejaculation. • In women, very little information exists as to whether sexual function is equally seriously disrupted at an early stage of the disease, but a single report shows that women with multiple system atrophy may have reduced genital sensitivity as an early symptom (Oertel et al., 2003).

SPINAL DISEASE

Definition: The impact of spinal disease on sexual dysfunction is determined by the level and completeness of a lesion. In men the main feature is erectile dysfunction, whereas the analogous process of vaginal lubrication dysfunction predominates in women. It is determined by psychogenic and reflex pathways (Sipski and Behnegar, 2001), and thus the level and completeness of a spinal cord injury determines what responses are preserved.

Spinal Cord Injury	• Main presentation: This is usually secondary to orgasmic or lubrication failure. • Aetiology: Failure of arousal may be secondary to audiovisual stimuli, fantasy or genital stimulation (Sipski and Behnegar, 2001). Failure to reach orgasm is common in women with spinal cord injury and correlates poorly with the type of injury (Sipski and Behnegar, 2001).
Multiple Sclerosis	• In men: The main presentation is erectile dysfunction (Betts et al., 1994; Fowler et al., 2005; Zivadinov et al., 1999). • In women: Sexual dysfunction is less frequently noted than in men (Mattson et al., 1995; Zorzon et al., 1999), but nevertheless it is a problem that is thought to affect more than 50% (Lundberg, 1981; Minderhoud et al., 1984), with the incidence increasing with increasing disability. From a questionnaire which allowed anonymous answering, a survey of a large number of women with multiple sclerosis showed loss of orgasm in 33%, loss of libido in 27% and spasticity in 12% (Lilius et al., 1996). Similar figures were obtained in a more recent case–control study which found that in women with multiple sclerosis, anorgasmia or hyporgasmia affected 37%, and there was decreased vaginal lubrication in 36% and reduced libido in 31.4% (Zorzon et al., 1999). Loss of orgasmic capacity (Yang et al., 2000) is the complaint for which women seek treatment (Dasgupta et al., 2004; Fowler et al., 2005).
Conus/Cauda Equina	• The cauda equina contains the sacral parasympathetic outflow together with the somatic efferent and afferent fibres. A lesion of the cauda equina therefore results in sensory loss as well as a parasympathetic defect. Following such a lesion, both men and women complain of perineal sensory loss and loss of erotic genital sensation—for which there is no effective treatment. In men, ED is also a complaint.

PERIPHERAL INNERVATION

Diabetes is the most common cause of erectile dysfunction. Surveys of andrology clinics have found between 20% and 31% of men attending to be diabetic. Age-matched studies of women with and without diabetes suggest that diabetic women may also be affected by specific disorders of sexual function including decreased vaginal lubrication and capacity for orgasm.

By contrast, neuropathies which selectively involve the small and unmyelinated nerve fibres (e.g., amyloid and other rare inherited neuropathies) have urogenital symptoms as prominent features, including sexual dysfunction in men and women (Villaplana et al., 1997).

TABLE 7.4.2	**Non-Neurological Causes of Female Sexual Dysfunction**
Physical	Physical conditions can decrease sexual desire and the body's ability to experience orgasm. These include: • Multiple medical conditions, such as heart disease, pelvic floor dysfunction (including bladder and bowel dysfunction), renal/liver failure and cancer. • Medications, such as blood pressure medication, antidepressants/antihistamines and chemotherapy drugs.
Hormonal	The impact of oestrogen on genital tissues and sexual responsiveness is well known to impact on women's quality of life. A decrease in oestrogen leads to decreased blood flow to the pelvic region, which can result in less genital sensation, as well as needing more time to build arousal and reach orgasm. The mode of action differs at different phases of women's lives: • Menopause: During menopause, the vaginal lining becomes thinner and less flexible, which can lead to painful intercourse (dyspareunia). Sexual desire also tends to decrease when hormonal levels decrease. • Postpartum: During postpartum, the hormonal shift after giving birth and during breastfeeding can lead to vaginal dryness and affect the desire to have sex.
Psychological	The impact of psychological conditions, such as untreated anxiety, depression or long-term stress (including the worries of marriage, relationships, pregnancy and the demands of being a new mother) can cause or contribute to female sexual dysfunction. This also includes chronic pain states.
Social	Cultural and religious issues and problems with body image also can contribute to sexual dysfunction. Most recently the issues surrounding female genital mutilation have made this a significant group issue to be addressed. Women from communities that practice female genital mutilation suffer from the combined impact of social taboo of the practice, psychological impact of the practice and the physical component of the practice which affect their bodies with a resultant loss of libido, dyspareunia and difficulty in achieving orgasms.

Female Sexual Dysfunction in Female Genital Mutilation

In women with FGM, there is no defined prevalence and much of what is known comes from anecdotal information provided by health workers in the field. It is known from the literature that many women suffer trouble with desire, arousability, satisfaction and ability to achieve orgasm in the general population. Thus it is not surprising that women with FGM, with the history of complications outlined previously, would tend to have problems with sexual intercourse and thus avoid sexual contact, as it exacerbates all of these problems (Ashimi et al., 2014; Elnashar et al., 2007).

As FSD is a multifactorial problem that may be exacerbated by external factors, such as chronic pain (Achtari & Dwyer, 2005a, 2005b), it is not surprising that in women with FGM it would be even more complex due to the anatomical distortion. There is a paucity of literature in this field, but if we draw on our knowledge of FSD in chronic urogenital pain we may begin to have a hint of the severity of the problem in women with FGM. Clearly, chronic urogenital pain and FGM coexist, and thus its impact on FSD cannot be underestimated (Ladjali et al., 1993; Lightfoot-Klein, 1993; Jaleel et al., 2002).

In an important work by Meltzer-Brody and Leserman (2011), the authors described that women were more likely to report antecedent stressful events, such as higher rates of physical and sexual abuse and post-traumatic stress disorder, when they were diagnosed with both major depression and chronic pain syndromes. They also reported symptoms of dyspareunia, dysmenorrhea and vulvar pain. The site and severity of pain, when compounded by depression and physical disability, impacted greatly on sexual dysfunction (Heinberg et al., 2004; Vloeberghs et al., 2012). Irrespective of the site of the pain, patients were depressed equally, with higher pain scores being associated with greater depression. It is important to draw from this experience to understand the situation seen in women with FGM.

MANAGEMENT OF FEMALE SEXUAL DYSFUNCTION

FSD needs to be managed in the context of the couple, as male sexual dysfunction often affects the female partner. The approach to treatment of both male sexual dysfunction and FSD must be holistic and multidisciplinary.

Overview of Therapeutic Options

The first step is to establish normal versus abnormal sexual functioning in women, as it is not usually well understood. A complete history combined with a physical examination is needed for a complete evaluation. Although laboratory tests are not always helpful in make a diagnosis, they may be indicated in women with abnormal physical examination findings or suspected comorbidities. It is important to identify and treat any underlying medical condition, as that in the first instance may alleviate most of the symptoms.

The main basis of sexual therapy and education remains cognitive behavioural therapy, individual and couples therapy, physiotherapy, and hormonal and non-hormonal medication. In postmenopausal women, hormonal medication such as testosterone (which improves sexual function in those with hypoactive sexual desire disorder, although data on its long-term safety and effectiveness are lacking) and oestrogen (which improves dyspareunia associated with vulvovaginal atrophy) are both thought to have a role in restoring function. However, the mainstay therapy for FSD remains physiotherapy.

Role of Physiotherapy

Physiotherapy in Men and Its Role in Female Sexual Dysfunction

Pelvic floor exercises in both men and women have been shown to improve symptoms. In one study of 55 men older than 20 years who had experienced ED for at least 6 months were recruited for a randomized controlled study with a crossover arm. The men were treated with either pelvic floor muscle exercises (taught by a physiotherapist) with biofeedback and lifestyle changes (intervention group) or were advised on lifestyle changes only (control group). Control patients who did not respond after 3 months were treated with the intervention. All men were given home exercises for a further 3 months. Outcomes were measured using the International Index of Erectile Function (IIEF), anal pressure measurements and independent (blinded) assessments. After 6 months, blind assessment showed that 40% of men had regained normal erectile function and 35.5% improved but 24.5% failed to improve. This study concluded that pelvic floor exercises should be considered as a first-line approach for men seeking long-term resolution of their ED. Further studies have mirrored findings of this study (Rosenbaum, 2007).

Role of Physiotherapy in Female Sexual Dysfunction in Neurological Conditions

Similarly, in women, trained physiotherapists were able to provide treatment and to restore/improve sexual function in women with sexual pain disorders, such as vaginismus and dyspareunia, by treating the associated musculoskeletal and neurological disorders.

In both men and women with neurological disease, pelvic floor exercises have been shown to improve symptoms but within the context of full physical rehabilitation. In a study looking at the role of sexual rehabilitation in patients with different experiences of sexuality after stroke, it was apparent that including sexual rehabilitation as part of holistic, person-centred stroke rehabilitation had the best outcomes overall (Nilsson et al., 2017).

In patients with multiple sclerosis, several studies have demonstrated that pelvic floor muscle therapy alone or in combination with electrical stimulation, such as transdermal tibial nerve stimulation, contributes to the improvement of sexual dysfunction (Lúcio et al., 2014). In a systematic review looking at improving sexuality of women with multiple sclerosis, pelvic floor muscles exercises alone or combined with electrostimulations, sexual therapy, administration of onabotulinumtoxinA and the use of clitoral devices were the most recommended interventions (Esteve-Rios et al., 2020). Thus, physiotherapy's role is well defined in this group, although not usually in isolation.

Role of Physiotherapy in Female Sexual Dysfunction in Non-Neurological Conditions

Within this group are several subgroups, including physical, hormonal, psychological and social aspects.

Physical: pelvic floor disorders. Interestingly, physiotherapy is routinely instituted in women with pelvic floor dysfunction, such as bladder and bowel dysfunction.

In the treatment of overactive bladder with physiotherapy, there was a secondary response in restoration of sexual function (Brækken et al., 2015). Similarly, in women with uterovaginal prolapse, when pelvic floor muscle therapy was instituted there was also improvement in sexual function, particularly in those who demonstrated the greatest increase in pelvic floor muscle strength and endurance (Brækken et al., 2015).

Hormonal: postpartum disorders. In young women, pelvic floor dysfunction is usually the primary problem, particularly after childbirth. In this group, a multidisciplinary approach between the physiotherapist, general practitioner and surgeons in the disciplines of urology, gynaecology and colorectal surgery should be engaged. By rectifying the anatomical problems, the functional problems can also be resolved. But physiotherapy on its own can have a positive and reaffirming role.

In a randomized controlled trial performed between 2007 and 2009, 90 patients aged 25 to 55 years with previous delivery and positive history of sexual dysfunction with less than stage 3 pelvic organ prolapse were divided into a surgical reconstruction group and a physiotherapy group (having received dedicated sessions for 8 weeks). The findings showed that libido and arousal were improved in both groups (p = 0.007 and p = 0.001, respectively), but orgasm and dyspareunia were improved mainly in the physiotherapy group (p = 0.001), indicating that physiotherapy works well in sexual disorders (Eftekhar et al., 2014).

Hormonal: menopause and perimenopause. In older women, menopause is a significant factor in affecting sexual intercourse (Graziottin and Leiblum, 2005). Although hormone replacement therapy has been used extensively and effectively, there is still a small subset of women in whom this is not enough. In this group the libido is affected greatly and the use of testosterone products has been found to be valuable (Graziottin and Leiblum, 2005). Pharmacotherapy, like use of phosphodiesterase type 5 inhibitors in men, has not been found to be useful in women, although a great deal of research is being pursued in finding the 'pink Viagra'.

Thus menopause-related sexual dysfunction may not be reversible without medical therapy. However, as hormonal deficiency does not usually decrease in severity over time, other therapeutic options must be considered, including psychosocial therapy which incorporates basic counselling, physiotherapy and psychosexual intervention (Al-Azzawi et al., 2010). Non-pharmacological approaches should be encouraged in all women, as their focus on lifestyle and non-medical therapy often results in better compliance over the long term (Ward et al., 2020), which may obviate the need for hormonal medication.

Psychological: chronic pain disorders. Chronic pelvic pain in women with sexual dysfunction is a complex syndrome, with the pain sensation and intensity often not corresponding to a specific location but usually associated with musculoskeletal and myofascial disorders. In this realm, physiotherapy is a widely underused and untapped resource, which has its place in the multidisciplinary approach to these health problems.

Social. Despite the lack of published data, many women in an FGM clinic treating complex urogynaecological issues will admit to avoiding sex due to pain and inability to achieve physical coitus due to scarring (Alsibiani and Rouzi, 2010; Elneil, 2016) resulting in superficial dyspareunia. In those women in whom scarring and dyspareunia persist, reconstructive surgery may be required. Deep dyspareunia may also occur, but it is often more difficult to treat and may require long-term pharmacological and possibly surgical treatment (Fox et al., 1997). Some women may complain of lack of sexual enjoyment (Fahmy et al., 2010), which may be a direct result of a clitoridectomy or because of the anxiety associated with the sexual act.

There is a paucity of literature regarding FGM and managing its long-term effects. Thus, to improve pelvic floor function, many women with FGM will need to be treated in the context of chronic vulval pain management, where physiotherapy has a critical role in holistic improvement. This is well demonstrated in a multicentre randomized study by Morin et al. (2021) looking at multimodal physical therapy versus topical lidocaine for provoked vestibulodynia, where there was strong evidence that the former was not only effective for pain but also in sexual function, as well as sexual distress. This supported the recommendation that physical therapy was the treatment of choice.

It is important to understand that FGM is complex. The FGM factors that contribute to the FSD include not only physical and social components but also psychological ones (Andersson, 2001; El-Defrawi et al., 2001; Knight et al., 1999), including low self-esteem, disturbed self-identity, psychosexual dysfunction and psychopathology, which is often under-reported (Alsibiani and Rouzi, 2010; Catania et al., 2007; Krause et al., 2001; Mohammed et al., 2014). The impact of FGM on FSD is yet to be properly quantified and qualified fully. But it is equally important to remember that sexual problems encountered with FGM need to be considered holistically. Thus both physical and psychological components need to always be considered and managed (El-Defrawi et al., 2001).

CONCLUSION

FSD clearly is a multifactorial problem that requires a multifaceted approach to care. Once the underlying cause is determined, a plan of action can be put in place. Although medications have a role, it is the non-medical interventions, particularly physiotherapy, that appear to have a more long-lasting holistic effect on both sexual function and other pelvic floor disorders.

REFERENCES

Achtari, C., & Dwyer, P. L. (2005). Sexual function and pelvic floor disorders. *Best Practice & Research Clinical Obstetrics & Gynaecology, 19*(6), 993–1008 quiz A1–A8.

Addis, I. B., Van Den Eeden, S. K., Wassel-Fyr, C. L., et al. (2006). Sexual activity and function in middle-aged and older women. *Obstetrics & Gynecology, 107*(4), 755–764.

Aimaretti, G., Ambrosio, M. R., Di Somma, C., et al. (2004). Traumatic brain injury and subarachnoid haemorrhage are conditions at high risk for hypopituitarism: Screening study at 3 months after the brain injury. *Clinical Endocrinology, 61*(3), 320–326.

Al-Azzawi, F., Bitzer, J., Brandenburg, U., et al. (2010). Therapeutic options for postmenopausal female sexual dysfunction. *Climacteric, 13*(2), 103–120.

Alsibiani, S. A., & Rouzi, A. A. (2010). Sexual function in women with female genital mutilation. *Fertility and Sterility, 93*(3), 722–724.

Andersson, C. (2001). [Female genital mutilation—a complex phenomenon]. *Lakartidningen, 98*(20), 2463–2468.

Andersson, K. E. (2001). Neurophysiology/pharmacology of erection. *International Journal of Impotence Research, 13*(Suppl. 3), 8–17.

Arnow, B. A., Desmond, J. E., Banner, L. L., et al. (2002). Brain activation and sexual arousal in healthy, heterosexual males. *Brain, 125*, 1014–1023.

Ashimi, A., Aliyu, L., Shittu, M., et al. (2014). A multicentre study on knowledge and attitude of nurses in northern Nigeria concerning female genital mutilation. *The European Journal of Contraception and Reproductive Health Care, 19*(2), 134–140.

Baessler, K., Bircher, M. D., & Stanton, S. L. (2004). Pelvic floor dysfunction in women after pelvic trauma. *BJOG, 111*(5), 499–502.

Betts, C. D., D'Mellow, M. T., & Fowler, C. J. (1994). Erectile dysfunction in multiple sclerosis: Associated neurological and neurophysiological deficits, and treatment of the condition. *Brain, 117*, 1303–1310.

Blumer, D. (1970). Hypersexual episodes in temporal lobe epilepsy. *American Journal Psychiatry, 126*, 1099.

Bondanelli, M., De Marinis, L., Ambrosio, M. R., et al. (2004). Occurrence of pituitary dysfunction following traumatic brain injury. *Journal of Neurotrauma, 21*(6), 685–696.

Borello-France, D., Leng, W., O'Leary, M., et al. (2004). Bladder and sexual function among women with multiple sclerosis. *Multiple Sclerosis, 10*(4), 455–461.

Bors, E., & Comarr, A. (1960). Neurological disturbances of sexual function with special references to 529 patients with spinal cord injury. *Urological Survey, 10*, 191–222.

Brækken, I. H., Majida, M., Engh, M. E., et al. (2015). Can pelvic floor muscle training improve sexual function in women with pelvic organ prolapse? A randomized controlled trial. *The Journal of Sexual Medicine, 12*(2), 470–480.

Burina, A., & Sinanovic, O. (2006). [Bladder, bowel and sexual dysfunction in patient with multiple sclerosis]. *Medicinski Arhiv, 60*(3), 182–184.

Catania, L., Abdulcadir, O., Puppo, V., et al. (2007). Pleasure and orgasm in women with female genital mutilation/cutting (FGM/C). *The Journal of Sexual Medicine, 4*(6), 1666–1678.

Dalpiaz, O., Kerschbaumer, A., Mitterberger, M., et al. (2008). Female sexual dysfunction: A new urogynaecological research field. *BJU International, 101*(6), 717–721.

Dasgupta, R., Wiseman, O. J., Kanabar, G., et al. (2004). Efficacy of sildenafil in the treatment of female sexual dysfunction due to multiple sclerosis. *Journal Urology, 171*(3), 1189–1193 discussion 1193.

Dobesberger, J., Walser, G., Unterberger, I., et al. (2004). Genital automatisms: A video-EEG study in patients with medically refractory seizures. *Epilepsia, 45*(7), 777–780.

Eftekhar, T., Sohrabi, M., Haghollahi, F., et al. (2014). Comparison effect of physiotherapy with surgery on sexual function in patients with pelvic floor disorder: A randomized clinical trial. *Iran Journal Reprod Medicine, 12*(1), 7–14.

El-Defrawi, M. H., Lotfy, G., Dandash, K. F., et al. (2001). Female genital mutilation and its psychosexual impact. *Journal of Sex & Marital Therapy, 27*(5), 465–473.

Elnashar, A. M., El-Dien Ibrahim, M., Eldesoky, M. M., et al. (2007). Sexual abuse experienced by married Egyptian women. *International Journal of Gynecology & Obstetrics*, *99*(3), 216–220.

Elneil, S. (2016). Female sexual dysfunction in female genital mutilation. *Tropical Doctor*, *46*(1), 2–11.

Esteve-Rios, A., Garcia-Sanjuan, S., Oliver-Roig, A., et al. (2020). Effectiveness of interventions aimed at improving the sexuality of women with multiple sclerosis: A systematic review. *Clinical Rehabilitation*, *34*(4), 438–449.

Fahmy, A., El-Mouelhy, M. T., & Ragab, A. R. (2010). Female genital mutilation/cutting and issues of sexuality in Egypt. *Reproductive Health Matters*, *18*(36), 181–190.

Feldman, H., Goldstein, I., Hatzichristou, D. G., et al. (1994). Impotence and its medical and psychosocial correlates: Results of the Massachusetts male aging study. *Journal Urology*, *151*, 54–61.

Fowler, C. J., Miller, J., Sharief, M., et al. (2005). A double blind, randomised study of sildenafil citrate for erectile dysfunction in men with multiple sclerosis. *Journal of Neurology Neurosurgery and Psychiatry*, *76*(5), 700–705.

Fox, E. F., de Ruiter, A., & Bingham, J. S. (1997). Female genital mutilation. *International Journal of STD & AIDS*, *8*(10), 599–601.

Georgiadis, J. R., & Holstege, G. (2005). Human brain activation during sexual stimulation of the penis. *Journal Comparactive Neurology*, *493*(1), 33–38.

Graziottin, A., & Leiblum, S. R. (2005). Biological and psychosocial pathophysiology of female sexual dysfunction during the menopausal transition. *The Journal of Sexual Medicine*, *2*(Suppl. 3), 133–145.

Hamann, S., Herman, R. A., Nolan, C. L., et al. (2004). Men and women differ in amygdala response to visual sexual stimuli. *Nature Neuroscience*, *7*(4), 411–416.

Hauser-Kronberger, C., Cheung, A., Hacker, G. W., et al. (1999). Peptidergic innervation of the human clitoris. *Peptides*, *20*(5), 539–543.

Heinberg, L. J., Fisher, B. J., Wesselmann, U., et al. (2004). Psychological factors in pelvic/urogenital pain: The influence of site of pain versus sex. *Pain*, *108*, 88–94.

Hibbard, M. R., Gordon, W. A., Flanagan, S., et al. (2000). Sexual dysfunction after traumatic brain injury. *NeuroRehabilitation*, *15*(2), 107–120.

Holstege, G., Georgiadis, J. R., Paans, A. M. J., et al. (2003). Brain activation during human male ejaculation. *Journal of Neuroscience*, *23*(27), 9185–9193.

Jacobs, H., Vieregge, A., & Vieregge, P. (2000). Sexuality in young patients with Parkinson's disease: A population based comparison with healthy controls. *Journal of Neurology Neurosurgery and Psychiatry*, *69*(4), 550–552.

Jaleel, H., Huengsberg, M., & Luesley, D. (2002). Female genital mutilation—case report and discussion. *International Journal of STD & AIDS*, *13*(12), 850–851.

Karama, S., Lecours, A. R., Leroux, J.-M., et al. (2002). Areas of brain activation in males and females during viewing of erotic film excerpts. *Human Brain Mapping*, *16*(1), 1–13.

Knight, R., Hotchin, A., Bayly, C., et al. (1999). Female genital mutilation—experience of the Royal women's Hospital, Melbourne. *The Australian and New Zealand Journal of Obstetrics and Gynaecology*, *39*(1), 50–54.

Korpelainen, J. T., Nieminen, P., & Myllyla, V. V. (1999). Sexual functioning among stroke patients and their spouses. *Stroke*, *30*(4), 715–719.

Krause, E., Brandner, S., Mueller, M. D., et al. (2011). Out of Eastern Africa: Defibulation and sexual function in woman with female genital mutilation. *The Journal of Sexual Medicine*, *8*(5), 1420–1425.

Ladjali, M., Rattray, T. W., & Walder, R. J. (1993). Female genital mutilation. *BMJ*, *307*(6902), 460.

Levin, R. J. (2002). The physiology of sexual arousal in the human female: A recreational and procreational synthesis. *Archives of Sexual Behavior*, *31*(5) 405–111.

Levy, G., & Lowenstein, L. (2020). Overactive bladder syndrome treatments and their effect on female sexual function: A review. *Sexual Medicine*, *8*(1), 1–7.

Lightfoot-Klein, H. (1993). Disability in female immigrants with ritually inflicted genital mutilation. *Women & Therapy*, *14*(3–4), 187–194.

Lilius, H. G., Valtonen, E. J., & Wikstrom, J. (1996). Sexual problems in patients suffering from multiple sclerosis. *Scandinavian Journal of Social Medicine*, *4*(1), 41–44.

Lúcio, A. C., D'Ancona, C. A. L., Lopes, M. H. B. M., et al. (2014). The effect of pelvic floor muscle training alone or in combination with electrostimulation in the treatment of sexual dysfunction in women with multiple sclerosis. *Multiple Sclerosis*, *20*(13), 1761–1768.

Lundberg, P. O. (1981). Sexual dysfunction in female patients with multiple sclerosis. *International Rehabilitation Medicine*, *3*, 32–34.

Marthol, H., & Hilz, M. J. (2004). [Female sexual dysfunction: A systematic overview of classification, pathophysiology, diagnosis and treatment]. *Fortschritte der Neurologie - Psychiatrie*, *72*(3), 121–135.

Mattson, D., Petrie, M., Srivastava, D. K., et al. (1995). Multiple sclerosis. Sexual dysfunction and its response to medications. *Archives of Neurology*, *52*(9), 862–868.

Meltzer-Brody, S., & Leserman, J. (2011). Psychiatric comorbidity in women with chronic pelvic pain. *CNS Spectrums*, *16*(2), 29–35.

Miller, B., Cummings, J., & McIntyre, H. (1986). Hypersexuality or altered sexual preference following brain injury. *Journal of Neurology Neurosurgery and Psychiatry*, *49*, 867–873.

Minderhoud, J. M., Leemhuis, J. G., Kremer, J., et al. (1984). Sexual disturbances arising from multiple sclerosis. *Acta Neurologica Scandinavica, 70*(4), 299–306.

Mohammed, G. F., Hassan, M. M., & Eyada, M. M. (2014). Female genital mutilation/cutting: Will it continue? *The Journal of Sexual Medicine, 11*(11), 2756–2763.

Morin, M., Dumoulin, C., Bergeron, S., et al. (2021). Multimodal physical therapy versus topical lidocaine for provoked vestibulodynia: A multicenter, randomized trial. *American Journal of Obstetrics and Gynecology, 224*(2), 189.e1–189.e12.

Mouras, H., Stoleru, S., Bittoun, J., et al. (2003). Brain processing of visual sexual stimuli in healthy men: A functional magnetic resonance imaging study. *NeuroImage, 20*(2), 855–869.

Nilsson, M. I., Fugl-Meyer, K., von Koch, L., et al. (2017). Experiences of sexuality six years after stroke: A qualitative study. *The Journal of Sexual Medicine, 14*(6), 797–803.

O'Carroll, R., Woodrow, J., & Maroun, F. (1991). Psychosexual and psychosocial sequelae of closed head injury. *Brain Injury, 5*, 303–313.

O'Connell, H. E., Hutson, J. M., Anderson, C. R., et al. (1998). Anatomical relationship between urethra and clitoris. *Journal Urology, 159*(6), 1892–1897.

Oertel, W. H., Wachter, T., Quinn, N. P., et al. (2003). Reduced genital sensitivity in female patients with multiple system atrophy of Parkinsonian type. *Movement Disorders, 18*(4), 430–432.

Park, K., Seo, J. J., Kang, H. K., et al. (2001). A new potential of blood oxygenation level dependent (BOLD) functional MRI for evaluating cerebral centers of penile erection. *International Journal of Impotence Research, 13*(2), 73–81.

Remillard, G. M., Andermann, F., Testa, G. F., et al. (1983). Sexual ictal manifestations predominate in women with temporal lobe epilepsy: A finding suggesting sexual dimorphism in the human brain. *Neurology, 33*(3), 323–330.

Rosenbaum, T. Y. (2007). Pelvic floor involvement in male and female sexual dysfunction and the role of pelvic floor rehabilitation in treatment: A literature review. *The Journal of Sexual Medicine, 4*(1), 4–13.

Sandel, M., Williams, K. S., Dellapietra, L., et al. (1996). Sexual functioning following traumatic brain injury. *Brain Injury, 10*, 719–728.

Scott, D. F., & Prior, F. P. (1984). Temporal lobe epilepsy and hyposexuality. *Lancet, 1*, 743.

Sipski, M. L., Alexander, C. J., & Rosen, R. (2001). Sexual arousal and orgasm in women: Effects of spinal cord injury. *Annals of Neurology, 49*(1), 35–44.

Sipski, M. L., & Behnegar, A. (2001). Neurogenic female sexual dysfunction: A review. *Clinical Autonomic Research, 11*(5), 279–283.

Sjogren, K., & Fugl-Meyer, A. R. (1981). Sexual problems in hemiplegia. *International Rehabilitation Medicine, 3*(1), 26–31.

Spark, R. F., Wills, C. A., & Royal, H. (1984). Hypogonadism, hyperprolacinaemia, and temporal lobe epilepsy in hyposexual men. *Lancet, 1*, 413–417.

Srivastava, R., Thakar, R., & Sultan, A. (2008). Female sexual dysfunction in obstetrics and gynecology. *Obstetrical and Gynecological Survey, 63*(8), 527–537.

Villaplana, G., Rosino, E. H., Cubillana, P. L., et al. (1997). Corino-andrade disease (familial amyloidotic polyneuropathy type I) in Spain: Urological and andrological disorders. *Neurourology and Urodynamics, 16*, 55–61.

Vloeberghs, E., van der Kwaak, A., Knipscheer, J., et al. (2012). Coping and chronic psychosocial consequences of female genital mutilation in The Netherlands. *Ethnicity and Health, 17*(6), 677–695.

Ward, L. J., Nilsson, S., Hammar, M., et al. (2020). Resistance training decreases plasma levels of adipokines in postmenopausal women. *Scientific Reports, 10*(1) Art. No. 19837.

Welsh, M., Hung, L., & Waters, C. H. (1997). Sexuality in women with Parkinson's disease. *Movement Disorders, 12*(6), 923–927.

Wermuth, L., & Stenager, E. (1995). Sexual problems in young patients with Parkinson's disease. *Acta Neurologica Scandinavica, 91*(6), 453–455.

Yang, C., Bowen, J. R., Kraft, G. H., et al. (2000). Cortical evoked potentials of the dorsal nerve of the clitoris and female sexual dysfunction in multiple sclerosis. *Journal Urology, 164*(6), 2010–2013.

Zivadinov, R., Zorzon, M., Bosco, A., et al. (1999). Sexual dysfunction in multiple sclerosis: II. Correlation analysis. *Multiple Sclerosis, 5*, 428–431.

Zorzon, M., Zivadinov, R., Bosco, A., et al. (1999). Sexual dysfunction in multiple sclerosis: A case–control study. I. Frequency and comparison of groups. *Multiple Sclerosis, 5*(6), 418–427.

The Complexity of Sexuality

INTRODUCTION

Sexuality is an important aspect throughout life, influenced by the interaction of biological, social, psychological, cultural and many other factors. It includes gender identities, sex, reproduction, roles, sexual orientation, eroticism, intimacy and pleasure. Sexuality is experienced and expressed in thoughts, fantasies, desires, beliefs, attitudes, values, behaviours, practices, roles and relationships (World Health Organization [WHO], 2006). Although sexuality can include all of these dimensions, not all of them are always experienced or expressed.

Sexual function and dysfunction was first studied by Masters and Johnson (1966) and described as a four-phase model of excitement, plateau, orgasm and resolution. Later understanding of female sexual function has expanded from the linear model proposed by Masters and Johnson to a more circular model, more suitable for the female sexual response, incorporating intimacy and emotional satisfaction as well as sexual desire and physical satisfaction (Basson, 2001).

Why Are Women More at Risk of Sexual Dysfunction Than Men?

Male sexual physiology is typically stable due to the lifelong and relatively constant production of testosterone; however, female sexual physiology is highly discontinuous throughout the menstrual cycle, as well as the reproductive life events of pregnancy, puerperium and menopause (Graziottin, 2006). There are therefore many complex barriers to optimal sexual health outcomes for women (Fig. 7.4.1).

The prevalence of female sexual dysfunction (FSD) is high across a woman's life cycle, with rates up to 45% among women in the general population (McCabe et al., 2016b). Prevalence of FSD has also shown to increase with increasing age (McCabe et al., 2016b). These high numbers require that health professionals, including physiotherapists, consider FSD in their clinical practice. The literature has further indicated that the most frequent sexual dysfunction for women is female sexual arousal dysfunction and hypoactive sexual desire dysfunctions, and that women often have multiple sexual dysfunctions as a vicious cycle to one problem (McCabe et al., 2016b, McCool et al., 2016).

Ageing, the partner's sexual health and the presence of pelvic floor disorder (PFD) are all independent predictors of FSD (Kanter et al., 2015). Furthermore, a recent systematic review and meta-analysis concluded that lifestyle habits including smoking, physical inactivity and diet could all contribute to FSD (Allen and Walter, 2018). The relationship between physical activity and sexual function may be due to an increase in levels of testosterone, but also more psychosocial effects impacting on self-esteem and body appreciation. This effect may also be explained by weight and people engaging in lower levels of physical activity. For physiotherapists, lifestyle interventions must be kept in mind as an important mediator of FSD.

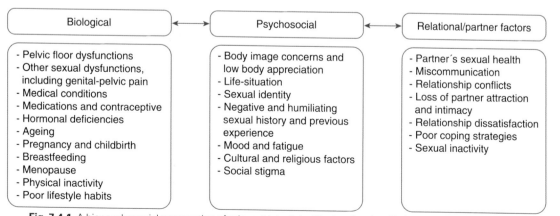

Fig. 7.4.1 A biopsychosocial perspective of relevant interlinked factors involved in female sexual dysfunction.

During pregnancy and following vaginal delivery, changes in pelvic organ support and an increase in the area surrounding the pelvic openings (levator hiatus area) have been shown, suggesting reduced support to the pelvic organs (Reimers et al., 2016; Staer-Jensen et al., 2015). A link between these physiological changes and FSD has been hypothesized, but a newly published study does not support an association between an increased hiatal area and a feeling of vaginal looseness (Roos et al., 2020). Furthermore, the loss of pelvic floor muscle (PFM) strength and muscular endurance following vaginal delivery (Hilde et al., 2013) may in itself lead to symptoms that may be associated with FSD, such as a feeling of vaginal looseness (Haylen et al., 2010; Tennfjord et al., 2015). Postpartum sexual functioning is also influenced by psychological changes associated with the transition into parenthood (Leeman and Rogers, 2012). Furthermore, according to the American College of Obstetricians and Gynecologists (ACOG), hormonal changes as a result of breastfeeding may cause vaginal dryness and subsequent dyspareunia (ACOG Committee on Practice Bulletins—Gynecology, 2019).

Strong PFMs have been associated with a higher level of sexual function including desire, lubrication and orgasm among middle-aged women with PFD (De Menezes Franco et al., 2017; Kanter et al., 2015). A possible explanation has been that during a strong voluntary PFM contraction, the bulbocavernosus may further exacerbate erection of the clitoris (Shafik, 2000a, 2000b) equivalent to the penile erection (Hoffman et al., 2012), intensifying orgasm. The increased blood flow to the clitoris, vagina and labia leads to engorgement of these organs (Achtari & Dwyer, 2005a, 2005b; Jha and Thakar, 2010; Shafik, 2000a, 2000b). Hypoactive PFMs have also been found to be associated with reduced desire among women aged 50 to 60 years, with age being a strong predictor of sexual activity and function (Grzybowska and Wydra, 2019).

International Recommendations

Understanding of the cause of FSD is far from complete, probably due to the complexity of their multifactorial nature and the overlapping of symptoms (Delancey et al., 2008). Focus on a single factor or single bodily area will therefore narrow our perspective in the understanding of FSD. The International consultation on Sexual Medicine (ICSM), Commitee three has also highlighted this complexity by shifting focus from an organic, psychogenic or mixed point of view to more of a biopsychosocial approach that aims to synthesize rather than categorize etiologic and contributing factors (Hatzichristou et al., 2016). Since FSD is multifactorial, there is often a need for an interdisciplinary approach addressing the different aspects of the problems required for assessment and treatment (Fig. 7.4.2).

The Role of Physiotherapy in Women With Sexual Dysfunction

Despite the life expectancy of women being higher than men, women are at greater risk of having their health impacted by chronic diseases affecting their sexual health. Physical therapy is services provided by physical therapists to individuals and populations to develop, maintain and restore maximum movement and functional ability throughout the lifespan (The World Confederation for Physical Therapy, 2019). They can help people at any stage of life when movement and function are threatened by ageing, injury, diseases, disorders, conditions or environmental factors. Physiotherapists can contribute to women's sexual health by assessing women's movement impairments, functional capacity in general and related to the pelvic floor, performing the physiotherapy diagnosis and prescribing the adequate treatment. Furthermore, physiotherapists have an important role to contribute to general women's health by promoting and addressing sexual health issues in their practice (see Fig. 7.4.2).

Communicative and Ethical Considerations When Addressing Female Sexual Function

Due to the social stigma around female sexuality in Western culture, women often avoid or become embarrassed to discuss their sexual health with healthcare professionals (Kingsberg et al., 2019). Furthermore, menopausal women are typically unaware or have misconceptions about conditions that may negatively affect their sexual life, commonly being female sexual arousal dysfunction and hypoactive sexual desire dysfunctions. To address sexual health needs and concerns, healthcare professionals can be trained to initiate and maintain a sexual health conversation that is comfortable for the woman and/or her partner. Moreover, healthcare professionals must be trained to correctly identify, diagnose and treat the sexual problems of their female patients.

A mix of interpersonal, clinical and organizational factors are perceived to influence patient–therapist

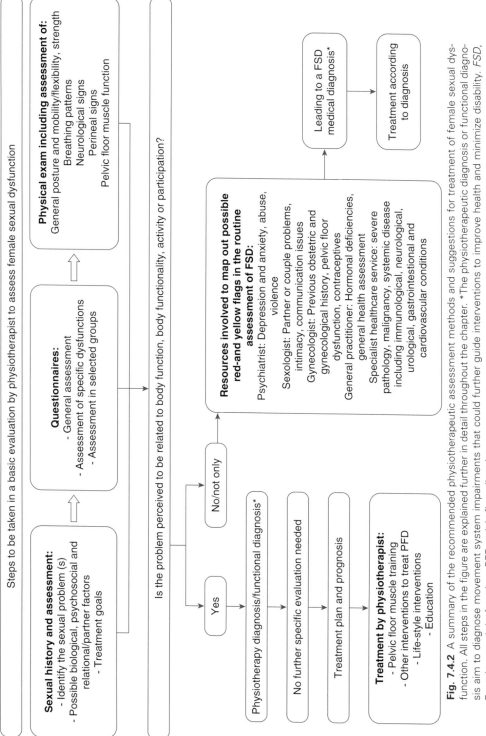

Steps to be taken in a basic evaluation by physiotherapist to assess female sexual dysfunction

Sexual history and assessment:
- Identify the sexual problem (s)
- Possible biological, psychosocial and relational/partner factors
- Treatment goals

Questionnaires:
- General assessment
- Assessment of specific dysfunctions
- Assessment in selected groups

Physical exam including assessment of:
General posture and mobility/flexibility, strength
Breathing patterns
Neurological signs
Perineal signs
Pelvic floor muscle function

Is the problem perceived to be related to body function, body functionality, activity or participation?

Yes

No/not only

Physiotherapy diagnosis/functional diagnosis*

No further specific evaluation needed

Treatment plan and prognosis

Treatment by physiotherapist:
- Pelvic floor muscle training
- Other interventions to treat PFD
- Life-style interventions
- Education

Resources involved to map out possible red-and yellow flags in the routine assessment of FSD:
Psychiatrist: Depression and anxiety, abuse, violence
Sexologist: Partner or couple problems, intimacy, communication issues
Gynecologist: Previous obstetric and gynecological history, pelvic floor dysfunction, contraceptives
General practitioner: Hormonal deficiencies, general health assessment
Specialist healthcare service: severe pathology, malignancy, systemic disease including immunological, neurological, urological, gastrointestional and cardiovascular conditions

Leading to a FSD medical diagnosis*

Treatment according to diagnosis

Fig. 7.4.2 A summary of the recommended physiotherapeutic assessment methods and suggestions for treatment of female sexual dysfunction. All steps in the figure are explained further in detail throughout the chapter. *The physiotherapeutic diagnosis or functional diagnosis aim to diagnose movement system impairments that could further guide interventions to improve health and minimize disability. *FSD,* Female sexual dysfunction; *PFD,* pelvic floor disorder.

BOX 7.4.1   A Model for Initiating Discussion and Treatment of Female Sexual Dysfunction—ALLOW

A – Ask the patient about her problem and sexual activity.

L – Legitimize the problem.

L – Identify limitations in the physiotherapeutic assessment and management methods (guided by patient-reported outcomes).

O – Open up for discussion, including referral to relevant disciplines (red and yellow flags).

W – Work together with the patient and/or partner to set realistic treatment goals.

Adapted from Sadovsky (2002) and Filamenco and Donato (2017).

BOX 7.4.2   Definitions of Female Sexual Dysfunction

Hypoactive Sexual Desire Dysfunction is characterised by absence or marked reduction in desire or motivation to engage in sexual activity as manifested by any of the following: 1) reduced or absent spontaneous desire (sexual thoughts or fantasies); 2) reduced or absent responsive desire to erotic cues and stimulation; or 3) inability to sustain desire or interest in sexual activity once initiated. The pattern of diminished or absent spontaneous or responsive desire or inability to sustain desire or interest in sexual activity has occurred episodically or persistently over a period at least several months, and is associated with clinically significant distress.

Sexual arousal dysfunctions include difficulties with the physiological or the subjective aspects of sexual arousal.

Orgasmic dysfunctions refer to difficulties related to the subjective experience of orgasm.

From WHO (2019).

interactions (O'Keeffe et al., 2016). Furthermore, the patient's own expectations for treatment are vital for success, and the development of treatment goals within a therapeutic setting is crucial. A model for initiating discussion and treatment of FSD (ALLOW) has been proposed (Sadovsky, 2002) and recently elaborated on (Filamenco and Donato, 2017). This model may be a useful tool for physiotherapists in their clinical practice treating women with sexual dysfunction (Box 7.4.1).

Aim of This Chapter

The aim of this chapter is to highlight the role of the physiotherapist in an interdisciplinary team. Furthermore, we provide an overview of physiotherapeutic assessment and treatment methods related to FSD, emphasizing their role related to body function and structure, activity, and participation. The levels of evidence of the different assessment methods and interventions were assessed, and recommendations were proposed. This chapter will not address assessment and interventions aiming to treat sexual pain penetration disorders, as this will be addressed in another chapter of this book.

Definitions and Classification of Sexual Function and Sexual Dysfunction Including Symptoms of Sexual Dysfunction
Sexual Function and Sexual Dysfunction

Sexual health is 'a state of physical, emotional, mental and social well-being in relation to sexuality; it is not merely the absence of disease, dysfunction or infirmity'

(WHO, 2006). *Sexual dysfunction*, however, is defined as syndromes that comprise the various ways in which adults may have difficulty experiencing personally satisfying, non-coercive sexual activities (WHO, 2019). A classic approach in medicine is to define disease by the aetiology. However, the aetiology of sexual dysfunction is often unknown or thought to be multifactorial, and in most cases the organic origin is difficult to separate from the non-organic origin, making the diagnosis of sexual dysfunction problematic.

Types of Sexual Dysfunction

There are two major systems of classifying sexual dysfunction: the International Classification of Diseases, 11th Edition (ICD-11) by the WHO (2019) and the Diagnostic and Statistical Manual of Mental Disorders, 5th Edition (DSM-5) by the American Psychiatric Association (APA, 2013). This chapter will focus on FSD, and the definitions adapted by the ICD-11 are explained in Box 7.4.2. To provide the best level of evidence we will concentrate on the following definitions which will be discussed further in the light of physiotherapy assessment and interventions:

- Hypoactive sexual desire dysfunction
- Female sexual arousal dysfunction
- Female orgasmic dysfunction

Pregnancy-related sexual dysfunction and menopause-related sexual dysfunction. Pregnancy-related sexual dysfunction and menopausal-related sexual dysfunction have been highlighted as a separate dysfunction by the ACOG (2019). However, no distinct criteria differ pregnancy-related sexual dysfunction and menopause-related sexual dysfunction from FSD in general and the same definitions apply (McCabe et al., 2016a).

Symptoms of sexual dysfunction. Symptoms of FSD have also been defined as 'a departure from normal sensation and/or function experienced by a woman during sexual activity' (Haylen et al., 2010).

Although symptoms of sexual dysfunction have been included as a pelvic floor dysfunction (Bø et al., 2017), some authors do not acknowledge symptoms of sexual dysfunction as part of pelvic floor dysfunction (Nygaard and Barber, 2008; Weber et al., 2001). In this chapter we will focus on sexual dysfunction rather than symptoms of sexual dysfunction as defined by Haylen et al. (2010), but we will briefly mention symptoms that we consider are of importance for women's health physiotherapists.

Symptoms of sexual dysfunction have been listed as:
- Dyspareunia: complaint of persistent or recurrent pain or discomfort associated with attempted or complete vaginal penetration

- Superficial (introital) dyspareunia: complaint of pain or discomfort on vaginal entry or at the vaginal introitus
- Deep dyspareunia: complaint of pain or discomfort on deeper penetration (mid or upper vagina)
- Obstructed intercourse: complaint that vaginal penetration is not possible due to obstruction
- Vaginal laxity: complaint of excessive vaginal laxity

Assessment

Physiotherapists base their clinical decisions on evaluating the patient's physical function. It is therefore important that the evaluation methods used are standardized and suitable for use in physiotherapy practice (Fitzpatrick et al., 1998). The physiotherapeutic diagnosis or functional diagnosis aim to diagnose movement system impairments that could further guide interventions to improve health and minimize disability (Jiandani and Mhatre, 2018). In other words, medical doctors primarily classify cause of disease, disorder and/or injury, whereas physical therapists primarily classify consequences that result from them. The International Classification of Functioning, Disability and Health (ICF) model is designed to categorize the patients' described activity problems into the areas of body function, activity or participation (WHO, 2001) (Fig. 7.4.3). Using the

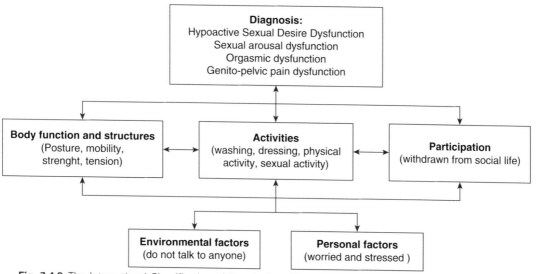

Fig. 7.4.3 The International Classification of Functioning, Disability and Health model (ICF). Body function and structure relates to loss of abnormality of psychological, physiological or anatomical structure or function at the organ level; activities relates to restriction or loss of ability of a person to perform activities of daily living; participation is the disadvantage due to impairment or disability that limits or restricts a person's normal functioning.

ICF model, physiotherapists try to influence the consequences of FSD on these areas. We will further discuss physiotherapeutic assessment methods in the light of a detailed history, use of questionnaires and clinical examination.

History

A sexual history aims to identify sexual problems, possible biological and psychosocial contributing factors, and the patient's and/or couple's treatment goals (Hatzichristou et al., 2016).

Updated guidelines for the assessment of FSD have been published (ACOG, 2019; Hatzichristou et al., 2016; Krakowsky and Grober, 2018), incorporating biological, cognitive, emotional and behavioural, contextual, and interpersonal contributing factors (Box 7.4.3). The

guidelines from the ACOG (2019) and the Canadian Urological Association (Krakowsky and Grober, 2018) are aimed towards gynaecologists and obstetricians, although these aspects would be relevant in a physiotherapeutic setting as well. However, the incorporation of aspects relevant to the ICF model has received less attention in the preceding guidelines and is therefore included in Box 7.4.3.

Questionnaire Data

A questionnaire can never replace a detailed sexual function history, but it can be used as an adjunct in the process of diagnosis and management (Kaminska et al., 2019). Questionnaires may also be used to answer more intimate questions that are not easily answered during a history. The use of validated questionnaires assures that

---

BOX 7.4.3   Important Considerations During History Taking in Female Sexual Dysfunction

History
(i) To identify the problem, ask:
Has the problem been lifelong? If not:
What caused the problem, onset, duration, location, frequency, intensity?
Is the problem primary or secondary?
Is the problem situational or generalized?
How is the woman's sexual and gender identity?
How is sexual history prior to the problem and context in which the problem arises?
What is the level of personnel distress about the condition?
What are past and current negative and humiliating sexual experiences, including abuse or violence?
Which factors trigger/relieve the problem?
(ii) Possible biological and psychosocial contributing factors
General medical history:
Self-care including hygiene, physical activity, nutrition
Medication including birth control and hormonal supplements
Previous injuries that could affect the condition (fall on the coccyx)
Previous obstetric and gynaecological history, including the presence of pelvic floor disorder
General health of self, partner and family/close friends
Psychosocial issues:
Life situation including work and social support

History of presenting illness including psychiatric history
Daily mood and fatigue
How are body image concerns, including change of body appearance and body self-esteem including genital appearance?
Personality characteristics: self-esteem, self-efficacy, sexual self-confidence
Previous relationships
Social skills including flirting and network
Relationship and partner problems:
How are partner factors including disease and relationship satisfaction?
Communication skills
Attraction to partner and physical intimacy
How does the couple cope with the problem?
Partner attitude and reaction to the problem?
Body function, activity and participation
Level of physical activity and training
Physical function and impairments
Problems with performance of activities of daily living
(iii)   Patient's and/or couple's treatment goals
The patient's and the partner's own expectations for treatment
'Is there anything else about your sexual life that I need to
know to ensure you receive good sexual healthcare?'

Adapted from the American College of Obstetricians and Gynecologists (ACOG 2019), the Canadian Urological Association (Krakowsky and Grober, 2018) and the International Consultation on Sexual Medicine (Hatzichristou et al., 2016).

data are responsive, reliable and quantifiable. Validated questionnaires utilized to assess FSD may be generalized or condition specific (Kammerer-Doak, 2009).

The following categorization of the included questionnaires has been adapted from Giraldi et al. (2011):
1. General assessment of FSD, including distress questionnaires
2. Assessment of specific dysfunctions/function (limited to FSD and PFD; urinary incontinence, anal incontinence and pelvic organ prolapse)
3. Assessment of sexual function in selected groups (limited to pregnancy-related sexual dysfunction and menopausal-related sexual dysfunction)

Due to the large number of questionnaires available to assess FSD, we have included those recommended by the International Continence Society (ICS) (Omotosho and Rogers, 2009), the ICSM (Hatzichristou et al., 2016) and the Fifth International Consultation

on Incontinence (Cherian et al., 2013). We have decided to include questionnaires that scored grade A (highly recommended with rigor) and grade B (recommended) (Cherian et al., 2013) and levels 1 and 2 (Hatzichristou et al., 2016). We additionally have included validated questionnaires covering important aspects of FSD (Box 7.4.4).

General Assessment of Female Sexual Dysfunction (Generalized Questionnaires)

Generalized questionnaires focus on evaluating sexual function in a general population and not specifically in women with sexual dysfunction or PFD. These types of questionnaires may not be sensitive enough to detect differences in sexual function due, for example, to incontinence and pelvic organ prolapse. To incorporate the ICF model of body function, activity or participation (WHO, 2001), we will first present questionnaires

---

BOX 7.4.4 Questionnaires Recommended to Include in the Assessment of Female Sexual Dysfunction

Questionnaire	Population	Level of Evidence
Goal Attainment Scale (GAS)	Generic	NA
Patient-Specific Functional Scale (PSFS)	Generic	NA
EuroQoL Health-Related Quality of Life (EQ-5D)	Generic	NA
Female Genital Self-Image Scale-7 (FGSIS-7)	Generic	A-1
Body Appreciation Scale 2 (BAS-2)	Generic	NA
International Physical Activity Questionnaire–Short Form (IPAQ-SF)	Generic	NA
Female Sexual Function Index (FSFI)	Generic/women with orgasmic disorder and HSDD	A-1
Brief Index of Sexual Functioning for Women (BISF-W)	Generic/surgically menopausal women	B
Female Sexual Distress Scale (FSDS/ FSDS-R)	Generic/HSDD in premenopausal women	A-1
The Pelvic Organ Prolapse/Urinary Incontinence Sexual Questionnaire (PISQ-12)	Women with urinary incontinence/pelvic organ prolapse	A
PISQ-IR (IUGA revised)	Women with faecal incontinence/sexually inactive women	A
Australian Pelvic Floor Questionnaire (APFQ)/ Pelvic Floor Questionnaire	Women with urogynaecological symptoms	NA
International Consultation on Incontinence Questionnaire (ICIQ)	Women with urinary incontinence/pelvic organ prolapse/faecal incontinence	A
Sexual Interest and Desire Inventory–Female (SIDI-F)	Women with HSDD	B-2
Screener for Hypoactive Sexual Desire Disorder (SHSDD)	Postmenopausal women with HSDD	NA

HSDD, Hypoactive sexual desire disorder; *NA,* not applicable.

used to assess more general impairment that can be used to individualize the treatment.

The Goal Attainment Scale (GAS) is a therapeutic method with follow-up of written attainment goals that is patient self-reported (Smith, 1976). The scale has shown satisfactory inter- and intra-rater reliability in goals related to chronic pain and excellent inter-rater reliability for goals related to self-esteem and romantic relations.

The Patient-Specific Functional Scale (PSFS) is used as a self-report outcome measure of function with a difficulty score from 0 to 10 that could be used in patients with varying levels of independence (Stratford et al., 1995). The PSFS is a valid, reliable and responsive outcome measure for patients with musculoskeletal problems.

The EuroQoL Health-Related Quality of Life (EQ-5D) is a self-report measure consisting of five items scored on a Likert scale covering walking, personal care, daily activities, pain/discomfort and anxiety/depression in addition to an overall score of general health problems (EuroQol Office, 2020). EQ-5D has been translated into several languages and has shown valid, responsive and reliable properties for a range of health problems.

The Female Genital Self-Image Scale 7 (FGSIS-7) consists of seven questions designed to evaluate feelings and beliefs about one's own genitals. The questionnaire has shown good internal consistency ($\alpha = 0.88$) and validity (concurrent validity as compared with the Female Sexual Function Index [FSFI]: $p < 0.001$). Recommendations for use by the ICSM (grade A-1) (Hatzichristou et al., 2016).

The Body Appreciation Scale 2 (BAS-2) is a development from the original BAS questionnaire assessing individuals' acceptance of, favourable opinions towards and respect for their bodies (Tylka and Wood-Barcalow, 2015). BAS-2 is a 10-item questionnaire that is valid and reliable in a general population of both men and women.

The International Physical Activity Questionnaire–Short Form (IPAQ-SF) (Craig et al., 2003) is used to assess the level of physical activity. IPAQ-SF is a reliable and valid questionnaire for adults containing three parts, where the first part consists of eight items covering the frequency and intensity of physical activity. IPAQ-SF has been used worldwide and has been translated into several languages.

Generic questionnaires focusing on sexual function. The Female Sexual Function Index (FSFI) is designed to measure FSD in a 19-item self-report measure which gives scores on six domains: sexual desire, arousal, lubrication, orgasm, satisfaction and pain (Rosen et al., 2000). The FSFI has shown adequate test–retest reliability ($r = 0.79$–0.88) and excellent internal consistency ($\alpha = 0.89$–0.97). The questionnaire is designed for women with a partner who are sexually active, and it has been translated into several languages. The FSFI should be combined with a measure of distress (Giraldi et al., 2011), such as the Female Sexual Distress Scale (FSDS). Recommendations for use are by the ICSM (grade A-1) (Hatzichristou et al., 2016).

The Brief Index of Sexual Functioning for Women (BISF-W) is a 22-item self-administered questionnaire designed to assess female sexual function and satisfaction in seven domains: thoughts/desire, arousal, frequency of sexual activity, receptivity/initiation, relationship satisfaction, pleasure/orgasm and problems (Taylor et al., 1994). The BISF-W has shown adequate test–retest reliability ($r = 0.68$–0.78) for the measurement of sexual function. Internal consistency ranges from low to acceptable ($\alpha = 0.39$–0.83). The BISF-W has been translated into several languages. The most notable strength of this scale is its neutrality with regards to women with different sexual preferences and partner status. Recommendations for use are by the ICS (grade B) (Omotosho and Rogers, 2009).

The Female Sexual Distress Scale (FSDS) was originally designed as a 12-item questionnaire to assess distress associated with impaired sexual function (Derogatis et al., 2002). The questionnaire addresses both intensity and frequency of distress on a 5-point Likert scale. A revised version (FSDS-R) was published as a 13-item questionnaire to cover sexual distress among women with hypoactive sexual desire disorder (Derogatis et al., 2008). Both versions show good internal consistency ($\alpha > 0.86$) and test–retest reliability ($r = 0.74$–0.91). The FSDS-R also demonstrates high discriminant validity, successfully identifying 92.7% of patients diagnosed independently with hypoactive sexual desire disorder. Recommendations for use of FSDS-R are by the ICSM (grade A-1) (Hatzichristou et al., 2016).

Assessment of Specific Dysfunctions/Function (Condition-Specific Questionnaires)

Questionnaires for women with sexual dysfunction. The FSFI has been validated among women with orgasmic disorder and in women with hypoactive sexual desire disorder (Meston, 2003). For more information, see the discussion on generic questionnaires.

There are no questionnaires recommended for use to assess female sexual arousal dysfunction (Cartagena-Ramos et al., 2018; Hatzichristou et al., 2016).

Questionnaires for women with pelvic floor dysfunction. The International Consultation on Incontinence Questionnaire (ICIQ) has several questionnaires that assess the impact of vaginal symptoms including prolapse (ICIQ-VS), sexual matters associated with urinary incontinence (ICIQ-FLUTSsex) and bowel symptoms (ICIQ-Bsex) on sexual life including a bother scale. The questionnaires have shown good validity, reliability and sensitivity to change. They have been translated into several languages and are available upon request at https://www.iciq.org. Recommendations for use are by the Fifth International Consultation on Incontinence (grade A) (Cherian et al., 2013).

The Pelvic Organ Prolapse/Urinary Incontinence Sexual Function Questionnaire (PISQ-12) is a validated short form of the original long form (Rogers et al., 2001) covering 12 items of behavioural and emotive, physical and partner-related domains. PISQ-12 is targeted for women with pelvic organ prolapse and urinary incontinence (Rogers et al., 2003). Recommendations for use are by the ICS (grade A) (Kaminska et al., 2019) and the ICSM (grade B-2) (Hatzichristou et al., 2016).

The The Pelvic Organ Prolapse/Urinary Incontinence Sexual Function Questionnaire–International Urogynecological Association (IUGA) Revised (PISQ-IR) has been validated and enables the assessment of sexual function in women who are not sexually active and in women with faecal incontinence (Rogers et al., 2013). Recommendations for use are by the ICS (grade A) (Kaminska et al., 2019). Both PISQ-12 and PISQ-IR are available in several languages and are the only questionnaires that comprehensively assess sexual function in women with PFD.

The Australian Pelvic Floor Questionnaire (APFQ)/Pelvic Floor Questionnaire is a reliable and valid interviewer-administered pelvic floor questionnaire that integrates bladder, bowel and prolapse symptoms and questions on sexual function in an urogynaecological population (Baessler et al., 2009). The sexual function domain gives a separate score on 11 items related to vaginal looseness, tightness, lubrication, sensation, pain and reasons for not being sexually active. The questionnaire has not been included for recommendations in the previous reviews on FSD (Hatzichristou et al., 2016).

Assessment of Sexual Function in Selected Groups

Menopause-related sexual dysfunction. The BISF-W has been validated in menopausal women undergoing surgery (Mazer et al., 2000). For more information, see the discussion on generic questionnaires.

The FSDS-R has been validated as a 13-item questionnaire to cover sexual distress among premenopausal women with hypoactive sexual desire disorder (Derogatis et al., 2008). For more information, see the discussion on generic questionnaires.

The Sexual Interest and Desire Inventory–Female (SIDI-F) is an administrator-based 13-item questionnaire focusing on measuring severity and change in response to the treatment of hypoactive sexual desire disorder in premenopausal women (Sills et al., 2005). SIDI-F shows excellent internal consistency ($\alpha = 0.90$) and good to very good reliability ($r = 0.85$–0.90); however, measures of validity have been weaker, showing conflicting and limited evidence (Cartagena-Ramos et al., 2018). Recommendations for use are by the ICSM (grade B-2) (Hatzichristou et al., 2016), although the instrument recommends that further robustness and contemporary techniques are taken (Cartagena-Ramos et al., 2018).

The Screener for Hypoactive Sexual Desire Disorder (SHSDD) is a self-report instrument developed to screen postmenopausal women for hypoactive sexual desire disorder using four questions (Hatzichristou et al., 2016). The SHSDD has demonstrated good internal consistency and test–retest reliability ($r = 0.70$) and good content and structural validity in determining the presence versus absence of hypoactive sexual desire disorder in a group of postmenopausal women. The instrument recommends that further robustness and contemporary techniques are taken (Cartagena-Ramos et al., 2018).

Pregnancy-related sexual dysfunction. There are no questionnaires recommended for use to assess pregnancy-related sexual dysfunction (ACOG, 2019; Hatzichristou et al., 2016; Tennfjord, 2017).

CLINICAL EXAMINATION AND METHODS

A physical examination is highly recommended in the assessment of FSD (ACOG, 2019; Hatzichristou et al., 2016; Krakowsky and Grober, 2018), and a gynaecological examination focused on the areas of concern can detect possible gynaecological pathologies responsible for sexual dysfunction. A list of what a general gynaecological examination should include for the assessment of FSD is given in Box 7.4.5.

Based on the condition or underlying factors that are reviled in the history, physiotherapists must be aware of possible red and yellow flags that require referral to other resources involved in the assessment of FSD (see Fig. 7.4.2).

Assessment of Body Function and Structure

It must be noted that although the available guidelines for the assessment and treatment of FSD include physiotherapy, there is no detailed overview of different physiotherapeutic assessment methods or tools in these reviews (ACOG, 2019; Hatzichristou et al., 2016; Krakowsky and Grober, 2018). The following description of assessment methods is therefore based on the scientific framework explained in the introduction of this chapter.

BOX 7.4.5   Details in a Gynaecological Examination to Assess Female Sexual Dysfunction (This Overview Does Not Include Specialized Tests)

General appearance of the vulva and vulvar area
  Vulvoscopy
  Cue tip testing for vulvodynia
  Vaginal pH for atrophic vaginitis
  Hormonal status: thyroid stimulating hormone, prolactin, sex hormone-binding globulin, estradiol, total testosterone and calculated free testosterone
  Abdominal examination
  Transperineal ultrasound/vaginal ultrasound
  Vaginal examination and palpation of the inner reproductive organs
  Note: Laboratory testing is often not necessary in the initial evaluation of female sexual dysfunction unless an undiagnosed medical aetiology is suspected.

Adapted from the American College of Obstetricians and Gynecologists (ACOG 2019), the Canadian Urological Association (Krakowsky and Grober, 2018) and the International Consultation on Sexual Medicine (Hatzichristou et al., 2016).

For a detailed description of the various assessment methods, and their reliability and validity, we refer the reader to the ICS/IUGA reports from Bø et al. (2017) and Haylen et al. (2010), as well as Chapter 5.

The physiotherapeutic assessment will start off by examining general movement when the woman enters the room, her posture and how she is sitting (Berghmans, 2018). Further assessment includes examining active movement of the spine and testing for range of motion on the hips and nearby joints. Assessment for breathing patterns, mobility, tension, strength and pain is essential (Tennfjord et al., 2017). Abdominal signs to look for include bladder fullness/retention by abdominal palpation. The perineal region is then examined looking for symptoms and signs associated with PFD (Bø et al. 2017; Haylen et al., 2010). If PFD is suspected, look for its signs and symptoms (Haylen et al., 2010). Assessment for perineal descent, trophic or atrophic signs of the perineum, scars, color and irregularities is important. Look for neurological signs including altered sensation (allodynia and hyperalgesia), muscle tone, especially the S2-S4 dermatome (pudendal), (further description will follow) and/or reflexes.

Assessment of Pelvic Floor Muscle Function

A physiotherapeutic approach in relation to PFD and FSD should include inspection, palpation, and preferably the use of electromyography, dynamometry, perineometry, dynamometry or ultrasound of the contractile components of the PFMs (Bø et al., 2017; Haylen et al., 2010). Furthermore, a description of patient position (supine or side-lying) is important in addition to a description of the depth and location of your palpation, the amount of pressure applied and how many fingers used for palpation. First assess for normal PFM contractile function, observed and palpated as a constriction and inward movement of the pelvic opening. Normally functioning PFMs should also include a voluntary and involuntary relaxation after a PFM contraction (Messelink et al., 2005). The modified Oxford scale is commonly used among physiotherapists to quantify PFM strength in terms of a maximal voluntary contraction ranging from 0 (meaning no contraction) to 5 (a strong contraction with lift of the muscle) (Bø et al., 2017; Laycock, 1994). However, its ability to differentiate between weak, moderate, good or strong contractions has been questioned (Bø and Finckenhagen, 2001; Morin et al.,

2004). A vaginal and rectal examination may be part of this investigation. Assess and look for extrapelvic muscle activity, such as that of the abdominals, gluteal muscles and adductors.

Another commonly used measure of PFM function is the measure of tone, tension and stiffness, and is the state of the muscle at rest and has been presented in several grading systems using palpation (Bø et al., 2017; Davidson et al., 2020; Devreese et al., 2004; Dietz and Shek, 2008; Haylen et al., 2010). There have also been attempts of measuring PFM stiffness with an elastometer on a scale ranging from +3 (very firm resistance and minimal movement of the muscle to palpation) down to −3 (no resistance and muscle not palpable), with 0 being normal (Davidson et al., 2020). It must be noted that there are no single accepted or standardized ways of measuring tone, tension or stiffness, and there are no normative values, making comparison difficult (Bø et al., 2017). The ICS recommends using the terms *increased tone*, which is an increase in muscle tone related to the contractile or the viscoelastic components of the pelvic floor, and *decreased tone*, which is a decrease in muscle tone related to the contractile or the viscoelastic components of the pelvic floor (Frawley et al., 2021).

REFERENCES

Achtari, C., & Dwyer, P. L. (2005). Sexual function and pelvic floor disorders. *Best Practice & Research Clinical Obstetrics & Gynaecology*, 19(6), 993–1008 quiz A1001–A1008.

Allen, M. S., & Walter, E. E. (2018). Health-related lifestyle factors and sexual dysfunction: A meta-analysis of population-based research. *The Journal of Sexual Medicine*, 15(4), 458–475.

American College of Obstetricians and Gynecologists (ACOG) Committee on Practice Bulletins—Gynecology. (2019). Female sexual dysfunction: ACOG practice bulletin clinical management guidelines for obstetrician-gynecologists, number 213. *Obstetrics & Gynecology*, 134(1), e1–e18.

American Psychiatric Association (APA). (2013). Diagnostic and statistical manual of mental disorders (5th ed.). Washington, DC: American Psychiatric Press.

Baessler, K., O'Neill, S. M., Maher, C. F., et al. (2009). Australian Pelvic Floor Questionnaire: A validated interviewer-administered pelvic floor questionnaire for routine clinic and research. *International Urogynecology Journal and Pelvic Floor Dysfunction*, 20, 149–158.

Basson, R. (2001). Using a different model for female sexual response to address women's problematic low sexual desire. *Journal of Sex & Marital Therapy*, 27(5), 395–403.

Berghmans, B. (2018). Physiotherapy for pelvic pain and female sexual dysfunction: An untapped resource. *International Urogynecology Journal*, 29(5), 631–638.

Bø, K., & Finckenhagen, H. B. (2001). Vaginal palpation of pelvic floor muscle strength: Inter-test reproducibility and comparison between palpation and vaginal squeeze pressure. *Acta Obstetricia et Gynecologica Scandinavica*, 80, 883–887.

Bø, K., Frawley, H. C., Haylen, B. T., et al. (2017). An International Urogynecological Association (IUGA)/International Continence Society (ICS) joint report on the terminology for the conservative and nonpharmacological management of female pelvic floor dysfunction. *Neurourology and Urodynamics*, 36(2), 221–244.

Cartagena-Ramos, D., Fuentealba-Torres, M., Rebustini, F., et al. (2018). Systematic review of the psychometric properties of instruments to measure sexual desire. *BMC Medical Research Methodology*, 18(1), 109.

Cherian, P., Cotterill, N., & Coyne, K. (2013). Patient-reported outcome assessment. In P. Abrams, L. Cardozo, S. Khoury, et al. (Eds.), *Incontinence*. Paris: European Association of Urology pp. 389–428.

Craig, C. L., Marshall, A. L., Sjostrom, M., et al. (2003). International Physical Activity Questionnaire: 12-country reliability and validity. *Medicine & Science in Sports & Exercise*, 35(8), 1381–1395.

Davidson, M. J., Nielsen, P. M. F., Taberner, A. J., et al. (2020). Is it time to rethink using digital palpation for assessment of muscle stiffness? *Neurourology and Urodynamics*, 39(1), 279–285.

De Menezes Franco, M., Driusso, P., Bø, K., et al. (2017). Relationship between pelvic floor muscle strength and sexual dysfunction in postmenopausal women: A cross-sectional study. *International Urogynecology Journal*, 28(6), 931–936.

Delancey, J. O., Kane Low, L., Miller, J. M., et al. (2008). Graphic integration of causal factors of pelvic floor disorders: An integrated life span model. *American Journal of Obstetrics and Gynecology*, 199(6), 610.e1–610.e5.

Derogatis, L., Clayton, A., & Lewis-D'Agostino, D. (2008). Validation of the Female Sexual Distress Scale–Revised for assessing distress in women with hypoactive sexual desire disorder. *The Journal of Sexual Medicine*, 5(2), 357–364.

Derogatis, L. R., Rosen, R., Leiblum, S., et al. (2002). The Female Sexual Distress Scale (FSDS): Initial validation of a standardized scale for assessment of sexually related personal distress in women. *Journal of Sex & Marital Therapy*, 28(4), 317–330.

Devreese, A., Staes, F., De Weerdt, W., et al. (2004). Clinical evaluation of pelvic floor muscle function in continent and incontinent women. *Neurourology and Urodynamics*, *23*(3), 190–197.

Dietz, H. P., & Shek, K. L. (2008). The quantification of levator muscle resting tone by digital assessment. *International Urogynecology Journal and Pelvic Floor Dysfunction*, *19*(11), 1489–1493.

EuroQol Office. (2020). *EQ-5D [online]*. Available: https://euroqol.org/euroqol/ (accessed 01.10.20).

Frawley, H., Shelly, B., Morin, M., et al. (2021). An International Continence Society (ICS) report on the terminology for pelvic floor muscle assessment. *Neurourol Urodyn*, *40*(5), 1217–1260.

Filamenco, M. T., & Donato, N. D. (2017). Evaluation systems of female sexual function. In E. Constantini, D. Villari, & N. T. Filacamo (Eds.), *Female sexual function and dysfunction* (pp. 33–46). Cham, Switzerland: Springer.

Fitzpatrick, R., Davey, C., Buxton, M. J., et al. (1998). Evaluating patient-based outcome measures for use in clinical trials. *Health Technology Assessment*, *2*(14), 1–74 i–iv.

Giraldi, A., Rellini, A., Pfaus, J. G., et al. (2011). Questionnaires for assessment of female sexual dysfunction: A review and proposal for a standardized screener. *The Journal of Sexual Medicine*, *8*(10), 2681–2706.

Graziottin, A. (2004). Similarities and differences between male and female sexual dysfunction. *The Journal of Men's Health & Gender*, *1*(1), 71–76.

Grzybowska, M. E., & Wydra, D. G. (2019). Is voluntary pelvic floor muscles contraction important for sexual function in women with pelvic floor disorders? *Neurourology and Urodynamics*, *38*(7), 2001–2009.

Hatzichristou, D., Kirana, P. S., Banner, L., et al. (2016). Diagnosing sexual dysfunction in men and women: Sexual history taking and the role of symptom scales and questionnaires. *The Journal of Sexual Medicine*, *13*(8), 1166–1182.

Haylen, B. T., de Ridder, D., & Freeman, R. M. (2010). An International Urogynecological Association (IUGA)/International Continence Society (ICS) joint report on the terminology for female pelvic floor dysfunction. *International Urogynecology Journal*, *21*(1), 5–26.

Hilde, G., Staer-Jensen, J., Siafarikas, F., et al. (2013). Impact of childbirth and mode of delivery on vaginal resting pressure and on pelvic floor muscle strength and endurance. *American Journal of Obstetrics and Gynecology*, *208*(1), 50.e1–50.e7.

Hoffman, B. L., Schorge, J. O., Schaffer, J. I., et al. (2012). *Williams Gynecology*. New York: McGraw Hill Medical.

IsHak, W. W., & Tobia, G. (2013). DSM-5 changes in diagnostic criteria of sexual dysfunctions. *Reproductive System & Sexual Disorders*, *2*(2), 122.

Jha, S., & Thakar, R. (2010). Female sexual dysfunction. *European Journal of Obstetrics & Gynecology and Reproductive Biology*, *153*, 117–123.

Jiandani, M. P., & Mhatre, B. S. (2018). Physical therapy diagnosis: How is it different? *Journal of Postgraduate Medicine*, *64*(2), 69–72.

Kaminska, A., Futyma, K., Romanek-Piva, K., et al. (2019). Sexual function specific questionnaires as a useful tool in management of urogynecological patients—review. *European Journal of Obstetrics & Gynecology and Reproductive Biology*, *234*, 126–130.

Kammerer-Doak, D. (2009). Assessment of sexual function in women with pelvic floor dysfunction. *International Urogynecology Journal*, *20*(Suppl. 1), 45–50.

Kanter, G., Rogers, R. G., Pauls, R. N., et al. (2015). A strong pelvic floor is associated with higher rates of sexual activity in women with pelvic floor disorders. *International Urogynecology Journal*, *26*(7), 991–996.

Kingsberg, S. A., Schaffir, J., & Faught, B. M. (2019). Female sexual health: Barriers to optimal outcomes and a roadmap for improved patient–clinician communications. *Journal Womens Health (Larchmt.)*, *28*(4), 432–443.

Krakowsky, Y., & Grober, E. D. (2018). A practical guide to female sexual dysfunction: An evidence-based review for physicians in Canada. *Can Urology Associate Journal*, *12*(6), 211–216.

Laycock, J. (1994). Clinical evaluation of the pelvic floor. In B. Schussler, J. Laycock, P. A. Norton, et al. (Eds.), *Pelvic floor Re-education: Principles and practice* (pp. 42–48). London: Springer Verlag.

Leeman, L. M., & Rogers, R. G. (2012). Sex after childbirth: Postpartum sexual function. *Obstetrics & Gynecology*, *119*(3), 647–655.

Masters, W. H., & Johnson, V. E. (1966). *Human sexual response*. Boston: Little Brown.

Mazer, N. A., Leiblum, S. R., & Rosen, R. C. (2000). The Brief Index of Sexual Functioning for Women (BISF-W): A new scoring algorithm and comparison of normative and surgically menopausal populations. *Menopause*, *7*(5), 350–363.

McCabe, M. P., Sharlip, I. D., Atalla, E., et al. (2016). Definitions of sexual dysfunctions in women and men: A consensus statement from the Fourth International Consultation on Sexual Medicine 2015. *The Journal of Sexual Medicine*, *13*(2), 135–143.

McCabe, M. P., Sharlip, I. D., Lewis, R., et al. (2016). Incidence and prevalence of sexual dysfunction in women and men: A consensus statement from the Fourth International Consultation on Sexual Medicine 2015. *The Journal of Sexual Medicine*, *13*(2), 144–152.

McCool, M. E., Zuelke, A., Theurich, M. A., et al. (2016). Prevalence of female sexual dysfunction among premenopausal women: A systematic review and meta-analysis of observational studies. *Sex. Med. Rev.*, *4*(3), 197–212.

Messelink, B., Benson, T., Berghmans, B., et al. (2005). Standardization of terminology of pelvic floor muscle function and dysfunction: Report from the pelvic floor clinical assessment group of the International Continence Society. *Neurourology and Urodynamics, 24*(4), 374–380.

Meston, C. M. (2003). Validation of the Female Sexual Function Index (FSFI) in women with female orgasmic disorder and in women with hypoactive sexual desire disorder. *Journal of Sex & Marital Therapy, 29*, 36–46.

Morin, M., Bourbonnais, D., Gravel, D., et al. (2004). Pelvic floor maximal strength using vaginal digital assessment compared to dynamometric measurements. *Neurourology and Urodynamics, 23*(4), 336–341.

Nygaard, I., & Barber, M. D. (2008). Prevalence of symptomatic pelvic floor disorders in US women. *JAMA, 17*, 1311–1316.

O'Keeffe, M., Cullinane, P., Hurley, J., et al. (2016). What influences patient–therapist interactions in musculoskeletal physical therapy? Qualitative systematic review and meta-synthesis. *Physical Therapy, 96*(5), 609–622.

Omotosho, T. B., & Rogers, R. G. (2009). Shortcomings/strengths of specific sexual function questionnaires currently used in urogynecology: A literature review. *International Urogynecology Journal and Pelvic Floor Dysfunction, 20*(Suppl. 1), 51–56.

Reimers, C., Staer-Jensen, J., & Siafarikas, F. (2016). Change in pelvic organ support during pregnancy and the first year postpartum: A longitudinal study. *British Journal of Obstetrics and Gynaecology, 123*(5), 821–829.

Rogers, R. G., Coates, K. W., Kammerer-Doak, D. N., et al. (2003). A short form of the Pelvic Organ Prolapse/Urinary Incontinence Sexual Questionnaire (PISQ-12). *International Urogynecology Journal and Pelvic Floor Dysfunction, 14*, 164–168.

Rogers, R. G., Kammerer-Doak, D. N., Villarreal, A., et al. (2001). A new instrument to measure sexual function in women with urinary incontinence or pelvic organ prolapse. *American Journal of Obstetrics and Gynecology, 184*, 552–558.

Rogers, R. G., Rockwood, T. H., Constantine, M. L., et al. (2013). A new measure of sexual function in women with Pelvic Organ Prolapse/Incontinence Sexual Questionnaire, IUGA–Revised (PISQ-IR). *International Urogynecology Journal, 24*(7), 1091–1103.

Roos, A. M., Speksnijder, L., & Steensma, A. B. (2020). Postpartum sexual function; the importance of the levator ani muscle. *International Urogynecology Journal, 31*(11), 2261–2267.

Rosen, R. C., Brown, C., Heiman, J., et al. (2000). The Female Sexual Function Index (FSFI): A multidimensional self-report instrument for the assessment of female sexual function. *Journal of Sex & Marital Therapy, 26*, 191–208.

Sadovsky, R. (2002). The role of the primary care clinician in the management of erectile dysfunction. *Reviews in Urology, 4*(Suppl. 3), 54–63.

Shafik, A. (2000). The role of the levator ani muscle in evacuation, sexual performance and pelvic floor disorders. *International Urogynecology Journal and Pelvic Floor Dysfunction, 11*(6), 361–376.

Sills, T., Wunderlich, G., Pyke, R., et al. (2005). The Sexual Interest and Desire Inventory–Female (SIDI-F): Item response analyses of data from women diagnosed with hypoactive sexual desire disorder. *The Journal of Sexual Medicine, 2*(6), 801–818.

Smith, D. L. (1976). Goal attainment scaling as an adjunct to counseling. *Journal Counseling Psychology, 23*(1), 22–27.

Staer-Jensen, J., Siafarikas, F., Hilde, G., et al. (2015). Postpartum recovery of levator hiatus and bladder neck mobility in relation to pregnancy. *Obstetrics & Gynecology, 125*(3), 531–539.

Stratford, P., Gill, C., & Westaway, M. (1995). Assessing disability and change on individual patients Physiother. *Can, 47*(4), 258–263.

Taylor, J. F., Rosen, R. C., & Leiblum, S. R. (1994). Self-report assessment of female sexual function: Psychometric evaluation of the Brief Index of Sexual Functioning for Women. *Archives of Sexual Behavior, 23*(6), 627–643.

Tennfjord, M. K. (2017). *Pelvic floor muscle function, vaginal symptoms and symptoms of sexual dysfunction in first time mothers: A cohort and a randomised controlled trial. Doctoral thesis.* Norwegian School of Sport Sciences.

Tennfjord, M. K., Ellström Engh, M., & Bø, K. (2017). Role of physical therapy in the treatment of female sexual dysfunction. In: Female sexual function and dysfunction. In E. Costantini, D. Villari, M. Filocamo, et al. (Eds.), *Female sexual function and dysfunction.* Cham, Switzerland: Springer. 289–204.

Tennfjord, M. K., Hilde, G., Staer-Jensen, J., et al. (2014). Dyspareunia and pelvic floor muscle function before and during pregnancy and after childbirth. *International Urogynecology Journal, 25*, 1227–1235.

Tennfjord, M. K., Hilde, G., Staer-Jensen, J., et al. (2015). Coital incontinence and vaginal symptoms and the relationship to pelvic floor muscle function in primiparous women at 12 months postpartum: A cross-sectional study. *The Journal of Sexual Medicine, 12*(4), 994–1003.

Tylka, T. L., & Wood-Barcalow, N. L. (2015). The Body Appreciation Scale −2: Item refinement and psychometric evaluation. *Body Image, 12*, 53–67.

Weber, A. M., Abrams, P., Brubaker, L., et al. (2001). The standardization of terminology for researchers in female pelvic floor disorders. *International Urogynecology Journal, 12*, 178–186.

World Health Organization. (2001). *International classification of functioning, disability and health (ICF) [online].* Available: https://www.who.int/classifications/icf/en/ (accessed 10.07.20).

World Health Organization. (2019). *ICD-11: International classification of diseases 11th revision. The global standard for Diagnostic health information [online].* Available: https://icd.who.int/en (accessed 28.10.20).

Pelvic Floor Muscle Training as an Intervention to Treat Female Sexual Dysfunction

Cristine Homsi Jorge and Merete Kolberg Tennfjord

Although several physiotherapy interventions for female sexual dysfunction can be found in the literature, almost all randomized controlled trials (RCTs) aiming to improve sexual function or treat non-painful sexual complaints investigated pelvic floor muscle training (PFMT). This chapter will focus on the evidence of PFMT from RCTs including PFMT alone or combined with other interventions.

RATIONALE FOR THE EFFECT OF PELVIC FLOOR MUSCLE TRAINING ON FEMALE SEXUAL FUNCTION

The different mechanisms by which PFMT could improve women's sexual function have been postulated. Back in 1952, Kegel advocated that PFMT could improve pelvic floor muscle (PFM) strength impacting women's capacity to achieve orgasm. Other authors have highlighted the ability of the PFMs to contract and their tone and strength as important factors to provide pleasure for both partners during intercourse. More than one study in the literature has shown an association between better PFM function and better sexual function in women (De Menezes Franco et al., 2017; Lowenstein et al., 2010; Martinez et al., 2014). According to Shafik (2000a, 2000b) the strength of the muscles attached to the corpus cavernous of the clitoris could increase the arousal and orgasmic response provided by a better involuntary contraction of the PFMs. A vascular hypothesis claims that PFMT could contribute to improvement in arousal, lubrication and orgasm by increased blood flow to the pelvis and clitoral sensitivity (Graber and Kline-Graber, 1979; Ma and Qin, 2009). Other possibilities include better body self-perception and PFM control favouring women's ability to relax the muscle and contract, providing a vaginal receptivity to the penis and more pleasure for both partners. It is possible that PFMT can increase orgasm intensity, maybe more than women's capacity to achieve orgasm. The levator ani muscles and the bulbocavernosus muscle play an active role in sexual response, providing rhythmic contractions during orgasm. Theoretically, if these muscles are stronger, they could provide more intense orgasms or a higher number of PFM rhythmic contractions during orgasm. However, women's capacity to achieve orgasm depends on many other variables not necessarily associated to PFM function.

RESEARCH METHODS

The literature search included the following databases: PubMed (from 1946 to October 2020, Ovid MEDLINE (from 1946 to October 2020), Scopus and Cochrane Central Register of Controlled Trials (CENTRAL), the Physiotherapy Evidence Database (PEDro) and Cochrane Database of Systematic Reviews (Issue 10 of 12, October 2020). The keywords used in different combinations in the search were as follows: *physiotherapy, women, female, sexual function, sexual dysfunction, exercise, PFMT*. Inclusion criteria were full text articles or abstracts of RCTs published in English addressing pelvic floor interventions or rehabilitation programmes including the PFMT in at least one arm, aiming to improve female sexual function or treat sexual dysfunction in women. All abstracts were read to identify RCTs according to the inclusion criteria. Two reviewers analysed the eligibility of articles, and any disagreement was resolved by consensus.

Risk of Bias

The risk of bias of included studies was assessed using the PEDro scale, which is a valid and reliable tool consisting of an 11-item checklist (Macedo et al., 2010). The score given in the database was used in this chapter.

Scientific Evidence

The search yielded a total of 3457 studies. After exclusions were applied and the removal of duplicate studies, 25 studies were included for qualitative synthesis. The outcome measures, content of the intervention and results of the studies are presented in Table 7.4.3.

There is a great heterogeneity of outcome measures and interventions, as the studies were published between 1983 and 2019. The size of the studies varied from 12 (Trudel and Saint-Laurent, 1983) to 477 participants (Hagen et al., 2014). The samples comprised heterogeneous populations in relation to the absence or presence of pelvic floor disorder (PFD). Most of the

TABLE 7.4.3 Randomized Controlled Trials Investigating the Effect of Pelvic Floor Muscle Training (Alone or in Combined With Other Intervention) on Female Sexual Function

Author	**Jha et al. (2018)**
Design	2-arm RCT Control (PFMT): n = 57 Intervention (PFMT + electrical stimulation): n = 57
Study population	114 women age >18 years presenting with urinary incontinence and sexual dysfunction
Control/intervention protocol	Control: 8 contractions performed 3×/day Intervention: 8 contractions performed 3×/day + electrical stimulation
Study withdrawals, n (% of full cohort)	Adverse effect: intervention, 1 (1%); control, 4 (7%) Lost to follow-up: intervention, 18 (31%); control, 12 (21%) Discontinued intervention: intervention, 6 (10%); control, 4 (7%) Excluded from analysis: intervention, 2 (3%); control, 3 (5%)
Outcomes	Completers' results: intervention, n = 30; control, n = 34 PISQ physical function dimension at post-treatment (primary), other dimensions of PISQ, SF-36, EQ-5D, EPAQ, resource use, adverse events and cost effectiveness (secondary outcomes) Primary outcomes: mean difference of PISQ domains between control and intervention PISQ: p = 0.474 SF-36: p = 0.345 EQ-5D: p = 0.412 EPAQ: p = 0.748 No differences between groups in any of the secondary outcomes at follow-up
Author	**Hwang et al. (2019)**
Design	2-arm RCT Intervention (electrical stimulation of PFM): n = 17 Control (PFMT): n = 17
Study population	34 women with SUI (mean age 41.7 years)
Control/intervention protocol	Intervention: Subjects were asked to use the device once a day (15-min session), 5 or 6 days/week for 8 weeks. In addition, subjects performed an EasyK7 session with a possible increase in stimulation amplitude. The device delivered asymmetric and biphasic impulses of 25 Hz, with a mean intensity of 19.37 ± 6.29 mA (range: 2.5e30 mA) during sessions lasting 15 min; pulses were delivered for 11 s, with 11-s rest periods in between. Control: The control group walked for 10 min and underwent restricted PFMT with regards to PFM or abdominal muscle contraction. After 8 weeks, each subject in the control group was given an EasyK7 unit and was trained in its use as a reward for participating in the experiment.
Study withdrawals, n (% of full cohort)	Lost to follow-up: intervention, 1 (5%); control, 1 (5%)
Outcomes	Completers' results: intervention, n = 16; control, n = 16 PFM parameters (strength, power, and endurance) and female sexual function were assessed using a perineometer and the FSFI. There were significant differences in PFM strength, power, and endurance and FSFI domain scores (desire, arousal, orgasm, satisfaction and total score) in both between-group analyses (intervention vs control group) and within-group analyses (pre-intervention vs post-intervention). Change in PFM endurance had the highest association with change in FSFI total score (r = 0.437, p = 0.006), and change in PFM power had the highest association with change in FSFI satisfaction (r = 0.420, p = 0.008).

Continued

TABLE 7.4.3   **Randomized Controlled Trials Investigating the Effect of Pelvic Floor Muscle Training (Alone or in Combined With Other Intervention) on Female Sexual Function—cont'd**

Author	**Mosalanejad et al. (2018)**
Design	3-arm RCT Control (mindfulness): n = 25 Intervention 1 (PFMT): n = 25 Intervention 2 (group combining the preceding groups): n = 25
Study population	75 patients with multiple sclerosis (mean age 35.7 years)
Control/intervention protocol	Control: each session lasted 90 min and practice was performed once a week over 8 weeks Intervention 1: 10 pelvic floor and perineal muscle contractions, each lasting 5–10 s in the lying, sitting and standing positions, followed by 10 s of rest; in total, 60–100 contractions/day were performed; protocol 2×/day over 8 weeks Intervention 2: performed both mindfulness and PFM exercise for 8 weeks
Study withdrawals, n (% of full cohort)	Unable to regularly participate: control, 1 (4%); intervention 1, 2 (8%); intervention 2, 1 (4%) Disease relapses: control, 1 (4 %), intervention 1, 0 (0%), intervention 2, 0 (0%)
Outcomes	Completers' results: control, n = 23; intervention 1, n = 23; intervention 2, n = 24 FSFI The total mean scores of participants' sexual function in the PFM exercise group before interventions (i.e., baseline), 8 weeks after baseline and 12 weeks after baseline were 18.8 ± 6.3, 23.7 ± 5.1 and 22.3 ± 4.7, respectively, whereas the total mean scores obtained for sexual function of the mindfulness group were 19.5 ± 6.4, 26.9 ± 4.8 and 25.6 ± 4.5, respectively. Moreover, mean scores obtained for PFM exercise along with mindfulness were 19.6 ± 5.9, 25.3 ± 5.4 and 25 ± 4.8, respectively. There was no significant difference in their effects on sexual function ($p > 0.05$).
Author	**Weidner et al. (2017)**
Design	Secondary report of 2 × 2 factorial RCT Intervention (perioperative BPMT/later ULS or SSLF): 200/186 Control (usual perioperative care/later ULS or SSLF): 208/188
Study population	374 women with stage 2–4 POP and SUI
Control/intervention protocol	Intervention: The protocol included 5 in-person visits in the office setting, including 1 preoperative visit 2–4 weeks prior to surgery and 4 postoperative visits (2, 4–6, 8 and 12 weeks after surgery) with PFM examination and training, individualized progressive PFMT and education on behavioural strategies to reduce urinary and colorectal symptoms. These behavioural strategies included one-on-one in-person instructions on ways to prevent or reduce urinary incontinence, obstructed defaecation or voiding dysfunction such as proper toileting posture and muscular relaxation during defaecations. Control: Routine perioperative instructions were used at each clinical site (e.g., on diet, postoperative pain medications and lifting restrictions). All participants received this information.
Study withdrawals, n (% of full cohort)	Pre-randomization (surgical) withdraw: intervention, 14 (8.8%); control, 20 (10.5%) Post-randomization withdraw: intervention, 34 (18%); control, 24 (13%) No completed questionnaires: intervention, 15 (7.5%); control, 8 (4%)
Outcomes	Completers' results: intervention, n = 137; control, n = 146 Change in body image and in PFIQ short form subscale, PISQ-12 short form, PGII and Brink scores No statistically significant differences between groups in PFIQ, SF-36, PGII, PISQ-12 or body image scale measures
Author	**Golmakani et al. (2015)**
Design	2-arm RCT: intervention 52; control 52
Study population	104 primiparous women after delivery (mean age 25.88 years)

TABLE 7.4.3 Randomized Controlled Trials Investigating the Effect of Pelvic Floor Muscle Training (Alone or in Combined With Other Intervention) on Female Sexual Function—cont'd

Control/intervention protocol	Intervention: The intervention group was given face-to-face training about the anatomy and function of the PFMs and how to do Kegel exercises. A pamphlet and an audio CD about how to do Kegel exercises were presented to this group. They were asked to do these exercises twice daily, each time 15–20 times depending on ability to contract their PFMs for 5–10 s and relax for 5–10 s, then repeating this exercise 20 times (for 5 min). After 2 min of rest, they again had to perform this exercise 3 times for 5 min so that a total of 20 min of exercise was performed each time. Control: The control group had no intervention.
Losses to follow-up/ adherence	Lost to follow-up: intervention 12 (23%); control 13 (25%)
Outcomes	Completers' results: intervention, n = 40; control, n = 39 Bailes Sexual Self-Efficacy Questionnaire (desire, sensuality, arousal, orgasm, emotion, communication, body acceptance and rejection) and PFM strength There was a statistically significant difference between the two groups in terms of mean strength of PFMs 8 weeks after beginning the study ($p < 0.0001$). In the intervention group, the mean score of all aspects of sexual self-efficacy was significantly increased 8 weeks after the study compared to baseline: desire ($p < 0.0001$), sensuality ($p = 0.002$), arousal ($p < 0.0001$), orgasm ($p < 0.0001$), emotions ($p < 0.0001$), communication ($p < 0.0001$), body acceptance ($p < 0.0001$) and refusing sex ($p < 0.0001$). In the control group, only sexual desire ($p = 0.01$) showed significant differences 8 weeks after the study compared to baseline. The two groups had statistically significant differences at the end of the study in terms of sexual desire ($p = 0.001$), arousal ($p = 0.001$), orgasm ($p < 0.0001$) and body acceptance ($p = 0.001$).
Author	**Nazarpour et al. (2018)**
Design	2-arm RCT: Intervention (PFMT): 52 Control (information): 52
Study population	104 postmenopausal women age 40–60 years (mean age 52.98)
Control/intervention protocol	12 weeks Intervention: comprehensive instructions on the ways of identifying the PFMs and PFM exercises (contraction of the muscles for 10 s, relaxation for 10 s and repetition 10 times in 3–4 sessions/day) were provided using written material, images and videos. Control: General information regarding menopause and postmenopause was provided.
Losses to follow-up/ adherence	Intervention 5 (9%); control 2 (4%)
Outcomes	Completers' results: intervention, n = 47; control, n = 50 FSFI domains and total score: Desire: $p = 0.536$ Arousal: $p = 0.034$ Lubrication: $p = 0.600$ Orgasm: $p = 0.028$ Satisfaction: $p = 0.011$ Pain: $p = 0.693$ Total score: $p = 0.167$ After the intervention, the scores of arousal, orgasm and satisfaction were significantly higher in the intervention group (3.10, 4.36 and 4.84 vs 2.75, 3.89 and 4.36, respectively; $p < 0.05$).

Continued

TABLE 7.4.3 Randomized Controlled Trials Investigating the Effect of Pelvic Floor Muscle Training (Alone or in Combined With Other Intervention) on Female Sexual Function—cont'd

Author	**Liebergall-Wischnitzer et al. (2012)**
Design	2-arm RCT: Intervention (Paula method + PFMT): n = 119 Control (PFMT): n = 126
Study population	245 women with SUI (mean age 46.65 years)
Control/intervention protocol	Intervention: Private 45-min session/week for 12 weeks using the Paula method. Control: Groups which included 1–10 people for 30 min; once a week for 4 weeks. After the first month, there were 2 more meetings, 3 weeks apart, for a total of 6 sessions over 12 weeks. The instructors followed a predetermined frame of exercises to promote consistency in instruction. PFMT exercise included the following: identifying the levator ani by raising the vagina from the chair the person is sitting on, and contracting and releasing the levator ani muscle with prolonged contractions or rapid contractions or gradual contractions. Exercises were performed 10 s apart between contractions and 1–2 min apart between exercises. All exercises could be done by sitting, lying, standing or walking.
Losses to follow-up/ adherence	Did not receive allocated intervention - Intervention: n = 2 (1%) Control: n = 3 (2%) Not met inclusion criteria for SF questionnaire - Intervention: n = 28 (23%) Control :n = 25 (19%) Lost to follow up - Intervention: n = 23 (19%) Control: n = 38 (30%)
Outcomes	Completers' results: intervention, n = 47; control, n = 50 (PISQ-12) SF score improvement was found to be significant in both groups (Paula, p = 0.01; PFMT, p = 0.05) with no significant difference between groups.
Author	**Brækken et al. (2015)**
Design	2-arm RCT Intervention (PFMT + lifestyle advice) : n = 50 Control (lifestyle advice): n = 59
Study Population	109 women with stage 1–3 POP, regardless of POP symptoms (mean age 48.85 years)
Control/Intervention protocol	Both groups were taught how to contract their PFM before and during increases in abdominal pressure, such as with coughing, sneezing, and heavy lifting. Intervention: Three sets of 8–12 repetitions of near maximal PFM contractions daily. Exercise sessions were individually supervised by a physical therapist (PT) once a week during the first 3 months and every second week during the last 3 months. They also received a booklet and a DVD of the exercise programme. Control: Asked not to commence or alter preexisting PFMT regimes during the intervention period.
Losses to follow-up/ Adherence	Lost to follow up: intervention, n = 1 (2%); control, n = 1 (1.6%) Baseline values carried forward
Outcomes	Completers' results: intervention, n = 50; control, n = 59 POP-specific questionnaire 12 women in the intervention group reported their sexual difficulties resolved as compared with 4 women in the control group (p = 0.06). No significant differences were found between groups regarding change in satisfaction with the frequency of sexual intercourse. Significantly more women in the intervention group reported an improvement in sexual function (n = 19 [39%]) compared with the control group (n = 2 [5%], p < 0.01).
Author	**Basgol and Oskay (2016)**
Design	2-arm RCT: Intervention (PFMT): 18 Control (no treatment): 18
Study population	36 women with sexual dysfunction (mean age 34.5 years)

TABLE 7.4.3 Randomized Controlled Trials Investigating the Effect of Pelvic Floor Muscle Training (Alone or in Combined With Other Intervention) on Female Sexual Function—cont'd

Control/intervention protocol	Intervention: PFMT with biofeedback. Participants were asked to do the exercise programme recorded on the device (three 5-s contractions with 10-s intervals) for 5 days/week, twice a day and for a period of 10 weeks, except during menstruation. Control: The control group received no treatment.
Losses to follow-up/ adherence	Intervention 0 (0%); control 0 (0%)
Outcomes	Completers' results: intervention, n = 18; control, n = 18 FSFI Desire: p = 0.000 Arousal: p = 0.000 Lubrication: p = 0.000 Orgasm: p = 0.000 Satisfaction: p = 0.000 Pain: p = 0.001 Total score: p = 0.000 It was found that the improvement in the total score and 6 dimensions of the FSFI 10 weeks after the conclusion of biofeedback treatment were statistically significant (p = 0.000), whereas no statistical significance was detected in the control group before and after the treatment (p < 0.19).
Author	**Citak et al. (2010)**
Design	Single-blinded RCT
Study population	118 primiparous women (mean age 22.6 years)
Control/intervention protocol	Intervention (PFMT): 10 repetitions increasing to 15 repetitions daily, 2-s contraction increasing to 5 and 10 s Control: no treatment
Losses to follow-up/ adherence	Total: 43 (36.4%) Intervention: 21 (17.8%) Control: 22 (18.6%)
Outcomes	FSFI; PFM strength assessed by digital palpation and manometer Positive effect in favour of training group on arousal, lubrication and orgasm; improvement in PFM strength
Author	**Wilson and Herbison (1998)**
Design	RCT
Study population	230 incontinent primi-/multiparous women
Control/intervention protocol	Intervention: subgroup 1, 80–100 repetitions 8–10×/day; subgroup 2, vaginal cones 20–100 g 15 min daily; subgroup 3: PFMT and cones Control: standard treatment as recommended at the hospital, but no follow-up
Losses to follow-up/ adherence	Total: n = 85 (36.9%) Intervention: n = 59 (25.7%) Control: n = 26 (11.3%)
Outcomes	Postal questionnaire: pain, interest in and satisfaction with sex, arousal, ability to orgasm, adequacy of vaginal tone and general feeling; PFM strength and endurance assessed by perineometer No difference between groups
Author	**Bø et al. (2000)**
Design	RCT
Study population	59 women with SUI (mean age 50.65 years)
Control/intervention protocol	Intervention: 8–12 (near-maximum PFM contractions) 3×/day Control: no treatment

Continued

TABLE 7.4.3   Randomized Controlled Trials Investigating the Effect of Pelvic Floor Muscle Training (Alone or in Combined With Other Intervention) on Female Sexual Function—cont'd

Losses to follow-up/ adherence	Total: 4 (6.8%) Intervention: 4 (6.8%) Control: 0 (0%)
Outcomes	QoLS-N and B-FLUTS; PFM strength assessed with a manometer; fewer problems with sex life spoiled by urinary symptoms in favour of training group; improved PFM strength
Author	**Yang et al. (2012)**
Design	RCT (pilot)
Study population	34 women with gynaecological cancer (mean age 52.4 years)
Control/intervention protocol	Intervention: 20-min biofeedback with 40 cycles with 10 sec of maximum activity followed by 20 sec of relaxation; 20 min with an intensive core exercise session; home training 10 repetitions 2×/day Control: no treatment
Losses to follow-up/ adherence	Total: 10 (29.4%) Intervention: 5 (14.7%) Control: 5 (14.7%)
Outcomes	APFQ on sexual function; PFM strength assessed with perineometer Improved sexual function, numbers being sexually active and PFM strength increased in favour of the training group; improved PFM strength
Author	**Hagen et al. (2014)**
Design	Parallel-group, multicentre RCT
Study population	477 women with symptomatic POP (mean age 56.85 years)
Control/intervention protocol	Intervention (PFMT): individualized, 10-sec maximum hold 10 times and 50 fast contractions 3×/day Control: no treatment
Losses to follow-up/ adherence	6 months: Intervention: 36 (16%) Control: 36 (16%) 12 months: Intervention: 75 (33.3%) Control: 77 (34.7%)
Outcomes	PISQ-12 Sexual scores (interference of prolapse symptoms with sex life) improved at 6 months after intervention in favour of training group; 12 months after intervention no difference
Author	**Wiegersma et al. (2014)**
Design	RCT
Study population	287 women with symptomatic, mild POP (mean age 64.25 years)
Control/intervention protocol	Intervention: PFMT (2–3×/day, 3–5×/week), myofeedback, electrical stimulation, the Knack, lifestyle advice (diet, body weight, toilet habits), PFM relaxation and general relaxation Control: no treatment
Losses to follow-up/ adherence	Total: 48 (16.7%) Intervention: 31 (10.8%) Control: 17 (5.9%)
Outcomes	PISQ 12 PFM function (ability to contract and relax) measured by digital palpation No effect and no improvement of PFM function

TABLE 7.4.3   Randomized Controlled Trials Investigating the Effect of Pelvic Floor Muscle Training (Alone or in Combined With Other Intervention) on Female Sexual Function—cont'd

Author	**Trudel and Saint-Laurent (1983)**
Design	RCT
Study population	12 women with orgasmic disorder
Control/intervention protocol	Intervention: PFMT, 3-s contract and 3-s relax with increasing intensity for 20 min/day Control: sexual awareness, relaxation, breathing; different exercises for 20 min/day
Losses to follow-up/adherence	0%
Outcomes	SAI, SII, clinical questionnaire (sexual reactions, stimuli needed to reach orgasm) No effect in main outcome: orgasmic responsivity between groups; higher scores for control group on sexual satisfaction, self-acceptance and perceptual accuracy scale, but no between-group differences
Author	**Handa et al. (2011)**
Design	RCT
Study population	445 women with SUI (mean age 49.76 years)
Control/intervention protocol	Control: continence pessary Intervention 1: behavioural therapy (pelvic floor muscle training and continence strategies) Intervention 2: combination therapy
Losses to follow-up/adherence	Total: 100 (22.5%)
Outcomes	SPEQ (libido, arousal and dyspareunia) and PISQ-12 PFM function were measured. Change in measured aspects of sexual function did not differ among treatment groups. In those with improved SUI, the combined therapy group had improved sexual function compared to a pessary group. In those with improved SUI, the behavioural therapy group had improved sexual function compared to the pessary group. In those with no improved SUI, groups were similar. Change in PFM strength was associated with improved SUI but not improved sexual function.
Author	**Kolberg Tennfjord et al. (2016)**
Design	RCT
Study population	175 women (mean age 29.8 years) with and without symptoms of sexual dysfunction
Control/intervention protocol	Intervention: PFMT with 3 sets of 8–12 close to maximum PFM contractions Control: standard treatment as recommended at the hospital but no follow-up
Losses to follow-up/adherence	Total: 15 (8.6%) Intervention: 12 (13.8%) Control: 3 (3.4%)
Outcomes	ICIQ-FLUTSsex and ICIQ-VS PFM function assessed with manometer Unadjusted subgroup analysis of women with a major defect of the levator ani muscle showed that women in the training group had 45% less risk of having the symptom 'vagina feels loose or lax' compared with the control group. No association with this symptom and change in PFM variables was found.
Author	**Chambless et al. (1984)**
Design	RCT
Study population	36 women with orgasmic disorder
Control/intervention protocol	Intervention: PFMT 10 min daily Placebo: 10 non-sexual images concerning vaginal sensations 10 min daily Control: no treatment

Continued

TABLE 7.4.3 Randomized Controlled Trials Investigating the Effect of Pelvic Floor Muscle Training (Alone or in Combined With Other Intervention) on Female Sexual Function—cont'd

Losses to follow-up/ adherence	Total: 21 (58.3%) Intervention: 8 (22.2%) Placebo: 10 (27.7%) Control: 3 (8.3%)
Outcomes	SAI-E (arousal, anxiety, satisfaction), WSQ (orgasmic responsiveness, frequency of orgasm, stimulation) and expectancy due to treatment or assessment only; PFM strength assessed with perineometer; higher expectancy scores in PFMT and placebo, but no between-group differences; all groups improved in orgasm, but no between-group differences; no improvement in strength
Author	**Panman et al. (2016)**
Design	RCT
Study population	287 women (age ≥55 years) with symptomatic mild prolapse, identified by screening (mean age 64.25) Intervention: 145 Control: 142
Control/intervention protocol	Intervention: Everyone started with the same PFMT programme, which was subsequently tailored to individuals. Participants were encouraged to continue practicing at home 3–5×/week for 2–3×/day. Control: Watchful waiting was used. Women received information on pelvic anatomy and PFM function by using illustrated leaflets. In addition, they were informed about the degree of their prolapse and the function of their PFMs.
Losses to follow-up/ adherence	Intervention 53 (36.5%); control 17 (11.9%)
Outcomes	PFDI-20, POPDI-6, CRADI-8, UDI-6, MOS-SF-12, PISQ-12 No differences in change observed between the groups in sexual functioning (PISQ-12) $p = 0.64$, with adjustment $p = 0.75$
Author	**Panman et al. (2017)**
Design	RCT
Study population	162 women (age ≥55 years) with symptomatic POP (mean age 65.25) Control: 82 Intervention: 80
Control/intervention protocol	Control (pessary): The first choice was an open ring pessary, followed by a ring pessary with support. Intervention (PFMT): Training was started by doing exercises during face-to-face contact and at home (3–5×/week, 2 or 3 times/day). All participants started with the same exercise regime, which was later tailored to the needs of each participant by adding specific exercises based on findings during the pelvic floor examination.
Losses to follow-up/ adherence	Control: 55 (67%) Intervention: 23 (28.75%) Intention-to-treat analysis AND per-protocol analysis
Outcomes	PISQ-12: secondary Significant difference between groups in favour of the pessary group for sexual functioning PISQ-12 Per protocol: $p = 0.99$ $p = 0.028$ *adjusted

TABLE 7.4.3 Randomized Controlled Trials Investigating the Effect of Pelvic Floor Muscle Training (Alone or in Combined With Other Intervention) on Female Sexual Function—cont'd

Author	Due et al. (2015)
Design	RCT
Study population	109 women with symptomatic POP stage ≥2 (mean age 59.3 years) Control: 53 Intervention: 56
Control/intervention protocol	Control: no information about PFMT during their sessions Intervention: received an appointment with a specialized pelvic floor physical therapist for visual and digital assessment of their PFM function and individual instruction in PFMT before starting group sessions to assure that they could perform the PFMT programme correctly All participants received 6 group sessions within 12 weeks; intervention and control group sessions were held on separate days, and the 2 groups never met
Losses to follow-up/ adherence	Control: 6 (11%) Intervention: 14 (25%) Intention-to-treat analysis*
Outcomes	PISQ-12: secondary None of the women obtained significant improvement in the PISQ-12.
Author	**Lúcio et al. (2014)**
Design	RCT
Study population	30 women with multiple sclerosis (mean age 46.1 years) Intervention 1: 10 Intervention 2: 10 Intervention 3: 10
Intervention/control protocol	Intervention 1: PFMT with electromyographic biofeedback and sham neuromuscular electrostimulation was used with 30 slow, maximal PFM contractions followed by 3 min of fast, maximal-effort PFM contractions in the supine position. Intervention 2: Patients underwent intravaginal electrical stimulation. A vaginal stimulating probe (Quark, Brazil) was used to deliver electrical pulses of a width of 200 μs to the vaginal wall at the level of the levator ani at a frequency of 10 Hz for 30 min (Dualpex 961; Quark). The stimulation was delivered at the participant's maximum-tolerated intensity. During each treatment session the stimulation intensity was increased as the patient acclimatized to the stimulus. Following the electrical stimulation protocol, PFMT performed with the assistance of electromyographic biofeedback was performed as described above for G1. Intervention 3: Patients underwent transcutaneous electrical stimulation. A pair of self-adhesive electrodes was used for stimulation. One electrode was applied below the left medial malleolus, and the other was located 5 cm cephalad to the distal electrode and delivered pulses of width 200 μs at a frequency of 10 Hz for 30 min (Dualpex 961; Quark). After the appropriate electrode site was confirmed (by the presence of great toe plantar flexion) the stimulation amplitude was reduced to a level just below the somatic sensory threshold. Following the electrical stimulation protocol, PFMT with the assistance of electromyographic biofeedback was performed as described earlier for interventions 1 and 2.
Losses to follow-up/ adherence	Intervention 1: 4 (40%) Intervention 2: 3 (30%) Intervention 3: 3 (30%)

Continued

TABLE 7.4.3   Randomized Controlled Trials Investigating the Effect of Pelvic Floor Muscle Training (Alone or in Combined With Other Intervention) on Female Sexual Function—cont'd

Outcomes	FSFI Desire: $p = 0.06$ Arousal: $p = 0.58$ Lubrication: $p = 0.46$ Orgasm: $p = 0.48$ Satisfaction: $p = 0.67$ Pain: $p = 0.29$ Total score: $p < 0.01$ Results show that intervention 1 improved in all domains of the questionnaire except for the desire, orgasm and pain domains. Intervention 2 improved in all FSFI variables, and intervention 3 patients also had their sexual function improve except for the pain domain. Intervention 2 improved more than intervention 3 in terms of pain measured by the FSFI tool.
Author	**Hagen et al. (2017)**
Design	RCT
Study population	414 participants involved in a longitudinal study of women after an index birth occurring between October 1993 and September 1994 (mean age 46.5 years) Intervention: 207 Control: 207
Control/intervention protocol	Intervention: PFMT with 5 appointments with a specialist women's health physiotherapist over 16 weeks (weeks 0, 2, 6, 11 and 16). The physiotherapist assessed PFMs, taught correct exercise technique, prescribed an individualized home PFMT programme (3 sets of exercises daily and completion of exercise diaries) and provided a prolapse lifestyle advice leaflet (with a focus on weight loss, avoidance of heavy lifting, constipation, coughing and high-impact exercise) and tailored lifestyle advice (phase 1). Women in the intervention group were then offered modified Pilates classes (with PFM exercises as a key distinct element and an exercise DVD for home use) and a one-on-one physiotherapy review appointment at years 1 and 2 after randomization (phase 2). Control: Women in the control group received, by post, the same prolapse lifestyle advice leaflet as did women in the intervention group.
Losses to follow-up/ adherence	After 1 year: Intervention: 46 (22%) Control: 42 (20%) After 2 years: Intervention: 44 (21%) Control: 25 (12%)
Outcomes	PISQ-12 Sexual symptoms did not differ between groups at 2 years
Author	**Eftekhar et al. (2014)**
Design	RCT
Study population	90 patients age 25–55 years with previous delivery, positive history of sexual dysfunction with less than stage 3 POP (mean age 36.55) Control: 45 Intervention: 45
Control/intervention protocol	Control: The control group received standard rectocele repair and perineorrhaphy. Intervention: The intervention group received physiotherapy for 8 weeks, 2×/week (electrical stimulation, Kegel exercises). Kegel exercises included slow and quick contractions 3×/day. The Kegel exercise was taught to patients (by the investigator) and consisted of 6–8 s of contractions with a 6-s rest in between for 15 min, 3×/day, for a total duration of 8 weeks.

TABLE 7.4.3 Randomized Controlled Trials Investigating the Effect of Pelvic Floor Muscle Training (Alone or in Combined With Other Intervention) on Female Sexual Function—cont'd

Losses to follow-up/ adherence	Control: 0 Intervention: 0
Outcomes	FSFI Libido and arousal were improved in both groups (p = 0.007 and p = 0.001, respectively). Orgasm and dyspareunia were improved in group B (p = 0.001). Dyspareunia was more painful in group A. There was significant difference between the 2 groups (improvement of orgasm and dyspareunia in group B) (p = 0.001).

APFQ, Australian Pelvic Floor Questionnaire; *B-FLUTS*, Bristol Female Lower Urinary Tract Symptoms; *BPMT*, behavioural therapy with pelvic floor muscle training; *CRADI-8*, Colorectal/Anal Distress Inventory 8; *EQ-5D*, EuroQoL Health-Related Quality of Life; *EPAQ*, Extended Personal Attitude Questionnaire; *FSFI*, Female Sexual Function Index; *ICIQ-FLUTSsex*, International Consultation on Incontinence Questionnaire-Female Sexual Matters Associated With Lower Urinary Tract Symptoms; *ICIQ-VS*, International Consultation on Incontinence Questionnaire-Vaginal Symptoms; *MOS-SF-12*, Medical Outcomes Study Short Form Health Survey 12; *PFDI-20*, Pelvic Floor Distress Inventory-Short Form; *PFIQ*, Pelvic Floor Impact Questionnaire; *PFIQ-SF*, Pelvic Floor Impact Questionnaire-Short Form; *PFM*, pelvic floor muscle; *PFMT*, pelvic floor muscle training; *PGII*, Patient Global Impression of Improvement; *PISQ*, Prolapse and Incontinence Sexual Function Questionnaire; *PISQ-12*, Pelvic Organ Prolapse/Urinary Incontinence Sexual Function Questionnaire; *POP*, pelvic organ prolapse; *POPDI-6*, Pelvic Organ Prolapse Distress Inventory 6; *QoLS-N*, Quality of Life Scale; *RCT*, randomized controlled trial; *SAI*, Sexual Arousal Inventory; *SAI-E*, Sexual Arousal Inventory-Expanded; *SF-36*, Short Form 36 Health Survey Questionnaire; *SII*, Sexual Interaction Inventory; *SPEQ*, Short Form Personal Experiences Questionnaire; *SSLF*, sacrospinous ligament fixation; *SUI*, stress urinary incontinence; *UDI-6*, Urinary Distress Inventory 6; *ULS*, uterosacral ligament suspension; *WSQ*, Women's Sexuality Questionnaire.

studies (69.2%) included only women with PFD. Only three small studies included only women with sexual dysfunction (Basgol and Oskay, 2016; Chambless et al., 1984; Trudel and Saint-Laurent, 1983). Ages in the included studies ranged from 18 to 65 years. Types of control and active intervention varied in the studies. Sexual function was the primary outcome in 17 (65.38) of the RCTs.

Control conditions included no intervention (Basgol and Oskay, 2016; Bø et al., 2000; Chambless et al., 1984; Citak et al., 2010; Golmakani et al., 2015; Hagen et al., 2017; Panman et al., 2016; Wiegersma et al., 2014; Yang et al., 2012); usual care/ only information (Kolberg Tennfjord et al., 2016; Weidner et al., 2017; Wilson and Herbison, 1998); lifestyle advice/information (Brækken et al., 2015; Due et al., 2015; Hagen et al., 2017; Nazarpour et al., 2018); continence pessary (Handa et al., 2011; Panman et al., 2017); pelvic organ prolapse (POP) surgery (Eftekhar et al., 2014); other exercises, relaxation, breathing or mindfulness (Liebergall-Wischnitzer et al., 2012; Mosalanejad et al., 2018; Trudel and Saint-Laurent, 1983); and electrical stimulation (Hwang et al., 2019; Lúcio et al., 2014).

Details of the interventions are shown in Table 7.4.3. The interventions ranged from individualized supervised PFM strength training alone (Chambless et al.,

1984; Citak et al., 2010; Golmakani et al., 2015; Hagen et al., 2014; Kolberg Tennfjord et al., 2016; Liebergall-Wischnitzer et al., 2012; Mosalanejad et al., 2018; Nazarpour et al., 2018; Panman et al., 2016; Panman et al., 2017; Trudel and Saint-Laurent, 1983; Wilson and Herbison, 1998) to PFMT added to other therapies (Eftekhar et al., 2014; Handa et al., 2011; Hwang et al., 2019; Lúcio et al., 2014; Wiegersma et al., 2014; Yang et al., 2012), lifestyle strategies (Brækken et al., 2015; Hagen et al., 2017; Handa et al., 2011; Weidner et al., 2017) and other extra non–pelvic muscle exercises (Bø et al., 2000; Hagen et al., 2017; Hwang et al., 2019; Yang et al., 2012). The intensity of PFM contraction was near-maximal or maximal in three studies (Bø et al., 2000; Brækken et al., 2015; Hagen et al., 2014; Kolberg Tennfjord et al., 2016; Lúcio et al., 2014; Yang et al. 2012), and most of the studies did not report the intensity of PFM contractions. Training duration varied from 1 month to 2 years. The amount of supervision ranged from only one session of instructions on PFMT over 3 months (Citak et al., 2010) to maximal weekly sessions over 6 months (Bø et al., 2000).

The statistical comparison between groups was not presented in all studies. Eleven (44%) of the 25 RCTs found a statistical difference between groups in favour of PFMT in at least one aspect of sexual function.

These studies found an improvement between group in arousal (Basgol and Oskay, 2016; Brækken et al., 2015; Citak et al. 2010; Golmakani et al., 2015; Nazarpour et al., 2018), desire (Basgol and Oskay, 2016), lubrication (Basgol and Oskay, 2016; Citak et al., 2010), orgasm (Basgol and Oskay, 2016; Brækken et al., 2015; Citak et al., 2010), pain (Brækken et al., 2015), satisfaction (Basgol and Oskay, 2016; Mørkved et al., 2007), gratification for partners (Brækken et al., 2015), number being sexual active (Yang et al., 2012), sexual worry (Yang et al., 2012), sexual vaginal function/vaginal laxity sensation (Kolberg Tennfjord et al., 2016; Yang et al., 2012), sensuality (Golmakani et al., 2015), emotion (Golmakani et al., 2015), communication (Golmakani et al., 2015), body acceptance and rejection (Golmakani et al., 2015), risk of sex life spoiled by urinary symptoms (Bø et al., 2000) and interference of POP symptoms in sexual life (Hagen et al., 2014). Nine of the 11 RCTs presenting between-group analysis used validated tools to assess sexual function. Four studies used the Female Sexual Function Index (FSFI) (Basgol and Oskay, 2016; Citak et al., 2010, Eftekhar et al., 2014, Nazarpour et al., 2018). One study used a sexual self-efficacy questionnaire to assess desire, sensuality, arousal, orgasm, emotion, communication, body acceptance and rejection (Golmakani et al., 2015). Some studies used validated questionnaires to assess sexual dysfunction related to PFD such as the Australian Pelvic Floor Questionnaire (APFQ) (Yang et al., 2012), to urinary incontinence such as the International Consultation on Incontinence Questionnaire–Female Sexual Matters Associated With Lower Urinary Tract Symptoms (ICIQ-FLUTSsex) and the International Consultation on Incontinence Questionnaire–Vaginal Symptoms (ICIQ-VS) (Kolberg Tennfjord et al., 2016), and to POP (Hagen et al., 2014). Miscellaneous aspects related to sexual function not validated and validated were used as outcome measures in the other studies that presented only pre- and post-intervention analysis.

The study conducted by Handa et al. (2011) compared the impact of three different conservative treatments on sexual function in women with mixed urinary incontinence or stress urinary incontinence alone. The authors found statistical improvement in sexual function only in the subgroups of women who obtained improvement in urinary incontinence. However, nearly 40% of participants lacked a sexual partner at enrolment and the power of the study was low. One trial including women with multiple sclerosis did not show any effect of PFMT on sexual function (Mosalanejad et al., 2018). Another trial including women with multiple sclerosis observed an improvement in sexual function from pre- to post-intervention in the three arms of the study, but unfortunately there was lack of an arm without PFMT to confirm its efficacy (Lúcio et al., 2014). The studies including women in the postpartum period (Golmakani et al., 2015; Hagen et al., 2017) found contradictory results. Golmakani et al. (2015) found an improvement in sexual desire, arousal, orgasm and body acceptance in the group receiving PFMT, whereas the study by Hagen et al. (2017) did not find statistical difference in the Pelvic Organ Prolapse/Urinary Incontinence Sexual Function Questionnaire (PISQ-12) 1 and 2 years after birth.

The study by Yang et al. (2012) was the only one to include cancer survivors. Although a clinically meaningful difference was reported, the between-group results for the European Organization for Research and Treatment of Cancer (EORTC) QLQ-CX24 were not presented, compromising the findings. In addition to a very small sample, the study had high withdrawal rates and a lack of an intention-to-treat analysis. Although the study conducted by Eftekhar et al. (2014) found an improvement in orgasm dyspareunia in the group receiving PFMT, the original domain and total scores of the FSFI were not presented at baseline and after intervention. The authors modified the specific original response options for each domain of the FSFI without presenting any validation of this adaptation. Two studies that obtained a positive effect of PFMT on sexual function in women with POP were secondary analysis (Brækken et al., 2015; Hagen et al., 2014). Contradictory results were obtained in another two secondary analyses of large RCTs including women with POP and women with POP and SUI, respectively (Weidner et al., 2017; Wiegersma et al., 2014).

Only two studies showed an association between sexual function and PFM function (Brækken et al., 2015; Yang et al., 2012), although nine studies found an improvement in PFM function in favour of the PFMT group (Basgol and Oskay 2016; Bø et al., 2000, Brækken et al., 2015; Citak et al., 2010; Golmakani et al., 2015; Handa et al., 2011; Kolberg Tennfjord et al., 2016; Mørkved et al., 2007; Yang et al., 2012).

Adherence to PFMT was described only in seven studies measuring the number of attendance at appointments, exercise training diaries during the treatment phase and post-intervention based on self-report of PFMT adherence recorded on postal questionnaires. Adherence ranged from low (19% [Liebergall-Wischnitzer et al. 2012]) to high (97% [Brækken et al., 2015]).

Although most studies indicated an improvement of at least one sexual variable, results need to be interpreted with caution, as fewer than half of the studies found a statistically significant difference between groups. Some of the trials that did not find any effect of PFMT on sexual function had a high drop-out rate (Chambless et al., 1984; Liebergall-Wischnitzer et al., 2012; Wilson and Herbison, 1998) and low adherence to the treatment protocol (Wiegersma et al., 2014).

The lack of any effect in some of the trials might be related to sexual function being influenced by many interpersonal, contextual, personal, psychological and biological factors. According to Ferreira et al. (2015), future RCTs should consider these variables in developing research questions and hypotheses, and specific groups of women with certain disorders would benefit more than others from PFMT. They highlighted that gynaecological pathology and partner factors may adversely affect sexual function and diminish the benefit of PFMT.

Quality of Intervention

As we do not know about a gold standard PFMT protocol to improve women's sexual function or treat specific sexual dysfunction, it is difficult to analyse the quality of PFMT in the available RCTs. However, it is established in the literature that successful treatment of pelvic floor dysfunction improves women's sexual functions (Ferreira et al., 2015). This indicates that a PFMT programme should follow the exercise science principles to be successful, increasing the chances to impact positively on women's sexual function. The training protocols in the RCTs were highly heterogeneous, and in many studies the details of them were not provided.

Risk of Bias Within Studies

The risk of bias according to PEDro scoring is shown in Table 7.4.4. Eleven (44%) of 25 trials scored 4 or 5 on the PEDro scale, representing only a fair methodological quality. The lowest score of 4 was given to six RCTs (Chambless et al., 1984; Citak et al., 2010; Golmakani et al., 2015; Nazarpour et al., 2018; Weidner et al., 2017;

Wilson and Herbison, 1998). Eight trials had a good internal validity, with a score of 7 or 8 (Bø et al., 2000; Brækken et al., 2015; Due et al., 2015; Ghaderi et al., 2019; Hagen et al., 2014; Kolberg Tennfjord et al., 2016; Panman et al., 2016; Wiegersma et al., 2014). However, most of these trials did not have sexual function as the primary outcome.

KEY MESSAGES FOR CLINICIANS

- It is essential to perform a complete assessment of women using validated tools, considering biopsychosocial aspects related to body function (movement impairments, body posture and PFM function), activity and participation.
- The clinician should be able to identify the red and yellow flags to refer patients to other healthcare providers and to work in a team to address all aspects necessary to improve women's sexual function and treat specific sexual dysfunctions.
- PFD should be effectively treated by the physical therapist to provide improvement in women's sexual function.
- There is level 2 evidence that PFMT can improve at least some aspects of sexual function in women.
- An intensive and supervised PFMT programme should be offered to women with PFD (urinary incontinence and POP).
- Exercises to improve body appreciation/awareness and education of body anatomy and physiology related to female sexual response should be provided.
- Information should be provided to encourage women to perform moderate resistance and aerobic exercises to improve general health and sexual function.

KEY MESSAGES FOR RESEARCHERS

Research recommendations:
- High-quality RCTs are required to investigate the effect of PFMT and other physiotherapy intervention in women with a specific diagnosis of sexual dysfunction and special groups of women such as those during pregnancy, postpartum and the climacteric period, as well as cancer survivors and others.
- It would be important to conduct studies to establish the effect of physiotherapy interventions in women with sexual dysfunction independently of PFD.

TABLE 7.4.4 PEDro Quality Scores of Randomized Controlled Trials

E – Eligibility criteria specified
1 – Subjects randomly allocated to groups
2 – Allocation concealed
3 – Groups similar at baseline
4 – Subjects blinded
5 – Therapist administering treatment blinded
6 – Assessors blinded
7 – Measures of key outcomes obtained from >85% of subjects
8 – Data analysed by intention to treat
9 – Statistical comparison between groups conducted
10 – Point measures and measures of variability provided

Study	E	1	2	3[a]	4	5	6[b]	7	8	9	10[b]	Total Score
Basgol and Oskay (2016)	+	+	−	+	−	−	−	+	−	+	+	5
Bø et al. (2000)	+	+	+	+	−	−	+	−	−	+	+	7
Brækken et al. (2015)	+	+	+	+	−	−	−	+	+	+	+	7
Chambless et al. (1984)	+	+	−	−	−	−	+	−	−	+	+	4
Citak et al. (2010)	+	+	−	+	−	−	−	−	−	+	+	4
Nazarpour et al. (2018)	+	+	−	−	−	−	+	−	−	+	+	4
Golmakani et al. (2015)	+	+	−	+	−	−	−	−	−	+	+	4
Hagen et al. (2014)	+	+	+	+	−	−	+	−	+	+	+	7
Handa et al. (2011)	+	+	+	+	−	−	+	−	−	+	+	6
Hwang et al. (2019)	+	+	−	+	−	−	−	+	−	+	+	5
Jha et al. (2018)	+	+	−	−	−	−	+	−	+	+	+	5
Liebergall-Wischnitzer et al. (2012)	+	+	−	+	−	−	+	−	−	+	+	5
Mosalanejad et al. (2018)	+	+	−	+	−	−	+	+	−	+	+	6
Kolberg Tennfjord et al. (2016)	+	+	+	+	−	−	+	+	+	+	+	8
Trudel and Saint-Laurent (1983)	+	+	−	+	−	−	−	+	−	+	+	5
Weidner et al. (2017)	+	+	+	+	−	−	−	−	−	+	−	4
Wiegersma et al. (2014)	+	+	+	+	−	−	+	+	+	+	+	8
Wilson and Herbison (1998)	+	+	−	+	−	−	−	−	−	+	+	4
Yang et al. (2012)	+	+	−	+	−	−	+	+	−	+	+	6
Panman et al. (2016)	+	+	+	+	−	−	+	+	+	+	+	8
Panman et al. (2017)	+	+	+	+	−	−	−	+	+	+	+	6
Due et al. (2015)	+	+	+	+	−	−	+	−	+	+	+	7
Lúcio et al. (2014)	−	+	−	+	+	−	+	−	−	+	+	6
Hagen et al. (2017)	+	+	+	+	−	−	−	−	+	+	+	6
Eftekhar et al. (2014)	−	+	−	+	−	−	−	+	+	+	+	6

+, Criterion is clearly satisfied; −, criterion is not satisfied; ?, not clear if the criterion was satisfied.
The total score is determined by counting the number of criteria that are satisfied, except the 'eligibility criteria specified' score is not used to generate the total score. Total scores are out of 10.

- Validated outcome measures should be carefully selected considering the range of variables known to affect sexual function, including the assessment of women's distress related to sexual function.
- The protocols investigated should be carefully planned considering plausible mechanisms for an effect and adequate dose–response.
- Women in the postpartum period, those in the climacteric period or cancer survivors are in a special group and should be investigated, taking into account specific outcome measures and protocols addressing their needs.

CONCLUSION

Physical therapists have an important role in the assessment and treatment of female sexual dysfunction, and a complete evaluation of the woman must be carried out considering the various aspects that influence her functionality. Several validated instruments can be used by physical therapists. This professional must be able to recognize and refer cases that require evaluation and treatment to another health professional. Teamwork is essential because complaints are often multifactorial. It is also of utmost importance that PFD is treated effectively by the physical therapist. The physical therapy intervention with the highest level of evidence to improve female sexual function is PFMT. Other specific interventions should be prescribed in view of the findings observed through the evaluation of each patient. A healthy lifestyle and physical exercise should always be encouraged, considering their positive impact on general health, including the woman's sexual health.

REFERENCES

Basgol, S., & Oskay, Ü. (2016). Examining the effectiveness of home-based pelvic floor muscle training in treating orgasmic dysfunction in women. *International Journal of Caring Sciences, 9*(1), 135–143.

Bø, K., Talseth, T., & Vinsnes, A. (2000). Randomized controlled trial on the effect of pelvic floor muscle training on quality of life and sexual problems in genuine stress incontinent women. *Acta Obstetricia et Gynecologica Scandinavica, 79*(7), 598–603.

Brækken, I. H., Majida, M., Ellström Engh, M., et al. (2015). Can pelvic floor muscle training improve sexual function in women with pelvic organ prolapse? A randomized controlled trial. *The Journal of Sexual Medicine, 12*(2), 470–480.

Chambless, D. L., Sultan, F. E., Stern, T. E., et al. (1984). Effect of pubococcygeal exercise on coital orgasm in women. *Journal of Consulting and Clinical Psychology, 52*(1), 114–118.

Citak, N., Cam, C., Arslan, H., et al. (2010). Postpartum sexual function of women and the effects of early pelvic floor muscle exercises. *Acta Obstetricia et Gynecologica Scandinavica, 89*(6), 817–822.

De Menezes Franco, M., Driusso, P., Bø, K., et al. (2015). Lifestyle advice with or without pelvic floor muscle training for pelvic organ prolapse: A randomized controlled trial. *International Urogynecology Journal, 27*(4), 555–563.

De Menezes Franco, M., Rosa, E., Silva, A. C. J., et al. (2017). Relationship between pelvic floor muscle strength and sexual dysfunction in postmenopausal women: A cross-sectional study. *International Urogynecology Journal, 28*(6), 931–936.

Due, U., Brostrøm, S., & Lose, G. (2016). Lifestyle advice with or without pelvic floor muscle training for pelvic organ prolapse: a randomized controlled trial. *Int Urogynecol J, 27*(4), 555–563.

Eftekhar, T., Teimoory, N., Miri, E., et al. (2014). Posterior tibial nerve stimulation for treating neurologic bladder in women: A randomized clinical trial. *Acta Medica Iranica, 52*(11), 816–821.

Ferreira, C. H., Dwyer, P. L., Davidson, M., et al. (2015). Does pelvic floor muscle training improve female sexual function? A systematic review. *International Urogynecology Journal, 26*(12), 1735–1750.

Golmakani, N., Zare, Z., Khadem, N., et al. (2015). The effect of pelvic floor muscle exercises program on sexual self-efficacy in primiparous women after delivery. *Iranian Journal of Nursing and Midwifery Research, 20*(3), 347–353.

Graber, B., & Kline-Graber, G. (1979). Female orgasm: Role of pubococcygeus muscle. *Journal Clinical Psychiatry, 40*, 348–351.

Hagen, S., Glazener, C., McClurg, D., et al. (2017). Pelvic floor muscle training for secondary prevention of pelvic organ prolapse (PREVPROL): A multicentre randomised controlled trial. *Lancet, 389*(10067), 393–402.

Hagen, S., Stark, D., Glazener, C., et al. (2014). Individualised pelvic floor muscle training in women with pelvic organ prolapse (POPPY): A multicentre randomised controlled trial. *Lancet, 383*, 796–806.

Handa, V. L., Whitcomb, E., Weidner, A. C., et al. (2011). Sexual function before and after non-surgical treatment for stress urinary incontinence. *Female Pelvic Medicine & Reconstructive Surgery, 17*(1), 30–35.

Hwang, U. J., Lee, M. S., Jung, S. H., et al. (2019). Pelvic floor muscle parameters affect sexual function after 8 weeks of transcutaneous electrical stimulation in women with stress urinary incontinence. *Sexual Medicine, 7*(4), 505–513.

Jha, S., Walters, S. J., Bortolami, O., et al. (2018). Impact of pelvic floor muscle training on sexual function of women with urinary incontinence and a comparison of electrical stimulation versus standard treatment (IPSU trial): A randomised controlled trial. *Physiotherapy, 104*(1), 91–97.

Kolberg Tennfjord, M., Hilde, G., Staer-Jensen, J., et al. (2016). Effect of postpartum pelvic floor muscle training on vaginal symptoms and sexual dysfunction-secondary analysis of a randomised trial. *BJOG, 123*(4), 634–642.

Liebergall-Wischnitzer, M., Paltiel, O., Hochner Celnikier, D., et al. (2012). Sexual function and quality of life of women with stress urinary incontinence: A randomized controlled trial comparing the Paula method (circular muscle exercises) to pelvic floor muscle training (PFMT) exercises. *The Journal of Sexual Medicine, 9*, 1613–1623.

Lowenstein, L., Gruenwald, I., Gartman, I., et al. (2010). Can stronger pelvic muscle floor improve sexual function? *International Urogynecology Journal, 21*(5), 553–556.

Lúcio, A. C., D'Ancona, C. A., Lopes, M. H., et al. (2014). The effect of pelvic floor muscle training alone or in combination with electrostimulation in the treatment of sexual dysfunction in women with multiple sclerosis. *Multiple Sclerosis, 20*(13), 1761–1768.

Ma, Y., & Qin, H. (2009). Pelvic floor muscle exercises may improve female sexual function. *Medical Hypotheses, 72*(2), 223.

Macedo, L. G., Elkins, M. R., Maher, C. G., et al. (2010). There was evidence of convergent and construct validity of Physiotherapy Evidence Database quality scale for physiotherapy trials. *Journal of Clinical Epidemiology, 63*, 920–925.

Martinez, C. S., Ferreira, F. V., Castro, A. A. M., et al. (2014). Women with greater pelvic floor muscle strength have better sexual function. *Acta Obstetricia et Gynecologica Scandinavica, 93*, 457–502.

Mørkved, S., Rommen, K., Schei, B., et al. (2007). No difference in urinary incontinence between training and control group six years after cessation of a randomized controlled trial, but improved sexual satisfaction in the training group. *Neurourology and Urodynamics, 26*(5), 667.

Mosalanejad, F., Afrasiabifar, A., & Zoladl, M. (2018). Investigating the combined effect of pelvic floor muscle exercise and mindfulness on sexual function in women with multiple sclerosis: A randomized controlled trial. *Clinical Rehabilitation, 32*(10), 1340–1347.

Nazarpour, S., Simbar, M., Majd, H. A., et al. (2018). Beneficial effects of pelvic floor muscle exercises on sexual function among postmenopausal women: A randomised clinical trial. *Sexual Health, 15*(5), 396–402.

Panman, C. M., Wiegersma, M., Kollen, B. J., et al. (2016). Effectiveness and cost-effectiveness of pessary treatment compared with pelvic floor muscle training in older women with pelvic organ prolapse: 2-year follow-up of a randomized controlled trial in primary care. *Menopause, 23*(12), 1307–1318.

Panman, C. M., Wiegersma, M., Kollen, B. J., et al. (2017). Two-year effects and cost-effectiveness of pelvic floor muscle training in mild pelvic organ prolapse: A randomised controlled trial in primary care. *BJOG, 124*(3), 511–520.

Shafik, A. (2000). The role of the levator ani muscle in evacuation, sexual performance and pelvic floor disorders. *International Urogynecology Journal and Pelvic Floor Dysfunction, 11*, 361–376.

Trudel, G., & Saint-Laurent, S. (1983). A comparison between the effects of Kegel's exercises and a combination of sexual awareness relaxation and breathing on situational orgasmic dysfunction in women. *Journal of Sex & Marital Therapy, 9*(3), 204–209.

Weidner, A. C., Barber, M. D., Markland, A., et al. (2017). Perioperative behavioral therapy and pelvic muscle strengthening do not enhance quality of life after pelvic surgery: Secondary report of a randomized controlled trial. *Physical Therapy, 97*(11), 1075–1083.

Wiegersma, M., Panman, C. M., Kollen, B. J., et al. (2014). Effect of pelvic floor muscle training compared with watchful waiting in older women with symptomatic mild pelvic organ prolapse: Randomised controlled trial in primary care. *BMJ, 349*, g7378.

Wilson, P. D., & Herbison, G. P. (1998). A randomized controlled trial of pelvic floor muscle exercises to treat postnatal urinary incontinence. *International Urogynecology Journal and Pelvic Floor Dysfunction, 9*(5), 257–264.

Yang, E. J., Lim, J. Y., Rah, U. W., et al. (2012). Effect of a pelvic floor muscle training program on gynecologic cancer survivors with pelvic floor dysfunction: A randomized controlled trial. *Gynecologic Oncology, 125*(3), 705–711.

7.5 Pregnancy and Childbirth: Pathophysiology and Injuries

John O.L. DeLancey and Fernanda Pipitone

INTRODUCTION

Vaginal birth is one of the most important causes of pelvic organ prolapse, as well as urinary and faecal incontinence—problems collectively known as pelvic floor disorders (López-López et al., 2020; Mant et al., 1997; Nygaard et al., 2008; Rortveit et al., 2003)—and physical therapy plays an important role in pelvic floor recovery after birth (Woodley, Lawrenson, Boyle, & et al., 2020a, 2020b, 2020c). If rehabilitation is to achieve its best results, it must be based on a firm, evidence-based understanding of the injuries involved, their biology, and the process of successful and failed recovery. In considering the role of childbirth in causing different pelvic floor disorders, it is important to emphasize that there are several different anatomical structures involved and each of these structures can be affected by birth in different ways. The anatomy is reviewed in Chapter 3.

HOW DOES CHILDBIRTH FIT INTO THE OVERALL PATHOPHYSIOLOGY OF PELVIC FLOOR DISORDERS?

During a woman's life, many things can impact pelvic floor function. Genetic, nutritional and hormonal factors affect an individual's eventual growth to adulthood. One woman may develop a strong pelvic floor, whereas another woman's might be more delicate. After reaching full maturity, childbirth, age and other factors can lead to damage or deterioration. In addition, the demands that a woman's lifestyle places on the pelvic floor, ranging from a sedentary individual to someone who competes in Ironman competitions, influence pelvic floor function. Depending on the status of the pelvic floor and the demands placed upon it, a point can be reached when symptoms occur.

A simple display of factors that affect the pelvic floor illustrates the different impairments at play and how they interact (Fig. 7.5.1). The graph shown in Fig. 7.5.1 has a theoretical y-axis variable representing 'pelvic floor function'. This variable could indicate any single factor, such as strength of the levator ani muscles, or it might represent the coordinated actions of several structures, such as the urethral support apparatus that involves muscles, their neural control system and attaching fascial structures. The x-axis represents age.

The basic concept is shown in Fig. 7.5.1A, where growth to maturity occurs and during which predisposing factors such as genetics and nutrition play a role. Childbirth and other inciting factors with variable recovery are shown. Finally, intervening factors, most notably age-related deterioration, occur until a symptom threshold is reached, at which demands placed on the pelvic organs exceed the capacity to resist and symptoms occur. Fig. 7.5.1B shows three examples of how different genetic and nutritional factors that affect initial growth can influence when a woman reaches a threshold where she is symptomatic.

Childbirth is shown in Fig. 7.5.1C and D. In Fig. 7.5.1C, two births are shown without significant injuries. Fig. 7.5.1D considers different degrees of pelvic floor injury during birth. For simplicity, only one birth is shown with three different levels of injury. An easy birth (line 1) may cause brief, temporary dysfunction with no long-term consequence. A birth with moderate injury that is partly recovered is not apparent for many years (line 2). There are also individuals with such significant damage that the body cannot repair it and immediate problems occur (line 3).

Women's bodies change at different rates over their lifespan. Development of sarcopenia varies, and accelerated loss may result in a woman becoming symptomatic at a younger age (Fig. 7.5.1E). Finally, the demands placed on the pelvic floor vary by an individual's activity level (Fig. 7.5.1F). An active woman who engages in high-impact aerobic exercise that places significant loads on the pelvic floor is more likely to experience incontinence than one with a sedentary lifestyle. The increased occurrence of stress incontinence in individuals with a high body mass index that results from them coughing harder than their normal body mass index counterparts (Swenson et al., 2017) would be another example, and disappearance of incontinence with weight loss confirms its cause (Subak et al., 2009).

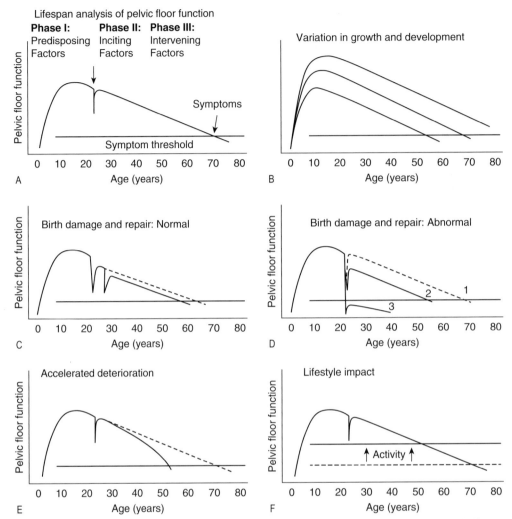

Fig. 7.5.1 Graphical display of the concept of pelvic floor function considering phases of a woman's lifespan (A), different degrees of functional reserve (B), variations in birth damage and repair (C, D), accelerated deterioration (E), and lifestyle impact (F). © *DeLancey*.

PELVIC FLOOR DISORDERS: SEPARATE ENTITIES, DISTINCT CAUSES

Each pelvic floor disorder has its own unique causal factors, so they cannot be lumped together. Although the focus of this chapter is on childbirth, a brief description of the evidence behind specific structural failures and specific symptom complexes is necessary. This is especially true because recent evidence has proven that many long- and widely held opinions are wrong.

Pelvic Organ Prolapse

Of the three pelvic floor disorders, pelvic organ prolapse is the most strongly tied to birth. It is rare in nulliparas and quite common in women who have given birth. This is not to say that it is the number of births, (one, two, three, etc.) that is the primary factor, but that having any vaginal birth versus being nulliparous plays a large role. Data from the Oxford Family Planning Cohort showed that the odds of having prolapse was 4 for one birth and 8 for two (Mant et al., 1997). At four births, the

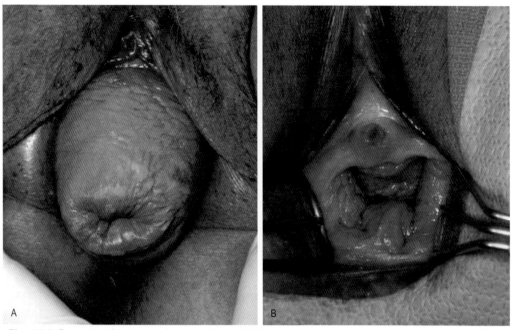

Fig. 7.5.2 Examples of enlarged urogenital hiatus. (A) A large uterovaginal prolapse seen in the clinic. (B) An enlarged hiatus (level III) once the prolapse has been reduced as seen in the operating room. © *DeLancey*.

increased odds were 12, and there did not seem to be an increase after that.

Although it has been traditional to say, especially among surgeons, that prolapse is caused by defective connective tissue, damage to the levator ani muscle and enlargement of the pelvic floor hiatuses are now well established as primary aetiological factors (Fig. 7.5.2). Muscle tearing, often referred to as avulsion, occurs during at least 15% of vaginal deliveries (Dietz and Lanzarone, 2005; Tunn et al., 1999). Large case–control studies indicate that 55% of women with prolapse have levator tears, whereas tears are seen in only 16% of women of similar age and parity who do not have prolapse—an odds ratio (OR) greater than 7 (DeLancey et al., 2007). The women with prolapse generated 37% less vaginal closure force during pelvic muscle contraction than controls (2 vs 3.2 newtons), whereas those with major levator defects generated 35% less force than women without defects. In addition, the genital hiatus was 50% longer in cases than controls. Similar findings have been seen using a pressure-based device to compare women with and without prolapse, when pelvic floor muscle strength was associated with prolapse (OR: 7.5) and endurance (OR: 11.5) (Brækken et al., 2009).

Stress Urinary Incontinence

Stress incontinence is primarily caused by failure of the muscles in the urethra itself to maintain adequate closure to prevent leakage. Although it was believed for many years that stress incontinence was due to poor urethral support, carefully conducted studies disprove this hypothesis. By comparing multiple urethral and support factors between women with stress incontinence and continent volunteers, urethral closure pressure was found to be, by far, the single factor that is most important in determining continence (DeLancey et al., 2008). Women with stress incontinence have a maximal urethral closure pressure that is 42% lower than normal. Closure pressure alone correctly classified 50% of cases. Urethral support does contribute, but analysis of how much urethral support only added 10% of predictive ability.

Faecal Incontinence

Faecal continence is determined by several factors, including stool consistency and volume, the rectum's ability to accommodate it, and anal sphincter function. Various neurological reflexes and muscle coordination mechanisms are in place to ensure retention of stool until it is deemed socially convenient to have a bowel movement (Rao, 2004). Ultimately, the ability of an individual to retain rectal contents depends on the anal canal pressure being higher than rectal pressure (Rasmussen et al., 1992; Stojkovic et al., 2002). This pressure gradient is ensured by adequate function and coordination of different structures: the external and internal anal sphincters, rectum (capacity and compliance), mucosal folds and vascular cushions, and puborectal muscle.

The internal anal sphincter is responsible for up to 70% of resting tone, and its dysfunction is usually translated clinically as flatus or liquid stool incontinence. The external anal sphincter is composed of striated muscle, contributes to up to 30% of the resting tone and is the main structure responsible for the squeeze pressure (Sultan and Nugent, 2004). The pubic portion of the levator ani muscle forms a sling behind the anorectal junction and may play a role as well ('flap-valve' effect) (Azpiroz et al., 2005).

WHAT INJURIES DOES BIRTH CAUSE THAT RESULT IN PELVIC FLOOR DISORDERS?

Levator Ani Injury and Prolapse

Details about levator injury during birth and the mechanisms of that injury are covered in Chapter 5.

The vaginal high-pressure zone (Raizada et al., 2010) closes the hiatuses in the pelvic floor through which prolapse occurs. The perineal closure complex that creates this zone includes complex interactions between the levator ani muscles with their neural control mechanism, perineal membrane and perineal body (Fig. 7.5.3). There are two hiatuses, the urogenital (=genital) and levator hiatuses, which are the largest hiatuses in the body. Both have the pubic bones as their anterior margin and the levator ani muscles as their lateral margins. The urogenital hiatus is bounded posteriorly by the perineal body, whereas the levator hiatus extends behind the rectum at the anorectal angle.

An enlarged hiatus is associated with prolapse (DeLancey and Hurd, 1998). In addition, hiatal enlargement precedes the occurrence of prolapse, indicating a causal relationship (Handa et al., 2019). During the first 20 years after birth, approximately 25% of women with an enlarged hiatus followed prospectively developed prolapse at least 1 cm below the hymenal ring. For

a woman with a 3-cm hiatus on physical examination (distance from the urethra to the perineal body), the estimated median time to develop prolapse would be 33 years, whereas for women with a hiatus of 4.5, it would be 6 years (Handa et al., 2020). Prolapse also is more common with reduced muscle strength (OR: 0.87 per 5 cmH_2O). Prolapse was associated with levator avulsion (OR: 4.2), and hiatus area and strength mediated 61% of the association between avulsion and prolapse.

It is important to recognize that visible levator muscle damage is not the only factor leading to an enlarged hiatus. The degree of muscle damage only explains less than a quarter of the variation in hiatus size (Nandikanti et al., 2018). This is probably an underestimate of the relationship between muscle dysfunction and prolapse because it includes minor variation in damage, but the point that it is not the only factor is important. When several aspects of pelvic floor closure are all examined (muscle strength, perineal elevation with muscle contraction, descent during Valsalva and visible muscle on magnetic resonance imaging), they are each independent factors (English et al., 2021). Correlations between these factors reveals that no one factor explains more than 20% of the variation in others. The only significant association was between levator defect status and both resting urogenital hiatus and change in urogenital hiatus with straining. But these were weak associations only explaining 13% of variation in hiatus size.

The key point is that the factors determining hiatus size at rest, during Valsalva and with maximal contraction are complex, and much more needs to be done to understand their inter-relationships, especially neural control. Muscle injury unquestionably plays an important role. However, it would be wrong to assume that this was the only factor. Connective tissue changes to the perineal body and perineal membrane also play a major role, and we must accept the challenge to determine all factors involved and not look at this as an overly simplistic question.

Mechanisms of Levator Ani Muscle Injury

Details of the injury to the pubococcygeal (=pubovisceral) portion of the levator ani are provided in Chapter 5, and the anatomy is defined in Chapter 3. It bears repeating that it is only the pubococcygeal portion of the levator that is injured (DeLancey et al., 2012).

Briefly, during vaginal birth, the levator ani muscle undergoes a degree of lengthening that is many times

Normal Closure   Failed Closure

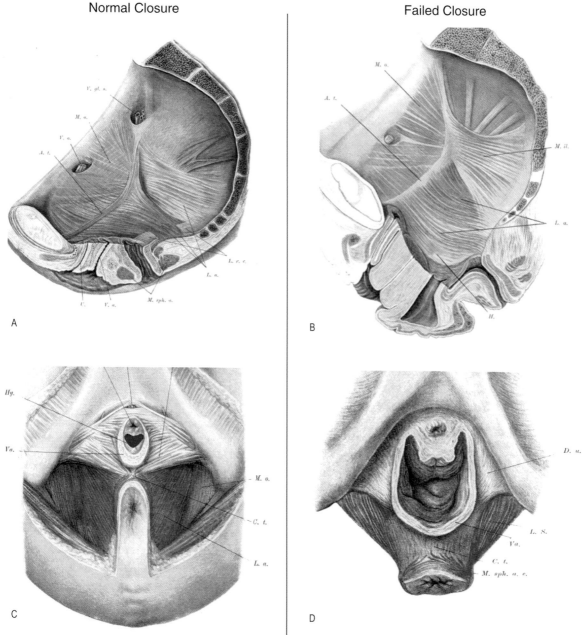

Fig. 7.5.3 Normal and failed perineal closure complexes. (A, B) Midsagittal view. (C, D) Caudal view. (*From Halban and Tandler (1907).*)

greater than any other muscle in the body (Lien et al., 2004) (Fig. 7.5.4). The pubococcygeal portion undergoes the greatest degree of lengthening. In approximately 15% of women during their first birth, more than 50% of the muscle is torn ('avulsion'), with the most severe cases having detachment of the muscle from its origin (Dietz and Lanzarone, 2005). Most women show significant oedema in the muscle that resolves by 6 months (Miller et al., 2010). This probably represents trauma within the muscle similar to a 'pulled muscle' or muscle strain. There is also denervation and re-innervation evident in the connective tissues that attach the muscles to the pelvic organs and pelvic outlet (perineal membrane, perineal body) (Snooks et al., 1984; South et al., 2009).

Pelvic Floor Changes in Preparation for Birth

Having a baby with a head diameter of 10 cm coming through a 2.5-cm diameter opening in the pelvic floor is one of the most remarkable phenomena in all human

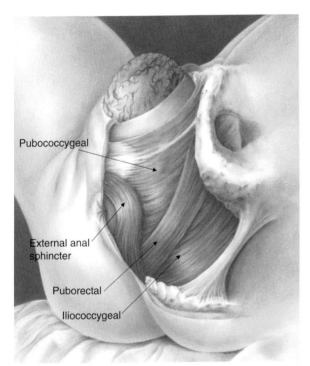

Pubococcygeal

External anal sphincter

Puborectal

Iliococcygeal

Fig. 7.5.4 Levator ani muscle subdivisions and external anal sphincter (as labeled) at crowning of the foetal head showing the massive changes needed for the head to emerge. © DeLancey.

biology. This would not be possible unless there are major changes to the pelvic floor. There is a 17% to 29% increase in the size of the levator hiatus area between 21 and 37 weeks of gestation at rest and 13% to 26% increase during maximal contraction (Bø, Hilde, Stær-Jensen, & et al., 2015a, 2015b). In addition, there is evidence from experimental studies in rats that shows that muscles around the birth canal add sarcomeres late in pregnancy with 20% to 30% fibre elongation (Alperin et al., 2015). Connective tissue in the extracellular matrix also increases 50% to 140% in these muscles. These changes would reduce how much the muscles would have to lengthen and play a role in decreasing stretch-induced injury.

Perhaps the most remarkable changes occur in the 'stretchiness' of the connective tissues. During labour, even before the head dilates the pelvic floor, it is possible for someone examining the woman to put an entire hand into the vagina—something that would not be possible in the non-pregnant state. Biomechanical studies have documented these changes (Jing, 2010), but the hormonal factors responsible have not yet been established. How this happens and how the connective tissue recovers remain a mystery.

Neuropathy

Injury to the nerves supplying the levator ani and urethral sphincter was one of the earliest changes to be specifically documented with direct physiological measurements. Electrodiagnostic techniques demonstrated that birth causes changes in mean motor unit duration after vaginal birth in the levator ani (Allen et al., 1991). This fact is explained by the great deal of pelvic floor descent that occurs during birth which can result in nerve stretching and possible detachment from some muscle segments (Fig. 7.5.5). In addition, abnormal turns/amplitude

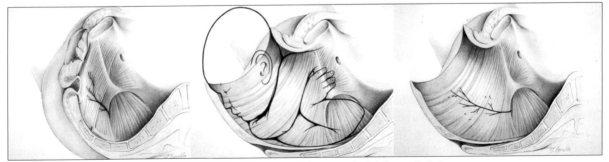

Fig. 7.5.5 The pudendal nerve in relation to vaginal delivery. © DeLancey.

findings were found in 29% of women at 6 months post-partum (Weidner et al., 2006). These changes are similar to findings in both prolapse and stress incontinence (Weidner et al., 2000). Although the pudendal nerve innervates the voluntary urethral and anal sphincters, it does not innervate the levator ani muscles, which receive their own nerve supply from the sacral plexus (Barber et al., 2002), so injury mechanisms may differ.

Pelvic Floor Status and Recovery After Birth

Soon after delivery the pelvic floor sags and the urogenital hiatus is wider than normal (Fairchild et al., 2020). Muscle recovery results in resumption of the near-normal position in most women over the course of the first 6 months—the time when normal pelvic muscle strength also returns to normal (Sampselle, Miller, Mims, & et al., 1998a, 1998b). In women 6 weeks after birth, those with major levator ani defects had 47% lower pelvic floor muscle strength and 47% lower endurance when compared with women without major levator defects (Hilde et al., 2013). No difference was found regarding resting pressures.

Urethral Pressure Differences and Stress Incontinence

Stress urinary incontinence is the most birth-related type of incontinence. In studies, primiparous women with new stress incontinence that persisted at least 9 months had 25% lower urethral closure pressures (47 cmH$_2$O) than women who did not (63 cmH$_2$0, d 0.91). Vesical neck movement on ultrasound during cough was 16 mm in incontinent women compared with 11 mm in primiparous continent women. Major injuries to the levator ani muscles may have contributed because they were twice as common (28%) in the incontinent group compared with the parous group (12%). Increased urethral mobility was also shown in a large prospective longitudinal study that compared urethral mobility in the third trimester to 4 months postpartum (Shek et al., 2010). Interestingly, the women who developed de novo stress incontinence did not have more mobility than those who did not. Women who have a major levator defect after vaginal birth have similar urethral closure pressures both at rest and during maximal contraction, indicating the independent nature of levator injury and urethral function (Brincat et al., 2011). It is also relevant to note that evidence does not indicate that pelvic floor muscle training increases urethral closure pressure at rest (Zubieta et al., 2016).

There is useful evidence about whether pregnancy changes urethral function. A longitudinal study of urethral function in healthy primigravidae showed that urethral function did not change throughout pregnancy and was similar to values seen in nulligravid women. In addition, values in women delivered by caesarean section were similar to pre-pregnancy values (Van Geelen et al., 1982). Thus this indicates that women who inherently have poor urethral function leak during pregnancy when the increased mechanical loads reveal the sphincter weakness.

These findings are consistent with the following hypothesis: women with weak sphincters are more prone to have stress incontinence symptoms during and persistently after pregnancy. Vaginal birth results in worse urethral support, contributed to by injury to the levator ani muscles. It should be noted that in middle-aged women presenting for treatment of stress urinary incontinence, there is no difference in levator injury and the difference in urethral function is greater (Delancey et al., 2008), indicating that the well-known decrease in urethral pressure over time (Rud, 1980; Trowbridge et al., 2007) becomes the dominant factor later in life.

Anal Incontinence

Although less strongly associated than urinary incontinence and pelvic organ prolapse, anal incontinence is certainly linked to childbirth (Blomquist et al., 2018; Sultan, Kamm, Hudson, & et al., 1993a, 1993b). Two separate and overlapping aetiologies have been discussed: (1) direct injury to the anal sphincter complex and (2) damage to the pudendal nerve. Obstetrical anal sphincter injury occurs in 3%, with primiparous women at 3.6-fold higher risk than multiparous women (Thiagamoorthy et al., 2014), and 10% to 50% will develop faecal incontinence symptoms later in life (Mous et al., 2008; Pollack, Nordenstam, Brismar, & et al., 2004a, 2004b; Samarasekera et al., 2008; Sangalli et al., 2000). Ultrasound studies done 15 to 24 years after delivery reported ORs of 2.5 and 4 for faecal incontinence if external and internal anal sphincter defects are seen on imaging (Guzman Rojas, 2018). Pudendal nerve damage probably is attributable to the fact that the inferior rectal branch of the pudendal nerve is stretched the most during vaginal birth (Lien et al., 2005). Pudendal terminal motor latency was increased in women who delivered vaginally when compared to nulliparas and those delivered by caesarean section (Snooks et al., 1984, 1986).

REFERENCES

Allen, R. E., Hosker, G. L., Smith, A. R. B., et al. (1991). Pelvic floor damage and childbirth: A neurophysiological study. *Obstetrical and Gynecological Survey, 46,* 209–210.

Alperin, M., Lawley, D. M., Esparza, M. C., et al. (2015). Pregnancy-induced adaptations in the intrinsic structure of rat pelvic floor muscles. *American Journal of Obstetrics and Gynecology, 213,* 191.e1–191.e7.

Azpiroz, F., Fernandez-Fraga, X., Merletti, R., et al. (2005). The puborectalis muscle. *Neuro-Gastroenterology and Motility, 17*(Suppl. 1), 68–72.

Barber, M. D., Bremer, R. E., Thor, K. B., et al. (2002). Innervation of the female levator ani muscles. *American Journal of Obstetrics and Gynecology, 187,* 64–71.

Blomquist, J. L., Muñoz, A., Carroll, M., et al. (2018). Association of delivery mode with pelvic floor disorders after childbirth. *JAMA, 320,* 2438–2447.

Bø, K., Hilde, G., Stær-Jensen, J., et al. (2015). Does general exercise training before and during pregnancy influence the pelvic floor "opening" and delivery outcome? A 3D/4D ultrasound study following nulliparous pregnant women from mid-pregnancy to childbirth. *British Journal of Sports Medicine, 49,* 196–199.

Brækken, I. H., Majida, M., Ellström Engh, M., et al. (2009). Pelvic floor function is independently associated with pelvic organ prolapse. *British Journal of Obstetrics and Gynaecology, 116,* 1706–1714.

Brincat, C. A., DeLancey, J. O. L., & Miller, J. M. (2011). Urethral closure pressures among primiparous women with and without levator ani muscle defects. *International Urogynecology Journal, 22,* 1491–1495.

DeLancey, J. O. L., & Hurd, W. W. (1998). Size of the urogenital hiatus in the levator ani muscles in normal women and women with pelvic organ prolapse. *Obstetrics & Gynecology, 91,* 364–368.

DeLancey, J. O. L., Morgan, D. M., Fenner, D. E., et al. (2007). Comparison of levator ani muscle defects and function in women with and without pelvic organ prolaps. *Obstetrical and Gynecological Survey, 62,* 374–375.

DeLancey, J. O. L., Sørensen, H. C., Lewicky-Gaupp, C., et al. (2012). Comparison of the puborectal muscle on MRI in women with POP and levator ani defects with those with normal support and no defect. *International Urogynecology Journal, 23*(1), 73–77.

DeLancey, J. O. L., Trowbridge, E. R., Miller, J. M., et al. (2008). Stress urinary incontinence: Relative importance of urethral support and urethral closure pressure. *Journal Urology, 179,* 2286–2290.

Dietz, H. P., & Lanzarone, V. (2005). Levator trauma after vaginal delivery. *Obstetrics & Gynecology, 106,* 707–712.

English, E. M., Chen, L., Sammarco, A. G., et al. (2021). Mechanisms of hiatus failure in prolapse: A multifaceted evaluation. *International Urogynecology Journal, 32*(6), 1545–1553.

Fairchild, P. S., Low, L. K., Kowalk, K. M., et al. (2020). Defining "normal recovery" of pelvic floor function and appearance in a high-risk vaginal delivery cohort. *International Urogynecology Journal, 31,* 495–504.

Guzmán Rojas, R. A., Salvesen, K. Å., Volløyhaug, I. (2018). Anal sphincter defects and fecal incontinence 15–24 years after first delivery: a cross-sectional study. *Ultrasound Obstet Gynecol, 51*(5), 677–683.

Handa, V. L., Blomquist, J. L., Carroll, M., et al. (2020). Genital hiatus size and the development of prolapse among parous women. *Female Pelvic Medicine & Reconstructive Surgery, 26,* 287–298.

Handa, V. L., Roem, J., Blomquist, J. L., et al. (2019). Pelvic organ prolapse as a function of levator ani avulsion, hiatus size, and strength. *American Journal of Obstetrics and Gynecology, 221,* 41.e1–41.e7.

Hilde, G., Stær-Jensen, J., Siafarikas, F., et al. (2013). How well can pelvic floor muscles with major defects contract? A cross-sectional comparative study 6 weeks after delivery using transperineal 3D/4D ultrasound and manometer. *British Journal of Obstetrics and Gynaecology, 120,* 1423–1429.

Jing, D. (2010). *Experimental and theoretical biomechanical analyses of the second stage of labor. Doctoral thesis.* University of Michigan.

Lien, K. C., Mooney, B., DeLancey, J. O. L., et al. (2004). Levator ani muscle stretch induced by simulated vaginal birth. *Obstetrics & Gynecology, 103,* 31–40.

Lien, K. C., Morgan, D. M., Delancey, J. O. L., et al. (2005). Pudendal nerve stretch during vaginal birth: A 3D computer simulation. *American Journal of Obstetrics and Gynecology, 192,* 1669–1676.

López-López, A. I., Sanz-Valero, J., Gómez-Pérez, L., et al. (2020). Pelvic floor: Vaginal or caesarean delivery? A review of systematic reviews. *International Urogynecology Journal, 32*(7), 1663–1673.

Mant, J., Painter, R., & Vessey, M. (1997). Epidemiology of genital prolapse: Observations from the Oxford family planning association study. *British Journal of Obstetrics and Gynaecology, 104*(5), 579–585.

Miller, J. M., Brandon, C., Jacobson, J. A., et al. (2010). MRI findings in patients considered high risk for pelvic floor injury studied serially after vaginal childbirth. *American Journal of Roentgenology, 195,* 786–791.

Mous, M., Muller, S. A., & De Leeuw, J. W. (2008). Long-term effects of anal sphincter rupture during vaginal delivery: Faecal incontinence and sexual complaints. *British Journal of Obstetrics and Gynaecology, 115,* 234–238.

Nandikanti, L., Sammarco, A. G., Kobernik, E. K., et al. (2018). Levator ani defect severity and its association with enlarged hiatus size, levator bowl depth, and prolapse size. *American Journal of Obstetrics and Gynecology, 218,* 537–539.

Nygaard, I., Barber, M. D., Burgio, K. L., et al. (2008). Prevalence of symptomatic pelvic floor disorders in US women. *JAMA, 300,* 1311–1316.

Pollack, J., Nordenstam, J., Brismar, S., et al. (2004). Anal incontinence after vaginal delivery: A five-year prospective cohort study. *Obstetrics & Gynecology, 104,* 1397–1402.

Raizada, V., Bhargava, V., Jung, S. A., et al. (2010). Dynamic assessment of the vaginal high-pressure zone using high-definition manometery, 3-dimensional ultrasound, and magnetic resonance imaging of the pelvic floor muscles. *American Journal of Obstetrics and Gynecology, 203,* 172.e1–172.e8.

Rao, S. S. C. (2004). Pathophysiology of adult fecal incontinence. *Gastroenterology, 126*(1 Suppl. 1), 14–22.

Rasmussen, O., Sørensen, M., Tetzschner, T., et al. (1992). Anorectal pressure gradient in patients with anal incontinence. *Diseases of the Colon & Rectum, 35,* 8–11.

Rortveit, G., Daltveit, A. K., Hannestad, Y. S., et al. (2003). Urinary incontinence after vaginal delivery or cesarean section. *New England Journal of Medicine, 348,* 900–907.

Rud, T. (1980). Urethral pressure profile in continent women from childhood to old age. *Acta Obstetricia et Gynecologica Scandinavica, 59,* 331–335.

Samarasekera, D. N., Bekhit, M. T., Wright, Y., et al. (2008). Long-term anal continence and quality of life following postpartum anal sphincter injury. *Colorectal Disease, 10,* 793–799.

Sampselle, C. M., Miller, J. M., Mims, B. L., et al. (1998). Effect of pelvic muscle exercise on transient incontinence during pregnancy and after birth. *Obstetrics & Gynecology, 91,* 406–412.

Sangalli, M. R., Floris, L., Faltin, D., et al. (2000). Anal incontinence in women with third or fourth degree perineal tears and subsequent vaginal deliveries. *The Australian and New Zealand Journal of Obstetrics and Gynaecology, 40,* 244–248.

Shek, K. L., Dietz, H. P., & Kirby, A. (2010). The effect of childbirth on urethral mobility: A prospective observational study. *Journal Urology, 184*(2), 629–634.

Snooks, S. J., Swash, M., Henry, M. M., et al. (1986). Risk factors in childbirth causing damage to the pelvic floor innervation. *International Journal of Colorectal Disease, 1*(1), 20–24.

Snooks, S. J., Swash, M., Setchell, M., et al. (1984). Injury to innervation of pelvic floor sphincter musculature in childbirth. *Lancet, 324,* 546–550.

South, M. M. T., Stinnett, S. S., Sanders, D. B., et al. (2009). Levator ani denervation and reinnervation 6 months after childbirth. *American Journal of Obstetrics and Gynecology, 200*(5), 519.e1–519.e7.

Stojkovic, S. G., Balfour, L., Burke, D., et al. (2002). Role of resting pressure gradient in the investigation of idiopathic fecal incontinence. *Diseases of the Colon & Rectum, 45,* 668–673.

Subak, L. L., Wing, R., Smith West, D., et al. (2009). Weight loss to treat urinary incontinence in overweight and obese women. *New England Journal of Medicine, 360,* 481–490.

Sultan, A. H., Kamm, M. A., Hudson, C. N., et al. (1993). Anal-sphincter disruption during vaginal delivery. *New England Journal of Medicine, 329*(26), 1905–1911.

Sultan, A. H., & Nugent, K. (2004). Pathophysiology and non-surgical treatment of anal incontinence. *British Journal of Obstetrics and Gynaecology, 111*(Suppl. 1), 84–90.

Swenson, C. W., Kolenic, G. E., Trowbridge, E. R., et al. (2017). Obesity and stress urinary incontinence in women: Compromised continence mechanism or excess bladder pressure during cough? *International Urogynecology Journal, 28,* 1377–1385.

Thiagamoorthy, G., Johnson, A., Thakar, R., et al. (2014). National survey of perineal trauma and its subsequent management in the United Kingdom. *International Urogynecology Journal and Pelvic Floor Dysfunction, 25,* 1621–1627.

Trowbridge, E. R., Wei, J. T., Fenner, D. E., et al. (2007). Effects of aging on lower urinary tract and pelvic floor function in nulliparous women. *Obstetrics & Gynecology, 109,* 715–720.

Tunn, R., DeLancey, J. O. L., Howard, D., et al. (1999). MR imaging of levator ani muscle recovery following vaginal delivery. *International Urogynecology Journal, 10,* 300–307.

Van Geelen, J. M., Lemmens, W., Eskes, T., et al. (1982). The urethral pressure profile in pregnancy and after delivery in healthy nulliparous women. *American Journal of Obstetrics and Gynecology, 144,* 636–649.

Weidner, A. C., Barber, M. D., Visco, A. G., et al. (2000). Pelvic muscle electromyography of levator ani and external anal sphincter in nulliparous women and women with pelvic floor dysfunction. *American Journal of Obstetrics and Gynecology, 183*(6), 1390–1399 discussion 1399–1401.

Weidner, A. C., Jamison, M. G., Branham, V., et al. (2006). Neuropathic injury to the levator ani occurs in 1 in 4 primiparous women. *American Journal of Obstetrics and Gynecology, 195,* 1851–1857.

Woodley, S. J., Lawrenson, P., Boyle, R., et al. (2020). Pelvic floor muscle training for preventing and treating urinary and faecal incontinence in antenatal and postnatal women. *Cochrane Database of Systematic Reviews* Issue 5, Art. No. CD007471.

Zubieta, M., Carr, R. L., Drake, M. J., et al. (2016). Influence of voluntary pelvic floor muscle contraction and pelvic floor muscle training on urethral closure pressures: A systematic literature review. *International Urogynecology Journal, 27,* 687–696.

Obstetric Anal Sphincter Injuries

Ruwan J. Fernando and Abdul H. Sultan

PREVALENCE

Obstetric anal sphincter injuries (OASIS) are defined as perineal trauma involving the anal sphincter complex during childbirth. There has been considerable variation in the classification of perineal tears in the literature leading to suboptimal treatment (Sultan and Thakar, 2002). A more descriptive classification was introduced by Sultan (1999). This Sultan classification (Table 7.5.1 and Fig. 7.5.6) is now accepted globally including the International Continence Society (Abrams et al., 2017), the Royal College of Obstetricians and Gynaecologists (RCOG; 2015), and the American College of Obstetricians and Gynecologists (2018).

The important change in this classification is that for the first time it includes a tear of the internal sphincter. It has been shown that if injuries to the internal sphincter persist after childbirth, there is a significant worsening of symptoms of anal incontinence (Mahony et al., 2007). If the tear involves the rectal mucosa with an intact anal sphincter complex, by definition it is not a fourth-degree tear. This must be documented as a rectal buttonhole tear (Fig. 7.5.7). However, OASIS can occur in combination with a rectal buttonhole tear when there

is an intervening island of anorectal epithelium between the two injuries, in which case it should be described as such. If not recognized and repaired, this type of tear may lead to a rectovaginal fistula (Roper, Amber, Wan, & et al., 2020a, 2020b).

Sultan et al. (1993a, 1993b) reported that 35% of primiparous women and 44% of multiparous women developed 'occult' anal sphincter defects during vaginal delivery. A total of 13% of these women developed subsequent anal incontinence. Further prospective studies showed that between 20% and 41% of women sustained occult sphincter injuries (Abramowitz et al., 2000; Belmonte-Montes et al., 2001; Chaliha et al., 2001; Donnelly et al., 1998; Faltin et al., 2000; Nazir et al., 2002; Rieger et al., 1998; Zetterstrom et al., 1999).

The term *occult anal sphincter injury* was used because in these studies there were no clinically detectable OASIS following vaginal delivery in most of the women. However, a subsequent study by Andrews et al. (2006) showed that these occult defects were clinically undiagnosed OASIS at the time of delivery that were subsequently detected by endoanal ultrasound scan.

Over the past decade, there has been an increase in the reported incidence of OASIS worldwide. In the UK, this has increased in primiparous vaginal deliveries from 1.8% in 2000 to 5.9% in 2012 (Gurol-Urganci et al., 2013). However, this apparent increase is probably a reflection of improved identification and diagnosis of OASIS following hands-on perineal and anal sphincter courses (Croyden Urogynaecology and Pelvic Floor Reconstruction Unit, 2017) rather than an increase in the incidence. These training workshops have been shown to have a beneficial effect in education and change of practice (Andrews et al., 2005).

CAUSES AND RISK FACTORS FOR OASIS

Causes and risk factors for OASIS are inter-related.

Parity

Primiparas carry a higher risk of sustaining OASIS compared to multiparas. As nulliparous women have a relatively inelastic perineum (Combs et al., 1990), it

TABLE 7.5.1	Sultan Classification of Obstetric Perineal Tears
First Degree	Injury only to the perineal skin with intact perineal muscles
Second Degree	Injury to the perineum involving perineal muscles but not involving the anal sphincter
Third Degree	Injury to the perineum involving the anal sphincter complex (EAS and IAS) 3a: <50% of EAS thickness torn 3b: >50% of EAS thickness torn 3c: both EAS and IAS torn
Fourth Degree	Injury to the perineum involving the anal sphincter complex (EAS and IAS) and rectal mucosa

EAS, External anal sphincter; *IAS,* internal anal sphincter.
From Sultan (1999).

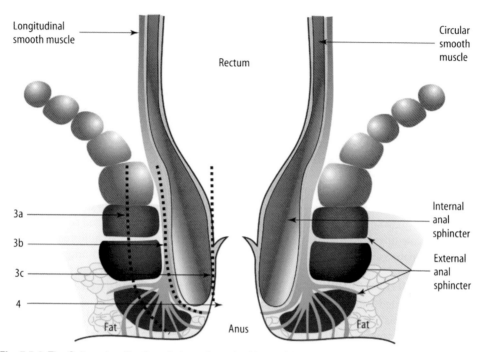

Fig. 7.5.6 The Sultan classification of obstetric anal sphincter injuries. *(Permission granted from Springer.)*

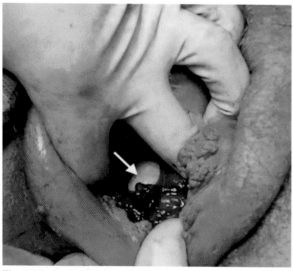

Fig. 7.5.7 A rectal buttonhole tear (arrow) during a digital rectal examination. *(From Roper et al. (2020b).)*

can lead to inadequate perineal stretching during the second stage of labour and predisposing to a higher incidence of perineal trauma. In addition, compared to multiparas, nulliparous women have a longer duration of labour, receive more episiotomies to prevent perineal trauma and also have a higher incidence of instrumental delivery. The combination of these risk factors increases the risk of OASIS in nulliparous women (McLeod et al., 2003).

Increased Birth Weight

Birth weight of more than 4 kg is associated with increased maternal perineal injury, especially OASIS (Beta et al., 2019). This may be attributed to a larger head circumference, prolonged labour and a difficult delivery, particularly when associated with instrumental delivery. A large baby is also likely to disrupt the fascial supports of the pelvic floor and cause a stretch injury to the pelvic and pudendal nerves (Sultan et al., 1994). Macrosomic babies are more likely to develop shoulder dystocia, and the different manoeuvres used during shoulder dystocia increase the risk of OASIS (Beta et al., 2019).

Malposition and Malpresentation

An occipitoposterior position (OPP) is reported to be associated with an increased incidence of OASIS (Beta et al., 2019; De Leew et al., 2001; Green and Soohoo, 1989; Pearl et al., 1993). This increase may be associated with several factors. Incomplete flexion of the foetal head in OPP increases the presenting diameter. In addition, OPP is associated with a prolonged second stage of labour which results in persistent pressure on the perineum leading to oedematous and friable tissues, making it more vulnerable to lacerations. OPPs are also associated with an increased rate of instrumental deliveries compared to occipitoanterior positions, which also contribute to an increased risk of OASIS.

Malpresentations such as face presentation are also associated with larger presenting diameters causing an increased risk of OASIS (Arsène et al., 2019; De Leeuw et al., 2001). However, breech deliveries do not appear to increase the risk, but this may be attributed to stringent selection criteria and a low threshold for caesarean section during labour (Hannah et al., 2000).

Duration of Labour and Rate of Delivery

Precipitate labour is associated with cervical, perineal, labial and urethral injury. This is due to the lack of time available for the maternal tissues to adjust to delivery forces and hence allow a controlled delivery with an episiotomy if necessary. Furthermore, delivery following precipitate labour is more likely to occur under less favourable circumstances, such as during transit to the hospital, in a standing position and quite often without experienced assistance. Several studies have reported that a second stage of labour lasting more than 60 minutes is associated with an increased incidence of OASIS (Beta et al., 2019; Bodner-Adler et al., 2001; De Leeuw et al., 2001; McLeod et al., 2003). There is evidence to suggest that a prolonged active second stage of labour causes pudendal nerve damage. It has been suggested that this may occur in the advanced first stage of labour, and therefore a caesarean section performed after the onset of labour resulting in cervical dilatation of more than 8 cm can be associated with pudendal nerve damage (Fynes et al., 1999; Sultan et al., 1994). It has also been suggested that the passive second stage of labour should be accelerated with oxytocics, particularly in women who have an epidural rather than resorting to instrumental delivery, which in itself can cause more trauma (Sultan et al., 1994).

Episiotomy

The Cochrane review by Carroli and Belizan (2009), which analysed six randomized controlled trials, concluded that compared to the use of routine episiotomy, restrictive episiotomy was associated with less posterior perineal trauma (risk ratio [RR]: 0.88, 95% CI: 0.84–0.92). But the restrictive episiotomy group reported a higher incidence of anterior perineal trauma compared to the routine episiotomy group (RR: 1.02, 95% CI: 0.90–1.16). This review concluded that there was no difference in terms of severe vaginal or perineal trauma between routine and restrictive episiotomy groups. The reviewers also concluded that the results for mediolateral versus median episiotomy were also similar to the overall comparison. The retrospective study by Bodner-Adler et al. (2001) reported a sixfold increase in OASIS with midline episiotomy compared to mediolateral episiotomy. A prospective non-randomized controlled study by Combs et al. (1990) reported an adjusted odds ratio of 5.92 for OASIS with midline episiotomy compared to mediolateral episiotomy. A more recent Cochrane review by Jiang et al. (2017) which analysed 12 randomized controlled studies concluded that for women where an unassisted vaginal birth was anticipated, a policy of selective episiotomy may result in 30% fewer women experiencing severe perineal/vaginal trauma (RR: 0.70, 95% CI: 0.52–0.94).

Although previous large observational studies warrant the liberal use of an adequate mediolateral or lateral episiotomy during operative vaginal delivery to reduce the risk of women sustaining OASIS, a recent review by Sultan et al. (2019) suggested that the angle of episiotomy of 60 degrees from the midline is also important in preventing OASIS.

Instrumental Delivery

Forceps delivery is more likely to cause injury because it occupies almost 12% more space in the pelvis and the shanks of the forceps stretch the perineum, causing injury particularly to the anal sphincter when pulling in the posterolateral direction to encourage flexion of the head. Unlike the ventouse extractor that can detach, the forceps does not have such a fail-safe mechanism, and therefore excessive force can be applied particularly under epidural anaesthesia.

Studies have consistently demonstrated that women with instrumental deliveries have higher rates of anal sphincter tears and that forceps deliveries carry the highest risk of third- or fourth-degree perineal tears. The risk of having a severe perineal injury has been reported to be 1.5 to 14 times higher with forceps, and up to 4 times higher with ventouse, than with spontaneous vaginal delivery (Pergialiotis et al., 2020).

MANAGEMENT OF OASIS

The RCOG (2015) has produced guidelines on the identification, repair and follow-up after the repair of OASIS. A recent review by Roper et al. (2020a, 2020b) on guidelines regarding the management of OASIS in different countries has shown that there was a wide variation in methodological quality and evidence used for recommendations, indicating that there is a need for an agreed-on international guideline. This will enable healthcare practitioners to follow the same recommendations and provide evidence-based care to all women globally.

Identification of OASIS

All women having a vaginal birth are at risk of sustaining an OASIS or buttonhole tear. They should therefore be examined systematically, including a digital vaginal and rectal examination, to assess the severity of damage, particularly prior to suturing (RCOG, 2015).

Before assessing for perineal trauma, healthcare professionals should do the following (National Institute for Health and Clinical Excellence, 2017):
1. Explain to the woman what they plan to do and why.
2. Offer analgesia if the patient has not already had regional analgesia.
3. Ensure good lighting.
4. Position the woman so that she is comfortable and so that the genital structures can be seen clearly.

Examination

The examination should be performed gently, preferably immediately after the delivery. If perineal trauma is identified following birth, further systematic assessment should be carried out, including a rectal examination. Systematic assessment of genital trauma should include the following (Sultan and Kettle, 2007):
1. Further explain what the healthcare professional plans to do and why.
2. Confirm that effective local or regional analgesia is in place.
3. Visually assess the extent of perineal trauma, preferably including the structures involved, the apex of the injury and assessment of bleeding.
4. Carefully examine the labia, clitoris and urethra, which is essential to identify any injury and structures needing repair prior to the perineal repair.

5. If uncertainty exists as to the nature or extent of the trauma sustained, a more experienced healthcare professional should review the extent of the trauma.
6. The systematic assessment and its results should be fully documented, preferably pictorially.

Diagnosis of OASIS

Sultan and Kettle (2007) described the following steps to make an accurate clinical diagnosis.

To diagnose OASIS, clear visualization is necessary, and the injury should be confirmed by palpation. By inserting the index finger in the anal canal and the thumb in the vagina, the anal sphincter can be palpated by performing a pill rolling movement. If there is still uncertainty, the woman should be asked to contract her anal sphincter, and if the anal sphincter is disrupted, a distinct gap will be felt anteriorly.

If the perineal skin is intact, there will be an absence of puckering on the perineal skin anteriorly. This may not be evident under regional or general anaesthesia. As the external anal sphincter (EAS) is in a state of tonic contraction, disruption results in retraction of the sphincter ends. Therefore, the sphincter ends need to be grasped and retrieved. The internal anal sphincter (IAS) should be identified and repaired separately.

Repair of OASIS

1. Immediate repair of the perineal injury compared to delayed repair is advisable, as the immediate repair will reduce bleeding and pain associated with the injury, which may in turn affect early breastfeeding and bonding. Immediate repair also prevents the development of oedema, which may affect the subsequent recognition of structures involved and reduce the possibility of infection (RCOG, 2015).
2. The repair should be performed only by a healthcare professional experienced in anal sphincter repair or by a trainee under direct supervision (RCOG, 2015).
3. Repair should be conducted in the operating theatre, where there is access to good lighting, appropriate equipment and aseptic conditions (RCOG, 2015).
4. Regional or general anaesthesia is an important prerequisite, as the inherent tone in the sphincter muscle can cause the torn muscle ends to retract within its sheath. Muscle relaxation is necessary to retrieve the ends and overlap without tension (Sultan and Thakar, 2007a).

5. In the presence of a fourth-degree tear, the torn anal epithelium is repaired with interrupted 3/0 Polyglactin sutures with the knots tied in the anal lumen. Use of PDS sutures for repair of the anorectal mucosa should be avoided, as they take longer to dissolve and may cause discomfort and irritation in the anal canal (RCOG, 2015; Sultan and Thakar, 2007a).

6. The IAS (which is the continuation of the longitudinal smooth muscle of the large intestine) appears paler than EAS. This should be identified. Any IAS tear should be repaired separately from the EAS with either interrupted or mattress sutures using 3/0 PDS without any attempt to overlap (RCOG, 2015; Sultan and Thakar, 2007a).

7. The EAS should be repaired with either 3/0 PDS or 2/0 Polyglactin sutures with an either end-to-end or overlapping technique. However, an overlap repair can only be performed if the full thickness of the external sphincter is torn (e.g., 3c and fourth-degree tears. Therefore, all 3a and partial-thickness 3b tears must only be repaired by an end-to-end technique (RCOG, 2015; Sultan and Thakar, 2007a).

8. Great care should be exercised in reconstructing the perineal muscles to provide support to the sphincter repair and maintain the vagino-anal distance. Burying of surgical knots beneath the superficial perineal muscles is recommended to minimize the risk of knot and suture migration to the skin (RCOG, 2015; Sultan and Thakar, 2007a).

9. A vaginal and rectal examination must be performed after the repair to ensure that no suture has been inadvertently inserted into the rectum; if a stitch is identified, the repair should be undone and the stitch removed to minimize the risk of a rectovaginal fistula (RCOG, 2015; Sultan and Thakar, 2007a).

10. The count of swabs and needles should be checked.

Postoperative Care

1. The use of broad-spectrum antibiotics is recommended following repair of OASIS to reduce the risk of postoperative infections and wound dehiscence. Type of antibiotics should be based on local antibiotics guidelines in keeping with advice from microbiologists (RCOG, 2015). A Cochrane review addressing antibiotic prophylaxis for third- and fourth-degree perineal tears, comparing prophylactic antibiotics against placebo or no antibiotics, included only one randomized controlled trial of 147 participants. Although the data suggested that prophylactic antibiotics help prevent perineal wound complications following third- or fourth-degree perineal tears, loss to follow-up was quite high (Buppasiri et al., 2014).

2. The use of postoperative laxatives is recommended to reduce the risk of wound dehiscence (RCOG, 2015). There is only one randomized controlled trial that compared codeine phosphate (constipation group) and lactulose (laxative group), which showed that the patients in the laxative group had significantly earlier and less painful bowel motion and earlier postnatal discharge. There was no difference in the symptomatic or functional outcome of repair between the two regimens (Mahony et al., 2004). The use of a stool-bulking agent in addition to a laxative has not been shown to be beneficial (Eogan et al., 2007).

3. A comprehensive record should be documented together with a diagram to demonstrate the injury. This is vital for audit and risk management purposes (RCOG, 2015).

4. A Foley catheter should be inserted for about 24 hours unless the midwifery staff can ensure that spontaneous voiding occurs at least every 3 to 4 hours to prevent bladder overdistention (Sultan and Thakar, 2007b).

5. Postoperative analgesia such as rectal or oral non-steroidal anti-inflammatory agents are recommended after the repair of OASIS. Codeine-based preparations are best avoided, as they may cause constipation, leading to excessive straining and possible disruption of the repair (Sultan and Thakar, 2007c).

Role of the Physiotherapist

The physiotherapist has a vital role to play in the management of OASIS, which is discussed in subsequent sections. In most healthcare settings a women's health physiotherapist would follow up with patients who had repair of OASIS before being discharged home and later after about 6 to 8 weeks. Physiotherapists must pay attention to the following aspects.

Immediate Examination (Within 24–48 Hours)

1. Examine for the presence of perineal bruising (Fig. 7.5.8) and extent. A minor degree of bruising is not

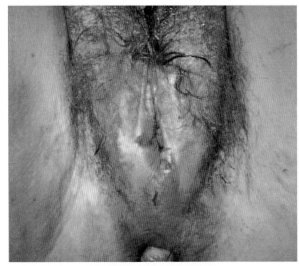

Fig. 7.5.8 Perineal bruising.

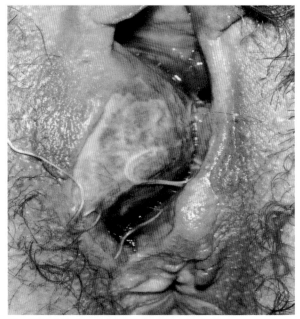

Fig. 7.5.10 Perineal wound infection and dehiscence.

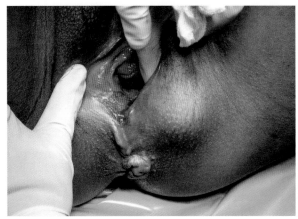

Fig. 7.5.9 Left vulval haematoma measuring more than 5 cm.

uncommon after the repair of OASIS due to dissection of underlying tissue. If the perineal bruising is expanding, it may be the first sign of an underlying haematoma which needs medical review.

2. Examine for the presence of a haematoma (Fig. 7.5.9). If less than 5 cm, the haematoma can be managed conservatively with analgesics. If the haematoma is more than 5 cm or expanding, it may need surgical drainage.

3. Evidence of urinary retention and voiding dysfunction (caused by pain following OASIS repair and effect of spinal, epidural or opioid analgesics) should be elicited from any history of passing a small amount of urine, inability to pass urine or overflow incontinence. The bladder can be palpable on abdominal examination.

4. Evidence of constipation and stool impaction should be elicited from the history. This can have an impact on the repair and need to be treated with appropriate laxatives.

If any of the preceding are significant, a discussion should be held with the medical team and managed appropriately.

Follow-Up Examination (Within 6–8 Weeks)

The physiotherapist may see women around 6 to 8 weeks separately or as the part of a perineal clinic depending on local guidelines and availability. This is a vital part of the follow-up, as it may be the first opportunity to assess the perineum and bowel symptoms, especially if there is no established perineal clinic. Use of validated questionnaires and systematic examination is important. Some of the complications seen at this stage are perineal wound dehiscence (Fig. 7.5.10), granulation tissue (Fig. 7.5.11), faecal soiling suggestive of anal incontinence, lack of anal puckering (Fig. 7.5.12) suggestive of residual sphincter damage or inadequate repair, and shortening of perineal body (Fig. 7.5.13) suggestive of inadequate repair.

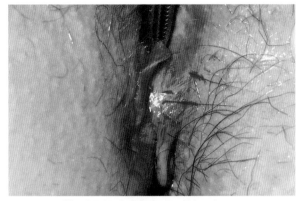

Fig. 7.5.11 Perineal granulation tissue.

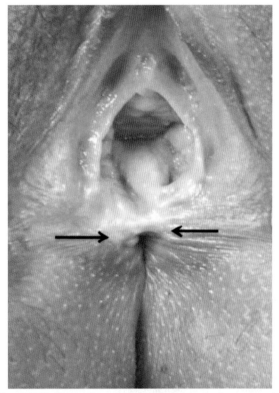

Fig. 7.5.13 Shortening of the perineal body (between the arrows) suggestive of an inadequate repair.

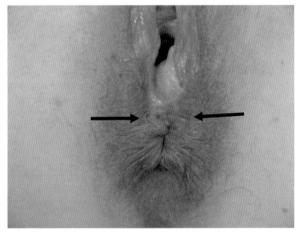

Fig. 7.5.12 Absence of anal puckering (arrows).

Absence of puckering of the anal skin between arrows in Figs 7.5.12 and 7.5.13 is suggestive of residual damage to the subcutaneous part of the EAS.

Role of a Perineal Clinic

It has been recommended that all women sustaining OASIS should have an assessment around 6 to 12 weeks postpartum by clinicians with a special interest in such injury where possible (RCOG, 2015). Different models of perineal clinics have been reported depending on the facilities and expertise available. These include clinics led by consultant urogynaecologists or consultant obstetricians and gynaecologists, with some triaged or assisted by specialized midwives or nurses and clinics led by a specialist midwife. Some clinics are designed as a one-stop clinic which offers a detailed history including the use of a validated bladder and bowel symptom questionnaire, an examination and investigations including endoanal ultrasound and anal manometry (Wan, Taithongchai, Veiga, & et al., 2020a, 2020b).

Endoanal Ultrasound

Endoanal ultrasound scanning using a 360-degree rotating transducer is the gold standard for assessing anal sphincter anatomy. This enables the identification of any defects in the anal sphincter complex (Figs 7.5.14–7.5.16).

Anal Manometry

Anal manometry assesses the resting and squeeze pressures of the anal sphincter complex. The IAS generates most of the resting pressure, whereas the EAS generates most of the squeeze pressure. Incremental squeeze pressure should be greater than 20 mmHg (Fig. 7.5.17). Patients who have had both EAS and IAS defects tend to have low resting and squeeze pressures (Fig. 7.5.18). Patients who have had an

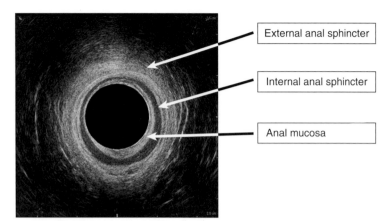

External anal sphincter

Internal anal sphincter

Anal mucosa

Fig. 7.5.14 Endoanal ultrasound scan of a normal anal sphincter complex.

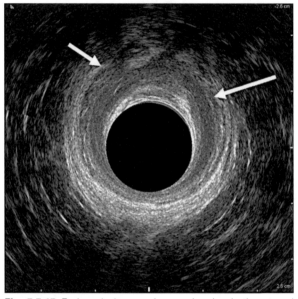

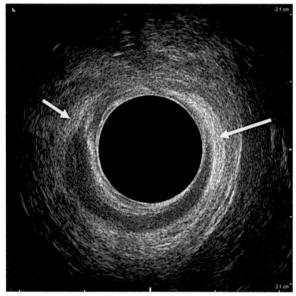

Fig. 7.5.15 Endoanal ultrasound scan showing both external anal sphincter and internal anal sphincter defects between the 11 and 2 o'clock position (arrows).

Fig. 7.5.16 Endoanal ultrasound showing an isolated internal anal sphincter defect between the 9 and 3 o'clock position with evidence showing a repaired external anal sphincter between the 11 and 12 o'clock position (arrows).

isolated IAS defect tend to have low resting pressure with normal squeeze pressure (Fig. 7.5.19).

MANAGEMENT OF SUBSEQUENT PREGNANCY AFTER OASIS

It has been recommended that all women who have sustained OASIS in a previous pregnancy and who are symptomatic or have abnormal endoanal ultrasonography and/or manometry should be counselled regarding the option of elective caesarean birth (RCOG, 2015).

A large cohort study showed the rate of recurrent OASIS to be 7.2% for women who had previously sustained OASIS during their first vaginal delivery compared with a rate of 1.3% for women who did not sustain OASIS (Endozien et al., 2014).

In a recently published randomized controlled trial, 222 women who had a third-degree tear and/

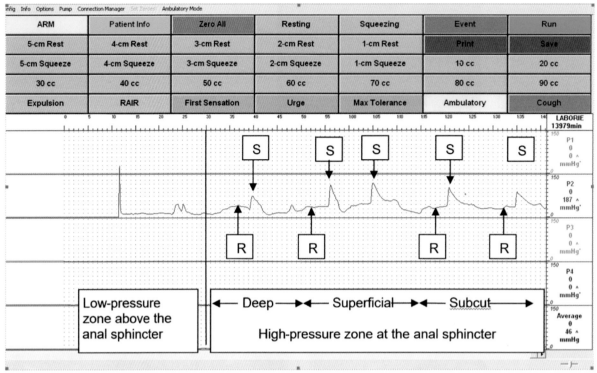

Fig. 7.5.17 Normal manometry. *R*, Resting pressure; *S*, squeeze pressure.

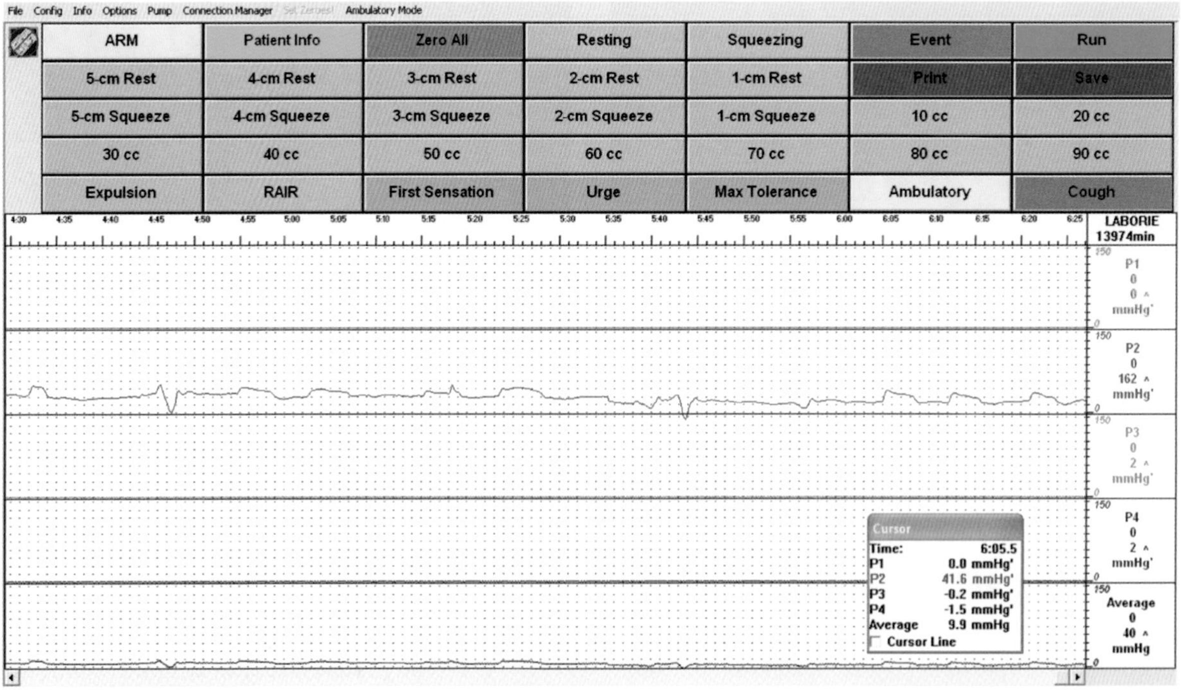

Fig. 7.5.18 Low resting pressure and low squeeze pressure in a patient who had both external and internal sphincter defects.

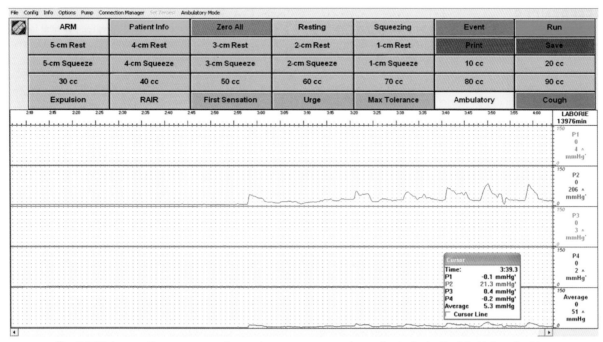

Fig. 7.5.19 Low resting pressure and normal squeeze pressure in a patient who had isolated internal sphincter defect.

or a forceps delivery in their first pregnancy with no symptoms of anal incontinence were randomized to have a vaginal birth or a planned caesarean section. The authors concluded that in women with asymptomatic obstetric anal sphincter lesions diagnosed by ultrasound, planning a caesarean section had no significant impact on anal continence 6 months after the second delivery, and the results do not support advising systematic caesarean section for this indication (Abramowitz et al., 2020). However, in this study, 49 of 222 women had OASIS diagnosed and repaired at the time of delivery, and the rest were detected by endoanal ultrasound scan subsequently. In addition, the patients did not undergo anal manometry. In effect, the randomized controlled trial by Abramowitz et al. (2020) does not fit in to the criteria recommended by the RCOG, and it is difficult to make any recommendations.

There are few observational studies where women were offered a vaginal birth or a caesarean section based on their symptoms, endoanal scan findings and anal manometry (Jordan et al., 2018; Karmarkar et al., 2015; Scheer et al., 2009).

These studies showed no significant worsening of bowel symptoms and sphincter integrity postpartum in the vaginal birth group if they were asymptomatic and had a normal endoanal scan and anal manometry prior to the second pregnancy.

▌ KEY POINTS

- OASIS are associated with significant maternal morbidity, including anal incontinence.
- Immediate identification, correct classification, appropriate repair and subsequent follow-up reduces the morbidity.
- A dedicated perineal clinic with facilities for endoanal ultrasound scanning and anal manometry is vital in early identification of complications, treatment and the decision of subsequent delivery.
- The physiotherapist plays a vital role in early recognition of haematoma, associated urinary retention and bowel symptoms.
- Follow-up assessment by a physiotherapist is also important in recognizing perineal wound infection, granulation tissue and bowel symptoms.

REFERENCES

Abramowitz, L., Mandelbrot, L., Bourgeois Moine, A., et al. (2020). Cesarean section in the second delivery to prevent anal incontinence after asymptomatic obstetric anal sphincter injury: The EPIC multicenter randomized trial. *British Journal of Obstetrics and Gynaecology*, *128*(4), 685–693.

Abramowitz, L., Sobhani, I., Ganasia, R., et al. (2000). Are sphincter defects the cause of anal incontinence after vaginal delivery? Results of a prospective study. *Diseases of the Colon & Rectum*, *43*, 590–598.

Abrams, P., Cardozo, L., Wagg, A., et al. (Eds.). (2017). *Incontinence* (6th ed.) Bristol, UK: International Continence Society.

American College of Obstetricians and Gynecologists. (2018). Practice Bulletin No. 198: Prevention and management of obstetric lacerations at vaginal delivery. *Obstetrics & Gynecology*, *132*(3), e87–e102.

Andrews, V., Thakar, R., Sultan, A. H., et al. (2005). Can hands-on perineal repair courses affect clinical practice. *British Journal of Midwifery*, *13*(9), 562–566.

Andrews, V., Thakar, R., Sultan, A. H., et al. (2006). Occult anal sphincter injuries—myth or reality? *British Journal of Obstetrics and Gynaecology*, *113*, 195–200.

Arsène, E., Langlois, C., Clouqueur, E., et al. (2019). Prognosis for deliveries in face presentation: A case–control study. *Archives of Gynecology and Obstetrics*, *300*(4), 869–874.

Belmonte-Montes, C., Hagerman, G., Vega-Yepez, P. A., et al. (2001). Anal sphincter injury after vaginal delivery in primiparous females. *Diseases of the Colon & Rectum*, *44*(9), 1244–1248.

Beta, J., Khan, N., Khalil, A., et al. (2019). Maternal and neonatal complications of fetal macrosomia: Systematic review and meta-analysis. *Ultrasound in Obstetrics and Gynecology*, *54*(3), 308–318.

Bodner-Adler, B., Bodner, K., Kaider, A., et al. (2001). Risk factors for third degree perineal tears in vaginal delivery with an analysis of episiotomy types. *Journal of Reproductive Medicine*, *46*, 752–756.

Buppasiri, P., Lumbiganon, P., Thinkhamrop, J., et al. (2014). Antibiotic prophylaxis for third- and fourth-degree perineal tear during vaginal birth. *Cochrane Database of Systematic Reviews* Issue 10, Art. No. CD005125.

Carroli, G., & Belizan, J. (2009). Episiotomy for vaginal birth. *Cochrane Database of Systematic Reviews* Issue 1, Art. No. CD000081.

Chaliha, C., Sultan, A. H., Kalia, V., et al. (2001). Anal function: Effect of pregnancy and delivery. *American Journal of Obstetrics and Gynecology*, *185*, 427–432.

Combs, C. A., Robertson, P. A., & Laros, R. K. (1990). Risk factors for third-degree and fourth-degree perineal lacerations in forceps and vacuum deliveries. *American Journal of Obstetrics and Gynecology*, *163*, 100–104.

Croydon Urogynaecology and Pelvic Floor Reconstruction Unit. (2017). *Home page [online]*. Available: https://www.perineum.net (accessed 21.07.22).

De Leeuw, J. W., Sruijk, P. C., Vierhout, M. E., et al. (2001). Risk factors for third degree perineal ruptures during delivery. *British Journal of Obstetrics and Gynaecology*, *108*, 383–387.

Donnelly, V., Fynes, M., Campbell, D., et al. (1998). Obstetric events leading to anal sphincter damage. *Obstetrics & Gynecology*, *92*, 955–961.

Edozien, L. C., Gurol-Urganci, I., Cromwell, D. A., et al. (2014). Impact of third- and fourth-degree perineal tears at first birth on subsequent pregnancy outcomes: A cohort study. *British Journal of Obstetrics and Gynaecology*, *121*(13), 1695–1703.

Eogan, M., Daly, L., Behan, M., et al. (2007). Randomised clinical trial of a laxative alone versus a laxative and a bulking agent after primary repair of obstetric anal sphincter injury. *British Journal of Obstetrics and Gynaecology*, *114*(6), 736–740.

Faltin, D., Boulvain, M., Irion, O., et al. (2000). Diagnosis of anal sphincter tears by postpartum endosonography to predict fecal incontinence. *Obstetrics & Gynecology*, *95*(5), 643–647.

Fynes, M., Donnelly, V., Behan, M., et al. (1999). Effect of second vaginal delivery on anorectal physiology and faecal continence: A prospective study. *Lancet*, *354*(9183), 983–986.

Green, J. R., & Soohoo, S. L. (1989). Factors associated with rectal injury in spontaneous delivery. *Obstetrics & Gynecology*, *73*, 732–738.

Gurol-Urganci, I., Cromwell, D., Edozien, L., et al. (2013). Third- and fourth-degree perineal tears among primiparous women in England between 2000 and 2012: Time trends and risk factors. *British Journal of Obstetrics and Gynaecology*, *120*, 1516–1525.

Hannah, M. E., Hannah, W. J., Hewson, S. A., et al. (2000). Planned caesarean section versus planned vaginal birth for breech presentation at term; a randomised multicentre trial. *Lancet*, *356*, 1375–1383.

Jiang, H., Qian, X., Carroli, G., et al. (2017). Selective versus routine use of episiotomy for vaginal birth. *Cochrane Database of Systematic Reviews* Issue 2, Art. No. CD000081.

Jordan, P. A., Naidu, M., Thakar, R., et al. (2018). Effect of subsequent vaginal delivery on bowel symptoms and anorectal function in women who sustained a previous obstetric anal sphincter injury. *International Urogynecology Journal*, *29*, 1579–1588.

Karmarkar, R., Bhide, A., Digesu, A., et al. (2015). Mode of delivery after obstetric anal sphincter injury. *European Journal of Obstetrics & Gynecology and Reproductive Biology*, 194, 7–10.

Mahony, R., Behan, M., Daly, L., et al. (2007). Internal anal sphincter defect influences continence outcome following obstetric anal sphincter injury. *American Journal of Obstetrics and Gynecology*, 196, 217.

Mahony, R., Behan, M., O'Herlihy, C., et al. (2004). Randomized, clinical trial of bowel confinement vs. laxative use after primary repair of a third-degree obstetric anal sphincter tear. *Diseases of the Colon & Rectum*, 47(1), 12–17.

McLeod, N. L., Gilmour, D. T., Joseph, K. S., et al. (2003). Trends in major risk factors for anal sphincter lacerations: A 10 year study. *Journal of Obstetrics and Gynaecology Canada*, 25, 586–593.

National Institute for Health and Clinical Excellence. (2017). *Intrapartum care: Care of healthy women and their babies during childbirth. Clinical guideline 190.* Manchester, UK: National Institute for Health and Clinical Excellence.

Nazir, M., Carlsen, E., & Nesheim, B. (2002). Do occult anal sphincter injuries, vector volume manometry and delivery variables have any predictive value for bowel symptoms after first time vaginal delivery without third and fourth degree rupture? A prospective study. *Acta Obstetricia et Gynecologica Scandinavica*, 81(8), 720–726.

Pearl, M. L., Roberts, J. M., Laros, R. K., et al. (1993). Vaginal delivery from persistent occiput posterior position. Influence on maternal and neonatal morbidity. *Journal of Reproductive Medicine*, 38(12), 955–961.

Pergialiotis, V., Bellos, I., Fanaki, M., et al. (2020). Risk factors for severe perineal trauma during childbirth: An updated meta-analysis. *European Journal of Obstetrics & Gynecology and Reproductive Biology*, 247, 94–100.

Rieger, N., Schloithe, A., Saccone, G., et al. (1998). A prospective study of anal sphincter injury due to childbirth. *Scandinavian Journal of Gastroenterology*, 33, 950–955.

Roper, J. C., Amber, N., Wan, O. Y. K., et al. (2020a). Review of available national guidelines for obstetric anal sphincter injury. *International Urogynecology Journal*, 31(11), 2247–2259.

Roper, J. C., Thakar, R., & Sultan, A. H. (2020b). Isolated rectal buttonhole tears in obstetrics: Case series and review of the literature. *International Urogynecology Journal*, 32(7), 1761–1769.

Royal College of Obstetricians and Gynaecologists (RCOG). (2015). *RCOG green top guideline 29: Management of third- and fourth-degree perineal tears following vaginal delivery.* London: Royal College of Obstetricians and Gynaecologists.

Scheer, I., Thakar, R., & Sultan, A. H. (2009). Mode of delivery after previous obstetric anal sphincter injuries (OASIS)—a reappraisal? *International Urogynecology Journal and Pelvic Floor Dysfunction*, 20(9), 1095–1101.

Sultan, A. H. (1999). Editorial: Obstetric perineal injury and anal incontinence. *Clinical Risk*, 5, 193–196.

Sultan, A. H., Kamm, M. A., Hudson, C. N., et al. (1993). Anal sphincter disruption during vaginal delivery. *New England Journal of Medicine*, 329, 1905–1911.

Sultan, A. H., Kamm, M. A., & Hudson, C. N. (1994). Pudendal nerve damage during labour: Prospective study before and after childbirth. *British Journal of Obstetrics and Gynaecology*, 101, 22–28.

Sultan, A. H., & Kettle, C. (2007). Diagnosis of perineal trauma. In A. H. Sultan, R. Thakar, & D. E. Fenner (Eds.), *Perineal and anal sphincter trauma: Diagnosis and clinical management* (pp. 13–19). London: Springer.

Sultan, A. H., & Thakar, R. (2002). Lower genital tract and anal sphincter trauma. *Best Practice & Research Clinical Obstetrics & Gynaecology*, 16, 99–115.

Sultan, A. H., & Thakar, R. (2007). Third and fourth degree tears. In A. H. Sultan, R. Thakar, & D. E. Fenner (Eds.), *Perineal and anal sphincter trauma: Diagnosis and clinical management* (p. 38). London: Springer.

Sultan, A. H., & Thakar, R. (2007). Third and fourth degree tears. In A. H. Sultan, R. Thakar, & D. E. Fenner (Eds.), *Perineal and anal sphincter trauma: Diagnosis and clinical management* (p. 40). London: Springer.

Sultan, A. H., & Thakar, R. (2007). Third and fourth degree tears. In A. H. Sultan, R. Thakar, & D. E. Fenner (Eds.), *Perineal and anal sphincter trauma: Diagnosis and clinical management* (pp. 41–42). London: Springer.

Sultan, A. H., Thakar, R., Ismail, K. M., et al. (2019). The role of mediolateral episiotomy during operative vaginal delivery. *European Journal of Obstetrics & Gynecology and Reproductive Biology*, 240, 192–196.

Wan, O. Y. K., Taithongchai, A., Veiga, S. I., et al. (2020). A one-stop perineal clinic: Our eleven-year experience. *International Urogynecology Journal*, 31(11), 2317–2326.

Zetterstrom, J., Mellgren, A., Jensen, L. J., et al. (1999). Effect of delivery on anal sphincter morphology and function. *Diseases of the Colon & Rectum*, 42, 1253–1260.

Evidence for Pelvic Floor Muscle Training for Urinary Incontinence Related to the Peripartum Period

Siv Mørkved

INTRODUCTION

Two important questions for pelvic floor muscle training (PFMT) for urinary incontinence (UI) are (1) whether UI can be prevented by training the pelvic floor muscles (PFMs) before problems arise (primary prevention) or (2) whether women at risk at an early stage can be identified with a view to secondary prevention using PFMT.

Reviews on PFMT in prevention and treatment of UI report inconsistent results (Brostrøm and Lose, 2008; Mørkved & Bø, 2014; Schreiner et al., 2018; Woodley et al., 2020). This may be due to the use of different inclusion criteria of studies and different criteria to classify studies as either prevention or treatment interventions. Some authors do not separate between antenatal or postpartum interventions (Brostrøm and Lose, 2008), and there seems to be little attention towards dose–response issues in the training protocols. The aims of this chapter are to answer the following questions:

- Is there evidence that pregnant women should be advised to do PFMT to prevent or treat UI?
- Is there evidence that postnatal women should be advised to do PFMT to prevent or treat UI?
- What is the most optimal training dosage for effective antenatal and postnatal PFMT in prevention and treatment of UI?
- What is the long-term effect of PFMT during pregnancy and after childbirth?

RESEARCH METHODS

We used searches from the Cochrane Incontinence Specialised Register, which contains trials identified from the Cochrane Central Register of Controlled Trials (CENTRAL), MEDLINE, MEDLINE In-Process, MEDLINE Epub Ahead of Print, CINAHL, ClinicalTrials.gov and the World Health Organization's International Clinical Trials Registry Platform (ICTRP), and hand-searched journals and the reference lists of retrieved studies.

Selection Criteria

We included only randomized controlled trials (RCTs) aiming to measure the effect of peripartum PFMT in the prevention or treatment of UI. Thus one arm had to include PFMT and the other arm(s) was no PFMT, usual antenatal or postnatal care, another control condition, or an alternative PFMT intervention. UI, prevalence or severity, had to be explicitly described as an outcome measure. Only full publications written in English or translated into English were included.

Populations included women who, at randomization, were continent (PFMT for prevention) or incontinent (PFMT for treatment), and a mixed population of women who were one or the other (PFMT for prevention or treatment).

Scoring of methodological quality was done according to the PEDro rating scale, giving 1 point for each of the following factors for internal validity: random allocation, concealed allocation, baseline comparability, blinded assessor, blinded subjects, blinded therapists, adequate follow up (≥85%), intention-to-treat analysis, between-group comparison, report of point estimates and variability (Mahler et al., 2003) (Table 7.5.2).

Seven studies included in the previous version of this chapter were excluded in the present version due to their design (Meyer, et al., 2001; Mørkved & Bø, 1997, 2000; Sangsawang and Serisathien, 2012), internal inconsistencies in the data (Mason et al., 2010) and outcome measure (Kim et al., 2012), and two because they only have been published as abstracts (Dias et al., 2011; Hughes et al., 2001).

Tables 7.5.3 to 7.5.7 show the variation in intervention period, training protocol, adherence, contrast between the intervention and control groups, and outcome measures used. No adverse effects of the interventions were reported.

TABLE 7.5.2   PEDro quality score of RCTs in systematic review of studies assessing the effect of pelvic floor muscle exercises during pregnancy (to prevent/treat urinary incontinence)

E – Eligibility criteria specified
1 – Subjects randomly allocated to groups
2 – Allocation concealed
3 – Groups similar at baseline
4 – Subjects blinded
5 – Therapist administering treatment blinded
6 – Assessors blinded
7 – Measures of key outcomes obtained from > 85% of subjects
8 – Data analysed by intention to treat
9 – Statistical comparison between groups conducted
10 – Point measures and measures of variability provided

Study	E	1	2	3	4	5	6	7	8	9	10	Total score
Sleep and Grant, 1987	?	+	?	?	–	–	–	+	–	+	+	4
Wilson et al., 1998	+	+	+	+	–	–	–	–	–	+	+	5
Sampselle et al., 1998	+	+	+	+	–	–	+	–	+	+	+	7
Glazener et al., 2001	+	+	+	+	–	–	+	–	+	+	+	7
Chiarelli et al., 2002	+	+	+	+	–	–	?	+	+	+	+	7
Reilly et al., 2002	+	+	+	+	–	–	+	+	+	+	+	8
Mørkved et al., 2003	+	+	+	+	–	–	+	+	+	+	+	8
Dumoulin et al., 2004	+	+	+	+	–	–	+	+	+	+	+	8
Ewings et al., 2005	+	+	+	+	–	–	–	–	+	+	+	6
Gorbea et al., 2004	+	+	+	+	–	–	–	+	+	+	?	6
Woldringh et al., 2007	+	+	–	+	–	–	?	–	+	+	+	5
Dinc et al., 2009	+	+	+	+	–	–	–	?	+	+	+	6
Wen et al., 2010	+	+	?	+	–	–	–	?	?	+	+	4
Bø et al., 2011	+	+	+	+	–	–	+	–	–	+	+	6
Ko et al., 2011	+	+	+	+	–	–	?	+	?	+	+	6
Liu et al., 2011	?	+	?	?	–	–	–	?	–	+	+	3
Stafne et al., 2012	+	+	+	+	–	–	+	+	+	+	+	8
Hilde et al., 2013	+	+	+	+	–	–	?	+	+	+	+	7
Kou et al., 2013	?	+	?	?	–	–	–	?	?	+	+	3
Miguelutti et al., 2013	+	+	+	+	–	–	–	+	+	+	+	7
Pelarez et al., 2014	+	+	?	+	–	–	–	+	?	+	+	5
Fritel et al., 2015	+	+	+	+	–	–	–	–	+	+	+	6
Assis et al., 2015	+	+	+	+	–	–	–	+	–	+	+	6
Sangsawang et al., 2016	+	+	+	+	–	–	–	+	?	+	+	6
Sut et al., 2016	+	+	?	+	–	–	–	+	–	+	+	5
Yang et al., 2017	+	+	?	+	–	–	–	–	?	+	+	4
Sacomori et al., 2019	+	+	+	+	–	–	–	–	+	+	+	6
Sigurdadottir et al., 2020	+	+	+	+	–	–	+	+	–	+	+	7

+, Criterion is clearly satisfied; –, criterion is not satisfied; ?, not clear if the criterion was satisfied. Total score is determined by counting the number of criteria that are satisfied, except that 'eligibility criteria specified' score is not used to generate the total score. Total scores are out of 10.

TABLE 7.5.3 Studies assessing the effect of antenatal pelvic floor muscle training (PFMT) for prevention (primary and secondary) of urinary incontinence (UI), including only women without urinary incontinence at inclusion

Author	Reilly et al., 2002
	Agur et al., 2008: 8-year follow-up
Design	2 arm RCT
	Control (C): n = 129
	Intervention (I): n = 139
Study population	268 primigravid, continent women with increased bladder neck mobility recruited at 20 weeks of pregnancy.
	Single centre, UK
	8 year follow up: 164/268 (61%) of the original group. C: n = 85, I: n = 79
Training protocol	C: Routine antenatal care (verbal advice).
	I: Individual PFMT with PT at monthly intervals from 20 weeks until delivery, with additional home exercises 3 sets of 8 contractions (each held for 6 seconds) repeated twice daily. Instructed to contract the PFM when coughing or sneezing
Drop-out/Adherence	Losses to follow-up at 12 mth: 14%
	Adherence PFMT: − 11% completed less than 28 days of PFMT; − 46% completed 28 days or more of PFMT. Adverse events not stated. ITT analysis: − 38% in the intervention group were doing PFMT twice or more per week
Results	Self-reported UI at 3 mth post partum:
	C 36/110 (32.7%); I 23/120 (19.2%); RR (95% CI) 0.59 (0.37–0.92); p = 0.023
	QoL: Higher score in the exercise group (p = 0.004)
	Pad-test: NS
	Bladder neck mobility: NS difference
	PFM strength: NS difference
	Self-reported UI at 8 yr follow-up:
	C 38.8%; I 35.4%; p = 0.75
Author	**Gorbea et al., 2004**
Design	2 arm RCT
	Control (C): n = 34 after drop outs
	Intervention (I): n = 38 after drop-outs
Study population	75 pregnant nulliparous continent women recruited at 20 weeks of pregnancy.
	Single setting, Mexico
Training protocol	C: Requested not to perform PFMT during pregnancy or post partum
	I: Individual PFMT with PT, 10 VPFMC each held for 8 s each followed by 3 fast 1-s contractions; 6 s rest. Clinic appointments weekly for 8 weeks, then weekly phone calls up to 20 weeks. Biofeedback and training diary. Correct VPFMC checked
Drop-out/Adherence	Losses to follow up 3/75 (4%)
	Adherence to PFMT: 84% attended 7 or 8 physical therapy appointments. ITT analyses
Results	UI:
	28 wk pregnancy: C 17%; I 0%; p = < 0.05
	35 wk pregnancy: C 47%; I: 0%; p = < 0.05
	6 wk post partum: C 47%; I 15%; p = < 0.05
Author	**Pelaez et al., 2014**
Design	2-arm RCT
	Control (C): n = 96
	Intervention (I): n = 73

TABLE 7.5.3 Studies assessing the effect of antenatal pelvic floor muscle training (PFMT) for prevention (primary and secondary) of urinary incontinence (UI), including only women without urinary incontinence at inclusion—cont'd

Study population	169 healthy, primiparous women recruited in gestational week 10–14. Single centre, Spain
Training protocol	C: Standard antenatal education about PFM. I: 12–16 weeks of aerobic fitness class including PFMT. PFMT program, 3 times per week for ≥ 22 weeks. Started with 1 set of 8 contractions increasing to 100, divided in sets of slow (6 sec) and fast contractions. Daily PFMT at home, 100 contractions in different sets. Instructed in correct contraction, and how to test themselves.
Drop-out/Adherence	Losses to follow up: 16% C:7/96; I:10/73 Adherence to training sessions: ≥80%.
Results	Self-reported UI at 36 weeks of pregnancy: Statistically significant (p = 0.001) difference in frequency of UI and in ICIQ-UI SF score in favor of the intervention group. CG: 2.7 (SD 4.1) IG: 0.2 (SD 1.2)
Author	**Sangsawang et al., 2016**
Design	2-arm RCT Control group (C): n = 35 Intervention group (I): n = 35
Study population	70 primiparous women recruited at 20–30 weeks of pregnancy. Single centre, Thailand
Training protocol	C: usual antenatal care including information about PFMT I: supervised group sessions 45 minutes every second week (total 3 sessions), with midwife. Home training: 20 sets of exercises slow and fast contractions) twice per day, at least 5 days per week. Digital palpation was not used to assess correct contraction.
Drop-out/Adherence	Losses to follow up: 10% C: 5/35; I: 2/35 No women were excluded for failing to perform the PFMT for < 28/42 days
Results	Self-reported UI at 38 weeks of pregnancy: Fewer women in the intervention group reported SUI than the control group: 27.3% versus 53.3% OR 3.05, 95% CI 1.07–8.70, P = 0.018.

ITT, Intention-to-treat analysis; *NS,* not statistically significant; *OR,* odds ratio; *RR,* relative risk; *SD,* standard deviation; *VPFMC,* voluntary pelvic floor muscle contraction. For other abbreviations, see text.

RESULTS

Is There Evidence That Pregnant Women Should Be Advised to Do Pelvic Floor Muscle Training to Prevent or Treat Urinary Incontinence?

Antenatal Pelvic Floor Muscle Training for Prevention (Primary and Secondary) of Urinary Incontinence (see Table 7.5.3)

Four RCTs including only continent pregnant women and assessing the preventive effect of PFMT have been published (Gorbea Chàvez et al., 2004; Pelaez et al., 2014; Reilly et al., 2002; Sangsawang and Sansawang, 2016).

They recruited nulliparous or primiparous women (Gorbea Chàvez et al., 2004; Pelaez et al., 2014; Reilly et al., 2002; Sangsawang and Sangsawang, 2016). One trial was a secondary prevention trial and included only women at risk of developing UI (with increased bladder neck mobility [Reilly et al., 2002]) and had a long-term follow-up study (Agur et al., 2008).

Most trials recruited the women before week 24 of gestation and started the PFMT period during pregnancy.

PEDro scores were from 3 to 8 (see Table 7.5.2).

Quality of the intervention. Pelaez et al. (2014) and Sangsawang and Sangsawang (2016) gave some information, although not enough to be categorized. Gorbea Chàvez et al. (2004) and Reilly et al. (2002) used a PFMT program that was characteristic of strength training. Adherence was registered in all trials.

The control groups were asked not to do PFMT in one trial (Gorbea Chàvez et al., 2004). In the other trials, the control group did not receive instructions in PFMT, received standard care that might have included PFMT or lacked information on control conditions.

Outcomes. Self-reported UI was the primary outcome in all trials.

Results. The results from all trials showed that women randomized to PFMT were significantly less likely to report UI in late pregnancy (Gorbea Chàvez et al., 2004; Pelaez et al., 2014; Sangsawang and Sangsawang, 2016), 0 to 3 months after delivery (Gorbea Chàvez et al., 2004; Pelaez et al., 2014) and 3 to 6 months after delivery (Reilly et al., 2002). Eight years of follow-up data from the trial of Reilly et al. (2002) showed no significant difference in UI between the original intervention and control groups (Agur et al., 2008).

Antenatal Pelvic Floor Muscle Training for Mixed Prevention and Treatment of Urinary Incontinence (Table 7.5.4)

Nine trials including pregnant women with and without UI assessing the effect of PFMT for mixed prevention and treatment of UI have been published (Assis et al., 2015; Bø and Haakstad, 2011; Fritel et al., 2015; Ko et al., 2011; Miquelutti et al., 2013; Mørkved et al., 2003; Sampselle et al., 1998; Stafne et al., 2012; Sut and Kaplan, 2016) (see Table 7.5.4).

All trials except two (Stafne et al., 2012; Sut and Kaplan, 2016) included only primigravid/nulliparous women (Assis et al., 2015; Bø and Haakstad, 2011; Fritel et al., 2015; Ko et al., 2011; Miquelutti et al., 2013; Mørkved et al., 2003; Sampselle et al., 1998; Sut and Kaplan, 2016).

Among the trials, one trial assessed the effect of doing PFMT both during pregnancy and after delivery, with the primary endpoint in the early postpartum period and also reported outcome in late pregnancy (Sut and Kaplan, 2016). A postnatal follow-up of the trial by Stafne et al. (2012) was published by Johannessen et al. (2021).

PEDro scores varied between 5 and 8 (see Table 7.5.2).

Quality of the intervention. The exercise period was during pregnancy and started between 16 and 26 weeks in seven trials (Assis et al., 2015; Bø and Haakstad, 2011; Ko et al., 2011; Miquelutti et al., 2013; Mørkved et al., 2003; Sampselle et al., 1998; Stafne et al. 2012), at 28 weeks gestation in two (Fritel et al., 2015; Sut and Kaplan, 2016) and also continued after delivery in one (Sut and Kaplan, 2016). The length of the training period, follow-up by health professionals, training intensity and frequency varied. The training protocol in all studies addressed both regular home training and follow-up (at different intervals) by a physical therapist (PT) or specialized healthcare worker. The PFMT programs included mostly few (up to 30 per day) and strong (near-maximal) contractions.

Adherence to the PFMT protocol was reported in most trials (Bø and Haakstad, 2011; Ko et al., 2011; Miquelutti et al., 2013; Mørkved et al., 2003; Sampselle et al., 1998; Stafne et al., 2012). No specific questionnaires/instruments to report adherence were used, although some studies used exercise diaries (Mørkved et al., 2003; Stafne et al., 2012). In six trials, the control group received usual care (Bø and Haakstad, 2011; Fritel et al., 2015; Miquelutti et al., 2013; Mørkved et al., 2003; Sampselle et al., 1998; Stafne et al., 2012) that might have included information about PFMT. Three trials reported specifically that the control group received no instructions in PFMT (Assis et al., 2015; Ko et al., 2011; Sut and Kaplan, 2016).

Outcomes. Primary outcome was self-reported UI (Bø and Haakstad, 2011; Fritel et al., 2015; Ko et al., 2011; Mørkved et al., 2003; Sampselle et al., 1998; Stafne et al., 2012 and the 3 month follow up by Johannessen et al., 2021). Others did not specify UI as the primary outcome (Miquelutti et al., 2013), or had urinary symptoms as secondary outcomes registered by the International Consultation on Incontinence Questionnaire–Short Form (ICIQ-SF) (Assis et al., 2015) and the Urinary Distress Inventory 6 (UDI-6) (Sut and Kaplan, 2016).

Results. Clinically relevant and statistically significant effects of the interventions were documented in seven trials and in one 3-months follow up (Johannessen et al. 2021). The results from the following trials showed that women randomized to PFMT were significantly less

TABLE 7.5.4 Studies assessing the effect of antenatal pelvic floor muscle training (PFMT) for mixed prevention and treatment of urinary incontinence (UI), including both women with and without urinary incontinence at inclusion

Author	**Sampselle et al., 1998**
Design	2 arm RCT Control (C): n = 38 Intervention (I): n = 34
Study population	72 primigravid women recruited at 20 weeks of pregnancy. Some women had existing UI. Groups comparable at baseline. Single centre, USA
Training protocol	C: Routine care I: Tailored PFMT programme beginning with muscle identification, progressing to strengthening. 30 contractions per day at max or near max intensity from 20 weeks of pregnancy. Correct VPFMC checked
Drop-out/Adherence	Losses to follow-up: 36% Adherence PFMT: 35 weeks of pregnancy 85%; 1 year post partum 62–90% Adverse events not stated. Self-reported adherence. Partial ITT analysis
Results	Change in mean UI symptom score: 35 wk pregnancy: C 0.20; I − 0.02; p = 0.07 6 wk post partum: C 0.25; I − 0.06; p = 0.03 6 mth post partum: C 0.15; I − 0.11; p = 0.05 12 mth post partum: C 0.06; I 0.00; p = 0.74 PFM strength: difference NS (low numbers)
Author	**Mørkved et al., 2003**
Design	2-arm RCT Control (C): n = 153 Intervention (I): n = 148
Study population	301 primigravid women recruited at 20 weeks of pregnancy. Some women had existing UI. Three outpatient physical clinics in Norway
Training protocol	C: Customary information from general practitioner/midwife. Not discouraged from PFMT. Correct PFM contraction checked at enrolment I: 12 weeks of intensive PFMT (in a group) led by PT, with additional home exercises 10 max contractions (each held for 6 s) and to the last 4 were 3–4 fast contractions added, repeated twice daily, between 20 and 36 weeks of pregnancy. Correct VPFMC checked at enrolment
Drop-out/Adherence	Losses to follow-up 12/301(5 I and 7 C) Adherence to PFMT: 81% adherence to PFMT in I group. Adverse events not stated. ITT analysis
Results	Self-reported UI at 36 weeks of pregnancy: C 48%; I 32%; RR (95% CI) 0.67 (0.50–0.89); p = 0.007 UI at 3 mth post partum: C 32%; I 19.6%; RR (95% CI) 0.61(0.40–.90); p = 0.018 PFM strength: significantly higher in I group
Author	**Bø et al., 2011**
Design	2-arm RCT Control (C): n = 53 Intervention (I): n = 52

Continued

TABLE 7.5.4   Studies assessing the effect of antenatal pelvic floor muscle training (PFMT) for mixed prevention and treatment of urinary incontinence (UI), including both women with and without urinary incontinence at inclusion—cont'd

Study population	105 nulliparous women recruited within 24 weeks of pregnancy. Some women had existing UI. Single centre, Norway
Training protocol	C: Usual care I: 12–16 weeks of aerobic exercise classes twice per week during pregnancy, including intensive PFMT (in a group) led by aerobic instructor. Additional home exercises 10 max contractions (each held for 6 s) and to the last 4 were added 3–4 fast contractions x 3, per day. Correct VPFMC was not checked at enrolment
Drop-out/Adherence	Losses to follow up: 21/105 (10 I and 11 C) Adherence to training sessions: 40%. Adverse events not stated. Not ITT analysis
Results	Self-reported UI: 36–38 wk pregnancy: C 7/53; I 9/52 3 months post partum: C 6/53; I 5/52; NS
Author	**Ko et al., 2011**
Design	2-arm RCT Control (C): n = 150 Intervention (I): n = 150
Study population	300 nulliparous women recruited at 16–24 weeks of pregnancy. Some women had existing UI. Single centre, Taiwan
Training protocol	C: Routine antenatal care. I: Individual PFMT with PT once per week between 20 and 36 weeks of pregnancy, with additional home exercises 3 sets of 8 contractions (each held for 6 s) repeated twice daily. Instructed to contract the PFM when coughing or sneezing
Drop-out/Adherence	Losses to follow up: 0%. Adherence PFMT: 87% practised PFMT at least 75% of the time. Adverse events not stated. ITT analysis
Results	Self-reported UI: 36 wk pregnancy: C 51%; I 34%; p = < 0.01 3 days post partum: C 41%; I 30%; p = 0.06 6 wk post partum: C 35%; I 25%; p = 0.06 6 mth post partum: C 27%; I 16%; p = 0.04 Significant improvement in I group in scores on IIQ-7 and UDI-6 in late pregnancy and up to 6 mth post partum
Author	**Stafne et al., 2012** **Johannessen et al., 2021** (3 months follow up)
Design	2-arm RCT Control (C): n = 426 Intervention (I): n = 429
Study population	855 pregnant women recruited at 20 weeks of pregnancy. Some women had existing UI. Two hospitals in Norway
Training protocol	C: customary information from general practitioner/midwife and written information. Not discouraged from PFMT I: 12 weeks of exercise class including led by PT, with additional home exercises 3 x 10 max contractions (each held for 6 s and to the last 4 were added 3–4 fast contractions) at least 3 times per week between 20 and 36 weeks of pregnancy. Correct VPFMC checked at enrolment

TABLE 7.5.4 **Studies assessing the effect of antenatal pelvic floor muscle training (PFMT) for mixed prevention and treatment of urinary incontinence (UI), including both women with and without urinary incontinence at inclusion—cont'd**

Drop-out/Adherence	Losses to follow-up: 93/855 (32 intervention and 61 controls)
	Adherence to PFMT:
	67% adherence to PFMT in I group
	40% adherence to PFMT in C group.
	No adverse events. ITT analysis
Results	Self-reported UI at 34–38 weeks pregnancy:
	Any UI: C 53%; I 42%; $p = 0.004$
	UI once per week or more: C 19%; I 11%;
	$p = 0.004$
	3 months follow up:
	Any UI: C 38%; I 29%; $p = 0.01$
Author	**Miquelutti et al., 2013**
Design	2-arm (parallel groups) RCT
	Control (C): n = 102
	Intervention (I): n = 103
Study population	205 nulliparous women with a single fetus, aged 16–40 years, and gestational age of 18–24 weeks. UI at recruitment: C 52.0%, I 50.4%.
	Women's Integral Health Care Hospital, University of Campinas and 4 municipal primary healthcare centres in Campinas, São Paulo, Brazil.
Training protocol	C: usual care
	I: Either in groups or on an individual basis (50 min, median 5 (range 2-10)) depending on the number of women present, supervised by a physiotherapist between 18–24 weeks' and 36–38 weeks' gestation. PFMT was additional to the routine activities offered at the antenatal clinic. Each session included non-aerobic exercises designed to reduce back pain, help venous return, prevent UI and minimise anxiety. Women also received standard antenatal education, and were instructed to perform daily PFMT at home as well as ≥ 30 min of aerobic exercise daily. Instructions were provided on performance of correct PFM contraction, but this was not evaluated (due to the pragmatic nature of the study). Women were given an exercise guide (PFMT and general stretching) and asked to complete an exercise diary.
Drop-out/Adherence	Exclusions post-randomisation: 3.9% I 6/103; C 2/102
	Discontinuation at 28–30 weeks' gestation: 2% I 3/103; C 1/102
	Discontinuation after delivery: 23%
	I 19/103; C 29/103
	Data on losses to follow-up (reported on CONSORT flowchart, text and tables) were incongruent.
	Adverse events: no adverse events associated with exercise were reported.
	Adherence not reported.
Results	Measured at baseline (18–24 weeks' gestation), 28-30 weeks' gestation, and 36–38 weeks' gestation.
	The risk of self reported UI was significantly lower in the intervention group at 30 weeks of pregnancy:
	C 62%; I 43% RR 0.69 (95% CI 0.51–0.93)
	and at 36 weeks of pregnancy:
	C 68%; I 41% RR 0.60 (95% CI 0.45–0.81)

Continued

TABLE 7.5.4   Studies assessing the effect of antenatal pelvic floor muscle training (PFMT) for mixed prevention and treatment of urinary incontinence (UI), including both women with and without urinary incontinence at inclusion—cont'd

Author	Assis et al., 2015
Design	3-arm (parallel groups) RCT. Control (C): n = 29 Intervention (I,1): n = 29 Intervention (I,2): n = 29
Study population	87 primiparous women ≤ 18 weeks' pregnant; no UI prior to pregnancy. Basic Health Units, Assis (Sao Paulo), Brazil. UI at recruitment: I (1) 58.6%; I (2) 51.7%; C 48.3%.
Training protocol	C: No manual or supervision, and no exercise and leakage diaries. Unclear if instructed not to perform PFMT. I (1): Supervised home exercise programme, daily exercise at home, with up to 5 monthly visits from a physiotherapist (at 22, 26, 30, 34, and 38 weeks' gestation). Women received a manual of home exercises and were instructed on how to use it, as well as exercise and leakage diaries. I (2): unsupervised PFMT, daily exercise at home as per the supervised group. Women received a manual of home exercises and were instructed on how to use it, as well as exercise and leakage diaries. Note: groups PFMT 1 and PFMT 2 were combined as the intervention group for comparison with controls.
Drop-out/Adherence	No drop outs Adherence not reported
Results	Primary outcome: self-reported UI. The risk of UI in late pregnancy was significantly lower in the intervention group: C 28/29, I (1+2) 4/58; RR 0.07 (95% CI 0.03-0.18)
Author	Fritel et al., 2015
Design	2-arm (parallel groups) RCT. Control (C): n = 142 Intervention (I): n = 140
Study population	282 nulliparous, pregnant women, 20-28 weeks' gestation. 5 university teaching hospitals (Nîmes, Poissy-Saint-Germain, Clermont-Ferrand, Clamart and Saint-Denis-de-la-Réunion), France. Incontinence at recruitment: I 32.9%; C 37.3%
Training protocol	C: written information on pelvic floor anatomy and PFM contraction exercises, at the time of inclusion. These instructions were also given to the PFMT group. I: 1-to-1 sessions, 20–30 min once per week, between 6th and 8th month of pregnancy (total of 8). An evaluation of PFM contraction was performed at each session through vaginal examination. PFMT supervised physiotherapists and midwives. Encouraged to perform daily PFM exercises at home. No specific instructions provided on the number or intensity of the contractions.
Drop-out/Adherence	Losses to follow-up 12 months postpartum: 3% I 47/140; C 45/142. Adherence: 69.3% completed all sessions. At the end of pregnancy, women in both groups reported a similar frequency and duration of PFMT.

TABLE 7.5.4 Studies assessing the effect of antenatal pelvic floor muscle training (PFMT) for mixed prevention and treatment of urinary incontinence (UI), including both women with and without urinary incontinence at inclusion—cont'd

Results	Measured at baseline (inclusion visit, 20–28 weeks' gestation), end of pregnancy, and 2 and 12 months' postpartum (primary endpoint).
	No significant difference between groups in UI severity (ICIQ-SF) and prevalence at 2 and 12 postpartum:
	Severity at 2 months (mean, SD):
	C 2.3 (± 3.4); I 1.9 ((2±2.9)
	12 months:
	C 2.1 (± 3.3); I 1.9 (± 3.7)
Author	**Sut et al., 2016**
Design	2-arm (parallel groups) RCT
	Control (C): n = 32
	Intervention (I): n = 32
Study population	64 pregnant women in their third trimester (28 weeks' gestation), aged > 18 years and attending the Gynaecology and Obstetrics. Urogynaecology Unit of the Gynaecology and Obstetrics Department of Trakya University Faculty of Medicine, Turkey.
	Statistically significant difference (P = 0.018) in vaginal deliveries between groups. UI at recruitment was not explicitly stated.
Training protocol	C: No instructions to the patients in C group
	I: Home exercise programme during pregnancy and postpartum, 3 sets of 10 exercises, 3 times per day. Instructions provided by researcher on how to perform Kegel exercises, but not reported if correct performance of contractions was confirmed. Women were phoned at two-week intervals to remind them to perform their exercises.
Drop-out/Adherence	Losses to follow-up: 5.4%
	I 2/32; C 2/32
	Adherence not reported
Results	Severity of UI.
	There were no significant difference in severity of UI (3-day voiding diary) in late pregnancy between the groups. Mean difference 0.2 (95% CI -0.35 to 0.75).

ITT, Intention-to-treat analysis; *NS,* not statistically significant; *OR,* odds ratio; *RR,* relative risk; *SD,* standard deviation; *VPFMC,* voluntary pelvic floor muscle contraction. For other abbreviations, see text.

likely to report UI in late pregnancy (Assis et al., 2015; Ko et al., 2011; Miquelutti et al., 2013; Mørkved et al., 2003; Stafne et al., 2012), 0 to 3 months after delivery (Ko et al., 2011) and 3 to 6 months after delivery (Ko et al., 2011; Mørkved et al., 2003; Johannessen et al., 2021). However, conflicting results were found in some studies (Bø and Haakstad, 2011; Fritel et al., 2015; Sampselle et al., 1998).

Antenatal Pelvic Floor Muscle Training for Treatment of Urinary Incontinence (Table 7.5.5)

PFMT for the treatment of UI was reported in two trials (Dinc et al., 2009; Woldringh et al., 2007). Both recruited primi- and multiparous women.

PEDro scores were 5 and 6 (see Table 7.5.2).

Quality of the intervention. The training protocols and follow-up varied. In the trial by Woldringh et al. (2007), the program consisted of three individual sessions during pregnancy weeks 23 to 30 and one 6 weeks after delivery, whereas the control group received routine care including instruction on PFMT. The drop-out rate was about 50%, and the adherence to regular PFMT among the women who stayed in the training group was 77%. Dinc et al. (2009) addressed both regular home training and follow-up between 20 and 36 weeks of pregnancy, and few (up to 30 contractions per day) and close-to-maximum contractions.

TABLE 7.5.5   Studies assessing the effect of antenatal pelvic floor muscle training (PFMT) for treatment of urinary incontinence (UI), including only women with urinary incontinence at inclusion

Author	**Woldringh et al., 2007**
Design	2-arm RCT Control (C): n = 152 Intervention (I): n = 112
Study population	264 women with UI at 22 weeks of pregnancy. Multicentre, The Netherlands
Training protocol	C: routine care; nearly 2/3 received some instruction on PFMT I: 3 sessions of individual therapy during week 23–30 of pregnancy and one 6 weeks after delivery, combined with written information
Losses to follow-up/ Adherence	Losses to follow up (C/I): 35 wk 17/14; 8 wk post partum 25/18; 6 mth post partum 30/29; 12 mth post partum: 42/35 Adherence to PFMT: I; 54% participated during the whole study period, and 77% of these women reported regular PFMT at 35 weeks of pregnancy; C; 50% participated during the whole study period, and 40% of these women reported regular PFMT at 35 weeks of pregnancy. Adverse events not stated. ITT analysis
Results	Self-reported severity of any UI: 35 wk pregnancy: C 93%; I 88%; p = 0.33 8 wk post partum: C 68%; I 62%; p = 0.44 6 mth post partum: C 60%; I 56%; p = 0.63 12 mth post partum: C 63%; I 58%; p = 0.61 12 mth post partum: negative correlation between training intensity and severity of UI
Author	**Dinc et al., 2009**
Design	2-arm RCT Control (C): n = 46 Intervention (I): n = 46
Study population	92 pregnant women recruited at 20–34 weeks of pregnancy. All women had existing UI. Primi- and multiparous. Single centre, Turkey
Training protocol	C: No treatment I: 3–16 weeks of intensive PFMT, with thorough instruction and additional home exercises between 20 and 36 weeks of pregnancy. 3 sets of 10–15 contractions 2–3 times per day. Both fast and slow (3–10 s) contractions Correct VPFMC checked at enrolment in both groups
Losses to follow-up/ Adherence	Losses to follow-up: 24/92 (6 in both groups) after first evaluation; 12 lost to follow-up at second (5 I and 7 C) Adherence to PFMT: Not reported. Not ITT analysis
Results	Self-reported UI: at 36–38 wk pregnancy: C 71.4%; I 43.2% at 6–8 wk post partum: C 38.4%; I 17.1% Significant difference in episodes of UI, urgency, number of voids and amount of urine in pad-test in favour of I group both at 36–38 weeks pregnancy and at 6–8 weeks post partum PFM strength: significant difference (p = 0.00) in favour of I both at 36–38 weeks pregnancy and at 6–8 weeks post partum

ITT, Intention-to-treat analysis; *NS,* not statistically significant; *OR,* odds ratio; *VPFMC,* voluntary pelvic floor muscle contraction; *RR,* relative risk; *SD,* standard deviation. For other abbreviations, see text.

Outcomes. Self-reported severity of UI was the primary outcome in the trial by Woldringh et al. (2007), whereas Dinc et al. (2009) did not specify primary outcome but reported several outcomes describing self-reported UI.

Results. Woldringh et al. (2007) found no difference in UI between the intervention and control groups during pregnancy and at the follow-up at 6 and 12 months postpartum. Conversely, Dinc et al. (2009) demonstrated a significant difference in UI after the intervention period in favour of the training group, both in late pregnancy and 6 to 8 weeks postpartum.

Is There Evidence That Postnatal Women Should Be Advised to Do Pelvic Floor Muscle Training to Prevent or Treat Urinary Incontinence?

Postnatal Pelvic Floor Muscle Training for Prevention (Primary and Secondary) of Urinary Incontinence

No trials including only continent women and assessing the effect of postnatal PFMT in primary or secondary prevention of UI were found.

Postnatal Pelvic Floor Muscle Training for Mixed Prevention and Treatment of Urinary Incontinence (Table 7.5.6)

Nine trials reported postnatal PFMT for mixed prevention and treatment of incontinence (Chiarelli & Cockburn, 2002a, 2002b; Ewings et al., 2005; Hilde et al., 2013; Kou et al., 2013; Liu, 2011; Sacomori et al., 2019; Sleep & Grant, 1987; Wen et al., 2010; Yang et al., 2017). The trials recruited women during their first pregnancy (Hilde et al., 2013; Liu, 2011) or postnatal women of mixed parity (Chiarelli & Cockburn, 2002a, 2002b; Ewings et al., 2005; Sacomori et al., 2019; Sleep & Grant, 1987; Yang et al., 2017). Two trials did not report this information (Kou et al., 2013; Wen et al., 2010). Only women with forceps or ventouse delivery or birth of a baby weighing 4000 g or more were included in one trial (Chiarelli & Cockburn, 2002a, 2002b).

Women were randomized to postnatal PFMT versus usual care, and in two trials the controls were explicitly instructed not to do PFMT (Sacomori et al., 2019; Yang et al., 2017).

PEDro scores were between 3 and 7 (see Table 7.5.2).

Quality of the intervention. In six studies, the training period most likely started while the women were still at the hospital (Chiarelli & Cockburn, 2002; Ewings et al., 2005; Liu, 2011; Sleep & Grant, 1987; Wen et al., 2010; Yang et al., 2017). The training started 8 weeks after delivery in the other studies. Length of the training period, follow-up by health professionals, training intensity and frequency varied. In three trials (Ewings et al., 2005; Sleep & Grant, 1987; Yang et al., 2017), no specific details about the PFMT program were reported, whereas in two (Kou et al., 2013; Liu, 2011), some information was given but not enough to be categorized. A PFMT program that was characteristic of strength training was used in four trials (Chiarelli & Cockburn, 2002a, 2002b; Hilde et al., 2013; Sacomori et al., 2019; Wen et al., 2010). Adherence was registered by Hilde et al. (2013), Chiarelli and Cockburn (2002), Ewings et al. (2005), Sleep and Grant (1987) and Yang et al. (2017). In the study by Ewings et al. (2005), the adherence rate was quite low (21 of 117).

The control group received standard care that might have included PFMT in all, except for two trials (Sacomori et al., 2019; Yang et al., 2017) where the control condition was no PFMT.

Outcomes. Primary outcome was self-reported UI (Chiarelli & Cockburn, 2002; Hilde et al., 2013; Kou et al., 2013; Sleep & Grant, 1987). Others did not specify UI as the primary outcome (Ewings et al., 2005; Liu, 2011; Wen et al., 2010), or had urinary symptoms as secondary outcomes or 'other' reported by the ICIQ-SF (Sacomori et al., 2019) and the incontinence severity score (Yang et al., 2017).

Results. Outcomes in the period 0 to 3 months after delivery were reported by Sacomori et al. (2019) and Yang et al. (2017), and the total risk estimates were significantly in favour of the PFMT group. Five trials (Chiarelli & Cockburn, 2002; Ewings et al., 2005; Hilde et al., 2013; Kou et al., 2013; Sleep & Grant, 1987) reported UI in the period between 3 and 6 months. Chiarelli and Cockburn (2002) and Kou et al. (2013) showed significant reduction in symptoms or frequency of UI after the intervention period, whereas conflicting results were reported from the other trials. The total risk estimate including all trials showed no significant risk reduction, and similar results were found in the trials assessing UI in period from 6 to 12 months after delivery, according to Woodley et al. (2020a, 2020b, 2020c). However, Chiarelli et al. (2004) reported that continued adherence to PFMT at 12 months was predictive of UI at that time, with less UI among women training the PFMs.

TABLE 7.5.6 Studies assessing the effect of postnatal pelvic floor muscle training (PFMT) for mixed prevention and treatment of urinary incontinence (UI), including both women with and without urinary incontinence at inclusion

Author	Sleep et al., 1987
Design	2-arm RCT Control (C): n = 900 Intervention (I): n = 900
Study population	1800 postpartum women recruited within 24 hours of vaginal delivery. Some women had existing UI. Single centre, England
Training protocol	C: current standard antenatal and postnatal care. Recommended to do PFM contractions as often as remembered and mid-stream urine stop. 4-week health diary I: as above plus one individual session daily while in hospital with midwifery coordinator. 4-week health diary including section recommending a specific PFMT task each week
Losses to follow-up/ Adherence	Losses to follow-up at 3 months: 84/900 in C group and 107/900 in I group Adherence to PFMT: 3 months post partum 58% in I group and 42% in C group. Adverse events not stated. Not ITT analysis
Results	Self-reported UI 3 mth post partum: C 22%; I 22%; RR (95% CI) 1 (0.83, 1.20)
Author	**Chiarelli and Cockburn, 2002** **Chiarelli et al., 2004**
Design	2-arm RCT Control (C): n = 350 Intervention (I): n = 370 Follow up Control (C): n = 294 Intervention (I): n = 275
Study population	720 postnatal women following forceps or ventouse delivery, or delivered a baby ≥ 4000 g. Some women had existing UI. Recruited at postnatal ward. Multicentre (3), Australia
Training protocol	C: usual care I: continence promotion: one contact with physiotherapist on postnatal ward and another at 8 weeks post partum (correct PFM contraction checked at second visit). Intervention included individually tailored PFMT, use of transversus abdominus contraction, the 'Knack', techniques to minimize perineal descent, post partum wound management. Written and verbal information. Adherence strategies
Losses to follow-up/ Adherence	Losses to follow-up: 6% in each group Adherence to PFMT: C 57.6%; I 83.9% Adverse events not stated. ITT analysis Losses to follow-up: 30% ITT analysis
Results	Self-reported UI 3 mth post partum: C 38.4%; I 31.0%, p = 0.044 OR of incontinence for the women in the I group compared with C group: 0.65 (0.46–0.91), p = 0.01 Self-reported UI 12 mth post partum: difference between groups NS Practice of PFMT at 12 mth promotes continence at this time
Author	**Ewings et al., 2005**
Design	Nested RCT Control (C): n = 117 Intervention (I): n = 117

TABLE 7.5.6   Studies assessing the effect of postnatal pelvic floor muscle training (PFMT) for mixed prevention and treatment of urinary incontinence (UI), including both women with and without urinary incontinence at inclusion—cont'd

Study population	n = 234 women in risk or with UI recruited from postnatal wards. Two centres, UK
Training protocol	C: usual postnatal care including verbal promotion of postnatal PFMT and leaflet explaining how to do PFMT I: taught one to one with PT in hospital, with intervention to attend PFMT group at 2 and 4 mth after delivery. No details of PFMT programme given
Losses to follow-up/ Adherence	Losses to follow-up: total 19%. C 17/100; I 27/90 Adherence to PFMT in I group: 5/90 (5.6%). ITT analysis
Results	UI at 6 mth post partum (Numbers and percentage): C 47/117 (47%); I 54/117 (60%); RR (95% CI) 1.28 (0.98–1.67), p = 0.10
Author	**Wen et al., 2010**
Design	2-arm (parallel groups) RCT. Control (C): n = 73 Intervention (I): n = 75
Study population	148 primiparous postpartum women. One hospital, China.
Training protocol	C: No details provided other than "conventional guidance". I : Twice per day, 15–30 min each set (anal contraction for at least 3 sec hold when inhaling, followed by relaxation with 3–5 faster contractions at the end of each time), for > 6-8 weeks. Exercises taught by experienced midwives but it was unclear who supervised the programme or the number and type of contacts/visits. An obstetrician assessed participants PFM strength and contraction (no further details provided).
Losses to follow-up/ Adherence	Losses to follow-up not reported. Adherence not reported.
Results	Severity of UI: Significant difference in favour of the intervention group at 12 months: SUI: Mean difference –1.04 (95% CI 1-16 to –0.92) Amount of leakage: RR 0.29 (95% CI 0.11 to 0.75)
Author	**Liu, 2011** Translation (Chinese)
Design	2-arm (parallel groups) RCT Control (C): n = 86 Intervention (I): n = 106
Study population	192 primiparous postpartum women. Yeyang Maternity and Child Health Care, China. Incontinence at recruitment not reported.
Training protocol	C: standard postpartum information. Unclear if this included PFMT I: 2–3 times per day, 15–30 min each set, started after birth and continued for ≥ 10 weeks. Exercises taught by experienced midwives who also supervised the programme (number and type of contacts/visits unclear). Not specified if a correct PFM contraction was confirmed.
Losses to follow-up/ Adherence	Losses to follow up not reported. Adherence not reported.
Results	Urinary condition score in favour of the intervention group: 3 months: Mean difference –0.60 (95% CI –0.69 to –0.51) 6 months: Mean difference –0.50 (95% CI –0.61 to –0.39)

Continued

TABLE 7.5.6 **Studies assessing the effect of postnatal pelvic floor muscle training (PFMT) for mixed prevention and treatment of urinary incontinence (UI), including both women with and without urinary incontinence at inclusion—cont'd**

Author	Hilde et al., 2013
Design	2-arm (parallel groups) RCT. Control (C): n = 88 Intervention (I): n = 87
Study population	175 Singleton primiparous women who delivered vaginally after more than 32 weeks of gestation. Single centre, Norway
Training protocol	C: Receiving instructions in correct PFM contractions and written information I: PFMT in groups supervised by physiotherapist once per week in 16 weeks (starting 6-8 weeks after delivery) and daily home training with three sets of 8-10 contractions close to maximum
Losses to follow-up/ Adherence	Loss to follow up: 9% C: 3/88 I: 12/87 96% of the women in the intervention group adhered to 80% of the class and daily home training.
Results	Self reported UI 6 months postpartum: Control: 39% Intervention: 35% NS
Author	**Kou et al., 2013** Translation (Chinese)
Design	2-arm (parallel groups) RCT. Control (C): n = 70 Intervention (I): n = 80
Study population	150 women, 6 weeks' postpartum. People's Hospital of Kenli County, China.
Training protocol	C: Standardized postpartum information I: PFMT combined with biofeedback. Biofeedback was used twice per week and PFMT (Kegel exercises) were undertaken 2-3 times per day for 20-30 min or 150-200 contractions (3 sec hold then relax), performed until women were 12 months' postpartum. Not specified if a correct PFM contraction was confirmed, who supervised the programme, or the number and type of contacts with health professional(s).
Losses to follow-up/ Adherence	Losses to follow-up not reported. Adherence not reported
Results	Self-reported UI in favour of the intervention group. 6 months' postpartum: RR 0.19 (0.04, 0.87) 12 months' postpartum: RR 0.28 (0.04, 0.92)
Author	**Yang et al., 2017**
Design	3-arm (parallel groups) RCT Control (C): n = 80 Intervention (I1): n = 80 Intervention (I2): n = 80 Note: groups PFMT 1 and PFMT 2 were combined as the intervention group for comparison with controls
Study population	240 primiparous women, with an episiotomy or second degree episiotomy tear. Shijiazhuang Maternal and Child Health Care Hospital, Shijiazhuang, China.

TABLE 7.5.6	Studies assessing the effect of postnatal pelvic floor muscle training (PFMT) for mixed prevention and treatment of urinary incontinence (UI), including both women with and without urinary incontinence at inclusion—cont'd
Training protocol	C: No PFMT, unclear if instructed not to perform PFMT. At two hours post-delivery, two specialized training stuff provided 1 hour of routine postpartum guidance. I 1: Unsupervised home exercise programme from 2 days to 3 months postpartum, 2-3 times per day. Kegel exercises and pelvic movements (Jonasson 1989) were taught by two specialised staff members at 2 days' postpartum (each training session went for 20 min with the exercises perform 6 times per min), with vaginal palpation used to confirm correct PFM contraction. I 2: In addition to home PFMT this group received electrical stimulation administered by two specialised staf, 30 min, 3 times per week, beginning at 6 weeks' postpartum (15 sessions in total). Note: groups PFMT 1 and PFMT 2 were combined as the intervention group for comparison with controls
Losses to follow-up/ Adherence	Losses to follow up: 21.3% C 60/80; I 1 66/80; I 2 70/80 No adverse events reported Adherence: three cases failed to complete the PFMT in accordance with the prescribed frequency and timing in the training group.
Results	UI early postnatal period (0-3 months). I: 66/129, C: 56/60 RR 0.55[0.46,0.66] Severity of UI related to PFMT Continence severity score (number of leakage episodes per week; 0=none, 1=once or fewer times per week; 2=2-3 times per week; 3=3-7 times per week, 4=>7 times per week, 5=leaking all the time) I: scored 0: 63/129 scored 1: 52/129 scored 2: 13/129 scored 3: 1/129 scored 4: 0/129 scored 5 0/129 C: scored 0: 4/60 scored 1: 4/60 scored 2: 25/60 scored 3: 25/60 scored 4: 2/60 scored 5: 0/60 Relative risk 0; 7.33 (95% CI 2.80 to 19.19) 1; 6.05 (95% CI 2.29 to 15.95) 2; 0.24 (95% CI 0.13 to 0.44) 3; 0.02 (95% CI 0.00 to 0.13) 4; 0.09 (95% CI 0.00 to 1.93) 5; not estimable Loss of urine under stress test postpartum. PFMT: 17/129 CG: 15/60 35.77% OR: 0.46[0.21,0.99]
Author	**Sacomori et al., 2019**
Design	2-arm (parallel groups) cluster-RCT. Control (C): n = 104 Intervention (I): n = 98

TABLE 7.5.6 **Studies assessing the effect of postnatal pelvic floor muscle training (PFMT) for mixed prevention and treatment of urinary incontinence (UI), including both women with and without urinary incontinence at inclusion—cont'd**

Study population	202 primiparous and multiparous postpartum women included immediately after giving birth to a live child. Carmela Dutra Maternity Hospital, Florianopolis, Santa Catarina, Brazil. Primiparous: I 49.3%, C 41.5%. Multiparous: I 50.7%, C 58.5%. Both continent and incontinence prior to pregnancy and by third trimester.
Training protocol	C: no PFMT. Women did not receive any kind of intervention or information regarding PFMT as this is not usual practice in Brazil. I: Postnatal home exercise; 10 repetitions of 10 sec holds (increasing intensity of contractions; strength and endurance training), 10 repetitions of 5 fast and strong contractions (strength training), and 'the knack' (a contraction before and during a sneeze or cough) to be performed 2 times per day (without supervision). Women received verbal and written (brochure) educational information provided by 'pelvic floor specialists' on PF structure, physiological changes, common problems during pregnancy, PF dysfunction, how to localise the PF and perform PFME. Correct PFM contraction was ascertained through visual assessment.
Losses to follow-up/ Adherence	Losses to follow-up: 34.7% I 31/98; C 39/104 Have presented complete case analysis imputed for missing data but no indication of the methods of imputation. A cluster-RCT with no apparent adjustment for the effect of cluster. Adherence to PFMT assessed via phone survey at 3 months postpartum: 55 (85.1%) women reported overall adherence to PFMT. 22 (32.3%) performed exercises 1-2 times per week and 33 (49.3%) did so 3-7 times per week. 33 (49.3%) performed both strength and endurance training, 14 (20.9%) only strength training and 10 (14.9%) focused only on endurance training. 21 (31.3%) performed PFMT for 3 months postpartum, others for around 2 months 38 (39.2%) multiparous and 23 (31.9%) primiparous women adhered to PFMT
Results	Urinary incontinence early postnatal period (0-3 months). RR 0.46 [0.15,1.41] I: 4/65 C: 9/67 Severity of incontinence: NS
Author	**Lin, 2020**
Design	2-arm (parallel groups) RCT Control (C): n = 48 Intervention (I): n = 49
Study population	97 puerperae with singleton pregnancy at Fujian Provincial Hospital, Fujian, China. Incontinence at recruitment not reported.
Training protocol	C: routine postpartum rehabilitation nursing. Unclear if this included PFMT I: one-to-one nursing intervention in postpartum PFM rehabilitation and more for 6-8 weeks. PFME 3 times per day, 30 min each set (number and type of contacts/visits unclear). Not specified if a correct PFM contraction was confirmed.
Losses to follow-up/ Adherence	Losses to follow up not reported. Adherence not reported.
Results	Primary endpoint was 6 months Lower incidence of SUI in I than in C, p<0.05 Significantly lower ICIQ-SF scores in I than C, and higher I-QOL scores in I than C. (P<0.05)

VPFMC, Voluntary pelvic floor muscle contraction; *NS,* not statistically significant; *CI,* confidence interval; *OR,* odds ratio; *RR,* risk ratio; *SD,* standard differentiation. For other abbreviations, see text.

Postnatal Pelvic Floor Muscle Training for Treatment of Incontinence (Table 7.5.7)

Four RCTs have been conducted aiming to treat UI with postnatal PFMT in women with persistent UI symptoms (Dumoulin et al., 2004; Glazener et al., 2001; Sigurdardottir et al., 2020; Wilson & Herbison, 1998). One trial recruited only primiparous women 6 to 10 weeks after delivery (Sigurdardottir et al., 2020), whereas others recruited both primi- and multiparous women from 3 months (Glazener et al., 2001; Wilson & Herbison, 1998a, 1998b or later (Dumoulin et al., 2004) after

delivery. In addition, one long-term follow-up study has been published (Glazener et al., 2005).

PEDro scores were between 5 and 8 (see Table 7.5.2).

Quality of the intervention. All trials provided supervised PFMT beginning at between 6 weeks and 3 months or later after delivery. The interventions included individual instructions in PFMT but followed different training protocols. Wilson and Herbison (1998) and Glazener et al. (2001) advised the women to perform 80 to 100 contractions per day and introduced three to four follow-up sessions in the period

TABLE 7.5.7 **Studies assessing the effect of postnatal pelvic floor muscle training for treatment of urinary incontinence (UI), including only women with urinary incontinence at inclusion**

Author	**Wilson and Herbison, 1998**
Design	2-arm RCT Control (C): n = 117 Intervention (I): n = 113
Study population	230 women with UI 3 mth post partum. Single centre, New Zealand
Training protocol	C: standard postnatal PFM exercises I: instructions by PTs (80–100 fast/slow contractions daily for 12 weeks) 3, 4, 6 and 9 mth post partum. Use of perineometer to teach awareness of VPFMC. Three groups: (a) 39 women performed only PFMT; (b) 36 women only trained with vaginal cones 15 mins per day; (c) 38 women used both (a) and (b)
Losses to follow-up/ Adherence	Losses to follow-up 12 mth outcome assessment: 36.9%. C 91/117; I 54/113 Adherence to PFMT: last month 89%; every day 48% 12 mth postnatally mean number of VPFMC 86 in I group and 35 in C group
Results	Self-reported UI at 12 mth post partum: C 69/91 (76%); I 27/54 (50%); p = 0.003 Pad-test: difference NS; perineometry: difference NS
Author	**Glazener et al., 2001** **Glazener et al., 2005, 2014**
Design	2-arm RCT Control (C): n = 6 Intervention (I): n = 371 3 centres: Aberdeen, Birmingham, Dunedin 6-year follow-up Control (C): n = 253 Intervention (I): n = 263
Study population	n = 747 women with UI 3 mth postnatally Multi-centre trial: New Zealand, UK n = 516
Training protocol	C: no visit I: advice + visit. Assessment of UI, with advice on PFMT (80–100 fast/slow contractions daily) followed up 5, 7 and 9 months after delivery supplemented by bladder training if appropriate at 7 and 9 mths

Continued

TABLE 7.5.7   Studies assessing the effect of postnatal pelvic floor muscle training for treatment of urinary incontinence (UI), including only women with urinary incontinence at inclusion—cont'd

Losses to follow-up/ Adherence	Lost to follow-up 12 mth: 31%. C 35%; I 25% Adherence to PFMT: in the 11th postnatal mth, 78% in I group (mean 20 VPFMC) and 48% in C group (mean 5 VPFMC) had done some PFMT. ITT analysis Lost to follow-up: 30%. Adherence (performing any PFMT): C 50%; I 50%
Results	Self-reported UI at 12 mth post partum: Any UI: C 69%; I 59.9%; p = 0.037 Severe UI: C 31.8%; I 19.7%; p = 0.002 Severe UI at 6 years follow up: C 39%; I 38%; p = 0.867
Author	**Dumoulin et al., 2004**
Design	3-arm RCT: (1) Control (C): n = 20 (2) PFM rehabilitation: n = 21 (3) PFM rehabilitation + training of deep abdominal muscles: n = 23 7-year follow-up. Combination of the previous two PFM rehabilitation groups (n = 35)
Study population	64 parous women under 45 years, still presenting symptoms of SUI at least once per week 3 months or more after their last delivery. Recruited during annual gynaecological visit at an obstetric clinic, Canada
Training protocol	(1) 8 weekly sessions of massage (2) PFM rehabilitation: weekly sessions supervised by physiotherapist for 8 weeks; 15 min ES + 25 min PFMT with BF + home training 5 days per week (3) PFM rehabilitation as group 2 + 30 mins of deep abdominal muscle training
Losses to follow-up/ Adherence	Losses to follow up: 3%. Adherence rate not stated. Adverse events not stated. ITT analysis.
Results	Self-reported UI after the intervention period: Objective cure (less than 2 g urine on pad-test): (1) Control: 0/19; (2) PFM rehabilitation: 14/20; (3) PFM rehabilitation + training of deep abdominal muscles: 17/23. Significant difference in favour of the intervention groups, p = 0.001
Author	**Sigurdadottir et al., 2020**
Design	2-arm RCT Control (C): n = 43 no instructions after initial assessment Intervention (I): n = 41 12 weekly sessions with physical therapist from 9 weeks postpartum
Study population	N = 84 with UI symptoms at 9 weeks postpartum Single hospital setting, Iceland
Training protocol	12x 45-60 minutes sessions with physical therapist with gradual progression of PFMT-exercises + home exercises 3x10 close to maximal VPFMC (exercise diary) 12x 45-60 minutes sessions with physical therapist with gradual progression of PFMT-exercises + home exercises 3x10 close to maximal VPFMC (exercise diary)
Losses to follow up / Adherence	Total loss to follow up:13/84 C:5/43, I:8/41 I:33/41 attended all 12 PFMT sessions. Adherence to exercise protocol, endpoint, 6 months postpartum: I:11/36 Adherence to exercise protocol, follow up, 12 months postpartum: I:8/38 No adverse effects were reported.
Results	Primary outcome measure UI postpartum: Endpoint, 6 months postpartum: C:31/38, I:21/37 (p = 0.03) Follow up, 12 months postpartum: C:34/42, I:28/38 (p = 0.6)

ITT, Intention to treat analysis; *NS*, no statistically significant difference; *OR*, odds ratio; *VPFMC*, voluntary pelvic floor muscle contraction; *RR*, relative risk; *SD*, standard deviation. For other abbreviations, see text.

up to 9 months after delivery. Dumoulin et al. (2004) addressed close follow-up (weekly) by a PT and used a training protocol including a lower number of high-intensity contractions. In the 8 weekly physical therapy appointments, they included biofeedback and electrical stimulation in the training program. Sigurdardottir et al. (2020) started the intervention at approximately 9 weeks postpartum, and it consisted of 12 weekly sessions of strength training of the PFMs with a PT. Adherence to the PFMT protocol was reported in three trials (Glazener et al., 2001; Sigurdardottir et al., 2020; Wilson & Herbison, 1998), but only Sigurdardottir et al. (2020) used exercise diaries.

Only Dumoulin et al. (2004) introduced an intervention in the control group (massage), whereas the two other trials compared PFMT with current standard care, allowing self-managed PFMT but no control intervention.

Outcomes. Outcomes were measured at different timing after delivery. The primary outcome in the trial by Dumoulin et al. (2004) was a standardized pad test, and the secondary outcome was the Urogenital Distress Inventory. Glazener et al. (2001) reported UI as the primary outcome, whereas Wilson et al. (1998) did not specify the primary outcome but used self-reported UI as an outcome measure. The rate of UI was the primary outcome in the trial by Sigurdardottir et al. (2020).

Results. A statistically significant reduction in symptoms or frequency of UI was found in all trials at 6 months after delivery and at 12 months in all but the trial by Sigurdardottir et al. (2020). No adverse effects of the interventions were reported. In the 6- and 12-year follow-up of the trial of Glazener et al. (2001), no difference in UI between groups was found.

DISCUSSION

In the present review of studies assessing the effect of PFMT in the prevention or treatment of peripartum UI, only full publications of RCTs that explicitly have chosen self-reported UI or severity of UI as an outcome measure have been included.

The studies remain heterogeneous regarding the content of the PFMT interventions and the control conditions in the trials that have been reviewed.

In a 2020 Cochrane review (Woodley et al., 2020), data from 46 different studies were pooled and treatment effects were reported as the risk ratio (RR). The methodological quality differed, as well as the quality of the PFMT protocols used in the trials. Several included studies have not been published as full papers and thus had not been exposed to the review process that is mandatory to be accepted in high-quality journals. The results presented in the Cochrane review are based on the analysis of these merged heterogeneous data (Woodley et al., 2020): key results were that pregnant women without UI who did PFMT to prevent leakage reported less urine leakage in late pregnancy (62% less; RR: 0.38, 95% CI: 0.20–0.72) and had less risk at 3 to 6 months after childbirth (29% less; RR: 0.71, 95% CI: 0.54–0.95). There was no evidence that doing PFMT as a treatment during pregnancy reduced UI (RR: 0.94, 95% CI: 0.70–1.24); however, groups of women with or without UI who began PFMT during pregnancy had less leakage in late pregnancy (22% less; RR: 0.78, 95% CI: 0.64–0.94) and up to 6 months after delivery (RR: 0.73, 95% CI: 0.55–0.97). For PFMT starting after delivery, there was uncertainty about the preventive and treatment effect on UI risk in the late postnatal period. Quality of the evidence varied.

Systematic reviews report that published studies on PFMT in general are small, underpowered and of uneven quality, and the available evidence suggests a lack of long-term efficacy of peripartum PFMT (Brostrøm and Lose, 2008; Davenport et al., 2018). In this chapter, we focus on the methodological quality of the included studies, dose–response issues in exercise trials and challenges in long-term assessment of PFMT during pregnancy and after childbirth.

Methodological Quality

Using the PEDro rating scale to assess, 10 is the top score. However, in exercise trials, 7 to 8 out of 10 reflects high quality, accepting that the two criteria related to blinding of the therapist and patient are almost impossible to meet in this kind of intervention. In this review, 9 of 28 studies received a PEDro score of 7 or 8, as detailed in Table 7.5.2.

In addition to the PEDro criteria, sample size is a crucial factor in RCTs. Small sample size may cause type II error, meaning that a possible effect is not revealed because of low power. On the other side, it is also well known that a large sample size may overestimate results in clinical trials, as small and clinically irrelevant effect sizes may reach statistical significance. One large trial reported (see Table 7.5.6) with 1169 participants (Sleep & Grant, 1987), is of great concern when judging the effect of postnatal PFMT for mixed prevention and treatment of UI. This trial has applied a very weak intervention, with few visits with either a PT or a midwife and a minimal training dosage with little potential for bringing significant effects. In addition, the training period in this trial was only 4 weeks (Sleep & Grant, 1987a, 1987b). Herbert and Bø (2005) have shown how another trial (Hughes et al., 2001) with huge numbers clearly dilutes the effect of smaller high-quality studies when pooling them in a meta-analysis.

What Is the Most Optimal Training Dosage for Effective Antenatal and Postnatal Pelvic Floor Muscle Training in Prevention and Treatment of Urinary Incontinence?

Quality of the Intervention: Dose–Response Issues

There is a strong dose–response relationship in exercise training. The type of exercise and frequency, intensity and duration of the training, as well as adherence to the exercise protocol, will decide the effect size (Bø, Hagen, Kvarstein, & et al., 1990; Imamura et al., 2010). In the area of PFMT, some trials with no or little effect have either used inadequate training dosages and left the participants alone to train (Sleep & Grant, 1987; Hughes et al., 2001) or have huge drop-outs and/or low adherence to the training protocol (Bø and Haakstad, 2011; Ewings et al., 2005; Fritel et al., 2015; Sleep & Grant, 1987; Woldringh et al., 2007). If the patients are not following the training protocol, we cannot evaluate the effect of PFMT. A conclusion can only be drawn on the feasibility of the program, which is another research question. Different classification systems of adherence were used, and none of the studies used specific questionnaires or instruments to assess adherence. Questions about home exercise were either asked in general questionnaires or in a personal interview, and some studies used exercise diaries. Those providing the supervision did registration of adherence to the supervised training sessions. Self-report by the

participants may overestimate actual adherence, and we recommend that future studies improve the methods used to register adherence.

Several RCTs in the PFMT literature support the early finding by Bø et al. (1990) that there is a very large difference in the effect size between programs with more or less intensive training and follow-up (Imamura et al., 2010). The term *intensive training* comes from the RCT of Bø et al. (1990), but the interpretation of this term can be questioned. The general recommendations for effective strength training to increase muscle cross-sectional area and strength are three sets of 8 to 12 close-to-maximum contractions three to four times a week (Haskell, 1994). Intensity in the exercise science literature on strength training is defined as the percentage of one repetition maximum, meaning how close the contraction is to the maximal contraction (Fleck and Kraemer, 2004). Bø et al. (1990) emphasized that close-to-maximum contractions and strength measurements were done throughout the training period. The same protocol has been used in several peripartum studies, which shows clinically relevant and statistically significant effect (Dinc et al., 2009; Dumoulin et al., 2004; Gorbea Chàvez et al., 2004; Ko et al., 2011; Mørkved and Bø, 1997, 2000; Mørkved et al., 2003; Reilly et al., 2002; Sangsawang and Sangsawang, 2016; Sigurdardottir et al., 2020; Stafne et al. 2012).

In an assessor-blinded RCT of PFMT to reduce pelvic organ prolapse, Brækken et al. (2010) found that this protocol significantly increased PFM strength and muscle thickness, reduced muscle length and area of the levator hiatus, in addition to lifting the position of the bladder neck and rectal ampulla. Hence PFMT is changing muscle morphology, working in the same way as strength training of general skeletal muscles. Nevertheless, surprisingly Hilde et al. (2013) found no significant difference in UI between a group of postnatal women following the same PFMT program and a control group. In this trial the control group was instructed in correct PFM contractions and not stopped from doing PFMT on their own. However, opposite results were found in the first controlled study assessing the effect of postnatal PFMT, using this specific PFMT protocol (Mørkved and Bø, 1997, 2000). One explanation of different results from these two trials using similar training protocols may be that the study of Hilde et al. (2013) intentionally recruited women with major levator ani defects, and this may have diluted the effect.

Training volume is the total workload of training (Kraemer and Ratamess, 2004). In the PFMT literature, exercise programs with only one supervised individual or group training session per week are named *intensive*. Some physicians suggest that follow-up once a week does not translate into clinical reality (Brostrøm and Lose, 2008). However, it is common to offer physical therapy at least two to three times a week for other conditions such as neck and low back pain; injured athletes are given supervised training at least once a day; and in rehabilitation centres, patients are exercising several hours per day. There are no pharmaceutical companies that would allow treatment or research with their drugs with an ineffective dosage. Nor would anyone suggest that surgeons should do suboptimal surgery. In the long run, there is no money to be saved on low or suboptimal training dosages in physical therapy because treating a large number of patients with ineffective interventions can be quite costly. Furthermore, by recommending low dosage or unsupervised training, the patients with no or little effect believe that they have tried PFMT and may not be motivated for conducting a new period of more optimal dosage and supervised training before choosing other treatment options. Evidence-based practice means to use protocols from high-quality RCTs showing worthwhile effect sizes (Bø and Herbert, 2009; Herbert and Bø, 2005).

Another specific problem in studies evaluating the effect of antenatal and postpartum PFMT is that in most countries it is established practice to advise all women to do PFMT. Hence most of the PFMT studies have compared PFMT with 'usual care'. Usual care can vary between thorough individual instruction with clinical assessment and motivation for training to providing women with written information only. In some studies the control group has done substantial PFMT (Fritel et al., 2015; Woldringh et al., 2007). Gorbea Chàvez et al. (2004) compared the effect of PFMT with a group specifically asked not to train the PFMs, and the difference between groups was highly significant with no women reporting UI in the PFMT group compared to 47% in the control group. To date, there are no studies comparing the effect of usual care with no exercise. For some women being able to perform strong contractions and being highly motivated for training, such initiatives may be enough, and there will be difficulties showing differences between the intervention and the control group. However, studies have shown that few women exercise regularly with a recommended dosage during pregnancy and after childbirth without supervision (Bø et al., 2007a; Bø et al., 2007b).

PTs, nurses, midwifes or physicians conducted the PFMT in most of the trials included in the present review, and to date there has been no comparison of the effects of interventions given by different professionals. Given the widespread prevalence of UI in the female population and the evidence for PFMT, we suggest that PFMT should be part of general strength training programs for women. This would imply that proper teaching of PFM function and dysfunction and how to teach PFMT correctly should be part of the curricula in exercise science, fitness and sports' educational programs.

What Is the Long-Term Effect of Pelvic Floor Muscle Training During Pregnancy and After Childbirth?

Another general critique of the effect of PFMT is a possible lack of long-term benefit, especially in the peripartum studies (Brostrøm and Lose, 2008). However, the effect of any training program will diminish with time if not continued (Garber et al., 2011). Strength training is described in detail in Chapter 6.2.

So far, no studies have evaluated how many contractions subjects have to perform to maintain PFM strength after cessation of organized training. However, a long-term effect cannot be expected if the women stop exercising. In addition, long-term effect, meaning for more than 1 year, in pregnant and postpartum women is almost impossible to evaluate, as many women would be pregnant again during the follow-up period. This is likely to interfere negatively with the short-term effect. Furthermore, in most trials the control groups receive information or supervised training after cessation of the RCT. This was shown in the follow-up study by Mørkved et al. (2007), where the control group received the training protocol after the results of the RCT were published. In the following period up to 6 years, the adherence to the PFMT protocol was similar in the original control and training groups. The continence rate in the training group was nearly the same at 3 months and 6 years of follow-up, whereas the number of incontinent women in the control group had decreased in the period. However, in another study by Mørkved and Bø (1997, 2000), the initial effect of postpartum PFMT was maintained 1 year later. In addition, the 7-year follow-up after the trial by Dumoulin et al. (2004) showed that more than 50% of the women in the PFMT groups were still continent according to pad test and incontinence-specific signs and symptoms. Quality of life remained better than before treatment, although not as good as immediately after cessation of the supervised training (Elliott et al., 2009).

Hence the demand for long-term follow-up studies of PFMT in general can be questioned, and longer follow-up periods of more than 1 year after birth, in our opinion, are not warranted.

CONCLUSION

Based on studies with relevant sample size, high adherence to a strength training protocol and close follow-up, peripartum PFMT can prevent and treat UI, and have no adverse effects. The most optimal dosage for effective PFMT is still not known. However, a training protocol following general strength training principles, emphasizing close-to-maximum contractions and at least an 8-week training period, can be recommended. Evidence-based practice of PFMT during pregnancy and after delivery implies using protocols from high-quality RCTs showing clinically relevant and statistically significant results. Given the detrimental negative effect of a non-functioning pelvic floor on women's participation in sport and physical activity, guidelines for exercise during pregnancy and after childbirth should include detailed recommendations for effective PFMT, and we provide an outline in Box 7.5.1.

BOX 7.5.1 How to tell if you are contracting the pelvic floor muscles correctly

- Sit on the arm of a chair or the edge of a table. Lift the pelvic floor up from the surface you are sitting on by pulling up and contracting around the urethra, vagina and rectum. Squeeze so hard that you feel a slight trembling in your vagina. When you squeeze hard enough, you can feel the lower part of the stomach being pulled in slightly at the same time. Release the contraction without pressing downward. Try to feel the difference between relaxing and tightening the pelvic floor.
- Try to stop the flow when you are urinating. If these muscles are weak, it may be difficult to stop the flow when it is strongest. You can then test yourself towards the end of urination, which is much easier. This is only a test to see whether you are using the muscles correctly. Do not use urination for training, as this can interfere with the ability to empty your bladder completely.
- If you are not sure about whether you are doing it correctly, contact your doctor and ask for a referral to a physical therapist with special training in women's health.

Training programme

Lift up and inward around your urethra, vagina and rectum. Squeeze as hard as you can during each contraction and try to hold it for 6–8 seconds before you gently relax. Relax and breathe with a slow, regular and gentle rhythm out and in both during and between the muscle contractions. Do 8–12 repetitions in three sets. If this seems too difficult, start with fewer repetitions. Choose one or more of these starting positions:

1. Sit with your legs apart and your back straight. Lift upwards and inwards around the openings in the pelvic floor.
2. Stand with your legs apart, and check that the buttock muscles are relaxed while you squeeze the pelvic floor muscles.
3. Kneel on all fours with your knees out to the side and feet together. Lift the pelvic floor upwards and inwards.

REFERENCES

Agur, W. I., Steggles, P., Waterfield, M., et al. (2008). The long-term effectiveness of antenatal pelvic floor muscle training: Eight-year follow up of a randomised controlled trial. *British Journal of Obstetrics and Gynaecology, 115*(8), 985–990.

Assis, L. C., Bernardes, J. M., Barbosa, A. M., et al. (2015). [Effectiveness of an illustrated home exercise guide on promoting urinary continence during pregnancy: A pragmatic randomized clinical trial]. *Revista Brasileira de Ginecologia e Obstetrícia, 37*(10), 460–466.

Bø, K., & Haakstad, L. A. (2011). Is pelvic floor muscle training effective when taught in a general fitness class in pregnancy? A randomised controlled trial. *Physiotherapy, 97*(3), 190–195.

Bø, K., Hagen, R. H., Kvarstein, B., et al. (1990). Pelvic floor muscle exercise for the treatment of female stress urinary incontinence: III. Effects of two different degrees of pelvic floor muscle exercises. *Neurourology and Urodynamics, 9*, 489–502.

Bø, K., & Herbert, R. D. (2009). When and how should new therapies become routine clinical practice? *Physiotherapy, 95*(1), 51–57.

Bø, K., Haakstad, A. H., & Voldner, N. (2007). Do pregnant women exercise their pelvic floor muscles? *International Urogynecology Journal and Pelvic Floor Dysfunction, 18*(7), 733–736.

Bø, K., Owe, K. M., & Nystad, W. (2007). Which women do pelvic floor muscle exercises six months' postpartum? *American Journal of Obstetrics and Gynecology, 197*(1), 49. e1–49.e5.

Brækken, I. H., Majida, M., Engh, M. E., et al. (2010). Morphological changes after pelvic floor muscle training measured by 3-dimensional ultrasonography: A randomized controlled trial. *Obstetrics & Gynecology, 115*(2 Pt. 1), 317–324.

Brostrøm, S., & Lose, G. (2008). Pelvic floor muscle training in the prevention and treatment of urinary incontinence in women—what is the evidence? *Acta Obstetricia et Gynecologica Scandinavica, 87*(4), 384–402.

Chiarelli, P., & Cockburn, J. (2002). Promoting urinary continence in women after delivery: Randomised controlled trial. *British Medicine Journal, 324*, 1241–1246.

Chiarelli, P., Murphy, B., & Cockburn, J. (2004). Promoting urinary continence in postpartum women: 12-month follow-up data from a randomised controlled trial. *International Urogynecology Journal and Pelvic Floor Dysfunction, 15*(2), 99–105.

Davenport, M. H., Nagpal, T. S., Mottola, M. F., et al. (2018). Prenatal exercise (including but not limited to pelvic floor muscle training) and urinary incontinence during and following pregnancy: A systematic review and meta-analysis. *British Journal of Sports Medicine, 52*(21), 1397–1404.

Dias, A., Assis, L., Barbosa, A., et al. (2011). Effectiveness of perineal exercises in controlling urinary incontinence and improving pelvic floor muscle function during pregnancy (abstract). *Neurourology and Urodynamics, 30*(6), 968.

Dinc, A., Kizilkaya Beji, N., & Yalcin, O. (2009). Effect of pelvic floor muscle exercises in the treatment of urinary incontinence during pregnancy and the postpartum period. *International Urogynecology Journal and Pelvic Floor Dysfunction, 20*(10), 1223–1231.

Dumoulin, C., Lemieux, M. C., Bourbonnais, D., et al. (2004). Physiotherapy for persistent postnatal stress urinary incontinence: A randomized controlled trial. *Obstetrics & Gynecology, 104*(3), 504–510.

Elliott, V., Dumoulin, C., Martin, C., et al. (2009). Physical therapy for persistent postpartum stress urinary incontinence: A seven year follow-up study (abstract). *Neurourology and Urodynamics, 28*(7), 820.

Ewings, P., Spencer, S., Marsh, H., et al. (2005). Obstetric risk factors for urinary incontinence and preventative pelvic floor exercises: Cohort study and nested randomized controlled trial. *Journal Obstetrics Gynaecological, 25*(6), 558–564.

Fleck, S. J., & Kraemer, W. J. (2004). *Designing resistance training programs* (3rd ed.). Champaign, IL: Human Kinetics.

Fritel, X., de Tayrac, R., Bader, G., et al. (2015). Preventing urinary incontinence with supervised prenatal pelvic floor exercises: A randomized controlled trial. *Obstetrics & Gynecology, 126*(2), 370–377.

Garber, C. E., Blissmer, B., Deschenes, M. R., et al. (2011). Quantity and quality of exercise for developing and maintaining cardiorespiratory, musculoskeletal, and neuromotor fitness in apparently healthy adults: Guidance for prescribing exercise. *Medicine & Science in Sports & Exercise, 43*(7), 1334–1359.

Glazener, C. M., Herbison, G. P., MacArthur, C., et al. (2005). Randomised controlled trial of conservative management of postnatal urinary and faecal incontinence: Six year follow up. *British Medicine Journal, 330*(7487), 337.

Glazener, C. M., Herbison, G. P., Wilson, P. D., et al. (2001). Conservative management of persistent postnatal urinary and faecal incontinence: Randomised controlled trial. *British Medicine Journal, 323*(7313), 593–596.

Glazener, C. M., MacArthur, C., Hagen, et al. (2014). Twelve-year follow-up of conservative management of postnatal urinary and faecal incontinence and prolapse outcomes: Randomized controlled trial. *British Journal of Obstetrics and Gynecology, 121*(1), 112–120.

Gorbea Chàvez, V., Velàzquez Sanchez, M. D. P., & Kunhardt Rasch, J. R. (2004). [Effect of pelvic floor exercise during pregnancy and puerperium on prevention of urinary stress incontinence]. *Ginecologia Obstetrics Mexico, 72*, 628–636.

Haskell, W. L. (1994). Dose–response issues. From a biological perspective. In C. Bouchard, R. J. Shephard, & T. Stephens (Eds.), *Physical activity, fitness, and health* (pp. 1030–1039). Champaign, IL: Human Kinetics.

Herbert, R. D., & Bø, K. (2005). Analysis of quality of interventions in systematic reviews. *British Medicine Journal, 331*, 507–509.

Hilde, G., Stær-Jensen, J., Siafarikas, F., et al. (2013). Postpartum pelvic floor muscle training and urinary incontinence: A randomized controlled trial [erratum appears in: Obstet. Gynecol. 124 (3), 639]. *Obstetrics & Gynecology, 122*(6), 1231–1238.

Hughes, P., Jackson, S., Smith, A., et al. (2001). Can antenatal pelvic floor exercises prevent postnatal incontinence (abstract)? *Neurourology and Urodynamics, 20*, 447–448.

Imamura, M., Abrams, P., Bain, C., et al. (2010). Systematic review and economic modelling of the effectiveness and cost-effectiveness of non-surgical treatments for women with stress urinary incontinence. *Health Technology Assessment, 14*(40), 1–188 iii–iv.

Johannessen, H. J., Frøshaug, B. E., Lysåker, P. J. G., et al. (2021). Regular antenatal exercise including pelvic floor muscle training reduces urinary incontinence 3 months postpartum: Follow up of a randomized controlled trial. *Acta Obstetricia et Gynecologica Scandinavica, 100*(2), 294–301.

Kim, E. Y., Kim, S. Y., & Oh, D. W. (2012). Pelvic floor muscle exercises utilizing trunk stabilization for treating postpartum urinary incontinence: Randomized controlled pilot trial of supervised versus unsupervised training. *Clinical Rehabilitation, 26*(2), 132–141.

Ko, P. C., Liang, C. C., Chang, S. D., et al. (2011). A randomized controlled trial of antenatal pelvic floor exercises to prevent and treat urinary incontinence. *International Urogynecology Journal and Pelvic Floor Dysfunction, 22*(1), 17–22.

Kou, J.-L., Dang, L.-J., & Feng, X.-Q. (2013). Clinical study on the treatment of postpartum rehabilitation to improve the pelvic floor function. *Medicine Innovations China, 10*(25), 55–57.

Kraemer, W. J., & Ratamess, N. A. (2004). Fundamentals of resistance training: Progression and exercise prescription. *Medicine & Science in Sports & Exercise, 36*(4), 674–688.

Liu, X.-B. (2011). Pelvic floor muscle training for prevention and treatment of postpartum urinary incontinence clinical observation. *Guide China Med, 9*(2), 21–22.

Mahler, C. G., Sherrington, C., Herbert, R. D., et al. (2003). Reliability of the PEDro scale for rating quality of randomized controlled trials. *Physical Therapy, 83*(8), 713–721.

Meyer, S., Hohlfeld, P., Achtari, C., et al. (2001). Pelvic floor education after vaginal delivery. *Obstetrics & Gynecology, 97*(5 Pt. 1), 673–677.

Miquelutti, M. A., Cecatti, J. G., & Makuch, M. Y. (2013). Evaluation of a birth preparation program on lumbopelvic pain, urinary incontinence, anxiety and exercise: A randomized controlled trial. *BMC Pregnancy and Childbirth, 13*, 154.

Mørkved, S., & Bø, K. (1997). The effect of postpartum pelvic floor muscle exercise in the prevention and treatment of urinary incontinence. *International Urogynecology Journal and Pelvic Floor Dysfunction, 8*(4), 217–222.

Mørkved, S., & Bø, K. (2000). Effect of postpartum pelvic floor muscle training in prevention and treatment of urinary incontinence: A one-year follow up. *British Journal of Obstetrics and Gynaecology, 107*(8), 1022–1028.

Mørkved, S., & Bø, K. (2014). Effect of pelvic floor muscle training during pregnancy and after childbirth on prevention and treatment of urinary incontinence: A systematic review. *British Journal of Sports Medicine, 48*(4), 299–310.

Mørkved, S., Bø, K., Schei, B., et al. (2003). Pelvic floor muscle training during pregnancy to prevent urinary incontinence: A single-blind randomized controlled trial. *Obstetrics & Gynecology, 101*(2), 313–319.

Mørkved, S., Rømmen, K., Schei, B., et al. (2007). No difference in urinary incontinence between training and control group six years after cessation of a randomized controlled trial, but improvement in sexual satisfaction in the training group (abstract). *Neurourology and Urodynamics, 26*(5), 667.

Pelaez, M., Gonzalez-Cerron, S., Montejo, R., et al. (2014). Pelvic floor muscle training included in a pregnancy exercise program is effective in primary prevention of urinary incontinence: A randomized controlled trial. *Neurourology and Urodynamics, 33*(1), 67–71.

Reilly, E. T., Freeman, R. M., Waterfield, M. R., et al. (2002). Prevention of postpartum stress incontinence in primigravidae with increased bladder neck mobility: A randomised controlled trial of antenatal pelvic floor exercises. *British Journal of Obstetrics and Gynaecology, 109*(1), 68–76.

Sacomori, C., Zomkowski, K., dos Passos Porto, I., et al. (2019). Adherence and effectiveness of a single instruction of pelvic floor exercises: A randomized clinical trial. *International Urogynecology Journal, 31*(5), 951–959.

Sampselle, C. M., Miller, J. M., Mims, B. L., et al. (1998). Effect of pelvic muscle exercise on transient incontinence during pregnancy and after birth. *Obstetrics & Gynecology, 91*(3), 406–412.

Sangsawang, B., & Sangsawang, N. (2016). Is a 6-week supervised pelvic floor muscle exercise program effective in preventing stress urinary incontinence in late pregnancy in primigravid women?: A randomized controlled trial. *European Journal of Obstetrics & Gynecology and Reproductive Biology, 197*, 103–110.

Sangsawang, B., & Serisathien, Y. (2012). Effect of pelvic floor muscle exercise programme on stress urinary incontinence among pregnant women. *Journal of Advanced Nursing, 68*(9), 1997–2007.

Schreiner, L., Crivelatti, I., de Oliveira, J. M., et al. (2018). Systematic review of pelvic floor interventions during pregnancy. *International Journal of Gynaecology & Obstetrics, 143*(1), 10–18.

Sigurdardottir, T., Steingrimsdottir, T., Geirsson, R. T., et al. (2020). Can postpartum pelvic floor muscle training reduce urinary and anal incontinence?: An assessor-blinded randomized controlled trial. *American Journal of Obstetrics and Gynecology, 222*(3), 247.e1–247.e8.

Sleep, J., & Grant, A. (1987). Pelvic floor exercises in postnatal care. *Midwifery, 3*(4), 158–164.

Stafne, S., Salvesen, K., Romundstad, P., et al. (2012). Does regular exercise including pelvic floor muscle training prevent urinary and anal incontinence during pregnancy? A randomised controlled trial. *British Journal of Obstetrics and Gynaecology, 119*(10), 1270–1280.

Sut, H. K., & Kaplan, P. B. (2016). Effect of pelvic floor muscle exercise on pelvic floor muscle activity and voiding functions during pregnancy and the postpartum period. *Neurourology and Urodynamics, 35*(3), 417–422.

Wen, X.-H., Shi, S.-Q., & Wang, J.-Y. (2010). Pelvic muscles exercise for postpartum stress urinary incontinence. *China Practical Medicine, 5*(15), 72–73.

Wilson, P. D., & Herbison, G. P. (1998). A randomized controlled trial of pelvic floor muscle exercises to treat postnatal urinary incontinence. *International Urogynecology Journal and Pelvic Floor Dysfunction, 9*(5), 257–264.

Woldringh, C., van den Wijngaart, M., Albers-Heitner, P., et al. (2007). Pelvic floor muscle training is not effective in women with UI in pregnancy: A randomised controlled trial. *International Urogynecology Journal and Pelvic Floor Dysfunction, 18*(4), 383–390.

Woodley, S. J., Lawrenson, P., Boyle, R., et al. (2020). Pelvic floor muscle training for preventing and treating urinary and faecal incontinence in antenatal and postnatal women. *Cochrane Database of Systematic Reviews* Issue 5, Art. No. CD007471.

Yang, S., Sang, W., & Feng, J. (2017). The effect of rehabilitation exercises combined with direct vagina low voltage low frequency electric stimulation on pelvic nerve electrophysiology and tissue function in primiparous women: A randomised controlled trial. *Journal of Clinical Nursing, 26*, 4537–4547.

Evidence for Pelvic Floor Muscle Training for Pelvic Organ Prolapse Related to the Peripartum Period

Kari Bø

As pregnancy and childbirth may cause damage to the pelvic floor, early intervention to prevent and treat pelvic organ prolapse (POP) should optimally start in the peripartum period.

METHODS

A search on PubMed was conducted using the search strategy of pelvic floor muscle training (PFMT) *and* POP *and* (pregnancy *or* postpartum) with limitation of randomized controlled trials (RCTs).

RESULTS

Only two RCTs were found evaluating the effect of PFMT in the peripartum period. In addition, a 12-year follow-up study of a brief nurse-led intervention of 747 women with urinary incontinence starting at 3 months postpartum (response rate at 12 years: 471 [63%]) was found (Glazener et al., 2014). This RCT only assessed POP at the follow-up with no report of POP in the original study or at 6-year follow-up.

In an assessor-blinded RCT including 175 primiparous women, no effect was found on symptoms of bulging, bladder neck position or POP stage after 4 months of group PFMT starting at 6 weeks postpartum (Bø et al., 2015). The study included women with and without POP, and the women presenting with POP had Pelvic Organ Prolapse Quantification (POP-Q) stages 1 and 2. The primary outcome of this RCT was urinary incontinence, and since the study included women with and without POP, the sample size may have been too small to detect differences in POP symptoms. The study included vaginal palpation and assessment of pelvic floor muscle strength and supervised group training with a physical therapist once a week plus daily home PFMT (3 × 8–12 maximal contractions).

In an RCT with 189 primiparous women aged 20 to 35 years and with an episiotomy or second-degree episiotomy tear (Yang et al., 2017), the women received either routine postpartum care (control group, n = 60) at 2 hours postpartum, rehabilitation exercises including PFMT after vaginal palpation plus 'pelvic movements' (n = 63) from 2 days until 3 months postpartum, or a combination of the rehabilitation program and 'direct vagina low-voltage, low-frequency electric stimulation' (combination group, n = 66). Electrical stimulation was given 15 times (30 min 3 times a week) beginning at 6 weeks postpartum. The results showed a statistically significant difference between groups post-intervention in the number of women with POP in favour of both PFMT and combination therapy. Results were not compared pairwise between the two intervention groups, but the conclusion was that combination therapy was more effective than PFMT/pelvic movements.

The 12-year follow-up of women who had participated in one-to-one home PFMT (instructed by nurses) on three occasions (5, 7 and 8 months postpartum) compared to usual care did not find any differences between the PFMT group and the control group in the prevalence of prolapse symptoms, severity of symptoms or objectively measured POP (assessed in 35% of those participating at 12 years). Neither was there any difference in the number of women performing PFMT at 6 or 12 years post-intervention (Glazener et al., 2014).

Further RCTs are warranted to test early prevention and treatment of POP in the peripartum period.

REFERENCES

Bø, K., Hilde, G., Stær-Jensen, J., et al. (2015). Postpartum pelvic floor muscle training and pelvic organ prolapse—a randomized trial of primiparous women. *American Journal of Obstetrics and Gynecology, 212*(1), 38.e1–38.e7.

Glazener, C. M. A., MacArthur, C., Hagen, S., et al. (2014). Twelve-year follow-up of conservative management of postnatal urinary and faecal incontinence and prolapse outcomes: Randomised controlled trial. *British Journal of Obstetrics and Gynaecology, 121*(1), 112–120.

Yang, S., Wenshu, S., Feng, J., et al. (2017). The effect of rehabilitation exercises combined with direct vagina low voltage low frequency electric stimulation on pelvic nerve electrophysiology and tissue function in primiparous women: A randomised controlled trial. *Journal of Clinical Nursing, 26*(23–24), 4537–4547.

Evidence for Pelvic Floor Muscle Training for Anal Incontinence Related to the Peripartum Period

Hege Hølmo Johannessen

INTRODUCTION

Anal incontinence (AI) is the involuntary loss of solid or liquid stool, and/or gas, whereas faecal urgency involves having difficulty or being unable to defer a sudden or compelling desire to defaecate (Sultan et al., 2017). In women, AI is associated with pregnancy, vaginal delivery, damage to the pudendal nerves, pelvic floor muscle (PFM) injuries and obstetric anal sphincter injuries (OASIS) during delivery (Bols et al., 2010; Eogan et al., 2011; Espuña-Pons et al., 2012; Johannessen et al., 2014b; Johannessen et al., 2019; MacArthur et al., 2013; Solans-Domènech et al., 2010; Van Brummen et al., 2006). Potentially, AI may lead to devastating and disabling effects on quality of life (QoL) and sexual dysfunction in both the short and long term (Dean et al., 2008; Johannessen et al., 2014a; MacArthur et al., 2013), and incontinence of gas in particular is reported to be the most embarrassing symptom (Johannessen et al., 2014a; Keighley et al., 2016). Studies suggest that those who experience the combination of urinary incontinence (UI) and AI, referred to as double incontinence (DI), tend to report more severe symptoms compared to patients reporting UI or AI alone (Espuña-Pons et al., 2012). Moreover, DI has a greater impact on psychosocial well-being, QoL and physical activity than UI or AI symptoms alone (Fialkow et al., 2003). However, few AI or DI sufferers volunteer information about their incontinence problems unless asked directly, and there is reason to believe that as few as one in four AI sufferers seek medical care mainly due to embarrassment (Bartlett et al., 2007; Brown et al., 2012a; Brown et al., 2012b). Many women believe that AI is a normal consequence of pregnancy and childbirth, and later report the onset of their AI symptoms in relation to the delivery of their first child or on return to work after maternity leave (Guise et al., 2007; MacLennan et al., 2000).

SEARCH METHODS

We used searches from Academic Search Premier, CINAHL, PubMed and the Physiotherapy Evidence Database (PEDro), and in addition to database searches, reference lists of selected papers were searched manually. Keywords used in different combinations in the search were *pregnancy, pelvic floor muscle, exercise, training, faecal/fecal incontinence, anal incontinence, postpartum/ postnatal, puerperium, perinatal/peri-partum, antenatal/ prenatal/pre-pregnancy.*

SELECTION CRITERIA

We included randomized and quasi-randomized controlled trials written in English aiming to measure the effect of peripartum pelvic floor muscle training (PFMT) in the prevention or treatment of AI. Thus one study arm had to include PFMT, and the other study arm(s) included no PFMT, usual antenatal or postnatal care, other conservative control condition or an alternative PFMT intervention. AI had to explicitly be described as an outcome measure, and only full publications were included. Abstracts were not included. Populations included women who at randomization were continent (PFMT for prevention) or incontinent (PFMT for treatment), and a mixed population of continent and incontinent (PFMT for prevention or treatment).

Scoring of methodological criteria was conducted according to the PEDro rating scale and assigning 1 point for each of the following factors of internal validity: random allocation, concealed allocation, baseline comparability, blinded assessor, blinded subjects, blinded therapist, adequate follow-up (≥85%), intention-to-treat analysis, between-group comparison, report of point estimates and variability (Maher et al., 2003). Due to the nature of PFMT as an active intervention based on instructions, feedback and communication between subjects and therapists, blinding is usually not possible. Thus the maximum score for most PFMT studies is 8 points on the PEDro rating scale (Table 7.5.8).

EVIDENCE FOR PREVENTION AND TREATMENT

Is There Evidence That Pregnant Women Should Be Advised to Do Pelvic Floor Muscle Training to Prevent or Treat Anal Incontinence? (Table 7.5.9)

We identified no randomized or quasi-randomized studies with AI as the primary outcome reporting on the effect of PFMT as prevention or treatment of AI during pregnancy. However, a few studies have reported AI as a secondary outcome. Bø and Haakstad (2011) found no differences in AI symptoms in late pregnancy between intervention and control group women following PFMT included in a general fitness class for pregnant women with and without AI at inclusion. Similar to their results during pregnancy, there was no difference in AI at 6 to 8 weeks postpartum (Bø and Haakstad, 2011). In the study by Stafne et al. (2012), fewer women reported faecal incontinence in the intervention group in late pregnancy, although this did not reach statistical significance. In a subgroup analysis, multiparous women performing regular PFMT in the second half of pregnancy had reduced risk of late pregnancy faecal incontinence. This protective effect was not seen among primiparous women (Stafne et al., 2012). However, these findings may indicate that even among women with previous pregnancies potentially weakening the PFMs and deliveries that may have resulted in perineal injuries, specific PFMT during pregnancy may prevent or reduce AI in subsequent pregnancies. As AI was not the primary outcome measure in these studies, they were not powered to evaluate differences in AI, and thus the results must be interpreted with caution.

Is There Evidence That Postnatal Women Should Be Advised to Do Pelvic Floor Muscle Training to Prevent or Treat Anal Incontinence?
Studies With Urinary Incontinence as the Primary Outcome Measure or Basis for Sample Size Estimation (Table 7.5.10)

We found no evidence favouring PFMT over standard or usual care in the two studies reporting on postpartum AI including women with and without AI at enrolment (prevention or treatment) (Meyer et al., 2001a, 2001b; Sleep & Grant, 1987).

TABLE 7.5.8 PEDro Quality Score of Randomized Controlled Trials in Systematic Reviews of Studies Assessing the Effects of Pelvic Floor Muscle Training During Pregnancy or Postpartum to Prevent or Treat Anal Incontinence

E – Eligibility criteria specified
1 – Subjects randomly allocated to groups
2 – Allocation concealed
3 – Groups similar at baseline
4 – Subjects blinded
5 – Therapist administering treatment blinded
6 – Assessor blinded
7 – Measures of key outcomes obtained from ≥85% of subjects
8 – Data analysed by intention to treat
9 – Statistical comparison between groups conducted
10 - Point measures and measures of variability

Study	E	1	2	3	4	5	6	7	8	9	10	Total Score
Sleep and Grant (1987)	?	+	?	?	–	–	–	+	–	+	+	4
Wilson and Herbison (1998)	+	+	+	+	–	–	–	–	–	+	+	5
Fynes et al. (1999)	–	+	?	+	–	–	+	+	+	+	+	7
Meyer et al. (2001a, 2001b)	+	?	–	?	–	–	?	+	?	+	+	3
Glazener et al. (2001)	+	+	+	+	–	–	+	-	+	+	+	7
Mahoney et al. (2004)	+	+	+	+	–	–	+	+	+	+	+	8
Bø and Haakstad (2011)	+	+	+	+	–	–	+	–	–	+	+	6
Stafne et al. (2012)	+	+	+	+	–	–	+	+	+	+	+	8
Peirce et al. (2013)	+	+	+	+	–	–	–	+	+	+	+	7
Oakley et al. (2016)	+	+	+	+	–	–	–	–	+	+	+	6
Johannessen et al. (2017)	+	+	+	+	–	–	–	–	+	+	+	6
Sigurdadottir et al. (2020)	+	+	+	+	–	–	+	+	–	+	+	7

+, Criterion is clearly satisfied; –, criterion is not satisfied; ?, not clear if the criterion is satisfied.
The total score is determined by counting the number of satisfied criteria, except 'eligibility criteria specified'. The total score is 10. Due to the nature of PFMT, blinding is usually not possible. Thus the maximum score for most PFMT studies is 8 points.

Sleep and Grant (1987) compared the effect of standard postpartum instructions of home PFMT prior to discharge from the hospital after delivery with reinforced instructions of home PFMT during home visits from community midwives during the first 4 weeks postpartum. Two months after delivery, there was no difference in UI or AI between groups (Sleep & Grant, 1987). Meyer et al. (2001a, 2001b) evaluated the effect of 12 sessions of PFMT with biofeedback and standardized electrical stimulation between 2 and 10 months postpartum among the 107 included women. One in three had UI during pregnancy, but no participants reported AI before index delivery. At pre- and post-intervention, only three (5%) and two (4%) participants reported AI

in the control and intervention groups, respectively (Meyer et al., 2001a, 2001b). None of these studies were designed with AI as the main outcome measure, and the reported confidence intervals related to postpartum AI tended to be wide, indicating that these studies may have been underpowered to evaluate the effect of the interventions on postpartum AI.

We identified three studies including women with UI at enrolment reporting on the prevalence of postpartum AI after the intervention period (prevention or treatment). In the study by Wilson and Herbison (1998), women with UI at 3 months postpartum were randomized to either a control group receiving standard care with instruction of PFMT before discharge home

TABLE 7.5.9 Studies Assessing the Effect of Pelvic Floor Muscle Exercises During Pregnancy to Prevent or Treat Anal Incontinence, Including Women With and Without Anal Incontinence at Inclusion, With Urinary Incontinence as the Primary Outcome Measure

Author	**Stafne et al. (2012)**
Design	2-arm RCT Control: n = 426 (15 reporting AI at inclusion) Intervention: n = 429 (21 reporting AI at inclusion); 12 weeks of aerobic fitness including intensive PFMT
Study population	N = 855 pregnant women recruited at 18–22 weeks of pregnancy; some had existing AI 2 centres in Norway
Training protocol	Control: routine antenatal care from midwife/general practitioner, written information; not discouraged from PFMT Intervention: 12 weeks of aerobic exercise class including PFMT led by physical therapist, with additional home exercises at least 3×/week between enrolment and pregnancy week 36; 3 × 10 max contractions (each held for 6 s), and 3–4 fast contractions were added to the last 4 contractions; correct VPFMC was checked at enrolment
Drop-out/adherence	Total loss to follow-up: 93/855; control 61/426, intervention 32/429 Adherence to PFMT: control 79%, intervention 95%; no adverse events reported; ITT analyses
Outcomes	Self-reported AI at pregnancy weeks 34–38 Reporting FI at follow-up: control 18/365, intervention 12/397
Author	**Bø and Haakstad (2011)**
Design	2-arm RCT Control: n = 53 (usual care) Intervention: n = 52; 12–16 weeks of aerobic fitness class including PFMT
Study population	N = 105 nulliparous women recruited within 24 weeks of pregnancy; some women had existing UI Single centre in Norway
Training protocol	Control: usual care Intervention: 12–16 weeks of aerobic exercise classes 2×/week during pregnancy, including intensive PFMT (group) led by an aerobics instructor; additional home exercises 10 max contractions (each held for 6 s), and 3–4 fast contractions were added to the last 4 contractions; correct VPFMC was not checked at enrolment
Drop-out/adherence	Total loss to follow-up post-intervention: 21/105; control 11/53, intervention 10/52; 6–8 weeks postpartum: control 6/53, intervention 9/52 Adherence to training sessions: 40%; adverse events not stated; no ITT analyses
Outcomes	Self-reported flatus incontinence post-intervention: control 9/42, intervention 11/42 (p = 0.61); 6–8 weeks postpartum: control 8/47, intervention 10/43 (p = 0.46) Self-reported FI post-intervention: control 1/42, intervention 1/42; 6–8 weeks postpartum: control 3/47, intervention 1/43 (p = 0.62)

AI, Anal incontinence; *FI,* faecal incontinence; *ITT,* intention to treat; *PFMT,* pelvic floor muscle training; *RCT,* randomized controlled trial; *UI,* urinary incontinence; *VPFMC,* voluntary pelvic floor muscle contraction.

TABLE 7.5.10 Studies Assessing the Effect of Postpartum Pelvic Floor Muscle Exercises to Prevent or Treat Anal Incontinence, Including Both Women With and Without Anal Incontinence at Inclusion, With Urinary Incontinence or Another Variable as the Primary Outcome Measure

Author	Sigurdadottir et al. (2020)
Design	2-arm RCT Control: n = 43; no instructions after initial assessment Intervention: n = 41; 12 weekly sessions with physical therapist from 9 weeks postpartum
Study population	N = 84 with UI symptoms at 9 weeks postpartum Single hospital setting, Iceland
Training protocol	45–60-min sessions 12×/week with physical therapist with gradual progression of PFMT exercises + home exercises 3 × 10 close-to-maximum VPFMC (exercise diary)
Drop-out/adherence	Total loss to follow-up: 13/84; control 5/43, intervention 8/41; intervention: 33/41 attended all 12 PFMT sessions Adherence to exercise protocol, endpoint, 6 months postpartum: intervention 11/36 Adherence to exercise protocol, follow-up, 12 months postpartum: intervention 8/38 No adverse effects reported
Outcomes	Primary outcome measure AI postpartum: Endpoint, 6 months postpartum: control 19/37, intervention 17/36 (p = 0.33) Follow-up, 12 months postpartum: control 26/42, intervention 23/38 (p = 1) Bowel-related bother: Endpoint, 6 months postpartum: control 19/37, intervention 17/36 (p = 0.83) Follow-up, 12 months postpartum: control 20/42, intervention 11/38 (p = 0.11) Changes in anal sphincter strength (S) and endurance (E): Endpoint, 6 months postpartum: S: control 71(34) hPa, intervention 84(31) (p = 0.01); E: control 450(237) hPa/s, intervention 578(272) (p = 0.02) Follow up, 12 months postpartum: S: control 77(35) hPa, intervention 91(34) (p = 0.08); E: control 504(266) hPa/s, intervention 618(267) (p = 0.04)
Author	**Oakley et al. (2016)**
Design	2-arm RCT Control: n = 25; usual postpartum care Intervention: n = 29; 6 weeks of physical therapist–led PFMT in combination with behavioural therapy
Study population	N = 54 with third- or fourth-degree obstetric anal sphincter injury requiring primary repair; 2/50 reported soiling at enrolment Single hospital setting, USA
Training protocol	4 × 60-min PFMT sessions with physical therapist (weeks 6, 8, 10, and 12 postpartum), number and type of PFMT contractions not reported + behavioural instructions on diet, perineal hygiene and level of activity at baseline, during PMFT sessions and leaflet + usual postpartum care Correct VPFMC checked for participants at enrolment, instruction on VPFMC not reported
Drop-out/adherence	Total loss to follow-up: control 2/25, intervention 2/29 Adherence to PFMT not reported
Outcomes	Primary outcome measure Fecal Incontinence Quality of Life Scale: NS difference Secondary outcome measure: AI as measured by the Fecal Incontinence Severity Index (0–61 points); NS difference (p = 0.058)

TABLE 7.5.10 Studies Assessing the Effect of Postpartum Pelvic Floor Muscle Exercises to Prevent or Treat Anal Incontinence, Including Both Women With and Without Anal Incontinence at Inclusion, With Urinary Incontinence or Another Variable as the Primary Outcome Measure—cont'd

Author	**Glazener et al. (2001, 2005, 2014)**
Design	2-arm RCT Control: n = 376; FI: 54 Intervention: n = 371; FI: 57; conservative advice on daily PFMT + bladder training if appropriate
Study population	2001: n = 747 primi/multiparas with UI at 3 months postpartum 2005: n = 516 (69%) 6 years postpartum 2014: n = 471 (63%) 12 years postpartum 3 centres: Dunedin, New Zealand, and Aberdeen and Birmingham in the UK
Training protocol	Control: usual care Intervention: conservative advice on PFMT (daily 80–100 fast/slow contractions) at 5, 7, and 9 months postpartum + bladder training if appropriate at 7 and 9 months postpartum
Drop-out/adherence	2001: Loss to follow-up 12 months postpartum: control 131/376 (35%), intervention 92/371 (25%) Adherence to PFMT 12 months postpartum: control 118/244, intervention 218/278 2005: Loss to follow-up 6 years postpartum: control 123/376 (33%), intervention 108/371 (29%) Adherence to any PFMT 6 years postpartum: control 126/253 (50%), intervention 131/263 (50%); daily PFMT: control 17 (6%), intervention 29 (12%) 2014: Loss to follow-up 6 years postpartum: control 135/376 (36%), intervention 141/371 (38%) Adherence to PFMT 6 years postpartum: control 118/241 (49%), intervention 118/228 (52%); daily PFMT: control 20/241 (8%), intervention 15/227 (7%)
Outcomes	2001: self-reported FI 12 months postpartum: control 25/237, intervention 12/273 (p = 0.012) 2005: self-reported FI 6 years postpartum: any FI, control 32/248, intervention 32/261 (p = 0.932); new-onset FI, control 15/248, intervention 12/261 (p = 0.598); persistent FI, control 13/248, intervention 15/261 (p = 0.965) 2014: self-reported FI 12 years postpartum: any FI, control 35/240, intervention 43/228 (p = 0.215); new-onset FI, control 19/240, intervention 26/228 (p = 0.183); persistent FI, control 12/240, intervention 14/228 (p = 0.987)
Author	**Meyer et al. (2001a, 2001b)**
Design	2-arm (R)CT* assigned in publication, randomly assigned in abstract Control: n = 56; no postpartum PFMT until 10 months postpartum Intervention: n = 51; PFMT, biofeedback and electrical stimulation
Study population	N = 107 pregnant nulliparous women recruited at 12–39 weeks of gestation; some had incontinence at enrolment Multiple clinics in single centre in Switzerland
Training protocol	Control: no postpartum PFMT until after intervention period Intervention: 12 sessions over 6 weeks in PFMT programme instructed by physical therapist between 2 and 10 months postpartum + 20 min of biofeedback + 15 min of electrical stimulation
Drop-out/adherence	No loss to follow-up Adherence not reported
Outcomes	Self-reported FI 10 months postpartum: control 5%, intervention 5%

Continued

TABLE 7.5.10 **Studies Assessing the Effect of Postpartum Pelvic Floor Muscle Exercises to Prevent or Treat Anal Incontinence, Including Both Women With and Without Anal Incontinence at Inclusion, With Urinary Incontinence or Another Variable as the Primary Outcome Measure—cont'd**

Author	**Wilson and Herbison (1998)**
Design	2-arm/4-arm RCT Control: n = 117; standard PFMT taught before discharge home from hospital Intervention: n = 113; daily PFMT and/or training with cone weights
Study population	N = 230 primi/multiparas with UI 3 months postpartum, stratified by parity, UI severity and mode of delivery; all women had UI at enrolment 3 months postpartum Single centre in New Zealand
Training protocol	Control: n = 117; standard postpartum PFMT taught by physical therapist while in hospital Intervention: 4 sessions (3, 4, 6, 9 months postpartum) with PFM exercises instructed by physical therapist, further randomized into 3 groups: i. PFiMT: n = 39; 8–10 daily sessions of a total of 80–100 VPFMC + biofeedback with vaginal perionometer ii. PiFMT and cone weights: n = 38; daily PFMT + 15 min of training with vaginal cone weight iii. Cone weights group: n = 36; daily 15 min of training with vaginal cones
Drop-out/adherence	Total loss to follow-up: control 26/117, intervention 59/113; i, 20/38, ii, 24/38, iii, 15/36 *Significantly less UI in intervention group; however, due to the high drop-out rate in the intervention group, results must be interpreted with caution. Adherence last months: control 77%, intervention 79% Adherence 12 months postpartum: control 65%, intervention 89%
Outcomes	Self-reported AI during the last month: control 20/91, intervention 12/54 (p = 0.86) Number of PFM contractions during the last month: control 35, intervention 59 (p < 0.01)
Author	**Sleep and Grant (1987)**
Design	2-arm RCT Control: n = 900; usual care including standard PFMT advice at maternity ward prior to discharge home Intervention: n = 900; 4 weeks of reinforced standard PFMT advice with health diary, telephone prompts and active participation by community midwives and health visitors
Study population	N = 1800 primi/multiparas recruited within 24 h of vaginal delivery Single centre in the UK
Training protocol	Control: current standard antenatal and postnatal care, including PFMT; recommended to do VPFMC as often as remembered and stop urine mid-stream; 4-week health diary Intervention: As control group + 1 daily individual session before discharge home with midwifery coordinator; 4-week health diary including additional section recommending specific PFMT task each week (all tasks related to integrating VPFMC with daily activities)
Drop-out/adherence	Total loss to follow-up: 191/1800 (11%); control 107/900 (12%), intervention 84/900 (9%) Adherence to PFMT: 10 days postpartum: control 68%, intervention 78% 3 months postpartum: control 42%, intervention 58%
Outcomes	Self-reported faecal loss: overall 3%, control 22/783, intervention 21/816

AI, Anal incontinence; *FI,* faecal incontinence; *NS,* not statistically significant; *PFM,* pelvic floor muscle; *PFMT,* pelvic floor muscle training; *RCT,* randomized controlled trial; *UI,* urinary incontinence; *VPFMC,* voluntary pelvic floor muscle contraction.

from the hospital (n = 117), or one of three intervention groups receiving PFMT alone (n = 39), PFMT in combination with cone weights (n = 38) or cone weights alone (n = 36). At 1 year after delivery, there was no difference in AI symptoms between the control and intervention groups or between intervention groups. A total of 48% of the intervention group women reported performing daily PFMT at follow-up. However, more than half of the women randomized to the intervention groups withdrew from the study for various reasons during the intervention period. Prevalence of AI symptoms was not reported at follow-up 24 to 44 months after index delivery, and only 8% of women in either group reported regular PFMT (Wilson & Herbison, 1998).

Women reporting UI at 3 months postpartum in the study by Glazener et al. (2001) were randomized to either a control group receiving standard postpartum care or an intervention group receiving four home visits including education on pelvic floor anatomy, instructions on PFMT and bladder training during the first year after delivery. Findings suggest that in patients with DI, PFMT may reduce the prevalence of coexisting AI at 12 months postpartum (Glazener et al., 2001). In addition, significantly more intervention group women (79%) performed regular PFMT compared to women in the control group (48%). However, women reporting AI alone at enrolment were excluded, and fewer women reporting severe UI at enrolment responded at follow-up. In the long-term follow-up studies, the group differences in incontinence symptoms did not persist, showing similar but increasing prevalence of AI in both groups at 6 years postpartum (Glazener et al., 2005) and 12 years postpartum (Glazener et al., 2014), and 40% of women reporting DI at enrolment had persistent symptoms at 12 years. Only 50% reported performing any PFMT in either group at 6 and 12 years, and at 12 years less than 10% reported daily PFMT.

In the recent study by Sigurdardottir et al. (2020), women with UI at 9 weeks postpartum were randomized to either a control group receiving no active treatment or an intervention group receiving 12 weekly individual sessions with gradual progression of PFMT exercises instructed by a physical therapist (Sigurdardottir et al., 2020a, 2020b). Approximately one in seven of the recruited women also reported coexisting symptoms of AI and bowel-related bother at baseline. Even though there was a significant reduction in UI, there

were no significant differences in AI symptoms or bowel-related bother between groups at 6 or 12 months postpartum. However, significantly more women in the intervention group had higher anal sphincter strength and endurance than control group women at both 6 and 12 months postpartum, but only one in four intervention group women reported PFMT during this 6-month period.

Studies With Health-Related Quality of Life as the Primary Outcome Measure

Two studies have explored the effect of PFMT on health-related QoL and PFM strength following OASIS. The main focus in the study by Oakley et al. (2016) was to explore whether four sessions of PFMT reinforced by biofeedback would improve health-related QoL following OASIS. The primary outcome was measured using the Fecal Incontinence Quality of Life Scale, which measures the impact of AI in four domains: lifestyle, coping, depression and embarrassment. The results show that there were no significant post-intervention differences in AI prevalence or clinical impact on QoL between groups 12 weeks after delivery (Oakley et al., 2016).

Women in the study by Peirce et al. (2013) were randomized to either instruction on PFMT for home use (n = 90) or home PFMT and additional early use of intra-anal biofeedback (n = 30) before discharge home from the hospital after delivery. Participants received no follow-up or further instructions during the intervention period, and there were no differences in PFM strength as measured by anal manometry, the Fecal Incontinence Quality of Life Scale or AI at follow-up 3 months postpartum (Peirce et al., 2013).

Neither study was powered to detect differences in AI between groups, nor did the included women have AI symptoms at enrolment. Using a condition-specific QoL measure may not have been the optimal method to evaluate the effect of PFMT among women with no AI symptoms in these studies, and the results must be interpreted with caution.

Studies With Anal Incontinence as the Primary Outcome Measure (Table 7.5.11)

Three studies with AI as the primary outcome measure have explored the effect of postpartum PFMT among women reporting postpartum AI. Two studies including women following obstetric injuries only have compared

TABLE 7.5.11   Studies Assessing the Effect of Pelvic Floor Muscle Exercises After Delivery to Prevent or Treat Postpartum Anal Incontinence, Including Women With or Without Anal Incontinence at Inclusion, With Anal Incontinence as the Primary Outcome Measure

Author	Johannessen et al. (2017)
Design	2-arm RCT Control: n = 55; written information only Intervention: n = 54; 6 months of individual physical therapist–led PFMT
Study population	N = 109 primi/multiparas recruited approximately 1 year postpartum; all had self-reported AI at enrolment Two hospitals in Norway
Training protocol	4–6 individual appointments with specialist physical therapist and individually adapted PFMT programme; 3 × 8–10 close-to-maximum contractions (held for 3 s and progressing to 10–12 s) and adding 3 fast contractions at the end of VPFMC, and progression in starting positions; participants unable to perform VPFMC were offered ES for home use until able to perform VPFMC and commence PFMT Correct VPFMC checked for all participants at enrolment
Drop-out/adherence	Total loss to follow-up: control 12/55, intervention 12/54 Adherence to PFMT: control not reported, intervention 32/54; no adverse events reported; ITT analyses
Outcomes	Change in self-reported AI St. Mark's Incontinence Score from baseline to post-intervention: control –0.7 points, intervention –2.4 points (p = 0.029) Change in prevalence of urgency (15 min): control NS, intervention 7/21 (p = 0.033); leakage of flatus: control 11/32 (p < 0.01), intervention 14/38 (p < 0.01); leakage of stool: NS differences
Author	**Peirce et al. (2013)**
Design	2-arm RCT Intervention 1 (home PFMT): n = 90; educated before discharge home to perform 3 months of standard home PFMT 5 min twice daily (written instructions) Intervention 2 (early BF + PFMT): n = 30; 3 months of standard home PFMT 5 min + EMG BF twice daily
Study population	N = 120 primiparas recruited prior to discharge home from hospital postpartum, all with third-degree perineal tear with primary repair Single centre in Ireland
Training protocol	Home PFMT: 3 months of standard home PFMT 5 min twice daily Early BF + PFMT: instruction to perform 3 months of standard home PFMT 5 min + EMG BF (VPFMC held for 5 s, 10 s relax × 10) twice daily
Drop-out/adherence	Total loss to follow-up: 0 Adherence to PFMT not reported in the home PFMT group Adherence to ES: 7/30 did not use ES as per protocol due to lack of time and/or absence of FI symptoms; no adverse events reported.
Outcomes	Self-reported AI (Wexner score): NS difference (p = 0.88) Quality of life (Fecal Incontinence Quality of Life Scale): NS difference Anal squeeze and resting pressures (manometry): NS difference (resting pressures p = 0.22; squeeze pressures p = 0.24)

TABLE 7.5.11	**Studies Assessing the Effect of Pelvic Floor Muscle Exercises After Delivery to Prevent or Treat Postpartum Anal Incontinence, Including Women With or Without Anal Incontinence at Inclusion, With Anal Incontinence as the Primary Outcome Measure—cont'd**
Author	**Mahoney et al. (2004)**
Design	2-arm, single blind RCT Intervention 1 (BF): n = 30; 12 weeks of weekly intra-anal BF with PFMT for 10 min with physical therapist Intervention 2 (BF + ES): n = 30; 12 weeks of weekly intra-anal BF with PFMT (as for group 1) + intra-anal ES
Study population	N = 60 primi/multiparas recruited 12 weeks following obstetric anal sphincter injury; all had AI at enrolment Hospital in Ireland
Training protocol	BF: 12 weeks of weekly intra-anal BF (alternating slow twitch VPFMC held for 5 s, relax 8 s/3 rapid maximum fast twitch VPFMC for 5 s, relax 8 s) for 10 min with physical therapist; daily PFMT home exercises BF + ES: 12 weeks of weekly intra-anal BF with PFMT (as for group 1) for 12 weeks + intra-anal ES (35 Hz, 20% ramp modulation, 20 min of 5 s on/8 s off, intensity eliciting contraction of the external anal sphincter muscle)
Drop-out/adherence	Total loss to follow-up: BF 4/30, BF + ES 2/30 Adherence to PFMT not reported
Outcomes	Self-reported AI (Wexner score): median change: BF 2.5 points, BF + ES 2 points; asymptomatic: BF 6/30, BF + ES 8/30 (p = 0.583) Quality of life (Fecal Incontinence Quality of Life Scale): significant reductions in all domains in both groups except embarrassment (p = 0.12) Mean maximal anal squeeze: NS difference between groups; mean maximal resting pressures: NS difference between groups
Author	**Fynes et al. (1999)**
Design	2-arm RCT Intervention 1 (sensory BF): n = 20; 12 weeks of vaginal BF with PFMT Intervention 2 (augmented BF): n = 20; 12 weeks of EMG BF with PFMT + intra-anal ES
Study population	N = 40 primi/multiparas consecutively recruited from perineal clinic following obstetric anal sphincter injury; all had AI at enrolment
Training protocol	Sensory BF: 12 weeks of weekly sensory vaginal BF PFMT (20 short maximum VPFMCs held for 6–8 s, 10 s relax and VPFMC held for 30 s) + standard home PFMT Augmented BF: 12 weeks of weekly anal ES (20% ramp modulation and 10 min 20 Hz, 5-s on/8-s off + 10 min 50 Hz, 8 s on/30 s off) and EMG BF (15 min alternating between VPFMC held for 5 s and rapid maximum squeezes held for 5 s and 8 s relax) + standard home PFMT
Drop-out/adherence	Total loss to follow-up: sensory BF 1/20, augmented BF 0/20 Adherence to PFMT not reported
Outcomes	Self-reported AI symptoms modified Pescatori questionnaire (0–12), median score (median change) at follow-up: sensory BF 4.2 (–3) points, augmented BF 0 (–10) points PFM strength (manometry): sensory BF NS difference, augmented BF increased mean maximal resting pressures (p = 0.01); mean maximal squeeze pressures p < 0.01 and squeeze increment p < 0.01

AI, Anal incontinence; *BF,* biofeedback; *EMG,* electromyography; *ES,* electrical stimulation; *FI,* faecal incontinence; *ITT,* intention to treat; *NS,* not statistically significant; *PFM,* pelvic floor muscle; *PFMT,* pelvic floor muscle training; *RCT,* randomized controlled trial; *VPFMC,* voluntary pelvic floor muscle contraction.

postpartum PFMT in combination with either bio-feedback or electrical stimulation (Fynes et al., 1999; Mahony et al., 2004), and one study has offered electrical stimulation in addition to PFMT in a small selection of participants (Johannessen et al., 2017). In an Irish study, 85% of women with obstetric injury reported improvements in AI symptoms, and one in four were asymptomatic after 12 weeks of receiving either PFMT with biofeedback or PFMT, biofeedback and additional electrical stimulation. Furthermore, participants in both groups reported significant improvements on the incontinence scores, anal squeeze pressures and QoL. Only two participants had normal ultrasound scans, and for ethical reasons the studies included no control group (Mahony et al., 2004). Similarly, Fynes et al. (1999) compared a group receiving 12 weeks of PFMT in combination with sensory vaginal biofeedback to a group receiving PFMT and anal biofeedback augmented by standardized electrical stimulation. All included women reported AI within 2 years of obstetric injury. Even though women in both groups showed improvements on the incontinence scores, more women were asymptomatic at follow-up in the group receiving PFMT augmented by electrical stimulation. Moreover, larger improvements in squeeze and resting pressures were seen in the group receiving PFMT without electrical stimulation compared to sensory biofeedback with no electrical stimulation (Fynes et al., 1999). Women with persistent full-thickness defects in the external anal sphincter muscle reported significantly lower improvement rates. In both studies, the drop-out rates were low, and the results show an increased ability to perform a voluntary pelvic floor muscle contraction (VPFMC) (Fynes et al., 1999; Mahony et al., 2004). However, for ethical reasons, none of these studies included control groups receiving no active treatment or standard care, and even though PFMT may seem to reduce AI postpartum, the actual effect of PFMT and biofeedback with or without electrical stimulation is difficult to determine.

In the study by Johannessen et al. (2017), intervention group women received four to six sessions with an individualized PFMT programme for home use on average between 12 and 18 months postpartum. Women unable to perform a VPFMC received additional electrical stimulation until able to perform VPFMC and PFMT at home. Findings show that the reduction in postpartum AI symptoms, and urgency

in particular, favoured the intervention group, and that women performing PFMT weekly or more often reduced their AI symptoms more than women performing PFMT less regularly. In addition, at follow-up, women with low anal sphincter defect scores reported fewer AI symptoms compared to women with larger, persistent sphincter defects (Johannessen et al., 2017). The study had a 22% drop-out rate, and included women with and without known OASIS.

The reported improvements in AI symptoms may appear to be relatively minor in all three studies compared to studies evaluating changes in continence scores in patients with moderate to severe long-standing AI symptoms (Bols et al., 2012). However, the included participants were healthy, young postpartum women reporting mostly light to moderate AI symptoms during the first year after delivery, which may explain the minor improvements.

Quality of the Pelvic Floor Muscle Training Interventions and Clinical Recommendations

Recent systematic reviews have concluded that there is limited evidence available on the effect of PFMT and the role of physical therapy after OASIS (Arkel et al., 2017; Woodley et al., 2020a, 2020b, 2020c; Wu et al., 2018). However, a few of the studies reporting on the effect of PFMT for AI included in these reviews were actually powered to detect differences in AI between groups (Glazener et al., 2001; Glazener et al., 2005; Glazener et al., 2014; Sleep & Grant, 1987; Stafne et al., 2012; Wilson & Herbison, 1998). In addition, others have evaluated condition-specific QoL in women with no symptoms (Oakley et al., 2016; Peirce et al., 2013). Findings in the three studies with AI as the primary outcome measure reporting on the effect of PFMT and biofeedback with and without electrical stimulation indicate that systematic PFMT may reduce postpartum AI symptoms in both the intermediate term (Mahony et al., 2004) and long term (Fynes et al., 1999; Johannessen et al., 2017). Two of the studies did not include a control group receiving no active intervention or standard care for ethical reasons, resulting in problems evaluating the reported effects of PFMT compared to no PFMT. Despite this, there is some evidence that women performing PFMT weekly or more often reduce their AI to a larger extent than women performing PFMT less often (Johannessen et al., 2017). Common factors for studies reporting positive effects of PFMT in the peripartum period are assessments of participants' ability to perform VPFMC and high adherence to exercise protocols based on recommendations for strength training. Studies with inadequate training dosage, insufficient duration (<8 weeks), low adherence to the intervention, and infrequent or no follow-up during the intervention period tend to report less favourable results with regards to reducing pelvic floor disorders (PFDs). Considering that spontaneous changes in the female body occur up to 6 months postpartum, timing of the intervention may also influence the results (Mørkved & Bø, 2014; Mørkved et al., 2017; Nazir et al., 2003). Assessment of PFDs and introduction of PFMT too soon after delivery may result in spontaneous clinical improvements in all participants, potentially diluting the effect of PFMT.

In the present evaluation of the evidence of PMFT in the prevention or treatment of AI in the peripartum period, studies showing no effect of PFMT on AI in the peripartum period tend to be flawed in that they were not designed for AI as the primary outcome measure and thus not powered to detect differences in AI after intervention. Moreover, the interventions provided in most studies are weak in that there are few visits or follow-up with the healthcare professional (physical therapist or nurse), and instruction on VPFMC is mostly given verbally. The patients' ability to perform VPFMC is not evaluated when the intervention is commenced, and few studies offer treatment according to the patients' individual needs (standardized PFMT or electrical stimulation). In general, there is little or no focus on dose–response issues (exercise frequency, duration, adherence to the recommended training), progression or how to improve PFM strength and function over time based on the recommendations for endurance and strength training (American College of Sports Medicine, 2009; Bø, 2011; Bø et al., 1990a, 1990b). However, studies show that DI has a greater impact on psychosocial well-being, physical activity and QoL than experiencing AI or UI alone (Fialkow et al., 2003). The prevalence of DI during the peripartum period in the studies presented varies between 10% (Johannessen et al., 2018) and 77% (Sigurdardottir et al., 2020a, 2020b). The underlying mechanisms of AI involve the complex interplay between factors such as stool consistency, rectal compliance, inter-related sensory and motor pathways, spinal reflexes, and anal sphincter muscle function. Moreover, symptoms of AI include leakage of stool (loose and/or formed stool consistency), flatus and urgency (Sultan et al., 2017), and some women also experience soiling and leakage of small amounts of stool between bowel movements. These symptoms may to some extent have varying aetiology and may thus require different treatment approaches. In addition, AI is found to be associated with constipation and bowel evacuation problems (Johannessen et al., 2018; van Brummen et al., 2006). In the study by Sigurdardottir et al. (2020a, 2020b), nearly one in seven reported DI symptoms. Even though they found increases in anal sphincter strength and endurance during and beyond the intervention period in women performing regular PFMT, these increases in strength did not result in reduced postpartum AI (Sigurdardottir et al., 2020a, 2020b). Thus, considering the evidence on the effect of PFMT on UI in the peripartum period, PFMT may reduce the symptom burden in women with reduced strength of the PFMs and anal sphincter muscles (Glazener et al., 2001), but not in women with AI symptoms related to stool consistency, problems with spinal reflexes or rectal compliance. In a recent Cochrane review, Woodley et al. (2020a, 2020b, 2020c) argue that targeted PFMT among women at risk or experiencing incontinence symptoms in the peripartum period may be more effective than population approaches and recruitment of pregnant or postpartum women regardless of incontinence status. Further research on the effect of PFMT in the prevention and treatment of pelvic floor dysfunction is needed. There especially is a need for studies focusing on, and designed for, women with AI, or DI, with appropriate protocols for PFMT dosage, timing and duration, as well as the effect of combining PFMT with approaches to modify stool consistency and bowel compliance (Cotterill et al., 2018; Menees, 2017; Woodley et al., 2020a, 2020b, 2020c).

The Role of Physical Therapy and Pelvic Floor Muscle Training Following OASIS: What Advice Should Be Given?

Despite limited knowledge of the role of physical therapy and PFMT following OASIS, several national guidelines recommend that women are referred for follow-up with women's health physical therapists (Roper et al., 2020a, 2020b), and the American College of Obstetricians and Gynecologists recommends that women are followed up with a comprehensive postpartum consultation within the first 12 weeks of delivery (McKinney et al., 2018). A recent systematic review concluded that despite limited evidence of the effect of PFMT for postpartum AI, targeted PFMT may be of benefit to women following OASIS (Wu et al., 2018). Moreover, in an overview of clinical physical therapy practice, Tan et al. (2013) suggest that management in the early and late postpartum period should follow the physiological principles for rehabilitation after soft tissue injury (Tan et al., 2013), with the aim to maximize soft tissue healing and subsequent restoration of full muscle strength and function (American College of Sports Medicine, 2009).

Early Management 1 to 21 Days Following OASIS

The repair phase starts approximately 24 hours after obstetrical injury and subsequent primary suturing. During the repair phase, scar tissue is laid down, complemented by formation of new myofibrils and tissue regeneration. Through macrophagic phagocytosis of necrotic tissue the ends of the injured myofibrils are brought closer together. From 48 hours after injury, proliferation and differentiation of satellite cells dominate the regeneration of myofibrils. For the next 20 days, connective scar tissue is formed with simultaneous revascularization of the injured pelvic area by way of capillary in-growth. Twelve days after injury, re-rupture is more likely in the adjacent myofibrils than in the newly formed and relatively strong scar tissue (Tan et al., 2013).

For most soft tissue injuries, recommendations for early management during the repair phase usually follows the RICE principles of Rest, Ice, Compression and Elevation. The rationale behind RICE during the repair phase is to facilitate scar tissue formation between the ends of the torn myofibrils. Moreover, avoiding excessive strain to the healing tissues to minimize the risk of re-rupture of the adjacent myofibrils or newly formed scar tissue is important during the tissue repair and regeneration phase in the first 21 days postpartum. Prolonged immobilization and inactivity (≥2 weeks) has been found to result in muscle atrophy, loss of muscle strength and functional deficits (Hendy et al., 2012). However, all functional activities affect the PFMs and surrounding soft tissues. Complete rest of the anal sphincter muscles is therefore not possible, and it is

unlikely that disuse atrophy presents a major problem following anal sphincter injury. There is no evidence on the effect of PFMT on AI during the first 3 weeks postpartum; however, promotion of pain-free, low-force voluntary activation of the PFMs in the early postpartum period may enhance revascularization and facilitate optimal orientation of the regenerating muscle fibres (Hendy et al., 2012; Tan et al., 2013). In a retrospective study comparing initiation of physical therapy intervention including PFMT within 30 days and 6 to 8 weeks postpartum of delivery among women with OASIS, Mathé et al. (2016) found that early intervention was effective in reducing AI and UI symptoms. Furthermore, in an Australian study, PFMT initiated prior to discharge home from the hospital after delivery reduced the prevalence of UI at 8 weeks postpartum (Chiarelli & Cockburn, 2002).

Constipation following obstetric anal injury may result in impaction and subsequent breakdown of the repair (Roper et al., 2020a, 2020b). Thus laxatives, manipulation of stool consistency and promotion of defaecation with minimal strain on the perineum may protect the healing tissues after obstetric injury. In addition, Tan et al. (2013) recommend regular rests in the horizontal position to protect the healing tissues during the first 2 weeks following delivery. There is no evidence that elevation of the pelvic area to above the level of the heart or compression is beneficial during the postpartum period (Tan et al., 2013).

Ice and moderate cooling of inflamed or injured soft tissues may reduce oedema (Collins, 2008), and some low-quality evidence indicates that cold therapy may be effective as pain relief during the first days postpartum (East et al., 2020). Furthermore, it is suggested that cold therapy and reduced pain may potentially reduce the inflammatory process and encourage functional use of the PFMs during the first days after delivery (Tan et al., 2013).

Overview of Physical Therapy Management 1 to 21 Days After OASIS

1. Provide information about OASIS and a management plan for the first year postpartum before discharge home from the hospital.
2. Rest in a horizontal position when possible.
3. Use ice for pain relief, if tolerated.
4. Perform pain-free, low-force active PFM contractions.

5. Provide advice on manipulation of stool consistency and defaecation techniques that minimize strain on the pelvic floor.

Management 3 Weeks to 6 Months Following OASIS

The most common PFDs following OASIS are UI, AI and perineal pain (Wan et al., 2020a, 2020b), and women who have sustained OASIS are at increased risk of PFDs in both the short and long term following delivery (Evans et al., 2020; Jango et al., 2016; Johannessen et al., 2014b; Johannessen et al., 2019). Spontaneous improvement in pelvic floor function may occur up to 6 months postpartum (Nazir et al., 2003); however, some studies suggest that PFDs present in the intermediate period 3 to 9 months postpartum may persist in the long term (Glazener et al., 2014; MacArthur et al., 2013; Pollack et al., 2004a, 2004b). In a recent review of national guidelines for OASIS, eight guidelines recommend physical therapy follow-up after OASIS, and one recommended physical therapy for women with symptoms of AI only (Roper et al., 2020a, 2020b). However, there is little evidence on what physical therapy follow-up should include. Considering the evidence in studies with an adequate sample size, in training protocols based on principles of strength training and efficient dose–response issues such as frequency, duration, progression and close follow up, PFMT is recommended as first-line prevention and treatment for postpartum UI (Woodley et al., 2020a, 2020b, 2020c). Although the evidence is less clear, it is likely that PFMT may be beneficial for women with AI symptoms following OASIS (Fynes et al., 1999; Johannessen et al., 2017; Mahony et al., 2004), and potentially even more beneficial for women with AI and coexisting UI symptoms (Glazener et al., 2001).

Overview of Physical Therapy Management 3 Weeks to 6 Months After OASIS

1. Provide information about OASIS and a management plan for the first year postpartum.
2. Use PFMT, if able, and alternatively electrical stimulation
   a. 3 × 10 contractions daily, progression as able (Mørkved & Bø, 2014), with progressively more challenging positions from lying, sitting, standing and walking to jogging and jumping on the trampoline
3. Address pain management.

4. Provide advice on manipulation of stool consistency and defaecation techniques that minimize strain on the pelvic floor.

Management Beyond 6 Months Following OASIS

There is limited evidence on the effect of PFMT in preventing or treating AI beyond 6 months after delivery. Johannessen et al. (2017) found that women with and without OASIS reporting postpartum AI who performed PFMT more than weekly between 12 and 18 months postpartum reduced their AI symptoms more than women who performed PFMT less regularly. However, fewer women with major persistent defects of the anal sphincter muscles on ultrasound reported reduced AI symptoms compared to women with only minor or no persistent defects on ultrasound (Johannessen et al., 2017).

PFMT is recommended as first-line treatment for UI among women in any age group (Cacciari et al., 2019). Some studies suggest that the short-term effects of PFMT may be maintained beyond 12 months postpartum in women with stress urinary incontinence (Bø and Hilde, 2013). However, considering all of the changes that happen in a woman's life from the first pregnancy and delivery through to, and beyond, menopause, it may not be realistic to expect the effect of PFMT during pregnancy or in the postpartum phase to last in the long term unless the reported adherence to PFMT in the long term is improved (Glazener et al., 2014). Some suggest that effective PFMT requires both physical and behavioral changes, and that an increased focus on the cognitive and behavioral perspectives may result in a more effective implementation of, and adherence to, PFMT in the long term (Frawley et al., 2017). In addition, studies suggest that during the early postpartum period when the focus may be more on the new infant and managing life as a new mother rather than on the mother's well-being, women may tolerate the embarrassment and bother of incontinence symptoms better than if the incontinence symptoms persist in the long term. This may especially apply when these women resume their working and social lives, and existing incontinence symptoms may become more embarrassing and difficult to manage on a day-to-day basis even though they may have improved since the early postpartum period (Mahony et al., 2004). Among women sustaining OASIS at delivery, this may be particularly important because they are at increased risk of AI in the long term (Jango et al., 2016; Roos et al., 2010).

Overview of Physical Therapy Management Beyond 6 Months After OASIS

1. Provide information about OASIS and a management plan for the long term.
2. Use PFMT, if able, and alternatively electrical stimulation.
   a. 3 × 10 contractions daily, progression as able (Mørkved & Bø, 2014), with progressively more challenging positions from lying, sitting, standing and walking to jogging and jumping on the trampoline
3. Provide advice on manipulation of stool consistency and defaecation techniques that minimize strain on the pelvic floor.

REFERENCES

American College of Sports Medicine. (2009). American College of Sports Medicine position stand. Progression models in resistance training for healthy adults. *Medicine & Science in Sports & Exercise, 41*, 687–708.

Arkel, E., Torell, K., Rydhög, S., et al. (2017). Effects of physiotherapy treatment for patients with obstetric anal sphincter rupture: A systematic review. *European Journal Physiotheraphy., 19*, 90–96.

Bartlett, L., Nowak, M., & Ho, Y. H. (2007). Reasons for non-disclosure of faecal incontinence: A comparison between two survey methods. *Techniques in Coloproctology, 11*, 251–257.

Bø, K. (2011). Evidence for pelvic floor muscle training during pregnancy and after childbirth: To do or not to do? *Australian and New Zealand Continence Journal, 17*, 121–122.

Bø, K., & Haakstad, I. A. (2011). Is pelvic floor muscle training effective when taught in a general fitness class in pregnancy? A randomised controlled trial. *Physiotherapy, 97*, 190–195.

Bø, K., Hagen, R. H., Kvarstein, B., et al. (1990). Pelvic floor muscle exercise for the treatment of female stress urinary incontinence: III. Effects of two different degrees of pelvic floor muscle exercises. *Neurourology and Urodynamics, 9*, 489–502.

Bø, K., & Hilde, G. (2013). Does it work in the long term?—a systematic review on pelvic floor muscle training for female stress urinary incontinence. *Neurourology and Urodynamics, 32*, 215–223.

Bols, E., Berghmans, B., De Bie, R., et al. (2012). Rectal balloon training as add-on therapy to pelvic floor muscle training in adults with fecal incontinence: A randomized controlled trial. *Neurourology and Urodynamics, 31*, 132–138.

Bols, E. M., Hendriks, E. J., Berghmans, B. C., et al. (2010). A systematic review of etiological factors for postpartum fecal incontinence. *Acta Obstetricia et Gynecologica Scandinavica, 89*, 302–314.

Brown, H. W., Wexner, S. D., Segall, M. M., et al. (2012). Accidental bowel leakage in the mature women's health study: Prevalence and predictors. *International Journal of Clinical Practice, 66*, 1101–1108.

Brown, S. J., Gartland, D., Donath, S., et al. (2012). Fecal incontinence during the first 12 months postpartum: Complex causal pathways and implications for clinical practice. *Obstetrics & Gynecology, 119*, 240–249.

Cacciari, I. P., Dumoulin, C., & Hay-Smith, E. J. (2019). Pelvic floor muscle training versus no treatment, or inactive control treatments, for urinary incontinence in women: A Cochrane systematic review abridged republication. *Brazilian Journal of Physical Therapy, 23*, 93–107.

Chiarelli, P., & Cockburn, J. (2002). Promoting urinary continence in women after delivery: Randomised controlled trial. *BMJ, 324*, 1241.

Collins, N. (2008). Is ice right? Does cryotherapy improve outcome for acute soft tissue injury? *Emergency Medicine Journal, 25*, 65–68.

Cotterill, N., Madersbacher, H., Wyndaele, J. J., et al. (2018). Neurogenic bowel dysfunction: Clinical management recommendations of the neurologic incontinence Committee of the Fifth international consultation on incontinence 2013. *Neurourology and Urodynamics, 37*, 46–53.

Dean, N., Wilson, D., Herbison, P., et al. (2008). Sexual function, delivery mode history, pelvic floor muscle exercises and incontinence: A cross-sectional study six years post-partum. *The Australian and New Zealand Journal of Obstetrics and Gynaecology, 48*, 302–311.

East, C. E., Dorward, E. D., Whale, R. E., et al. (2020). Local cooling for relieving pain from perineal trauma sustained during childbirth. *Cochrane Database of Systematic Reviews* Issue 10, Art. No. CD006304.

Eogan, M., O'Brien, C., Daly, L., et al. (2011). The dual influences of age and obstetric history on fecal continence in parous women. *International Journal of Gynaecology & Obstetrics, 112*, 93–97.

Espuña-Pons, M., Solans-Domènech, M., & Sánchez, E. (2012). Double incontinence in a cohort of nulliparous pregnant women. *Neurourology and Urodynamics, 31*, 1236–1241.

Evans, E., Falivene, C., Briffa, K., et al. (2020). What is the total impact of an obstetric anal sphincter injury? An Australian retrospective study. *International Urogynecology Journal, 31*, 557–566.

Fialkow, M. F., Melville, J. L., Lentz, G. M., et al. (2003). The functional and psychosocial impact of fecal incontinence on women with urinary incontinence. *American Journal of Obstetrics and Gynecology, 189,* 127–129.

Frawley, H. C., Dean, S. G., Slade, S. C., et al. (2017). Is pelvic-floor muscle training a physical therapy or a behavioral therapy? A call to name and report the physical, cognitive, and behavioral elements. *Physical Therapy, 97,* 425–437.

Fynes, M. M., Marshall, K., Cassidy, M., et al. (1999). A prospective, randomized study comparing the effect of augmented biofeedback with sensory biofeedback alone on fecal incontinence after obstetric trauma. *Diseases of the Colon & Rectum, 42,* 753–758 discussion 758–761.

Glazener, C., Herbison, G. P., MacArthur, C., et al. (2005). Randomised controlled trial of conservative management of postnatal urinary and faecal incontinence: Six year follow up. *BMJ, 330,* 337.

Glazener, C., Herbison, G. P., Wilson, P. D., et al. (2001). Conservative management of persistent postnatal urinary and faecal incontinence: Randomised controlled trial. *BMJ, 323,* 593–596.

Glazener, C., MacArthur, C., Hagen, S., et al. (2014). Twelve-year follow-up of conservative management of postnatal urinary and faecal incontinence and prolapse outcomes: Randomised controlled trial. *British Journal of Obstetrics and Gynaecology, 121,* 112–120.

Guise, J. M., Morris, C., Osterweil, P., et al. (2007). Incidence of fecal incontinence after childbirth. *Obstetrics & Gynecology, 109,* 281–288.

Hendy, A. M., Spittle, M., & Kidgell, D. J. (2012). Cross education and immobilisation: Mechanisms and implications for injury rehabilitation. *Journal of Science and Medicine in Sport, 15,* 94–101.

Jango, H., Langhoff-Roos, J., Rosthoj, S., et al. (2016). Mode of delivery after obstetric anal sphincter injury and the risk of long-term anal incontinence. *American Journal of Obstetrics and Gynecology, 214,* 733.e1–733.e13.

Johannessen, H. H., Mørkved, S., Stordahl, A., et al. (2014). Anal incontinence and quality of life in late pregnancy: A cross-sectional study. *British Journal of Obstetrics and Gynaecology, 121,* 978–987.

Johannessen, H. H., Stafne, S. N., Falk, R. S., et al. (2018). Prevalence and predictors of double incontinence 1 year after first delivery. *International Urogynecology Journal, 29,* 1529–1535.

Johannessen, H. H., Stafne, S. N., Falk, R. S., et al. (2019). Prevalence and predictors of anal incontinence 6 years after first delivery. *Neurourology and Urodynamics, 38,* 310–319.

Johannessen, H. H., Wibe, A., Stordahl, A., et al. (2014). Prevalence and predictors of anal incontinence during pregnancy and 1 year after delivery: A prospective cohort study. *British Journal of Obstetrics and Gynaecology, 121,* 269–279.

Johannessen, H. H., Wibe, A., Stordahl, A., et al. (2017). Do pelvic floor muscle exercises reduce postpartum anal incontinence? A randomised controlled trial. *British Journal of Obstetrics and Gynaecology, 124,* 686–694.

Keighley, M. R., Perston, Y., Bradshaw, E., et al. (2016). The social, psychological, emotional morbidity and adjustment techniques for women with anal incontinence following obstetric anal sphincter injury: Use of a word picture to identify a hidden syndrome. *BMC Pregnancy and Childbirth, 16,* 275.

MacArthur, C., Wilson, D., Herbison, P., et al. (2013). Faecal incontinence persisting after childbirth: A 12 year longitudinal study. *British Journal of Obstetrics and Gynaecology, 120,* 169–179.

MacLennan, A. H., Taylor, A. W., Wilson, D. H., et al. (2000). The prevalence of pelvic floor disorders and their relationship to gender, age, parity and mode of delivery. *British Journal of Obstetrics and Gynaecology, 107,* 1460–1470.

Maher, C. G., Sherrington, C., Herbert, R. D., et al. (2003). Reliability of the PEDro scale for rating quality of randomized controlled trials. *Physical Therapy, 83,* 713–721.

Mahony, R. T., Malone, P. A., Nalty, J., et al. (2004). Randomized clinical trial of intra-anal electromyographic biofeedback physiotherapy with intra-anal electromyographic biofeedback augmented with electrical stimulation of the anal sphincter in the early treatment of postpartum fecal incontinence. *American Journal of Obstetrics and Gynecology, 191,* 885–890.

Mason, L., Roe, B., Wong, H., et al. (2010). The role of antenatal pelvic floor muscle exercises in prevention of postpartum stress incontinence: a randomised controlled trial. *J Clin Nurs, 19*(19–20), 2777–2786.

Mathe, M., Valancogne, G., Atallah, A., et al. (2016). Early pelvic floor muscle training after obstetrical anal sphincter injuries for the reduction of anal incontinence. *European Journal of Obstetrics & Gynecology and Reproductive Biology, 199,* 201–206.

McKinney, J., Keyser, L., Clinton, S., et al. (2018). ACOG committee opinion No. 736: Optimizing postpartum care. *Obstetrics & Gynecology, 132,* 784–785.

Menees, S. B. (2017). My approach to fecal incontinence: it's all about consistency (stool, that is). *American Journal of Gastroenterology, 112,* 977–980.

Meyer, S., Hohlfeld, P., Achtari, C., et al. (2001). Pelvic floor education after vaginal delivery. *Obstetrics & Gynecology, 97,* 673–677.

Mørkved, S., & Bø, K. (2014). Effect of pelvic floor muscle training during pregnancy and after childbirth on prevention and treatment of urinary incontinence: A systematic review. *British Journal of Sports Medicine, 48,* 299–310.

Mørkved, S., Stafne, S. N., & Johannessen, H. H. (2017). Pelvic floor physiotherapy for the prevention and management of childbirth trauma. In S. K. Doumouchtsis (Ed.), *Childbirth trauma* (pp. 271–302). London: Springer.

Nazir, M., Stien, R., Carlsen, E., et al. (2003). Early evaluation of bowel symptoms after primary repair of obstetric perineal rupture is misleading. *Diseases of the Colon & Rectum, 46,* 1245–1250.

Oakley, S. H., Ghodsi, V. C., Crisp, C. C., et al. (2016). Impact of pelvic floor physical therapy on quality of life and function after obstetric anal sphincter injury: A randomized controlled trial. *Female Pelvic Medicine & Reconstructive Surgery, 22,* 205–213.

Peirce, C., Murphy, C., Fitzpatrick, M., et al. (2013). Randomised controlled trial comparing early home biofeedback physiotherapy with pelvic floor exercises for the treatment of third-degree tears (EBAPT trial). *British Journal of Obstetrics and Gynaecology, 120,* 1240–1247 discussion 1246.

Pollack, J., Nordenstam, J., Brismar, S., et al. (2004). Anal incontinence after vaginal delivery: A five-year prospective cohort study. *Obstetrics & Gynecology, 104,* 1397–1402.

Roos, A. M., Thakar, R., & Sultan, A. H. (2010). Outcome of primary repair of obstetric anal sphincter injuries (OASIS): Does the grade of tear matter? *Ultrasound in Obstetrics and Gynecology, 36,* 368–374.

Roper, J. C., Amber, N., Wan, O. Y. K., et al. (2020). Review of available national guidelines for obstetric anal sphincter injury. *International Urogynecology Journal, 31,* 2247–2259.

Sigurdardottir, T., Steingrimsdottir, T., Geirsson, R. T., et al. (2020). Can postpartum pelvic floor muscle training reduce urinary and anal incontinence?: An assessor-blinded randomized controlled trial. *American Journal of Obstetrics and Gynecology, 222,* 247.e1–247.e8.

Sleep, J., & Grant, A. (1987). Pelvic floor exercises in postnatal care. *Midwifery, 3,* 158–164.

Solans-Domènech, M., Sánchez, E., & Espuña-Pons, M. (2010). Urinary and anal incontinence during pregnancy and postpartum: Incidence, severity, and risk factors. *Obstetrics & Gynecology, 115,* 618–628.

Stafne, S. N., Salvesen, K., Romundstad, P. R., et al. (2012). Does regular exercise including pelvic floor muscle training prevent urinary and anal incontinence during pregnancy? A randomised controlled trial. *British Journal of Obstetrics and Gynaecology, 119,* 1270–1280.

Sultan, A. H., Monga, A., Lee, J., et al. (2017). An International Urogynecological Association (IUGA)/International Continence Society (ICS) joint report on the terminology for female anorectal dysfunction. *Neurourology and Urodynamics, 36,* 10–34.

Tan, J.-L., Ruane, T., & Sherburn, M. (2013). The role of physiotherapy after obstetric anal sphincter injury: An overview of current clinical practice. *Australian and New Zealand Continence Journal, 19,* 6.

Van Brummen, H. J., Bruinse, H. W., van de Pol, G., et al. (2006). Defecatory symptoms during and after the first pregnancy: Prevalences and associated factors. *International Urogynecology Journal and Pelvic Floor Dysfunction, 17,* 224–230.

Wan, O. Y. K., Taithongchai, A., Veiga, S. I., et al. (2020). A one-stop perineal clinic: Our eleven-year experience. *International Urogynecology Journal, 31,* 2317–2326.

Wilson, P. D., & Herbison, G. P. (1998). A randomized controlled trial of pelvic floor muscle exercises to treat postnatal urinary incontinence. *International Urogynecology Journal, 9,* 257–264.

Woodley, S. J., Lawrenson, P., Boyle, R., et al. (2020). Pelvic floor muscle training for preventing and treating urinary and faecal incontinence in antenatal and postnatal women. *Cochrane Database of Systematic Reviews* Issue 5, Art. No. CD007471.

Wu, Y. M., McInnes, N., & Leong, Y. (2018). Pelvic floor muscle training versus watchful waiting and pelvic floor disorders in postpartum women: A systematic review and meta-analysis. *Female Pelvic Medicine & Reconstructive Surgery, 24,* 142–149.

Female Genital Fistula

Sandhya Gupta, Usama Shahid and Ajay Rane

DEFINITION

A genital fistula is an abnormal communication between two epithelial surfaces in the female genital tract. Genital fistulae can involve the bladder, ureters, urethra or bowel.

PREVALENCE

In the developing world, obstetric causes from prolonged, obstructed labour remain the most common aetiology of fistula formation (Hilton and Cromwell, 2012). Limited access to obstetric services, poverty and a general lack of medical literacy have kept the prevalence high (Tahzib, 2005). A systematic review over three and a half decades reported obstetric complications to be responsible for 95.2% of fistulae in developing countries (Hillary et al., 2016). The World Health Organization (2018) estimates that two million women worldwide live with untreated obstetric fistulae and suffer social ostracism. It remains reasonable to assume that due to economic constraints and scarcity of treatment facilities in geographical areas where obstetric fistulae are common, there is likely a gross under-reporting of prevalence numbers.

In the developed world, pelvic surgery remains the most prominent cause of genital fistulae formation. This can be in the form of iatrogenic injury from surgical management of pelvic pathology or radiation therapy for the management of pelvic malignancies. A study in the UK showed a 0.12% incidence of vesicovaginal fistula following all types of hysterectomy (Hilton and Cromwell, 2012). It has been speculated that due to the rise of laparoscopic and robotic surgical techniques, overall fistula incidence may be increasing (Kobayashi et al., 2012). Even in the developing world, the incidence of iatrogenic fistulae are on the rise (Raassen et al., 2014).

There are two types of female genital fistulae: vecisovaginal and rectovaginal. Vesicovaginal fistulae are the most common type, accounting for roughly 80% of cases. Rectovaginal fistulae are rare in isolation (5% of cases), whereas the remaining 15% of patients have concomitant vesicovaginal and rectovaginal fistulae (Kelly, 1992).

PATHOPHYSIOLOGY

The pathophysiology of obstetric fistulae is both simple and preventable. As labour obstructs, the relentless pressure from the impacted foetal skull against the maternal pelvis results in ischaemic necrosis and eventual fistula formation (Ahmad et al., 2005). A lack of access to obstetric services means that these women labour for days and eventually present with either a stillborn baby, genital fistula or both (Hancock and Browning, 2009). The location and extent of the fistula is dependent upon the position of the obstructed foetal head and the overall duration of the obstruction.

DIAGNOSIS

The correct diagnosis of the number, size and exact location of the genital fistula is critical towards establishing the optimal treatment plan for the patient (Stamatakos et al., 2014). The correct diagnosis will determine the triaging of care, decision to refer to a specialized centre, surgical approach of repair and preoperative counselling regarding long-term prognosis.

- History taking:
  - A routine medical/surgical history along with a detailed obstetric history of the birth and any previous gynaecological issues is important.
  - To best elucidate patient concerns, a robust understanding of both the short- and long-term complications of genital fistulae is essential.
- Short-term complications:
  - Uterine rupture
  - Foetal loss
  - Postpartum sepsis
  - Ischaemic processes in pelvic organ tissues
  - Spontaneous symphysiolysis
- Long-term complications:
  - Urinary incontinence
  - Haematometra
  - Recurrent urinary tract infection
  - Gastrointestinal damage, anal sphincter damage, hydronephrosis (from obstructed ureters)
  - Nerve damage (foot drop from the L5 root)
- Secondary consequences:
  - Malnutrition
  - Dyspareunia/apareunia
  - Chronic pelvic pain
  - Infertility (Asherman's syndrome)
  - Social stigma
  - Depression, post-traumatic stress disorder
- Physical examination and classification:
  - Perform a routine general inspection (malnutrition) and assess vitals and mental status.
  - Perform a systemic cardiovascular, respiratory and abdominal examination.
  - Pelvic examination:
    - With a chaperone present, examine the external genitalia in a well-lit room for ulceration or excoriation (from urinary incontinence).
    - Perform a speculum and digital examination, in which the primary aim is to establish the

anatomical site, size and scarring of the fistula (Hancock and Browning, 2009).

- Site:
  1. Juxta-urethral: most common site, at the urethrovesical junction
  2. Mid-vaginal: 4 cm or more from the external urethral orifice
  3. Juxta-cervical: more common in multiparous women and following caesarean section
  4. Intra-cervical: rare, between the bladder and the cervical canal; almost always follows a caesarean section
  5. Circumferential: bladder completely separates from the urethra and back of the pubic bone can be easily palpated through the vagina
  6. Miscellaneous: ureterovaginal during a caesarean section or hysterectomy and vault fistulae during elective or emergency hysterectomy
- Size:
  1. Tiny: admitting only a small probe
  2. Small: 0.5 to 1.5 cm
  3. Medium: 1.5 to 3 cm
  4. Large: greater than 3 cm, may involve loss of most of the anterior vaginal wall and a circumferential loss of the urethrovesical junction
  5. Extensive: major loss of bladder and urethra with a large gap in between
- Scarring:
  1. Minimal: fistula margins that are soft and mobile
  2. Extreme: fistula margins that are rigid and fixed
  - A scarred, fixed fistula is associated with a poor postoperative prognosis (Maroyi et al., 2021).
  - If no fistula if visualized, then ask the patient to cough to gauge for stress urinary incontinence.
  - A dye test can be performed when there is no visible or palpable fistula:
    - A dye test is performed by inserting dry cotton swabs into the vagina (classically, three are inserted) and instilling methylene blue or other sterile coloured solution into the bladder by means of a catheter. The swabs are removed after a few minutes. If the swab that was the lowest in the vagina is stained, the patient has a urethrovaginal fistula (care should be taken to exclude urethral spilling of the dye); if the middle swab is stained, the patient has a vesicovaginal fistula; and if the upper swab is stained, the patient has a juxta-cervical fistula, a vault

fistula, a ureterovesical fistula or a cervicovesical fistula. If the upper swab is stained with urine but not with dye, the patient has a ureterovaginal fistula.

- Of note: there are other fistula classification systems in place (Goh and Waaldijk being the common ones).
- Imaging in the form of ultrasound can aid in the detection of stones or hydronephrosis. Cystoscopy can be used, if available, to further clarify the exact anatomical location of the fistula.

MANAGEMENT

- Conservative:
  The following steps should be considered if the vesicovaginal fistula is discovered within 1 month of the trauma:
  - Catheterize the bladder: continuous drainage for 2 to 3 weeks may help the fistula heal.
  - Increase fluid intake: Up to 3 to 5 L of fluid per day is recommended due to a tropical environment.
  - Institute perineal hygiene: sitz or salt baths twice daily help heal the perineum.
  - Re-assess the clinical situation: the vagina and perineum should be regularly assessed, preferably once a week.
  - Determine timing of surgery after careful clinical assessment and excision of necrotic tissue, if necessary.
- Preoperative:
  - Treat anaemia and consider cross matching blood.
  - Opportunistically manage comorbidities (hepatitis B/C, HIV).
  - Obtain informed consent and have a discussion on the prognosis.
  - Consider an enema (essential for rectovaginal fistula repairs).
  - Assess the need for antibiotic prophylaxis.
- Surgical principles:
  - Ensure adequate anaesthesia.
  - Position the patient in exaggerated lithotomy with appropriate lighting.
  - Decide on the approach (vaginal or abdominal).
  - Expose the fistula with the help of an assistant (labial suture, vaginal speculum, Lone Star retractor, episiotomy).

- Incise around the edges of the fistula looking for the ureteric orifices, if necessary.
- Mobilize the bladder and trim the edges of the fistula, if needed.
- Close the fistula without tension in one (or two) layers with 2-0 Vicryl in a horizontal or vertical fashion.
- Introduce an indwelling catheter (14F or 16F), and perform a dye test to check the closure and reveal any missed vesicovaginal fistula.
- Measure the lengths of the urethra and bladder, and record the values.
- Close the vaginal mucosa.
- A vaginal pack can be inserted at the end.
- Surgical complications:
  - Haemorrhage
  - Urethral strictures (may require intermittent self-catherization or dilatation)
  - Vaginal strictures
  - Cervical stenosis causing haematometra
  - Dyspareunia
  - Infertility (Asherman's or Sheehan's syndrome)
  - Bladder stones
- Postoperative care:
  - Encourage the patient to drink at least 3 L of water daily.
  - Encourage a normal diet once bowels have opened.
  - Encourage early mobilization.
  - Physical therapy:
    - Physical therapy is an essential postoperative component of fistula management. Physical therapists specializing in the management of fistula patients provide exercises to improve the strength, function and coordination of injured or weak muscles. In addition, manual therapy is provided to improve tissue mobility or function. Furthermore, the patient's holistic cares are accommodated for with patient education including bladder training, fluid schedule and hydration.
    - Consideration is also given to logistical aspects of care following fistula repairs including incontinence management with pads and mobility devices like walkers/crutches.
    - Unique physical therapy challenges with genital fistulae (Hancock and Browning, 2009):

- Foot drop or neuropathy:
  - In extreme cases, ischaemia to the lumbosacral plexus may lead to saddle anaesthesia or a complete inability to walk (due to damage to the L5 root).
  - Physical therapy in this case is of utmost importance.
  - Through guided active and passive movements of joints, motor power and sensory loss will improve.
  - Residual foot drop can be a debilitating barrier towards the patient returning to a functioning life.
- Contractures:
  - Social stigma and the general taboo nature of genital fistulae mean that women often significantly delay seeking medical attention.
  - During this time, patients can lie in one position for days on end, forming severe muscle contractures.
  - For these to be treated, months of passive stretching exercises can help alleviate immobility.
  - Often, this needs to be done preoperatively.
- Malnutrition:
  - Similarly, neglect, social isolation and the mental health sequalae of genital fistulae can lead to malnutrition.
  - Malnourishment in itself not only impedes the physical therapy rehabilitation process but is also associated with anaemia, worsening muscle condition and poorer surgical outcomes.
  - A high-protein and high-calorie diet with iron supplementation where required should be undertaken.
- Sexual function and pelvic pain:
  - There is limited evidence on the incidence and management of sexual dysfunction and pelvic pain in the genital fistula context.
  - With that in mind, it is well understood that these issues involve a complex interplay of anatomical, psychological and cultural factors.
  - Physical therapy, particularly in the presence of postoperative vaginal stenosis or a shortened vagina, can help tackle these issues.
  - Upon discharge, remove the indwelling catheter and perform a dye test to ensure an adequately repaired fistula.
- Follow-up:
  - Overall, the success rate of surgical repairs of female genital fistulae remains high. In specialized

fistula centres, a greater than 95% postoperative success rate (no incontinence) can be expected (Maroyi et al., 2021). Furthermore, qualitative studies have established a significant improvement in the quality of life of patients following surgical repair. Improved relationships with family/friends, increased community participation and reduced stigma have all been established following fistula repair (Drew et al., 2016).

CHALLENGES

Despite increasing awareness and education about genital fistulae, they remain a prominent cause of gynaecological morbidity. There are several challenges that need to be addressed for this trend to be effectively reversed.

Primary Prevention

- The most important factor in this context is preventing genital fistulae from occurring in the first place.
- This can only be achieved through the provision of competent maternal care with improved access to emergency obstetric services. This includes increasing the efficiency of intrapartum care with surveillance of labour and the adequate use of partograms.
- In addition, patient education and raising awareness are key components towards shifting public perception and mobilizing resources.
- Similarly, safe and ease of access to contraception and family planning services play an important role in the prevention of obstetric genital fistulae.
- Finally, there needs to be a push to train surgeons to perform better caesarean sections with the aim of decreasing iatrogenic genital fistulae. This can be achieved through anatomical courses and increased supervision.

Secondary Prevention

- Once a woman has had a prolonged or obstructed labour, there are a few management steps that may prevent the formation of a genital fistula:
  - Insertion of an indwelling catheter for 2 weeks
  - Sitz baths twice a day
  - Encouraging the patient to drink 3 to 5 L of fluid daily
  - Excising grossly necrotic vaginal tissue as soon as possible

- Treating inter-current infections with antibiotics
- Ensuring that pelvic floor physical therapy is in place
- Setting up appointments for regular postpartum follow-up

Governance (Slinger et al., 2018)

- The International Federation of Gynaecology and Obstetrics (FIGO) has set up robust systems in the global context towards achieving the World Health Organization's Sustainable Development Goals.
- In the absence of adequately trained fistula surgeons the likelihood of most genital fistulae resolving are slim. FIGO has addressed this with the Fistula Surgery Training Initiative. Through the appointment of supervised fistula Fellows, FIGO has increased the number and quality of fistula surgeons to some of the most remote places on Earth.
- Through the systematic grading of competency and certification, a high level of standardized fistula surgical skill sets has been laid out.
- As of 2017, these FIGO fistula Fellows have now completed more than 6000 fistula surgeries with an overall continence success rate of 82%.
- Furthermore, FIGO has enjoined a holistic multidisciplinary approach (involving psychologists, physical therapists and lawyers), thereby placing the patient at the centre of the management ethos.
- Particular note needs to be made to the need for further regulation and governance of medical tourism 'fistula camps'. Although well intended, the varying surgical skillset, lack of multidisciplinary involvement and limited patient follow-up often leads to suboptimal outcomes.

CONCLUSION

Female genital fistulae remain a prominent cause of gynaecological morbidity in the developing world. Ideally, these patients should be managed in specialized fistula centres providing sensitive and holistic patient care. Although a complex interplay of factors affect management outcomes, a positive course overall can be expected in most clinical cases, thereby empowering the woman and facilitating her re-integration to society beyond the stigma and disability that comes with genital fistulae.

REFERENCES

Ahmad, S., Nishtar, A., & Hafeez, G. A. (2005). Management of vesico-vaginal fistula in women. *International Journal of Gynaecology & Obstetrics*, 88(1), 71–75.

Drew, L. B., Wilkinson, J. P., Nundwe, W., et al. (2016). Long-term outcomes for women after obstetric fistula repair in Lilongwe, Malawi: A qualitative study. *BMC Pregnancy and Childbirth*, 16(1) Art. No. 2.

Hancock, B., & Browning, A. (2009). *Practical obstetric fistula surgery*. London: Royal Society of Medicine Press.

Hillary, C. J., Osman, N. I., Hilton, P., et al. (2016). The aetiology, treatment, and outcome of urogenital fistulae managed in well- and low-resourced countries: A systematic review. *European Urology*, 70(3), 478–492.

Hilton, P., & Cromwell, D. (2012). The risk of vesicovaginal and urethrovaginal fistula after hysterectomy performed in the English National Health Service—a retrospective cohort study examining patterns of care between 2000 and 2008. *British Journal of Obstetrics and Gynaecology*, 119(12), 1447–1454.

Kelly, J. (1992). Vesico-vaginal and recto-vaginal fistulae. *Journal of the Royal Society of Medicine*, 85(5), 257–258.

Kobayashi, E., Nagase, T., Fujiwara, K., et al. (2012). Total laparoscopic hysterectomy in 1253 patients using an early ureteral identification technique. *Journal of Obstetrics and Gynaecology Research*, 38(9), 1194–1200.

Maroyi, R., Shahid, U., Vangaveti, V., Rane, A., & Mukwege, D. (2021). Obstetric vesico-vaginal fistulas: midvaginal and juxtacervical fistula repair outcomes in the Democratic Republic of Congo. *Int J Gynecol Obstet*, 1–6.

Maroyi, R., Shahid, U., Vangaveti, V., et al. (2021). Obstetric vesico-vaginal fistulas: Midvaginal and juxtacervical fistula repair outcomes in the Democratic Republic of Congo. *International Journal of Gynecology & Obstetrics*, 00, 1–6.

Raassen, T. J., Ngongo, C. J., & Mahendek, M. M. (2014). Iatrogenic genitourinary fistula: An 18 year retrospective review of 805 injuries. *International Urogynecology Journal*, 25(12), 1699–1706.

Slinger, G., Trautvetter, L., Browning, A., et al. (2018). Out of the shadows and 6000 reasons to celebrate: An update from FIGO's fistula surgery training initiative. *International Journal of Gynecology & Obstetrics*, 141, 280–283.

Stamatakos, M., Sargedi, C., Stasinou, T., et al. (2014). Vesico-vaginal fistula: Diagnosis and management. *Indian J. Surg*, 76(2), 131–136.

Tahzib, F. (2005). Epidemiological determinants of vesico-vaginal fistula. *British Journal of Obstetrics and Gynaecology*, 9(5), 387–439.

World Health Organization. (2018). *Obstetric fistula [online]*. Available: https://www.who.int/news-room/facts-in-pictures/detail/10-facts-on-obstetric-fistula (accessed 22.07.22).

Evidence-Based Physical Therapy for Pelvic Floor
Dysfunctions Affecting Both Women and Men

OUTLINE

8.1 Anal Incontinence: Prevalence, Causes and Pathophysiology

Bary Berghmans, Esther Bols, Patrizia Pelizzo, Abdul H Sultan and Giulio A Santoro

Continence depends on several anatomical and physiological entities: anal sphincter function, pelvic floor function, rectal distensibility, anorectal sensation, anorectal reflexes, intact nervous system, mental function, stool volume, stool consistency and colonic transit. Deficiency of one or more of these factors can lead to anal incontinence (AI). This chapter will focus on the prevalence, causes and pathophysiology of this pathological condition.

INTRODUCTION AND DEFINITION

AI is a major healthcare problem that can be particularly embarrassing and affects 2% to 24% of community-dwelling adults, with 1% to 2% experiencing significant impact on daily activities (Farage et al., 2008). The actual prevalence is likely to be higher due to under-reporting (Markland et al., 2008). The prevalence of AI increases to 57% in older people living in care homes (Pretlove et al., 2006) .

AI as a symptom of anorectal dysfunction can be defined as the complaint of involuntary loss of faeces or flatus (Haylen et al., 2010). AI covers a wide spectrum including involuntary but recognized passage liquid or solid stool (urgency incontinence); loss of flatus (flatus incontinence); unrecognized anal leakage of mucus, fluid or stool (passive incontinence); seepage of stool due to faecal impaction (overflow faecal incontinence [FI]); and compliance of both AI and urinary incontinence (double incontinence). Anal continence is based on a synergy between faeces consistency, sensory and motor nervous system, reservoir functions and mental component (Madoff et al., 2004). Incontinence occurs if one or more of these components fail and when compensatory mechanisms fall short. Vaginal delivery has been reported to be one of the major causes of AI in women (Bohle et al., 2011), and in accordance with this finding, Bols et al. (2013) found that risk factors for postpartum AI appeared to be a third- or fourth-degree sphincter rupture and AI during pregnancy. Several colorectal, urological or gynaecological interventions can cause AI as well. Specific neurological diseases associated with AI include diabetes, multiple sclerosis, Parkinson's disease, stroke and spinal cord injury. AI is mostly associated with advancing age and disability (Potter et al., 2003). However, younger patients are often affected as well, resulting in difficulties participating in school, work or social life. It is not hard to imagine what it is like to experience loss of faeces in the middle of a shop, workplace, bus or school. Often, it is difficult to explain the problem to others, like family or a partner. The implications of AI are huge, and the social restriction in many patients is severe: staying at home nearby a toilet, having to avoid social contacts including relationships or sexual contact, having feelings of depression and low self-confidence (Nelson et al., 1995; Saldana Ruiz and Kaiser, 2017). A lot of these implications are due to the unpredictable character of AI and the fear of odour. Despite this huge impact, it is striking that only one-third of all patients with FI (incontinence of stool only) report their problem to a doctor, because of fear, embarrassment and insufficient knowledge that their problem can be treated (Kalantar et al., 2002; Lehto et al., 2014).

AI often coincides with other pelvic floor, pelvic or abdominal health problems, such as constipation, prolapse or urinary incontinence (Macmillan et al., 2004; Adelborg et al., 2019).

EPIDEMIOLOGY

Prevalence figures of AI are often influenced by the use of different definitions and target populations. In a systematic review based on cross-sectional studies, the prevalence in the general population was estimated to be 2% to 24% for AI and 0.4% to 18% for FI (Macmillan et al., 2004). Another systematic review reported prevalence of AI to be 0.8% and 1.6% for men and women younger than 60 years, respectively, and 5.1% and 6.2% for men and women 60 years or older (Pretlove et al., 2006). Based on clinical studies, AI seems to be more prevalent among women, although epidemiological studies report a more equal distribution. This discrepancy might be related to the age and gender of individuals who actively seek help (Haylen et al., 2010; Madoff et al., 2004). Moreover, the prevalence is higher in postpartum women and patients with cognitive problems or a neurological disease (Giu-gale et al., 2021; Tjandra et al., 2007). Approximately 47% of FI patients also suffer from urinary incontinence, most likely based on a dysfunctional levator ani muscle (Musa et al., 2019; Teunissen et al., 2004). Only a few studies report on FI incidence rates. The 5- and 10-year incidence rate among community-dwelling persons is 5.3% to 7% (women) and 4.1% to 5.3% (men) and increases with age: 13% to 15.3% (women) and 13.2% to 20% (men) (Lehto et al., 2014; Rey et al., 2010). Among elderly persons living in nursing homes, the 10-month incidence rate was 20% (Chassagne et al., 1999).

ANATOMY AND PATHOPHYSIOLOGY

The anal sphincter muscles are located in the distal part of the anal canal, which arises from the sigmoid colon and rectum. The anal sphincter mechanism involves the internal anal sphincter (IAS), external anal sphincter (EAS) and puborectalis (PR) muscle.

The IAS is a circular smooth muscle layer under involuntary control and is mainly contracted in rest. This sphincter represents 80% of the basal resting pressure (Rey et al., 2010). IAS dysfunction is often associated with faecal seepage (passive AI). The sphincter can be damaged during childbirth, anorectal surgery (sphincterotomy or fistulotomy) and anal stretch (Cariati, 2013) or affected by primary degeneration (Vaizey et al., 1997).

The EAS is a striated muscle, innervated by the pudendal nerve (S2–S4) and comprising three parts: subcutaneous, superficial and deep. At rest, the EAS is submaximally contracted and only modestly contributing to basal pressure. Basal pressure normally redoubles in case of voluntary sphincter contraction (Dunivan et al., 2010). A sudden increase of the intra-abdominal pressure initiates a spinal reflex which causes the EAS to contract. In addition, the haemorrhoidal plexus contributes to basal pressure (15%).

The PR muscle is part of the levator ani muscle, joined with the pubococcygeus and ileococcygeus muscles. This muscle is anatomically and functionally closely related to the EAS. The PR muscle forms a muscular sling around the anorectal junction and creates an angulation between the anal canal and rectum due to its attachment anterior to the pubic bone. At rest, the anorectal angle is 90 degrees, increasing during straining and defaecation to about 135 degrees, which facilitates the passage of stool (Lucas et al., 1999). The PR muscle sling and anorectal angle seem to contribute to maintain continence, although uncertainty exists as to what extent (Madoff et al., 1992; Skardoon et al., 2017).

In response to rectal distension, the EAS contracts, which coincides with reflex inhibition of the IAS (Whitehead et al., 1982). Further accommodation of the rectum occurs when defaecation is not appropriate and the IAS regains its tone. Consequently, the possibility to postpone defaecation is dependent on rectum distensibility, reservoir function and efficiency of the anal sphincter mechanism. Adequate rectal sensation is necessary to notice rectal contents. The presence of a small amount results in some relaxation of the IAS, and the sensitive nerves in the anal mucosa are able to discriminate gas, solid or liquid faeces. Rectal sensation is often impaired in patients with diabetes, spinal disease or constipation (Madoff et al., 1992). Voluntary relaxation of the EAS and puborectal sling causes opening of the anal canal. Straining further decreases anal pressure due to relaxation of the IAS, and defaecation becomes possible.

AETIOLOGY AND RISK FACTORS

Many aetiological factors can be associated with AI (Uludağ et al., 2002; Van Lanschot, 1999). The most important causes of AI are summarized in Table 8.1.1. Often, a multifactorial aetiology is present (Wald, 1995).

Obstetric Trauma

Obstetric trauma is one of the major causes of AI in women. After delivery, a post-sphincter defect and/or pudendal neuropathy following excessive straining can occur (Sultan et al., 2017). The true prevalence of AI related to obstetric anal sphincter injury (OASIS) may be underestimated. The reported rates of AI following the primary repair of OASIS range between 15% and 61%, with a mean of 39% (Sultan and Thakar, 2007). It has also been shown that in the majority of these women, the cause can be attributed to persistent anal sphincter defects. A pudendal/pelvic neuropathy may coexist but in the majority recovers with time.

Endoanal ultrasonography revealed that 35% of women after delivery had a defect of the EAS, the IAS or both (Sultan et al., 1993). OASIS is reported to occur in 0.5% to 14% of vaginal deliveries (2.9%–19% of primiparous vaginal deliveries). In a prospective study, it has been shown that about one-third of OASIS can be

TABLE 8.1.1	Aetiology of Anal Incontinence		
Trauma	**Congenital Abnormalities**	**Neurological**	**Colorectal Causes**
Obstetric trauma	Imperforate anus	*Cerebral:*	Atrophy due to ageing
Direct trauma	Hirschsprung's disease	Stroke	Inflammatory bowel disease
Surgery	Spina bifida	Parkinson's disease	Impaction
		Dementia	Procidentia
		Tumour	Diarrhoea
		Psychological causes	Fistulas
		Brain injury	Rectal prolapse/rectocele/enterocele
		Spinal:	
		Spinal cord injury	
		Paraplegia	
		Cauda equina syndrome	
		Multiple sclerosis	
		Peripheral:	
		Pudendopathy	
		Diabetes mellitus	

diagnosed 8 weeks after delivery by endoanal ultrasonography alone. As these sonographic injuries were not identified clinically, they were believed to be 'occult' but have subsequently been shown to be clinically apparent but missed injuries at the time of vaginal delivery (Andrews et al., 2006). It is therefore now established that sonographic anal sphincter defects are usually clinically missed injuries and are not 'occult' injuries.

Perineal trauma is classified into four degrees, and the Sultan classification provides a quantified description. Many women present with symptoms later in life, presumably because cumulative effects of multiple deliveries, progressive neuropathy, ageing and menopause overcome compensatory mechanisms (Eason et al., 2002; Santoro et al., 2021). Risk factors for a ruptured sphincter are vaginal birth, midline episiotomy, forceps delivery, vacuum-assisted delivery, induced labour, high birth weight and epidural anaesthesia (Eason et al., 2002; Wald, 1995).

OTHER AETIOLOGICAL FACTORS

Several colorectal, urological or gynaecological interventions can also cause AI. The surgical procedures most related to AI are sphincterotomy for anal fissure, sphincter dilatation, haemorrhoidectomy, fistulotomy, ileal pouch reconstruction and hysterectomy (Cortez et al., 2011; Madoff et al., 1992).

Children with congenital abnormalities, such as imperforate anus or Hirschsprung's disease (encopresis), often experience lifelong problems with incomplete evacuation of faeces and soiling despite anatomical correction (Nelson, 2004).

Specific neurological diseases associated with AI include stroke, Parkinson's disease, spinal cord injury, multiple sclerosis and diabetes. Denervation or neuropathy is frequently present in patients with diabetes, vaginal delivery, descending perineum syndrome, chronic straining at stool and rectal prolapse (Rao, 2004). AI disproportionately affects individuals with physical and mental disabilities, especially in nursing homes. Characteristics associated with the development of AI in the institutionalized elderly are history of urinary incontinence, impaired mobility, poor cognitive function, older age, neurological disease, core stability problems, non-Caucasian race and problems with daily living activities (Chassagne et al., 1999; Madoff et al., 2004). In these settings, the association between urinary incontinence and AI is also well known. This so-called 'double incontinence' can be explained by the same underlying causes of poor mobility and cognitive impairment (Chassagne et al., 1999).

Residents with dementia are at high risk of developing faecal impaction because of neglect of the call to stool, impaired awareness of rectal fullness and coexistent limited mobility (Gallagher and O'Mahony, 2009; Tobin and

Brocklehurst, 1986). An association between poor health and chronic AI has also been demonstrated (Chassagne et al., 1999). Furthermore, AI is often related to irritable bowel syndrome and constipation, which is thought to be more prevalent among women (Palsson et al., 2004).

Symptoms associated with AI are sometimes related to other causes, known as pseudo-incontinence (Madoff et al., 1992). Clinically significant AI should be differentiated from perianal leakage of material other than stool (due to fistulas, prolapsing haemorrhoids, anorectal neoplasms, sexually transmitted diseases and poor hygiene), increased frequency of defaecation and urge sensations without loss of anal contents (due to inflammatory bowel disease, pelvic irradiation, irritable bowel syndrome and low anterior resection of the rectum). Appropriate diagnostic tests should enable differentiation between pseudo-incontinence and clinically important AI (Madoff et al., 1992).

Men aged 85 years and older or suffering from kidney problems have a higher risk of developing AI (Lucas et al., 1999). Radiotherapy following prostate cancer increases the risk of flatus incontinence. Lower radiotherapy doses do not seem to prevent the development of AI. In both men and women, kidney problems, diarrhoea, feeling of incomplete evacuation, pelvic radiation in the past, development of urgency complaints (Rey et al., 2010) and urinary incontinence (Markland et al., 2010) contribute to the development of AI.

REFERENCES

Adelborg, K., Veres, K., Sundbøll, J., et al. (2019). Risk of cancer in patients with fecal incontinence. *Cancer Medicine*, 8(14), 6449–6457.

Andrews, V., Thakar, R., Sultan, A. H., et al. (2006). Occult anal sphincter injuries—myth or reality? *BJOG, 113*, 195–200.

Bohle, B., Belvis, F., Vial, M., et al. (2011). Menopause and obstetric history as risk factors for fecal incontinence in women. *Diseases of the Colon & Rectum, 54*(8), 975–981.

Bols, E. M., Hendriks, H. J., Berghmans, L. C., et al. (2013). Responsiveness and interpretability of incontinence severity scores and FIQL in patients with fecal incontinence: A secondary analysis from a randomized controlled trial. *International Urogynecology Journal, 24*(3), 469–478.

Cariati, A. (2013). Anal stretch plus fissurectomy for chronic anal fissure. *Acta Chirurgica Belgica, 113*(5), 322–324.

Chassagne, P., Landrin, I., Neveu, C., et al. (1999). Fecal incontinence in the institutionalized elderly: Incidence, risk factors, and prognosis. *The American Journal of Medicine, 106*(2), 185–190.

Cortez, K. D., Mendonca, S. D. S., Figueiroa, M. D. S., et al. (2011). Fecal incontinence as consequence of anorectal surgeries and the physiotherapeutic approach. *Revista Brasileira de Coloproctologia, 31*(3), 248–256.

Dunivan, G. C., Heymen, S., Palsson, O. S., et al. (2010). Fecal incontinence in primary care: Prevalence, diagnosis, and health care utilization. *American Journal of Obstetrics and Gynecology, 202*(5), 493.e1–493.e6.

Eason, E., Labrecque, M., Marcoux, S., et al. (2002). Anal incontinence after childbirth. *Canadian Medical Association Journal, 166*(3), 326–330.

Farage, M. A., Miller, K. W., Berardesca, E., et al. (2008). Psychosocial and societal burden of incontinence in the aged population: A review. *Archives of Gynecology and Obstetrics, 277*(4), 285–290.

Gallagher, P., & O'Mahony, D. (2009). Constipation in old age. *Best Practice & Research Clinical Gastroenterology, 23*(6), 875–887.

Giugale, L. E., Moalli, P. A., & Canavan, T. P. (2021). Prevalence and predictors of urinary incontinence at 1 year postpartum. *Female Pelvic Medicine & Reconstructive Surgery, 27*(2), e436–e441.

Haylen, B. T., De Ridder, D., Freeman, R. M., et al. (2010). An International Urogynecological Association (IUGA)/International Continence Society (ICS) joint report on the terminology for female pelvic floor dysfunction. *International Urogynecology Journal and Pelvic Floor Dysfunction, 21*(1), 5–26.

Ihnát, P., Kozáková, R., Vávra, P., et al. (2016). Fekální inkontinence—závažný medicínský a společenský problém [Faecal incontinence—serious medical and social issue]. *Casopis Lékaru Ceských, 155*(3), 25–30.

Kalantar, J. S., Howell, S., & Talley, N. J. (2002). Prevalence of faecal incontinence and associated risk factors; an underdiagnosed problem in the Australian community? *Medical Journal, 176*(2), 54–57.

Lehto, K., Ylönen, K., Hyöty, M., et al. (2014). Anal incontinence: Long-term alterations in the incidence and healthcare usage. *Scandinavian Journal of Gastroenterology, 49*(7), 790–793.

Lucas, M., Emery, S., Beynon, J., et al. (1999). *Incontinence.* Oxford: Blackwell Scientific.

Macmillan, A. K., Merrie, A. E., Marshall, R. J., et al. (2004). The prevalence of fecal incontinence in community-dwelling adults: A systematic review of the literature. *Diseases of the Colon & Rectum, 47*(8), 1341–1349.

Madoff, R. D., Parker, S. C., Varma, M. G., et al. (2004). Faecal incontinence in adults. *Lancet, 364*(9434), 621–632.

Madoff, R. D., Williams, J. G., & Caushaj, P. F. (1992). Fecal incontinence. *New England Journal of Medicine, 326*(15), 1002–1007.

Markland, A. D., Goode, P. S., Burgio, K. L., et al. (2008). Correlates of urinary, fecal, and dual incontinence in older African-American and white men and women. *Journal of the American Geriatrics Society, 56*(2), 285–290.

Markland, A. D., Goode, P. S., Burgio, K. L., et al. (2010). Incidence and risk factors for fecal incontinence in black and white older adults: A population-based study. *Journal of the American Geriatrics Society, 58*(7), 1341–1346.

Musa, M. K., Saga, S., Blekken, L. E., et al. (2019). The prevalence, incidence, and correlates of fecal incontinence among older people residing in care homes: A systematic review. *Journal of the American Medical Directors Association, 20*(8), 956–962 e8.

Nelson, R. (2004). Epidemiology of fecal incontinence. *Gastroenterology, 126*(1 Suppl. 1), 3–7.

Nelson, R., Norton, N., Cautley, E., et al. (1995). Community-based prevalence of anal incontinence. *The Journal of the American Medical Association, 274*(7), 559–561.

Østbye, T., Seim, A., Krause, K., et al. (2004). A 10-year follow-up of urinary and fecal incontinence among the oldest old in the community: The Canadian study of health and aging. *Canadian Journal on Aging, 23*(4), 319–331.

Palsson, O. S., Heymen, S., & Whitehead, W. E. (2004). Biofeedback treatment for functional anorectal disorders: A comprehensive efficacy review. *Applied Psychophysiology and Biofeedback, 29*(3), 153–174.

Potter, J., Norton, C., & Cottenden, A. (2003). Bowel care in older people. *Clinical Medicine, 3*(1), 48–51.

Pretlove, S. J., Radley, S., Toozs-Hobson, P. M., et al. (2006). Prevalence of anal incontinence according to age and gender: A systematic review and meta-regression analysis. *International Urogynecology Journal and Pelvic Floor Dysfunction, 17*(4), 407–417.

Rao, S. S. (2004). Diagnosis and management of fecal incontinence. American College of Gastroenterology practice parameters Committee. *American Journal of Gastroenterology, 99*(8), 1585–1604.

Rey, E., Choung, R. S., Schleck, C. D., et al. (2010). Onset and risk factors for fecal incontinence in a US community. *American Journal of Gastroenterology, 105*(2), 412–419.

Saldana Ruiz, N., & Kaiser, A. M. (2017). Fecal incontinence—challenges and solutions. *World Journal of Gastroenterology, 23*(1), 11–24.

Santoro, G. A., Wieczorek, A. P., & Sultan, A. H. (2021). *Pelvic floor disorders: a multidisciplinary textbook* (2nd ed.). Cham, Switzerland: Springer Nature.

Skardoon, G. R., Khera, A. J., Emmanuel, A. V., et al. (2017). Review article: Dyssynergic defaecation and biofeedback therapy in the pathophysiology and management of functional constipation. *Alimentary Pharmacology & Therapeutics, 46*(4), 410–423.

Slieker-Ten Hove, M. C., Pool-Goudzwaard, A. L., Eijkemans, M. J., et al. (2010). Prevalence of double incontinence, risks and influence on quality of life in a general female population. *Neurourology and Urodynamics, 29*(4), 545–550.

Sultan, A. H., Kamm, M. A., Hudson, C. N., et al. (1993). Anal sphincter disruption during vaginal delivery. *New England Journal of Medicine, 329*, 1905–1911.

Sultan, A. H., Monga, A., Lee, J., et al. (2017). An International Urogynecological Association (IUGA)/International Continence Society (ICS) joint report on the terminology for female anorectal dysfunction. *International Urogynecology Journal, 28*(1), 5–31.

Sultan, A. H., & Thakar, R. (2007). Third and fourth degree tears. In A. H. Sultan, R. Thakar, & D. Fenner (Eds.), *Perineal and anal sphincter trauma* (pp. 33–51). London: Springer.

Teunissen, T. A. M., Van den Bosch, W. J. H. M., Van den Hoogen, H. J. M., et al. (2004). Prevalence of urinary, fecal and double incontinence in the elderly living at home. *International Urogynecology Journal and Pelvic Floor Dysfunction, 150*(44), 2430–2434.

Tjandra, J. J., Dykes, S. L., Kumar, R. R., et al. (2007). Standards Practice Task Force of the American Society of Colon and Rectal Surgeons. Practice parameters for the treatment of fecal incontinence. *Diseases of the Colon & Rectum, 50*(10), 1497–1507.

Tobin, G. W., & Brocklehurst, J. C. (1986). Faecal incontinence in residential homes for the elderly: Prevalence, aetiology and management. *Age and Ageing, 15*(1), 41–46.

Uludağ, O., Darby, M., Dejong, C. H., et al. (2002). [Sacral neuromodulation is effective in the treatment of fecal incontinence with intact sphincter muscles; a prospective study]. *Nederlands Tijdschrift voor Geneeskunde, 146*(21), 989–993.

Vaizey, C. J., Kamm, M. A., & Bartram, C. I. (1997). Primary degeneration of the internal anal sphincter as a cause of passive faecal incontinence. *Lancet, 349*(9052), 612–615.

Van Lanschot, J. J. B. (1999). In *Gastro-intestinale chirurgie en gastro-enterologie in onderling verband*. Houtem/Diegem: Bohn Stafleu Van Loghum.

Wald, A. (1995). Incontinence and anorectal dysfunction in patients with diabetes mellitus. *European Journal of Gastroenterology and Hepatology, 7*(8), 737–739.

Whitehead, W. E., Orr, W. C., Engel, B. T., et al. (1982). External anal sphincter response to rectal distention: Learned response or reflex. *Psychophysiology, 19*(1), 57–62.

Assessment of the Nature and Severity of Anal Incontinence

Bary Berghmans, and Esther Bols

To determine the nature and severity of anal incontinence (AI), different subjective and objective diagnostic procedures are available. Inquiry on some aspects of AI can be obtained by a defaecation or stool diary. A diary is useful to determine the severity of AI, regarding frequency of unintentional bowel movements and constitution of lost faeces. Unfortunately, the use of diaries in patient management is often uncommon, despite the fact that it can offer important information to guide selection of diagnostics or treatment. It is important to promote and stimulate the patient to keep a record of their stool behaviour and to provide the physician with this information, as the results can contribute to the treatment of AI. History taking and physical examination precede the additional diagnostic investigations of the rectum, anus and pelvic floor. Additional diagnostic investigations, performed by or within the physician's area of responsibility, are anal manometry, rectal capacity measurement, endoanal sonography, anorectal sensation, neurophysiological testing, defaecography and magnetic resonance imaging.

DIAGNOSTIC ASSESSMENT

In the diagnostic assessment process, the pelvic physiotherapist examines the nature, severity (assessed on the basis of the International Classification of Functioning, Disability and Health [ICF] [World Health Organization, 2018]) and degree of modifiability of the patient's health problem (general and local impeding factors). This information is derived from history taking, self-report by the patient, the defaecation diary as indicated before, measurement instruments (e.g., questionnaires) and the pelvic physiotherapy examination. Intake assessment focuses on patient's request for help; red flags (i.e., clinical indicators of possible serious underlying conditions); proctological, gynaecological, obstetric, urological and sexological history in relation to the musculoskeletal system; comorbidities; coping strategies; psychosocial problems; defaecation and micturition patterns; nutrient and fluid intake; status of the components of the continence mechanism (muscle function, reservoir function, consistency of stools, awareness and

acknowledgement of health problem, and their interactions); and the patient's pattern of expectations. This process can be integrated with education and advice.

History Taking

During history taking, the following topics should be addressed specifically:

- Nature and severity of AI, where the nature of AI is classified as either passive incontinence, urgency (Haylen et al., 2010) or a combination of both (mixed incontinence) (Baeten, 2003; Rao, 2004; Soffer and Hull, 2000; Teunissen et al., 2004)
- Proctological, gynaecological, obstetric (number of deliveries, duration of birth, birth weight, instrumental delivery, episiotomy or sphincter rupture), urological and sexological history
- Comorbidity
- Coping strategies (e.g., pad and medication use)
- Psychosocial complaints
- Defaecation and micturition pattern
- Diet and fluid intake
- Local and/or general barriers
- Above all, the physician should specifically ask in what way the patient is socially disabled, as relevant social and personal limitations caused by AI are a main focus in the intervention programme (Madoff et al., 1992; Lucas et al., 1999).

Measurement Instruments

Measuring the severity of a patient's AI and its consequences for their everyday life and sense of self-respect is important for the patient's perception of the health problem, and serves a diagnostic and prognostic purpose. Moreover, they are essential to evaluate and monitor the effects of (pelvic) physiotherapy interventions. The Wexner (Cleveland Clinic) score is a suitable instrument to assess the severity of AI as a health problem and how well the patient is coping (Jorge and Wexner, 1993). In view of its simplicity and manageability, the Global Perceived Effect (GPE) questionnaire can be used to evaluate patient-perceived changes in health status (Jaeschke et al., 1989). The International Consultation on Incontinence Questionnaire–Bowels (ICIQ-B) is a validated questionnaire for use in individuals with AI of varying causes (Cotterill et al., 2011). It also provides assessment of the impact of these symptoms on quality of life (QoL). The findings of psychometric studies and systematic reviews suggest that the Fecal Incontinence Quality of Life Scale (FIQL) (Rockwood et al., 2000) might be recommended as an instrument to assess disease-specific QoL (Avery et al., 2007; Bols et al., 2013a; Castro-Diaz et al., 2016; Fallon et al., 2008). A patient's defaecation diary enables the therapist to determine the defaecation frequency and the severity of the AI (Bharucha et al., 2008; Fallon et al., 2008). It is recommended to keep a defaecation diary until the consistency and frequency of defaecation have normalized and certain regularity has been established. The Bristol Stool Form Scale (BSFS) is an adequate instrument to monitor the consistency of the stool and can be included in a defaecation diary (Lewis and Heaton, 1997). An example of a defaecation diary including the BSFS is available elsewhere (Bols et al., 2013).

Physical Examination

- General inspection: to assess breathing, spinal column, pelvis, hips, mobility and gait analysis.
- Local inspection of the perianal area in rest: to assess presence of faecal matter, scars, fistulas, dermatitis, gapping anus, keyhole deformity, haemorrhoids and skin tags. Scars can be indicative of previous episiotomies or perianal lacerations and a gapping anus for major loss of sphincter function. A gapping anus is often associated with rectal prolapse (Madoff et al., 2004). Deformities in the anal region may be due to previous haemorrhoidectomy, fistulotomy or fissurectomy. Sometimes, chronic skin irritation is present.
- Local inspection of the perianal area during voluntary contraction (lifting and inward movement of the pelvic floor), relaxation (observe any co-contractions, breathing) and involuntary contraction (coughing and pushing [Valsalva] or straining: to assess the performance of contracting/relaxing and to demonstrate mucosal or rectal prolapse, perineal descent or paradoxal straining).
- Rectal palpation: to assess perianal sensation, anal pressure at rest, during contraction and endurance, presence of precontraction, straining, Valsalva and coughing, relaxation and reflexive contraction (anocutaneous reflex). Sphincter defects can be located

and palpated, especially during contraction. In women, the presence of a rectocele can be established. External anal sphincter and puborectal muscle strength can be assessed by digital rectal examination and graded according to the joined International Continence Society (ICS)/International Urogynecological Association (IUGA) standardization report (Haylen et al., 2010) as 'strong', 'normal', 'weak' or 'absent'. Another possibility is the assessment according to the modified Oxford grading system (Enck and Klosterhafen, 2005; Laycock and Jerwood, 2001; Madoff et al., 1992) (Table 8.1.2). The Oxford scale is an internationally accepted and most frequently used muscle grading method, with the intra-observer variability reported to be high (Messelink et al., 2005). The score ranges from 0 (no muscle contraction) to 5 (strong contraction). Endurance of submaximal strength and exhaustion of these muscles are also determined.

- Vaginal examination: provides a good impression of the pelvic floor musculature and may detect abnormalities of the rectovaginal wall (Madoff et al., 1992).

The PERFECT assessment is often used during rectal palpation and vaginal examination to direct a patient-specific treatment protocol, although its use is somewhat hampered due to validity issues (Laycock and Jerwood, 2001). Table 8.1.2 explains the characters of the PERFECT acronym. The power represents the strength of the pelvic floor muscles and is measured using the modified Oxford grading system, as mentioned earlier. Assessment of endurance strength and peak force

---

TABLE 8.1.2   The PERFECT Assessment Scheme and Modified Oxford Scale

P Power (pressure)
0 – No muscle contraction
1 – Flickering contraction
2 – Weak contraction
3 – Moderate contraction
4 – Good contraction
5 – Strong contraction
E Endurance
R Repetitions
F Number of fast maximum, 1-s contractions
E Elevation of the pelvic floor
C Co-contractions
T Timing and coordination

strength helps to prescribe an appropriate exercise programme. For example, patients graded 0, 1 or 2 on the modified Oxford scale seem to be more suitable for rectal balloon training and/or electrical stimulation instead of pelvic floor muscle training (Lucas et al., 1999; Terra et al., 2006).

ADDITIONAL DIAGNOSTIC TESTS

After history taking and physical examination, additional tests for the assessment of the anorectal region in relation to AI might be performed.

Additional Tests Performed by Either the Physician or the Pelvic Physiotherapist

Discrepancy exists between the perception of the patient and the clinician regarding severity of symptoms (De Backer, 1998). Therefore, it is recommended during screening, diagnostic and prognostic assessment or evaluation to use at least one patient-reported outcome that enables the patient to report severity of symptoms and consequences of the health problem (Avery et al., 2007).

Defaecation Diary

As stated before, the use of a defaecation diary is important at the onset of assessment and makes it possible to assess the defaecation pattern (De Backer, 1998). It is recommended to fill out a diary until the point that consistency and frequency are normalized. The BSFS (Lewis and Heaton, 1997; Rogers et al., 2006) seems to be an adequate instrument to map out faeces consistency and can be integrated in a defaecation diary (Table 8.1.3).

Wexner and Vaizey Scores

Severity of AI, including social impact, can be assessed with the frequently used grading system of Wexner (Cleveland Clinic score), ranging from 0 (perfect continence) to 20 (complete incontinence) (Jorge and Wexner, 1993) and of Vaizey (St Mark's score), which is a modification of the Wexner score (with the items 'urgency' and 'medication use' and a lower weighting for 'pad use', ranging from 0 (perfect continence) to 24 (complete incontinence) (Bols et al., 2010; Vaizey et al., 1999) (Table 8.1.4).

TABLE 8.1.3 Bristol Stool Form Scale
Type 1 Separate hard lumps, like nuts
Type 2 Sausage-shaped but lumpy
Type 3 Like a sausage or snake but with cracks on its surface
Type 4 Like a sausage or snake, smooth and soft
Type 5 Soft blobs with clear-cut edges
Type 6 Fluffy pieces with ragged edges, a mushy stool
Type 7 Watery, no solid pieces

TABLE 8.1.4 Grading System According to Wexner and Vaizey

Incontinent	Never	Rarely	Sometimes	Weekly/Usually	Daily/Always
Solid stool[a]	0	1	2	3	4
Liquid stool[a]	0	1	2	3	4
Gas[a]	0	1	2	3	4
Alteration in lifestyle[a]	0	1	2	3	4
Wears pad[b]	0	1	2	3	4
		No		**Yes**	
Need to wear a pad or plug[c]		0		2	
Taking constipating medication[c]		0		2	
Lack of ability to defer defaecation for 15 min[c]		0		4	

[a]Vaizey and Wexner items.
[b]Only Wexner item.
[c]Only Vaizey item.
Wexner: never, 0; rarely, <1/month; sometimes, <1/week and ≥1/month; usually, ≥1/week and <1/day; always, ≥1/day.
Vaizey: never, no episodes in the past 4 weeks; rarely, 1 episode in the past 4 weeks; sometimes, >1 episode in the past 4 weeks but <1 a week; weekly, ≥1 episodes a week but <1 a day; daily, ≥1 episodes a day.

Quality of Life Evaluation

The FIQL is designed for use in clinical trials and outcome research in adults with AI. Furthermore, it has been developed to be responsive to the condition in question and is based on a clearly described conceptual framework (Rockwood, 2004; Rockwood et al., 2000). Rockwood et al. (2000) concluded that the FIQL subscales demonstrated acceptable internal consistency, test–retest reliability, and adequate discriminate and convergent validity. Another psychometric study (Bols et al., 2012b) showed that the depression subscale had inadequate responsiveness. The FIQL total score had acceptable responsiveness, test–retest reliability and longitudinal construct validity. Practical issues related to the 29-item FIQL include the complicated addition of items and time-consuming completion, which holds consequences for clinical use. Based on these results and in the absence of other recommendable disease-specific QoL scales, the International Consultation on Incontinence (ICI) suggests a grade A recommendation to use the FIQL for evaluating QoL of patients with AI (Avery et al., 2007; Castro-Diaz et al., 2016).

Global Perceived Effect

The Global Perceived Effect (GPE) questionnaire, reflecting patients' global perceived change or extent of improvement of subjective health status, is attractive due to its simplicity and practicality (Castro-Diaz et al., 2016; Jaeschke et al., 1989; Veldhuyzen-van Zanten et al., 1999).

Biofeedback

Electromyography/Pressure. An intra-anal electromyography sensor, a perianal surface electromyography electrode (both measuring change of motor unit activity) or an anal manometric probe (measuring intra-anal pressure change), connected to a biofeedback device/machine, is used to inform the patient about the activity of the pelvic floor and sphincter ani muscles by way of a visual display and/or an auditory signal. This (feedback) data can be collected and stored for further counselling and evaluation (Norton, 2004).

Rectal balloon. A rectal balloon, attached to a syringe, can be introduced into the rectum and slowly inflated with air while the patient is lying in lateral position. This enables assessment of sensory threshold, urge sensation, change in distinction of and response to rectal volume related to distension, maximal tolerated volume, and rectoanal inhibitory reflex (Bols et al., 2012a; Norton and Chelvanayagam, 2004).

Additional Tests Performed by the Physician

The following diagnostic tests should be performed according to a standard procedure by physicians (or technicians) specialized in performing the specific tests.

Anal manometry determines resting pressure (mmHg) and maximal squeeze pressure (mmHg) of the anal sphincter and puborectalis muscle and rectal capacity can be measured (Diamant et al., 1999). With endoanal sonography (Stoker et al., 2001, 2002), the integrity of the anal sphincter complex can be demonstrated. Neurophysiological testing, in casu pudendus nerve terminal motor latencies (PNTML), measures the conduction time of the left and right pudendal nerves. Uncertainty exists on the accuracy of PNTML and its predictive value on outcome (Heitmann et al., 2019; Kiff and Swash, 1984; Madoff et al., 2004).

Defaecography is a dynamic radiologic study of attempted defaecation. Abnormalities can be detected during rest, straining and squeezing, such as rectocele and rectal intussusception (incomplete rectal prolapse) (Terra et al., 2008). Endoanal magnetic resonance imaging provides an impression of the anatomy of the anus and pelvic floor and can adequately demonstrate sphincter defects (Stoker et al., 2001, 2002).

The pelvic physiotherapist should receive the conclusions from all diagnostic tests to gain more insight into the aetiology and prognosis of improvement or recovery of AI.

Physiotherapy Analysis/Diagnosis

It is important to analyze whether and to what extent there is sufficient balance between strain and patients' physical condition. The physical condition may be affected by dysfunctions of the continence mechanisms:

- Damage to or weakness of the pelvic floor muscles (external anal sphincter and levator ani muscle)
- Damage to or weakness of the internal anal sphincter
- A neurological problem: nuclear/infranuclear dysfunction, peripheral innervation, spinal cord, brainstem or awareness.

The physical condition partly depends on other factors, such as general mobility, diet, the intestinal system (peristalsis or faecal composition), medication, problematic history (e.g., adverse sexual experiences, physical violence) and comorbidity. The patient's physical condition (at the local, personal and participation level) determines how much they can bear.

The analysis process is used to determine the nature, severity and modifiability of the problem. The Dutch guideline development team, in consultation with a feedback group of experts in the field, has distinguished four problem categories for patients with AI (for further subdivision, consult the full-text Evidence Statement of the original document and flowchart at https://www.fysionet-evidencebased.nl (Bols et al., 2013):

I: AI with pelvic floor dysfunction and awareness of loss of stools (urgency). The treatment plan is developed based on the presence or absence of a neurological problem, anorectal sensation, voluntary or involuntary control, and factors that adversely affect pelvic floor function.

II: AI with pelvic floor dysfunction without awareness of loss of stools (passive). The treatment plan is developed based on the presence or absence of a neurological problem and anorectal sensation.

III: AI without pelvic floor dysfunction.

IV: AI with or without pelvic floor dysfunction, in combination with general factors impeding the recovery or adjustment processes. The treatment plan is developed based on the presence or absence of comorbidity.

The nature and severity of any pain symptoms must be taken into consideration for all four problem categories, as these represent a complicating factor.

REFERENCES

Avery, K. N., Bosch, J. L., Gotoh, M., et al. (2007). Questionnaires to assess urinary and anal incontinence: Review and recommendations. *The Journal of Urology*, 177(1), 39–49.

Baeten, C. G. M. I. (2003). Reoperative surgery for persistent fecal incontinence. In W. E. Longo, & J. M. Northover (Eds.), *Reoperative colon and rectal surgery* (pp. 17–132). London: Martin Dunitz, Taylor & Francis.

Bharucha, A. E., Seide, B. M., Zinsmeister, A. R., et al. (2008). Insights into normal and disordered bowel habits from bowel diaries. *American Journal of Gastroenterology*, 103(3), 692–698.

Bols, E., Berghmans, B., de Bie, R., et al. (2012). Rectal balloon training as add-on therapy to pelvic floor muscle training in adults with fecal incontinence: A randomized controlled trial. *Neurourology and Urodynamics*, 31(1), 132–138.

Bols, E., Groot, J., Van Heeswijk-Faasse, I., et al. (2013). *KNGF evidence statement anal incontinence*. Royal Dutch Society for Physical Therapy. Amersfoort, the Netherlands [Online]. Available: http://www.kngfrichtlijnen.nl/index.php/kngf-guidelines-in-english (Accessed 02.11.22).

Bols, E., Hendriks, E., de Bie, R., et al. (2012). Predictors of a favorable outcome of physiotherapy in fecal incontinence: Secondary analysis of a randomized trial. *Neurourology and Urodynamics*, 31(7), 1156–1160.

Bols, E., Hendriks, E., Deutekom, M., et al. (2010). Inconclusive psychometric properties of the Vaizey score in fecally incontinent patients: A prospective cohort study. *Neurourology and Urodynamics*, 29(3), 370–377.

Bols, E., Hendriks, H., Berghmans, L., et al. (2013). Responsiveness and interpretability of incontinence severity scores and FIQL in patients with fecal incontinence: A secondary analysis from a randomized controlled trial. *International Urogynecology Journal*, 24(3), 469–478.

Castro-Diaz, D., Robinson, D., Bosch, R., et al. (2016). Patient-reported outcome assessment. In P. Abrams, L. Cardozo, A. Wagg, et al. (Eds.), *Incontinence: Sixth international consultation on incontinence* (pp. 497–541). Bristol, UK: ICUD.

Cotterill, N., Norton, C., Avery, K. N., et al. (2011). Psychometric evaluation of a new patient-completed questionnaire for evaluating anal incontinence symptoms and impact on quality of life: The ICIQ-B. *Diseases of the Colon & Rectum*, 54(10), 1235–1250.

De Backer, J. (1998). Bekkenbodemreëducatie bij anale problematiek. In B. C. M. Smits-Engelsman, I. Van Ham, P. Vaes, et al. (Eds.), *Jaarboek Fysiotherapie/kinesitherapie* (pp. 16–37). Houten: Bohn Stafleu Van Loghum.

Diamant, N. E., Kamm, M. A., Wald, A., et al. (1999). AGA technical review on anorectal testing techniques. *Gastroenterology*, 116, 735–760.

Enck, P., & Klosterhafen, S. (2005). Perception of incontinence in and by society. In H.-D. Becker, A. Stenzl, D. Wallwiener, et al. (Eds.), *Urinary and fecal incontinence* (pp. 33–39). Heidelberg: Springer-Verlag.

Fallon, A., Westaway, J., & Moloney, C. (2008). A systematic review of psychometric evidence and expert opinion regarding the assessment of faecal incontinence in older community-dwelling adults. *International Journal of Evidence-Based Healthcare*, 6(2), 225–259.

Haylen, B. T., de Ridder, D., Freeman, R. M., et al. (2010). An International Urogynecological Association (IUGA)/ International Continence Society (ICS) joint report on the terminology for female pelvic floor dysfunction. *International Urogynecology Journal and Pelvic Floor Dysfunction, 21*(1), 5–26.

Heitmann, P. T., Rabbitt, P., Schloithe, A., et al. (2019). Relationships between the results of anorectal investigations and symptom severity in patients with faecal incontinence. *International Journal of Colorectal Disease, 34*(8), 1445–1454.

Jaeschke, R., Singer, J., & Guyatt, G. H. (1989). Measurement of health status. Ascertaining the minimally important difference. Control. *Clinical Trials, 10*(4), 407–415.

Jorge, J. M., & Wexner, S. D. (1993). Etiology and management of fecal incontinence. *Diseases of the Colon & Rectum, 36*(1), 77–97.

Kiff, E. S., & Swash, M. (1984). Slowed conduction in the pudendal nerves in idiopathic (neurogenic) faecal incontinence. *British Journal of Surgery, 71*, 614–616.

Laycock, J., & Jerwood, D. (2001). Pelvic floor assessment: The PERFECT scheme. *Physiotherapy, 87*(12), 631–642.

Lewis, S. J., & Heaton, K. W. (1997). Stool form scale as a useful guide to intestinal transit time. *Scandinavian Journal of Gastroenterology, 32*(9), 920–924.

Lucas, M., Emery, S., & Beynon, J. (1999). *Incontinence*. Oxford: Blackwell Scientific.

Madoff, R. D., Parker, S. C., Varma, M. G., et al. (2004). Faecal incontinence in adults. *Lancet, 364*(9434), 621–632.

Madoff, R. D., Williams, J. G., & Caushaj, P. F. (1992). Fecal incontinence. *New England Journal of Medicine, 326*(15), 1002–1007.

Messelink, B., Benson, T., Berghmans, B., et al. (2005). Standardization of terminology of pelvic floor muscle function and dysfunction: Report from the pelvic floor clinical assessment group of the international continence society. *Neurourology and Urodynamics, 24*(4), 374–380.

Norton, C. (2004). Nurses, bowel continence, stigma and taboos. *Journal of Wound Ostomy & Continence Nursing, 31*(2), 85–94.

Norton, C., & Chelvanayagam, S. (2004). *Bowel continence nursing*. Beaconsfield, England: Beaconsfield Publishers.

Rao, S. S. (2004). Diagnosis and management of fecal incontinence. American College of Gastroenterology practice parameters Committee. *American Journal of Gastroenterology, 99*(8), 1585–1604.

Rockwood, T. H. (2004). Incontinence severity and QOL scales for fecal incontinence. *Gastroenterology, 126*(1 Suppl. 1), 106–113.

Rockwood, T. H., Church, J. M., Fleshman, J. W., et al. (2000). Fecal incontinence quality of life scale: Quality of life instrument for patients with fecal incontinence. *Diseases of the Colon & Rectum, 43*(1), 9–16; discussion 7.

Rogers, R. G., Abed, H., & Fenner, D. E. (2006). Current diagnosis and treatment algorithms for anal incontinence. *BJU International, 98*(Suppl. 1), 97–106; discussion 7–9.

Soffer, E. E., & Hull, T. (2000). Fecal incontinence: A practical approach to evaluation and treatment. *American Journal of Gastroenterology, 95*(8), 1873–1880.

Stoker, J., Bartram, C. I., & Halligan, S. (2002). Imaging of the posterior pelvic floor. *European Radiology, 12*, 779–788.

Stoker, J., Halligan, S., & Bartram, C. I. (2001). Pelvic floor imaging. *Radiology, 218*, 621–641.

Terra, M. P., Deutekom, M., Dobben, A. C., et al. (2008). Can the outcome of pelvic-floor rehabilitation in patients with fecal incontinence be predicted? *International Journal of Colorectal Disease, 23*(5), 503–511.

Terra, M. P., Dobben, A. C., Berghmans, B., et al. (2006). Electrical stimulation and pelvic floor muscle training with biofeedback in patients with fecal incontinence: A cohort study of 281 patients. *Diseases of the Colon & Rectum, 49*(8), 1149–1159.

Teunissen, T. A., van den Bosch, W. J., van den Hoogen, H. J., et al. (2004). Prevalence of urinary, fecal and double incontinence in the elderly living at home. *International Urogynecology Journal and Pelvic Floor Dysfunction, 15*(1), 10–13 , discussion 3.

Vaizey, C. J., Carapeti, E., Cahill, J. A., et al. (1999). Prospective comparison of faecal incontinence grading systems. *Gut, 44*(1), 77–80.

Veldhuyzen-van Zanten, S. J., Talley, N. J., Bytzer, P., et al. (1999). Design of treatment trials for functional gastrointestinal disorders. *Gut, 45*(Suppl. II), 1169–1177.

World Health Organization. (2018). *International classification of functioning, disability and health (ICF)*. Geneva: World Health Organization.

Conservative Interventions for Treatment of Anal Incontinence

Bary Berghmans, and Esther Bols

Treatment of patients with anal incontinence (AI) consists of both conservative and surgical interventions. Conservative interventions incorporate lifestyle interventions like dietary adaptations, medication, bowel management, smoking behaviour, absorbent materials and physiotherapy. Table 8.1.5 summarizes the therapeutic options and goals regarding conservative treatment of AI.

The physiotherapeutic process includes the actual treatment, evaluation and conclusion of treatment. The treatment plan relates to the identified problem category, and the objective is to improve one or more of the following components of continence: muscle function, reservoir function, consistency of stools, awareness and acknowledgement of the health problem, or interactions between these components. No adverse effects or worsening of symptoms have been reported for any of the forms of therapy discussed in the following.

The International Consultation on Incontinence (ICI) (Bliss et al., 2016) states that physiotherapy should be tried before any surgical treatment. Moreover, national guidelines in the UK and the Netherlands recommend maximal education, lifestyle and dietary interventions preceding pelvic floor muscle training (PFMT) or biofeedback (BF) (Berghmans et al., 2015; Norton et al., 2007).

Patients with an embarrassing condition such as AI must be treated carefully. Therefore, prior to physiotherapy, education and information should be given about the disorder. One determinant in success of

TABLE 8.1.5   Therapeutic Options and Goals Regarding Conservative Treatment of Anal Incontinence

Therapy	Goal
A. Dietary	Altering stool consistency, stool volume and transit time, regularization of timing of defaecation
B. Pharmacological	Altering stool consistency, stool volume and transit time, regularization of timing of defaecation
C. Bowel management	Colonic cleansing
D. Products and appliances	Prevention of faecal passage or soiling
E. Physiotherapy	
E1 Education and information	On general health, and more specific advice and teaching about lifestyle changes related to toilet behaviour, toilet facilities, bowel function and coping (strategies)
E2 Pelvic floor muscle training	Improve coordination of muscle contractions
	Improve muscular strength, endurance and relaxation
	Increase awareness and isolated contraction of pelvic floor muscles and anal sphincter
E3 Biofeedback	Information on activity anal sphincters and puborectalis muscle (EMG-BF)
	Increase awareness and isolated contraction of anal sphincter and pelvic floor muscles (EMG-BF); accent on timing and coordination
E4 Rectal balloon training	Decrease sensory threshold in case of passive FI (P-BF)
	Increase sensory threshold in case of urge FI (P-BF)
	Improve rectoanal inhibitory reflex (P-BF)
E5 Electrical stimulation	Increase awareness and isolated contraction of pelvic floor muscles and anal sphincter

EMG-BF, Electromyographic biofeedback using intra-anal electromyographic sensor/probe or perianal surface electromyography; *FI,* faecal incontinence; *P-BF,* pressure biofeedback using rectal balloon.

physiotherapy is a reliable relationship with the therapist and motivation of both the therapist and the patient (Norton and Cody, 2012). After diagnostic assessment, manually directed techniques or specifically designed equipment are used to treat the motor, sensory or reservoir component of the disorder.

LIFESTYLE INTERVENTIONS

Information and Education

Patients with AI often lack knowledge about bowel function, working mechanism and the anatomy of pelvic organs related to stool and bowel function. Many of them have an inefficient or wrong toilet behaviour or defaecation pattern and are not well educated or trained. They have developed attitudes towards defaecation based on what they learned from their family and societal environment (Damon et al., 2014; Norton, 2004).

Therefore, every treatment programme should start with information and education on general health, and more specific advice and teaching about lifestyle changes related to toilet behaviour and bowel function (Norton and Chelvanayagam, 2004). Although the literature does not consistently report on the strength of association of relevant risk factors for AI (e.g., weight loss; toilet behaviour, use and facilities; and smoking), patient and healthcare provider attitudes, information and education should incorporate these topics.

Weight Loss

Although obesity is considered a risk factor for AI by some authors, others did not find a significant correlation between obesity and AI (Bliss et al., 2016). Markland et al. (2010) found improvement on reducing AI comparing weight loss (i.e., dieting) versus a control (i.e., education) intervention in a subgroup of 80 of 291 women with double (AI and urinary incontinence [UI]) incontinence who participated in an 18-month intervention examining the ability of weight loss to improve UI. There was no significant difference in the Faecal Incontinence Severity Index (FISI) or AI type (i.e., consistency) between the weight loss and control groups. Women who showed improvement in AI had a lower weight at baseline (89 kg) than those with no improvement in AI severity or no AI symptoms (97 kg).

Smoking

Anecdotally, smoking has been claimed to stimulate the onset of defaecation. This might be due to stimulation of distal colonic motility and faecal urgency (Bliss et al., 2016; Rausch et al., 1998). The scientific evidence for such an association is weak. No association has been found between antenatal smoking and postnatal AI (Chaliha et al., 1999). In another study, involving twin sisters, no significant association was found between smoking and AI (Abramov et al., 2005). In a longitudinal observational study of community-living elderly men and women, smoking was not predictive of prevalence or incidence of FI (Ostbye et al., 2004).

EVIDENCE FOR EFFECTIVENESS OF PATIENT EDUCATION

In a randomized controlled trial (RCT), nurse-led education and advice about conservative AI management (e.g., advice on diet, medication titration and bowel retraining) alone, and as part of a combined intervention that added exercises and/or BF, were compared (Norton et al., 2003). All four study groups showed an effect in reducing frequency of AI, but there were no statistical differences between the groups (Norton et al., 2003). Another study, reported as an abstract only, underlined the benefits of systematic education and standard medical care for a group of AI patients who had failed prior attempts at medical management, leading to a successful outcome in 38% (Heymen et al., 2001). Success was defined as self-reported adequate relief of bowel symptoms.

The overall conclusion of the Sixth International Consultation on Incontinence (ICI 6) (Bliss et al., 2016) is that there is insufficient evidence to recommend or discourage most lifestyle modifications either for the prevention or treatment of AI. The ICI recommends patient education about the causes of AI and a systematic effort to remove barriers to effective toileting as an intervention that is likely to be beneficial based on the consensus of experts (Bliss et al., 2016). This may be provided at relatively low cost and involves no significant risk to the patient.

Apart from education and information on lifestyle interventions, some other relevant subjects to discuss with the patient are the following:
- Influence of stress and relaxation on pressure resilience of the pelvic floor
- General and local relaxation exercises
- Relation with other pelvic floor–related symptoms, such as prolapse and UI
- Optimization of defaecation frequency, consistency and position during toileting.

PELVIC PHYSIOTHERAPY

Pelvic physiotherapy for AI includes PFMT, BF (including rectal balloon training [RBT]) and electrical stimulation (ES), and is offered by pelvic physiotherapists (see Table 8.1.5). Often, one or more physiotherapy interventions are combined, depending on the underlying cause of AI.

As pelvic physiotherapy, in general, is simple, inexpensive and mostly without unfavourable physical side effects, it is an appealing conservative treatment option in patients with AI (Bliss et al., 2016; Madoff et al., 2004).

Pelvic Floor Muscle and Sphincter Training

Pelvic floor muscle and sphincter training are recommended as an early intervention in the treatment of AI as part of an integrated conservative management approach (Bliss et al., 2016; Norton et al., 2006, 2009).

The pelvic floor muscles support the abdominal organs and work tonically and reflexively to maintain continence. Approximately 70% slow-twitch and 30% fast-twitch fibres are present in the pelvic floor muscles to serve this purpose (Laycock and Jerwood, 2001). Patients suffering from AI often show weakened muscle function. PFMT aims to restore the muscular strength, relaxation, coordination and timing of contractions.

Exercises consist of selective (maximal) voluntary contractions and relaxations of the pelvic floor muscles and external anal sphincter with a repetitive character. Exercises can activate latent motor units to the point that the muscle becomes functional again (MacLeod, 1983). Exercises in a progressive resistance programme adhere to the basic muscle training principles. The principle of 'overload' is based on stimulation of the muscle beyond its normal level of performance. To evaluate this principle, a physiotherapeutic diagnostic assessment prior to training is necessary (Berghmans et al., 2020). The principle of 'specificity' refers to training a muscle in the way the muscle needs to be used. Exercises are adapted to slow-twitch fibres (endurance exercises) and fast-twitch fibres (power and speed exercises). The principles 'maintenance' and 'reversibility' alert the patient to train regularly, sometimes lifelong. Inactivity will convert the muscle to its pretrained status, and symptoms can occur again (Kuijpers, 1997). Awareness of the different muscles involved in maintaining continence is necessary to be sure of avoidance of co-contractions of surrounding muscles (abdominals, buttocks, thighs and back) and activation of the relevant muscles. Sometimes, when patients find and use the relevant muscles at the appropriate time, symptoms can reduce at once (Norton, 2004). Ultimately, exercises should be practised in different starting positions, from lying to sitting to standing, simulating everyday situations as much as possible (Berghmans, 2017; Bols et al., 2012a; Lucas et al., 1999).

Biofeedback and Rectal Balloon Training

Haskell and Rovner made the first attempt at BF for AI in 1967 (MacLeod, 1983). They reported the successful use of electrodes and electromyography in 71% of patients treated for AI. Cerulli et al. (1979) were the first to use BF by way of insertion of three balloons: one intrarectal (to allow rectal distension) and two intra-anal (to record internal and external sphincter contractions separately).

Many authors estimate BF to be a useful adjunct to PFMT or ES in patients with AI (Bliss et al., 2016; Norton and Kamm, 2001). BF is a technique that monitors biological signals and electrically amplifies these to provide feedback to the patient. BF intends to control physiological processes, normally being under involuntary control.

Today, three modalities of BF in the treatment of AI can be recognized (Norton and Cody, 2012):

1. An intra-anal electromyography sensor, an anal manometric probe (measuring intra-anal pressure change) or perianal surface electromyography electrode is used to inform the patient about the activity of the pelvic floor muscles by way of a visual display and/or an auditory signal. The patient attempts to align the response (the patient's pelvic floor muscle activity) to the ideal response (preset, visualized on screen). The goal of this treatment modality is to create awareness of the squeezing musculature and strengthen it without rectal distension. In addition, the correct muscle response and progress of the patient can be demonstrated. Training can focus on endurance force (a submaximal contraction sustained for prolonged time) or increase of squeeze amplitude (peak force). The exercises are based on exercise programmes originally used for UI (Schüssler et al., 1994).

2. The second modality involves the use of a manometric rectal balloon (RBT). The rectal balloon is filled with air to imitate rectal contents. The patient with an elevated sensory threshold is trained to discriminate smaller rectal volumes, resulting in an earlier

warning from stool entering the rectum and earlier external sphincter response to counteract reflex inhibition of the internal sphincter (Heymen et al., 2009; Miner et al., 1990). However, progressive distension of the rectal balloon is used in patients with a hypersensitive rectum to resist feelings of urgency.

3. The third modality is a three-balloon system (3T = triplet: a balloon-tipped water-perfused catheter or a Schuster-type three-balloon probe) used for coordination training (Engel et al., 1974; Heymen et al., 2000). One balloon is inserted into the rectum. Two other, smaller, pressure-recording balloons are introduced into the upper and lower parts of the anal canal. As the rectal balloon is filled, it elicits the rectoanal inhibition reflex. This causes anal relaxation, which is visualized by the two recording balloons, and which the patient must become aware of and must learn to counteract by means of a voluntary anal sphincter contraction. This contraction must be long and powerful enough to allow the resting pressure to return to its initial value.

Overall, BF provides feedback about the possibility, degree and quality of contracting and relaxing the pelvic floor, and gives feedback on the coordination between rectal distension and contracting the anal closing system (Bols et al., 2012a; Heymen et al., 2009).

The use of BF as a treatment for AI is recommended by the ICI when other behavioural and medical management has been tried and inadequate symptom relief obtained (Bliss et al., 2016). Moreover, its use is promoted given the numerous positive outcomes from uncontrolled trials, limitations in the current RCTs and low morbidity associated with its application. Patients most likely to benefit from BF include those who have motivation, intact cognitive skills, some rectal sensation, and nearly intact sphincters and innervation (Heymen et al., 2000; Jorge and Wexner, 1993; Loening-Baucke, 1990; Schwandner et al., 2010). It is reported that patients with neurological deficits (diabetes, spina bifida, multiple sclerosis) are less likely to be treated successfully (Heymen et al., 2000).

Even though continence is achieved after pelvic physiotherapy, the rectosphincteric reflexes sometimes remain abnormal, implicating that the external sphincter response to rectal distension is an unreliable predictor of treatment outcome (Latimer et al., 1984).

Electrical Stimulation

The use of ES for the treatment of UI and AI spans more than 35 years with apparent success (Hosker et al., 2007).

ES is the application of an electrical current, thereby passively stimulating the pelvic floor muscles, sphincters and accompanying nerve structures. The purpose of ES is to re-educate weakened and poorly functioning pelvic floor muscles by means of increasing awareness and isolated contraction of the stimulated structures (Hosker et al., 2007). ES is often used as an adjunct to pelvic floor muscle and sphincter exercises and BF to assist with identification and isolation of pelvic floor muscles and to increase contraction strength.

In ES, the number of motor units recruited is dependent on several factors. These include the parameters of the electrical stimulus, impedance (resistance to the flow of the current), and the size and orientation of the electrodes. The electrodes should be placed as close as possible to the pelvic floor muscles. The electrical stimulus should be stimulating enough to depolarize the nerve, whereas uncomfortable sensations should be avoided (Bliss et al., 2016; Laycock et al., 1994).

A specific type of ES is tibial nerve stimulation. This is a form of ES in which a surface electrode is placed on the skin over the tibial nerve on one ankle and referenced to another electrode on the ipsilateral foot (transcutaneous tibial nerve stimulation) or a needle inserted beneath the skin close to the tibial nerve on one side and is referenced to an electrode on the ipsilateral foot (percutaneous tibial nerve stimulation [PTNS]) (Horrocks et al., 2014). Typical transcutaneous tibial nerve stimulation parameters are 250-µs pulses at a frequency of 10 Hz and current of up to 30 mA. Typical PTNS stimulation parameters are 200- to 250-µs pulses at a frequency of 10 to 20 Hz and up to 9 mA.

The precise mechanisms by which ES can restore faecal control are not well understood: Salmons and Vrbova (1969) suggested that ES improves muscle function by transforming fatigable fast-twitch muscle fibres to less fatigable slow-twitch fibres, and Hudlicka et al. (1982) reported an increase of capillary density, which supports the efficient working of these slow-twitch, oxidative fibres. Some studies have shown an increase in axonal budding following denervation (Laycock et al., 1994). Changes in fibre diameter may be important. However, apart from physiological changes, it may be that the predominant mechanism of improved faecal control is an enhanced awareness of the anal sphincter (Haskell and Rovner, 1967). A possible working mechanism of neuromodulation through efferent or afferent nerve stimulation needs to be further investigated.

Contraindications for ES are anal infections, rectal bleeding, complete denervation of the pelvic floor (will not respond), swollen/painful haemorrhoids, deficient sensation, atrophy of mucosa, the 6-week period after surgery, pacemaker, dementia, pregnancy and pain during palpation (Newman and Giovannini, 2002).

Evaluation

The physiotherapist should evaluate the treatment with the measurement instruments used during assessment and should also evaluate the modifiable components of the continence mechanism that emerged from the physical examination. The therapist and patient may jointly consider arranging a re-evaluation, in the form of a check-up or reminder therapy, at predefined dates after the conclusion of the treatment.

EVIDENCE FOR EFFECTIVENESS OF PELVIC PHYSIOTHERAPY

A literature review was undertaken to ascertain the effectiveness of different pelvic physiotherapy interventions (i.e., PFMT, BF and ES) as conservative treatment for AI.

Literature Search Strategy

The ICI Committee 16 updated recommendations on assessment and conservative management of AI and quality of life in adults for the Sixth Consultation on Incontinence by reviewing in detail relevant literature published up to March 2016 (Bliss et al., 2016). For this update, a search was conducted in the electronic databases of the Cochrane Library, PubMed, Embase, PEDro and CINAHL. A search of the same computerized databases from April 2016 to June 2020 was undertaken. Furthermore, reference lists of included studies were screened for unidentified articles. Only randomized trials were included, with full reports in English, German or Dutch reporting on PFMT, BF or ES as conservative treatment in adults with AI. Because PTNS requires insertion of a needle near the malleolus medialis of the tibia, this procedure is not allowed for physiotherapists in most countries. Therefore, RCTs including PTNS as the intervention arm were excluded. Characteristics of the 28 included RCTs are detailed in Table 8.1.6.

Methodological Quality

The PEDro rating score was used to classify the methodological quality of all included trials (Table 8.1.7), resulting in low (2/10) to high (8/10) methodological quality. It should be noted that the two criteria related to blinding of the therapist and patient are almost impossible to meet in physiotherapy trials.

Pelvic Floor Muscle Training

PFMT has been proven to be effective in the treatment of stress UI (Berghmans et al., 1998). Since the anal sphincter and puborectalis muscle form a part of the same pelvic floor as the closing urethral system, expectations are raised for the same positive results of pelvic floor muscle re-educative techniques in AI. Hay-Smith et al. (2009) concluded that PFMT, properly taught, is still the mainstay of physiotherapy.

Norton and Cody (2012) compared a group receiving PFMT with advice with a group with only advice, finding no statistical difference between the groups posttreatment and at 1-year follow-up. However, this study was executed by specialized nurses who were not pelvic physiotherapists. Moreover, the PFMT programme left doubts about adequacy of the dose–response relationship.

Bartlett et al. (2011) found no difference between BF either combined with a PFMT programme of prolonged submaximal pelvic floor muscle contractions or combined with the same contractions and quick repetitive maximal pelvic floor muscle contractions. Glazener et al. (2001) found that PFMT 3 months after delivery in women with UI did not significantly decrease the risk of AI at 1 year postpartum. At 6-year follow-up, AI rates were similar between the active PFMT group and the standard care group (Glazener et al., 2005). Four studies published since 2012 evaluated PFMT as the primary treatment (Glazener et al., 2014; Lin et al., 2015; Peirce et al., 2013; Ussing et al., 2019). Glazener et al. (2014) reported the long-term follow-up of the former study comparing PFMT to standard medical care. All 747 women included in this study had UI 3 months after vaginal delivery, and 15.7% of them also reported faecal incontinence (FI). PFMT had a significantly greater impact on FI than standard medical care at the 1-year follow-up but not at 12 years. Limitations of this study include that comparisons at 12 years are confounded by some patients undergoing additional treatments, especially if they had an inadequate response to the initial treatment, together with progression of underlying disease. Peirce et al. (2013) compared PFMT alone to PFMT supplemented by clinic-based BF in 120 women

TABLE 8.1.6 Characteristics of Included Randomized Controlled Trials

Author (Year)	Mean Age (Range)	Sample Size (F/M)	Study Population	Methods	Training Protocol	Outcome	Results (Between Group Analyses)
Bartlett et al. (2011)	62.1 (32–82)	72	Adults with AI after failure of conservative treatment	1. BF + PFMT (sustained exercises) + home exercises 2. BF + PFMT (sustained exercises + rapid exercises) + home exercises	1x/week over 4 weeks. Quick maximal contractions: repeated short and strong contractions, 1-s rest between contractions. Long-duration contractions: submax, 10-s rest between contractions	CRO: manometry, first sensation, first feeling of urge, rectal/anal sensation MTV PRO: FI questionnaire, Wexner, FIQL	PI, 2 years: NS PI, 2 years: NS
Bols et al. (2012)	1. 58.3 2. 60.2	80	Adults with moderate to severe AI after failing treatment of dietary measures and medication	1. PFMT + RBT + education 2. PFMT + education	2x/week for 3 weeks, then 1x/week for 6 weeks. PFMT: 1 cycle: 8–12 max contractions 1–3 s (expand to 6–8 s, from 1 to 3 series, and from 1 to 3 cycles); 1-min rest between cycles; 3 submax contractions 3 × 30 s. RBT: sensoric and coordination protocol	CRO: manometry, first sensation, first feeling of urge, rectal/anal sensation, Oxford EAS/PF, endurance EAS/PF, fatigue PF. MTV, fatigue EAS. PRO: GPE, FIQL subscale 'Lifestyle' Vaizey, remaining subscales FIQL	PI: NS PI: 1 better PI: 1 better PI: NS
Davis et al. (2004)	60.5	38	FI (liquid and solid stool over ≥12 min) and scheduled for sphincter repair	1. Sphincter repair 2 Sphincter repair + BF (manometry balloon) + PFMT at home	Start 3 min after surgery, 1x/week 30 min over 6 weeks (5 series max long-duration contractions 10 s, submax 5 s, and series quick contractions) PFMT at home: 2x/day	CRO: manometry PRO: VAS, FIQL, Wexner	PI: NS

Continued

TABLE 8.1.6 Characteristics of Included Randomized Controlled Trials—cont'd

Author (Year)	Mean Age (Range)	Sample Size (F/M)	Study Population	Methods	Training Protocol	Outcome	Results (Between Group Analyses)
Fynes et al. (1999)	32 (18-48)	40	AI after obstetric anal sphincter damage	1. Vaginal manometry BF (perineometer) + PFMT at home 2. Anal EMG-BF + ES + PFMT at home	1. 1x/week 30 min over 12 weeks (20 short max contractions of 6-8 s, 10-s rest + long-duration contractions 30 s) + PFMT at home (standard Kegel PFMT, instructions not reported) 2. 1x/week over 12 weeks (audiovisual EMG feedback + ES + PFMT at home (standard Kegel PFMT, instructions not reported)	CRO: manometry, vector symmetry index PRO: modified Pescatori scale	PI (12 weeks): 2 better PI (12 weeks): 2 better
Glazener et al. (2001)	1. 29.6 2. 29.4	747	Self-reported AI 3 months postnatal	1. Education + PFMT + visit nurse 2. Standard care	Advice PFMT at 5, 7 and 9 months postnatal (8-10 sessions daily 80-100 short- and long-duration contractions + bladder training in case indicated)	PRO: symptom questionnaire	12 months: 1 better AI 4% vs 10%
Glazener et al. (2005)	1. 29.6 2. 29.4	747	Self-reported AI 3 months postnatal	1. Education + PFMT + visit nurse 2. Standard care	Advice PFMT at 5, 7 and 9 months postnatal (8-10 sessions daily 80-100 short- and long-duration contractions + bladder training in case indicated)	PRO: symptom questionnaire	6 years: NS, AI 12% vs 13%
Healy et al. (2006)	1. 25 (41-68) 2. 23 (40-74)	58	AI without severe sphincter damage	1. Endoanal ES at home 2. ES + EMG-BF (supervised)	Treatment duration: 3 months 1. Daily 1 h with portable device; different frequencies 3, 10, 20, 30, 40 Hz 2. 30 min/week: (1) = alternated ES + EMG-BF supervised, 30 min/week; (2) = ES 2x 15 min: 15 min at 10 Hz and 15 min at 40 Hz, both without EMG	CRO: manometry, PNTML PRO: Wexner, RAND-36	PI: NS

Study	Age	N	Population	Intervention	Protocol	Outcome	Result
Heyman et al. (2000)	74 (36–88)	40	Patients not suitable for surgery	1. EMG-BF + education 2. EMG-BF + RBT (sensoric) 3. EMG-BF + EMG-BF at home 4. EMG-BF + RBT (sensoric) + EMG-BF at home	BF: 1x/week 1 h EMG at home: 5 sets/day (1 set = 20 cycles of 10-s contraction followed by 10-s rest)	PRO: incontinence episodes	PI: NS
Heyman et al. (2009)	59.6	108	Weekly FI after failure of education, medication and lifestyle changes	1. PFMT + manometry BF (coordination training + sensoric) 2. PFMT	1x/2 weeks 1 h over 12 weeks PFMT at home: 5x/day + during ADLs	CRO: squeeze pressure, first sensation PRO: FISI, subjective improvement diary FIQL, BDI, STAI-1, STAI-2	3 months: 1 better NS 3 months, 1 year: 1 better 3 months: 1 better NS
Ilnyckyj et al. (2005)	59 (26–75)	54	Chronic and weekly idiopathic FI	1. Education + PFMT 2. Education + PFMT + BF (manometry balloon)	3x/week over 1 week, followed by 2 weeks PFMT at home, then fourth treatment session (first, 45 min- second and through fourth, 30 min)	PRO: incontinence episodes	PI: NS
Mahony et al. (2004)	1. 35 (23–39) 2. 32 (22–42)	60	FI symptoms after obstetric traumas	1. Intra-anal EMG-BF + PFMT at home 2. Intra-anal EMG-BF + PFMT at home + ES	Over 12 weeks: intra-anal BF: 10 min of 3 quick max contractions in 5 s and 8-s rest, and long-duration contractions of 5 s and 8-s rest ES: 35 Hz, 20% ramp modulation. 20 min of 5-s stimulation and 8-s rest; intensity resulting in EAS contraction	CRO: manometry PRO: Wexner, FIQL	PI: NS PI: NS
Miner et al. (1990)	M: 17–64 F: 30–76	25	FI	Phase 1: 1. BF (sensoric) with feedback 2. BF (sensoric) without feedback Phase 2: crossover of strength and coordination training: analysis not possible	3 x 20 min over 3 days	CRO: rectal sensation manometry PRO: diary (number incontinence episodes, achieving continence)	PI: 1 better PI: NS PI: 1 better

Continued

TABLE 8.1.6   Characteristics of Included Randomized Controlled Trials—cont'd

Author (Year)	Mean Age (Range)	Sample Size (F/M)	Study Population	Methods	Training Protocol	Outcome	Results (Between Group Analyses)
Naimy et al. (2007)	36 (22–44)	49	AI after third/fourth-grade rupture	1. EMG-BF (anal electrode) 2. ES (anal electrode)	1. 2x instructional session 30 min; at home: 5 × 3 s, 10 s and submax as long as possible contractions 20 min, 2x/day over 8 weeks 2. 2x instructional session 30 min; at home: 30–40 Hz, <80 mAmp (max tolerance), 3-s stimulation, 3-s rest, 20 min, 2x/day over 8 weeks	PRO: Wexner, FIQL, RQL, VAS	PI: NS
Norton et al. (2003)	56 (26–85)	171	FI	1. Standard care (advice) 2. 1 + PFMT 3. 2 + clinical manometry BF 4. 3 + intra-anal EMG-BF at home	PFMT: 50 max sustained sphincter contractions + 50 fast-twitch contractions/day Manometry BF: sensoric, coordination and strength training protocol. 9 × 40–60-min sessions over 3–6 months	CRO: manometry PRO: subjective improvement (range, 0–11), diary, Vaizey, SF-36, HADS and disease-specific questionnaire	PI, 1 year: NS
Norton et al. (2006)	55 (30–77)	90	FI and on waiting list for BF	1. ES (35 Hz) 2. Placebo ES (1 Hz)	3 weeks, 20 min/day; weeks 4–8, 40 min/day	CRO: manometry PRO: subjective improvement VAS, diary, symptom questionnaire PRO: FIQL	PI: NS PI: NS
Osterberg et al. (2004)	F: 68 (52–80) M: 64 (43–81)	59	Idiopathic (neurogenic) AI, despite dietary advice	1. Levatorplasty 2. ES (anal electrode)	2–7 weeks (median, 4), 12 sessions 20 min; 25 Hz, duration 1.5 s, pulse-train interval 3 s, up to max tolerance	CRO: physiological variables PRO: Miller's incontinence score Physical and social limitations	3, 12, 24 months: NS 3 months: 1 better 3, 12, 24 months: 1 better

Study	N	Age	Population	Intervention	Dose	Outcomes	Results
Schwandner et al. (2010)	158	1. 62 2. 63.6	AI	3T (triple target regimen): amplitude-modulated middle-frequency ES (AM-MF) + EMG-BF EMG-BF	3T: 25 KHz + biphasic modulations of 40 Hz; 1 pulse = 5–8 s with pause of 10–15 s, ≥80–100 mA, 20 min, 2x/day over 9 months EMG-BF: 20 min, 2x/day over 9 months, contraction 3–8 s, pause 10–15 s	PRO: Vaizey, Wexner FIQL Park score Continence	9 months: 1 better 9 months: NS 9 months (PP): 1 better 9 months (PP): 1 better (50% vs 25.8%)
Solomon et al. (2003)	120	62	Self-reported mild to severe FI with at least mild neuropathy and no defect of EAS	1. PFMT + BF with anal manometry 2. PFMT + BF with transanal ultrasound 3. BBST + feedback using digital palpation	1x/month 30 min over 5 months PFMT at home: 10 sessions 10 x 5-s sphincter contractions	CRO: manometry, fatigue time, fatigue contractions PRO: Pescatori, St. Mark's Hospital FI score, VAS, questionnaire results of preset aims	PI: NS
Cohen-Zubary et al. (2015)	36	68 (61–75)	Chronic FI referred for pelvic floor disorders with intact anal sphincter	1. Standardized BF 2. Home ES	24) 1x/week 30–45 min over 6 weeks 2x/day 25 min over 6 weeks, 50 Hz, ramp-up/down time 1/1 s, 20-s off cycle, pulse width 200 ms; no additional PFME	CRO: muscle strength by intra-anal surface EMG, maximal contraction, $\delta\delta$ >4 ok PRO: VIS; VAS, HADS RESULTS: CRO: NS PRO: NS	
Bartlett et al. (2015)	75 (63/12)	61 (59–63)	FI not responding to conservative treatment	1. Standard PFMT + BF 2. Standard PFMT + BF with home BF (perineometer)	Start with 3–4 rapid squeezes and 2–3 sustained squeezes, lasting 3–4 s, practicing 6–10 sets daily up to 10 rapid squeezes + 6 x 10-s sustained squeezes for both anal and pelvic floor practiced 5x/day	CRO: perineometer; anorectal function PRO: exercise regimen, bowel charts/food diary; symptom severity and QoL, patient satisfaction	Results: younger (18/36) over older (7/23) participants had significant benefits using home BF (perineometer)

Continued

TABLE 8.1.6 **Characteristics of Included Randomized Controlled Trials—cont'd**

Author (Year)	Mean Age (Range)	Sample Size (F/M)	Study Population	Methods	Training Protocol	Outcome	Results (Between Group Analyses)
Damon et al. (2014)	60 (47–73)	157 (121/36) randomized but analysis per protocol in 142 who did not drop out	AI	1. Standard medical care + 20 sessions home BF 2. Standard medical care	1. 20 sessions 30 min home BF; BF training protocol developed by consensus physical therapists, 4 months, 4 (weeks 2–3 sessions/week, thereafter 1–2 sessions/week) 2. A tandard medical care only followed French national guidelines	CRO: manometry PRO: primary outcome self-rating of improvement (–5 to 5); secondary measures diary and questionnaires	Results: home BF significantly better compared to standard medical care only group (57% vs 37%); home BF self-reported very improved in 15 cases (22%), improved in 35 (52%), stable in 17 (25%), none worsened
Dehli et al. (2013)	57.5 (54–61)	126 (117/9)	Adults with FI, minimum severity of 4 on St Mark's scale; patients with any prior treatment for FI were excluded	1. BF 2. Intra-anal injection (dextranomer)	1. BF 5 days/week for 6 months at home using a portable device; BF patients met with physical therapist 5–6x and 28/62 received supplemental ES 2. Intra-anal injections of 4 mL of bulking agents repeated in 21/64 at 3 months	CRO: St Mark's score for incontinence (0–24) at 2 years after starting treatment PRO: FIQL, EQ-5D	Primary assessment at 6 months showed significant improvement in both groups but no between-group difference; also, no difference at 24 months; QoL also showed no between-group difference; more adverse events seen in the anal injection group, but most could be prevented with antibiotic prophy-

Study	Age	n	Population	Design	Intervention	Outcomes/Results
Glazener et al. (2014)	1. 29.6 2. 29.4	117	747 women with UI 3 months after vaginal delivery; 15.7% also reported FI at study initiation	Assess 12-year follow-up of study of Glazener et al. (2001, 2005) comparing brief PFMT to standard care for UI and FI	Nurses taught PFMT in 3 home visits 5, 7 and 9 months after delivery; controls received standard medical care; FU at 1, 6 and 12 years	PRO: symptom questionnaire Results: PRO: NS FI rate significantly lower after PFMT at 1 year (4% vs 11%) but not at 12 years (19% vs 15%); 52% still using PFMT after 12 years
Lin et al. (2015)	64 (27–79)	60	FI patients in Taiwan with rectal cancer	1. PFMT instructional DVD pamphlet 2. Pamphlet alone	PFMT taught just before hospital discharge; appropriate PFME performance confirmed by physical examination before discharge and at the first follow-up visit; PFMT patients were given the DVD to remind them how to perform PFMT and instructed to practice 20 squeezes 4x/day; weekly phone calls for the first month in both groups; FU at 1, 3, 6 and 9 months	PRO: CCI score Results: PRO: FI severity (CCI scale) decreased over time and significantly less in PFMT group vs controls at 1-, 3- and 6-month follow-up; no difference at 9 months
Peirce et al. (2013)	Not provided	120	Postpartum women with third-degree obstetric tears	1. Home EMG-BF 2. PFMT prior to discharge from hospital	PFMT taught in hospital before discharge from hospital Both groups told to practice 2x/day	CRO: anal canal resting and squeeze pressures PRO: CCI scale, QoL Results: CRO: NS PRO: NS

Continued

TABLE 8.1.6   **Characteristics of Included Randomized Controlled Trials—cont'd**

Author (Year)	Mean Age (Range)	Sample Size (F/M)	Study Population	Methods	Training Protocol	Outcome	Results (Between Group Analyses)
Schwandner et al. (2011)	63 (51–75)	80	Patients with FI of any severity including gas only	1. EMG-BF (3T) + ES 2. EMG-BF (3T) only	Two 20-min sessions/day for 6 months; for 3T group, morning BF session included alternating between ES and voluntary contraction, and afternoon session involved medium-frequency ES triggered by voluntary contractions above a threshold determined by ability; control group received low-frequency ES in both sessions each day	PRO: CCI scale, QoL Results: PRO: CCI scores higher in 3T vs low-frequency ES at 3 and 6 months; QoL was also significantly better in 3T group; 54% of 3T group continent at 6 months vs none in ES group; attrition rate was low in this trial (8% in 3T group vs 15% in ES group)	
Sjodahl et al. (2015)	60 (41–68)	64	≥1 episode FI in 2 weeks; excluded patients with any disease explanation for FI but allowed those with sphincter tears	1. EMG-BF 2. Loperamide 3. EMG-BF and loperamide	Crossover design: patients randomized to either BF or medical treatment in phase 1; second treatment added in phase 2; anorectal manometry tested at baseline and after each treatment phase	CRO: anal canal resting and squeeze pressures PRO: diary Results: CRO: anal resting and squeeze pressures did not change significantly in either study phase PRO: FI frequency no different between groups in phase 1 but decreased significantly for both groups following combined treatment	

| Ussing et al. (2019) | 62 (27–90) | 98 (89/9) | FI | 1. Supervised PFMT +BF + conservative treatment 2. Attention-control treatment + conservative treatment | 25) PFMT group received 6 individual treatments distributed over 16 weeks; each treatment lasted 45 min and consisted of individually supervised PFMT and home training program daily of 3 sets of 10 PFM contractions sustained for up to 10 s and 2 sets of 3 contractions sustained for up to 30 s; training diary The attention-control group had 6 individual treatments performed over 16 weeks; each treatment lasted 30 min of massage of neck and back; participants received no instructions on PFMT | CRO: secondary anal canal resting and squeeze pressures, rectal capacity PRO: primary PGI-I; secondary Vaizey score, FISI, FIQL, bowel diary Results: CRO: NS PRO: supervised PFMT + BF + conservative treatment superior effect (1) compared with (2) |

ADLs, Activities of daily living; AI, anal incontinence; BBST, XX; BDI, Beck Depression Inventory; BF, biofeedback; CCI, Cleveland Clinic Incontinence; CRO, clinician-reported outcome; EAS, external anal sphincter; EMG, electromyography; EMG-BF, electromyographic biofeedback using intra-anal electromyographic sensor/probe or perianal surface electromyography; EQ-5D, EuroQOL Health-Related Quality of Life; ES, electrical stimulation; F, female; FI, faecal incontinence; FIQL, Fecal Incontinence Quality of Life scale; FISI, Faecal Incontinence Severity Index; GPE, Global Perceived Effect; HADS, Hospital Anxiety and Depression Scale; M, male; max, maximum; MTV, maximal tolerable volume; NS, no significant difference; PF, pelvic floor; PFM, pelvic floor muscle; PFME, pelvic floor muscle exercise; PFMT, pelvic floor muscle training; PI, post-intervention; PNTML, pudendus nerve terminal motor latency; PP, per protocol; PRO, patient-reported outcome measures; QoL, quality of life; RBT, rectal balloon training; RQL, reduced Quality of Life scale; SF-36, 36-item Short Form Health Survey Questionnaire; STAI, Speilberger State-Trait Anxiety Inventory; UI, urinary incontinence; VAS, visual analogue scale; VIS, Vaizey incontinence score.

TABLE 8.1.7　PEDro Quality Score of Randomized Controlled Trials in Systematic Review

Study	E	1	2	3	4	5	6	7	8	9	10	Total Score
Bartlett et al. (2011)	Y	Y	Y	Y	Y	N	N	Y	N	Y	Y	7/10
Bols et al. (2012)	Y	Y	Y	Y	N	N	Y	Y	Y	Y	Y	8/10
Davis et al. (2004)	Y	Y	?	Y	N	N	Y	N	N	Y	Y	5/10
Fynes et al. (1999)	Y	Y	?	Y	N	N	Y	Y	N	Y	Y	6/10
Glazener et al. (2001)	Y	Y	Y	Y	N	N	Y	N	Y	Y	Y	7/10
Glazener et al. (2005)	Y	Y	Y	Y	N	N	?	N	N	Y	Y	5/10
Healy et al. (2006)	N	Y	?	N	N	N	?	N	N	Y	Y	3/10
Heymen et al. (2000)	N	Y	?	Y	N	N	?	Y	N	Y	Y	5/10
Heymen et al. (2009)	Y	Y	?	Y	N	N	?	Y	Y	Y	Y	6/10
Ilnyckyj et al. (2005)	Y	Y	?	?	N	N	?	N	N	Y	N	2/10
Mahony et al. (2004)	Y	Y	?	Y	N	N	Y	Y	N	Y	Y	6/10
Miner et al. (1990)	Y	Y	?	?	N	?	?	Y	Y	Y	Y	5/10
Naimy et al. (2007)	Y	Y	?	?	N	N	?	N	N	Y	Y	3/10
Norton et al. (2003)	Y	Y	Y	Y	N	N	Y	N	Y	Y	Y	7/10
Norton et al. (2006)	Y	Y	Y	Y	Y	N	Y	N	Y	Y	Y	8/10
Osterberg et al. (2004)	Y	Y	?	Y	N	N	?	Y	N	Y	Y	5/10
Schwandner et al. (2010)	Y	Y	Y	Y	N	Y	Y	N	Y	Y	Y	7/10
Solomon et al. (2003)	Y	Y	Y	Y	N	N	Y	Y	Y	Y	Y	8/10

Y, Criterion is clearly satisfied; N, criterion is not satisfied; ?, not clear if the criterion was satisfied.

The total score is determined by counting the number of criteria that are satisfied, except E (eligibility criteria specified) is not used to generate the total score. Total scores are out of 10.

E – Eligibility criteria specified

1 – Random allocation

2 – Allocation concealed

3 – Groups similar at baseline

4 – Patients blinded

5 – Therapists blinded

6 – Assessors blinded

7 – Measures of key outcomes obtained from >85% of subjects

8 – Intention to treat analysis

9 – Comparison between groups conducted

10 – Point estimates and measures of variability provided

Study	E	1	2	3	4	5	6	7	8	9	10	Total Score
Cohen-Zubary et al. (2015)	Y	Y	Y	Y	N	N	N	Y	N	Y	Y	6/10
Bartlett et al. (2015)	Y	Y	Y	?	N	N	Y	Y	Y	Y	Y	7/10
Damon et al. (2014)	Y	Y	Y	Y	N	N	Y	Y	N	Y	Y	7/10
Dehli et al. (2013)	Y	Y	Y	Y	N	N	Y	Y	N	Y	Y	7/10
Glazener et al. (2014)	Y	Y	Y	Y	N	N	?	N	N	Y	Y	5/10
Lin et al. (2015)	Y	Y	Y	Y	N	N	Y	Y	N	Y	Y	7/10
Peirce et al. (2013)	Y	Y	Y	Y	Y	N	N	N	Y	Y	Y	6/10
Schwandner et al. (2011)	Y	Y	Y	Y	N	N	Y	Y	Y	Y	Y	8/10
Sjodahl et al. (2015)	Y	Y	Y	Y	N	N	N	Y	N	Y	Y	6/10
Ussing et al. (2019)	Y	Y	Y	Y	N	N	Y	Y	Y	Y	Y	8/10

with a third-degree sphincter laceration during vaginal delivery to determine whether supplemental BF is more effective at preventing FI. No differences were seen, but the study was underpowered to detect a difference in incident cases of FI. Lin et al. (2016) evaluated whether PFMT combined with an instructional PFMT DVD as a reminder was more effective than no treatment in reducing FI following low anterior resection for cancer. This (very low dosage) PFMT, taught by a research assistant prior to discharge from the hospital, was associated with lower rates of FI at 1-, 3- and 6-month follow-up. An unanswered question remains whether PFMT taught by digital palpation of pelvic floor muscles rather than by verbal or printed instructions is as effective as BF augmented by PFMT, as some earlier studies suggested (Norton et al., 2003; Solomon et al., 2003).

In another RCT, Ussing et al. (2019) provided support for a superior effect of supervised PFMT in combination with conservative treatment compared with attention-control massage treatment, which consisted of six individual 30-minutes sessions of massage of the neck and back over 16 weeks and conservative treatment. They found that participants who received supervised PFMT had fivefold higher odds of reporting improvements in FI symptoms and had a larger mean reduction of incontinence severity based on the Vaizey score compared with attention-control massage treatment.

No definite statement was available in the latest ICI recommendations on the role of anal sphincter and pelvic floor muscle exercises as an intervention for AI patients (Bliss et al., 2016).

Currently, with the availability of additional evidence, PFMT and anal sphincter exercises might be recommended as part of an integral approach based on all treatable components, such as education/advice, awareness, BF and RBT (Bliss et al., 2016; Ussing et al., 2019). This recommendation is also based on the low costs and lack of side effects of this intervention.

Biofeedback

Success rates of physiotherapy in AI are generally based on numerous uncontrolled trials, mainly focusing on BF therapy. There are more than 60 uncontrolled trial reports in the literature on the use of BF for the management of AI (Norton and Cody, 2012). Some authors conclude that BF is the treatment of choice for AI on the basis of these observational studies (Enck et al., 1994) and controlled clinical trials (Enck et al., 1994;

Guillemot et al., 1995; Heymen et al., 2009). An overall cure and improvement rate of about 70% has been reported (Norton et al., 2003; Solomon et al., 2003).

With regard to controlled trials, some authors report on the hypothesis that BF together with another intervention is more effective than another intervention alone. Healy et al. (2006) found no statistical difference in effect of supervised electromyographic biofeedback using intra-anal electromyographic sensor/probe or perianal surface electromyography (EMG-BF) and endoanal ES in comparison with endoanal ES at home. Naimy et al. (2007) compared EMG-BF with ES (anal probe) in patients with AI after third/fourth-degree sphincter rupture. After treatment, there were no differences between the study groups. It should be noted that the intervention lasted no more than 2 months.

Heymen et al. (2009) concluded that manometric BF as add-on therapy to PFMT significantly improved squeeze pressure, FISI scores and subjective improvement post intervention compared to PFMT alone. Bols et al. (2010) compared PFMT alone against PFMT and RBT. Adding RBT significantly improved maximal tolerable volume, subjective improvement and the subscale 'Lifestyle' of the FIQL, although loss of power in this study should be taken into account.

Davis et al. (2004) compared anal sphincter repair with and without subsequent manometric BF and home-based PFMT commenced 3 months postoperatively in a small group of women with obstetric sphincter trauma over 6 weeks only. There were no statistically significant differences between both groups. Ilnyckyj et al. (2005) found no difference between a group with PFMT and manometric BF and a group with PFMT only. This intervention contained only four treatment sessions over 4 weeks.

Some authors studied whether one BF modality would be more effective than other BF modalities. Solomon et al. (2003) found no difference between groups using PFMT (feedback by digital palpation) combined with anal manometric BF or PFMT combined with transanal ultrasound BF. Heymen et al. (2000) found no difference between clinical EMG-BF, clinical EMG-BF with RBT, clinical EMG-BF with EMG-BF at home, and clinical EMG-BF with RBT and EMG-BF at home. Miner et al. (1990) compared a group with sensory BF with feedback and without feedback. The group with feedback significantly improved more regarding rectal sensation, incontinence episodes frequency and regaining continence.

There is little evidence as to which method of BF is superior due to the small study samples and the doubtful training intensity, especially in the two last-mentioned studies. Already in the year 2006, the results of a Cochrane review on the effects of BF and/or PFMT for the treatment of AI in adults, based on 21 RCTs, showed that some elements of BF therapy, like RBT and sphincter exercises, might have a therapeutic effect (Norton et al., 2006). However, a few years later, a meta-analysis by Enck et al. (2009) concluded that BF for AI was not different in efficacy from non-BF therapy, and no differences were observed comparing various modes of BF.

In the past decade, new evidence has been published comparing BF with standard medical care and home BF compared with other treatment modalities. Two RCTs followed a traditional design by comparing BF to standard medical care, defined as dietary counselling and use of antidiarrhoeal drugs or laxatives to normalize stool consistency. Damon et al. (2014) randomized patients to receive either standard medical care alone or standard medical care plus 20 sessions of BF, finding that significantly more of the BF-treated patients met the responder definition compared to the standard medical care only group. Sjodahl et al. (2015) used a crossover design in which patients were initially randomized to receive either standard medical care or three sessions of EMG-BF in phase 1 and the combination of standard medical care and BF in phase 2. There was no evidence of differential effects in phase 1, but the combined treatment was associated with significant improvement compared to baseline. Since most patients had tried standard medical care prior to the study and the BF training was less than is usually employed in phase 1, this study may also be seen as supporting the efficacy of BF.

The efficacy of home-based BF, which allows for more frequent BF training and reduces the amount of professional time required, was the focus of six studies (Bartlett et al., 2015; Damon et al., 2014; Dehli et al., 2013; Peirce et al., 2013; Schwandner et al., 2010; Schwandner et al., 2011). Two studies, in which 3T was provided twice daily for 6 to 9 months, both supported the efficacy of 3T (Schwandner et al., 2010; Schwandner et al., 2011). Dehli et al. (2013) compared intra-anal injections of a bulking agent to 6 months of twice-daily BF, finding that both treatments improved AI severity and quality of life with no significant difference between treatments. Damon et al. (2014) compared 4 months of home BF

to standard medical care and reported that significantly more patients in the BF group were responders. Bartlett et al. (2015) assessed whether the addition of home BF to clinic BF improved outcomes compared to clinic BF alone: for the whole group, supplementation with home BF did not significantly improve outcomes, but a post hoc analysis showed that the youngest half of the patients (below the median age of 61 years) did benefit significantly more when clinic-based BF was augmented by home BF. A study by Peirce et al. (2013) compared daily home BF to daily PFMT at 3 months postpartum to determine whether either treatment could prevent AI in women with a third-degree sphincter laceration sustained during childbirth. There was no evidence that home-based BF training prevented the development of AI, but the study was underpowered to show a difference in incident cases of AI.

The six studies of home BF described earlier suggest that home practice one to two times daily with a battery-operated BF device is more beneficial than either ES or BF in the clinic, or standard medical care. Home BF may also be less costly to provide. However, these studies also suggests that home BF has possible limitations: (1) longer periods of BF training may be required (at least 6 months according to one investigator); (2) on average, younger patients benefit more than older patients, so older patients profit less; and (3) daily practice is a burden which may increase the drop-out rate.

In summary, the use of BF as a treatment for AI is recommended after other behavioural and medical management have been tried and if inadequate symptom relief has been obtained. This recommendation is based on the numerous positive outcomes from (un)controlled trials, limitations in the current RCTs and low morbidity associated with its application (Bliss et al., 2016; Norton et al., 2010).

Electrical Stimulation

A second Cochrane review by Hosker et al. (2007) evaluated ES in adult patients with AI. Four eligible trials with 260 participants were identified. Findings from one trial suggested that ES with anal BF and exercises provides more short-term benefits than vaginal BF and exercises for women with obstetric-related AI (Fynes et al., 1999). Other studies found contradictory results, with no added benefit from ES over BF and exercises alone (Mahony et al., 2004; Naimy et al., 2007; Osterberg et al., 2004). Although all trials included in this

Cochrane review reported that patients' symptoms were generally improved, it was not clear that this was the effect of ES. No further conclusions could be drawn from the data available (Hosker et al., 2007). Norton et al. (2006) examined in an RCT whether anal ES, using an anal probe electrode in the absence of any adjunctive exercises or advice, would improve symptoms of AI and anal sphincter pressures when compared with 'sham' ES. Patients rated that their bowel control had improved to a modest extent. However, there was no statistically significant difference detected between the groups, suggesting that 1 Hz was as effective as 35 Hz. This raises the possibility that the main effect is not sphincter contraction but sensitization of the patient to the anal area, or simply the effect of intervening per se (Norton et al., 2006). This result is in agreement with Mahony et al. (2004), who concluded that the addition of ES did not enhance symptomatic outcome. Schwandner et al. (2010) compared amplitude-modulated middle-frequency ES as adjunct to EMG-BF and PFMT/anal sphincter training (3T) with EMG-BF and PFMT/anal sphincter training only. The 3T appeared superior on all outcome measures except for quality of life.

Schwandner et al. (2011) also evaluated the efficacy of a 3T protocol in which medium-frequency ES (3000 Hz, 500 µV) plus EMG-BF was compared to low-frequency ES (100 Hz, 50 µV) alone. The protocol for 3T is complex, in which patients are directed to practice during two 20-minute sessions each day at home. In the morning session, they received EMG-BF and alternately contracted their pelvic floor muscles voluntarily or stimulated contractions with medium-frequency ES. In the afternoon session, they received EMG-BF and were also provided with medium-frequency ES contingent on voluntary contractions that exceeded an individually determined threshold. The threshold required to trigger ES was progressively raised as performance improved in an effort to encourage stronger contractions. Triple therapy was provided by battery-operated devices at home. A minimum of 6 months of twice-daily sessions was required to improve AI. There were few drop-outs: 92% of the 3T group and 84% of the EMG-BF group completed the 6-month trial. The 3T group showed significant improvement by 3 months, whereas the low-frequency ES group showed no change from baseline at 3 or 6 months.

Two other studies tested low-frequency ES alone (Cohen-Zubary et al., 2015) or combined ES with BF (Dehli et al., 2013). The aim of the first study was to compare daily home ES to standard BF training in six weekly sessions provided in the clinic. There was no difference between these two treatments in overall improvements in AI, although there was a significant decrease in AI frequency from baseline to the end of treatment for the ES group. Home ES was less costly than BF provided in the clinic (Cohen-Zubary et al., 2015).

In the second study, ES was combined with BF but only in half of patients (28/62), and then only if, in the opinion of the investigators, ES was needed to 'help the patient identify and contract their sphincter'. There was no difference in AI severity or AI quality of life between the BF/ES group and the group receiving anal injections of dextranomer at the 6-month assessment (Dehli et al., 2013).

Overall, patients seem to benefit from physiotherapy interventions and results are promising (Norton et al., 2009). However, uncertainty exists on the effectiveness of physiotherapy interventions in AI, and therefore it needs to be further elucidated which intervention is superior, which (treatment) parameters provoke optimal results and which intervention is suitable for a particular patient.

PREDICTIVE FACTORS FOR SUCCESS OF PELVIC PHYSIOTHERAPY

Evaluation of predictive factors for success of pelvic physiotherapy is hindered by the heterogeneity of studies, especially regarding study population, type of interventions and intensity of therapy.

In general:
- An adequate training dose (train specific muscles, three times per day, two to three times per week during at least 5 months, 8–12 nearly maximal contractions) and adherence to therapy increases the likelihood of recovery (Bliss et al., 2016; Bø and Aschehoug, 2007).

BF with PFMT:
- Longer time since AI onset decreases the chance of recovery after BF with PFMT (Bols et al., 2012b).
- Experiencing minor embarrassment, the use of constipation medication and presence of at least one delivery-related risk factor (including high birth weight/episiotomy/instrumental delivery/prolonged second stage of labour/breech delivery) increase the chance of recovery after BF with PFMT (Bliss et al., 2016; Bols et al., 2012b).

- Necessity of more than three BF sessions is predictive for deterioration during follow-up (Ryn et al., 2000).

BF with PFMT and ES:

- Having passive AI, diarrhoea, primary repair of a rupture after vaginal delivery, and perineal and/or perianal scar tissue decreases the chance of recovery (Terra et al., 2008).

Electrical stimulation:

- Less severe FI symptoms and the loss of liquid stool instead of solid stool increases the chance of recovery after ES (Govaert et al., 2009; Osterberg et al., 1999).

REFERENCES

Abramov, Y., Sand, P. K., Botros, S. M., et al. (2005). Risk factors for female anal incontinence: New insight through the Evanston–Northwestern twin sisters study. *Obstetrics & Gynecology, 106*(4), 726–732

Bartlett, L., Sloots, K., Nowak, M., et al. (2011). Biofeedback for fecal incontinence: A randomized study comparing exercise regimens. *Diseases of the Colon & Rectum, 54*(7), 846–856.

Bartlett, L., Sloots, K., Nowak, M., Ho, Y. (2015). Supplementary home biofeedback improves quality of life in younger patients with fecal incontinence. *J Clin Gastroenterol, 49*, 419–428.

Berghmans, B. (2017). Pelvic floor muscle training: What is important? A mini-review. *International Journal of Gynecology & Obstetrics, 6*(4), 99.

Berghmans, B., Seleme, M. R., & Bernards, A. T. M. (2020). Physiotherapy assessment for female urinary incontinence. *International Urogynecology Journal, 31*(5), 917–931.

Berghmans, L. C., Groot, J. A. M., & van Heeswijk-Faase, I. (2015). Dutch evidence statement for pelvic physical therapy in patients with anal incontinence. *International Urogynecology Journal, 26*(4), 487–496.

Berghmans, L. C., Hendriks, H. J., Bø, K., et al. (1998). Conservative treatment of stress urinary incontinence in women: A systematic review of randomized clinical trials. *British Journal of Urology, 82*(2), 181–191.

Black, C. J., & Ford, A. C. (2018). Chronic idiopathic constipation in adults: Epidemiology, pathophysiology, diagnosis and clinical management. *Medical Journal of Australia, 209*(2), 86–91.

Bliss, D. Z., Mimura, T., Berghmans, B., et al. (2016). Assessment and conservative management of faecal incontinence and quality of life in adults. In P. Abrams, L. Cardozo, A. Wagg, et al. (Eds.), *Incontinence: Sixth international consultation on incontinence* (pp. 1993–2087). Bristol, UK: ICUD.

Bø, K., & Aschehoug, A. (2007). Strength training. In K. Bø, B. Berghmans, S. Mørkved, et al. (Eds.), *Evidence-based physical therapy for the pelvic floor* (pp. 119–132). London: Elsevier.

Bols, E., Berghmans, B., de Bie, R., et al. (2012). Rectal balloon training as add-on therapy to pelvic floor muscle training in adults with fecal incontinence: A randomized controlled trial. *Neurourology and Urodynamics, 31*(1), 132–138.

Bols, E., Hendriks, E., de Bie, R., et al. (2012). Predictors of a favorable outcome of physiotherapy in fecal incontinence: Secondary analysis of a randomized trial. *Neurourology and Urodynamics, 31*, 1156–1160.

Bols, E. M., Hendriks, E. J., Deutekom, M., et al. (2010). Inconclusive psychometric properties of the Vaizey score in fecally incontinent patients: A prospective cohort study. *Neurourology and Urodynamics, 29*(3), 370–377.

Borre, M., Qvist, N., Raahave, D., et al. (2015). [The effect of lifestyle modification on chronic constipation]. *Ugeskr Laeger, 177*(15), V09140498.

Cerulli, M. A., Nikoomanesh, P., & Schuster, M. M. (1979). Progress in biofeedback conditioning for fecal incontinence. *Gastroenterology, 76*(4), 742–746.

Chaliha, C., Kalia, V., Stanton, S. L., et al. (1999). Antenatal prediction of postpartum urinary and fecal incontinence. *Obstetrics & Gynecology, 94*(5), 689–694.

Cohen-Zubary, N., Gingold-Belfer, R., Lambort, I., et al. (2015). Home electrical stimulation for women with fecal incontinence: a preliminary randomized controlled trial. *Int J Colorectal Dis, 30*, 521–Õ28.

Damon, H., Siproudhis, L., Faucheron, J., et al. (2014). Perineal retraining improves conservative treatment for faecal incontinence: A multicentre randomized study. *Digestive and Liver Disease, 46*(3), 237–242.

Davis, K. J., Kumar, D., & Poloniecki, J. (2004). Adjuvant biofeedback following anal sphincter repair: A randomized study. *Alimentary Pharmacology & Therapeutics, 20*(5), 539–549.

Dehli, T., Stordahl, A., Vatten, L. J., et al. (2013). Sphincter training or anal injections of dextranomer for treatment of anal incontinence: A randomized trial. *Scand J Gastroenterol, 48*, 302–310.

Enck, P., Daublin, G., Lubke, H. J., et al. (1994). Long-term efficacy of biofeedback training for fecal incontinence. *Diseases of the Colon & Rectum, 37*(10), 997–1001.

Enck, P., Van der Voort, I. R., & Klosterhalfen, S. (2009). Biofeedback therapy in fecal incontinence and constipation. *Neuro-Gastroenterology and Motility, 21*, 1133–1141.

Engel, B. T., Nikoomanesh, P., & Schuster, M. M. (1974). Operant conditioning of rectosphincteric responses in the treatment of fecal incontinence. *New England Journal of Medicine, 290*, 646–649.

Fynes, M., Marshall, K., Cassidy, M., et al. (1999). A prospective, randomized study comparing the effect of augmented biofeedback with sensory biofeedback alone on fecal incontinence after obstetric trauma. *Invited Editorial—the authors' reply. Dis. Colon Rectum, 42*(6), 760–761.

Glazener, C., Herbison, G., MacArthur, C., et al. (2005). Randomised controlled trial of conservative management of postnatal urinary and faecal incontinence: Six year follow up. *British Medical Journal, 330*, 337.

Glazener, C., Herbison, G., Wilson, P., et al. (2001). Conservative management of persistent postnatal urinary and faecal incontinence: Randomised controlled trial. *British Medical Journal, 323*, 593–596.

Glazener, C., MacArthur, C., Hagen, S., et al. (2014). Twelve-year follow-up of conservative management of postnatal urinary and faecal incontinence and prolapse outcomes: Randomised controlled trial. *BJOG, 121*, 112–120.

Govaert, B., Melenhorst, J., Nieman, F. H. M., et al. (2009). Factors associated with percutaneous nerve evaluation and permanent sacral nerve modulation outcome in patients with fecal incontinence. *Diseases of the Colon & Rectum, 52*, 1688–1694.

Guillemot, F., Bouche, B., Gower-Rousseau, C., et al. (1995). Biofeedback for the treatment of fecal incontinence. Long-term clinical results. *Diseases of the Colon & Rectum, 38*(4), 393–397.

Haskell, B., & Rovner, H. (1967). Electromyography in the management of the incompetent anal sphincter. *Diseases of the Colon & Rectum, 10*(2), 81–84.

Hay-Smith, J., Berghmans, B., Burgio, K., et al. (2009). Committee 12: Adult conservative management. In P. Abrams, L. Cardozo, S. Khoury, et al. (Eds.), *Incontinence: Fourth international consultation on incontinence* (pp. 1025–1120). Paris: Health Publication/Editions 21.

Healy, C. F., Brannigan, A. E., Connolly, E. M., et al. (2006). The effects of low-frequency endo-anal electrical stimulation on faecal incontinence: A prospective study. *International Journal of Colorectal Disease, 21*(8), 802–806.

Heyman, S., Jones, K. R., Ringel, Y., et al. (2001). Biofeedback for fecal incontinence and constipation: The role of medical management and education. *Gastroenterology, 120*(Suppl. 1), A397.

Heyman, S., Pikarsky, A., Weiss, E., et al. (2000). A prospective randomized trial comparing four biofeedback techniques for patients with fecal incontinence. *Colorectal Disease, 2*, 88–92.

Heyman, S., Scarlett, Y., Jones, K., et al. (2009). Randomized controlled trial shows biofeedback to be superior to pelvic floor exercises for fecal incontinence. *Diseases of the Colon & Rectum, 52*(10), 1730–1737.

Horrocks, E., Thin, N., Thaha, M., et al. (2014). Systematic review of tibial nerve stimulation to treat faecal incontinence. *British Journal of Surgery, 101*, 457–468.

Hosker, G., Cody, J. D., & Norton, C. C. (2007). Electrical stimulation for faecal incontinence in adults. *Cochrane Database of Systematic Reviews* (Issue 3) Art. No. CD001310.

Hudlicka, O., Dodd, L., Renkin, E. M., et al. (1982). Early changes in fiber profile and capillary density in long-term stimulated muscles. *American Journal of Physiology, 243*, 528–535.

Ilnyckyj, A., Fachnie, E., & Tougas, G. (2005). A randomized-controlled trial comparing an educational intervention alone vs education and biofeedback in the management of faecal incontinence in women. *Neuro-Gastroenterology and Motility, 17*(1), 58–63.

Jorge, J. M., & Wexner, S. D. (1993). Etiology and management of fecal incontinence. *Diseases of the Colon & Rectum, 36*(1), 77–97.

Kuijpers, H. (1997). In Wielrennen (Ed.), *Training in de praktijk* (pp. 60–80). Haarlem: De Vrieseborch.

Latimer, P. R., Campbell, D., Kasperski, J. (1984). A components analysis of biofeedback in the treatment of fecal incontinence. *Biofeedback Self Regul, 9*(3), 311–324.

Laycock, J., & Jerwood, D. (2001). Pelvic floor assessment: The PERFECT scheme. *Physiotherapy, 87*(12), 631–642.

Laycock, J., Plevnik, S., & Senn, E. (1994). Electrical stimulation. In B. Schüssler (Ed.), *Pelvic floor Re-education: Principles and practice* (pp. 143–153). London: Springer-Verlag.

Lin, Y., Yang, H., Hung, S., et al. (2015). Effects of pelvic floor muscle exercise on faecal incontinence in rectal cancer patients after stoma closure. *Eur J Cancer Care*, 449–457.

Loening-Baucke, V. (1990). Efficacy of biofeedback training in improving faecal incontinence and anorectal physiologic function. *Gut, 31*(12), 1395–1402.

Lucas, M., Emery, S., & Beynon, J. (1999). *Incontinence*. Oxford: Blackwell Scientific.

MacLeod, J. H. (1983). Biofeedback in the management of partial anal incontinence. *Diseases of the Colon & Rectum, 26*(4), 244–246.

Madoff, R. D., Parker, S. C., Varma, M. G., et al. (2004). Faecal incontinence in adults. *Lancet, 364*(9434), 621–632.

Mahony, R. T., Malone, P. A., Nalty, J., et al. (2004). Randomized clinical trial of intra-anal electromyographic biofeedback physiotherapy with intra-anal electromyographic biofeedback augmented with electrical stimulation of the anal sphincter in the early treatment of postpartum fecal incontinence. *American Journal of Obstetrics and Gynecology, 191*(3), 885–890.

Markland, A. D., Goode, P. S., Burgio, K. L., et al. (2010). Incidence and risk factors for fecal incontinence in black and white older adults: A population-based study. *Journal of the American Geriatrics Society, 58*(7), 1341–1346.

Miner, P. B., Donelly, T. C., Read, N. W. (1990). Investigation of mode of action of biofeedback in treatment of fecal Incontinence. *Dig Dis Sci, 35*(10), 1291–1298.

Naimy, N., Lindam, A. T., Bakka, A., et al. (2007). Biofeedback vs. electrostimulation in the treatment of postdelivery anal incontinence: A randomized, clinical trial. *Diseases of the Colon & Rectum, 50,* 2040–2046.

Newman, D. K., & Giovannini, D. (2002). The overactive bladder: A nursing perspective. *American Journal of Nursing, 102*(6), 36–45. quiz 46.

Norton, C. (2004). Nurses, bowel continence, stigma and taboos. *Journal of Wound Ostomy & Continence Nursing, 31*(2), 85–94.

Norton, C., & Chelvanayagam, S. (2004). *Bowel continence nursing.* Beaconsfield: Beaconsfield Publishers.

Norton, C., Chelvanayagam, S., Wilson-Barnett, J., et al. (2003). Randomized controlled trial of biofeedback for fecal incontinence. *Gastroenterology, 125,* 1320–1329.

Norton, C., & Cody, J. D. (2012). Biofeedback and/or sphincter exercises for the treatment of faecal incontinence in adults. *Cochrane Database of Systematic Reviews* (Issue 7) Art. No. CD002111.

Norton, C., Gibbs, A., & Kamm, M. A. (2006). Randomized, controlled trial of anal electrical stimulation for fecal incontinence. *Diseases of the Colon & Rectum, 49*(2), 190–196.

Norton, C., & Kamm, M. A. (2001). Anal sphincter biofeedback and pelvic floor exercises for faecal incontinence in adults—a systematic review. *Alimentary Pharmacology & Therapeutics, 15*(8), 1147–1154.

Norton, C., Thomas, L., & Hill, J. (2007). Management of faecal incontinence in adults: Summary of NICE guidance. *British Medical Journal, 334,* 1370–1371.

Norton, C., Whitehead, W. E., Bliss, D. Z., et al. (2009). Conservative and pharmacological management of faecal incontinence in adults. In P. Abrams, L. Cardozo, S. Khoury, et al. (Eds.), *Incontinence: Fourth international consultation on incontinence* (pp. 1321–1386). Paris: Health Publications/Editions 21.

Norton, C., Whitehead, W. E., Bliss, D. Z., et al. (2010). Management of fecal incontinence in adults. *Neurourology and Urodynamics, 29*(1), 199–206.

Ostbye, T., Seim, A., Krause, K. M., et al. (2004). A 10-year follow-up of urinary and fecal incontinence among the oldest old in the community: The Canadian study of health and aging. *Canadian Journal on Aging, 23*(4), 319–331.

Osterberg, A., Edebol Eeg-Olofsson, K., Hallden, M., et al. (2004). Randomized clinical trial comparing conservative and surgical treatment of neurogenic faecal incontinence. *British Journal of Surgery, 91*(9), 1131–1137.

Osterberg, A., Graf, W., Eeg-Olofsson, K., et al. (1999). Is electrostimulation of the pelvic floor an effective treatment for neurogenic faecal incontinence? *Scandinavian Journal of Gastroenterology, 34*(3), 319–324.

Peirce, C., Murphy, C., Fitzpatrick, M., et al. (2013). Randomised controlled trial comparing early home biofeedback physiotherapy with pelvic floor exercises for the treatment of third-degree tears (EBAPT Trial). *Br J Obstet Gynaecol, 120,* 1240–1247.

Rausch, T., Beglinger, C., Alam, N., et al. (1998). Effect of transdermal application of nicotine on colonic transit in healthy nonsmoking volunteers. *Neuro-Gastroenterology and Motility, 10,* 263–270.

Ryn, A.-K., Morren, G. I., Hallbook, O., et al. (2000). Long-term results of electromyographic biofeedback training for faecal incontinence. *Diseases of the Colon & Rectum, 43,* 1262–1266.

Salmons, S., & Vrbova, G. (1969). The influence of activity on some contractile characteristics of mammalian fast and slow muscles. *The Journal of Physiology, 201*(3), 535–549.

Schüssler, B., Laycock, J., Norton, P., et al. (1994). *Pelvic floor Re-education: Principles and practice.* Berlin: Springer-Verlag.

Schwandner, T., Hemmelmann, C., Heimerl, T., et al. (2011). Triple target treatment versus low-frequency electro-stimulation for anal incontinence. *Dtsch Arztebl Int, 108,* 653–660.

Schwandner, T., Konig, I. R., Heimerl, T., et al. (2010). Triple target treatment (3T) is more effective than biofeedback alone for anal incontinence: The 3T-AI study. *Diseases of the Colon & Rectum, 53*(7), 1007–1016.

Sjodahl, J., Walter, S. A., Johansson, E., Ingemansson, A., Ryn, A. K., Hallbook, O. (2015). Combination therapy with biofeedback, loperamide, and stoolbulking agents is effective for the treatment of fecal incontinence in women: A randomized controlled trial. *Scand J Gastroenterol, 50,* 965–974.

Solomon, M. J., Pager, C. K., Rex, J., et al. (2003). Randomized, controlled trial of biofeedback with anal manometry, transanal ultrasound, or pelvic floor retraining with digital guidance alone in the treatment of mild to moderate fecal incontinence. *Diseases of the Colon & Rectum, 46*(6), 703–710.

Terra, M. P., Deutekom, M., Dobben, A. C., et al. (2008). Can the outcome of pelvic floor rehabilitation in patients with fecal incontinence be predicted? *International Journal of Colorectal Disease, 23*(5), 503–511.

Ussing, A., Dahn, I., Due, U., Sørensen, M., Petersen, J., Bandholm, T. (2019). Efficacy of supervised pelvic floor muscle training and biofeedback vs attention-control treatment in adults with fecal incontinence. *Clinical Gastroenterology and Hepatology, 17,* 2253–2261.

8.2 Constipation: Prevalence, Causes and Pathophysiology

Giulio A Santoro, Patrizia Pelizzo, Esther Bols, Abdul H Sultan and Bary Berghmans

INTRODUCTION AND DEFINITION

Constipation is described as a common disease determined by difficult and/or rare passage of stool related to infrequent bowel movements, excessive straining, a sense of incomplete evacuation, failed or lengthy attempts to defaecate, use of digital manoeuvres for evacuation of stools, abdominal bloating and hard consistency of stools. The difference in the definition of constipation has led to a wide range of reported prevalence (ranging between 1% and 80%) (Forootan et al., 2018).

Constipation is a concept that has subjective and objective definitions. Subjectively, it is related to the feeling of inadequate or insufficient defaecation despite the possible nonconstipated bowel. Objectively, it was defined with Rome criteria in 1988. According to the updated Rome IV criteria, functional constipation is defined as the presence of two or more of the following criteria during the previous 3 months (Table 8.2.1): straining with more than 25% of defaecations, Bristol stool form types 1 and 2 for more than 25% of defaecations, sensation of incomplete evacuation for more than 25% of defaecations, sensation of anorectal obstruction or blockage for more than 25% of defaecations, manual manoeuvers to facilitate more than 25% of defaecations (e.g., digital manipulation) or less than three spontaneous bowel movements per week. The differential diagnosis is based on the absence of diarrhoea (except after laxative therapy) and the nonapplicability of the irritable bowel syndrome (IBS) criteria; symptoms must be present for at least 6 months before the diagnosis (Peppas et al., 2008; Simren et al., 2017) (Table 8.2.2).

EPIDEMIOLOGY

There is a huge variation in the literature regarding the prevalence of constipation, ranging from 2% to 30% Santoro et al. (2021). It depends on the population

TABLE 8.2.1   Rome IV Criteria for Functional Constipation

1	Straining to evacuate	>25% of defaecations
	Lumpy or hard stools	>25% of defaecations
	Sensation of incomplete evacuation	>25% of defaecations
	Sensation of anorectal obstruction/blockage	>25% of defaecations
	Manual manoeuvers to facilitate defaecations	>25% of defaecations
	<3 evacuations per week	Yes
2	Diarrhoea must not be present except after using a laxative	
3	Insufficient criteria for irritable bowel syndrome	

Note: Symptoms must be present ≥6 months before the diagnosis.

TABLE 8.2.2   Defaecatory and Post-Defaecatory Symptoms of Constipation

Feeling of incomplete bowel evacuation	Complaint that the rectum does not feel empty after defaecation and may be accompanied by a desire to defaecate again
Straining to defaecate	Complaint of the need to make an intensive effort (by abdominal straining or Valsalva) to either initiate, maintain or improve defaecation
Sensation of blockage	Complaint suggestive of anorectal obstruction
Digitation	Complaint of the need to make an intensive effort (by abdominal straining or Valsalva) to either initiate, maintain or improve defaecation Vaginal digitation: use of thumb or fingers in the vagina to assist in evacuation of stool
Splinting	Support perineum or buttocks manually (usually with thumb or fingers) to assist in evacuation of stool content
Post-defaecatory soiling	Soiling occurring after defaecation

studied and the diagnostic criteria used. A review by Peppas et al. (2008) reported that in Europe, constipation ranged widely from a low of 0.7% to a high of 81% (mean value of the reported constipation rates was 17.1%, and the median value was 16.6%). In Oceania (Australia and New Zealand), the mean value of constipation prevalence was 15.3%. A review from Black et al. (2018) confirmed that chronic idiopathic constipation (CIC) has a global prevalence of 14% and is one of the most common gastrointestinal disorders. Higgins and Johanson (2004) reported that constipation touches and compromises the quality of life of about 63 million people in the United States alone, between 2% and 27% of North Americans. Worldwide, this condition has socioeconomic issues in terms of healthcare (the constipation-related emergency department visits gained more than $1.5 billion in 2011, and purchasing of laxatives in the United States was more than $1 billion). These data are assumed using Rome II criteria for constipation (Ribas et al., 2011). The impact of constipation on quality of life is comparable in all countries. Constipated women reported more impaired quality of life than constipated men (Gudipally and Sharma, 2022), and constipation was often correlated with premenstrual syndrome (up to 48% of women of childbearing potential) (Poddar, 2016). Overall, the prevalence rates are lower in studies using the more stringent Rome criteria compared to studies based on self-reporting of constipation.

Childhood constipation is common, with a prevalence of 3% to 30% worldwide (Poddar, 2016). The majority (95%) of children with constipation have functional impairment related to behavioural withholding after an unpleasant stool event (Poddar, 2016). Males have a lower risk than females of developing severe constipation.

Ribas et al. (2011) evaluated 600 healthy young women and found that almost 29% met the Rome II criteria for constipation. Sandler et al. (1990) described that 12.8% of constipation events are self-reported. This study is poorly correlated with stool frequency. A total of 9% of subjects with daily evacuation and 30.6% with four to six bowel movements per week complained of symptoms of constipation. Constipation is more frequent in blacks (17.3%), women (18.2%) and those older than 60 years (23.3%) (Suares and Ford, 2011); after adjusting for age, sex and race, it is more prevalent in subjects with daily inactivity, little leisure exercise, low income and poor education. Constipation is

related to lower consumption of cheese, dry beans and peas, milk, meat and poultry, beverages (sweetened, carbonated and noncarbonated), and fruits and vegetables and higher consumption of coffee or tea (Sandler et al., 1990). Palsson et al. (2020) analysed the prevalence values of census-adjusted Rome IV faecal bowel diseases (FBDs) in the United States, Canada and the UK. These values were similar among the three countries, ranging from 4.4% to 4.8% for IBS, 7.9% to 8.6% for functional constipation, 3.6% to 5.3% for functional diarrhoea, 2% to 3.9% for functional bloating or distention, 1.1% to 1.9% for opioid-induced constipation, 7.5% to 10% for unspecified FBDs and 28.6% to 31.7% for any Rome IV FBD. Nellesen et al. (2013) found that patients with IBS-C (IBS with constipation) or CIC frequently experienced a wide range of comorbidities that contributed to their disease burden. Thus, it is advisable that medical professionals consider common comorbidities when diagnosing and treating patients with IBS-C or CIC. The total constipation prevalence worldwide (Suares and Ford, 2011) and the prevalence of most common bowel disorders in the United States, Canada and UK are shown in Figs. 8.2.1 and 8.2.2.

ANATOMY AND PATHOPHYSIOLOGY

The anal canal is about 4 cm in length and it is in continuous with the rectum at the anorectal junction. The puborectalis (PR) muscle surrounds the junction posteriorly, forming the anorectal angle (ARA), varying between 90 and 110 degrees at rest. At the anal canal level, muscularis propria of the gastrointestinal tract thickens and becomes the internal anal sphincter. The external anal sphincter is a somatic muscle continuous with the PR muscle posteriorly and the levator ani. The dentate line (which is a 'watershed area' and is the exact transition of epithelium to neurovascular supply) separates the anal canal into an upper and lower part, not only in structure but also for the neurovascular supply (reflecting the differing embryological origin). The dentate line is formed by the anal columns, which consists of a series of anal sinuses (which drain the anal glands) at approximately the midpoint of the anal canal. Above the dentate line, the epithelium is a mucous membrane like the rest of the gastrointestinal tract; below the dentate line, the epithelium is considered cutaneous (i.e., stratified squamous keratinized with hair and sebaceous glands). The internal anal sphincter and the mucosa

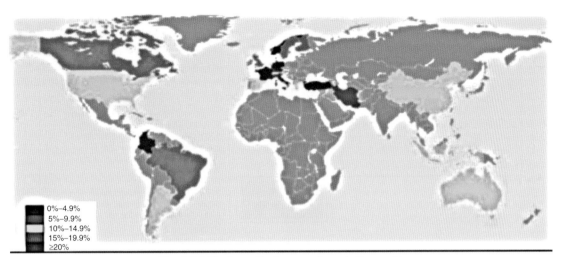

Fig. 8.2.1 Total constipation prevalence in the world.

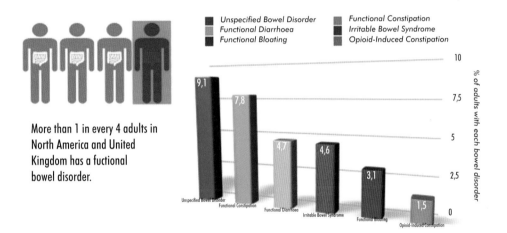

Fig. 8.2.2 Prevalence of functional bowel disorders among adults in the United States, Canada and the UK.

above the dentate line are innervated by sympathetic nerves, which are part of the pelvic plexus, whereas parasympathetic nerves and afferent sensory nerves derive from the pelvic splanchnic nerves. The external anal sphincter and the anal canal below the dentate line are innervated by the inferior rectal branches of the pudendal nerve (McMinn, 2003; Rosse and Gaddum-Rosse, 1997).

Normal Colonic Pathophysiology

The normal defaecatory process is quite complex, and it includes faecal dehydration, absorption of electrolytes, faecal storage, propagation and eventually coordinated

evacuation. Complex sensory and motor functions of the colon, rectum and pelvic floor musculature are involved. Any disturbance in this process might cause constipation.

Motility

The main mechanisms of propulsive motility of faeces are both peristalsis and mass movements, which occur a few times each day, until ending with defaecation (Holdstock et al., 1970). Mass movements become high-amplitude propagating contractions when they are joined to the primary motor pattern. They arise from the inhibition of distal haustral segments and

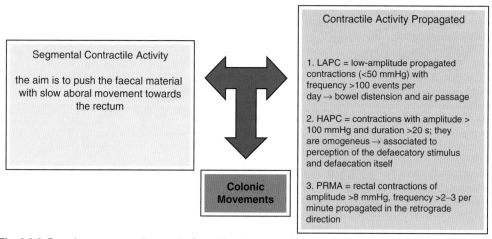

Fig. 8.2.3 Bowel movements: the result of combined segmental contractile activity and propagated contractile activity.

contractions of the proximal bowel wall (Smith et al., 2014). Even if the underlying neurophysiological mechanism is still misunderstood, high-amplitude propagating contractions arise from the contraction of colonic smooth muscle. Peristalsis is also stimulated by neuromodulator, a hormone (synthesized and released by enterochromaffin cells) (Spencer, 2015), serotonin or 5-hydroxytryptamine (5-HT), which, through the myenteric nerve plexus, is involved in the propagation of a wave of intestinal smooth muscle contraction and the propelling of luminal contents. The process is mediated by the cells of Cajal which act as a pacemaker (Radenkovic et al., 2018). On the other side, the colonic contents move in a retrograde direction. This happens moreover after a meal and potentially provides a 'brake' to prevent rapid rectal filling (Lin et al., 2017). The gastrocolic reflex increases the postprandial colonic movements (Fig. 8.2.3).

Fluid and Electrolytes

Abundant hydration has a key role for a good daily faecal routine. The pathophysiological mechanism is related with the preponderant role of the colon in managing intestinal fluid and electrolyte content. This contributes to the aetiology of chronic constipation and is relevant to pharmacological treatment. The colon reabsorbs approximately 1 to 2 L of fluid per day (Sandle, 1998). Prosecretory drugs can increase intestinal luminal fluid and electrolyte content sufficiently to saturate this process, thereby altering stool consistency and reducing colonic

transit time (Thomas and Luthin, 2015). Alternatively, osmotic laxatives increase luminal water content by creating an osmotic gradient across the intestinal epithelium, with similar effects (Krogh et al., 2017). The diet of constipated patients is characterized by a lot of processed grains, a low amount of fibre, inadequate intake of fluids and reduced physical activity. The recommended intake is 30 to 40 g per day of dietary fibre, with a hydration goal of more than 2 L of liquids daily. Dietary fibre counteracts constipation in several mechanisms: fibre increases stool bulk, allowing adequate colonic distension and more effective peristalsis and propulsion of stool; fibre fermentation generates short-chain fatty acids that increase the intraluminal osmotic pressure and aid stool propulsion; fibre absorbs water, which improves stool consistency; and fibre promotes bowel function, contributing to selection of the microbiome (Borre et al., 2015).

AETIOLOGY AND RISK FACTORS

The aetiology of constipation can be categorized into primary or secondary constipation.

Primary Constipation

CIC or primary constipation can be classified into constipation related to IBS-C, slow-transit constipation or constipation associated with obstructed defaecation syndrome (ODS). Other secondary causes of constipation must be excluded before the diagnosis (Yurtdas et al., 2020).

Normal Transit Constipation and Irritable Bowel Syndrome

This condition represents the most frequent type of CIC (up to 70% of cases). Problems associated with bowel habit affect 7% to 21% of the general population (Smith et al., 2014) and are often related to important stress conditions. Patients do not have abnormalities in bowel transit or pelvic floor dysfunctions.

Smith et al. (2014) reported that IBS may have the following pathophysiological mechanisms: genetic factors, abnormalities in serotonin metabolism (neurohormonal up-regulation) and alterations in brain function which could be primary or secondary factors, increased abnormal colonic motility or transit, intestinal or colorectal sensation, increased colonic bile acid concentration and superficial colonic mucosal inflammation, as well as epithelial barrier dysfunction and activation of secretory processes in the epithelial layer. IBS-related constipation can cause abdominal pain and discomfort, but it can also be associated with diarrhoea (Holtmann et al., 2016). This diagnosis is typically made by exclusion of secondary causes. Fig. 8.2.4 shows the worldwide prevalence of IBS (Lovell and Ford, 2012).

Slow Transit Constipation

The disorders of bowel motility are confirmed by radiologic evidence of increased colonic transit time (typically the markers are scattered throughout the colon). Slow transit constipation is characterized by neurodegeneration of myenteric plexus ganglia and a reduced number of the intestinal pacemaker cells of Cajal, reduced cholinergic response and accelerated adrenergic response, as well as abnormal levels of enteric neurotransmitters such as pancreatic polypeptide, peptide YY, neuropeptide Y, serotonin, vasoactive intestinal peptide, substance P and cholecystokinin. This produces an abnormal gastrocolic reflex. Indeed, the pelvic floor function is typically normal. Symptoms of this condition are a reduced urge to defaecate, and patients typically do not complain of rectal fullness, nausea and bloating (Frattini and Nogueras, 2008).

Obstructed Defaecation With Constipation

ODS is characterized by excessive straining at stool, incomplete rectal evacuation and the need for perineal splinting. This condition contributes to approximately 7% to 15% of all causes of constipation (D'Hoore and Penninckx, 2003). ODS is refractory to laxative use. Typically, the block is found in the rectosigmoid portion. The main causes are divided into mechanical and functional.

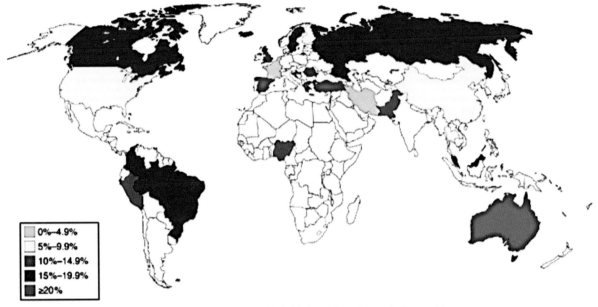

Legend:
- 0%–4.9%
- 5%–9.9%
- 10%–14.9%
- 15%–19.9%
- ≥20%

Fig. 8.2.4 Prevalence of irritable bowel syndrome in the world.

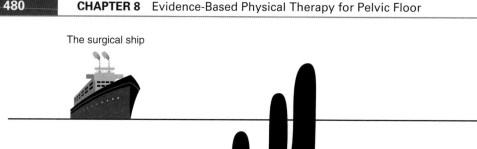

Fig. 8.2.5 The Iceberg diagram of obstructed defaecation syndrome. (Illustrator: Mario Pescatori) *IBS*, Irritable bowel syndrome.

Mechanical causes interfere with stool passage: colorectal cancer, extraintestinal masses, post-diverticulitis stenosis, post-ischemic stenosis, post-anastomosis stenosis, rectocele and rectal prolapse. Functional causes include various neurological or behavioral disorders, leading to pelvic floor dysfunction, discoordination of the defaecatory process and impaired rectal sensation. In dyssynergic defaecation, which affects up to one-half of patients with chronic constipation, there is an inability to coordinate the abdominal and pelvic floor muscles to evacuate stools. Paradoxical contraction of the pelvic floor muscles during defaecation hinders evacuation (Rao et al., 2016; Steele and Mellgren, 2007). ODS is characterized by a persistent sensation of rectal fullness and painful, prolonged defaecation or excessive straining, accompanied by a sensation of incomplete evacuation and clustering, often, digital manipulation.

Haemorrhoids and fissures are also related to functional ODS due to the psychological condition to avoid pain during defaecation.

A holistic approach is needed for patients with ODS, considering that most of them present with psychological distress, either anxiety or depression. Anismus, described as the absence of relaxation or paradoxical contraction during defaecation, plays a relevant role in ODS. It may affect nearly half of ODS patients (Pescatori, 2019; Rao et al., 2016) (Fig. 8.2.5).

Secondary Constipation

Secondary constipation includes both extraintestinal constipation and lifestyle-related factors. It can be due to systemic causes (endocrine and metabolic disorders like diabetes mellitus, hypothyroidism, hypercalcemia, chronic renal injury, pregnancy and other electrolyte imbalances), neurologic disorders (spinal cord injury, Parkinson's disease, multiple sclerosis), psychological issues (depression, anxiety, anorexia nervosa), connective tissue disease (scleroderma, amyloidosis) and pharmacological causes (opiates, anticholinergics, antidepressants, iron supplementation, etc.) (Rao et al., 2016; Wald et al., 2007).

OTHER AETIOLOGICAL FACTORS

There is no reliable evidence to support a genetic predisposition to constipation. Insufficient physical activity, decreasing fibre and water intake, obesity, advancing age and female gender are associated with increased constipation risks. Combining regular physical activity and increasing fibre and water intake may protect from constipation and relieve constipation symptoms (Sultan et al., 2017).

Borre et al. (2015) reported that daily intake of 2 L of water and adequate intake of fibre had positive effects on constipation. Moreover, at least 30 minutes per day of aerobic exercise also alleviated symptoms and increased the frequency of defaecation. The role of exercise was more important in the aged population than in young people.

REFERENCES

Black, C. J., & Ford, A. C. (2018). Chronic idiopathic constipation in adults: Epidemiology, pathophysiology, diagnosis and clinical management. *Medical Journal of Australia, 209*(2), 86–91

Borre, M., Qvist, N., Raahave, D., et al. (2015). [The effect of lifestyle modification on chronic constipation]. *Ugeskr Laeger, 177*(15), V09140498

D'Hoore, A., & Penninckx, F. (2003). Obstructed defaecation. *Colorectal Disease, 5*(4), 280–287.

Forootan, M., Bagheri, N., & Darvishi, M. (2018). Chronic constipation: A review of literature. *Medicine (Baltimore), 97*(20), e10631.

Frattini, J. C., & Nogueras, J. J. (2008). Slow transit constipation: A review of a colonic functional disorder. *Clinics in Colon and Rectal Surgery, 21*(2), 146–152.

Gazala, M. A., & Wexner, S. D. (2021). Epidemiology and etiology of constipation and obstructed defectaion: An overview. In G. A. Santoro, A. P. Wieczorek, & A. H. Sultan (Eds.), *Pelvic floor disorders: A Multidisciplinary Textbook* (2nd ed.) (pp. 737–741). Cham, Switzerland: Springer Nature.

Gudipally, P. R., & Sharma, G. K. (2022). In *Premenstrual syndrome [online]* Available at https://www.pubmed.ncbi.nlm.nih.gov/32809533/.

Higgins, P. D., & Johanson, J. F. (2004). Epidemiology of constipation in North America: A systematic review. *American Journal of Gastroenterology, 99*(4), 750–759.

Holdstock, D. J., Misiewicz, J. J., Smith, T., et al. (1970). Propulsion (mass movements) in the human colon and its relationship to meals and somatic activity. *Gut, 11*(2), 91–99.

Holtmann, G. J., Ford, A. C., & Talley, N. J. (2016). Pathophysiology of irritable bowel syndrome. *The Lancet Gastroenterology and Hepatology, 1*(2), 133–146.

Krogh, K., Chiarioni, G., & Whitehead, W. (2017). Management of chronic constipation in adults. *United European Gastroenterol. J, 5*(4), 465–472.

Lin, A. Y., Du, P., Dinning, P. G., et al. (2017). High-resolution anatomic correlation of cyclic motor patterns in the human colon: Evidence of a rectosigmoid brake. *American Journal of Physiology - Gastrointestinal and Liver Physiology, 312*(5), G508–G515.

Lovell, R. M., & Ford, A. C. (2012). Global prevalence of and risk factors for irritable bowel syndrome: A meta-analysis. *Clinical Gastroenterology and Hepatology, 10*(7), 712–721.e4.

McMinn, R. M. H. (Ed.). (2003). *Last's anatomy: Regional and applied.* London: Churchill Livingstone.

Nellesen, D., Chawla, A., Weissman, T., et al. (2013). Comorbidities in patients with irritable bowel syndrome with constipation or chronic idiopathic constipation: A review of the literature from the past decade. *Postgraduate Medical Journal, 125*(2), 40–50.

Palsson, O. S., Whitehead, W., Törnblom, H., et al. (2020). Prevalence of Rome IV functional bowel disorders among adults in the United States, Canada, and the United Kingdom. *Gastroenterology, 158*(5), 1262–1273.

Peppas, G., Alexiou, V. G., Mourtzoukou, E., et al. (2008). Epidemiology of constipation in Europe and Oceania: A systematic review. *BMC Gastroenterology, 8*, 5.

Pescatori, M. (2019). The Iceberg diagram for the treatment of obstructed defaecation. *Siccr - Società Italiana di Chirurgia Colo-Rettale, 50*, 430–439.

Poddar, U. (2016). Approach to constipation in children. *Indian Pediatrics, 53*(4), 319–327.

Radenkovic, G., Radenkovic, D., & Velickov, A. (2018). Development of interstitial cells of Cajal in the human digestive tract as the result of reciprocal induction of mesenchymal and neural crest cells. *Journal of Cellular and Molecular Medicine, 22*(2), 778–785.

Rao, S. S., & Patcharatrakul, T. (2016). Diagnosis and treatment of dyssynergic defaecation. *Journal of Neurogastroenterology and Motility, 22*(3), 423–435.

Rao, S. S., Rattanakovit, K., & Patcharatrakul, T. (2016). Diagnosis and management of chronic constipation in adults. *Nature Reviews Gastroenterology & Hepatology*, 13(5), 295–305.

Ribas, Y., Saldaña, E., Martí-Ragué, J., et al. (2011). Prevalence and pathophysiology of functional constipation among women in Catalonia. *Diseases of the Colon & Rectum*, 54(12), 1560–1569.

Rosse, C., & Gaddum-Rosse, P. (1997). *Hollinshead's Textbook of anatomy*. Philadelphia, PA: Lippincott Williams & Wilkins.

Sandle, G. I. (1998). Salt and water absorption in the human colon: A modern appraisal. *Gut*, 43(2), 294–299.

Sandler, R. S., Jordan, M. C., & Shelton, B. J. (1990). Demographic and dietary determinants of constipation in the US population. *The American Journal of Public Health*, 80(2), 185–189.

Simren, M., Palsson, O. S., & Whitehead, W. E. (2017). Update on Rome IV criteria for colorectal disorders: Implications for clinical practice. *Current Gastroenterology Reports*, 19(4), 15.

Smith, T. K., Park, K. J., & Henning, G. W. (2014). Colonic migrating motor complexes, high amplitude propagating contractions, neural reflexes and the importance of neuronal and mucosal serotonin. *Siccr - Società Italiana di Chirurgia Colo-Rettale*, 20(4), 423–446.

Spencer, N. J. (2015). Constitutively active 5-HT receptors: An explanation of how 5-HT antagonists inhibit gut motility in species where 5-HT is not an enteric neurotransmitter? *Frontiers in Cellular Neuroscience*, 9, 487.

Steele, S. R., & Mellgren, A. (2007). Constipation and obstructed defaecation. *Clinics in Colon and Rectal Surgery*, 20(2), 110–117.

Suares, N. C., & Ford, A. C. (2011). Prevalence of, and risk factors for, chronic idiopathic constipation in the community: Systematic review and meta-analysis. *American Journal of Gastroenterology*, 106(9), 1582–1591.

Sultan, A. H., & Monga, A. (2017). An International Urogynecological Association (IUGA)/International Continence Society (ICS) joint report on the terminology for female anorectal dysfunction. *Int Urogynecol J*, 28(1), 5–31 2017.

Thomas, R. H., & Luthin, D. R. (2015). Current and emerging treatments for irritable bowel syndrome with constipation and chronic idiopathic constipation: Focus on prosecretory agents. *Pharmacotherapy: The Journal of Human Pharmacology and Drug Therapy*, 35(6), 613–630.

Wald, A. (1995). Incontinence and anorectal dysfunction in patients with diabetes mellitus. *European Journal of Gastroenterology and Hepatology*, 7(8), 737–739.

Wald, A., Scarpignato, C., Kamm, M. A., et al. (2007). The burden of constipation on quality of life: Results of a multinational survey. *Alimentary Pharmacology & Therapeutics*, 26(2), 227–236.

Yurtdaş, G., Acar-Tek, N., Akbulut, G., et al. (2020). Risk factors for constipation in adults: A cross-sectional study. *Journal of the American College of Nutrition*, 39(8), 713–719.

Pain

OUTLINE

9.1 Pain Physiology

Bert Messelink and Bary Berghmans

PAIN DEFINITIONS

International Association for the Study of Pain

The International Association for the Study of Pain (IASP) is a multidisciplinary organization 'bringing together scientists, clinicians, health-care providers, and policymakers to stimulate and support the study of pain and to translate that knowledge into improved pain relief worldwide' (IASP, 2021). The first IASP definition on pain was set up in 1979. In 2020, they accepted a new version of their own definition. The new definition is: 'An unpleasant sensory and emotional experience associated with, or resembling that associated with, actual or potential tissue damage'. This definition is expanded upon by the addition of six key Notes and the etymology of the word *pain* for further valuable context (Raja et al., 2020):

- Pain is always a personal experience that is influenced to varying degrees by biological, psychological and social factors.
- Pain and nociception are different phenomena. Pain cannot be inferred solely from activity in sensory neurons.
- Through their life experiences, individuals learn the concept of pain.
- A person's report of an experience as pain should be respected.
- Although pain usually serves an adaptive role, it may have adverse effects on function and social and psychological well-being.
- Verbal description is only one of several behaviours to express pain; inability to communicate does not negate the possibility that a human or a non-human animal experiences pain.

In 2016, an alternative new definition of pain was proposed to IASP to update the old one. This new definition was: 'Pain is a distressing experience associated with actual or potential tissue damage with sensory, emotional, cognitive and social components' (Williams and Craig, 2016). The main background thought for change was the recognition of the psychosocial influences on pain.

Neuro Orthopaedic Institute

The Neuro Orthopaedic Institute is a neuroscience institute that has set up the Explain Pain programme. The idea behind Explain Pain is that pain is produced by the brain even if there is no (more) tissue or organ damage. Their mission is to translate (basic) neuroscience into clinical practice. By explaining the pain, people will become less frightened about their pain, and that helps in diminishing the pain. Their vision is based on pain as a 'spontaneous construction of the brain, in response to perceived threat and aimed at healing. This construction is influenced by several biological, psychological and social factors' (Moseley and Butler, 2015).

In their view, pain is a perceptual consequence, whereby the brain processes experience into consciousness that reflects the best guess estimate of what will be an advantageous response. And for the response, it can be said that the tendency will usually be to err on the

side of protection. This means that the brain produces pain to prevent the person from further damage.

European Association of Urology

The European Association of Urology (EAU) is an organization for urologists. The EAU produces the Guideline on Chronic Pelvic Pain, and it is one of the most cited ones in discussions about pelvic pain. The definition of chronic pelvic pain used by the EAU (2020) is: 'chronic or persistent pain perceived in structures related to the pelvis of either men or women' (https://uroweb.org/guideline/chronic-pelvic-pain/).

The EAU pays a lot of attention to the taxonomy of chronic pelvic pain.

Phenotyping is describing the condition. Example: In a patient with chronic bladder pain, you see either Hunner lesions or a normal bladder mucosa. These are two different phenotypes.

Terminology is the words that are used. Example: Words associated with bladder pain, such as interstitial cystitis and bladder pain syndrome.

Taxonomy places phenotypes into a relationship hierarchy. Example: The EAU guideline subdivides chronic pelvic pain into (1) non-pain syndromes, including well-recognized pathology like infections, and (2) pain syndromes where pain is a disease in its own right (Engeler et al., 2013).

International Classification of Diseases

For the first time in the history of the International Classification of Diseases (ICD), the diagnosis of chronic pain has been included as a separate disease. Within the most recent version (ICD-11), two sorts of chronic pain are outlined (Treede et al., 2019).

Chronic primary pain is characterized by disability or emotional distress and not better accounted for by another diagnosis of chronic pain. Here, you will find chronic widespread pain, chronic musculoskeletal pain, and conditions such as chronic pelvic pain and irritable bowel syndrome. They are recognized as a group of chronic pain syndromes for the first time in ICD-11.

Chronic secondary pain is organized into the following six categories: (1) chronic cancer-related pain; (2) chronic post-surgical or post-traumatic pain; (3) chronic neuropathic pain; (4) chronic secondary headache or orofacial pain; (5) chronic secondary visceral pain, including pain as a consequence of underlying conditions in the abdominal or pelvic regions, which can be caused by persistent inflammation, vascular mechanisms or mechanical factors; and (6) chronic secondary musculoskeletal pain.

Future of Terminology

As is clear from this summing up of (a few) definitions, there is a need for one taxonomy for all visceral pain (syndromes). In a recent topical review in Pain (the official journal of IASP), the strengths and limitations of different taxonomies for visceral pain were described with the following intention: '[T]o initiate collaborations between the different scientific associations, who have developed different classification systems. Ultimately, a unified and evidenced-based pain classification system will have to be widely adopted by patients and both the clinical and the research communities, as well as regulatory agencies and pharmaceutical companies to advance diagnosis, clinical pain management, clinical trial design and pain research in the field of visceral pain' (Häuser et al., 2020).

Therefore, there is a lot to do regarding definition and terminology in the world of chronic pelvic pain. Support from the ICD is a helpful step forward in this process.

PAIN THEORY

In the past 10 years we have learned a lot about pain. The most important new information comes from brain research (Reddan and Wager, 2018). In earlier years, the approach of pelvic pain was merely organ based, and in the new approach, the pain itself is the way to go. This is reflected in changing the terminology from prostatitis and interstitial cystitis to prostate pain syndrome and bladder pain syndrome. In discussing with the patient, instead of asking where the pain is coming from, we ask them where the pain is felt. Bladder pain syndrome means that the pain is felt in the bladder, but this does not say anything about whether the bladder is the origin of the pain.

Pain is an outgoing signal produced by the brain. As Fernando Cervero (at that time, chairman of IASP) once said: 'Transforming a sensory input into a behavioural meaningful output: that is how the brain works' (Cervero, 2014). Pain does not have its starting point in the organ or tissue; it originates from the brain in 100% of the cases. As mentioned in the definition paragraph, the brain is reacting on an input signal that is experienced as threatening, and the goal of the brain is to react in such

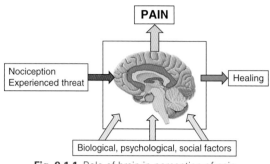

Fig. 9.1.1 Role of brain in perception of pain.

a way that a healing action is taken (Moseley and Butler, 2003) (Fig. 9.1.1). The way the brain does this also depends on biological, psychological and social factors. Neuroimaging studies have taught us that pain is a very personal experience (Apkarian et al., 2005; de Felice and Ossipov, 2016). It has also taught us the importance of realizing that tissue damage or dysfunction is not directly related to pain in a one-on-one relationship. There can be tissue damage without pain, and there can be pain without tissue damage. In other words, nociception and pain are not the same. If the tissue is damaged, 'danger receptors' will be activated and an alarm signal is sent to the spinal cord and upwards to the brain. The brain then responds with protective actions, including pain in the body part where the signal started. Urinary tract infections and pelvic surgery are examples of this mechanism. In case, there is nociceptive signalling but the environment demands that you go on with what you are doing, the brain can give priority to that demand and will not bother you with a pain signal. At that moment, continuing your work is then an advantageous response for the brain. However, if the brain judges normal input as threatening information, it may ask for your attention by giving the pain signal. For more detailed information on this theory, read Explain Pain Supercharged (Moseley and Butler, 2017a).

Thus, pain is a way to communicate between body and mind. There are different reasons why the brain makes pain (Baliki and Apkarian, 2015). You might have had pain before in the same region, based on an infection or surgery. You might be in fear for problems with an organ because you have bad experiences with that disfunction (pain during micturition) or because you think something dangerous is happening (fear of cancer). In these situations, the incoming signal is a non-nociceptive signal but nonetheless experienced by the brain as a threat, on which the brain responds with pain. That pain may itself be reassuring that something is wrong and demands action: searching for help, asking for diagnostics and so on. Research underpinning these phenomena was done by using functional magnetic resonance imaging of the brain. In the studies, it was found that maladaptive cognitive and emotional factors are associated with several brain regions involved in chronic pain (Malfliet et al., 2017). However, pain can be helpful if we listen to our brain and learn how to let the brain know that it is heard and listened to. This may give rest and reduce the pain. One of the options to do so is mindfulness or mindfulness-based cognitive behavioural therapy (CBT) (Hilton et al., 2017). And accepting the pain as something that is present can also help in lowering the pain. Acceptance, in its way, is a moderator of attention (Crombez et al., 2013).

PAIN MECHANISMS

Visceral Versus Somatic Pain

There are many differences between visceral and somatic pain. In pelvic pain, both mechanisms may play a role. Pain experienced in the organs is visceral pain, and pain experienced in the muscles or skin is somatic pain. In Fig. 9.1.2, the differences between the two mechanisms are illustrated. Talking about pelvic pain we will often deal with visceral pain, and being aware of the specific properties will help explain the pain and the combination with organ symptoms (Farquhar-Smith and Jaggar, 2008). Notably, the fact that visceral pain is poorly localized helps to get away from an organ-based approach. The fact that pain is felt in the bladder does not mean that there is something wrong with the bladder. The gut or the uterus can be the location of origin as well.

Our nervous system cannot differentiate between them (Pedersen et al., 2010; European Association of Urology, 2020). The appearance of referred pain is another item often seen in pelvic pain and also easy to explain by knowing the specific characters of visceral pain (Torstensson et al., 2015).

Peripheral Pain

Peripheral pain mechanisms can be well explained by neuroimmune phenomena (Moseley and Butler, 2017b; Matsuda et al., 2019). When there is tissue damage, such as an infection or a (surgical) wound, the body will produce a lot of substances at the location of damage, the so-called inflammatory soup. This soup contains substances like substance P, tumor necrosis factor alpha and interleukin (IL), all of which play a role in starting the healing process. The two most prominent mechanisms used for healing and repair are vasodilatation and inflammation. However, these substances also lead to nociceptive information to the central nervous system via afferent nerve fibres. Furthermore, we know that there are specific receptors called *Toll-like receptors* (TLRs) that play an important role, for instance, in cystitis-induced bladder pain (Cui et al., 2019). When TLRs are activated, they generate inflammatory reactions. The activation of these TLRs is mediated by associated molecular patterns (AMPs), and several types of these AMPs are identified, such as DAMP, which is damage-AMP made by damaged cells, and XAMP, which is xenobiotic-AMP, such as drugs used for treatment. TLR4 especially is related to pain generation. This receptor has a great amount of memory for the different AMPs, and it shows an increasing sensitivity for other AMPs, thereby playing a role in sensitization and expanding of the pain region (Lacagnina et al., 2018).

	Visceral	Somatic
✓ Stimuli	Stretching, distension, poorly localized	Mechanical, well localized
✓ Summation	Magnifying pain	Modest increase pain
✓ Referred pain	Common	Seldom
✓ Innervation	Unmyelinated C-fibres , thin Aδ fibers	Wide range of fibers
✓ Primary efferent	Intensity coding	Two fibre coding

Fig. 9.1.2 The characteristics of the visceral and somatic nerve system.

Central Pain

In the central nervous system we find the pain pathways, a huge network of neurons and cells that work together to process information and generate pain signals. The idea is that there are different pathways in different forms of chronic pain (Farmer et al., 2012). The brain not only receives information from lower centres but also sends information down by itself via spinal tracts (dorsal root ganglia and the dorsal horn) to the periphery. In the phase of acute pain, this descending modulation leads to inhibition of pain signalling. In chronic pain, the balance between ascending and descending signals may be distorted, and descending modulation may well exaggerate the pain. In chronic pain situations, the brain concludes that there is more danger in the tissue which needs healing (Ossipov et al., 2014). The process of healing involves the neuroinflammation processes mentioned previously that in themselves can worsen the pain. It is good to realize that the pain matrix processes both physical and emotional pain. We all know that one can have abdominal pain when something scary is happening or when one is in fear of something that may happen. Both physical and emotional pain can alter brain function, contributing to the transition from acute to chronic pain and to the comorbidity between chronic pain, depression and anxiety disorders (Crofford, 2015).

Psychosomatic Pain

Knowing how the nervous system works in chronic pain, the step to psychosomatic aspects of (pelvic) pain is just a small one. Several processes take place in the brain, and some of them we already know from the peripheral nervous system. TLR4 receptors are found in the brain (Trotta et al., 2014). There is a theory stating that these brain TLRs react on so-called BAMPs, which are behavioural-AMPs (facing danger), and CAMPs, which are cognitive-AMPs (thinking about pain) (Moseley and Butler, 2017a). If this is true, it makes clear how anxiety, thoughts and behaviour can influence the experience of pain. The existence of a danger-associated molecular pattern has been studied and found in people with depression (Franklin and Xu, 2018). From animal studies, we know that IL4 plays a role in cognitive processes: IL4 makes mice smarter. We also know that IL4 plays a role in the neuroimmunological processes and that it is reduced in patients with chronic pain. Animal experiments have also shown that if you put an animal in a threatening condition and then apply a noxious stimulus, the IL1 level will increase. If you apply the same stimulus to an animal in a friendly surrounding, the IL1 level does not change. Obviously, it is the combination of the surrounding and the noxious stimulus that leads to a chemical body reaction (Goshn et al., 2007).

The amount of knowledge gained about these mechanisms has increased, and is quite helpful for understanding the pain processes and especially illustrates the mutual relationship between pain and mind. All of these understandings will help us explain pain to our patients. It is quite beneficial to provide pain education and management strategies for pelvic pain (Wijma et al., 2016).

PAIN MANAGEMENT

Acute Pain

Acute pain will bring a patient to the general practitioner's office or the emergency room of a hospital. The pain started suddenly, is preventing the patient from carrying out any activities and often generates anxiety. In the case of physical trauma, the origin of the pain will be clear from the start. For example, in the case of pain felt in the pelvic area, such as painful voiding, frequency or change of urine, we can easily decide that a urinary tract infection is the most plausible explanation. A urine test is done and, if an infection is confirmed, antibiotics are started. In most cases, the pain will subside and micturition will return to normal. In acute pain, it is important to look for 'well-known diseases' that can explain the pain and subsequently treat them, not only for direct relief of the pain and improvement in comfort for patients, but also for potential long-term consequences. Imagine that the brain makes a dossier on the acute pain including time, location, activity, amount of nociception and what action was undertaken to find relief for the complaints (including the pain) (Mansour et al., 2014). Thus, treating the disease causing the acute pain is important because the brain will add this successful outcome to the dossier. The speed in which investigations are carried out in order to get a diagnosis of a well-known disease depends on the presence of red and yellow flags: things that are known to lead to bigger problems if not quickly and accurately treated. Red means that medical diagnostics should be done before any other treatment (such as physiotherapy) is started.

Yellow means that diagnostics are needed but can be done in parallel with starting the treatment.

Acute to Chronic Pain

If the outcome is not successful, then one should look further to find other clues about the origin of the pain. Neurobiology has clarified the mechanisms that play a role in moving from acute to chronic (Brodin et al., 2016). At this subacute stage, it is important to pay attention to the function of the pelvic floor muscles and to the psychosocial aspects. If the patient's father just died from bladder cancer, this will influence the perception of pain felt in the bladder. If the patient is known to have other pain conditions, this will also be a risk factor for prolonged pain, with the patient not reacting to the standard therapies that are given. If the patient has personality characteristics that amplify negative emotions and thoughts (catastrophizing), this will make the pain worse as well (Sewell et al., 2018). Establishing the factors that determine the risk of having prolonged or chronic pelvic pain may help in planning a further approach (Van Hecke et al., 2013). Examples of these risk factors are presented in Fig. 9.1.3. So far, there is no literature on the effect of using these factors to plan the next step. However, based on pain science and pain mechanisms, if there is low risk, the next step should be a short investigation into possible causes for the pain, basing these investigations on the 'organ history taking'. The results must be made clear to the patient and explained in a positive way. Telling the patient that although they have pain, the organ is in good health and that the focus needs to be on the pain is better than telling the patient that nothing wrong has been found and therefore help cannot be provided. Even worse is explaining that this type of pain is extremely difficult to treat, followed by referring to another organ specialist. This nocebo will confirm to the patient the idea that something is wrong but cannot be found. In addition, nocebos worsen the pain and slow down the process of getting better (Benedetti et al., 2020).

If the risk is estimated as high, the patient should preferably be referred to an expert centre in the field of pelvic pain, which includes a team of healthcare professionals experienced in treating pelvic pain. This team should address all aspects, biomedical, psychological and social, simultaneously, and not, for example, only looking at psychosocial factors once biomedical causes have been exhausted (Messelink, 2020). If a low-risk patient develops chronic pelvic pain, that patient should also be referred to an expert centre.

Chronic Pain

The most important task in the chronic phase is to get away from the organ itself and all cognitions about damage, organ failure and the future of living with pain. Pain should be put at the centre of all communication, and it should be clear for the patient that pain can be treated even if no underlying pathology is found. Pain education can help the patient understand what goes on in the mind and also helps the provider and patient stay in contact and work together on pain relief. It can also help to literally ask the patient permission to talk about pain from a different perspective. This is called *motivational interviewing* (Alperstein and Sharpe, 2016). Using this approach helps create a good atmosphere when talking about pain that cannot be explained by organ problems in a way that suits the patient and is in alignment with their own ideas. It may also improve adherence to pain treatments.

The idea is to use models that help get away from the linear 'organ damage cause based' model (Ploteau et al., 2015). For example, when taking a pain history, you can use a consequences model, in which you do not look at causes but primarily at the consequences of the pain and how it affects daily life.

- Multiple organ systems involved
- Previous periods of pain
- Chronic pain diagnoses
- Somatic unexplained complaints
- Multiple psychosocial consequences
- Expectation of permanent complaints

Fig. 9.1.3 Risk factors for developing chronic pain.

Conservative Management

Conservative options in treatment of pelvic pain are readily available. One of the options that should always be used is pelvic floor muscle therapy. Well-trained physiotherapists who know much about the pelvic floor, the pelvic organs and pelvic pain can be of great help to the patient. Because the pelvic floor muscles often play a role in persistent pelvic pain, optimization of pelvic floor muscle function is helpful. Physiotherapists can also help in other forms of therapy, such as moving and doing exercises which improve the patient's general condition and well-being. Furthermore, good function of the pelvic floor muscles helps eliminate complaints of organ dysfunction, such as urinary frequency, constipation and pain during sexual activity (Berghmans, 2018). This is in line with the activation contingent approach that physiotherapists use instead of a pain contingent intervention.

Psychologists also play an important role in conservative management. Several forms of CBT are used in treating patients with pelvic pain. Mindfulness-based CBT (Turnera et al., 2016) and acceptance and commitment therapy (Hughes et al., 2017) are examples of what a psychologist can offer as treatment. Special forms of psychological care include eye movement desensitization and reprocessing (EMDR) and hypnotherapy.

EMDR has been developed for trauma treatment and is first-line therapy in the field of psychology. In pelvic pain, it can educate patients to focus on the pain without feeling tension or anxiety (Grant, 2000; Tesarz et al., 2014). The 'flashforward' protocol (Logie and de Jongh, 2014) helps unload a disaster image that comes up during the experience of pain. By using 'resource development and installation' (Hornsveld et al., 2011), a resource is installed that can help when facing pain in the future. It is based on questions like 'What do you need to move without pain? To have sex without pain?' (Korn and Leeds, 2002).

Hypnotherapy has not been studied in the field of pelvic pain, but it has been studied in acute and chronic pain. Studies that have been done on the use of hypnosis in inflammatory bowel disease show encouraging results (Peters et al., 2015). Other studies have shown the efficacy of hypnosis in reducing chronic pain. Neurophysiologically, it seems clear that hypnotic treatments may have an effect on brain function (Jensen and Paterson, 2014). The idea is that the patient in hypnosis gains access to the subconscious part of the brain. This part is protected by the so-called critical factor. Passing the critical factor and capturing acceptable selective thoughts is what hypnosis does. In that subconscious part, the information about safety, earlier experiences and anger about pain is located (Vanhaudenhuyse et al., 2014). This information cannot be changed by just saying to oneself that you want to change it. In hypnosis, the positive suggestions proposed by the therapist can be put into the subconscious part of the brain by the patient.

Self-Management

We need to realise that not all pain journeys will have a happy ending. Not all patients will be completely pain free at the end of their journey through the healthcare system. If this is the case, we need to provide our patients with good instruments for self-management of their pain (Devan et al., 2018). Introducing and explaining self-management to patients is important because even if they visit a healthcare provider twice a year, they are on their own with their pain the other 363 days.

Physiotherapists play an important role here by educating the patient about what to do with their muscles when the pain returns or worsens. They can also address the effect of pain on personal factors, such as limitations and disabilities, and social factors, such as restriction in participation. A psychologist can help by paying attention to 'relapse prevention', meaning that they teach the patient to recognize the start of a new episode of pain and what to do when that happens. They can explain how to use the lessons they have learned about acceptance and commitment. Mindfulness exercises, meditation and self-hypnosis are techniques a patient can put in his backpack and have available at any time they are needed. The social environment can also be of help in supporting the patient when needed. Doctors can help by telling the patient in which situations they should arrange for a new visit. If pain persists, patients can make a yearly appointment to talk things over and hear what the actual situation is rather than what they imagine it to be. When this is well explained to the patient, it might yield a feeling of trust and certainty.

The following resources are available for further reading on backgrounds and practical options:
- Understanding Pain in Less Than 5 Minutes, and What to Do About It! (Hunter Integrated Pain

Service (HIPS), Newcastle, 2013; Available: https://youtu.be/C_3phB93rvI)

- Explain Pain Supercharged, by G. Lorimer Moseley and David S. Butler (Noigroup Publications, Adelaide, Australia, 2017)
- Abdominal and Pelvic Pain: From Definition to Best Practice, by Bert Messelink, Andrew Baranowski and John Hughes (Wolters Kluwer, New York, 2015)
- The European Association of Urology Guideline on Chronic Pelvic Pain (Available: https://uroweb.org/guideline/chronic-pelvic-pain/)

REFERENCES

Alperstein, D., & Sharpe, L. (2016). The efficacy of motivational interviewing in adults with chronic pain: A meta-analysis and systematic review. *The Journal of Pain*, 17(4), 393–403.

Apkarian, A. V., Bushnell, M. C., Treede, R. D., et al. (2005). Human brain mechanisms of pain perception and regulation in health and disease. *European Journal of Pain*, 9, 463–484.

Baliki, M. N., & Apkarian, A. V. (2015). Nociception, pain, negative moods, and behavior selection. *Neuron*, 87(3), 474–491.

Benedetti, F., Frisaldi, E., Barbiani, D., et al. (2020). Nocebo and the contribution of psychosocial factors to the generation of pain. *Neural Transmission*, 127(4), 687–696.

Berghmans, B. (2018). Physiotherapy for pelvic pain and female sexual dysfunction: An untapped resource. *International Urogynecology Journal*, 29, 631–638.

Brodin, E., Ernberg, M., & Olgart, L. (2016). Neurobiology: General considerations—from acute to chronic pain. *North Dentistry Journal*, 126, 28–33.

Cervero, F. (2014). *Understanding pain: Exploring the perception of pain*. Cambridge, MA: MIT Press.

Crofford, L. J. (2015). Chronic pain: Where the body meets the brain. *Transactions of the American Clinical & Climatological Association*, 126, 167–183.

Crombez, G., Viane, I., Eccleston, C., et al. (2013). Attention to pain and fear of pain in patients with chronic pain. *Journal of Behavioral Medicine*, 36, 371–378.

Cui, X., Jing, X., & Lutgendorf, S. K. (2019). Cystitis-induced bladder pain is Toll-like receptor 4 dependent in a transgenic autoimmune cystitis murine model: A MAPP research network animal study. *American Journal of Physiology Renal Physiology*, 317(1), 90–98.

De Felice, M., & Ossipov, M. H. (2016). Cortical and subcortical modulation of pain. *Pain Management*, 6(2), 111–120.

Devan, H., Hale, L., Hempel, D., et al. (2018). What works and does not work in a self-management intervention for people with chronic pain? Qualitative systematic review and meta-synthesis. *Physical Therapy*, 98(5), 381–397.

EAU. (2020). *Chronic pelvic pain [online]*. Available: https://uroweb.org/guideline/chronic-pelvic-pain/ (Accessed 10.16.22).

Engeler, D. S., Baranowski, A. P., Dinis-Oliveira, P., et al. (2013). The 2013 EAU guidelines on chronic pelvic pain: Is management of chronic pelvic pain a habit, a philosophy, or a science? 10 years of development. *European Urology*, 64, 431–439.

Farmer, M. A., Baliki, M. N., & Apkarian, A. V. (2012). A dynamic network perspective of chronic pain. *Neuroscience Letters*, 520(2), 197–203.

Farquhar-Smith, P., & Jaggar, S. (2008). Visceral pain mechanisms. In A. P. Baranowski (Ed.), *Urogenital pain in clinical practice*. New York: Informa Healthcare.

Franklin, T. C., & Xu, C. (2018). Depression and sterile inflammation: Essential role of danger associated molecular patterns. *Brain, Behavior, and Immunity*, 72, 2–13.

Goshn, I., Kreisel, T., Ounallah-Saad, H., et al. (2007). A dual role for IL-1 in hippocampal-dependent memory processes. *Psychoneuroendocrinology*, 32, 1106–1115.

Grant, M. (2000). EMDR: A new treatment for trauma and chronic pain. *Complement Theraphy Nursing Midwifery*, 6(2), 91–94.

Häuser, W., Baranowski, A., Messelink, E. J., et al. (2020). Taxonomies for chronic visceral pain. *Pain*, 161(6), 1129–1135.

Hilton, L., Hempel, S., & Ewing, B. A. (2017). Mindfulness meditation for chronic pain: Systematic review and meta-analysis. *Annals of Behavioral Medicine*, 51, 199–213.

Hornsveld, H., Joutveen, J. H., Vroomen, M., et al. (2011). Evaluating the effect of eye movements on positive memories such as those used in resource development and installation. *Journal of EMDR Practice and Research*, 5(4), 146–155.

Hughes, L. S., Clark, J., Colclough, J. A., et al. (2017). Acceptance and commitment therapy (ACT) for chronic pain: A systematic review and meta-analyses. *The Clinical Journal of Pain*, 33(6), 552–568.

International Association for the Study of Pain. (2021). *Home page [online]*. Available: https://www.iasp-pain.org/Mission?navItemNumber=586 (Accessed 10.16.22).

Jensen, M. P., & Patterson, D. R. (2014). Hypnotic approaches for chronic pain management clinical implications of recent research findings. *American Psychologist*, 69(2), 167–177.

Korn, D. L., & Leeds, A. M. (2002). Preliminary evidence of efficacy for EMDR resource development and installation in the stabilization phase of treatment of complex post-traumatic stress disorder. *Journal of Clinical Psychology*, *58*(12), 1465–1487.

Lacagnina, M. J., Watkins, L. R., & Grace, P. M. (2018). Toll-like receptors and their role in persistent pain. *Pharmacol Therapy.*, *184*, 145–158.

Logie, R. D. J., & de Jongh, A. (2014). The "flashforward procedure": Confronting the catastrophe. *Journal of EMDR Practice and Research*, *8*(1), 25–32.

Malfliet, A., Coppieters, I., & Van Wilgen, P. (2017). Brain changes associated with cognitive and emotional factors in chronic pain: A systematic review. *European Journal of Pain*, *21*(5), 769–786.

Mansour, A. R., Farmer, M. A., Baliki, M. N., et al. (2014). Chronic pain: The role of learning and brain plasticity. *Restorative Neurology and Neuroscience*, *32*(1), 129–139.

Matsuda, M., Huh, Y., & Ji, R. R. (2019). Roles of inflammation, neurogenic inflammation, and neuroinflammation in pain. *Journal of Anesthesia*, *33*(1), 131–139.

Messelink, B. (Ed.). (2020). *Dutch guideline on chronic pelvic pain*. Utrecht, Netherlands: Federation of Medical Specialists.

Moseley, L. G., & Butler, D. S. (2003). *Explain pain*. Adelaide, Australia: Noigroup Publications.

Moseley, L. G., & Butler, D. S. (2015). Fifteen years of explaining pain: The past, present, and future. *The Journal of Pain*, *16*(9), 807–813.

Moseley, L. G., & Butler, D. S. (2017). *Explain pain supercharged*. Adelaide, Australia: Noigroup Publications.

Moseley, L. G., & Butler, D. S. (2017). Part B. Time for neuroimmune coupling. In *Explain pain supercharged* (p. 55). Adelaide, Australia: Noigroup Publications.

Ossipov, M. H., Morimura, K., & Porreca, F. (2014). Descending pain modulation and chronification of pain. *Current Opinion in Supportive and Palliative Care*, *8*(2), 143–151.

Pedersen, K. V., Drewes, A. M., Frimodt-Moller, P. C., et al. (2010). Visceral pain originating from the upper urinary tract. *Urological Research*, *38*, 345–355.

Peters, S. L., Muir, J. G., & Gibson, P. R. (2015). Review article: Gut-directed hypnotherapy in the management of irritable bowel syndrome and inflammatory bowel disease. *Alimentary Pharmacology & Therapeutics*, *41*(11), 1104–1115.

Ploteau, S., Labat, J. J., & Riant, T. (2015). New concepts on functional chronic pelvic and perineal pain: Pathophys-iology and multidisciplinary management. *Discovery Medicine*, *19*(104), 185–192.

Raja, S. N., Carr, D. B., Cohen, M., et al. (2020). The revised International association for the study of pain definition of pain: Concepts, challenges, and compromises. *Pain*, *161*(9), 1976–1982.

Reddan, M. C., & Wager, T. D. (2018). Modeling pain using fMRI: From regions to biomarkers. *Neuroscience Bulletin*, *34*(1), 208–215.

Sewell, M., Churilov, L., Mooney, S., et al. (2018). Chronic pelvic pain—pain catastrophizing, pelvic pain and quality of life. *Scand Journal Pain*, *18*(3), 441–448.

Tesarz, J., Leisner, S., Gerhardt, A., et al. (2014). Effects of eye movement desensitization and reprocessing (EMDR) treatment in chronic pain patients: A systematic review. *Pain Medicine*, *15*, 247–263.

Torstensson, T., Butler, S., & Lindgren, A. (2015). Referred pain patterns provoked on intra-pelvic structures among women with and without chronic pelvic pain: A descriptive study. *PLoS One*, *10*(3), e0119542.

Treede, R. D., Rief, W., Aziz, Q., et al. (2019). Chronic pain as a symptom or a disease: The IASP classification of chronic pain for the international classification of diseases (ICD-11). *Pain*, *1600*(1), 19–27.

Trotta, T., Porro, C., Calvello, R., et al. (2014). Biological role of Toll-like receptor-4 in the brain. *Journal of Neuroimmunology*, *268*, 1–12.

Turnera, J. A., Anderson, M. L., Balderson, B. H., et al. (2016). Mindfulness-based stress reduction and cognitive-behavioral therapy for chronic low back pain: Similar effects on mindfulness, catastrophizing, self-efficacy, and acceptance in a randomized controlled trial. *Pain*, *157*(11), 2434–2444.

Vanhaudenhuyse, A., Laureys, S., & Faymonville, M. E. (2014). Neurophysiology of hypnosis. *Neurophysiologie Clinique*, *44*(4), 343–353.

Van Hecke, O., Torrance, N., Smith, B. H., et al. (2013). Chronic pain epidemiology and its clinical relevance. *British Journal of Anaesthesia*, *111*(1), 13–18.

Wijma, A. J., van Wilgen, C. P., Meeus, M., et al. (2016). Clinical biopsychosocial physiotherapy assessment of patients with chronic pain: The first step in pain neuroscience education. *Physiotherapy Theory and Practice*, *32*(5), 368–384.

Williams, A. C., & Craig, K. D. (2016). Updating the definition of pain. *Pain*, *157*(11), 2420–2423.

9.2 Chronic Pelvic Floor Pain

Helena Frawley and Mélanie Morin

BACKGROUND

Definitions

This chapter will focus on chronic pelvic floor (PF) pain in females and males. Our aim was to put chronic PF pain into the context of chronic pain generally to encourage a holistic perspective of the patient/person presenting with pain, and to learn from developments in research from areas of pain science beyond the PF. Where possible we have tried to refer to evidence that is inclusive of female and male PF pain or refers to each with specific differences, and to use images that are representative of both sexes; however, to reduce length and because female images were often more available, these may serve as examples to illustrate a concept.

Pain is defined by the International Association for the Study of Pain (IASP) as 'an unpleasant sensory and emotional experience associated with, or resembling that associated with, actual or potential tissue damage' (IASP, 2020). *Persistent*, or *chronic*, pain is defined as pain that persists or recurs for longer than 3 months (Treede et al., 2019). The terms *persistent pain* and *chronic pain* are often used interchangeably. The PF refers to structures located within the bony pelvis, such as urogenital and anorectal viscera, pelvic floor muscles (PFMs) and their connective tissues, and nerves and blood vessels (Bø et al., 2017), and all of these structures can contribute to PF pain (Doggweiler et al., 2017). Terminology related to PFM function and dysfunction follows the International Continence Society (ICS) terminology (Frawley et al., 2021). In this chapter, pain perceived in the perineal/vulval areas is included in the PF, which is also known as pelvi-perineal pain (Levesque et al., 2018). The PFMs and the urogenital structures in the perineum are clearly identifiable as PF structures, whereas the pelvic viscera and the entirety of the female and male reproductive organ systems are not. To help distinguish PF visceral pain from abdominopelvic visceral pain, it may be useful to consider the 'pelvic pain line' as a reference interface. From a theoretical perspective, anatomists have identified this line as the neural interface for visceral afferents conveying pain: visceral afferents from pelvic viscera located above the pelvic line accompany sympathetic fibres (T10–L2), whereas those below it accompany parasympathetic fibres (S2–S4) (Eizenberg, 2015), as illustrated in Fig. 9.2.1.

The pelvic pain line passes through the bladder (at the junction of the detrusor with the trigone), the cervix (at the junction of the supravaginal part with the vaginal part) in the female and the rectum (at its upper end) (Eizenberg, 2015). The pelvic pain line corresponds to the level of the peritoneal cavity, with intraperitoneal viscera being above the pelvic pain line and the subperitoneal viscera below it (Eizenberg, 2015). The pelvic pain line is coincidentally along the plane of least dimensions in the bony pelvis (passing obliquely upwards and backwards from the bottom of the pubic symphysis through the ischial spines to the sacrum). The pelvic pain line divides the bladder; although this line is a clear interface for visceral afferent nerves, from a clinical PF pain perspective, this may not be a functional division. Nevertheless, conceptually the line does help divide PF from

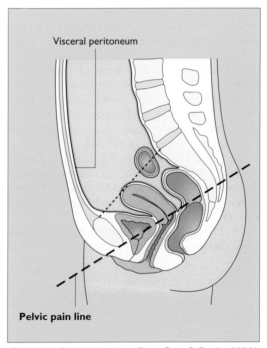

Fig. 9.2.1 Pelvic pain line. *(From Oats & Boyle, 2023)*

abdominopelvic pain conditions. Pain conditions perceived primarily in the abdominopelvic area, or primarily related to the major reproductive organs in females (e.g., endometriosis) and males lying above the pelvic pain line, have been excluded to limit the scope of this chapter to the PF.

Unlike other PF disorders that predominantly affect PF structures and function (e.g., incontinence, pelvic organ prolapse), pain as a disease state or disorder does not affect a single body system or location. As many knowledge gaps exist in our understanding of chronic PF pain and optimal management, it is important to place chronic PF pain into the context of chronic pain more generally, to guide our care. Indeed, some argue that chronic pain generally should be the primary focus in management of idiopathic chronic pelvic pain (CPP) syndromes, not the presumed end organ or perceived anatomical location of pain (Engeler et al., 2020).

Pain is a personal experience, influenced to varying degrees by biological, psychological and social factors (IASP, 2020), and therefore a focus on only biological tissues is incomplete in the consideration of PF pain. In 1977, Engel, a professor of psychiatry and medicine, felt the existing biomedical model of healthcare did not account for the social, psychological and behavioural dimensions of illness and proposed a 'bio-(medical)-psycho-social model' (Engel, 1977) which can be considered a conceptual framework or approach to management. The biopsychosocial framework focuses on both disease and illness, with illness being viewed as the complex interaction of biological, psychological and social factors (Gatchel, 2004), and is illustrated in Fig. 9.2.2. In 2011, the Institute of Medicine Pain Consensus Statement recommended interdisciplinary, biopsychosocial approaches as the most promising for treating patients with chronic pain, yet noted that 'for most patients (and clinicians), such care is a difficult-to-attain ideal, impeded by numerous structural barriers—institutional, educational, organizational, and reimbursement-related' (Institute of Medicine, 2011). Despite ongoing research and efforts to translate findings into clinical practice, large evidence–practice gaps remain in current management of chronic pain (Chalmers and Madden, 2019; Mardian et al., 2020). To add to the complexity of biopsychosocial factors, the respective contribution of each biopsychosocial factor may differ among different pain conditions (Perrot et al., 2019). In addition, it is possible that the complexity of PF pain conditions, which must include consideration of both visceral and somatic structures, and recognition that the PF is an intimate and sensitive part of the body, further impede our progress towards optimal clinical care.

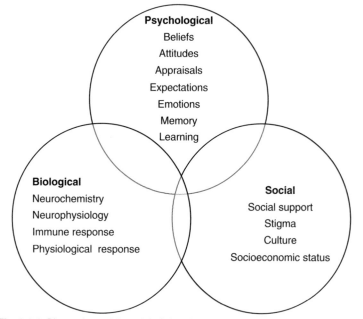

Fig. 9.2.2 Biopsychosocial model of chronic pain. *(From Adams and Turk (2015).)*

Chronic Pain Classification

Several different classification systems have been developed to describe chronic pain and CPP diagnoses/conditions/syndromes. The most recent classification and coding system for chronic pain is by the IASP for the upcoming International Classification of Diseases (ICD), 11th Edition (Treede et al., 2019). In this classification system, the organizing principle gives first priority to pain aetiology (primary pain syndromes, cancer-related pain, and postsurgical or post-traumatic pain), followed by underlying pathophysiological mechanisms (e.g., neuropathic pain), and finally the body site or affected organ system (e.g., visceral pain and musculoskeletal pain) (Treede et al., 2019). In this classification system, chronic pain is the 'parent code' for seven subcategory codes ('top-level' diagnoses) that comprise the most common clinically relevant groups of chronic pain conditions (Fig. 9.2.3).

As depicted in Fig. 9.2.3, in chronic primary pain syndromes (left), pain can be conceived as a disease, whereas in chronic secondary pain syndromes (right), pain initially manifests itself as a symptom of another disease such as breast cancer, a work accident, diabetic neuropathy, chronic caries, inflammatory bowel disease or rheumatoid arthritis. A differential diagnosis between primary and secondary pain conditions may sometimes be challenging (arrows), but in either case the patient's pain needs special care when it is moderate or severe. After spontaneous healing or successful management of the underlying disease, chronic pain may sometimes continue, and hence the chronic secondary pain diagnoses may remain and continue to guide treatment as well as healthcare statistics.

The first of these top-level diagnoses is *chronic primary pain*, which is pain that cannot be better accounted for by another chronic pain condition and can be viewed

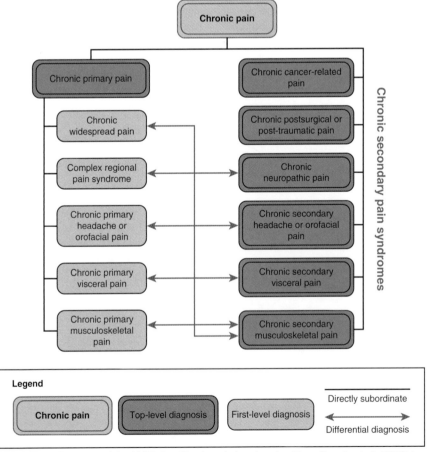

Fig. 9.2.3 Structure of the IASP classification of chronic pain. *(From Treede et al. (2019).)*

as a disease in its own right. This category is subdivided (first-level diagnoses) into chronic widespread pain, such as fibromyalgia, complex regional pain syndrome, chronic primary headache and orofacial pain, chronic primary visceral pain, and chronic primary musculoskeletal pain. In additional to chronic primary pain, there are six further top-level diagnoses, which are called *chronic secondary pain syndromes*, in which pain can be viewed at least initially as a symptom of another disease: chronic cancer-related pain, chronic postsurgical or post-traumatic pain, chronic neuropathic pain, chronic secondary headache or orofacial pain, chronic secondary visceral pain, and chronic secondary musculoskeletal pain. Chronic secondary visceral pain nociceptive mechanisms may include pain from persistent inflammation, vascular mechanisms or mechanical factors (Aziz et al., 2019), and chronic secondary musculoskeletal pain nociceptive mechanisms may include pain from persistent inflammation, pain associated with structural changes and pain associated with diseases of the nervous system (Perrot et al., 2019). In many chronic secondary pain syndromes, the chronic pain may continue beyond successful treatment of the initial cause; in this case the pain diagnosis will remain even after the diagnosis of the underlying disease is no longer relevant.

Within the field of pelvic pain, the European Association of Urology (EAU) classification system for CPP is widely known (Engeler et al., 2020). Many of the EAU-specific disease-associated pelvic pain conditions can be mapped against the IASP ICD-11 chronic primary pain syndromes, and many of the EAU pelvic pain syndromes can be mapped against the IASP ICD-11 chronic secondary pain syndromes. Similarly, using our definition of 'PF' listed previously, chronic PF pain conditions due to varying aetiology (e.g., following pelvic cancer treatments, mesh surgery and traumatic vaginal birth), varying pathophysiology (e.g., pudendal neuropathy) and varying PF sites (e.g., bladder pain syndrome [BPS], provoked vestibulodynia [PVD], irritable bowel syndrome [IBS]) could be classified within the IASP ICD-11 top-level or first-level pain diagnoses. In addition to the preceding classification systems, efforts have been made to standardize terminology, taxonomy and phenotyping of CPP conditions (Engeler et al., 2020; Doggweiler et al., 2017), such as the Rome criteria for IBS (Lacy and Patel, 2017), and the international consensus on criteria for vulvodynia (Bornstein et al., 2019) and interstitial cystitis (IC)/BPS. The new IASP classification of chronic

pain for ICD-11 is intended to provide an umbrella classification system for all chronic pain syndromes.

Once a pain condition has been identified, it can be further described according to pain phenotypes. Phenotypes are based upon mechanisms of pain, when they are known (Engeler et al., 2020). Considerable work in understanding phenotypes in CPP syndromes, with a focus on urological chronic pelvic pain syndromes (UCPPSs) in men and women has been undertaken by the Multidisciplinary Approach to the Study of Chronic Pelvic Pain (MAPP) Research Network (Landis et al., 2014; MAPP, 2021). Within gynaecological CPP conditions, phenotyping has proposed the role of both peripheral and central mechanisms in the modulation of pain (Yong et al., 2020).

Prevalence and Impact

As the structures in the PF include visceral and neuromyofascial tissues, there is no single chronic PF pain condition, and no single prevalence. Prevalence estimates vary according to definitions used and assessment methods to identify the presence of the condition; however, prevalence rates for pelvic pain conditions generally are higher for women than men (Table 9.2.1).

The impact of PF pain conditions can be debilitating, leading to significantly reduced quality of life. The impact of vulvodynia is well documented (Bergeron et al., 2020; Pukall et al., 2016), and quality of life for patients with IC/BPS can be worse than that of patients with end-stage renal disease (Clemens et al., 2019). Further, CPP is reported to have a significantly higher negative impact on quality of life in women than in men (Quaghebeur and Wyndaele, 2015).

Pain Mechanisms/Pathophysiology

Pain mechanism–based classifications have been developed to further understand the pathophysiology of chronic pain, to guide treatment and to inform the mechanisms underpinning the treatment effect. They can be applied to musculoskeletal pain (Shraim et al., 2020) and visceral pain (Kosek et al., 2016; Treede et al., 2019), and are therefore relevant to PF pain syndromes. Pain mechanisms as defined by the IASP are:
1. Nociceptive pain: pain that arises from actual or threatened damage to non-neural tissue and is due to the activation of nociceptors. The term is used to describe pain occurring with a normally functioning

TABLE 9.2.1   Prevalence Estimates of Chronic Pelvic Floor Pain Conditions

Condition	Prevalence: Females	Prevalence: Males
Vulvodynia, subtype: provoked vestibulodynia	7%–8% (Harlow et al. 2014; Lamvu et al., 2015)	—
Urological chronic pelvic pain syndromes: • Interstitial cystitis/Bladder pain syndrome	2.7%–6.5% (Morales-Solchaga et al., 2019; Berry et al., 2011)	1.9%–4.2% (Suskind et al., 2013)
• Chronic pelvic pain syndrome	—	8% (Suskind et al., 2013); up to 11.5% in men <50 years (Daniels et al., 2007)
Irritable bowel syndrome	9.2% (Rome III criteria) to 3.8% (Rome IV criteria) (Oka et al., 2020); prevalence higher in females (odds ratio: 1.46) (Oka et al., 2020)	
Pelvic floor tension myalgia (often coexists with several other pelvic floor pain conditions)	Unknown	Unknown

somatosensory nervous system to contrast with the abnormal function seen in neuropathic pain.

2. Neuropathic pain: pain caused by a lesion or disease of the somatosensory nervous system. This can be divided into central neuropathic pain, which is pain caused by a lesion or disease of the central somatosensory nervous system, or peripheral neuropathic pain, which is pain caused by a lesion or disease of the peripheral somatosensory nervous system.

3. Nociplastic pain: pain that arises from altered nociception despite no clear evidence of actual or threatened tissue damage causing the activation of peripheral nociceptors or evidence for disease or lesion of the somatosensory system causing the pain. Patients can have a combination of nociceptive and nociplastic pain.

Nociception involves the stimulation of nerves that convey information about potential tissue damage to the brain. In contrast, pain is the subjective perception that results from or resembles that associated with the transduction, transmission and modulation of sensory information (Gatchel et al., 2007). The new IASP classification (Treede et al., 2019) recognizes that nociplastic pain may be the mechanism underlying the chronic primary pain conditions (including visceral and musculoskeletal) (Kosek et al., 2016). The key critical process in nociplastic pain conditions is thought to be various sensitization processes and particularly facilitated central gain (i.e., amplification of central excitatory signalling) (Arendt-Nielsen et al., 2018; Woolf, 2011). *Sensitization* is defined as follows: 'Increased responsiveness of nociceptive neurons to their normal input, and/or recruitment

of a response to normally subthreshold inputs. Sensitization can include a drop in threshold and an increase in suprathreshold response. Spontaneous discharges and increases in receptive field size may also occur' (IASP, 2017). Sensitization can be subdivided into central sensitization, defined as increased responsiveness of nociceptive neurons in the central nervous system to their normal subthreshold afferent input or increased responsiveness due to dysfunction of endogenous pain control systems, and peripheral sensitization, defined as increased responsiveness and reduced threshold of nociceptive neurons in the periphery to the stimulation of their receptive fields (IASP, 2017). Neural activity in both ascending and descending pathways may influence the pain experience, as illustrated in Fig. 9.2.4.

A systematic review of central sensitization in urogynaecological CPP identified that generalized hyperalgesia is present in response to pressure and electrical stimuli in women with CPP, and that 'bottom-up' (excitatory) nociceptive mechanisms are overactive, as evidenced by enhanced reflex responses and temporal summation (Kaya et al., 2013). Evidence for central sensitization in this population was further supported by studies which demonstrated brain function and brain activation changes in women with CPP (Kaya et al., 2013). An expert consensus on pelvi-perineal pain proposed that central sensitization is the most important neural mechanism in chronic pelvic and perineal pain conditions (Levesque et al., 2018). MAPP data suggest the presence of a centralized pain phenotype in many patients with UCPPS, potentially characterized by central nervous system alterations or systemic pathologies

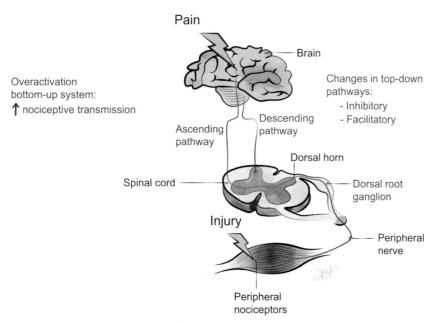

Fig. 9.2.4 Ascending and descending pathways that modulate the perception of pain.

(Clemens et al., 2019; Harte et al., 2019). However, in some patients with CPP the role of peripheral nervous system mechanisms appears important, with mechanisms including small fibre polyneuropathy (Chen et al., 2019). Efforts to understand the interplay between peripheral and central pain mechanisms in pelvic pain continue to emerge (Yong et al., 2020). Clearly, knowledge is evolving rapidly in this field.

As the IASP notes, *sensitization* is 'a neurophysiological term that can only be applied when both input and output of the neural system under study are known, [such as] by controlling the stimulus and measuring the neural event' (IASP, 2017). This is important to recognize, as the term *central sensitization* is currently applied to many patients who present with chronic pain who have not undergone neurophysiological testing. As direct electrophysiological recordings from central neurons are not an option in humans, it is advised that the term *central sensitization* should be used cautiously (Arendt-Nielsen et al., 2018). Nevertheless, Smart et al. (2011) have proposed that particular clusters of pain-related symptoms and clinical signs may be able to distinguish different pain mechanisms—nociceptive versus peripheral neuropathic versus central sensitization—as the primary pain mechanism in musculoskeletal pain. To acknowledge the uncertainty of the presence of central sensitization, some authors recommend alternative terms, such as *central sensitivity syndrome* or simply *nociplastic pain* (Van Griensven et al., 2020); further, Van Griensven et al. (2020) caution against using the term *central sensitization* synonymously with *psychological problems*, as the terms are not interchangeable. Depression and anxiety can have a direct influence on the nervous system and may influence central sensitization through descending modulation; however, central sensitization and psychology are distinct (Adams and Turk, 2015; van Griensven et al., 2020). This distinction is also recognized by pelvic pain researchers who identify hypersensitivity of the peripheral and central pain systems, dysfunctional pain modulation and psychological distress as different contributors to a dysfunctional pain system in patients with CPP syndromes (Grinberg et al., 2019), and the role of psychological factors in pain facilitation as uncertain (Kaya et al., 2013).

Measurement of Sensitization

In clinical practice, a variety of diagnostic surrogate markers, besides clinical history (e.g., intensity, character/modality, spatial and temporal characteristics, spontaneous/provoked, and possible exacerbating factors of the pain), are being used for assessment including questionnaires (e.g., neuropathic pain scales and pain features), simple bedside sensory testing (hypo- or hyper-phenomena, wind-up like pain and after-sensation) and mapping of areas with sensory abnormalities (Arendt-Nielsen et al., 2018). Although central sensitization screening questionnaires (e.g., the Central Sensitization Inventory [CSI] and Pain Sensitivity Questionnaire [PSQ]) have good clinical measurement properties, the construct validity of these tools as a measure of pain sensitivity has been questioned (Coronado and George, 2018), and therefore caution is required in the interpretation of these questionnaire results.

The nociceptive excitability of the nervous system may be measured by combining different quantitative assessment tools to achieve a proxy estimate of how the peripheral and central nervous system are functioning (gain or loss). Quantitative sensory testing is a way to evaluate the excitability of different pain pathways/mechanisms and involves a variety of stimulus modalities (Rolke et al., 2006). Positive findings from these tests are generally accepted as clinical correlates of central sensitization (Arendt-Nielsen et al., 2018), with hyperalgesia and allodynia frequently identified in patients with chronic pain conditions (Van Griensven et al., 2020). Hyperalgesia may be widespread, with contralateral and extrasegmental widespread pressure pain hyperalgesia found in chronic musculoskeletal (Staud et al., 2012) and visceral pain conditions (Xu et al., 2019). Hypersensitivity to both visceral (Fitzgerald et al., 2005; Giamberardino et al., 2014; Lowenstein et al., 2004) and somatic (Ness et al., 2005; Neziri et al., 2010) stimuli applied to referred and remote body areas have been reported in patients with BPS, together with impaired habituation to noxious stimuli at referred pain areas (Kaya et al., 2013; Lowenstein et al., 2009). Quantitative tools for assessing central gain in pain may also include measures of temporal summation, spatial summation and after-pain (Arendt-Nielsen et al., 2018). Prolonged pain 'after-sensation' has also been demonstrated in women with CPP and BPS compared to pain-free women (Hellman et al., 2015).

Pain Modulation

Conditioned pain modulation (CPM) is a measure of the efficacy of descending pain pathways, which have both facilitatory and inhibitory effects (Ramaswamy and Wodehouse, 2020). It is a central phenomenon and may be a surrogate measure of the central nervous system's capacity for activating endogenous analgesia, possibly via the descending tracts. Impaired descending

pain modulatory pathways are thought to contribute to the development and maintenance of central sensitization (Ramaswamy and Wodehouse, 2020). It has been proposed that pain modulation ranges from the inhibitory end (CPM) to the excitatory end, frequently measured by the repetition of a nociceptive stimuli to produce enhanced temporal summation responses (Yarnitsky et al., 2014). The differences in individuals in their inhibitory/facilitatory balance can be described on a clinical spectrum between 'pro-nociception' and 'antinociception' (Yarnitsky et al., 2014). An individual expressing low-efficiency CPM and/or enhanced temporal summation positioned on the pro-nociceptive side of the spectrum would express a higher pain phenotype, which may result in a higher risk to develop chronic pain (Ramaswamy and Wodehouse, 2020; Yarnitsky et al., 2014). A systematic review of central sensitization in women with CPP found that evidence for impaired CPM or 'top-down' mechanisms (pain inhibition or pain facilitation) was inconclusive, due to only two studies with conflicting results (Kaya et al., 2013). More recently however, a pro-nociceptive pain profile with both enhanced facilitation and inefficient inhibition, and which appeared to be common to both PVD and BPS, has been identified (Grinberg et al., 2017). Reduced CPM has been reported in patients with IC/BPS (Ness et al., 2014) and IBS (Wilder-Smith and Robert-Yap, 2007; Williams et al., 2013). However, the CPM paradigms show a large variability and are influenced by patient-related factors such as age, gender, hormones, race and genetic makeup; psychological factors including anxiety, depression and catastrophizing; methodological and procedural factors such as testing site, surface area/duration; nature of central sensitization and temporal summation; concurrent medications; and underlying medical problems including pre-existing chronic pain conditions (Ramaswamy and Wodehouse, 2020). Therefore, the clinical significance of these findings to the pain experience of the patient is not yet certain and further research is required.

Comorbidities and Cross-Talk

The term *chronic overlapping pain conditions* (COPCs) has been coined to describe the clinical state of significant overlap among chronic pain disorders (Maixner et al., 2016). The chronic visceral pain syndromes are the chronic pain conditions that are more frequently encountered in these clusters of COPCs (Aziz et al.,

2019). Clinical studies in patients with secondary visceral pain syndromes have demonstrated that comorbid pain conditions can potentially exacerbate each other; however, there is also evidence that in patients with COPCs, treatment of one chronic pain syndrome such as secondary visceral pain can result in improvement of another comorbid pain condition as well (Costantini et al., 2017; Giamberardino et al., 2015). It is therefore important, when evaluating patients presenting with chronic secondary visceral PF pain syndromes, to assess all concurrent chronic pain conditions as well. Prevalence studies indicate high overlap in pelvic visceral pain conditions such as BPS, PVD and IBS, as well as overlap between these visceral pain syndromes and PF myofascial pain syndromes (Bharucha and Trabuco, 2008; Chelimsky et al., 2019; Lai et al., 2019; Rodriguez et al., 2013). The shared characteristics of PFM abnormalities, a dysfunctional pain system and psychological distress observed in patients with PVD and BPS (Grinberg et al., 2017) may explain the common co-occurrence of CPP syndromes. The co-occurrence of visceral pelvic pain conditions may also be explained by pelvic organ cross-sensitization (Malykhina, 2007). Further, pelvic pain conditions may be modulated by both the visceral and somatic systems, making the differential diagnosis challenging. A model to describe the mechanisms behind the overlap between visceral and myofascial CPP syndromes has been proposed by Hoffman (2011). This model describes the inter-relationships among viscero-visceral convergence, viscero-somatic convergence, increased tone in the PFM creating visceral symptoms along with somato-visceral convergence and central sensitization with expansion of receptive fields, as illustrated in Fig. 9.2.5.

This neural complexity is appreciated when considering the dual innervation within the pelvis by the somatic (T12–S5) and visceral (T10–S5) nervous systems; together, these systems create a complex anatomical and neurobiological network (Origoni et al., 2014). The nerve supply to the female PFM and sphincters is illustrated in Fig. 9.2.6A, and the nerve supply to the female visceral organs is illustrated in Fig. 9.2.6B.

An additional characteristic that may further support the commonality of various CPP syndrome subgroups is psychological susceptibility to develop and maintain the pain condition. In one of the MAPP studies, participants with UCPPS reported more psychosocial difficulties, including higher levels of current and lifetime stress, poorer coping, and more self-reported cognitive deficits

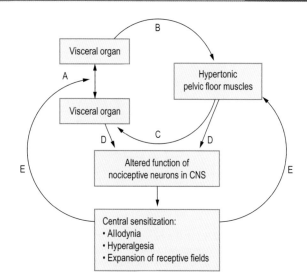

Fig. 9.2.5 Interconnected relationships of the viscera, pelvic floor muscles/myofascial structures and central nervous system (CNS) create the multisymptom presentation of chronic pelvic pain. Viscero-visceral, viscero-somatic and somato-visceral convergence are depicted by pathways A, B and C. Pathway D represents nociceptive inputs from viscera and/or myofascial sources leading to central sensitization. Pathway E represents central sensitization creating pain perception in either myofascial structures or a visceral organ. All can occur in a single patient, contributing to multiple seemingly unrelated symptoms. *(Reprinted from Hoffman (2011).)*

than healthy control individuals matched for age and sex who did not have pain (Naliboff et al., 2015). In addition, both sexes showed similar levels of psychosocial problems, although women had higher levels of childhood adversity and widespread discomfort than men (Naliboff et al., 2015). Further, the presence of non-urological COPCs in the UCPPS cohort was associated with higher rates of depression and anxiety, as well as greater UCPPS symptom severity (Krieger et al., 2015). Studies have reported that women with PVD experience impaired sexual functioning, increased pain catastrophizing, fear, hypervigilance, higher levels of depression and anxiety, and increased relationship dissatisfaction than controls (Desrochers et al., 2008; Pukall et al., 2016), and women with either CPP or BPS exhibit higher levels of psychological distress (Hellman et al., 2015).

Aetiological/Contributing or Associated Factors

Similar to many chronic pain conditions, the exact aetiology of chronic PF pain conditions is unknown. The

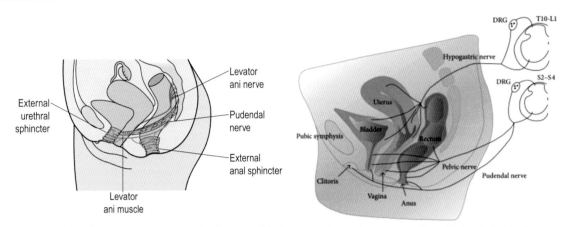

Fig. 9.2.6 (A) The nerve supply to the female pelvic floor muscles and sphincters. *From Vodusek (2014).* (B) The nerve supply to the female visceral organs. *DRG,* Dorsal root ganglion. *(Reprinted with permission from Jobling, P., O'Hara, K., & Hua, S. (2014). Female reproductive tract pain: targets, challenges, and outcomes. Frontiers in Pharmacology, vol. 5, article 17.)*

pain may persist following an acute presentation of idiopathic onset or persist after an initial identifiable disease/pathology has recovered yet the pain remains, as recognized in the IASP classification of chronic primary and chronic secondary pain syndromes. For this reason, many chronic PF pain syndromes are described according to their presumed contributing or associated factors, without certainty of causality. Chronic PF pain syndromes frequently share several characteristics, suggestive of musculoskeletal, neurological, urological, gynaecological, anorectal and psychological involvement. As the previous sections have addressed all of these except musculoskeletal, this next section will address properties related to PFM function, including PFM tenderness, pressure–pain thresholds, tone, contractility and relaxation (terms as defined elsewhere [Frawley et al., 2021]) that have been implicated as dysfunctional in patients with CPP syndromes. Only studies that compared cases with and without pelvic pain have been included, as normative data of PFM function are lacking.

When interpreting these findings, the reader needs to be aware of certain limitations in the certainty of the results: not all studies defined the CPP condition precisely, so the findings may not be generalizable to all chronic PF pain conditions; the clinimetric properties of the scales/tools used to measure PFM properties, particularly digital palpation, may be uncertain or may be surrogate measures of the property under measure, which may confound interpretation of the results; lack of blinding of patient pain status may introduce bias in assessor measures; and small sample sizes, which may fail to capture

the true 'normal' distribution of PFM properties and therefore fail to show a difference between groups. Further, despite evidence of statistical significance of differences between groups, it is important to know if clinically meaningful differences exist in these properties between patients with the CPP condition and pain-free controls before we consider the PFM finding dysfunctional, or whether differences are part of the spectrum of 'normal' PFM function with natural variation between individuals. Finally, no studies have yet determined whether the PFM properties observed pre-date the pelvic pain condition or are consequent to the onset of pelvic pain, and therefore the cause and effect of any observed changes are unknown. Much more research in this area is needed.

Pelvic Floor Muscle Tenderness

PF myofascial tenderness with palpation has been shown in numerous case–control studies, with results consistently indicating higher levels of tenderness in women with CPP than controls (Hellman et al., 2015; Loving et al., 2014; Montenegro et al., 2010; Tu et al., 2008) and men with CPP syndrome (Hetrick et al., 2003). Hellman et al. (2015) identified that digital palpation of PFM tenderness reasonably discriminated between women with CPP/BPS and pain-free controls.

The magnitude of palpation pain (tenderness on palpation) has been shown to correlate with pressure–pain thresholds and after-sensation, and therefore may be used by a physical therapist where quantitative sensory testing is unavailable (Hellman et al., 2015). Results of one of the MAPP studies that undertook

PFM examinations in cohorts of men and women with UCPPS demonstrated that PFM tenderness was more prevalent in cases with UCPPS (55%) than in patients with chronic fatigue syndrome (14.6%) or pain-free controls (10.5%), with no differences in PFM tenderness observed between men and women with UCPPS (Yang et al., 2018). This study indicated PFM tenderness as a phenotype, or characteristic of UCPPS. Several studies have found increased muscle tenderness throughout the pelvic muscles and PFMs in cases compared to controls, commonly obturator internus (Meister et al., 2018); for this reason, Meister et al. (2019) recommend a complete clinical assessment of myofascial pelvic pain that includes both levator ani and obturator internus muscle groups.

Pelvic Floor Muscle Pressure–Pain Threshold and Other Measures of Sensitization

Patient report of tenderness/sensitivity on digital palpation in response to a known quantum of applied pressure can be measured using algometry. Several studies have demonstrated higher sensitivity (lower pressure–pain threshold) in women with CPP compared to asymptomatic controls (Hellman et al., 2015; Loving et al., 2014). Cases with CPP also had prolonged pain sensation lasting after the pelvic examination (Hellman et al., 2015). This study found that the combination of pressure–pain thresholds and after-sensation were better than pressure–pain thresholds alone to discriminate between women with CPP/BPS and pain-free controls (Hellman et al., 2015). Pain lasting more than 10 minutes was observed in less than 2% of pain-free participants but in 20% of women with CPP/PBS. Differences were not found between CPP and BPS groups. The authors concluded that one-third of women with CPP/PBS have a phenotype of substantially reduced threshold for mechanical sensitivity ($0.8 \ kg/cm^2$) (Hellman et al., 2015). Lower pressure–pain thresholds have also been shown at body sites remote from the PFMs in women with CPP compared to controls (As-Sanie et al., 2013; Fuentes-Márquez et al., 2019), and in females and males with UCCPS compared to healthy controls (Harte et al., 2019). Deficits in endogenous pain modulation as measured by an objective physiological test have been shown in patients with BPS and PVD compared to controls, and these deficits were associated with pain on PFM palpation (Grinberg et al., 2017).

Pelvic Floor Muscle Tone

Understanding the involvement of increased PFM tone in CPP conditions is challenging because of the complexity of muscle tone physiology. In addition, the interpretation derived from each PFM tone assessment tool regarding the exact physiological property assessed is even more complex. Different tools may assess different properties of tone (e.g., passive resistance, stiffness, spasm, flexibility, relaxation), and each term has a slightly different meaning (Frawley et al., 2021). Further, different tools may assess different components of muscle tone (active/neurogenic vs passive/viscoelastic vs both) and different parts/layers of the PFM (superficial vs deep vs both), and some tools may measure a surrogate property of tone (e.g., morphometry) or intra-vaginal/anal pressure. The following studies are grouped by measurement method as an aid to interpreting homogeneity in findings. The pelvic pain population most frequently studied is PVD. Most studies have used electromyography (EMG) to assess the myoelectrical activity in the PFMs at rest, indicating the active component of resting tone. No difference between groups was found in three studies (Naess and Bø, 2015; Reissing et al., 2004; Van der Velde and Everaerd, 1999); however, all other studies detected higher resting tone or baseline instability using surface or intramuscular EMG in women with pelvic pain (Engman et al., 2004; Frasson et al., 2009; Gammoudi et al., 2016; Gentilcore-Saulnier et al., 2010; Glazer et al., 1998; Loving et al., 2014; Morin et al., 2017; Polpeta et al., 2012; Shafik and El-Sibai, 2002). One study investigated PFM tone in men with CPP syndrome and also demonstrated a higher resting baseline and increased instability at rest compared with pain-free men (Hetrick et al., 2006). It should be highlighted that these conflicting findings may be explained by the quality of the EMG system as well as confounding factors affecting the recorded signal amplitude, such as vaginal lubrication, positioning of electrodes relative to the muscles and properties of the vaginal tissues (Auchincloss and McLean, 2009; Besomi et al., 2020; Keshwani and McLean, 2015). For these reasons the comparison of absolute EMG amplitude values between subjects is not recommended (Auchincloss and McLean, 2009; Besomi et al., 2020; Keshwani and McLean, 2015).

Digital palpation is commonly used in clinical settings to assess PFM tone but has been criticized for its subjectivity and lack of sensitivity (Davidson et al., 2020). Assessment techniques commonly assess either passive resistance to compression or to stretch. Studies have referred to this property as hypertonicity, tension and spasm, among others. Studies using a variety of tone assessment scales all detected higher intra-vaginal resting tone in female patients with pain than pain-free controls (Dos Bispo et al., 2016; Gentilcore-Saulnier et al., 2010; Loving et al., 2014; Reissing et al., 2004; Reissing et al., 2005; Thibault-Gagnon et al., 2018), with the exception of one study that measured tone on a –9 to +9 scale (Hellman et al., 2015). In a study by Reissing et al. (2005), increased tone was found when using an intra-vaginal assessment but not using an intra-anal approach. In studies that defined the property of interest as 'flexibility' or 'relaxation', pelvic pain cases consistently demonstrated lower flexibility or reduced relaxation than controls (Gentilcore-Saulnier et al., 2010; Loving et al., 2014; Reissing et al., 2005; Thibault-Gagnon et al., 2018). One study assessed resting PFM tone in men with CPP syndrome and found increased resting tone and more frequent detection of spasm in levator ani and coccygeus muscles than in controls (Hetrick et al., 2003).

Dynamometry measurements of PFM stiffness, passive forces at fixed vaginal aperture and passive forces against the stretch of the speculum branches have shown higher initial passive resistance, higher passive elastic stiffness and reduced flexibility in women with PVD compared to controls (Morin et al., 2017). When using dynamometry alone, the resting parameters (e.g., forces and stiffness) reflect the summative contribution of the active and passive components of tone. Morin et al. (2017) combined dynamometry and EMG to investigate the relative contribution of the active and the passive components of tone in women with vulvodynia. They demonstrated that women with pain presented with higher EMG activation recorded during vaginal tissue elongation when compared to pain-free counterparts, providing evidence of neurogenic tone (Morin et al., 2017). This study also showed that women with pain who demonstrated a quiescent EMG signal during the tissue elongation phase had higher passive forces and greater tissue stiffness (Morin et al., 2017). Overall, these findings support the involvement of both active and passive components of PFM tone in women with pain. Myotonometry to assess the perineal layer of the PFMs showed higher stiffness values in women with PVD compared to controls in one study (Davidson et al., 2014). Intra-vaginal pressure manometry is a surrogate, or indirect, measure of PFM tone. One study detected a difference between women with and without PVD (Naess and Bø, 2015), whereas another study did not find a difference between groups (Polpeta et al., 2012). Imaging is also a surrogate measure of tone, reflecting the morphometry of the PFMs at rest. Various landmarks have been measured as indicators of PFM tone. As this tool uses an external probe on the perineum, it has a significant advantage in assessment of patients with pain, therefore preventing the potential bias due to pain elicited by the assessment. Using 4D ultrasound, a smaller levator hiatus area dimension at rest has been shown in two studies in women with vulvodynia compared to asymptomatic controls, suggestive of increased tone (Morin et al., 2014; Thibault-Gagnon et al., 2016). The smaller levator hiatus was related to a smaller anteroposterior hiatus diameter in two studies (McLean et al., 2016; Morin et al., 2014) and to a smaller transverse diameter in another study (Thibault-Gagnon et al., 2016). A larger levator plate angle was found in women with vulvodynia in two studies (McLean et al., 2016; Morin et al., 2014). A smaller anorectal angle was shown in women with pain compared to controls (Morin et al., 2014). However, this was not replicated in a smaller cohort (McLean et al., 2016; Thibault-Gagnon et al., 2016). One study found no differences in morphometry in nulliparous women with or without pelvic pain on any measure of 4D ultrasound at rest (Nesbitt-Hawes et al., 2018). The population targeted in this study may explain this discrepancy, as their sample may have included women with endometriosis, and chronicity of pain was not defined. One study used magnetic resonance imaging to investigate differences in morphometry between women with IC/BPS and controls, finding a smaller H-line and shorter puborectalis length (Ackerman et al., 2016).

Given the significant heterogeneity in assessment methods and complexities related to PFM tone, the results of a systematic review currently under way are eagerly awaited to further elucidate the involvement of PFM tone in women with pelvic pain (Kadah et al., 2020b). Further, the association between PFM tone and pelvic pain is also clinically relevant; the results of a systematic review currently under way on this topic will contribute important knowledge to this question (Kadah et al., 2020a).

Pelvic Floor Muscle Trigger Points

In the assessment of PF myofascial pain syndrome, several studies refer to the finding of 'trigger points' (Tough et al., 2007); however, there is no clear consensus of the definition and diagnostic criteria associated with trigger points (Bourgaize et al., 2019; Tough et al., 2007), and the theory of myofascial pain caused by trigger points is not universally accepted (Quintner et al., 2015). The paired criteria of tender points in taut bands and predicted or recognized pain referral form the most frequently cited combination of diagnostic criteria of a trigger point. Given that this is a 'composite' finding of two or more properties (tenderness/tender point, tone/tension at a specific location in the muscle, pain referral, etc.) that are quite different, and there is no scoring of how to rate the individual components into a combined score, we recommend rating all of the findings separately, using the terms *tenderness*, *tone* and so forth as defined in a recent standardization of terminology document (Frawley et al., 2021). This clarity of reporting findings will aid re-assessment following intervention, as tenderness may change but not muscle tone, and vice versa.

Pelvic Floor Muscle Contractility and Post-Contraction Relaxation Ability

The results of studies investigating PFM strength and post-contraction relaxation ability in patients with pelvic pain compared to pain-free controls are quite varied. Although used frequently in clinical practice, assessment using digital palpation and surface electromyography (sEMG) are limited in their ability to confirm between-patient comparisons. Poorer PFM contraction strength assessed using digital palpation was found in women with PVD (Reissing et al., 2004; Reissing et al., 2005) and in women with CPP (Loving et al., 2014) than in controls. In contrast, no difference in PFM strength, assessed using digital palpation, was found in women with CPP (Fitzgerald et al., 2011) or PVD (Gentilcore-Saulnier et al., 2010) and men with CPP syndrome (Hetrick et al., 2003) and controls. Using intra-vaginal pressure manometry, no difference in strength nor endurance was found in women with PVD compared to controls (Naess and Bø, 2015). Using sEMG, no difference was found at peak myoelectrical activity in women with PVD (Naess and Bø, 2015), vestibulitis or vaginismus (Engman et al., 2004), vulvodynia (Polpeta et al., 2012) and CPP (Tu et al., 2008). However, endurance

was found to be lower in several studies using sEMG in women with PVD (Naess and Bø, 2015), vulvodynia (Polpeta et al., 2012), vulvodynia/dyspareunia (Reissing et al., 2004), and vestibulitis or vaginismus (Engman et al., 2004). Poorer ability to relax or maintain relaxation in women with versus without pain was a consistent finding across studies, with the exception of one study in women with CPP that did not detect a difference in relaxation (Hellman et al., 2015).

Using dynamometry, an instrument that provides direct assessment of muscle contractile properties, reduced strength (10 seconds), endurance (60 seconds), decreased speed of contraction and an altered coordination as reflected by the number of contractions performed within 15 seconds were found in women with PVD compared to asymptomatic controls (Morin et al., 2017). Changes in levator ani morphology on PFM contraction have been shown using transperineal ultrasound, with smaller changes in levator hiatus area narrowing, displacement of the bladder neck, and changes of the anorectal and levator plate angles found in women with PVD compared with controls (Morin et al., 2014). In contrast, another study with a smaller sample size found no difference between levator plate length and levator plate angle assessed using transperineal ultrasound during maximum voluntary contraction in women with PVD compared to controls (McLean et al., 2016), possibly due to lack of statistical power for the comparisons undertaken.

Fewer studies have investigated PFM contractility and relaxation ability in men. Hetrick et al. (2006) observed reduced ability to maintain relaxation during the sEMG rest phase in males with CPP syndrome compared to pain-free males. Overall, findings of differences in PFM strength in patients with versus without pelvic pain are not consistent, and a systematic review would give clarity to this question.

The emerging understanding of the complexity of chronic PF pain conditions means that much more research is needed to inform clinical management of these conditions with greater certainty than we currently have. As there is considerable uncertainty regarding which patients, with which pain condition(s), with which pain profiles—alterations in either excitatory or inhibitory or both pathways—and which phenotypes, or with what degree of associated comorbidities, will respond to which type of treatment or combinations of treatments, a careful and comprehensive assessment of each patient presenting with chronic PF pain is required.

MANAGEMENT

An appreciation of the complexity of chronic PF pain as described previously provides the rationale for the application of a biopsychosocial approach to management of this condition. A biopsychosocial approach does not necessarily require a multidisciplinary team, but it does require a physical therapist to think beyond biomedical contributors to pain, to involve other disciplines in management when required and to ensure that the process is patient/person centred. Physical therapy management of PF pain includes assessment (history, physical examination and investigations), diagnosis, formulation of a treatment plan and prognosis, and ongoing reassessment, as presented in Box 9.2.1. Management should be undertaken by a physical therapist who is competent in PF physical therapy, include informed consent, and adhere to local policies and procedures that govern infection control and intimate assessment procedures (Frawley et al., 2019). In addition to pain, a patient may present with concomitant symptoms of PF dysfunction (i.e., bladder, bowel or sexual dysfunction). Physical therapists should be guided by evidence-based clinical practice guidelines, or best available evidence, in their management of all aspects of PF dysfunction.

Framework of Assessment Leading to Diagnostic Decision Making and Clinical Reasoning

Assessment follows a logical and comprehensive process and involves clinical reasoning at each step. Standardization of terminology documents provides a useful guide as to the breadth and depth of assessment and treatment aspects to consider (Bø et al., 2017; Doggweiler et al., 2017; Frawley et al., 2021; Rogers et al., 2018; Sultan et al., 2017). The history, an understanding of the experience of pain for that individual patient, an understanding of pain mechanisms, the findings of a biopsychosocial assessment and a knowledge of evidence to support different conservative therapies should inform treatment. Pre-assessment screening may indicate the need for referral to another healthcare provider before

physical therapy assessment commences, such as if psychosocial distress is significant and beyond the scope of practice of that physical therapist. Alternatively, multidisciplinary input may be required concurrently with physical therapy management to achieve the optimal outcome for the patient.

Assessment should include components of the International Classification of Functioning, Disability and Health framework (ICF), such as body functions, body structures, impairments, activity and participation (World Health Organization, 2001). The IASP has proposed a core set of functioning properties to assess in all patients with chronic primary and chronic secondary pain: energy and drive, emotional functions, sensation of pain, sleep, attention, exercise tolerance, joint mobility, muscle power, performing one's daily routine, walking, moving around, remunerative employment, lifting and carrying objects, intimate relationships, recreation and leisure, individual attitudes of immediate family members, social security services, systems, and policies (Nugraha et al., 2019).

Assessment of bladder, bowel and sexual dysfunction that may accompany chronic PF pain are covered elsewhere in this book. The following text will refer to assessment of musculoskeletal structures that may be implicated in the aetiology or contributing to the maintenance of chronic PF pain. These elements can be assessed within a general diagnostic decision-making framework as presented in Box 9.2.1, although it is acknowledged that experienced clinicians may take a more heuristic approach.

SUMMARY

Chronic PF pain is a complex condition or range of conditions/syndromes. The exact aetiology of each subset of chronic PF pain is unclear but may involve neurological, urological, gynaecological, anorectal and musculoskeletal causes. An understanding of chronic pain mechanisms and the contribution of psychosocial factors to the patient presentation is critical. Research is accumulating and requires the clinician to remain as informed as possible regarding new developments in this field. A patient presenting with chronic PF pain requires careful assessment to inform an evidence-based treatment plan to maximize patient outcome.

BOX 9.2.1 Framework for Management of Chronic Pelvic Floor Pain

A. Pre-consultation screening: A clinician may ask a patient to complete pre-attendance questionnaires for the purpose of triaging a referral or collecting patient-reported data. Often screening focuses on psychological and social factors, and the presence of significant psychological and social factors should be documented (Treede et al., 2019). Psychological factors include cognitive (e.g., catastrophizing or worry and rumination), behavioural (e.g., avoidance or endurance) and emotional (e.g., fear or anger). Social factors refer to the impact of chronic pain on the relationship with others and vice versa. Details of psychosocial distress should be recorded when psychological and social factors are judged to contribute to the onset, the maintenance or exacerbations of pain or are regarded as relevant consequences of the pain. Commonly used questionnaires to assess psychosocial distress and pain in pelvic floor (PF) pain studies include the Central Sensitization Inventory (CSI) (Neblett, 2018), Pain Sensitivity Questionnaire (PSQ) (Sellers et al., 2013), Pain Catastrophizing Scale (PCS) (Severeijns et al., 2001), Positive and Negative Affect Schedule (PANAS) (Watson et al., 1988), Pain Self-Efficacy Questionnaire (PSEQ-2) (Nicholas et al., 2015), Depression Anxiety Stress Scale 21 (DASS-21) (Osman et al., 2012), Brief Symptom Inventory (BSI) (Derogatis and Melisaratos, 1983) and Beck Depression Inventory-II (BDI-II) (Wang and Gorenstein, 2013), among others. Screening may also cover elements of general health and medical history, the core set of functioning properties (as described earlier [Nugraha et al., 2019]), quality of life and impact of pain measures (Ghai et al., 2020).

B. Assessment:

1. Symptoms and history: Include current symptoms, noting any PF-related symptoms predating the onset of pain, treatment sought and response to treatment. Include relevant patient-reported outcome measures to use in re-assessment. In all chronic pain conditions, the International Association for the Study of Pain recommends recording pain severity and its temporal course, as follows (Treede et al., 2019). The severity of chronic pain may be determined as a compound measure of pain intensity, as well as pain-related distress and task interference. Pain intensity denotes the strength of the patient's pain experience ('How much does it hurt?'). Pain-related distress is the multifactorial unpleasant emotional experience of a psychological (cognitive, behavioural and emotional), social or spiritual nature because of the persistent or recurrent experience of pain ('How distressed are you by the pain?'). Pain-related inter-

ference describes how much the pain interferes with daily activities and participation ('How much does the pain interfere with your life?'). Each of the severity determinants (intensity, pain-related distress and interference) is rated by the patient on a numerical rating scale from 0 to 10 and then transformed into severity stages of 'mild', 'moderate' and 'severe' (Treede et al., 2019). Temporal characteristics can be coded as continuous pain, episodic recurrent pain and continuous pain with pain attacks.

2. Details of current and past general health not included in section A:

   • At this point, the physical therapist may formulate differential diagnoses of the patient's main presenting problem, informed by clinical reasoning, to be further tested in clinical evaluation.

3. Clinical signs, detected via visual observation, physical inspection and simple tests: Care should be taken to ensure that the patient fully understands the components of the physical examination, and her or his right to withdraw consent. The examination will focus on the differential diagnoses the clinician suspects, based on the history and symptoms, and may include:

   a. PF assessment per perineal, per vaginal and/or per rectal examination, as indicated: Digital palpation must be performed gently, with due recognition of the presence of any sensitivity and patient apprehension which may limit assessment. Assessment will include aspects of pelvic floor muscle (PFM) function, such as tenderness/tender points, resting tone, contractility (strength, endurance), relaxation ability and organ support with rises in intra-abdominal pressure. Definitions of these terms and descriptions of how to assess and rate the finding were published recently (Frawley et al., 2021). All PFM properties should be measured very carefully, using a method/tool with the strongest clinimetric properties that the physical therapist has available. Include relevant clinician-reported outcome measures to use in re-assessment.

   b. Musculoskeletal structures beyond the PF, both intra- and extrapelvic: Details of these assessments are beyond the scope of this chapter.

      • At this point, the physical therapist will refine the differential diagnoses, informed by clinical reasoning, to be further tested with investigations, if available.

C. Investigations: These may include assessment of bladder, vaginal and bowel function where indicated or tolerated, and assessment of PFM function using quantitative sensory testing (e.g., algometry), electro-

Continued

BOX 9.2.1   Framework for Management of Chronic Pelvic Floor Pain—cont'd

myography, dynamometry, myotonometry, manometry or ultrasound imaging, as indicated or tolerated. Include relevant instrumented outcome measures to use in re-assessment.

- At this point, the physical therapist will identify a primary diagnosis, informed by clinical reasoning, which may change if further information becomes available or response to treatment does not support the primary diagnosis.

D. Diagnosis: The diagnosis is arrived at through a process of clinical reasoning and evidence-based decision making informed by knowledge of the condition and biopsychosocial assessment findings from that patient. Based on assessment findings, a particular PF pain condition/syndrome may be identifiable, such as provoked vestibulodynia, bladder pain syndrome, urological chronic pelvic pain syndrome, irritable bowel syndrome or PF tension myalgia. Alternatively, if the exact end organ is unclear, a higher-level diagnosis, such as chronic primary or chronic secondary PF pain, visceral or musculoskeletal (Treede et al., 2019), may be identified.

E. Treatment plan: Treatment underpinned by an evidence-based treatment plan (Haynes et al., 2002) will maximize the chance of a successful outcome. Evidence from randomized controlled trials to inform the choice of therapies to treat chronic PF pain is emerging (see Chapter 9.3), although many uncertainties remain. A collaborative approach will take into account patient preferences and, for the individual patient, will engender a sense of control over her own health. The quality of the patient–therapist relationship, often called *therapeutic alliance*, may confer therapeutic effects that are above and beyond the known influence of the therapies on pain (Bardin et al., 2020; Kinney et al., 2020). The patient may write a list of her or his own treatment goals, which the physical therapist can cross-check against the treatment plan, to ensure that the treatment plan is congruent with the patient's expectations. Treatment will likely include both in-clinic, therapist-supervised sessions and at home, patient-directed sessions. The physical therapist should try to formulate a prognosis of likely response to therapy, based on evidence from research, clinical expertise, and patient uptake and adherence to proposed therapy. Consider the role of other clinicians in the care of the patient (e.g., psychologist/pain physician).

F. Re-assessment: The physical therapist should re-assess progress and response to treatment to ensure that initial diagnosis is still correct and initial prognosis is achievable. Slow or non-response should trigger a re-assessment, and an alternative treatment plan may be required. In-clinic re-assessment frequency and length of supervised treatment will be determined by individual patient, therapist and health system factors.

REFERENCES

Ackerman, A. L., Lee, U. J., Jellison, F. C., et al. (2016). MRI suggests increased tonicity of the levator ani in women with interstitial cystitis/bladder pain syndrome. *International Urogynecology Journal, 27,* 77–83.

Adams, L. M., & Turk, D. C. (2015). Psychosocial factors and central sensitivity syndromes. *Current Rheumatology Reviews, 11,* 96–108.

An@tomedia. (2000). *An@tomedia: A new approach to medical education, developments in anatomy [online].* Available: https://anatomedia.com (Accessed 23.07.22).

Arendt-Nielsen, L., Morlion, B., Perrot, S., et al. (2018). Assessment and manifestation of central sensitisation across different chronic pain conditions. *European Journal of Pain, 22,* 216–241.

As-Sanie, S., Harris, R. E., Harte, S. E., et al. (2013). Increased pressure pain sensitivity in women with chronic pelvic pain. *Obstetrics & Gynecology, 122,* 1047–1055.

Auchincloss, C. C., & McLean, L. (2009). The reliability of surface EMG recorded from the pelvic floor muscles. *Journal of Neuroscience Methods, 182*(1), 85–96.

Aziz, Q., Giamberardino, M. A., Barke, A., et al. (2019). The IASP classification of chronic pain for ICD-11: Chronic secondary visceral pain. *Pain, 160,* 69–76.

Bardin, M., Brassard, A., Dumoulin, C., et al. (2020). Examining the role of the physiotherapist in treatment response of women with provoked vestibulodynia. *Neurourology and Urodynamics, 39,* 37–38.

Bergeron, S., Reed, B. D., Wesselmann, U., et al. (2020). Vulvodynia. *Nature Reviews Diseases Primers, 6,* 36.

Berry, S. H., Elliott, M. N., Suttorp, M., et al. (2011). Prevalence of symptoms of bladder pain syndrome/interstitial cystitis among adult females in the United States. *Journal Urology, 186,* 540–544.

Besomi, M., Hodges, P. W., Clancy, E. A., et al. (2020). Consensus for experimental design in electromyography (CEDE) project: Amplitude normalization matrix. *Journal of Electromyography and Kinesiology, 53,* 102438.

Bharucha, A. E., & Trabuco, E. (2008). Functional and chronic anorectal and pelvic pain disorders. *Gastroenterol. Clinical North American, 37* 685, ix.

Bø, K., Frawley, H. C., Haylen, B. T., et al. (2017). An International Urogynecological Association (IUGA)/

International Continence Society (ICS) joint report on the terminology for the conservative and nonpharmacological management of female pelvic floor dysfunction. *Neurourology and Urodynamics, 36,* 221–244.

Bornstein, J., Preti, M., Simon, J. A., et al. (2019). Descriptors of vulvodynia: A multisocietal definition consensus (international society for the study of vulvovaginal disease, the international society for the study of women sexual health, and the international pelvic pain society). *Journal of Lower Genital Tract Disease, 23,* 161–163.

Bourgaize, S., Janjua, I., Murnaghan, K., et al. (2019). Fibromyalgia and myofascial pain syndrome: Two sides of the same coin? A scoping review to determine the lexicon of the current diagnostic criteria. *Musculoskeletal Care, 17,* 3–12.

Chalmers, K. J., & Madden, V. J. (2019). Shifting beliefs across society would lay the foundation for truly biopsychosocial care. *Journal of Physiotherapy, 65,* 121–122.

Chelimsky, G. G., Yang, S., Sanses, T., et al. (2019). Autonomic neurophysiologic implications of disorders comorbid with bladder pain syndrome vs myofascial pelvic pain. *Neurourology and Urodynamics, 38,* 1370–1377.

Chen, A., De, E., & Argoff, C. (2019). Small fiber polyneuropathy is prevalent in patients experiencing complex chronic pelvic pain. *Pain Medicine, 20,* 521–527.

Clemens, J. Q., Mullins, C., Ackerman, A. L., et al. (2019). Urologic chronic pelvic pain syndrome: Insights from the MAPP research network. *Nature Reviews Urology, 16,* 187–200.

Coronado, R. A., & George, S. Z. (2018). The central sensitization inventory and pain sensitivity questionnaire: An exploration of construct validity and associations with widespread pain sensitivity among individuals with shoulder pain. *Musculoskeletal Science and Practice, 36,* 61–67.

Costantini, R., Affaitati, G., Wesselmann, U., et al. (2017). Visceral pain as a triggering factor for fibromyalgia symptoms in comorbid patients. *Pain, 158,* 1925–1937.

Daniels, N. A., Link, C. L., Barry, M. J., et al. (2007). Association between past urinary tract infections and current symptoms suggestive of chronic prostatitis/chronic pelvic pain syndrome. *Journal of the National Medical Association, 99,* 509–516.

Davidson, M., Bryant, A., & Frawley, H. (2014). Perineal muscle stiffness in women with and without vulvodynia: Reliability of measurement and differences in muscle stiffness. *Neurourology and Urodynamics, 33,* 709–710.

Davidson, M. J., Nielsen, P. M. F., Taberner, A. J., et al. (2020). Is it time to rethink using digital palpation for assessment of muscle stiffness? *Neurourology and Urodynamics, 39,* 279–285.

Derogatis, L. R., & Melisaratos, N. (1983). The brief symptom inventory: An introductory report. *Psychological Medicine, 13,* 595–605.

Desrochers, G., Bergeron, S., Landry, T., et al. (2008). Do psychosexual factors play a role in the etiology of provoked vestibulodynia? A critical review. *Journal of Sex & Marital Therapy, 34,* 198–226.

Doggweiler, R., Whitmore, K. E., Meijlink, J. M., et al. (2017). A standard for terminology in chronic pelvic pain syndromes: A report from the chronic pelvic pain working group of the international continence society. *Neurourology and Urodynamics, 36,* 984–1008.

Dos Bispo, A. P., Ploger, C., Loureiro, A. F., et al. (2016). Assessment of pelvic floor muscles in women with deep endometriosis. *Archives of Gynecology and Obstetrics, 294,* 519–523.

Eizenberg, N. (2015). *General anatomy: Principles and applications.* Sydney, Australia: McGraw-Hill Education.

Engel, G. L. (1977). The need for a new medical model: A challenge for biomedicine. *Science, 196,* 129–136.

Engeler, D., Baranowski, A., Berghmans, B., et al. (2020). *EAU guidelines on chronic pelvic pain [online].* Available: https://uroweb.org/guidelines/chronic-pelvic-pain (Accessed 23.07.22).

Engman, M., Lindehammar, H., & Wijma, B. (2004). Surface electromyography diagnostics in women with partial vaginismus with or without vulvar vestibulitis and in asymptomatic women. *Journal of Psychosomatic Obstetrics and Gynaecology, 25,* 281–294.

Fitzgerald, C. M., Neville, C. E., Mallinson, T., et al. (2011). Pelvic floor muscle examination in female chronic pelvic pain. *Journal of Reproductive Medicine, 56,* 117–122.

Fitzgerald, M. P., Koch, D., & Senka, J. (2005). Visceral and cutaneous sensory testing in patients with painful bladder syndrome. *Neurourology and Urodynamics, 24,* 627–632.

Frasson, E., Graziottin, A., Priori, A., et al. (2009). Central nervous system abnormalities in vaginismus. *Clinical Neurophysiology, 120,* 117–122.

Frawley, H., Neumann, P., & Delany, C. (2019). An argument for competency-based training in pelvic floor physiotherapy practice. *Physiotherapy Theory and Practice, 35,* 1117–1130.

Frawley, H., Shelly, B., Morin, M., et al. (2021). An International Continence Society (ICS) report on the terminology for pelvic floor muscle assessment. *Neurourology and Urodynamics, 40*(5), 1217–1260.

Fuentes-Márquez, P., Valenza, M. C., Cabrera-Martos, I., et al. (2019). Trigger points, pressure pain hyperalgesia, and mechanosensitivity of neural tissue in women with chronic pelvic pain. *Pain Medicine, 20,* 5–13.

Gammoudi, N., Affes, Z., Mellouli, S., et al. (2016). The diagnosis value of needle electrode electromyography in vaginismus. *Sexologies, 25,* e57–e60.

Gatchel, R. J. (2004). Comorbidity of chronic pain and mental health disorders: The biopsychosocial perspective. *American Psychologist, 59,* 795–805.

Gatchel, R. J., Peng, Y. B., Peters, M. L., et al. (2007). The bio-psychosocial approach to chronic pain: Scientific advances and future directions. *Psychological Bulletin, 133*, 581–624.

Gentilcore-Saulnier, E., McLean, L., Goldfinger, C., et al. (2010). Pelvic floor muscle assessment outcomes in women with and without provoked vestibulodynia and the impact of a physical therapy program. *The Journal of Sexual Medicine, 7*(2 Pt. 2), 1003–1022.

Ghai, V., Subramanian, V., Jan, H., et al. (2020). A systematic review on reported outcomes and outcome measures in female idiopathic chronic pelvic pain for the development of a core outcome set. *British Journal of Obstetrics and Gynaecology, 128*(4), 628–634.

Giamberardino, M. A., Affaitati, G., Martelletti, P., et al. (2015). Impact of migraine on fibromyalgia symptoms. *The Journal of Headache and Pain, 17*, 28.

Giamberardino, M. A., Tana, C., & Costantini, R. (2014). Pain thresholds in women with chronic pelvic pain. *Current Opinion in Obstetrics and Gynecology, 26*, 253–259.

Glazer, H. I., Jantos, M., Hartmann, E. H., et al. (1998). Electromyographic comparisons of the pelvic floor in women with dysesthetic vulvodynia and asymptomatic women. *Journal of Reproductive Medicine, 43*, 959–962.

Grinberg, K., Granot, M., Lowenstein, L., et al. (2017). A common pronociceptive pain modulation profile typifying subgroups of chronic pelvic pain syndromes is interrelated with enhanced clinical pain. *Pain, 158*, 1021–1029.

Grinberg, K., Weissman-Fogel, I., Lowenstein, L., et al. (2019). How does myofascial physical therapy attenuate pain in chronic pelvic pain syndrome? *Pain Research and Management, 2019*, 6091257.

Harlow, B. L., Kunitz, C. G., Nguyen, R. H., et al. (2014). Prevalence of symptoms consistent with a diagnosis of vulvodynia: Population-based estimates from 2 geographic regions. *American Journal of Obstetrics and Gynecology, 210*, 40.e1–40.e8.

Harte, S. E., Schrepf, A., Gallop, R., et al. (2019). Quantitative assessment of nonpelvic pressure pain sensitivity in urologic chronic pelvic pain syndrome: A MAPP research network study. *Pain, 160*, 1270–1280.

Haynes, R. B., Devereaux, P. J., & Guyatt, G. H. (2002). Clinical expertise in the era of evidence-based medicine and patient choice. *ACP Journal Club, 136*(2), A11–A14.

Hellman, K. M., Patanwala, I. Y., Pozolo, K. E., et al. (2015). Multimodal nociceptive mechanisms underlying chronic pelvic pain. *American Journal of Obstetrics and Gynecology, 213*(6), 827.e1–827.e9.

Hetrick, D. C. (2006). Pelvic floor electromyography in men with chronic pelvic pain syndrome: A case–control study. *Neurourology and Urodynamics, 25*, 46–49.

Hetrick, D. C., Ciol, M. A., Rothman, I., et al. (2003). Musculoskeletal dysfunction in men with chronic pelvic pain syndrome type III: A case–control study. *Journal Urology, 170*, 828–831.

Hetrick, D. C., Glazer, H., Liu, Y.-W., et al. (2006). Pelvic floor electromyography in men with chronic pelvic pain syndrome: A case–control study. *Neurourology and Urodynamics, 25*, 46–49.

Hoffman, D. (2011). Understanding multisymptom presentations in chronic pelvic pain: The inter-relationships between the viscera and myofascial pelvic floor dysfunction. *Current Pain and Headache Reports, 15*, 343–346.

Institute of Medicine. (2011). *Relieving pain in America: A blueprint for transforming prevention, care, education, and research*. Washington, DC: National Academies Press.

International Association for the Study of Pain. (2017). *IASP terminology*. Updated From Part III: December 14, 2017, Edition [Online]. Available: https://www.iasp-pain.org/resources/terminology/#Sensitisation. (Accessed 23.07.22).

Kadah, S., Schneider, M., Morin, M., et al. (2020a). *The association between pelvic pain and pelvic floor muscle tone in women: A systematic review* [online]. Available: https://www.crd.york.ac.uk/prospero/display_record.php?RecordID=139584. (Accessed 23.07.22).

Kadah, S., Schneider, M., Morin, M., et al. (2020b). *Differences in pelvic floor muscle tone between women with and without pelvic pain: A systematic review* [online]. Available: https://www.crd.york.ac.uk/prospero/display_record.php?RecordID=175785. (Accessed 23.07.22).

Kaya, S., Hermans, L., Willems, T., et al. (2013). Central sensitization in urogynecological chronic pelvic pain: A systematic literature review. *Pain Physician, 16*, 291–308.

Keshwani, N., & McLean, l. (2015). State of the art review: Intravaginal probes for recording electromyography from the pelvic floor muscles. *Neurourology and Urodynamics, 34*, 104–112.

Kinney, M., Seider, J., Beaty, A. F., et al. (2020). The impact of therapeutic alliance in physical therapy for chronic musculoskeletal pain: A systematic review of the literature. *Physiotherapy Theory and Practice, 36*, 886–898.

Kosek, E., Cohen, M., Baron, R., et al. (2016). Do we need a third mechanistic descriptor for chronic pain states? *Pain, 157*, 1382–1386.

Krieger, J. N., Stephens, A. J., Landis, J. R., et al. (2015). Relationship between chronic nonurological associated somatic syndromes and symptom severity in urological chronic pelvic pain syndromes: Baseline evaluation of the MAPP study. *Journal Urology, 193*, 1254–1262.

Lacy, B. E., & Patel, N. K. (2017). Rome criteria and a diagnostic approach to irritable bowel syndrome. *Journal of Clinical Medicine, 6*(11), 99.

Lai, H. H., Thu, J. H. L., Moh, F. V., et al. (2019). Clustering of patients with interstitial cystitis/bladder pain syndrome and chronic prostatitis/chronic pelvic pain syndrome. *Journal Urology*, 202, 546–551.

Lamvu, G., Nguyen, R. H., Burrows, L. J., et al. (2015). The evidence-based vulvodynia assessment project. A national registry for the study of vulvodynia. *Journal of Reproductive Medicine*, 60, 223–235.

Landis, J. R., Williams, D. A., Lucia, M. S., et al. (2014). The MAPP research network: Design, patient characterization and operations. *BMC Urology*, 14, 58.

Levesque, A., Riant, T., Ploteau, S., et al. (2018). Clinical criteria of central sensitization in chronic pelvic and perineal pain (convergences PP criteria): Elaboration of a clinical evaluation tool based on formal expert consensus. *Pain Medicine*, 19, 2009–2015.

Loving, S., Thomsen, T., Jaszczak, P., et al. (2014). Pelvic floor muscle dysfunctions are prevalent in female chronic pelvic pain: A cross-sectional population-based study. *European Journal of Pain*, 18, 1259–1270.

Lowenstein, L., Kenton, K., Mueller, E. R., et al. (2009). Patients with painful bladder syndrome have altered response to thermal stimuli and catastrophic reaction to painful experiences. *Neurourology and Urodynamics*, 28, 400–404.

Lowenstein, L., Vardi, Y., Deutsch, M., et al. (2004). Vulvar vestibulitis severity—assessment by sensory and pain testing modalities. *Pain*, 107, 47–53.

Maixner, W., Fillingim, R. B., Williams, D. A., et al. (2016). Overlapping chronic pain conditions: Implications for diagnosis and classification. *The Journal of Pain*, 17, t93–t107.

Malykhina, A. P. (2007). Neural mechanisms of pelvic organ cross-sensitization. *Neuroscience*, 149, 660–672.

MAPP. (2021). *Multi-disciplinary approach to the study of chronic pelvic pain research network [online]*. Available: http://www.mappnetwork.org/. (Accessed 23.07.21).

Mardian, A. S., Hanson, E. R., Villarroel, L., et al. (2020). Flipping the pain care model: A sociopsychobiological approach to high-value chronic pain care. *Pain Medicine*, 21, 1168–1180.

McLean, l., Thibault-Gagnon, S., Brooks, K., et al. (2016). Differences in pelvic morphology between women with and without provoked vestibulodynia. *The Journal of Sexual Medicine*, 13, 963–971.

Meister, M. R., Shivakumar, N., Sutcliffe, S., et al. (2018). Physical examination techniques for the assessment of pelvic floor myofascial pain: A systematic review. *American Journal of Obstetrics and Gynecology*, 219(5), 497.e1–497.e13.

Meister, M. R., Sutcliffe, S., Ghetti, C., et al. (2019). Development of a standardized, reproducible screening examination for assessment of pelvic floor myofascial pain. *American Journal of Obstetrics and Gynecology*, 220(3), 255.e1–255.e9.

Montenegro, M. L. L. D.S., Mateus-Vasconcelos, E. C. L., Rosa e Silva, J. C., et al. (2010). Importance of pelvic muscle tenderness evaluation in women with chronic pelvic pain. *Pain Medicine*, 11, 224–228.

Morales-Solchaga, G., Zubiaur-Libano, C., Peri-Cusi, L., et al. (2019). Bladder pain syndrome: Prevalence and routine clinical practice in women attending functional urology and urodynamics units in Spain. *Actas Urológicas Españolas*, 43, 62–70.

Morin, M., Bergeron, S., Khalife, S., et al. (2014). Morphometry of the pelvic floor muscles in women with and without provoked vestibulodynia using 4D ultrasound. *The Journal of Sexual Medicine*, 11, 776–785.

Morin, M., Binik, Y. M., Bourbonnais, D., et al. (2017). Heightened pelvic floor muscle tone and altered contractility in women with provoked vestibulodynia. *The Journal of Sexual Medicine*, 14, 592–600.

Naess, I., & Bø, K. (2015). Pelvic floor muscle function in women with provoked vestibulodynia and asymptomatic controls. *International Urogynecology Journal*, 26, 1467–1473.

Naliboff, B. D., Stephens, A. J., Afari, N., et al. (2015). Widespread psychosocial difficulties in men and women with urologic chronic pelvic pain syndromes: Case–control findings from the multidisciplinary approach to the study of chronic pelvic pain research network. *Urology*, 85(6), 1319–1327.

Neblett, R. (2018). The central sensitization inventory: A user's manual. *Journal of Applied Biobehavioral Research*, 23(2), e12123.

Nesbitt-Hawes, E. M., Dietz, H. P., & Abbott, J. A. (2018). Morphometry of the nulliparous pelvic floor. *Ultrasound in Obstetrics and Gynecology*, 52, 672–676.

Ness, T. J., Lloyd, L. K., & Fillingim, R. B. (2014). An endogenous pain control system is altered in subjects with interstitial cystitis. *Journal Urology*, 191, 364–370.

Ness, T. J., Powell-Boone, T., Cannon, R., et al. (2005). Psychophysical evidence of hypersensitivity in subjects with interstitial cystitis. *Journal Urology*, 173, 1983–1987.

Neziri, A. Y., Haesler, S., Petersen-Felix, S., et al. (2010). Generalized expansion of nociceptive reflex receptive fields in chronic pain patients. *Pain*, 151, 798–805.

Nicholas, M. K., McGuire, B. E., & Asghari, A. (2015). A 2-item short form of the pain self-efficacy questionnaire: Development and psychometric evaluation of PSEQ-2. *The Journal of Pain*, 16, 153–163.

Nugraha, B., Gutenbrunner, C., Barke, A., et al. (2019). The IASP classification of chronic pain for ICD-11: Functioning properties of chronic pain. *Pain*, 160, 88–94.

Oats, J, & Boyle, J. (2023). Llewellyn-Jones Fundamentals of Obstetrics and Gynaecology, Eleventh Edition. Elsevier Ltd.

Oka, P., Parr, H., Barberio, B., et al. (2020). Global prevalence of irritable bowel syndrome according to Rome III or IV criteria: A systematic review and meta-analysis. *Lancet Gastroenterol Hepatology*, 5, 908.

Origoni, M., Leone Roberti Maggiore, U., Salvatore, S., et al. (2014). Neurobiological mechanisms of pelvic pain. *BioMed Research International*, 2014, 903848.

Osman, A., Wong, J. L., Bagge, C. L., et al. (2012). The depression anxiety stress scales-21 (DASS-21): Further examination of dimensions, scale reliability, and correlates. *Journal of Clinical Psychology*, 68, 1322–1338.

Perrot, S., Cohen, M., Barke, A., et al. (2019). The IASP classification of chronic pain for ICD-11: Chronic secondary musculoskeletal pain. *Pain*, 160, 77–82.

Polpeta, N. C., Giraldo, P. C., Juliato, C. R., et al. (2012). Electromyography and vaginal pressure of the pelvic floor muscles in women with recurrent vulvovaginal candidiasis and vulvodynia. *Journal of Reproductive Medicine*, 57, 141–147.

Pukall, C. F., Goldstein, A. T., Bergeron, S., et al. (2016). Vulvodynia: Definition, prevalence, impact, and pathophysiological factors. *The Journal of Sexual Medicine*, 13, 291–304.

Quaghebeur, J., & Wyndaele, J. J. (2015). Prevalence of lower urinary tract symptoms and level of quality of life in men and women with chronic pelvic pain. *Scand Journal Urology*, 49, 242–249.

Quintner, J. L., Bove, G. M., & Cohen, M. L. (2015). A critical evaluation of the trigger point phenomenon. *Rheumatology*, 54, 392–399.

Raja, S. N., Carr, D. B., Cohen, M., et al. (2020). The revised International Association for the Study of Pain definition of pain: concepts, challenges, and compromises. *Pain*, 161, 1976–1982.

Ramaswamy, S., & Wodehouse, T. (2020). Conditioned pain modulation—a comprehensive review. *Neurophysiologie Clinique*, 51(3), 197–208.

Reissing, E. D., Binik, Y. M., Khalife, S., et al. (2004). Vaginal spasm, pain, and behavior: An empirical investigation of the diagnosis of vaginismus. *Archives of Sexual Behavior*, 33, 5–17.

Reissing, E. D., Brown, C., Lord, M. J., et al. (2005). Pelvic floor muscle functioning in women with vulvar vestibulitis syndrome. *Journal of Psychosomatic Obstetrics and Gynaecology*, 26, 107–113.

Rodriguez, M. A. B., Afari, N., Buchwald, D. S., et al. (2013). Evidence for overlap between urological and nonurological unexplained clinical conditions. *Journal Urology*, 189, S66–S74.

Rogers, R. G., Pauls, R. N., Thakar, R., et al. (2018). An International Urogynecological Association (IUGA)/

International Continence Society (ICS) joint report on the terminology for the assessment of sexual health of women with pelvic floor dysfunction. *Neurourology and Urodynamics*, 37, 1220–1240.

Rolke, R., Baron, R., Maier, C., et al. (2006). Quantitative sensory testing in the German research network on neuropathic pain (DFNS): Standardized protocol and reference values. *Pain*, 123, 231–243.

Sellers, A. B., Ruscheweyh, R., Kelley, B. J., et al. (2013). Validation of the English language pain sensitivity questionnaire. *Regional Anesthesia and Pain Medicine*, 38, 508–514.

Severeijns, R., Vlaeyen, J. W., Van Den Hout, M. A., et al. (2001). Pain catastrophizing predicts pain intensity, disability, and psychological distress independent of the level of physical impairment. *The Clinical Journal of Pain*, 17, 165–172.

Shafik, A., & El-Sibai, O. (2002). Study of the pelvic floor muscles in vaginismus: A concept of pathogenesis. *European Journal of Obstetrics & Gynecology and Reproductive Biology*, 105, 67–70.

Shraim, M. A., Masse-Alarie, H., Hall, L. M., et al. (2020). Systematic review and synthesis of mechanism-based classification systems for pain experienced in the musculoskeletal system. *The Clinical Journal of Pain*, 36, 793–812.

Smart, K. M., Blake, C., Staines, A., et al. (2011). The discriminative validity of "nociceptive," "peripheral neuropathic," and "central sensitization" as mechanisms-based classifications of musculoskeletal pain. *The Clinical Journal of Pain*, 27, 655–663.

Staud, R., Weyl, E. E., Price, D. D., et al. (2012). Mechanical and heat hyperalgesia highly predict clinical pain intensity in patients with chronic musculoskeletal pain syndromes. *The Journal of Pain*, 13, 725–735.

Sultan, A. H., Monga, A., Lee, J., et al. (2017). An International Urogynecological Association (IUGA)/International Continence Society (ICS) joint report on the terminology for female anorectal dysfunction. *Neurourology and Urodynamics*, 36, 10–34.

Suskind, A. M., Berry, S. H., Ewing, B. A., et al. (2013). The prevalence and overlap of interstitial cystitis/bladder pain syndrome and chronic prostatitis/chronic pelvic pain syndrome in men: Results of the Rand interstitial cystitis Epidemiology male study. *The Journal of Urology*, 189, 141.

Thibault-Gagnon, S., Goldfinger, C., Pukall, C., et al. (2018). Relationships between 3-dimensional transperineal ultrasound imaging and digital intravaginal palpation assessments of the pelvic floor muscles in women with and without provoked vestibulodynia. *The Journal of Sexual Medicine*, 15, 346–360.

Thibault-Gagnon, S., McLean, L., Goldfinger, C., et al. (2016). Differences in the biometry of the levator hiatus at rest, during contraction, and during Valsalva maneuver between women with and without provoked vestibulodynia assessed by transperineal ultrasound imaging. *The Journal of Sexual Medicine*, 13, 243–252.

Tough, E. A., White, A. R., Richards, S., et al. (2007). Variability of criteria used to diagnose myofascial trigger point pain syndrome—evidence from a review of the literature. *The Clinical Journal of Pain*, 23, 278–286.

Treede, R. D., Rief, W., Barke, A., et al. (2019). Chronic pain as a symptom or a disease: The IASP classification of chronic pain for the international classification of diseases (ICD-11). *Pain*, 160, 19–27.

Tu, F. F., Holt, J., Gonzales, J., et al. (2008). Physical therapy evaluation of patients with chronic pelvic pain: A controlled study. *American Journal of Obstetrics and Gynecology*, 198(3), 272.e1–272.e7.

Van der Velde, J., & Everaerd, W. (1999). Voluntary control over pelvic floor muscles in women with and without vaginistic reactions. *International Urogynecology Journal and Pelvic Floor Dysfunction*, 10, 230–236.

Van Griensven, H., Schmid, A., Trendafilova, T., et al. (2020). Central sensitization in musculoskeletal pain: Lost in translation? *Journal of Orthopaedic & Sports Physical Therapy*, 50, 592–596.

Vodusek, D. B. (2014). Neuroanatomy and neurophysiology of pelvic floor muscles. In K. Bo, L. C. M. Berghmans, M. Van Kampen, & S. Morkved (Eds.), *Evidence-Based Physical Therapy for the Pelvic Floor: Bridging Science and Clinical Practice*. London: Elsevier.

Wang, Y. P., & Gorenstein, C. (2013). Psychometric properties of the Beck depression Inventory-II: A comprehensive review. *Brazilian Journal Psychiatry*, 35, 416–431.

Watson, D., Clark, L. A., & Tellegen, A. (1988). Development and validation of brief measures of positive and negative affect: The PANAS scales. *Journal of Personality and Social Psychology*, 54, 1063–1070.

Wilder-Smith, C. H., & Robert-Yap, J. (2007). Abnormal endogenous pain modulation and somatic and visceral hypersensitivity in female patients with irritable bowel syndrome. *World Journal of Gastroenterology*, 13, 3699–3704.

Williams, A. E., Heitkemper, M., Self, M. M., et al. (2013). Endogenous inhibition of somatic pain is impaired in girls with irritable bowel syndrome compared with healthy girls. *The Journal of Pain*, 14, 921–930.

Woolf, C. J. (2011). Central sensitization: Implications for the diagnosis and treatment of pain. *Pain*, 152, S2–S15.

World Health Organization. (2001). *International classification of functioning, disability, and health: ICF*. Geneva: World Health Organization.

Xu, T., Lai, H. H., Pakpahan, R., et al. (2019). Changes in whole body pain intensity and widespreadness during urologic chronic pelvic pain syndrome flares—findings from one site of the MAPP study. *Neurourology and Urodynamics*, 38, 2333–2350.

Yang, C. C., Miller, J. L., Omidpanah, A., et al. (2018). Physical examination for men and women with urologic chronic pelvic pain syndrome: A MAPP (multidisciplinary approach to the study of chronic pelvic pain) network study. *Urology*, 116, 23–29.

Yarnitsky, D., Granot, M., & Granovsky, Y. (2014). Pain modulation profile and pain therapy: Between pro- and antinociception. *Pain*, 155, 663–665.

Yong, P. J., Williams, C., Bedaiwy, M. A., et al. (2020). A proposed platform for phenotyping endometriosis-associated pain: Unifying peripheral and central pain mechanisms. *Current Obstetrics Gynecology Report*, 9, 89–97.

9.3 Conservative Therapies to Treat Pelvic Floor Pain in Females

Helena Frawley and Mélanie Morin

INTRODUCTION

Physical therapy, which may deliver a range of biopsychosocial interventions, is recommended as an important discipline in the management of chronic pelvic pain (CPP) (American College of Obstetricians and Gynecologists, 2020; Jarrell et al., 2018) or CPP subtypes (Engeler et al., 2020) in women. However, recent systematic literature reviews have had limited scope and do not provide an overall review of the level of evidence for physical therapy treatment of CPP nor an in-depth review of the range of biopsychosocial treatments delivered. Recent reviews have limited their search to studies that included only CPP conditions considered to be of gynaecological origin (Armour et al., 2019; Bonocher et al., 2014; Brooks et al., 2020; Evans et al., 2019; Mira et al., 2018); excluded women presenting with dyspareunia, dyschezia or dysuria (Fuentes-Márquez et al., 2019);

provided either passive manual and/or active treatments but excluded physical or electro-therapeutic agents alone (Klotz et al., 2019); included electrical neuromodulation as the only intervention (Cottrell et al., 2020); included only psychological interventions (Brooks et al., 2020); included only acupuncture (Sung et al., 2018); included study designs other than randomized controlled trials (RCTs) (Brooks et al., 2020; Cottrell et al., 2020; Klotz et al., 2019); drew from a narrow date range (Fuentes-Márquez et al., 2019); or have combined men and women in their search (Cottrell et al., 2020; Fuentes-Márquez et al., 2019; Klotz et al., 2019). Therefore an updated review of the evidence synthesizing the findings from RCTs alone, in women with any type of chronic pelvic floor (PF) pain, using any biopsychosocial treatments, is lacking.

METHODS

We undertook a rapid systematic review of published trials. Our research question was this: What is the efficacy of conservative treatments therapies for women with persistent or chronic pelvi-perineal pain in comparison with no treatment, placebo, active treatment or 'treatment as usual' control? We searched the following databases from inception to September 2020: the Allied and Complementary Medicine Database (AMED), CINAHL, PsyINFO, SPORTDiscus, MEDLINE, Embase and Cochrane Central Register of Controlled Trials (CENTRAL). We did not apply any language restrictions to the search. We searched for RCTs that included adult women with pelvi-perineal pain of at least 3 months duration. Studies were required to report pain data. We excluded studies that included women with pelvic girdle pain or other musculoskeletal or extra-PF pain (e.g., women with endometriosis or endometriosis-associated pelvic pain) as the primary pain presentation. Interventions could include any conservative therapy, such as non-surgical or non-pharmacological therapy, with any body tissue, region or system as the target.

Two authors independently screened for eligibility of studies. The following details were extracted: design of the study, participant characteristics, primary diagnosis, intervention details, outcome measures used and detailed results of the studies. Authors of potentially eligible studies were contacted when clarity of data was required. Where available, we reported the findings of

between-group comparison to judge treatment efficacy. The PEDro rating score was used to classify the methodological quality of the included trials.

GROUPING OF INTERVENTIONS USED IN STUDIES

For interpretation of results we grouped studies according to the type of intervention provided. We did not group these according to PF pain condition, as there were few studies identified per pain condition/diagnosis; many studies combined conditions without specific diagnoses. In addition, for some populations, chronic pain may be the primary condition, without reference to the end organ, and therefore the intervention may be targeted to the experience of pain, not a specific visceral or musculoskeletal condition.

Based on the range of conservative therapies used to treat chronic PF pain, we divided the intervention categories into the following: (1) biologically focused or 'tissue-based' treatments (a traditional physical therapy structural/mechanical approach), (2) 'psychologically informed' treatments (cognitive behavioural approaches developed originally to treat psychological conditions, to which we have added pain education) (Main and George, 2011) and (3) multimodal care. We acknowledge the limitations of these groupings, as not all components of the treatment in the studies may have been reported with equivalent detail and rigour (Frawley et al., 2017). Such identification and reporting may be important to identify the treatment effect attributed to a particular component and to understand the mechanisms behind the response to each component so that future studies may maximize treatment success but minimize treatment burden (May et al., 2009). Furthermore, our understanding of the mechanisms behind each treatment, either alone or in combination with other treatments, and how a treatment works to reduce pain in chronic PF pain conditions, is incomplete. Biologically focused or tissue-based PF physical therapy has been shown to result in improvement in not just local pelvic floor muscle (PFM) outcomes but also psychological and social outcomes (Grinberg et al., 2019). Grinberg et al. (2019) proposed that the improvements observed were due not only to the effect myofascial-based therapies had on peripheral structures but also to the reduction in sensitivity in the spinal and supraspinal structures, including changes in the activity of the sympathetic nervous system and induction of pain inhibitory effects via supraspinal pathways. It may be that these central mechanisms resulted in reduction of psychological distress. Conversely, reduced psychological distress from a psychological intervention may influence peripheral or central sensitization. Nevertheless, the following grouping of different interventions is intended to broadly represent the method of application of therapies, not the presumed mechanism of effect.

RESULTS

Thirty-five studies were included in our review. They are grouped according to intervention type in Tables 9.3.1, 9.3.2 and 9.3.3.

TABLE 9.3.1	Randomised Controlled Trials That Provided Predominantly Biologically Focused Interventions to Treat Chronic Pelvic Floor Pain
Author	**Amin et al. (2015)**
Study design	RCT
Study population	127 women with CPP ≥6 months
Intervention	TG1: inferior hypogastric plexus blockade technique
	TG2: electroacupuncture technique with disposable stainless steel needles, applied to standardized set of acupuncture points delivered by trained doctors; electrical stimulation using low-intensity pulsed current at high frequencies (10–200 pulses/s) at the site of pain and at high intensity and low frequency (≤10 pulses/s, usually 2 pulses/s) into identified trigger points; applied 30 min twice daily for 6 weeks
Drop-out/adherence	TG1: 2/64
	TG2: 8/63
	Adherence not reported
Outcome (measure)	Pain intensity (VAS)
	Pain status (categorical scale: completely relieved, partially relieved, no change, not able to decide)
	Sample size sufficient for pain intensity (VAS) according to power calculation provided
	Primary time endpoint not stated
Results (between-group analyses)	Pain intensity lower in TG1 compared to TG2 at 1 h after treatment, as well as 2, 6 and 12 weeks post-treatment:
	1 h: 2.2 ± 0.88 vs 7.8 ± 0.24, $p = 0.001$
	2 weeks: 2.2 ± 0.88 vs 6.3 ± 0.14, $p < 0.05$
	6 weeks: 2.2 ± 0.88 vs 5.2 ± 0.06, $p < 0.05$
	12 weeks: 2.2 ± 0.88 vs 4.7 ± 0.11, $p < 0.05$
	TG1 and TG2 not significantly different for pain status at 4 and 12 weeks post-treatment (except for the 'no change' category):
	At 4 weeks post-treatment:
	Completely relieved: 61% vs 40%, $p = 0.6899$
	Partially relieved: 23% vs 24%, $p = 0.9149$
	No change: 10% vs 31%, $p = 0.0330$[a]
	Not able to decide: 6% vs 5%, $p = 1$
	At 12 weeks post-treatment:
	Completely relieved: 73% vs 54%, $p = 0.3737$
	Partially relieved: 18% vs 18%, $p = 0.9588$
	No change: 6% vs 25%, $p = 0.0294$[a]
	Not able to decide: 3% vs 2%, $p = 1$
	No complications reported.

[a]SD illustrated but numerical data not provided.

Continued

TABLE 9.3.1   Randomised Controlled Trials That Provided Predominantly Biologically Focused Interventions to Treat Chronic Pelvic Floor Pain—cont'd

Author	Bergeron et al. (2001)
Study design	RCT
Study population	87 women with PVD (pain during intercourse ≥6 months) and pain (VAS ≥4) in ≥1 locations of vestibule during cotton swab test
Intervention	TG1: vestibulectomy TG2: biofeedback according to Glazer protocol, 8 sessions of 45 min over 12 weeks, home biofeedback twice daily TG3: group cognitive behavioral therapy including education and information about vulvar pain, sexual anatomy, progressive muscle relaxation, abdominal breathing, PFM exercises, vaginal dilation
Drop-out/adherence	21 (TG1 10/29, TG2 11/29, TG3 1/29) Adherence to home exercises (frequency ratings of weekly practice of exercises): biofeedback 57%, group cognitive behavioural therapy 65%
Outcome (measure)	Pain intensity during cotton swab test (vestibular pain index) Pain intensity during intercourse (NRS) Pain quality (MPQ) Subjective improvement (scale of 0 [worse] to 5 [complete cure]) No sample size calculation provided
Results (between-group analyses)	Vestibular pain index (identified as primary outcome): At post-treatment, TG1 had significantly lower pain levels on cotton swab test than both TG2 (p = 0.01) and TG3 participants (p = 0.01) (1.89 ± 1.68 vs 4.55 ± 2.36 vs 5.26 ± 2). At 6-month follow-up, TG1 participants had significantly lower pain levels than TG2 participants only (p = 0.05) (1.90 ± 2.24 vs 4.42 ± 2.63 vs 3.89 ± 2.09). Pain intensity during intercourse: no between-group differences found in intention-to-treat analysis Pain quality: no between-group differences found in intention-to-treat analysis Subjective improvement (complete relief or great improvement of pain): TG1:15/22 (2 reported worsening) TG2: 10/28 (0 reported worsening) TG3: 11/28 (0 reported worsening)
Author	Bergeron et al. (2008)
Study design	RCT
Study population	78 women with PVD
Intervention	Same as Bergeron et al. (2001): TG1: vestibulectomy TG2: home biofeedback TG3: group cognitive behavioral therapy
Drop-out/adherence	Total 27/78, TG1 7/22, TG2 11/28, TG3 9/28 Adherence not assessed, as it is a follow-up study (i.e., not including an active phase of treatment) 78 participants contacted who completed treatment (Bergeron et al., 2001)
Outcome (measure)	Pain intensity during cotton swab test (vestibular pain index) Pain intensity during intercourse (NRS) Pain quality (MPQ) Sample size calculation provided based on large between-group difference for pain outcomes

TABLE 9.3.1 Randomised Controlled Trials That Provided Predominantly Biologically Focused Interventions to Treat Chronic Pelvic Floor Pain—cont'd

Results (between-group analyses)	Outcomes assessed at 6-month and 2.5-year follow-up (treatment group main effect considered in analysis) Vestibular pain index (primary outcome according to Bergeron et al. [2001]): TG1 (6 months: 1.90 ± 2.24; 2.5 years: 1.58 ± 1.91) was superior to TG2 (6 months: 4.42 ± 2.63; 2.5 years: 4.22 ± 2.54) and TG3 (6 months: 3.89 ± 2.09; 2.5 years: 3.66 ± 2.33) (p = 0.01). Statistical difference between TG2 and TG3 was not reported. Results obtained appear to reflect a small effect size between TG2 and TG3. Pain intensity during intercourse: TG1 (6 months: 3.41 ± 3.17; 2.5 years: 2.05 ± 1.87) was superior to TG2 (6 months: 4.5 ± 2.63; 2.5 years: 4.29 ± 2.66) (p < 0.05). TG1 and TG3 (6 months: 4.46 ± 2.47; 2.5 years: 3.3 ± 2.73) were not significantly different. Statistical difference between TG2 and TG3 was not reported. Pain quality: TG1 (6 months: 14.27 ± 13.06; 2.5 years: 7.95 ±8.95) was superior to TG2 (6 months: 20.43 ± 18.1; 2.5 years: 20.32 ± 18.31) and TG3 (6 months: 20.93 ± 14.18; 2.5 years: 19.96 ± 15.6) (p < 0.05). Statistical difference between TG2 and TG3 was not reported.
Author	**Bond et al. (2017)**
Study design	Pilot RCT
Study population	9 women with bladder pain syndrome
Intervention	TG: For the first 6 weeks, women had weekly sessions of myofascial release of PFMs (15 min) + TheraWand for 15 min, 3×/week between physical therapy sessions + daily PFM active release exercises in sitting or standing. For the subsequent 6 weeks, participants had TheraWand treatment for 15 min 3×/week + daily PFM active release exercises in sitting or standing. CG: For the first 6 weeks, participants had weekly sessions of myofascial release of PFMs (15 min) + daily PFM active release exercises in sitting or standing. For the subsequent 6 weeks, participants performed daily PFM active release exercises in sitting or standing.
Drop-out/adherence	Adherence not reported; no adverse events observed
Outcome (measure)	Interstitial cystitis symptom and problem (OSPI) comprising symptoms and problem subscale: MCID –4 = moderate improvement, –7 = great improvement, –9 = symptom resolution Genitourinary pain index: MCID –4 Pelvic Pain and Urinary Urgency Frequency Patient Symptom Scale: MCID reduction of 0.5 Bladder pain (VAS): MCID –10 mm Overall pain (VAS): MCID –10 mm PFM pain with palpation (NRS): MCID –5 = very effective, –2 = moderately effective, –1 = not effective No sample size calculation provided
Results (between-group analyses)	No statistical analyses were performed to assess change over time nor between-group difference. Data were interpreted subjectively using observed mean changes and known MCID. For all outcomes, changes occurring from baseline to 12 weeks in both CG and TG appeared to exceed MCID. Between-group differences are difficult to interpret due to absence of statistical analysis.
Author	**Chuang et al. (2020)**
Study design	RCT
Study population	54 patients with interstitial cystitis/bladder pain syndrome refractory to conventional treatments

Continued

TABLE 9.3.1 Randomised Controlled Trials That Provided Predominantly Biologically Focused Interventions to Treat Chronic Pelvic Floor Pain—cont'd

Intervention	TG: extracorporeal shock wave therapy (2000 shocks, frequency of 3 Hz, and maximum total energy flow density 0.25 mJ/mm^2) once a week for 4 weeks at suprapubic bladder area CG: shock wave setting without energy transmission
Drop-out/adherence	TG: 2/25 at 4 weeks and 4/25 at 12 weeks CG: 1/24 at 4 weeks and 3/24 at 12 weeks Adherence not reported
Outcome (measure)	Interstitial cystitis symptom (OSPI symptom subscale) Pain intensity (VAS), further categorized in responders as VAS reduction ≥3 Perceived improvement (GRA) Information incomplete for sample size calculation
Results (between-group analyses)	Non-significant between-group differences were found regarding changes in interstitial cystitis symptoms (OSPI symptoms) and pain intensity (VAS) from baseline to 4 weeks and to 12 weeks ($p < 0.05$). However, a significantly higher proportion of participants in TG reported being improved in VAS category ≥3 compared to placebo (TG 57.1% vs 19% (TG vs placebo, $p = 0.011$). The proportion of women with improvement on GRA (≥2) was not significant between groups.
Author	**Danielsson et al. (2006)**
Study design	RCT
Study population	46 women with PVD
Intervention	TG1: home PFM exercise with electromyography biofeedback; Glazer protocol used for 4 months; monthly supervised sessions and home biofeedback 3×/day TG2: topical lidocaine 2% and 5% for 4 months
Drop-out/adherence	TG1: 5/23 at 12 months TG2: 4/23 at 12 months Low adherence to TG1 reported: No participants did exercises 3×/day, 10/18 (56%) did them 2×/day and the rest did exercises 1×/day. For TG2: 18 of 19 (95%) women used an average number of ≥5 applications/day. Approximately 50% switched to 5% ointment after 2 months, whereas the rest continued with gel.
Outcome (measure)	Pain intensity during intercourse (VAS) Pain intensity during cotton swab test (VAS) Pressure pain threshold (vulvar algesiometer) Subjective perception of improvement (cured/improved/no change) Sample size calculation based on non-pain outcomes
Results (between-group analyses)	Significant reduction in pain (VAS) from baseline to follow-up for both groups; non-significant difference found between both groups Significant increase in pain thresholds at both vestibular sites and for both treatment groups from baseline to 12-month follow-up Non-significant difference found between both groups Self-reported perception of improvement: Biofeedback: 2/23 completely cured, 12/23 improved Lidocaine: 2/23 completed cured; 10/23 improved
Author	**De Bernardes et al. (2010)**
Study design	Crossover RCT
Study population	26 women with CPP ≥6 months; VAS >3; absence of well-defined pelvic pathologies

TABLE 9.3.1   Randomised Controlled Trials That Provided Predominantly Biologically Focused Interventions to Treat Chronic Pelvic Floor Pain—cont'd

Intervention	Both groups received 10 × 30 min, twice-weekly sessions of intravaginal electrical stimulation, followed by crossover period: TG phase: active intravaginal electrical stimulation (8 Hz, 1 msec pulse length, intensity adjusted for each individual) CG phase: sham intravaginal electrical delivered through inactive device
Drop-out/adherence	At completion of crossover phase: TG: 0/15 CG: 1/11 Adherence not reported
Outcome (measure)	Average daily pain intensity on VAS 0–10, further categorized as pain score ≤3 or >4. Dyspareunia (present, absent) Sample size calculation based on VAS 0–10, not binary pain category scale as reported in results
Results (between-group analyses)	Significantly higher proportion of women following active stimulation (TG 86.7%–90.9%) had pain scores ≤3 compared to sham phase (CG 54.5%–78.6%). No significant change was found in proportion of women presenting with dyspareunia from baseline to post-treatment in both phases ($p = 0.317$). It should be specified that a small number of women had dyspareunia at baseline, which may explain non-significant change.
Author	**Divandari et al. (2019)**
Study design	Crossover RCT; all participants were their own controls and randomly received both active and sham treatments
Study population	16 women with CPP based on definition from American College of Obstetricians and Gynecologists
Intervention	TG (phase), active tDCS: 1 session of 20-min 0.3 mA stimulation with current density of 0.1 mA/cm^2 CG (phase), sham tDCS: 30 s of active stimulation, which was then interrupted for the rest of the treatment; sham procedure demonstrated to be valid as a placebo intervention
Drop-out/adherence	No drop-outs reported All participants attended single stimulation session
Outcome (measure)	Pain intensity (VAS) Information incomplete for sample size calculation
Results (between-group analyses)	Mean change in pain intensity appears significantly higher in TG than CG (MD: 3.06 ± 1.69 vs 0.56 ± 1.26). It is uncertain that statistics provided assessed between-group differences. Further, it is not clear if baseline scores in pain were similar between TG and CG phases.
Author	**Fitzgerald et al. (2012)**
Study design	RCT
Study population	81 women with interstitial cystitis/bladder pain syndrome, ≤3 years duration, VAS pain rating ≥3, presenting with PFM tenderness on vaginal palpation
Intervention	10 sessions over 12 weeks with a physical therapist: TG: myofascial therapy treatments to internal and external pelvic myofascial structures CG: global therapeutic massage therapy

Continued

TABLE 9.3.1   Randomised Controlled Trials That Provided Predominantly Biologically Focused Interventions to Treat Chronic Pelvic Floor Pain—cont'd

Drop-out/adherence	TG: 1/39 post-treatment and 9/39 at 3-month follow-up CG: 2/42 post-treatment and 4/42 at 3-month follow-up 21 (55%) participants in TG and 15 (38%) in CG completed all 10 assigned treatments in 12-week study period
Outcome (measure)	Pain intensity (NRS) Interstitial cystitis symptom and problem (OSPI symptom and problem subscales) Patient perceived improvement (GRA) (primary outcome) Sample size sufficient for GRA according to power calculation provided
Results (between-group analyses)	Significant changes in pain intensity and OSPI from baseline to post-treatment not significantly different between groups Proportion of women reporting significant improvement on GRA significantly higher in TG compared to tCG at post-treatment: 59% vs 26%, p = 0.0012
Author	**Haugstad et al. (2006); follow-up study: Haugstad et al. (2008)**
Study design	RCT
Study population	40 women with CPP (deep pelvic pain) 1–10 years duration; PFM palpated as part of vaginal examination to exclude obvious pathology, but findings of PFM tenderness and tension not reported
Intervention	Standard gynaecological treatment (hormonal, analgesic treatment as required, dietary and bowel advice, sexological advice): TG: Mensendieck somatocognitive therapy (cognitive-based approach to increase awareness of body movements, tension, relaxation, posture, gait, respiration) for 3 months (10 treatment sessions) CG: nil additional treatment
Drop-out/adherence	1 from each group at 3 months; 1 further at 1 year Adherence not reported
Outcome (measure)	Therapist rating of Mensendieck score (in 5 domains) of motor function evaluated by video recording Pain intensity (VAS and GHQ-30) Information incomplete for sample size calculation
Results (between-group analyses)	Significant improvement in Mensendieck score, VAS and GHQ-30 in TG (VAS: 48% reduction in score, p < 0.001) Non-significant changes in CG (VAS: 8% reduction in score, p = 0.07) No between-group difference reported
Author	**Heyman et al. (2006)**
Study design	RCT
Study population	50 women with CPP >6 months; inclusion criterion of pain on firm palpation of PFMs (rated as present/absent)
Intervention	TG: 'forceful' distension of PFMs per rectal digital palpation; pressure applied for 60 s; procedure repeated after 2–3 weeks CG: counselling
Drop-out/adherence	TG: 3/25 CG: 3/25 With exception of women who dropped out, all women completed distension session (TG); attendance at counselling (CG) not reported

TABLE 9.3.1	**Randomised Controlled Trials That Provided Predominantly Biologically Focused Interventions to Treat Chronic Pelvic Floor Pain—cont'd**
Outcome (measure)	Pain intensity of pelvic pain (VAS) Pain intensity during intercourse (VAS) Information incomplete for sample size calculation
Results (between-group analyses)	Change in pain intensity of pelvic pain significantly higher in TG compared to CG (MD: 35 ± 31 vs −0.8 ± 9.2, p = 0.001) Change in pain intensity during intercourse significantly higher in TG compared to CG (MD: 19 ± 38 vs −0.13 ± 10.7, p = 0.001)
Author	**Hullender Rubin et al. (2019)**
Study design	Feasibility/acceptability RCT
Study population	19 women with PVD, diagnosed using Friedrich's criteria, pain ≥3 months and vestibular pain confirmed by tampon test pain (VAS ≥40/100) and cotton swab (VAS ≥40/100)
Intervention	TG1: traditional acupuncture; 20 visits for 4 weeks ê 18 interventions (twice weekly for 6 weeks, followed by once weekly for 6 weeks) and 2 assessment visits (weeks 12 and 24): Supine: acupuncture on 3 core points indicated for genital pain and with potential for 2 additional points based on traditional Chinese medicine diagnosis Prone: standardized treatment using mixed stimulation methods of manual and electroacupuncture (100-Hz continuous mA, mild intensity and localized over pudendal nerve and intended to treat pain in genitals) 15 min after insertion, needles manually stimulated using rotation or lifting/thrusting method to evoke mild 'de qi' sensation (supine) or adjustment of electroacupuncture intensity (prone) Lidocaine 5% cream for self-application to vestibule 4×/day TG2: non-traditional acupuncture; 20 visits for 4 weeks ê 18 interventions (twice weekly for 6 weeks, followed by once weekly for 6 weeks) and 2 assessment visits (weeks 12 and 24): Standardized intervention of 4 needles on non-specific points Superficial needling without stimulation; in prone, electroacupuncture lead taped to needles with machine turned on but no electricity emitted (sham current) Lidocaine 5% cream for self-application to vestibule 4×/day
Drop-out/adherence	TG1: 3/10 TG2: 2/9 Attendance to sessions: TG1 96% and TG2 97%
Outcome (measure)	Pain intensity (tampon test, 100-mm VAS) Vulvar pain sensitivity (cotton swab test) No sample size calculation provided
Results (between-group analyses)	Outcomes collected at baseline and 12 and 24 weeks Only descriptive data reported; no statistics performed to assess between-group differences Pain intensity with tampon test: Baseline: TG1 (68.0 ± 18.9) vs TG2 (61.5 ± 15.9) 12 weeks: TG1 (−42.4 ± 19.4) vs TG2 (−28.7 ± 28.5) compared to baseline 24 weeks: TG1 (−35.7 ± 17.8) vs TG2 (−36.7 ± 17.7) compared to baseline Vulvar pain sensitivity (cotton swab test): Baseline: TG1 (66.8 ± 17.0) vs TG2 (69.2 ± 15.8) 12 weeks: TG1 (−23.9 ± 28.7) vs TG2 (−25.9 ± 14.3) compared to baseline 24 weeks: TG1 (−18.5 ± 31.7) vs TG2 (−31.4 ± 18.3) compared to baseline 32 adverse events reported in TG1 and 36 in TG2; of all adverse events across both groups, 7 adverse events related to lidocaine use and 5 to acupuncture; all adverse events mild, and no patient discontinued study because of acupuncture

Continued

TABLE 9.3.1   Randomised Controlled Trials That Provided Predominantly Biologically Focused Interventions to Treat Chronic Pelvic Floor Pain—cont'd

Author	Hurt et al. (2020)
Study design	RCT
Study population	62 women with vulvodynia (vulvar pain ≥3 months) with positive cotton swab test
Intervention	TG: perineal application of extracorporeal shock wave therapy weekly (3000 pulses each for 4 consecutive weeks); position of shock wave transducer changed after every 500 pulses; 6 areas covering whole vulva and perineum treated; energy flux density 0.25 mJ/mm², frequency 4 Hz, focus zone 0–30 mm, therapeutic efficacy 0–90 mm, stand-off II; device used was standard electromagnetic shock wave unit with focused shock wave handpiece CG: same treatment procedure as extracorporeal shock wave therapy group, but handpiece provided with placebo stand-off that disabled energy transmission but enabled generation of sound and shaking to mimic treatment
Drop-out/adherence	TG: 0/31 CG: 1/31 Participants in both groups attended all treatment sessions
Outcome (measure)	Pain intensity (VAS) Vulvar pain sensitivity (cotton swab test, Goetsch scale 0–4: 0 indicating no pain and 4 severe pain) Sample size sufficient for VAS according to power calculation provided
Results (between-group analyses)	Significant differences in pain intensity found between TG and CG at 1 week (2.67 ± 0.71 vs 6.1 ± 0.78), 4 weeks (2.69 ± 0.92 vs 6.16 ± 0.92) and 12 weeks post-treatment (2.63 ± 0.93 vs 6.17 ± 0.93) (all $p < 0.01$) Significant differences in vulvar pain sensitivity found between TG and CG at 1 week (0.7 ± 0.65 vs 3.07 ± 0.86), 4 weeks (0.8 ± 0.61 vs 3.37 ± 0.76) and 12 weeks post-treatment (0.77 ± 0.62 vs 2.97 ± 0.8) (all $p < 0.01$)
Author	Istek et al. (2014)
Study design	RCT
Study population	33 women with CPP (non-cyclic pain persisting ≥ 6months; localized to pelvis, infraumbilical anterior abdominal wall, or lumbosacral back or buttocks, leading to degrees of functional disability)
Intervention	TG: PTNS once a week for 3 min; total treatment period 12 weeks; frequency 20 Hz, pulse duration 200 μs and amplitude of current between 0.5 and 10 mA; 34-gauge needle placed on point 1 cm posterior and 3 cm proximal to medial malleolus; stimulation amplitude set at maximum tolerable level according to subject under investigation; plantar flexion accepted as proof of effectiveness CG: oral analgesics but no PTNS throughout study
Drop-out/adherence	No dropouts Adherence not reported
Outcome (measure)	Subjective improvement/cured/worse (primary outcome) Present pain intensity (VAS) Pain quality (SF-MPQ including sensory pain subscale, affective pain subscale and total score) Pain (SF-36 pain subscale) Information incomplete for sample size calculation

TABLE 9.3.1 Randomised Controlled Trials That Provided Predominantly Biologically Focused Interventions to Treat Chronic Pelvic Floor Pain—cont'd

Results (between-group analyses)	9 patients (56.3 %) suggested either cured or much improved after 12 weeks of PTNS treatment at 6-month follow-up, whereas in CG, only 2 patients (11.8 %) improved; no statistical analysis provided
	Present pain intensity–VAS: no significant difference between groups at 12 weeks (TG 3.8 ± 3.5, CG 6.0 ± 1.5, p = 0.063) and at 6 months (TG 4.5 ± 3.7, CG 5.9 ± 2.2, p = 0.213)
	Significant improvement of TG group compared to CG for sensory subscale (TG 10.1 ± 6.1, CG 15.9 ± 4.1, p = 0.008), affective subscale (TG 2.6 ± 2.1, CG 4.6 ± 1.8, p = 0.004) and total score (TG 12.6 ± 8.1, CG 20.6 ± 5.6, p = 0.002) at 12 weeks post-treatment
	No significant differences between groups for sensory subscale, affective subscale and total score at 6-month follow-up
	No significant differences between groups for pain, as measured by the SF-36 pain subscale, at 12 weeks and 6 months
Author	**Lev-Sagie et al. (2017)**
Study design	Pilot RCT
Study population	35 women with PVD (≥3 months of dyspareunia and/or pain with tampon insertion and confirmation of vestibular tenderness by cotton swab test)
Intervention	TG: LLLT delivered twice weekly for 6 weeks, for a total of 12 LLLT sessions; pen-size probe transmitting irradiation applied to vestibule for 20 s at each point; irradiation parameters: wavelength of 820 nm, energy density of 32 J/cm² and pulsed light (alternating 73, 146 and 700 Hz); number of treatment points defined according to each woman's physical examination
	CG: placebo twice weekly for 6 weeks, for a total of 12 placebo sessions; same procedures than LLLT group but without emitting irradiation
Drop-out/adherence	TG: 0/18
	CG: 1/17
	Adherence not reported
Outcome (measure)	Vulvar pain sensitivity (cotton swab test, 5 points on vestibule, NRS)
	Pain during intercourse (NRS): further categorized as no improvement (pain reduction <30%), moderate improvement (pain reduction between 30% and 70%) and great improvement (pain reduction >70%)
	Severity of discomfort in daily activities and during sexual activity (VAS from 0 = 'no discomfort at all' and 10 = 'severe discomfort')
	Pain intensity (tampon test, NRS)
	Daily 24-h vulvar pain intensity including intercourse (NRS)
	No sample size calculation provided
Results (between-group analyses)	Changes in pain sensitivity and pain intensity (all outcomes) from baseline to post-treatment were not significantly different between groups.
	Only significant difference between both groups was pain intensity converted into a categorial variable. Significantly more women reported improvement in TG (n = 14/18, 2 for 'complete', 10 for 'great' and 2 for 'moderate') compared to placebo (n = 7/16, 5 for 'great' and 2 for 'moderate') (p = 0.042).
Author	**Morin et al. (2017)**
Study design	RCT
Study population	40 women diagnosed with PVD (pain intensity >5/10 in at least 90% of attempted sexual intercourse episodes for >6 months)

Continued

TABLE 9.3.1   Randomised Controlled Trials That Provided Predominantly Biologically Focused Interventions to Treat Chronic Pelvic Floor Pain—cont'd

Intervention	TG: active tDCS consisted of an intensity of 2 mA CG: sham tDCS consisted of a 30-s real stimulation, which was then interrupted for the rest of the session; sham procedure demonstrated to be valid as a placebo intervention; both active and sham tDCS consisted of 10 × 20-min sessions delivered over 2-week period with anode positioned over primary motor cortex and cathode over contralateral supraorbital area
Drop-out/adherence	TG: 1/20 (inability to assess outcomes due to absence of intercourse attempt) CG: 0/20 Participants in both groups attended all treatment sessions
Outcome (measure)	Pain intensity during intercourse (NRS) Pain quality (MPQ) Vestibular pain sensitivity (pressure pain threshold and pressure pain tolerance assessed with an algometer) Patient perceived improvement (patient global impression of change) Sample size sufficient for pain intensity according to power calculation provided
Results (between-group analyses)	Changes in pain intensity during sexual intercourse not significantly different between TG and CG from baseline to post-treatment and to follow-up Change in pain quality significant only from baseline to follow-up in favour of CG compared to TG Non-significant changes found in pain threshold and tolerance in both groups Non-significant differences found regarding patient-perceived improvement with 68% assigned to TG reported being very much, much or slightly improved at post-treatment compared to 65% assigned to CG; both groups also comparable at follow-up (42% vs 65%)
Author	**Murina et al. (2008)**
Study design	RCT
Study population	40 women with PVD (vulvar pain upon tampon insertion or attempted intercourse ≥6 months and positive cotton swab test) in absence of other causes
Intervention	TG: 20 TENS treatment sessions were administered twice per week. Electrical stimulation was in the form of a symmetrical biphasic wave. The stimulation was delivered through a commercially available plastic intra-vaginal probe, 20 mm in diameter and 110 mm in length, with 2 gold metallic transverse rings as electrodes. It was inserted into the vagina to a depth of 20 mm. There was alternation of low- and high-frequency stimulation. Protocol for active TENS was 15 min of 10-Hz frequency and pulse duration of 50 μs followed by 15 min of 50-Hz frequency and pulse duration of 100 μs. The intensity was set to as high as the woman could bear without discomfort. It was monitored throughout stimulation time and ranged between 10 and 100 mA peak to peak. CG: 20 treatment sessions on a twice per week basis. The placebo group received electrical stimulation considered to be non-active, which consisted of 2 sets of 3-s stimulation (frequency 2 Hz, pulse duration 2 μs) followed by 15-min pause.
Drop-out/adherence	No dropouts Adherence not reported
Outcome (measure)	Sensation of irritation and burning (VAS) Pain quality (MPQ) Pain intensity during intercourse (Marinoff Dyspareunia Scale, 0–3 score) Sample size calculation based on within-group changes

TABLE 9.3.1	**Randomised Controlled Trials That Provided Predominantly Biologically Focused Interventions to Treat Chronic Pelvic Floor Pain—cont'd**
Results (between-group analyses)	Significant improvement in TG from baseline to post-treatment found for VAS (pre: 6.2 ± 1.9, post: 2.1 ± 2.7, p = 0.004), pain quality (pre: 19.5 ± 11.9, post: 8.5 ± 10.7, p = 0.001) and Marinoff Dyspareunia Scale (pre: 2.7 ± 0.4, post: 1.1 ± 0.9, p = 0.001); changes from baseline to 3-month follow-up also significant for VAS (3-month follow-up: 2.8 ± 2.5, p = 0.004), SF-MPQ (3-month follow-up: 8.5 ± 10.7, p = 0.001) and Marinoff Dyspareunia Scale (3-month follow-up: 1.1 ± 0.9, p = 0.001) No significant change for placebo group in post-treatment and 3-month follow-up compared to baseline for VAS (pre: 6.7 ± 2.0, post: 5.7 ± 2.2, 3-month follow-up: 5.6 ± 2.1), SF-MPQ (pre: 18.4 ± 11.6, post: 15.1 ± 10.4, 3-month follow-up: 17.1 ± 8.4) and Marinoff Dyspareunia Scale (pre: 2.7 ± 0.4, post: 2.4 ± 0.8, 3-month follow-up: 2.4 ± 0.8) with all p ≥ 0.005 Between-group differences not assessed
Author	**Murina et al. (2018)**
Study design	RCT
Study population	42 women with PVD (confirmed diagnosis with cotton swab examination at 1, 3, 5, 7, 9 and 11 o'clock around vaginal opening at Hart's line) with diagnosis of moderate or severe pelvic floor hypertonic dysfunction (diagnosis established with empirical score grade 0 = no hypertonicity, grade 1 = mild hypertonicity, grade 2 = moderate hypertonicity and grade 3 = severe hypertonicity of levator ani complex)
Intervention	TG1 (diazepam + TENS): insert 1 vaginal tablet (5 mg of diazepam) daily before going to sleep for 60 days + vaginal TENS therapy in self-administered domiciliary protocol TG2: (placebo tablet + TENS): insert 1 vaginal tablet (5 mg of diazepam) daily before going to sleep for 60 days + vaginal TENS therapy in self-administered domiciliary protocol TENS protocol for all patients (2 customized programs set): standard protocol for TENS was 15 min of 100-Hz frequency and pulse duration of 50 ms (first program) followed by 15 min of 5-Hz frequency and pulse duration of 100 ms (second program); all patients received supervised trial consisting of 6–7 sessions to familiarize patient on use of TENS while allowing therapist to check that patient was using device properly; pulse was increased rapidly until patient reported onset of any sensation under electrodes; intensity was then increased slowly until this sensation reached a level described as maximum tolerable without experiencing pain
Drop-out/adherence	No dropouts Adherence not reported
Outcome (measure)	Pain intensity during intercourse (VAS) Pain during intercourse (dyspareunia with Marinoff Dyspareunia Scale) Sample size calculation based on proportion of participants cured, but results reported pain outcomes as continuous variable
Results (between-group analyses)	Pain intensity (VAS) decreased in both groups from baseline to post-treatment, but no significant difference found between TG1 and TG2 (p ≥ 0.05) Marinoff Dyspareunia Scale: improvement from baseline to post-treatment significantly higher in TG1 (mean at post-treatment: 1.6[a]) compared to TG2 (mean at post-treatment: 1.3[a]) (p < 0.01)
Author	**O'Reilly et al. (2004)**
Study design	RCT
Study population	56 women with interstitial cystitis (pain with bladder filling and relieved by emptying, present >12 months)
Intervention	TG: daily transdermal laser stimulation of posterior tibial nerve for 30 s over SP6 acupuncture point for 12 weeks CG: sham laser delivered with deactivated device
Drop-out/adherence	No drop-outs reported Adherence not reported

[a]SD illustrated but numerical data not provided.

Continued

TABLE 9.3.1 **Randomised Controlled Trials That Provided Predominantly Biologically Focused Interventions to Treat Chronic Pelvic Floor Pain—cont'd**

Outcome (measure)	Symptoms (Interstitial Cystitis Problem Index) Sample size calculation based on proportion of participants having significant improvement, but results reported pain outcomes as continuous variable
Results (between-group analyses)	Changes in symptom severity from baseline to post-treatment not significantly different between both groups
Author	**Schlaeger et al. (2015)**
Study design	Pilot RCT
Study population	36 women with vulvodynia
Intervention	TG: acupuncture 2×/week for 5 weeks for total of 10 sessions CG: waitlist (usual care for 5 weeks)
Drop-out/adherence	No drop-outs No adherence reported
Outcome (measure)	Pain intensity during intercourse (VAS) Pain quality (MPQ short form including total score, present pain intensity scale) Pain (FSFI pain subscale) Information incomplete for sample size calculation
Results (between-group analyses)	Change in pain intensity from baseline to post-treatment significantly higher in TG than CG (mean change score: 2.9 ± 2.1 vs 0.54 ± 2.4, p = 0.003) Changes in pain quality favoured TG (mean change of total score: 8.9 ± 8.1 vs 2.7 ± 6.6, p = 0.02; mean change of present pain intensity scale: 1.4 ± 0.8 vs 0.4 ± 1.1, p = 0.002) Changes in FSFI pain subscale also favoured TG (-1.3 ± 1.9 vs 0.3 ± 1.1, p = 0.003)
Author	**Schvartzman et al. (2019)**
Study design	RCT
Study population	42 peri- and postmenopausal women with dyspareunia
Intervention	TG: five 1-h sessions of thermotherapy for relaxation of PFMs, myofascial release and PFM training CG: five 1-h sessions during which heat applied to lower back with myofascial release of abdominal diaphragm, piriformis and iliopsoas muscles; no treatment directed at PFMs
Drop-out/adherence	No drop-outs Adherence not reported
Outcome (measure)	Pain intensity during intercourse (VAS) Pain (FSFI pain subscale) Sample size sufficient for pain (VAS) according to power calculation provided
Results (between-group analyses)	Change in pain intensity significantly higher in TG (7.77 ± 0.38 to 2.25 ± 0.30) than CG (7.62 ± 0.29 to 5.58 ± 0.49) from baseline to post-treatment (p = 0.005) Change in FSFI pain subscale also favoured TG (p = 0.002)
Author	**Zoorob et al. (2015)**
Study design	RCT
Study population	34 women with pelvic floor myalgia
Intervention	TG1: pelvic floor physical therapy including trigger point release techniques, massage and stretching (average of 7.3 ± 2.8 sessions) TG2: vaginal injection of 1 mL of triamcinolone (40 mg/mL) and 9 mL of bupivacaine 0.5 %; minimum of 5 mL of solution injected/site with up to 4 sites injected/patient (average of 4.4 ± 1.6 sessions)
Drop-out/adherence	TG1: 0/17 TG2: 5/17 Adherence not reported

TABLE 9.3.1 Randomised Controlled Trials That Provided Predominantly Biologically Focused Interventions to Treat Chronic Pelvic Floor Pain—cont'd

Outcome (measure)	Pain intensity (NRS) Perceived improvement (patient global impression of change) Pain (FSFI pain subscale) Sample size insufficient according to power calculation provided
Results (between-group analyses)	Non-significant differences between both groups for pain intensity and perceived improvement Changes in pain, as assessed with FSFI subscale, favoured TG1 compared to TG2 (2.4 ± 1.43 vs 0.8 ± 1.61, p = 0.02)

CG, Control group; *CPP*, chronic pelvic pain; *FSFI*, Female Sexual Function Index; *GHQ-30*, 30-item General Health Questionnaire; *GRA*, global response assessment; *LLLT*, low-level laser therapy; *MCID*, minimally clinically important difference; *MD*, mean difference; *MPQ*, McGill Pain Questionnaire; *NRS*, numerical rating scale; *OSPI*, O'Leary–Sant Symptom Problem Index; *PFM*, pelvic floor muscle; *PTNS*, percutaneous tibial nerve stimulation; *PVD*, provoked vestibulodynia; *RCT*, randomized controlled trial; *SF-MPQ*, Short-Form McGill Pain Questionnaire; *TENS*, transcutaneous electrical nerve stimulation; *TG*, treatment group; *VAS*, visual analogue scale.

TABLE 9.3.2 Randomized Controlled Trials That Provided Predominantly Psychological/Cognitive Interventions to Treat Chronic Pelvic Floor Pain

Author	**Brotto et al. (2019)**
Study design	Cohort study with nested RCT
Study population	130 women with PVD (diagnosis of PVD confirmed by both clinical history and by a cotton swab test, duration of PVD ≥6 months); 46/130 participants randomized
Intervention	8 weekly sessions, 2.25 h in length TG1: 8 sessions of mindfulness-based cognitive therapy TG2: 8 sessions of cognitive behavioral therapy
Drop-out/adherence	TG1 8/67, TG2 14/63 TG1: 75% attendance to treatment sessions TG2: 81% attendance to treatment sessions
Outcome (measure)	Pain during intercourse (NRS) Vulvar sensitivity (vulvalgesiometer) Global impression of change (patient global impression of change) Authors stated that sample size calculation was based on non-inferiority design; however, power analysis described does not allow for non-inferiority margin.
Results (between-group analyses)	Results presented are based on the whole sample (not limited to the randomized participants). The authors stated that randomization status did not significantly alter any findings. Changes in pain during intercourse were greater in TG1 compared to TG2 from baseline to post-treatment (p = 0.034) and to 6-month follow-up (p = 0.020) (baseline: 6.69 ± 1.91 vs 5.86 ± 2.13; post-treatment: 4.34 ± 2.22 vs 4.65 ± 2.21; 6-month follow-up: 3.39 ± 1.89 vs 4.03 ± 2.11). Reduction in vulvar pain sensitivity was not significantly different between both groups. Proportion of participants reporting moderate or great improvement in pain was not significantly different between both groups at post-treatment (TG1 35% vs TG2 51%) nor at 6-month follow-up (TG1 58% vs TG2 68%).
Author	**Carrico et al. (2008)**
Study design	Pilot RCT
Study population	30 women with interstitial cystitis presenting with PFM pain on palpation

Continued

TABLE 9.3.2 Randomized Controlled Trials That Provided Predominantly Psychological/Cognitive Interventions to Treat Chronic Pelvic Floor Pain—cont'd

Intervention	TG1: Guided imagery, where participants listened to a 25-min guided imagery CD (focused on healing bladder, relaxing PFMs and quieting nerves), 2×/day for 8 weeks TG2: Relaxation session, where participants rested in lying or sitting position for 25 min 2×/day for 8 weeks
Drop-out/adherence	TG1: 4/15 TG2: 1/15 Adherence not reported
Outcome (measure)	Interstitial cystitis symptom and problem (OSPI symptom and problem subscales) Pain intensity (VAS) Patient-perceived improvement (GRA) No sample size calculation provided
Results (between-group analyses)	OSPI (symptom and problem subscales) scores declined in both groups from baseline to post-treatment, but non-significant difference was found between groups. Pain scores significantly decreased in TG1, but no difference was found between groups. For patient's perceived improvement, 45% of women in TG1 reported moderate or marked improvement on GRA compared to 14% in TG2, but this difference was not significant.
Author	**Carty et al. (2019)**
Study design	RCT (randomization ratio: 2:1)
Study population	70 women with chronic urogenital pain (e.g., interstitial cystitis, pelvic floor dysfunction or dyspareunia)
Intervention	TG: 90-min life stress emotional awareness and expression interview that encouraged disclosure about stressors and used experiential techniques to increase awareness of links between stress, emotions and symptoms CG: no interview, usual care
Drop-out/adherence	TG: 8/45 CG: 4/25 All participants analysed completed single interview (TG)
Outcome (measure)	Pain severity (Brief Pain Inventory) This study included several non-pain outcomes. However, sample size calculation provided did not specify which outcome it referred to.
Results (between-group analyses)	Within-group changes were non-significant in both groups. Changes in pain severity were greater in TG compared to CG from baseline to 6-week follow-up (TG 3.87 ± 2.03 to 3.42 ± 0.26 vs CG 4.24 ± 1.65 to 4.33 ± 0.32; $p = 0.05$[b]).
Author	**Goldfinger et al. (2016)**
Study design	Pilot RCT
Study population	20 women with PVD
Intervention	Both treatments: 8 supervised sessions of 1.5-h duration delivered over 8–24 weeks TG1: Physical therapy, including education, PFM exercises, manual techniques, surface electromyographic biofeedback, progressive vaginal penetration exercises through use of 4 silicone vaginal dilators of varied diameter, stretches of hip muscles, deep breathing and global body relaxation exercises, and pain management techniques TG2: Cognitive behavioral therapy, including education, collaborative reconceptualization of PVD as a multifactorial pain condition, desensitization exercises including instructions on how to perform genital self-exploration at home, diaphragmatic breathing and other relaxation techniques, techniques for increasing sexual desire and arousal, sexual communication skills training, cognitive restructuring, and instructions on carrying out PFM exercises and using 4 silicone vaginal dilators to perform progressive vaginal penetration exercises at home (same dilators as used in TG1)

[b]Statistical analyses controlled for baseline imbalances between groups.

TABLE 9.3.2 **Randomized Controlled Trials That Provided Predominantly Psychological/ Cognitive Interventions to Treat Chronic Pelvic Floor Pain—cont'd**

Drop-out/adherence	No dropouts reported TG1: 90% attended all 8 sessions TG2: 80% attended all 8 sessions
Outcome (measure)	Pain intensity during intercourse (NRS), further categorized into women having or not having decrease of 30% and 50% in pain Pain during cotton swab test (NRS) Pain quality (MPQ) Degree of vulvar pain improvement from 1 (complete cure) to 6 (pain worse) No sample size calculation provided, but authors discussed lack of power
Results (between-group analyses)	Changes in pain intensity and pain quality were not significantly different between groups at post-treatment and 6-month follow-up. Percentages of women having decrease in pain of 30% and 50%, as well as degree of vulvar improvement, were not significantly different between groups at post-treatment and 6-month follow-up. Only TG1 group showed significant decreases in pain during cotton swab test from before to after treatment (baseline: 4.2 ± 1.5, post-treatment: 1.3 ± 1; 6-month follow-up: 1.9 ± 2.2), compared to TG2 (baseline: 3.9 ± 2.3; post-treatment: 3.3 ± 2.7; 6-month follow-up: 2.6 ± 2.9). By 6-month follow-up, both groups demonstrated non-significant difference.
Author	**Guillet et al. (2019)**
Study design	RCT
Study population	31 women with PVD (pain >6 months, diagnosed according to Friedrich's criteria)
Intervention	TG1: mindfulness-based group cognitive behavior therapy, 8 weekly sessions TG2: education support group, 8 weeks of online education with 3 in-person group visits
Drop-out/adherence	No drop-outs reported TG1: 10/14 women attended all visits; 4/14 attended 7 of 8 visits TG2: 12/17 women attended all visits; 5/17 attended 2 of 3 visits.
Outcome (measure)	Vaginal insertion pain during tampon test (NRS) Pain catastrophizing (Pain Catastrophizing Scale) Information incomplete for sample size calculation
Results (between-group analyses)	Vaginal insertion pain decreased in both groups, but changes were not statistically different between groups from baseline to post-treatment (difference between groups: 0.022; 95% CI: −1.272 to 1.316), to 3-month (−0.666; 95% CI: −2.035 to 0.703) and to 6-month follow-up (−0.557; 95% CI: −1.947 to 0.834). Change in pain catastrophizing was superior in TG1 compared to TG2 from baseline to post-treatment (difference between groups: −2.959; 95% CI −9.705 to 3.788), to 3-month (−3.591; 95% CI: −10.364 to 3.182) and to 6-month follow-up (−1.077; 95% CI: −8.016 to 5.862).
Author	**Kanter et al. (2016)**
Study design	RCT
Study population	20 women with interstitial cystitis/bladder pain syndrome (as defined by the AUA): an unpleasant sensation (pain, pressure, discomfort) perceived to be related to urinary bladder, associated with lower urinary tract symptoms >6 weeks duration, in absence of infection or other identifiable causes, and minimum score ≥8 on OSPI

Continued

TABLE 9.3.2	**Randomized Controlled Trials That Provided Predominantly Psychological/ Cognitive Interventions to Treat Chronic Pelvic Floor Pain—cont'd**
Intervention	TG: Mindfulness-based stress reduction class for 8 weeks + continuation of current care regimen. Classes were taught by a certified instructor. Standardized course included seven 2-h courses at weekly intervals with an all-day retreat in the fifth week. These sessions taught meditation, yoga and other relaxation techniques. In addition to class training, participants were given a 4-CD guide to meditation and a book to assist with home meditation practice. CG: Usual care including either first-line treatments (relaxation/stress management, pain management and self-care/behavioral modification) or second-line therapy (physical therapy in addition to oral or intravesical medications) Both groups received standardized education, including an educational handout.
Drop-out/adherence	TG: 1/9 CG: 0/11 8 patients who attended classes completed ≥50% of classes
Outcome (measure)	Pain intensity (VAS) Pain (FSFI pain subscale) Interstitial cystitis symptom and problem (OSPI symptoms and problem total subscale, as well as total score) Pain self-efficacy (Pain Self-Efficacy Questionnaire) Perceived improvement (GRA) Sample size sufficient for GRA according to power calculation provided
Results (between-group analyses)	Changes in pain intensity (VAS, FSFI pain subscale) and interstitial cystitis/bladder pain syndrome symptoms (OSPI symptoms subscale) from baseline to post-treatment did not differ between groups. Changes in interstitial cystitis/bladder pain syndrome problem (OSPI problem subscale and OSPI total score) from baseline to post-treatment were significantly higher in TG compared to CG (OSPI problem subscale TG from 10.3 ± 3.1 to 6.4 ± 4 vs CG from 10.2 ± 3.9 to 9.4 ± 3.6, $p = 0.04$; OSPI total score TG from 26.4 ± 8.1 to 18.9 ± 8.7 vs CG from 25.4 ± 6.6 to 24.4 ± 5.6, $p < 0.05$). Change in pain self-efficacy from baseline to post-treatment was significantly higher in TG (34.3 ± 7 to 45.8 ± 11.3) compared to CG (30.8 ± 10.7 to 33.5 ± 9.3) ($p = 0.04$). Significantly more women in TG rated post-treatment symptoms based on GRA as being improved compared to CG (TG 7/8 [87.5%] vs CG 4/11 [36.4%], $p = 0.03$).
Author	**Lee et al. (2018)**
Study design	RCT
Study population	60 women with interstitial cystitis/bladder pain syndrome
Intervention	TG: E-health intervention included video clips for health education and symptom self-management available on a smartphone application. Participants also received usual care in outpatient clinics. A total of 21 brief videos, including 13 for promoting healthy lifestyles and 8 for self-managing emergent symptom flares, were available over 8 weeks to promote healthy lifestyles and behaviours. CG: usual care in outpatient clinics
Drop-out/adherence	TG: 3/29 CG: 1/27 Access to video and adherence to educational content not documented
Outcome (measure)	Pain intensity (VAS) Pain (SF-36 QoL survey bodily pain subscale) Interstitial cystitis symptom and problem (OSPI symptom and problem subscales) Sample size calculation based on non-pain outcome

TABLE 9.3.2 Randomized Controlled Trials That Provided Predominantly Psychological/Cognitive Interventions to Treat Chronic Pelvic Floor Pain—cont'd

Results (between-group analyses)	Change in pain intensity from baseline to post-treatment not significantly different between groups (p = 0.418) Change in pain, as measured with SF-36 QoL survey bodily pain subscale, significantly higher in TG compared to CG (MD: 37.86 ± 30.11 vs −1.11 ± 14.76, p < 0.001) from baseline to post-treatment Change in symptoms and related problem significantly higher in TG compared to CG (symptom MD: −2.31 ± 3.54 vs −0.22 ± 2.97, p = 0.021 and problem MD: −4.48 ± 3.53 vs 0.00 ± 2.83, p < 0.001) from baseline to post-treatment
Author	**Nygaard et al. (2020)**
Study design	RCT
Study population	62 women with CPP ≥6 months and referred to physical therapy
Intervention	TG1: Group-based multimodal physical therapy, including a total of 16 days organized as 10 consecutive days followed by 2-day sessions after 3, 6 and 12 months. A 1-day program started at 8:30 am and finished at 3 pm, with a combination of movement classes, lectures and discussions. There was a preplanned schedule for all 16 days. Intervention was a combination of movement therapy, patient education and acceptance/commitment therapy. Program was given in a group setting with 5–10 women in each group. TG2: Physical therapy treatment was according to therapist academic competence and in consultation with woman.
Drop-out/adherence	TG1: 4 did not receive allocated treatment, 3 discontinued treatment and 6 were lost to follow-up ê 26/32 were analyzed at 12 months. TG2: 1 did not receive allocated treatment, 1 discontinued treatment and 3 were lost to follow-up ê 25/30 were analyzed at 12 months (2 excluded from analysis due to missing 12-month data). Most women in TG1 attended all sessions; 1 woman attended only first 10-day session, and 7 attended 12–14 days of total 16 treatment days (median: 16, interquartile range: 2). In TG2, median number of physical therapy consultations was 14 (interquartile range: 29).
Outcome (measure)	Pelvic pain intensity during previous 7 days (NRS) Worst and least pain intensities during last 7 days (NRS) Pain-related fear of physical movement and activity (Tampa scale for kinesiophobia) Pain during intercourse (yes/no) Pain intensity during intercourse (NRS) Sample size sufficient for mean pelvic pain intensity according to power calculation provided
Results (between-group analyses)	Mean pelvic pain intensity: TG1 significantly improved compared to TG2 from baseline to 12 months (MD between groups: −1.2; 95% CI: −2.3 to −0.1, p = 0.03). Worst and least pain intensities during last 7 days: no significant difference between TG1 compared to TG2 for worst (MD between groups: −1.4; 95% CI: −0.4 to 3.1, p = 0.117) and least (MD between groups: 0.3; 95% CI: −0.9 to 1.4, p = 0.651) from baseline to 12 months. Pain-related fear of physical movement and activity significantly improved in TG1 compared to TG2 from baseline to 12 months (MD between groups: −2.9; 95% CI: −5.5 to −0.3, p = 0.032). Pain during intercourse (yes/no): At baseline, 9 (75%, 4 missing) women in TG1 and 11 (73%, 1 missing) in TG2 reported painful intercourse. At 12 months, 6 (38%) women in TG1 and 10 (63%) in TG2 reported painful intercourse. No statistical analysis was performed. Changes in pain intensity during intercourse (NRS) were not significantly different between groups (MD between groups: −1.9; 95% CI: −5.6 to 2, p = 0.326).

Continued

TABLE 9.3.2 Randomized Controlled Trials That Provided Predominantly Psychological/Cognitive Interventions to Treat Chronic Pelvic Floor Pain—cont'd

Author	Poleshuck et al. (2014)
Study design	RCT
Study population	62 women with CPP co-occurring with depression as defined by Patient Health Questionnaire 2-item version (score >3); minimal pain intensity >3 and pain interference >2 assessed with SF-36
Intervention	TG1: interpersonal psychotherapy for 8 sessions; treatment tailored interpersonal issues associated with both onset and maintenance of depression TG2: research coordinator–facilitated psychotherapy referral to community mental health center and monthly phone call
Drop-out/adherence	TG1: 7/37 TG2: 4/28 TG1: 24/34 received ≥1 session and 6/34 received 0 sessions (mean number of sessions attended: 3.5 ± 0.7) TG2: 16/28 received ≥1 session and 12/28 received 0 sessions (mean number of sessions attended: 2.3 ± 1.9)
Outcome (measure)	Pain intensity (Multidimensional Pain Inventory) No sample size calculation provided
Results (between-group analyses)	Non-significant changes for pain intensity in both groups from baseline to 12, 24 and 26 weeks after randomization; non-significant between-group differences

AUA, American Urological Association; *CG,* control group; *CPP,* chronic pelvic pain; *FSFI,* Female Sexual Function Index; *GRA,* global response assessment; *MD,* mean difference; *MPQ,* McGill Pain Questionnaire; *NRS,* numerical rating scale; *OSPI,* O'Leary–Sant Symptom Problem Index; *PFM,* pelvic floor muscle; *PVD,* provoked vestibulodynia; *QoL,* quality of life; *RCT,* randomized controlled trial; *SF-36,* Short Form 36 Health Survey Questionnaire; *TG,* treatment group; *VAS,* visual analogue scale.

TABLE 9.3.3 Randomized Controlled Trials That Provided Multimodal Physical Therapy Intervention to Treat Chronic Pelvic Floor Pain

Author	Bardin et al. (2020b)
Study design	RCT
Study population	73 women with vulvodynia (provoked or mixed) for ≥3 months; participants included if they had positive cotton swab test and reported sexual pain for ≥50% of sexual intercourse episodes
Intervention	TG1: PFM physical therapy treatment combined with amitriptyline (25 mg orally 1×/day before bedtime for 8 weeks); 8 weeks of home exercise protocol including PFM contraction in 4 different positions (lying in supine + flexed knees, lying in supine with abducted hips, seated and standing) and stretching exercises; stretching exercises performed by physical therapist once a week and self-performed 1×/day by participant TG2: amitriptyline (25 mg orally 1×/day before bedtime for 8 weeks) + meeting with physical therapist 1×/week to discuss adherence.
Drop-out/adherence	TG1: 7/32 TG2: 9/27 Adherence assessed but not reported
Outcome (measure)	Pain intensity during the cotton swab test (NRS) Pain during intercourse (Friedrich score of 0–15, ranging from no symptoms to most intense clinical symptoms of vulvodynia); pain intensity during intercourse (NRS) Sample size calculated for non-pain outcome

TABLE 9.3.3 Randomized Controlled Trials That Provided Multimodal Physical Therapy Intervention to Treat Chronic Pelvic Floor Pain—cont'd

Results (between-group analyses)	TG1 resulted in significantly higher changes from baseline to post-treatment compared to TG2 for pain intensity during cotton swab test (MD: –3.7; 95% CI: –7 to –0.4, p = 0.018), Friedrich's criteria (MD: –1.9; 95% CI: –3.2 to –0.6, p = 0.003) and pain intensity during intercourse (MD: –1.7; 95% CI: –3.1 to –0.2, p = 0.01)
	Adverse event: n = 1 (skin rash) in TG1
Author	**Ghaderi et al. (2019)**
Study design	RCT
Study population	64 women with dyspareunia related to pelvic floor myalgia (women with vestibulodynia excluded)
Intervention	TG: Weekly physical therapy sessions for 3 months, each session entailing 15–20 min of manual techniques to release trigger points in pelvic floor using intravaginal myofascial soft tissue release and deep intravaginal massage, and 20–25 min of high-frequency TENS using intravaginal electrodes (at 110 Hz for 80-ms pulse duration and maximal tolerable intensity to relieve pain); participants also instructed to perform PFM exercises at home
	CG: no treatment
Drop-out/adherence	No dropouts reported
	Adherence measured in diary but not reported
Outcome (measure)	Pain during palpation of PFMs (VAS)
	Pain (FSFI pain subscale)
	Sample size sufficient for FSFI total score (but not pain subscale) according to power calculation provided
Results (between-group analyses)	Changes in pain intensity during palpation significantly higher in TG compared to CG from baseline to post-treatment (between-group MD: 7.32; 95% CI: 6.76–7.88, p < 0.05)[b] and 3-month follow-up (between-group MD: 7.57; 95% CI: 7.03–8.10, p < 0.05)[b]
	Changes in pain (as measured with FSFI subscale) significantly higher in TG compared to CG from baseline to post-treatment (between-group MD: 8.07; 95% CI: 7.26–8.89, p < 0.05)[b]
Author	**Morin et al. (2020)**
Study design	RCT
Study population	212 women diagnosed with PVD according to modified Friedrich's criteria; participants had average pain intensity >5/10 in ≥90% of attempted sexual intercourse episodes for >6 months
Intervention	TG1: physical therapy, consisting of 10 weeks of individual 1-h sessions entailing education, PFM exercises with biofeedback, manual therapy and vaginal dilation
	TG2: overnight application of topical lidocaine (5%) ointment according to protocol of Zolnoun et al. (2003)
Drop-out/adherence	TG1: 6/105 at post-treatment and 11/105 at 6-month follow-up
	TG2: 5/107 at post-treatment and 6/107 at 6-month follow-up
	All participants in TG1 attended 10 treatment sessions; median adherence to home exercises 85% (interquartile range: 75%–91%)
	For TG2, median adherence to lidocaine 91% (interquartile range: 83%–96%)
Outcome (measure)	Pain intensity during intercourse (NRS)
	Pain quality (McGill Pain Questionnaire)
	Patient perceived improvement (patient global impression of change)
	Sample size sufficient for pain intensity according to power calculation provided

[b]Statistical analyses adjusted for baseline group imbalance.

Continued

TABLE 9.3.3 **Randomized Controlled Trials That Provided Multimodal Physical Therapy Intervention to Treat Chronic Pelvic Floor Pain—cont'd**	
Results (between-group analyses)	TG1 was more effective than TG2 for reducing pain intensity during intercourse (MD between groups: 1.8; 95% CI: 1.2–2.3), and results were maintained at 6-month follow-up (MD between groups: 1.8; 95% CI: 1.2–2.5). TG1 was more effective than TG2 for pain quality (MD between groups: 7.8; 95% CI: 4.2–11.4), and results were maintained at 6-month follow-up (MD between groups: 7.8; 95% CI: 4.8–11.4). Regarding participants' impression of change, 79% of women in TG1 reported being very much or much improved compared with 39% in TG2 (p < 0.001).

CG, Control group; *FSFI,* Female Sexual Function Index; *MD,* mean difference; *NRS,* numerical rating scale; *PFM,* pelvic floor muscle; *PVD,* provoked vestibulodynia; *RCT,* randomized controlled trial; *TENS,* transcutaneous electrical nerve stimulation; *TG,* treatment group; *VAS,* visual analogue scale.

METHODOLOGICAL QUALITY

The PEDro rating scale was used to assess the methodological quality of the 35 included trials, as illustrated in Table 9.3.4.

For trials investigating the effectiveness of predominantly biological interventions, 9 of 22 studies rated fair quality (score 4–5), 10 of 22 rated good quality (score 6–8) and only 3 of 22 rated excellent quality. For trials assessing predominantly psychological interventions, 2 of 11 rated poor quality (score 0–3), 3 of 11 rated fair quality, and 6 of 11 rated good quality. Most of the trials evaluating multimodal physical therapy (4 of 5 studies) were rated as having a good-quality PEDro score. The overall trend is an improved quality of RCTs in recent years, probably related to the development and publication of consensus and expert opinion guides for optimal study design and methodologies (Boutron et al., 2017; Dworkin et al., 2008). The main source of bias across the trials was related to the blinding of participants, therapists and assessors, with 26 of 35, 29 of 35 and 25 of 35 studies not satisfying these criteria, respectively. As emphasized in the CONSORT statement for behavioural/non-pharmacological treatment (Boutron et al., 2017), masking these types of intervention is almost impossible to achieve given the inherent nature of these treatments (e.g., exercises, manual therapy, psychotherapy, comparison of two active treatments). For most of the studies included the use of a sham intervention would not have been credible nor feasible for the participants nor the therapist. The only exception was the studies using electrotherapy (8 of 35) (i.e., laser, electrical stimulation, electroacupuncture, extracorporeal shock wave therapy) for which a sham intervention,

and therefore blinding of the therapist and patients, was feasible (Chuang et al., 2020; Divandari et al., 2019; Hullender Rubin et al., 2019; Hurt et al., 2020; Lev-Sagie et al., 2017; Morin et al., 2017; Murina et al., 2008; Murina et al., 2018; O'Reilly et al., 2004). Moreover, given that pain is a subjective experience, it has been recommended that researchers use self-reported outcomes such as pain severity (intensity, distress and interference) as a primary outcome to capture the effects of an intervention (Dworkin et al., 2008; Treede et al., 2019). In such circumstances, the patient becomes the assessor of her own condition and therefore, when an intervention cannot be masked, a negative bias is automatically assigned to the criterion 'assessors blinded' (25 of 35 studies). The risk of bias tool used for assessing the quality of trials should consider these methodological challenges in behavioural/non-pharmacological intervention for chronic pain conditions and should instead assess the strategies used to mitigate this bias.

Other criteria that were frequently rated as 'not satisfied' on the PEDro scale in the included studies were non-report of the concealment method (15 of 35 studies) and the analyses not conducted by intention to treat (13 of 35). Furthermore, several studies (7 of 35) did not present the statistical comparison between groups, most often limiting their analyses to within-group changes (Bond et al., 2017; Divandari et al., 2019; Haugstad et al., 2006; Haugstad et al., 2008; Hullender Rubin et al., 2019; Istek et al., 2014; Murina et al., 2008). As the between-group difference is the required standard to establish treatment effectiveness (Moher et al., 2010), these studies are not further described in the following unless promising clinically meaningful findings emerged from these studies (Dworkin et al., 2008). Other frequent

TABLE 9.3.4 PEDro Quality Score of Randomized Clinical Trials on Conservative Therapy Treatments for Chronic Pelvic Floor Pain

E – Eligibility criteria specified
1 – Subjects randomly allocated to groups
2 – Allocation concealed
3 – Groups similar at baseline
4 – Subjects blinded
5 – Therapist administering treatment blinded
6 – Assessors blinded
7 – Measures of key outcomes obtained from >85% of subjects
8 – Data analysed by intention to treat
9 – Statistical comparison between groups conducted
10 – Point measures and measures of variability provided

Study	E	1	2	3	4	5	6	7	8	9	10	Total Score
Amin et al. (2015)	+	+	−	+	−	−	−	+	+	+	+	6
Bardin et al. (2020b)	+	+	+	+	−	−	−	−	−	+	+	5
Bergeron et al. (2001)	+	+	+	+	−	−	−	−	+	+	+	6
Bergeron et al. (2008)	+	+	+	+	−	−	−	−	+	+/−	+	6
Bond et al. (2017)	+	+	+	−	−	−	−	+	+	−	+	5
Brotto et al. (2019)	+	−	−	+	−	−	−	+	+	+	+	4
Carrico et al. (2008)	+	+	+	−	−	−	−	−	−	+	−	3
Carty et al. (2019)	+	+	+	+	−	−	−	−	+	+	+	6
Chuang et al. (2020)	−	+	−	+	+	+	+	+	+	+	+	9
Danielsson et al. (2006)	+	+	−	+	−	−	−	−	+	+	+	5
De Bernardes et al. (2010)	+	+	+	−	−	+	−	+	+	+	−	7
Divandari et al. (2019)	+	+	−	−	+	+	+	+	+	−	+	7
Fitzgerald et al. (2012)	+	+	−	+	−	−	−	+	−	+	+	5
Ghaderi et al. (2019)	+	+	+	+	−	−	−	+	+	+	+	7
Goldfinger et al. (2016)	+	+	−	+	−	−	−	+	+	+	+	6
Guillet et al. (2019)	+	+	+	+	−	−	−	+	+	+	+	7
Haugstad et al. (2006)	+	+	−	+	−	−	+	+	−	−	+	5
Haugstad et al. (2008)	−	+	−	+	−	−	−	+	−	−	+	4
Heyman et al. (2006)	+	+	−	−	−	−	−	+	−	+	+	4
Hullender Rubin et al. (2019)	+	+	+	−	+	−	+	−	−	−	+	5
Hurt et al. (2020)	+	+	+	−	+	−	+	+	−	+	+	7
Istek et al. (2014)	+	+	−	−	−	−	−	+	+	−	+	4
Kanter et al. (2016)	+	+	+	+	−	−	−	+	−	+	+	6
Lee et al. (2018)	−	−	−	−	−	−	−	+	−	+	+	3
Lev-Sagie et al. (2017)	+	+	−	+	+	+	+	+	−	+	+	8
Morin et al. (2017)	+	+	+	+	+	+	+	+	+	+	+	10
Morin et al. (2020)	+	+	+	+	−	−	−	+	+	+	+	7
Murina et al. (2008)	−	+	+	+	+	−	+	+	+	−	+	8
Murina et al. (2018)	−	+	+	+	+	+	+	+	+	+	+	10

Continued

TABLE 9.3.4 PEDro Quality Score of Randomized Clinical Trials on Conservative Therapy Treatments for Chronic Pelvic Floor Pain—cont'd

Study	E	1	2	3	4	5	6	7	8	9	10	Total Score
Nygaard et al. (2020)	+	+	+	+	−	−	−	−	−	+	+	5
O'Reilly et al. (2004)	+	+	−	−	+	−	+	+	+	+	+	7
Poleshuck et al. (2014)	+	+	−	−	−	−	−	+	+	+	4
Schlaeger et al. (2015)	+	+	+	+	−	−	−	+	+	+	+	7
Schvartzman et al. (2019)	+	+	+	+	−	−	−	+	+	+	+	7
Zoorob et al. (2015)	+	+	+	−	−	−	−	−	−	+	+	4

+, Criterion is clearly satisfied; −, criterion is not satisfied.
The total score is determined by counting the number of criteria that are satisfied, except the 'eligibility criteria specified' score is not used to generate the total score. Total scores are out of 10.

methodological aspects not captured by the PEDro scale include the very small sample size for a large proportion of the included studies. Indeed, 22 of 35 studies had very small sample sizes, less than 25 per treatment arm. Studies with small sample sizes are known to yield larger effect estimates than larger trials (Dechartres et al., 2013). In addition, very few studies (8 of 35) provided an adequate, sufficiently detailed, sample size calculation based on pain outcomes (Amin et al., 2015; Fitzgerald et al., 2012; Hurt et al., 2020; Kanter et al., 2016; Morin et al., 2020; Nygaard et al., 2020; Schvartzman et al., 2019). This is critical for interpreting the findings of RCTs, as it is not possible to judge if the non-significant results obtained from most of the trials (Bergeron et al., 2001; Bergeron et al., 2008; Bond et al., 2017; Brotto et al., 2019; Carrico et al., 2008; Chuang et al., 2020; Danielsson et al., 2006; Divandari et al., 2019; Goldfinger et al., 2016; Guillet et al., 2019; Hullender Rubin et al., 2019; Kanter et al., 2016; Lee et al., 2018; Lev-Sagie et al., 2017; Murina et al., 2018; O'Reilly et al., 2004; Poleshuck et al., 2014; Zoorob et al., 2015) represent a lack of statistical power or represent evidence against the intervention. Further, some studies (4 of 35) administered interventions with a very low dose, which may have been below the therapeutic dose for that intervention. Although the optimal dose for many of these interventions remains unknown, some studies provided only one or two treatment sessions (Carty et al., 2019; Poleshuck et al., 2014) or had low adherence, where participants completed less than half of the prescribed exercises (Bergeron et al., 2001; Danielsson et al., 2006).

EVIDENCE FOR EFFECTIVENESS OF PREDOMINANTLY BIOLOGICAL INTERVENTIONS

In this review, predominantly biological interventions represented the most frequent intervention tested. A total of 22 RCTs assessed the effectiveness of electrotherapies, acupuncture, PFM exercises with biofeedback, manual therapy and body awareness on pain outcomes in women with different subtypes of CPP (e.g., interstitial cystitis [IC]/bladder pain syndrome [BPS], provoked vestibulodynia [PVD], myalgia) or CPP not further defined.

Electrotherapies
Intra-Vaginal Electrical Stimulation
The effectiveness of intra-vaginal electrical stimulation in women with CPP was investigated in a crossover RCT by de Bernardes et al. (2010). They found a significantly higher proportion of women reporting a daily pain intensity score of 3 or less as measured with the visual analogue scale (VAS) following active stimulation compared to sham stimulation. The effect on dyspareunia was difficult to judge, as it was assessed using a binary outcome (present/absent) and few women presented with dyspareunia at baseline (De Bernardes et al., 2010). Murina et al. (2008) compared intravaginal transcutaneous electrical nerve stimulation (TENS) to sham in women with PVD. Significant reduction in irritation and burning sensation (VAS) and pain quality (McGill Pain Questionnaire [MPQ]) were shown in the TENS

group, whereas no changes were found in the sham group. Despite a lack of between-group differences presented, the within-group change in the treatment group may represent a clinically meaningful improvement. In another RCT, Murina et al. (2018) assessed the effects of adding either intra-vaginal diazepam or a placebo tablet to TENS. They showed that the addition of diazepam to TENS significantly improved the Marinoff dyspareunia scale but not the pain intensity as measured with the VAS.

Percutaneous Tibial Nerve Stimulation

Istek et al. (2014) assessed the effectiveness of 12 weeks of percutaneous tibial nerve stimulation (PTNS) in women with CPP compared to usual care including the use of analgesics. Nine patients (56.3%) reported that they were either cured or much improved, based on a non-validated outcome measure, after PTNS at 6-month follow-up, whereas in the control group, only two patients (11.8%) were improved. However, no statistical analysis was presented to determine a between-group difference for this outcome. Regarding secondary outcomes, PTNS was also superior to usual care for improving pain quality (MPQ) at 12 weeks post-treatment but not at 6-month follow-up. Further, the changes in pain intensity and quality of life were non-significant between the two groups (Istek et al., 2014). O'Reilly et al. (2004) used laser to perform stimulation of the tibial nerve in women with IC compared to a sham stimulation. The laser stimulation was not shown to be effective for improving symptom severity, as the between-group difference was not significant and the changes that occurred appeared below the margin of clinically meaningful improvement.

Transcranial Direct Current Stimulation

Morin et al. (2017) conducted a well-powered triple-blinded study comparing 10 sessions of transcranial direct current stimulation (tDCS) to sham in women with PVD. They found that tDCS was not effective compared to sham for all outcomes (pain intensity, quality of pain, vestibular sensitivity, perceived improvement) at immediate post-treatment and 3-month follow-up (Morin et al., 2017).

Extracorporeal Shock Wave Therapy

In the RCT of Chuang et al. (2020) the effectiveness of four weekly sessions of shockwave therapy (2000 pulses per session) applied suprapubically was assessed in women with IC/BPS refractory to conventional therapy compared to sham. Only the proportion of participants reporting improvement, defined as VAS reduction of 3 or more, significantly favoured shockwave therapy. All other outcomes including IC symptoms (O'Leary–Sant Symptom Problem Index [OSPI] symptom subscale) and perceived improvement (global response assessment) were not significantly different between the two groups. It is unclear if these findings relate to lack of statistical power. In contrast, the study of Hurt et al. (2020) supported the effectiveness of four weekly sessions of shockwave (3000 pulses per session) administered on the vulvar area in women with PVD. This study showed that shockwave was more effective than sham to reduce pain intensity and vulvar pain sensitivity at 1, 4 and 12 weeks post-treatment, and the changes observed appear to overcome the minimal clinically important differences.

Low-Level Laser Therapy

A pilot RCT was conducted by Lev-Sagie et al. (2017) to investigate the effect of laser in women with PVD in comparison to sham. The only significant difference between the two groups was the pain intensity when converted into a categorial variable. Non-significant differences were found between the two groups for all other outcomes (vulvar pain sensitivity, pain during intercourse, severity of discomfort in daily activities and during sexual activity, pain during the tampon test), which could be related to the small sample size.

Acupuncture

Amin et al. (2015) showed that electroacupuncture was less effective than inferior hypogastric nerve blockade for reducing pain intensity, assessed with the VAS, after 1 hour, 2 weeks, 6 weeks and 12 weeks post-treatment in women with CPP. However, non-significant difference between groups was found for pain status categorized as completely relieved, partially relieved, no change and not able to decide (Amin et al., 2015). In contrast, when comparing traditional acupuncture to a waitlist control in women with PVD, Schlaeger et al. (2015) showed that acupuncture was significantly more effective for all pain outcomes (VAS, MPQ, Female Sexual Function Index [FSFI] pain subscale), and the changes observed appeared to exceed minimal clinically important differences.

Pelvic Floor Muscle Exercises With Biofeedback

Bergeron et al. (2001) conducted an RCT comparing the effectiveness of vestibulectomy, PFM exercise using home biofeedback and cognitive behavioural therapy (CBT) in women with PVD. Significant improvements were shown in all treatment groups from pre- to post-treatment in pain intensity during intercourse, pain quality and subjective improvement. However, no between-group differences were found. The only outcome favouring the vestibulectomy group was the pain intensity during the cotton swab test (vestibular pain index). It is difficult to interpret these findings, as no sample size estimation was provided and an important lack of adherence was reported in the biofeedback group. The subsequent follow-up study (Bergeron et al., 2008) suggested that results were maintained over time in all groups, but vestibulectomy was found to be superior to biofeedback for pain intensity, vestibular pain index and pain quality at 6-month and 2.5-year follow-up. The statistical analysis comparing the biofeedback group and the CBT group was not presented. Danielsson et al. (2006) compared home biofeedback to topical lidocaine in women with PVD. Although they found significant improvements in both groups from pre- to post-treatment, the between-group comparisons revealed non-significant differences for pain intensity, vulvar pain sensitivity and perception of improvement. Once again, the interpretation of findings is hindered by a sample size calculation based on non-pain outcome and limited adherence to exercises.

Manual Therapy

Three RCTs examined different treatment protocols of manual therapy in women with IC/BPS, CPP and myalgia, revealing significant effects on pain, sexual function and perceived improvement (Fitzgerald et al., 2012; Heyman et al., 2006; Zoorob et al., 2015). Fitzgerald et al. (2012) compared myofascial therapy applied to the PFMs and the surrounding tissues to global therapeutic massage in women with IC/BPS. This study was sufficiently powered to examine the patient's perceived improvement as a primary outcome and found that myofascial therapy was superior to global massage. Non-significant between-group differences were found for pain intensity and IC symptoms, which could be related to lack of statistical power for these outcomes. In the study of Heyman et al. (2006), the effectiveness of stretching of the PFMs per rectal digital palpation was compared to counselling in women with CPP. Stretching applied for two sessions showed superior effects to counselling for reducing spontaneous pain and pain during intercourse, and the changes observed appeared to exceed minimal clinically important differences. In women with PF myalgia, Zoorob et al. (2015) evaluated the effectiveness of PFM trigger point release techniques, massage and stretching in comparison with the trigger point injection of a mixture of anaesthetics and steroids. Both groups showed statistically and clinically meaningful changes in pain from pre- to post-treatment. However, only the FSFI total score and pain subscale were significantly different between the two groups and favoured manual therapy (Zoorob et al., 2015).

Body Awareness

Haugstad et al. (2006, 2008) undertook an RCT and a follow-up study to investigate the addition of a body awareness program (e.g., awareness of body movements, tension, relaxation, posture, gait, respiration) to usual care in women with CPP. Significant improvement in motor control (Mensendieck score assessed by a therapist blinded to group allocation) and pain intensity were shown in the body awareness group, whereas no changes were found in the usual care group. No between-group differences were presented; however, the within-group changes appeared to show an effect in the treatment group that may represent a clinically meaningful improvement for pain intensity.

EVIDENCE FOR EFFECTIVENESS OF PREDOMINANTLY PSYCHOLOGICAL/ COGNITIVE INTERVENTIONS

A total of 12 RCTs investigated the effectiveness of predominantly psychological or cognitive interventions including CBT (Bergeron et al., 2001; Bergeron et al., 2008; Brotto et al., 2019; Goldfinger et al., 2016), mindfulness (Brotto et al., 2019; Guillet et al., 2019; Kanter et al., 2016), other types of psychotherapy (Carty et al., 2019; Poleshuck et al., 2014), mental imagery (Carrico et al., 2008) and different forms of an educational program (Lee et al., 2018; Nygaard et al., 2020).

Cognitive Behavioural Therapy

Four studies investigated the effectiveness of CBT in women with PVD. As discussed previously in the section on biofeedback, Bergeron et al. (2001) compared vestibulectomy, biofeedback and CBT, and no between-group differences were found for pain intensity, pain quality and subjective improvement. The only outcome favouring the vestibulectomy group was pain intensity during the cotton swab test (vestibular pain index). The follow-up study (Bergeron et al., 2008) suggested that results were maintained over time in all groups, but vestibulectomy was found to be superior to CBT for the vestibular pain index and pain quality at 6-month and 2.5-year follow-up. Vestibulectomy was not different from CBT for pain during intercourse. The pilot study of Goldfinger et al. (2016) showed improvements in both CBT and physical therapy groups regarding pain intensity during intercourse, pain quality and perceived improvement at post-treatment and 6-month follow-up, but it was not sufficiently powered to detect between-group differences. The only exception was the change in pain during the cotton swab test at post-treatment, which favoured the physical therapy group (Goldfinger et al., 2016). The study of Brotto et al. (2019) was a cohort study in which a third of the participants were randomized. They compared CBT to mindfulness treatment and found that the changes in pain intensity at post-treatment and at 6-month follow-up were significantly higher in the mindfulness group. Vulvar sensitivity and global impression of change were similar between the two groups.

Mindfulness

In addition to the study of Brotto et al. (2019) described earlier, two RCTs examined the effectiveness of mindfulness in women with PVD and IC/BPS. Guillet et al. (2019) compared mindfulness to education support group sessions in women with PVD. Significant improvements in pain during the tampon test and pain catastrophizing were shown in both groups from pre- to post-treatment, but only the latter showed a significant between-group difference in favour of the mindfulness group. Kanter et al. (2016) concluded that mindfulness was more effective than usual care in women with IC/BPS, as they found that mindfulness was superior in the primary outcome of perceived improvement. Mindfulness also yielded superior effects for IC/BPS-related problem (OSPI problem and total score) and pain self-efficacy. No significant between-group differences were found for pain intensity (VAS, FSFI pain subscale) and IC/BPS (OSPI symptoms), which may be explained by the lack of statistical power.

Other Types of Psychotherapy

Poleshuck et al. (2014) examined the effectiveness of psychotherapy tailored to interpersonal issues associated with the onset and maintenance of depression compared with referral to other subtypes of psychotherapy in women with CPP co-occurring with depression. No within- nor between-group changes were found for pain, which may be due to low attendance at therapy sessions. Likewise, the dosage may also have been insufficient in the study of Carty et al. (2019) given that neither statistically significant nor clinically meaningful changes were found in pain after a single stress emotional awareness and expression interview in women with chronic urogenital pain (e.g., IC, PF dysfunction or dyspareunia).

Mental Imagery

In a pilot study by Carrico et al. (2008), mental imagery focusing on healing the bladder, relaxing the PFMs and quieting the nerves) was compared to general relaxation in women with IC/BPS with PFM pain on palpation. Although imagery resulted in significant changes in pain intensity and IC symptoms and problems from pre- to post-treatment, the study was not powered to detect between-group differences (Carrico et al., 2008).

Education

The effectiveness of an app including educational video clips and symptom self-management advice was compared to usual care in women with IC/BPS (Lee et al., 2018). The app showed superior effects to usual care for pain (measured with the Short Form 36 Health Survey Questionnaire [SF-36] bodily pain subscale) and bladder cystitis symptoms (OSPI) but not pain assessed with the VAS. It is difficult to judge if these improvements exceeded clinically important changes. Nygaard et al. (2020) examined a physical therapy group-based treatment program including pain education, movement therapy (e.g., relaxation, yoga, mindfulness) and acceptance/commitment therapy offered over 16 intensive full days compared to regular physical therapy sessions in women with CPP. The educational program showed superior effects for mean pain intensity and pain-related fear of movement, but non-significant differences were found between groups for worst and least pain intensity during daily life and pain during intercourse. The authors also questioned the clinical relevance of the observed changes.

EVIDENCE FOR EFFECTIVENESS OF MULTIMODAL PHYSICAL THERAPY INTERVENTION

In addition to the pilot study of Goldfinger et al. (2016) described earlier comparing CBT and physical therapy, the effectiveness of multimodal physical therapy was investigated in four large RCTs in women with PVD and with dyspareunia of different aetiologies (Bardin et al., 2020b; Ghaderi et al., 2019; Morin et al., 2020; Schvartzman et al., 2019). The results of all of these studies support the effectiveness of multimodal physical therapy, as all showed statistically and clinically significant changes in pain intensity during intercourse. The large multicentre trial of Morin et al. (2020) compared multimodal physical therapy to overnight topical lidocaine in women with PVD. The 10-week physical therapy treatment, including education, PFM exercises with biofeedback, manual therapy and vaginal dilation, showed superior effects for pain intensity and pain quality at post-treatment, and the benefits were maintained at 6-month follow-up compared to lidocaine. The clinical relevance of these findings in the physical therapy group were confirmed by comparing the proportion of women presenting improvements that exceed clinically important changes. Regarding participant impression of change, 79% of women in the physical therapy group reported being very much or much improved compared with 39% in the lidocaine group.

Bardin et al. (2020b) examined the additional effect of multimodal physical therapy (e.g., PFM exercises and stretching) to amitriptyline in women with PVD. They found that the group receiving physical therapy had a superior reduction in the Friedrich score, pain during the cotton swab test and pain during intercourse compared to amitriptyline alone. The observed changes also appear to exceed minimal clinically important differences. In women with dyspareunia related to PF myalgia, Ghaderi et al. (2019) investigated physical therapy sessions including myofascial soft tissue release and deep intravaginal massage, PFM exercises and high-frequency intra-vaginal TENS compared to no treatment. Physical therapy was found to be more effective for reducing pain (measured with the VAS and the FSFI pain subscale). Likewise, using the same outcomes measures for assessing pain, Schvartzman et al. (2019) showed that multimodal physical therapy applied to the PFMs (thermotherapy for relaxation of PFMs, myofascial release and PFM exercises) was statistically and clinically superior to myofascial release applied to the abdominal diaphragm, the piriformis and the iliopsoas muscles in peri- and postmenopausal women with dyspareunia.

DISCUSSION

The studies in this review presented significant heterogeneity in population, intervention provided and methodological rigour. A strength of most studies was the use of validated outcome measures for pain. Unfortunately, many studies were underpowered for the outcome of pain and/or did not present between-group differences, which are necessary to interpret treatment effectiveness in RCTs.

Overall, it appears that multimodal physical therapy interventions to treat vulvodynia and dyspareunia demonstrated the strongest effect and provided the most certainty of effectiveness, due to the methodological rigour of the included studies (Bardin et al., 2020b; Ghaderi et al., 2019; Goldfinger et al., 2016; Morin et al., 2020; Schvartzman et al., 2019), and perhaps because multimodal therapies are more likely to address the complexity and multidimensionality of CPP. This is reassuring, as this approach more closely reflects current clinical practice (Hartmann et al., 2007). Nevertheless, studies that attempted to investigate the effectiveness of any single modality are to be applauded, as it is important to identify the 'active ingredients' of any intervention to minimize the treatment burden to patients and unnecessary use of healthcare resources. The attainment of this goal is perhaps more challenging with the application of a biopsychosocial approach to chronic pain management compared to other health conditions. Clinicians are aware of the importance of the patient–therapist relationship, often called *therapeutic alliance*, in maximizing patient gains from treatment. A positive and supportive relationship may confer therapeutic effects that are above and beyond the direct local influence on the muscular system (Bardin et al., 2020a; Kinney et al., 2020). Although many physical therapists have moved towards more biopsychosocial and person-centred approaches in their care of pain conditions, many do not feel confident in delivering all aspects of these approaches (Holopainen et al., 2020). Training is required to provide physical therapists with skills to judiciously apply treatment for chronic PF pain within an evidence-based practice framework (Haynes et al., 2002).

The effect of conservative therapies on pain in other chronic PF pain conditions was less certain, perhaps because fewer trials have been conducted in specific populations of chronic PF pain. The importance of this distinction is unknown. Thirty-five RCTs may seem to be a reasonable number of studies; however, it appears that much more research is needed to answer the questions of what works for whom and how (the mechanism of effect). In some of the included studies in this review, the effect of biologically focused treatment or psychologically informed treatment alone was promising, and future research may identify that a particular intervention has a worthwhile effect in a particular subtype of chronic PF pain or a particular phenotype within the population with the condition.

SUMMARY

Recommendations for clinicians:
- Multimodal physical therapy showed the strongest evidence in subtypes of women with CPP. More specifically, multimodal physical therapy is effective for reducing pain in women with vulvodynia and dyspareunia, as shown in large and sufficiently powered RCTs. These trials showed statistically significant results (e.g., between-group difference) and clinically meaningful changes in pain outcomes. They also found that the benefits were maintained at longer-term follow-up.
- Some evidence supports the following interventions, as statistically significant results (between-group difference) and clinically meaningful changes in pain outcomes were found in single trials:
  - Acupuncture in women with PVD
  - Manual therapy (stretching of the PFMs) in women with CPP or PFM trigger point therapy, massage and stretching in women with PF myalgia
  - Myofascial therapy in women with IC/BPS
  - Extracorporeal shockwave perineal therapy in women with PVD
- Encouraging outcomes (based on within-group changes) or clinically meaningful improvements may be obtained from the following interventions. However, treatment efficacy cannot be concluded

due to methodological limitations. The evidence for these interventions was gathered mostly from single small trials, which may have lacked power to detect between-group differences or did not present between-group comparisons:
  - Intra-vaginal electrical stimulation in women with CPP or PVD
  - Low-level laser therapy in women with PVD
  - PFM exercises with biofeedback in women with PVD
  - Body awareness in women with CPP
  - CBT in women with PVD
  - Mindfulness in women with PVD and IC/BPS
  - Mental imagery in women with IC/BPS
- Unclear or conflicting results were shown from small trials which assessed the following interventions, and therefore there is uncertainty related to their effect:
  - Extracorporeal shockwave suprapubic therapy in women with IC/BPS
  - Education in women with IC/BPS or CPP
- A lack of effect was seen in small trials which assessed the following interventions, and therefore they cannot be recommended at this time:
  - Laser stimulation of the tibial nerve in women with IC
  - tDCS in women with PVD
  - Electroacupuncture in women with CPP
  - Psychotherapy in women with CPP
- Until stronger evidence of treatment effectiveness and a clearer understanding of the mechanisms of pain reduction emerge to guide clinical practice, clinicians are urged to follow the principles of evidence-based practice closely, drawing from knowledge of the clinical condition the patient presents with (including relevant pathophysiology of the musculoskeletal or visceral structures, pain neurophysiology, psychosocial factors), the relevance of existing high-quality research to the patient and patient preferences for treatment (Haynes et al., 2002).

Directions for future research in chronic PF pain intervention trials:
- Studies must be based on a well-informed hypothesis and an a priori–stated minimum clinically important difference, as well as have sufficient power.
- Researchers must stay abreast of developments in pain neurophysiology and pain neuroscience when planning interventions and the presumed mechanism of effect.

- Studies must be designed and reported to provide the reader with clarity of the strengths and limitations of their findings. Close attention to the relevant CONSORT guideline (Boutron et al., 2017; Montgomery et al., 2018) and relevant intervention reporting checklists (Hoffmann et al., 2014; Slade et al., 2016) is essential.

REFERENCES

American College of Obstetricians and Gynecologists. (2020). Chronic pelvic pain: ACOG practice Bulletin, No. 218. *Obstetrics & Gynecology, 135*, e98–e109.

Amin, M. M., Ait-Allah, A. S., Ali Ael, S., et al. (2015). Inferior hypogastric plexus blockade versus acupuncture for the management of idiopathic chronic pelvic pain: A randomized clinical trial. *Biomedical Journal, 38*, 317–322.

Armour, M., Ee, C. C., Naidoo, D., et al. (2019). Exercise for dysmenorrhoea. *Cochrane Database of Systematic Reviews, 9*, CD004142.

Bardin, M., Brassard, A., Dumoulin, C., et al. (2020). Examining the role of the physiotherapist in treatment response of women with provoked vestibulodynia. *Neurourology and Urodynamics, 39*, 37–38.

Bardin, M. G., Giraldo, P. C., & Martinho, N. (2020). Pelvic floor biometric changes assessed by 4D translabial ultrasound in women with vulvodynia submitted to physical therapy: A pilot study of a randomized controlled trial. *The Journal of Sexual Medicine, 17*(11), 2236–2246.

Bergeron, S., Binik, Y. M., Khalifé, S., et al. (2001). A randomized comparison of group cognitive-behavioral therapy, surface electromyographic biofeedback, and vestibulectomy in the treatment of dyspareunia resulting from vulvar vestibulitis. *Pain, 91*, 297–306.

Bergeron, S., Khalifé, S., Glazer, H. I., et al. (2008). Surgical and behavioral treatments for vestibulodynia: Two-and-one-half year follow-up and predictors of outcome. *Obstetrics & Gynecology, 111*, 159–166.

Bond, J., Pape, H., & Ayre, C. (2017). Efficacy of a therapeutic wand in addition to physiotherapy for treating bladder pain syndrome in women: A pilot randomized controlled trial. *Journal Pelvic Obstetrique Gynaecologists Physiotherapy, 120*, 12–27.

Bonocher, C. M., Montenegro, M. L., Rosa, E. S. J. C., et al. (2014). Endometriosis and physical exercises: A systematic review. *Reproductive Biology and Endocrinology, 12*, 4.

Boutron, I., Altman, D. G., Moher, D., et al. (2017). Consort statement for randomized trials of nonpharmacologic treatments: A 2017 update and a consort extension for nonpharmacologic trial abstracts. *Annals of Internal Medicine, 167*, 40–47.

Brooks, T., Sharp, R., Evans, S., et al. (2020). Predictors of psychological outcomes and the effectiveness and experience of psychological interventions for adult women with chronic pelvic pain: A scoping review. *Journal of Pain Research, 13*, 1081–1102.

Brotto, L. A., Bergeron, S., Zdaniuk, B., et al. (2019). A comparison of mindfulness-based cognitive therapy vs cognitive behavioral therapy for the treatment of provoked vestibulodynia in a hospital clinic setting. *The Journal of Sexual Medicine, 16*, 909–923.

Carrico, D. J., Peters, K. M., & Diokno, A. C. (2008). Guided imagery for women with interstitial cystitis: Results of a prospective, randomized controlled pilot study. *Journal of Alternative and Complementary, 14*, 53–60.

Carty, J. N., Ziadni, M. S., Holmes, H. J., et al. (2019). The effects of a life stress emotional awareness and expression interview for women with chronic urogenital pain: A randomized controlled trial. *Pain Medicine, 20*, 1321–1329.

Chuang, Y. C., Meng, E., Chancellor, M., et al. (2020). Pain reduction realized with extracorporeal shock wave therapy for the treatment of symptoms associated with interstitial cystitis/bladder pain syndrome—a prospective, multicenter, randomized, double-blind, placebo-controlled study. *Neurourology and Urodynamics, 39*, 1505–1514.

Cottrell, A. M., Schneider, M. P., Goonewardene, S., et al. (2020). Benefits and harms of electrical neuromodulation for chronic pelvic pain: A systematic review. *European Urology Focus, 6*, 559–571.

Danielsson, I., Torstensson, T., Brodda-Jansen, G., et al. (2006). EMG biofeedback versus topical lidocaine gel: A randomized study for the treatment of women with vulvar vestibulitis. *Acta Obstetricia et Gynecologica Scandinavica, 85*, 1360–1367.

De Bernardes, N. O., Marques, A., Ganunny, C., et al. (2010). Use of intravaginal electrical stimulation for the treatment of chronic pelvic pain: A randomized, double-blind, crossover clinical trial. *Journal of Reproductive Medicine, 55*, 19–24.

Dechartres, A., Trinquart, L., Boutron, I., et al. (2013). Influence of trial sample size on treatment effect estimates: Meta-epidemiological study. *British Medicine Journal, 346*, f2304.

Divandari, N., Manshadi, F. D., Shokouhi, N., et al. (2019). Effect of one session of tDCS on the severity of pain in women with chronic pelvic pain. *Journal of Bodywork and Movement Therapies, 23*, 678–682.

Dworkin, R. H., Turk, D. C., Wyrwich, K. W., et al. (2008). Interpreting the clinical importance of treatment outcomes in chronic pain clinical trials: IMMPACT recommendations. *The Journal of Pain, 9*, 105–121.

Engeler, D., Baranowski, A., Berghmans, B., et al. (2020). *EAU guidelines on chronic pelvic pain [online]*. Available: http://www.uroweb.org/guidelines/online-guidelines/ (Accessed 24.07.22).

Evans, S., Fernandez, S., Olive, L., et al. (2019). Psychological and mind-body interventions for endometriosis: A systematic review. *Journal of Psychosomatic Research, 124,* 109756.

Fitzgerald, M. P., Payne, C. K., Lukacz, E. S., et al. (2012). Randomized multicenter clinical trial of myofascial physical therapy in women with interstitial cystitis/painful bladder syndrome and pelvic floor tenderness. *Journal Urology, 187,* 2113–2118.

Frawley, H. C., Dean, S. G., Slade, S. C., et al. (2017). Is pelvic-floor muscle training a physical therapy or a behavioral therapy? A call to name and report the physical, cognitive, and behavioral elements. *Physical Therapy, 97,* 425–437.

Fuentes-Márquez, P., Cabrera-Martos, I., & Valenza, M. C. (2019). Physiotherapy interventions for patients with chronic pelvic pain: A systematic review of the literature. *Physiotherapy Theory and Practice, 35,* 1131–1138.

Ghaderi, F., Bastani, P., Hajebrahimi, S., et al. (2019). Pelvic floor rehabilitation in the treatment of women with dyspareunia: A randomized controlled clinical trial. *International Urogynecology Journal, 30,* 1849–1855.

Goldfinger, C., Pukall, C. F., Thibault-Gagnon, S., et al. (2016). Effectiveness of cognitive-behavioral therapy and physical therapy for provoked vestibulodynia: A randomized pilot study. *The Journal of Sexual Medicine, 13,* 88–94.

Grinberg, K., Weissman-Fogel, I., Lowenstein, L., et al. (2019). How does myofascial physical therapy attenuate pain in chronic pelvic pain syndrome? *Pain Research and Management, 2019,* 6091257.

Guillet, A. D., Cirino, N. H., Hart, K. D., et al. (2019). Mindfulness-based group cognitive behavior therapy for provoked localized vulvodynia: A randomized controlled trial. *Journal Low Gent Tract Disease, 23,* 170–175.

Hartmann, D., Strauhal, M. J., & Nelson, C. A. (2007). Treatment of women in the United States with localized, provoked vulvodynia: Practice survey of women's health physical therapists. *Journal of Reproductive Medicine, 52,* 48–52.

Haugstad, G. K., Haugstad, T. S., Kirste, U. M., et al. (2006). Mensendieck somatocognitive therapy as treatment approach to chronic pelvic pain: Results of a randomized controlled intervention study. *American Journal of Obstetrics and Gynecology, 194,* 1303–1310.

Haugstad, G. K., Haugstad, T. S., Kirste, U. M., et al. (2008). Continuing improvement of chronic pelvic pain in women after short-term mensendieck somatocognitive therapy: Results of a 1-year follow-up study. *American Journal of Obstetrics and Gynecology, 199,* 615.e1–615.e8.

Haynes, R. B., Devereaux, P. J., & Guyatt, G. H. (2002). Clinical expertise in the era of evidence-based medicine and patient choice. *ACP Journal Club, 136*(2), A11–A14.

Heyman, J., Ohrvik, J., & Leppert, J. (2006). Distension of painful structures in the treatment for chronic pelvic pain in women. *Acta Obstetricia et Gynecologica Scandinavica, 85,* 599–603.

Hoffmann, T. C., Glasziou, P. P., Boutron, I., et al. (2014). Better reporting of interventions: Template for intervention description and replication (TIDieR) checklist and guide. *British Medicine Journal, 348,* g1687.

Holopainen, R., Simpson, P., Piirainen, A., et al. (2020). Physiotherapists' perceptions of learning and implementing a biopsychosocial intervention to treat musculoskeletal pain conditions: A systematic review and metasynthesis of qualitative studies. *Pain, 161,* 1150–1168.

Hullender Rubin, L. E., Mist, S. D., Schnyer, R. N., et al. (2019). Acupuncture augmentation of lidocaine for provoked, localized vulvodynia: A feasibility and acceptability study. *Journal of Lower Genital Tract Disease, 23,* 279–286.

Hurt, K., Zahalka, F., Halaska, M., et al. (2020). Extracorporeal shock wave therapy for treatment of vulvodynia: A prospective, randomized, double-blind, placebo-controlled study. *European Journal of Physical and Rehabilitation Medicine, 56,* 169–174.

Istek, A., Gungor Ugurlucan, F., Yasa, C., et al. (2014). Randomized trial of long-term effects of percutaneous tibial nerve stimulation on chronic pelvic pain. *Archives of Gynecology and Obstetrics, 290,* 291–298.

Jarrell, J. F., Vilos, G. A., Allaire, C., et al. (2018). No. 164—consensus guidelines for the management of chronic pelvic pain. *Journal of Obstetrics and Gynaecology Canada, 40,* e747–e787.

Kanter, G., Komesu, Y. M., Qaedan, F., et al. (2016). Mindfulness-based stress reduction as a novel treatment for interstitial cystitis/bladder pain syndrome: A randomized controlled trial. *International Urogynecology Journal, 27,* 1705–1711.

Kinney, M., Seider, J., Beaty, A. F., et al. (2020). The impact of therapeutic alliance in physical therapy for chronic musculoskeletal pain: A systematic review of the literature. *Physiotherapy Theory and Practice, 36,* 886–898.

Klotz, S. G. R., Schon, M., Ketels, G., et al. (2019). Physiotherapy management of patients with chronic pelvic pain (CPP): A systematic review. *Physiotherapy Theory and Practice, 35,* 516–532.

Lee, M.-H., Wu, H.-C., Tseng, C.-M., et al. (2018). Health education and symptom flare management using a video-based m-health system for caring women with IC/BPS. *Urology, 119,* 62–69.

Lev-Sagie, A., Kopitman, A., & Brzezinski, A. (2017). Low-level laser therapy for the treatment of provoked vestibulodynia—a randomized, placebo-controlled pilot trial. *The Journal of Sexual Medicine, 14,* 1403–1411.

Main, C. J., & George, S. Z. (2011). Psychologically informed practice for management of low back pain: Future directions in practice and research. *Physical Therapy, 91,* 820–824.

May, C., Montori, V. M., & Mair, F. S. (2009). We need minimally disruptive medicine. *British Medicine Journal, 339,* b2803.

Mira, T. A. A., Buen, M. M., Borges, M. G., et al. (2018). Systematic review and meta-analysis of complementary treatments for women with symptomatic endometriosis. *International Journal of Gynaecology & Obstetrics, 143,* 2–9.

Moher, D., Hopewell, S., Schulz, K. F., et al. (2010). CONSORT 2010 explanation and elaboration: Updated guidelines for reporting parallel group randomised trials. *British Medicine Journal, 340,* c869.

Montgomery, P., Grant, S., Mayo-Wilson, E., et al. (2018). *Reporting randomised trials of social and psychological interventions: The CONSORT-SPI 2018 extension.* Trials 19, Art. No. 407.

Morin, A., Léonard, G., Gougeon, V., et al. (2017). Efficacy of transcranial direct-current stimulation in women with provoked vestibulodynia. *American Journal of Obstetrics and Gynecology, 216,* 584.e1–584.e11.

Morin, M., Dumoulin, C., Bergeron, S., et al. (2020). Multimodal physical therapy versus topical lidocaine for provoked vestibulodynia: A prospective, multicenter, randomized trial. *American Journal of Obstetrics and Gynecology, 224*(2), 189.e1–189.e12.

Murina, F., Bianco, V., Radici, G., et al. (2008). Transcutaneous electrical nerve stimulation to treat vestibulodynia: A randomised controlled trial. *British Journal of Obstetrics and Gynaecology, 115,* 1165–1170.

Murina, F., Felice, R., Di Francesco, S., et al. (2018). Vaginal diazepam plus transcutaneous electrical nerve stimulation to treat vestibulodynia: A randomized controlled trial. *European Journal of Obstetrics & Gynecology and Reproductive Biology, 228,* 148–153.

Nygaard, A. S., Rydningen, M. B., Stedenfeldt, M., et al. (2020). Group-based multimodal physical therapy in women with chronic pelvic pain: A randomized controlled trial. *Acta Obstetricia et Gynecologica Scandinavica, 99,* 1320–1329.

O'Reilly, B. A., Dwyer, P. L., Hawthorne, G., et al. (2004). Transdermal posterior tibial nerve laser therapy is not effective in women with interstitial cystitis. *Journal Urology, 172,* 1880–1883.

Poleshuck, E. L., Gamble, S. A., Bellenger, K., et al. (2014). Randomized controlled trial of interpersonal psychotherapy versus enhanced treatment as usual for women with co-occurring depression and pelvic pain. *Journal of Psychosomatic Research, 77,* 264–272.

Schlaeger, J. M., Xu, N., Mejta, C. L., et al. (2015). Acupuncture for the treatment of vulvodynia: A randomized wait-list controlled pilot study. *Journal of Sexual Medicine, 12,* 1019–1027.

Schvartzman, R., Schvartzman, L., Ferreira, C. F., et al. (2019). Physical therapy intervention for women with dyspareunia: A randomized clinical trial. *Journal of Sex & Marital Therapy, 45,* 378–394.

Slade, S. C., Dionne, C. E., Underwood, M., et al. (2016). Consensus on exercise reporting template (CERT): Explanation and elaboration statement. *British Journal of Sports Medicine, 50,* 1428–1437.

Sung, S. H., Sung, A. D., Sung, H. K., et al. (2018). Acupuncture treatment for chronic pelvic pain in women: A systematic review and meta-analysis of randomized controlled trials. Evid. Based Complement. *Alternat Medicine, 2018,* 9415897.

Treede, R. D., Rief, W., Barke, A., et al. (2019). Chronic pain as a symptom or a disease: The IASP classification of chronic pain for the international classification of diseases (ICD-11). *Pain, 160,* 19–27.

Zolnoun, D. A., Hartmann, K. E., & Steege, J. F. (2003). Overnight 5% lidocaine ointment for treatment of vulvar vestibulitis. *Obstetrics & Gynecology, 102,* 84–87.

Zoorob, D., South, M., Karram, M., et al. (2015). A pilot randomized trial of levator injections versus physical therapy for treatment of pelvic floor myalgia and sexual pain. *International Urogynecology Journal, 26,* 845–852.

9.4 Conservative Therapies to Treat Pelvic Floor Pain in Males

Bary Berghmans and Bert Messelink

INTRODUCTION

Pain is a warning and unpleasant, but in general, it is a protection against noxious stimuli.

Chronic pelvic pain (CPP) is chronic or persistent pain perceived in structures related to the pelvis of—in this chapter—men. It is often associated with negative cognitive, behavioural, sexual and emotional consequences, as well as with symptoms suggestive of lower urinary tract, sexual, bowel or pelvic floor dysfunction (Engeler et al., 2020).

Chronic pelvic pain syndrome (CPPS) is the occurrence of CPP when there is no proven infection or other obvious local pathology that may account for the pain (Engeler et al., 2020). CPPS is pathology in itself, often persisting after the inciting stimulus has resolved.

Repeated or prolonged somatic and visceral sensory input of nociceptors results in lowering their activation threshold, as well as the sensitization of previously non-involved afferent nerve fibers. This so-called peripheral sensitization, expressed in greater stimulus intensities, generates a greater postsynaptic response (Willard et al., 2008). The intense afferent bombardment of noxious information through viscero-somatic convergence and ongoing somatosensorial input from muscle and skin at the dorsal horn of a segment in the spinal cord leads to central sensitization perceived in the brain as prolonged, intense pain (Hoffman, 2011). With central sensitization initiation, amplification and perpetuation of pain, perception will manifest as allodynia (a condition where pain is caused by a stimulus that does not normally elicit pain), hyperalgesia and referred pain (Berghmans, 2018).

This upregulation of the sensory system effects interneurons that connect to alpha and gamma motor neurons, leading to segmental overactivity of pelvic floor muscles (PFMs), spasm and contracture (Berghmans, 2018). These pelvic floor dysfunctions and myofascial pain can lead to sexual dysfunction, such as erectile dysfunction (Hoffman, 2011). Muscle tightness and shortness, inflexible tissues, incapacity to stretch and relax, and connective tissue problems may also be involved (Hartmann and Sarton, 2014).

Ultimately, these mechanisms result in functional and structural rearrangements of the central nervous system that both sustain the perception of pain and facilitate its expansion to distant regions (Berghmans, 2018).

Despite the relation between myofascial and musculoskeletal dysfunction, involving the pelvic floor, and CPPS (Aredo et al., 2017; Berghmans, 2018), the role and added value of a physical therapist's assessment and intervention in patients with CPPS remains widely unknown by healthcare professionals, including physical therapists and relevant medical doctors. This is partly because the biological rationale of the working mechanism of physical therapy for CPPS, including pelvic floor muscle training (PFMT) and/or other physiotherapy modalities, is not well understood and only sparsely studied and is rarely used in clinical practice. Besides PFMT, trigger point therapy, massage, PFMT with biofeedback, electrical stimulation and combinations have been introduced (Engeler et al., 2020).

CLINICAL MANIFESTATIONS

The most common *functional* disorders of the PFMs, accompanied by perineal pain, are PFM pain syndrome, proctalgia fugax, myofascial pain syndrome and coccygodynia (Andromanakos et al., 2011). The aetiology of chronic perineal pain is not well understood, and many terms or synonyms can be found in literature, such as chronic idiopathic pelvic pain and spastic pelvic floor syndrome (Andromanakos et al., 2011).

PFM syndrome, especially involving the levator ani muscle, goes hand-in-hand with chronic or recurrent anorectal pain. Patients have a foreign body feeling or describe it as a dull pressure sensation, worsened when sitting, with a duration from several hours to several days. Digital palpation of the levator ani muscle during a contraction gives a sore and tender feeling (Mazza et al., 2004).

Overactivity and spasm of PFMs, abnormal contractions of the internal anal sphincter and myopathic hypertrophy of the internal anal sphincter have been suggested to lead to proctalgia fugax, which is a sudden and heavy, sharp anorectal pain lasting for several seconds or minutes (<30 minutes) which then disappears completely until the next attack, occurring mostly at night (Thompson, 1981).

Myofascial pain is an expression of dysfunction in the muscle and surrounding myofascial/connective tissue (Aredo et al., 2017), manifesting in the pelvic region in the levator ani, piriformis, obturator internus and several hip muscles. According to Simons (1996), myofascial pain has a lifetime prevalence of up to 85% in the general population. Nevertheless, physicians traditionally underdiagnose and often overlook this issue. The presence of myofascial trigger points (MTrPs) in the symptomatic region is a distinctive feature (Zoorob et al., 2015). MTrPs are small, palpable, hyperirritable nodules located on taut bands of skeletal muscle in an area of sustained contracture (Simons et al., 1999) and can be active or latent. Active trigger points are spontaneously painful areas that do not require physical stimuli, whereas latent trigger points are painful only upon physical palpation. The identification and interpretation of MTrPs by physical examination has been challenged by Lucas et al. (2009), who evaluated the diagnostic reliability of MTrPs and came to the conclusion that, considering the lack of reliability data for clinically relevant and active MTrPs in symptomatic patients, physical examination cannot yet be recommended as a reliable

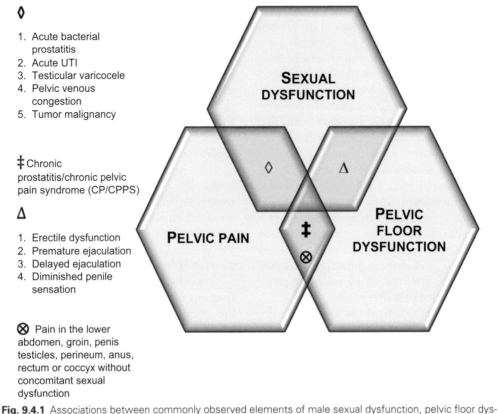

◊

1. Acute bacterial prostatitis
2. Acute UTI
3. Testicular varicocele
4. Pelvic venous congestion
5. Tumor malignancy

‡ Chronic prostatitis/chronic pelvic pain syndrome (CP/CPPS)

Δ

1. Erectile dysfunction
2. Premature ejaculation
3. Delayed ejaculation
4. Diminished penile sensation

⊗ Pain in the lower abdomen, groin, penis testicles, perineum, anus, rectum or coccyx without concomitant sexual dysfunction

Fig. 9.4.1 Associations between commonly observed elements of male sexual dysfunction, pelvic floor dysfunction and pelvic pain. *UTI,* Urinary tract infection. *(From Cohen et al. (2016).)*

test for the diagnosis of MTrPs. CPPS can be associated with overactivity and MTrPs in the PFMs (Zoorob et al., 2015), but MTrPs may also be localized in the abdominal muscles, adductor muscles and paraspinal muscles, and in muscles not directly related to the pelvis (Engeler et al., 2020).

Coccygodynia is pain in or around the coccyx, which is known as tailbone pain (Andromanakos et al., 2011).

The differential diagnosis of chronic perineal pain includes anorectal neoplasms, anal fissure, transphincteric abscess, thrombosed external haemorrhoids, prostatitis, cystitis, internal rectal prolapse, descending perineum syndrome, solitary rectal ulcer, leukaemia and bone or neurological disorder (spinal column, spinal cord) (Denneny et al., 2019).

Male sexual pain, sometimes called *male dyspareunia,* can occur as a stand-alone symptom in healthy men but can also arise as part of a wider symptom complex. Ejaculatory pain is frequently seen in patients with CPPS and is often not well understood (Luzzi and Law, 2006).

The relationship between male sexual function, pelvic floor function and pelvic pain is complex, with these three conditions often overlapping, and is only beginning to be appreciated (Fig. 9.4.1).

One of the imminent symptoms related to sexual dysfunction is pelvic pain (Rosenbaum and Owens, 2008). Rosenbaum and Owens (2008) stated that male pelvic pain is associated with premature ejaculation, erectile dysfunction and diminished desire and arousal. Discomfort or pain accompanying ejaculation or after ejaculation is common, as are the concurrent sexual dysfunctions mentioned earlier.

CPPS is strongly associated with both sexual and pelvic floor dysfunction and can significantly impact a man's quality of life and relationships (McNaughton et al., 2001). In one study, men with CPPS had greater rates of depression when compared with controls (Smith et al., 2007).

Men with CPPS show significantly more PFM tension and overactivity compared to healthy men. In about 50%, musculoskeletal dysfunction can be identified (Shoskes et al., 2008). Digital palpation of the PFMs and surrounding hip muscles demonstrates tenderness as well in these men (Hetrick et al., 2003). Zermann et al. (1999) reported that 9 of 10 men with CPPS had pathologic tenderness of PFMs and poor to absent PFM function.

PHYSICAL THERAPEUTIC ASSESSMENT PROCESS

The physical therapeutic assessment process, which is used to optimize patient selection and to formulate a specific treatment plan, investigates the nature of the pelvic pain and coexisting functional limitations that affect both the patient, the pain and its severity. These are examined in the context of whether the underlying pain and disorders and/or any identified unfavourable prognostic factors are modifiable by physical therapy.

Using the International Classification of Functioning, Disabilities and Health (ICF), the physical therapist tries to influence the *consequences* of pelvic pain and concurrent pelvic floor dysfunction on three different levels: the organ/local level (impairment/disorder level, e.g., intra-anorectal pain at penetration), personal level (disability level, e.g., inability to have intercourse) and social-societal level (restriction of participation, e.g., avoidance of social relationship–behavioural consequence) (World Health Organization, 2018).

All of these consequences are the basis for and the key elements to identify if and to what extent PFMT with or without another treatment modality and/or trigger point massage is feasible as an intervention for a particular patient suffering from CPPS.

The assessment of pelvic floor pain syndromes incorporates the following:
- History taking
- Physical examination
  - Observation in rest
  - Observation while moving
  - Digital palpation of painful spots/regions using a visual analogue scale (VAS) or numerical rating scale (tenderness, sensitive trigger points)
  - PFM functional assessment (leading to identification of parameters for the PFMT, with or without biofeedback/electrical stimulation, program)

- Pathological tests (electromyography, radiographs of the coccyx) and exclusion of the organic disease (anorectal or endopelvic) with pain, such as proctalgia (so-called red flags)

More detailed information about the physical therapist's physical examination techniques and interpretation can be found elsewhere (Berghmans et al., 2020) (Table 9.4.1).

REVIEWING THE LITERATURE RELATED TO CONSERVATIVE THERAPIES FOR MALE CPPS

For this chapter, in May 2020 we updated our search in the MEDLINE (via Ovid) and CINAHL (via Ebsco) databases with relevant search terms for systematic reviews and randomized controlled trials (RCTs) on conservative therapies, including PFMT and other treatment modalities, in patients with male CPPS. Selection criteria for inclusion in the evaluation were systematic reviews and RCTs comparing PFMT with or without biofeedback and/or electrical stimulation, electrical stimulation alone, trigger point massage or other kind of massage, behavioural therapy with a control group in adult males with CPPS, and at least one of the following outcome measures reported at more than 3 months after completion of the intervention: pain intensity, patient satisfaction, complications and quality of life.

Our literature search did not provide any systematic review or RCT on PFMT in adult males only.

The only other relevant RCT on *pelvic* physical therapy in males did not involve PFMT but transcutaneous electrical nerve stimulation (TENS). In an RCT graded 'low methodological quality', Tantawy et al. (2018) compared a 4-week treatment of analgesia and TENS (33 men, 26.6 ± 2.6 years, pain duration prior to study: 11.7 ± 2.3 months) with treatment with analgesia only (33 men, 26.3 ± 2.5 years, pain duration prior to study: 11.1 ± 1.6 months) (Tables 9.4.1 and 9.4.2). TENS was given five times a week for 30 minutes for 4 weeks. Electrodes were placed on the abdominal suprapubic region. The frequency of the stimulation signal was 100 Hz (pulse width: 100 μs). The patients had been diagnosed with idiopathic chronic testicular pain.

Tantawy et al. (2018) reported pain based on the mean VAS score. After 2 months of follow-up, there was a significant difference in pain score between the groups in favour of the intervention group (mean difference:

TABLE 9.4.1 PEDro Quality Score of Randomized Controlled Trials in Systematic Review of Conservative Treatment to Treat Chronic Pelvic Pain

E – Eligibility criteria specified

1 – Subjects randomly allocated to groups

2 – Allocation concealed

3 – Groups similar at baseline

4 – Subjects blinded

5 – Therapist administering treatment blinded

6 – Assessors blinded

7 – Measures of key outcomes obtained from >85% of subjects

8 – Data analysed by intention to treat

9 – Statistical comparison between groups conducted

10 – Point measures and measures of variability provided

Study	E	1	2	3	4	5	6	7	8	9	10	Total Score
Giubilei et al. (2007)	+	+	+	+	+	−	+	+	−	+	+	8
Tantawy et al. (2018)	+	+	+	+	−	−	+	+	−	+	+	7

+, Criterion is clearly satisfied; −, criterion is not satisfied.
The total score is determined by counting the number of criteria that are satisfied, except the 'eligibility criteria specified' score is not used to generate the total score. Total scores are out of 10.

−2.30; 95% CI: −2.81 to −1.79). The mean standardized difference was −2.2 SD, meaning that this was a clinically relevant difference.

In another RCT, Giubilei et al. (2007) compared aerobic exercises, consisting of isometric and strengthening exercises (no specific PFM exercises) combined with 40 minutes of fast-paced walking, with stretching and motion exercises as a placebo in a group of 103 males with a grand mean of 36.7 years (Tables 9.4.1 and 9.4.2).

The authors used the Italian version of the pain section of the National Institutes of Health Chronic Prostatitis Symptom Index (NIH-CPSI), a validated tool useful in assessing quality of life in men with CPPS for pain reduction as the primary outcome parameter (Litwin et al., 1999) and the VAS for pain measurement at baseline, after 6 weeks and post-treatment after 18 weeks. They performed a 'within' (pre-/post-treatment) comparison in both the treatment group and the control group and reported that both pain scales decreased significantly from baseline to post-treatment (both p < 0.001), stating that the improvements were higher in the treatment group. The 'in-between' comparisons were not statistically significant (NIH-CPSI: p < 0.94, State Anxiety Inventory-Y [SAI-Y]: p < 0.45). Despite the fact that they should have reported the in-between comparison

as primary analysis instead of the within comparison, they concluded that significant group differences in both pain scales could be found in favour of the treatment group (NIH-CPSI: p < 0.001, VAS: p < 0.01). This preliminary conclusion should be interpreted with caution. For the parameters 'anxiety' and 'depression', values improved significantly (p < 0.001) in both groups, but no significant group difference could be identified (p < 0.45 and p < 0.94, respectively). The study had a loss to post-treatment measurement of 21 (20%) participants (Giubilei et al., 2007).

PELVIC FLOOR MUSCLE TRAINING FOR CHRONIC PELVIC PAIN SYNDROMES

Despite the apparent lack of RCTs of sufficient high quality in this field, improvement of symptoms of CPPS may be realized effectively in programs involving treatment of pelvic floor dysfunction (Berghmans, 2018). Overactive and painful PFMs associated with abnormally high PFM tone is a significant component of pain and dysfunction in men with CPPS (Hetrick et al., 2003; Hetrick et al., 2006). Therefore neuromuscular re-education and PFMT including relaxation exercises have been considered to be an important part of recovery, fostering, for example, relaxation of overactive PFMs (Siegel, 2014).

TABLE 9.4.2   Randomized Controlled Trials to Treat Male Pelvic Pain

Author	Giubilei et al. (2007)
Design	2-arm RCT: AEG; P/FlexG
Sample size and age (years)	103 men age >50
Diagnosis	Sedentary, NIH type III chronic pelvic pain (NIH-CPSI:VAS)
Training protocol	AEG: warm-up/cool down, isometric + strengthening exercise, 40 min of fast-paced walking with 70%–80% of predicted age-adjusted max heart rate; 3×/week for 18 weeks Flexibilty and motion exercises program same period same frequency AEG; instruction to keep heart rate < 110 BPM during session
Drop-out	20%
Adherence	In equal participation
Results	BDI: AEG: baseline mean 12.1, post-treatment mean 8.3, p < 0.0001; P/FlexG: baseline mean 11.2, post-treatment mean 7.8, p < 0.0001, between-group difference p < 0.94 SAI-Y: AEG: baseline mean 44, post-treatment mean 37.8, p < 0.0001; P/FlexG: baseline mean 46.5, post-treatment mean 40.4, p < 0.0001, between-group difference p < 0.45
Author	**Tantawy et al. (2018)**
Design	2-arm RCT Pain sedation + TENS Pain sedation alone
Sample size and age (years)	33 men; mean age 26.6 ± 2.6
Diagnosis	Idiopathic chronic testicular pain; duration of pain before study: 11.7 ± 2.3 months
Training protocol	TENS 5×/week for 4 weeks, each session 30 min; electrodes placement on abdominal suprapubic region; frequency stimulation signal 100 Hz (pulse width 100 μs)
Drop-out	4.5%
Adherence	Not reported
Results	At end of intervention and after 2-month follow-up, significant difference in mean VAS pain score between groups in favour of intervention group (mean difference: –2.30; 95% CI: –2.81 to –1.79); mean standardized difference –2.2 SD, meaning that there was clinical relevant difference

AEG, Aerobic exercise group; *BDI,* Beck Depression Inventory; *CI,* confidence interval; *CPSI,* Chronic Pros–tatitis Symptom Index; *NIH,* National Institutes of Health; *P/FlexG,* placebo/stretching and motion exercise group; *RCT,* randomized controlled trial; *SAI-Y,* State Anxiety Inventory-Y; *TENS,* transcutaneous electrical nerve stimulation; *VAS,* visual analogue scale.
The BDI is a 21-item test presented in multiple choice format. It purports to measure the presence and degree of depression in adolescents and adults. The SAI-Y is a 20-item test measuring the level of current anxiety, such as calm, tension and worry, and is self-administered.

Neuromuscular re-education is the guided conscious retraining of muscle activation and deactivation and coordination of motor strategies in related muscle groups to accomplish a functional task, and it is a component of physical therapy treatments across many specializations, including pelvic floor health (Cohen et al., 2016).

In a non-randomized study in men with CPPS, PFMT and re-education with or without biofeedback reportedly reduced resting baseline tone of the PFMs

(Cornel et al., 2005) Moreover, reduced muscle activity led to reduction in pain ratings, as well as overall scores on the NIH-CPSI (Duclos et al., 2007).

Recent literature shows that pelvic floor physical therapy, including PFMT, may play an important role in improving symptoms in CPPS (Berghmans, 2018; Cheong et al., 2014; Engeler, 2020; Jarrell et al., 2005; Murina et al., 2018; Pazin et al., 2016; Rees et al., 2015; Tantawy et al., 2018).

A recent meta-analysis by Anderson et al. (2018) in non-randomized studies shows that the combination of therapies such as PFMT with and without biofeedback, and/or cognitive behavioral therapy, are associated with a clinically and statistically significant reduction in pain, improvement of micturition symptoms and quality of life in patients with CPP. Recent studies also indicate significant clinical effects of pelvic floor physical therapy in patients with CPP and sexual dysfunctions (Berghmans, 2018). Pelvic floor physical therapy can also play a positive role in chronic pelvic floor pain and anorectal dysfunctions (Bharucha and Lee, 2016).

However, the results should be interpreted with caution because of low to very low weight of evidence (Engeler et al., 2020). The current literature shows a wide range of methodological problems, ranging from small sample size to inadequate analysis to interpretation of results and to operational definition (Fuentes-Márquez et al., 2018).

According to the recent Dutch Guidelines on Chronic Pelvic Pain (Messelink et al., 2020), despite the fact that few or no studies of high methodological quality are known that have studied PFMT for CPP, with or without another treatment modality, based on positive experiences from the professional field, pelvic floor physical therapy, including PFMT, should be part of the multidisciplinary diagnosis and treatment of chronic pelvic floor pain. This is also stated by other authors (Berghmans, 2018; Engeler, 2020; Jarrell et al., 2005). It is recommended to set up further high-quality scientific research (including RCTs) to further substantiate the effectiveness of pelvic floor physical therapy, including PFMT, in CPP (Engeler et al., 2020).

REFERENCES

Anderson, R. U., Wise, D., & Nathanson, B. H. (2018). Chronic prostatitis and/or chronic pelvic pain as a psychoneuromuscular disorder—a meta-analysis. *Urology, 120*, 23–29.

Andromanakos, N. P., Kouraklis, G., & Alkiviadis, K. (2011). Chronic perineal pain: Current pathophysiological aspects, diagnostic approaches and treatment. *European Journal of Gastroenterology and Hepatology, 23*(1), 2–7.

Aredo, J. V., Heyrana, K. J., Karp, B. I., et al. (2017). Relating chronic pelvic pain and endometriosis to signs of sensitization and myofascial pain and dysfunction. *Seminars in Reproductive Medicine, 35*, 88–97.

Berghmans, B. (2018). Physiotherapy for pelvic pain and female sexual dysfunction: An untapped resource. *International Urogynecology Journal, 29*(5), 631–638.

Berghmans, B., Seleme, M. R., & Bernards, A. T. M. (2020). Physiotherapy assessment for female urinary incontinence. *International Urogynecology Journal, 31*(5), 917–931.

Bharucha, A. E., & Lee, T. H. (2016). Anorectal and pelvic pain. *Mayo Clinic Proceedings, 91*(10), 1471–1486.

Cheong, Y. C., Smotra, G., & Williams, A. C. (2014). Nonsurgical interventions for the management of chronic pelvic pain. *Cochrane Database of Systematic Reviews* , (3), CD008797.

Cohen, D., Gonzalez, J., & Goldstein, I. (2016). The role of pelvic floor muscles in male sexual dysfunction and pelvic pain. *Sexual Medicine Reviews, 4*, 53–62.

Cornel, E. B., van Haarst, E. P., Browning-Groote Schaarsberg, R. W. M., et al. (2005). The effect of biofeedback physical therapy in men with chronic pelvic pain syndrome type III. *European Urology, 47*, 607–611.

Denneny, D., Frawley, H. C., & Petersen, K. (2019). Trigger point manual therapy for the treatment of chronic noncancer pain in adults: A systematic review and meta-analysis. *Archives of Physical Medicine and Rehabilitation, 100*, 562–577.

Duclos, A. J., Lee, C. T., & Shoskes, D. A. (2007). Current treatment options in the management of chronic prostatitis. *Theraphy Clinical Risk Management, 3*, 507.

Engeler, D., Baranowski, A. P., & Berghmans, B. (2020). *EAU Guidelines on chronic pelvic pain.* Arnheim, Netherlands: European Association of Urology.

Fuentez-Marquez, P., Cabrera-Martos, I., Valenza, M., 2108. Physiotherapy interventions for patients with chronic pelvic pain: A systematic review of the literature. *Physiotherapy Theory and Practice, 35*(12), 1131–1138.

Giubilei, G., Mondaini, N., Minervini, A., et al. (2007). Physical activity of men with chronic prostatitis/chronic pelvic pain syndrome not satisfied with conventional treatments—could it represent a valid option? The physical activity and male pelvic pain trial: A double-blind, randomized study. *Journal Urology, 177*, 159–165.

Hartmann, D., & Sarton, J. (2014). Chronic pelvic floor dysfunction. *Best Practice & Research Clinical Obstetrics & Gynaecology, 28*, 977–990.

Hetrick, D. C., Ciol, M. A., Rothman, I., et al. (2003). Musculoskeletal dysfunction in men with chronic pelvic pain syndrome type III: A case–control study. *Journal Urology, 170*, 828.

Hetrick, D. C., Glazer, H., Liu, Y. W., et al. (2006). Pelvic floor electromyography in men with chronic pelvic pain syndrome: A case–control study. *Neurourology and Urodynamics, 25*, 46–49.

Hoffman, D. (2011). Understanding multisymptom presentations in chronic pelvic pain: The inter-relationships between the viscera and myofascial pelvic floor dysfunction. *Current Pain and Headache Reports, 15*, 343–346.

Jarrell, J. F., Vilos, G. A., Allaire, C., et al. (2005). Consensus guidelines for the management of chronic pelvic pain. *Journal of Obstetrics and Gynaecology Canada, 27*(9), 869–910.

Litwin, M. S., McNaughton-Collins, M., Fowler, F. J., et al. (1999). The National Institutes of Health Chronic Prostatitis Symptom Index: Development and validation of a new outcome measure. Chronic prostatitis collaborative research network. *Journal Urology, 162*, 369–375.

Lucas, N., Macaskill, P., Irwig, L., et al. (2009). Reliability of physical examination for diagnosis of myofascial trigger points: A systematic review of the literature. *The Clinical Journal of Pain, 25*(1), 80–89.

Luzzi, G. A., & Law, L. A. (2006). The male sexual pain syndromes. *International Journal of STD & AIDS, 17*, 720–726.

Mazza, L., Formento, E., & Fronda, G. (2004). Anorectal and perineal pain: New pathophysiological hypothesis. *Techniques in Coloproctology, 8*, 77–83.

McNaughton, C. M., Pontari, M. A., O'Leary, M. P., et al. (2001). Quality of life is impaired in men with chronic prostatitis: The chronic prostatitis collaborative research network. *Journal of General Internal Medicine, 16*, 656.

Messelink, B., Adamse, C., Felt-Bersma, R.J.F. Guideline chronic pelvic pain (Dutch). Dutch Urologic Association, 2020.

Murina, F., Felice, R., & Di Francesco, S. (2018). Vaginal diazepam plus transcutaneous electrical nerve stimulation to treat vestibulodynia: A randomized controlled trial. *European Journal of Obstetrics & Gynecology and Reproductive Biology, 228*, 148–153.

Pazin, C., de Souza Mitidieri, A. M., & Silva, A. P. (2016). Treatment of bladder pain syndrome and interstitial cystitis: A systematic review. *International Urogynecology Journal, 27*(5), 697–708.

Rees, J., Abrahams, M., Doble, A., et al. (2015). Diagnosis and treatment of chronic bacterial prostatitis and chronic prostatitis/chronic pelvic pain syndrome: A consensus guideline. *BJU International, 116*(4), 509–525.

Rosenbaum, T. Y., & Owens, A. (2008). The role of pelvic floor physical therapy in the treatment of pelvic and genital pain-related sexual dysfunction. *The Journal of Sexual Medicine, 5*, 513–523.

Shoskes, D. A., Berger, R., Elmi, A., et al. (2008). Muscle tenderness in men with chronic prostatitis/chronic pelvic pain syndrome: The chronic prostatitis cohort study. *Journal Urology, 179*, 556.

Siegel, A. L. (2014). Pelvic floor muscle training in males: Practical applications. *Urology, 84*, 1.

Simons, D. G. (1996). Clinical and etiological update of myofascial pain from trigger points. *Journal Musculoskelet Pain, 4*(1–2), 93–122.

Simons, D. G., Travell, J. G., & Simons, L. S. (1999). *Myofascial pain and dysfunction: The trigger point manual* (2nd ed.). Baltimore, MD: Williams & Wilkins.

Smith, K. B., Pukall, C. F., Tripp, D. A., et al. (2007). Sexual and relationship functioning in men with chronic prostatitis/chronic pelvic pain syndrome and their partners. *Archives of Sexual Behavior, 36*, 301.

Tantawy, S., Kamel, D., & Abdelbasset, W. (2018). Does transcutaneous electrical nerve stimulation reduce pain and improve quality of life in patients with idiopathic chronic orchialgia? A randomized controlled trial. *Journal of Pain Research, 11*, 77–82.

Thompson, W. G. (1981). Proctalgia fugax. *Digestive Diseases and Sciences, 26*, 1121–1124.

Willard, F. (2008). Basic mechanisms of pain. In J. F. Audette, & A. Bailey (Eds.), *Integrative pain medicine: The science and practice of complementary and alternative medicine in pain management* (pp. 19–61). Totowa, NJ: Humana Press.

World Health Organization. (2018). *International classification of functioning, disability and health*. Geneva: World Health Organization.

Zermann, D. H., Ishigooka, M., Doggweiler, R., et al. (1999). Neurourological insights into the etiology of genitourinary pain in men. *Journal Urology, 161*, 903.

Zoorob, D., South, M., Karram, M., et al. (2015). A pilot randomized trial of levator injections versus physical therapy for treatment of pelvic floor myalgia and sexual pain. *International Urogynecology Journal, 26*, 845–852.

10

The Prevalence and Consequences of Sexual Violence to the Pelvic Floor

Denis Mukwege, Raha Maroyi, Usama Shahid and Ajay Rane

INTRODUCTION

The World Health Organization (WHO) defines sexual violence as any sexual act ranging from verbal harassment to forced penetration done under coercion (WHO, 2012). For the purposes of this chapter we will focus on the forced penetration of rape and its impact on the pelvic floor. Being an unexpected and incidental event for the pelvic floor, rape leads to many traumatic complications, ranging from simple superficial injuries to complex lesions, altering the quality of life of the victim (Beck et al., 2009; Postmaet al., 2013). This chapter will focus on the experience of the Panzi Hospital (Democratic Republic of Congo) in the specialized medical and surgical management of sexual violence.

PREVALENCE

Sexual violence exists in all societies, affecting men and women of all ages and backgrounds. However, the primary victims of sexual violence remain girls and women. Due to the sensitive and taboo nature of the topic, exact prevalence numbers remain difficult to estimate. A national survey from the United States found that 14.8% of females older than 17 years had

been raped in their lifetime (Tjaden and Thoennes, 2000). The perpetrators of sexual violence can often be well known to the woman, with the act being conducted in settings like schools, healthcare facilities, or as part of cultural initiation. Unfortunately, sexual violence tends to be exacerbated during times of conflict and even employed as a weapon of war. Furthermore, a potential cause of rising female infanticide (Bongaarts and Guilmoto, 2015) could be rising sexual violence. At the Panzi Hospital, by the year 2019 we had treated 56,050 victims of sexual violence. An alarming trend during this time has been the increase in the rape of girls under the age of 10 years, which increased from 3% in 2008 to 6% in 2019.

ANATOMICAL BRIEFING OF SEXUALITY

The Pelvis

The pelvis or bony pelvis is an intermediate bone ring between the trunk and the lower limbs. It is formed by two coxal bones, sacrum and coccyx joined by the pubic symphysis anteriorly and the sacroiliac and sacrococcygeal joints posteriorly. Trauma to the bony pelvis that occurs as a result of sexual violence will not be discussed in this chapter.

The Pelvic-Perineal Wall

The pelvic-perineal wall is a musculotendinous hammock that extends from an insertion line in the plane of the middle strait, down and back towards the coccygeal region. This hammock closes the abdominopelvic cavity at the bottom. It is formed from two superposed structures: the perineum and the pelvic diaphragm. Several closely related organs pass through the pelvic wall, such as the urinary tract, genital tract and lower digestive tract.

In humans, the pelvic-perineal wall is strong in men and weaker in women due to a large urogenital hiatus that is subject to the constraints of childbirth. The pelvic diaphragm is formed from the anus elevator muscles and coccygeal muscles. On the other side, thanks to a bi-tuberositary line, the female perineum is divided into two regions: anterior to the urogenital perineum and posterior to the anal perineum. Between the two perineums on the median line is the tendinous centre of the perineum or the central fibrous core of the perineum, where the muscles are inserted. These anatomical structures may be injured, depending on the mechanism and type of sexual violence.

CONSEQUENCES AND TYPE OF INJURIES FROM SEXUAL VIOLENCE TO THE PELVIC FLOOR

The trauma from sexual violence to the pelvic wall may involve the skeleton, pelvic-perineal wall, lower digestive tract, genital tract, bladder or all of these areas at the same time. Hence there is need for a multidisciplinary team approach in the treatment of traumatic lesions of the pelvic-perineal region.

Mechanisms of Pelvic-Perineal Wall Trauma

Several mechanisms can be described to understand the lesions that are clinically observed in patients following sexual violence.

By Penetration or Introduction of a Blunt Object

The most common injury from sexual violence occurs secondary to blunt penetration with either a foreign body or penis. Due to the sheer force and brutality often involved in coerced penetration with sexual violence cases, the anatomy along the entire path of penetration is usually injured. This is especially true in cases of sexual violence against minors.

By Burning and Application of Chemicals

Thermal or chemical injury to external genitalia is also seen in cases of sexual violence. As expected, these injuries develop retractile scarring over time, requiring plastic surgical repair.

Type of Lesions

Due to a multitude of variables, the injuries seen in adult and minor sexual violence victims can be hard to predict. Bearing this in mind, there are certain patterns that we have established regarding the types of lesions and what to look for when managing adult and minor sexual violence victims. In the following section, we will discuss the interplay between the various anatomical lesions caused by sexual violence, the complexity in their management and patient factors.

In Adult Victims

Several types of lesions can be observed in adult victims of sexual violence (Fig. 10.1).

Superficial lesions. Vaginal lacerations are a common injury among cases of adult sexual violence. These are usually secondary to a penetrative insult. These lesions can simply be treated in the same way as lesions observed during vaginal birth with suturing in anatomical layers.

Sometimes women arrive at the hospital with burns caused by boiling water and chemicals (see Fig. 10.1). These burns are intentionally targeted towards the female genitalia by perpetrators of sexual violence, with the aim being prolonged suffering and subsequent dyspareunia or apareunia in an attempt the end the woman's reproductive capacity.

Deep lesions. Due to the degree of anatomical disruption, deeper lesions tend to be much more complex to manage. These can also be caused by penetrative injury, usually with a sharp object or even a firearm. These lesions lead to communication between the pelvic organs: the genital, urinary and digestive systems, or all three systems, thus creating various fistulae (see Fig. 10.1). It is worth noting that these injuries can also be caused by obstructed labour during childbirth. The issue can be significantly compounded in the case where very young patients (with an inadequately developed pelvis) become pregnant after rape. Not only are these girls vulnerable to injury from the sexual violence itself, but the fistulae themselves may occur in childbirth with obstructed labour. A lack of access to obstetric services

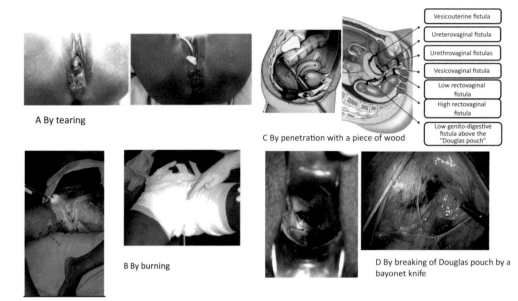

Figure 10.1 Pelvic-perineal wall injuries after sexual violence in adults.

often means that obstructed labour can cause compression and ischaemic necrosis of the pelvic organs, resulting in fistulae. Although these fistulae have their distant origin in rape, they are called *obstetric fistulae*. They develop in most fistula cases encountered.

We studied 604 fistula cases between 2005 and 2006 (Onsrud et al., 2008). Only 4% of these fistulae were post-rape, directly or indirectly. Five cases (0.8%) were directly related to rape. In these cases, the fistulae were the result of the introduction of an object into the genital tract. Paradoxically, traumatic fistulae are easier to operate on when compared to obstetric fistulae. Likewise, the outcomes are better since there is no significant fibrosis, as is often found in obstetric fistulae. But there can be traumatic injuries that affect several organs and require multiple, multidisciplinary surgeons (urologists, bowel surgeons). Despite these multiple lesions, the surgical outcome is often satisfactory. However, we have had significant difficulty at Panzi Hospital in treating high retrovaginal fistulae. The difficulty is in their anatomical location. When attempting to repair transvaginally, the fistulae are too high, and we simply are not able to reach them. Similarly, when adopting a transabdominal approach, it is impossible to reach the pelvis to access the retrovaginal fistula. This issue has been made substantially easier with the new technology of minimally invasive endoscopic surgery. In an article published in Surgical Endoscopy, we highlight three possible stages

of high rectovaginal traumatic fistulae (see Fig. 10.1). In the first stage, the rectum has remained healthy, but like the vagina, it has suffered a laceration that needs to be sutured. In the second stage, 2 cm of healthy rectum remains above the sphincter: this requires rectal resection and colorectal anastomosis. And finally, in the third stage, the laceration of the rectum continues to the sphincter: this will require the pull-through technique. The study involved 10 patients, from September 2012 to January 2014. Three patients were in stage 1, two were in stage 2 and three were in stage 3. Of this group, 9 of 10 patients were clinically cured.

In Rape of Children

We conducted another study that looked at 205 children and found that children older than 5 years, raped by penetration of an adult genital organ or introduction of a foreign object into the genital tract, had lesions similar to those found in adults. However, for children 5 years and younger, penetration of the male genital organ alone leads to genitourinary and lower digestive tract lesions (Mukwege D., 2014), which we describe as being one of five types (Fig. 10.2):

- Type I involves skin abrasions on the vulva and thighs, without muscular damage.
- Type II involves muscle, skin and mucous membrane lacerations unilaterally or bilaterally, without faecal or urinary incontinence.

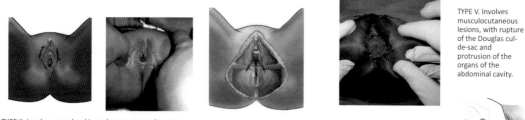

TYPE I. Involves skin abrasions on the vulva and thighs, without muscular damage.

TYPE III. Cutaneous-musculo-mucosal involvement, with tearing of the anal sphincter and faecal incontinence.

TYPE V. Involves musculocutaneous lesions, with rupture of the Douglas cul-de-sac and protrusion of the organs of the abdominal cavity.

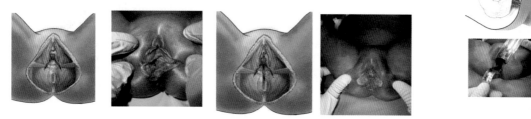

TYPE II. Involves muscle, skin and mucous membrane lacerations unilaterally or bilaterally, without faecal or urinary incontinence.

TYPE IV. A star-shaped cutaneo-musculo-mucosal tear, with tearing of the bladder and anal sphincters and urinary and faecal incontinence.

Figure 10.2 Types of pelvic-perineal wall injuries in children under 5 years of ages after sexual abuse.

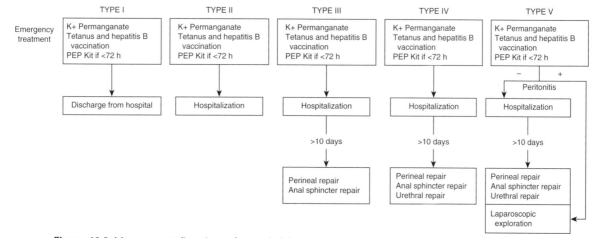

Figure 10.3 Management flowchart of sexual violence based on the type of pelvic-perineal wall trauma. *PEP,* Post-exposure prophylaxis.

- Type III has cutaneous-musculo-mucosal involvement, with tearing of the anal sphincter and faecal incontinence.
- Type IV has a star-shaped cutaneo-musculo-mucosal tear, with tearing of the bladder and anal sphincters and urinary and faecal incontinence.
- Type V involves musculocutaneous lesions, with rupture of the Douglas cul-de-sac and protrusion of the organs of the abdominal cavity.

The management of these lesions in children younger than 5 years can be done according to the algorithm shown in Fig. 10.3 (Mukwege, 2016).

All girls who have been raped must receive immediate medical treatment: antibiotics (if necessary), local hospital-based care, hepatitis B vaccination and tetanus vaccination (if there is no proof of this vaccination). For types I and II, it is not advisable to intervene surgically. It could in theory be done for type II, but children usually arrive at the hospital more than 6 hours after the rape, so an infectious process has already set in. If the surgeon cleans the wounds of the vulva and tries to close them, often the suture does not hold. By operating, the surgeon risks aggravating the problem, lengthening the hospital admission and even in some cases spreading the infection. However, when the wound is simply cleaned with ongoing medical treatment and sitz baths, it often heals without leaving any marks. This is quite different for type III, with damage to the anal sphincter. Here, it is necessary to be able to perform reconstructive surgery on the sphincter and try to restore continence. In types IV and V, it is necessary to repair the anal sphincter and restore the bladder closure mechanism, but also to perform a laparoscopy to remove the faecal matter brought back into the abdominal cavity by penetrating movements of the penis. The surgical outcomes are encouraging, both functionally and cosmetically: 91% of the girls in the study cited had good results.

CONCLUSION

Sexual violence remains a prominent yet poorly understood cause of gynaecological morbidity. The taboo nature of the injury, fear of further marginalization, vulnerability of patients and often complex anatomical disruption means that quality holistic services are required. A 'one-stop centre' framework should be adopted, developed from four pillars of care: medical, psychological, socioeconomic and legal (Mukwege, 2016). It will require a multidisciplinary approach involving gynaecologists, bowel surgeons, urologists, physical therapists, psychologists and lawyers. With sensitive, non-judgemental, evidence-based care, these women can effectively reintegrate into society.

REFERENCES

Beck, J. J., Elzevier, H. W., Pelger, R. C., et al. (2009). Multiple pelvic floor complaints are correlated with sexual abuse history. *The Journal of Sexual Medicine*, 6(1), 193–198.

Bongaarts, J., & Guilmoto, C. (2015). How many more missing women? *Lancet*, 386(9992), 427.

Mukwege, D., Alumeti, D., Himpens, J., et al. (2016). Treatment of rape-induced urogenital and lower gastrointestinal lesions among girls aged 5 years or younger. *International Journal of Gynaecology and Obstetrics*, 132(3), 292–296.

Mukwege D. Classification of gender-based genitourinary and rectovaginal trauma in girls under 5 years of age. *Int J Gynaecol Obstet*. 2014 Feb;124(2):97–8.

Mukwege, D., & Berg, M. (2016). A holistic, person-centred care model for victims of sexual violence in Democratic Republic of Congo: the Panzi Hospital One-Stop Centre model of care. *PLoS Medicine*, 13(10), e1002156.

Onsrud, M., Sjoveian, S., & Luhiriri, R. (2008). Sexual violence-related fistulas in the Democratic Republic of Congo. *International Journal of Gynaecology and Obstetrics*, 103, 265–269.

Postma, R., Bicanic, I., van der Vaart, H., et al. (2013). Pelvic floor muscle problems mediate sexual problems in young adult rape victims. *The Journal of Sexual Medicine*, 10(8), 1978–1987.

Tjaden, P., & Thoennes, N. (2000). *Full report of the prevalence, incidence and consequences of violence against women: Findings from the national violence against women survey. NCJ 183781*. Washington, DC: National Institute of Justice, Office of Justice Programs, United States Department of Justice and Centers for Disease Control and Prevention.

World Health Organization. (2012). *Understanding and addressing violence against women: Health consequences*. Available: https://who.int/publications/i/item/WHO-RHR-12.43. (Accessed 26.07.22).

11

Male Pelvic Floor Dysfunction and Evidence-Based Physical Therapy

11.1 Prevention, Causes and Pathophysiology of Urinary Incontinence in Males

Philip EV Van Kerrebroeck

INTRODUCTION

Lower urinary tract symptoms (LUTS), such as urinary incontinence, are a common problem in men that adversely and significantly affect health-related quality of life, as well as increase the risk of institutionalization (Burkhard et al., 2019). The prevalence of urinary incontinence in males increases with age, and it is estimated that more than one in four men older than 70 years have urinary incontinence (Burkhard et al., 2019). The presence of additional medical problems, such as poor general health, comorbidities, severe physical limitations, cognitive impairment, neurological conditions, recurrent urinary tract infection and prostatic diseases, has been associated with an increased risk for urinary incontinence in a male population (Burkhard et al., 2019).

In recent years, in most males with urinary incontinence the problem is secondary to sphincter weakness following prostatic surgery. As there is a rising elderly population and increasing numbers of surgical interventions for prostate cancer, the incidence of male incontinence is indeed rising. Hence male urinary incontinence has become a subject of growing interest, both because of the need for preventive measures and the increased therapeutic possibilities, conservative as well as surgical.

Persistent, non-neurogenic urinary incontinence in adult males can be classified as stress urinary incontinence (SUI), urgency urinary incontinence (UUI) eventually in the framework of overactive bladder (OAB) syndrome, mixed incontinence (a combination of SUI and UUI), overflow (paradoxical) incontinence, continuous urinary incontinence (as a consequence of a fistula) and functional incontinence (Abrams et al., 2002).

We will review the current understandings of the pathophysiological mechanisms and causes that can be responsible for SUI and UUI/OAB, and present, based on an analysis of these specific causes, some preventive measures that could reduce the risk for urinary incontinence in men.

STRESS URINARY INCONTINENCE

SUI in a male patient is most frequently caused by prostatectomy, more specifically radical retropubic prostatectomy (RPP), and is a devastating complication associated with significant alteration in quality of life.

The incidence of urinary incontinence following RRP, as reported in the literature, varied initially from 2.5% to 87% (Shamliyan et al., 2009). In more recent series, however, incidences tend to be lower and are documented in 2% to 10% of patients (Heesakkers et al., 2017). Yet SUI may also occur in patients undergoing surgical treatment for benign prostatic hypertrophy, and indeed incontinence after this type of surgery is estimated to be present in about 1% to 5% (Cornu et al., 2015).

Although the incidence of incontinence after radical prostatectomy has decreased with better understanding of the neurovascular bundles and modification of the operative technique, it continues to be one of the most feared complications after that type of surgery. Incontinence after RPP is related to the fact that the global urethral closure mechanism weakens with ageing and hence there is a risk of insufficient closure during times of physical stress in patients where the bladder neck has been removed simultaneously with the prostatic tissue as part of the standard technique of RPP (Hoyland et al., 2014).

The reason for the wide range in incidence of SUI after RPP is the use of different definitions of continence/incontinence, the variation in methods of assessment and the timing since surgery. The definition of incontinence depends also on who asks the question. Indeed, incontinence rates as reported by patients to independent observers exceed, in general, those reported to the surgeons who performed the prostatectomy.

Screening for and early detection of prostate cancer has led to a significant increase in the numbers of radical prostatectomy. Also, as increasing number of younger patients are undergoing radical prostatectomy, the impact of urinary incontinence on the quality of life following surgery assumes greater importance. Herr (1994) reported that 26% of men who underwent radical prostatectomy and suffered from urinary incontinence were extremely upset and limited their daily activities. Data from the largest multicentre trials and prostate cancer databases suggest that after RPP, 8% to 20% of patients have persistent significant incontinence problems, even if maximal conservative treatment has been applied (Sacco et al., 2006). In a review of complications in a sample of 757 Medicare patients who had undergone a radical prostatectomy, 41% of survey respondents stated that urine dripped daily, 31% needed pads, adult diapers or a penile clamp for protection; and 6% required another surgical intervention for urinary incontinence (Fowler et al., 1993). Despite these quite high figures, it appears that only 6% to 7% of patients currently undergo subsequent surgical treatment for post-prostatectomy incontinence (Bianco et al., 2005). The implication of this is that a significant number of men remain incontinent and essentially untreated.

Although post-prostatectomy incontinence may be caused by both sphincter dysfunction and/or bladder dysfunction, there is evidence that sphincter weakness is the most important contributing factor for incontinence (Majoros et al., 2006). Preservation of the functional integrity of the distal urethral sphincter mechanism therefore is germane for maintaining continence postoperatively. Direct surgical injury to the rhabdosphincter or its innervation are potentially the two factors responsible for postoperative incontinence.

However, sphincter denervation can also occur as a result of radical pelvic surgery, such as abdomino-perineal extirpation, transurethral resection of the prostate (TURP), removal of benign prostatic adenoma (open prostate adenomectomy), pelvic trauma, pelvic irradiation or neurological injury. During TURP, it is optimal to avoid resecting distal to the veru montanum, which represents the most proximal part of the rhabdosphincter. Damage to the sphincter during TURP occurs more commonly anteriorly where the landmark of the veru montanum is not visible.

Several mechanisms of sphincteric injury during or after radical prostatectomy have been suggested: ischemia and immobilization by scar formation, atrophy, direct pudendal nerve injury or shortening of the urethra below critical functional length (Kadono et al., 2016). Some studies have concluded that continent patients have longer functional urethral length than incontinent patients following RPP. It also has been postulated that preservation of continence following RPP requires a functional urethral length of at least 2.8 cm (Rudy et al., 1984). However, in another study, no statistical difference was found in maximum urethral closure pressure or functional urethral length measured pre- and postoperatively (Eastham et al., 1996).

Possible additional risk factors for incontinence after RPP include age, prostate volume, previous history of TURP, volume of urine leaked on removal of catheter and features of the surgical technique, including nerve sparing and the technique of bladder neck reconstruction, although each with contradictory results in the literature (Constantinou and Freiha, 1992).

Various technical modifications have been proposed to preserve as much of the external sphincter as possible after RPP. The US pioneer of radical prostatectomy Patrick Walsh described a modified apical dissection that may lead to earlier continence by incorporating the tissue posterior to the urethra in the vesicourethral anastomosis (Walsh et al., 1994). According to Walsh, anatomical factors rather than preservation of autonomic innervation are the major factors responsible for improved continence associated with an anatomical approach to radical prostatectomy. Additional radiation therapy after RPP may induce additional sphincteric damage and/or denervation in men, with subsequent sphincteric compromise. The expected benefits of robotic prostate surgery in reducing the urinary and sexual side effects following prostatectomy have not yet been demonstrated conclusively (Coughlin et al., 2018).

Although sphincteric weakness and subsequent SUI is recognized as the main factor for urinary incontinence after radical prostatectomy, detrusor overactivity or loss of bladder compliance is demonstrated to be present during urodynamics in up to 60% of incontinent patients after radical prostatectomy (Leach et al., 1996). The associated bladder dysfunction is often an important contributing factor even if SUI is present, and can result in urinary frequency and/or urgency incontinence. Therefore bladder disorders are important to recognize and treat before surgical management of sphincteric incompetence is considered. It has been shown that detrusor hyperactivity demonstrated in patients after radical prostatectomy often arises de novo, although it may already be present, symptomatically or not, before the operation. In addition, it is speculated that bladder overactivity may be a result of denervation of the bladder base as caused during surgery (Leach et al., 1996).

The pathophysiology of incontinence after radical prostatectomy was assessed in an interesting study by Groutz (2000). In this study the various mechanisms of incontinence were examined in 83 men using a combination of clinical and urodynamic parameters, including history, a voiding diary, the pad test, sophisticated video urodynamics and pressure flow studies. Intrinsic sphincter deficiency was the most common urodynamic finding and dominant cause of incontinence, occurring in 73 patients (88%). Bladder overactivity, demonstrated in 28 individuals (33.7%), was the only urodynamic finding in 3 patients (3.6%) and was determined to be the main cause of incontinence in 6 patients (7.2%). In addition, the authors concluded that low urethral compliance, presumably from urethral scarring, was a significant cause of intrinsic sphincter deficiency in 25 patients (30.1%). Overflow incontinence after RPP is most commonly due to a bladder neck contracture, and therefore this complication should be ruled out in patients with post-prostatectomy incontinence.

Although the main pathophysiology behind SUI in men relates to underlying dysfunction of the urethral sphincter complex and/or change in the urethral axis following prostate surgery, other causes of male SUI are iatrogenic sphincter injury (e.g., sphincterotomy in spinal patients), neurological conditions or trauma to the pelvic floor (e.g., pelvic trauma). The exact incidence of SUI may vary depending on the underlying pathology, definition of SUI and source of data (e.g., physician vs patient report) (Bauer et al., 2011).

Although sphincter deficiency is often the main causative factor, other bladder conditions, such as detrusor overactivity, poor bladder compliance and detrusor underactivity, can often coexist and contribute to the pathophysiology of SUI. Anastomotic stricture and scarring of the urethral tissue due to surgery and/or radiation should be considered in a patient complaining of the combination of urinary incontinence and decreased urine flow.

URGENCY URINARY INCONTINENCE

UUI in a male patient can be one of the symptoms of OAB syndrome. However, in view of the specific anatomy of the male lower urinary tract and the pathophysiological processes that this can cause, UUI can also be the consequence of specific pathology, such as bladder outlet obstruction (BOO). BOO may be caused by anatomical or functional benign prostatic pathology such as benign prostatic enlargement or an increased muscular tone at the level of the prostatic urethra (functional obstruction). The obstruction may cause detrusor hypertrophy to develop, and this anatomical change can alter detrusor behaviour that becomes overactive. This secondary detrusor overactivity can be an important cause of UUI in male patients. However, these mechanisms can also coexist with the intrinsic (idiopathic) processes that cause OAB and therefore can make the pathophysiology of UUI in males complex.

Detrusor overactivity occurs in about 75% of men with benign prostatic hyperplasia and can also be present in the absence of obstruction (Cornu et al., 2015). In most patients, relieving the outflow obstruction improves the detrusor overactivity, but in about 10% of patients, no improvement will be observed. This could possibly be related to the fact that the detrusor overactivity arose de novo and was not at all related to the obstruction. An alternative reason for persisting UUI may be some form of pre-existing occult neuropathy.

Moreover, several other distinct pathophysiological processes can cause abnormalities that lead to UUI, such as urinary tract infections, prostatitis, urethral strictures, neurological conditions and finally nocturnal polyuria that can cause nocturnal episodes of UUI. Furthermore, the simultaneous presence of detrusor underactivity can be responsible for post-void residuals that will limit the functional bladder capacity. This can be an important contributing factor to UUI or can at least aggravate the incontinence.

UUI in a male patient must be studied in the framework of global symptomatology summarized under the common umbrella of LUTS. This denominator includes three sets of symptoms: storage symptoms (related to filling of the bladder), voiding symptoms (related to emptying of the bladder) and post-micturition symptoms (occurring after finishing evacuation of urine). Part of the storage symptoms are indicated as OAB.

OAB is a clinical syndrome characterized by urinary urgency, with or without urgency incontinence, usually accompanied by frequency and nocturia (Abrams et al., 2002). The diagnosis of OAB as a clinical syndrome is made based on the exclusion of any specific pathology and hence is considered an idiopathic condition. However, several pathophysiological, but clinically undetectable, mechanisms are proposed that may lead to the symptoms of OAB. A very important causative element includes age-related changes in smooth muscle, leading to:

- hyperexcitability of muscarinic receptors in the detrusor smooth muscle, urothelium and neurovascular structures, and atropine resistance;
- increased afferent (sensory group C fibres) nerve activity and hypersensitivity of other ion channels; and
- denervation at the spinal and cortical levels, resulting in hyperactive voiding that is secondary to spinal micturition reflexes (Shamliyan et al., 2009).

These processes can be the consequence of age-related changes, both at the level of the lower urinary tract and surrounding structures including the pelvic floor, and also at the level of the peripheral and central innervations of the lower urinary tract. Furthermore, these changes may also be caused or aggravated by clinically detectable neurological conditions, such as Parkinson disease, multiple sclerosis or stroke. This pathology may cause loss of inhibitory neurons, resulting in neurogenic voiding dysfunction, including UUI (Chung, 2013).

Hence the global risk factors for UUI include neurological conditions, various inflammatory processes of the bladder, bladder outlet dysfunction, physiological ageing and psychosocial stressors, or the condition may be idiopathic in nature (Smith and Wein, 2011). Although it is accepted that OAB occurs more commonly in women, the true prevalence of OAB in men remains largely unknown. This is because most storage symptoms are frequently attributed to an enlarged prostate. The most common finding in patients with UUI is detrusor overactivity, which is a urodynamic observation of involuntary bladder contractions that are commonly associated with a corresponding sensation of urgency during bladder filling. An enlarged prostate and ensuing BOO can result in bladder adaptations and abnormal detrusor contractions (i.e., detrusor overactivity). It is also important to exclude other conditions that can simulate OAB-like symptoms, such as urinary tract infections, a distal ureteral stone, a bladder stone, an intravesical foreign body and even oncological processes at the level of the bladder (carcinoma in situ or urothelial cell carcinoma) (Miller and Miller, 2011).

MIXED INCONTINENCE

Ageing increases not only the risk for SUI but also can be a causative factor for UUI. Therefore both SUI and UUI can coexist, leading to mixed incontinence. Additional analysis will be necessary to elucidate the specific mechanisms of each of these types of incontinence, but attention should be paid to the subtle, but often complex, interplay of different mechanisms influencing each of the pathological processes.

CONCLUSON

Urinary incontinence in males is a rather frequent yet definitely disturbing symptom with a major impact on quality of life. Two types are prevalent: SUI and UUI.

The most frequent cause for SUI is iatrogenic, radical prostatectomy for prostate cancer. Weakness of the urethral closure during filling of the bladder as a consequence of removal of the prostate and the bladder neck, in combination with sphincter damage either by direct trauma or by damage to the innervation, is the most prominent mechanism. Reported extra risk factors for post-prostatectomy SUI include the patient's age, body mass index, preoperative bladder function, urinary continence status before urgery, prior radiation therapy, preoperative length of the membranous urethra, prior TURP, vascular comorbidities, stage of disease, surgical technique employed (including nerve sparing) and finally the surgeon's level of experience. Robotic techniques do not seem to reduce the risk of SUI after RRP.

UUI is reported in a significant proportion of men with urinary incontinence and can be one of the symptoms of OAB syndrome. In addition, BOO caused by anatomical or functional prostatic pathology may be responsible for secondary detrusor overactivity that can cause UUI. However, several other pathophysiological processes can lead to UUI in men, such as urinary tract infections, prostatitis, urethral strictures and neurological diseases. Finally, detrusor underactivity during voiding that can coexist with detrusor hyperactivity during filling can be responsible for post-void residuals that may cause or aggravate UUI.

REFERENCES

Abrams, P., Cardozo, L., Fall, M., et al. (2002). The standardisation of terminology of lower urinary tract function: Report from the standardisation sub-committee of the international continence society. *Neurourology and Urodynamics, 21*, 167–201.

Bauer, R., Gozzi, C., Hübner, W., et al. (2011). Contemporary management of postprostatectomy incontinence. *European Urology, 59*(6), 985–996.

Bianco, F., Jr., Riedel, E., Begg, C., et al. (2005). Variations among high volume surgeons in the rate of complications after radical prostatectomy: Further evidence that technique matters. *Journal of Urology, 173*, 2099–2103.

Burkhard, C., Bosch, J., Cruz, F., et al. (2019). *EAU guidelines on urinary incontinence.* Arnhem, Netherlands: European Association of Urology.

Medical treatments of overactive bladder: Current and future therapeutic applications. (2013). In E. Chung (Ed.), *Urinary incontinence: Causes, epidemiology and treatment* (pp. 101–111). New York: Nova Science Publishers.

Constantinou, L., & Freiha, F. (1992). Impact of radical prostatectomy on the characteristics of bladder and urethra. *Journal of Urology, 148*, 1215–1220.

Cornu, J., Ahyai, S., Bachmann, A., et al. (2015). A systematic review and meta-analysis of functional outcomes and complications following transurethral procedures for lower urinary tract symptoms resulting from benign prostatic obstruction: An update. *European Urology, 67*(6), 1066–1096.

Coughlin, G., Yaxley, J., Chambers, S., et al. (2018). Robot-assisted laparoscopic prostatectomy versus open radical retropubic prostatectomy: 24-month outcomes from a randomised controlled study. *The Lancet Oncology, 19*, 1051–1059.

Eastham, J., Kattan, M., Rogers, E., et al. (1996). Risk factors for urinary incontinence after radical prostatectomy. *The Journal of Urology, 156*, 1707–1713.

Fowler, F., Jr., Barry, M., Lu-Yao, G., et al. (1993). Patient-reported complications and follow-up treatment after radical prostatectomy: The national Medicare experience: 1988–1990 (updated June 1993) *Urology, 42*, 622–631.

Groutz, A., Blaivas, J., Chaikin, D., et al. (2000). The pathophysiology of post-radical prostatectomy incontinence: A clinical and video urodynamics study. *Journal of Urology., 163*, 1767–1770.

Heesakkers, J., Farag, F., Bauer, R., et al. (2017). Pathophysiology and contributing factors in postprostatectomy incontinence: A review. *European Urology, 71*(6), 936–944.

Herr, H. (1994). Quality of life of incontinent men after radical prostatectomy. *Journal of Urology, 151*, 652–654.

Hoyland, K., Vasdev, N., Abrof, A., et al. (2014). Post-radical prostatectomy incontinence: Etiology and prevention. *Reviews in Urology, 16*(4), 181–188.

Kadono, Y., Ueno, S., Kadomoto, S., et al. (2016). Use of preoperative factors including urodynamic evaluations and nerve-sparing status for predicting urinary continence recovery after robot-assisted radical prostatectomy: Nerve-sparing technique contributes to the reduction of postprostatectomy incontinence. *Neurourology and Urodynamics, 35*, 1034–1041.

Leach, G., Trockman, B., Wong, A., et al. (1996). Post-prostatectomy incontinence urodynamic findings and treatment outcomes. *Journal of Urology, 155*, 1256–1259.

Majoros, A., Bach, D., Keszthelyi, A., et al. (2006). Urinary incontinence and voiding dysfunction after radical retropubic prostatectomy (prospective urodynamic study). *Neurourology and Urodynamics, 25*, 2–7.

Miller, S., & Miller, M. (2011). Urological disorders in men: Urinary incontinence and benign prostatic hyperplasia. *Journal of Pharmacy Practice, 24*(4), 374–385.

Rudy, D., Woodside, J., & Crawford, E. (1984). Urodynamic evaluation of incontinence in patients undergoing modified campbell radical retropubic prostatectomy: A prospective study. *Journal of Urology, 132*, 708–712.

Sacco, E., Prayer-Galetti, T., Pinto, F., et al. (2006). Urinary incontinence after radical prostatectomy: Incidence by definition, risk factors and temporal trend in a large series with a long-term follow-up. *BJU International, 97*, 1234–1241.

Shamliyan, T., Wyman, J., Ping, R., et al. (2009). Male urinary incontinence: Prevalence, risk factors, and preventive interventions. *Reviews in Urology, 11*(3), 145–165.

Smith, A., & Wein, A. (2011). Urinary incontinence: Pharmacotherapy options. *Annals of Medicine, 43*(6), 461–476.

Walsh, P., Partin, A., & Epstein, J. (1994). Cancer control and quality of life following anatomical radical retropubic prostatectomy: Results at 10 years. *Journal of Urology, 152*, 1831–1836.

11.2 Pelvic Floor Muscle Training for Urinary Incontinence

Marijke Van Kampen, Inge Geraerts and Anne Asnong

INTRODUCTION

This chapter provides a summary of the current evidence for the physiotherapeutic treatment of urinary incontinence (UI) and other lower urinary tract symptoms in the male population.

Prostate surgery is one of the major causes of UI in the male population. Randomized controlled studies considering physical therapy for men with incontinence after prostatectomy have been published since the end of the 1990s (Ahmed et al., 2012; Bales et al., 2000; Burgio et al., 2006; Centemero et al., 2010; Dubbelman et al., 2010; Filocamo et al., 2005; Floratos et al., 2002; Franke et al., 2000; Geraerts et al., 2013; Glazener et al., 2011; Goode et al., 2011; Ip, 2004; Joseph et al., 2000; Manassero et al., 2007; Marchiori et al., 2010; Mariotti et al., 2009; Mathewson-Chapman, 1997; Moore et al., 1999; Moore et al., 2008; Nilssen et al., 2012; Overgard et al., 2008; Parekh et al., 2003; Park et al., 2012; Porru et al., 2001; Ribeiro et al., 2010; Robinson et al., 2008; Sueppel et al., 2001; Tibaek et al., 2007; Tienforti et al., 2012; Van Kampen et al., 2000; Wille et al., 2003; Yamanishi et al., 2010; Yokoyama et al., 2004; Zhang et al., 2007). Since the previous edition of this book, 19 new studies have focused on physical therapy and incontinence after prostatectomy (Anan et al., 2020; Au et al., 2020; Aydin Sayilan, 2018; de Lira et al., 2019; Dijkstra-Eshuis et al., 2015; Gomes et al., 2018; Heydenreich et al., 2020,

Hou et al., 2013; Jalalinia et al., 2020; Kongtragul et al., 2014; Laurienzo et al., 2013; Laurienzo et al., 2018; Milios et al., 2019; Ocampo-Trujillo et al., 2014; Oh et al., 2020; Pedriali et al., 2016; Santos et al., 2017; Tantawy et al., 2019; Zachovajeviene et al., 2019). A Cochrane review and clinical guidelines for incontinence after prostatectomy have described the evidence for physical therapy for male incontinence (Campbell et al., 2012; Lucas et al., 2012; Nambiar et al., 2018).

Besides UI, men may suffer from other lower urinary tract symptoms. These symptoms in males include filling symptoms or irritative symptoms, such as frequency, urgency, urgency incontinence and nocturia, and voiding symptoms or obstructive symptoms, such as hesitancy, weak stream, straining, incomplete emptying, intermittency, and terminal and post-voiding dribble (Abrams et al., 2003; D'Ancona et al., 2019; Dorey, 2001). Although physical therapy should have the potential to alleviate lower urinary tract symptoms, the number of studies concerning these symptoms is scarce. The efficacy of physical therapy for terminal and post-void dribble is investigated in three randomized controlled studies (Dorey et al., 2004; Paterson et al., 1997; Porru et al., 2001).

POST-PROSTATECTOMY INCONTINENCE

UI is a common consequence in many men undergoing prostate surgery (Diokno, 1998; Dorey, 2000; Peyromaure et al., 2002; Tienza et al., 2018).

The prostate gland is part of the male sex gland and can be divided into three zones: the central zone (25%, situated just under the bladder), the transition zone (5% around the urethra) and the peripheral zone (70% around the other zones). Benign prostatic hyperplasia mostly develops in the transition zone. Prostate hyperplasia (Fig. 11.2.1) was typically treated by a transurethral or transvesical resection (Fig. 11.2.2) of the prostatic adenoma.

Currently also holmium laser enucleation of the prostate (HoLEP; the bulky prostate tissue that is blocking the flow of urine is removed with a surgical laser) is gaining interest.

This procedure is minimally invasive and can be performed in patients with large-sized prostatic hyperplasia (Cornu et al., 2015). A total of 75% of all prostatic adenocarcinomas are situated in the peripheral zone. Localized prostate cancer can be treated by radical prostatectomy, and this treatment is commonly thought to be the most effective (Mottet et al., 2017) (see Fig. 11.2.1).

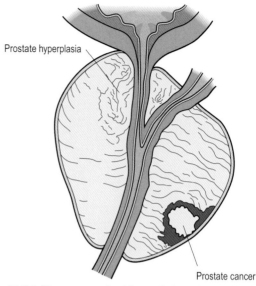

Fig. 11.2.1 The prostate gland, hyperplasia and prostate cancer.

Radical prostatectomy can be performed via an open, laparoscopic or robot-assisted laparoscopic approach (Fig. 11.2.3).

Removal of the prostate can lead to leakage of urine. The occurrence of incontinence, especially in the early recovery period after surgery, is hard to accept for all patients. Patients express fear of odour, shame, increased self-consciousness and embarrassment, and there is a trend that incontinent patients appear to benefit from support (Ko and Sawatzky, 2008; Moore et al., 1999).

Conservative management including pelvic floor muscle training (PFMT), biofeedback (BF) and electrical stimulation (ES) with a transcutaneous or a rectal electrode has been suggested to improve incontinence after prostate surgery in some trials (Anderson et al., 2015; Hunter et al., 2004). However, the latter did not find sufficient evidence as to whether or not conservative management is effective in treating or preventing postprostatectomy UI (Anderson et al., 2015). The rationale beyond this treatment is that pelvic floor contraction may improve the strength of the external urethral sphincter during periods of increased abdominal pressure. PFMT results in hypertrophy of the striated muscles, increasing the external mechanical pressure on the urethra. Moreover, contraction of the pelvic floor leads to inhibition of detrusor contraction, and therefore incontinence can be improved (Berghmans et al., 1998; Berghmans et al., 2002).

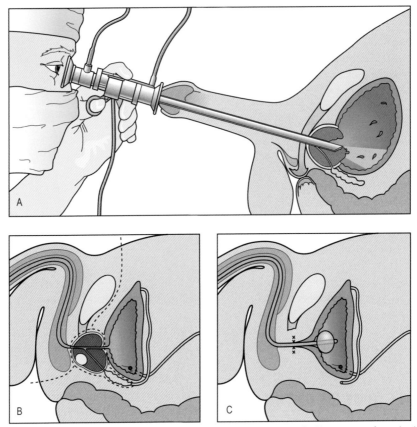

Fig. 11.2.2 (A) Transurethral prostatectomy. (B) Radical prostatectomy. (C) Placement of urethral catheter after radical prostatectomy.

Incidence and Pathophysiology

The incidence of incontinence after transurethral and open adenectomy is distinctly low, and incontinence resolves in a few days or months. Incontinence rates around 9% are reported initially and about 1% at 12 months postoperatively (Lourenco et al., 2008; Milsom et al., 2009). Only Glazener et al. (2011) found higher numbers, with 17% of patients with incontinence at 6 weeks after transurethral resection of the prostate (TURP) and 10% of patients still incontinent at 12 months. After HoLEP, postoperative transient incontinence has been reported as a bothersome complication in 16% to 44% of patients within 3 months (Anan et al., 2020). In general, it is believed that incontinence is a troubling long-term problem in only a small proportion of patients after TURP (Anderson et al., 2015; Van Kampen et al., 1997). The incidence of UI after radical prostatectomy varies widely. Immediately after catheter removal, the incontinence rate is reported to be 59% to 90% after open radical prostatectomy (Ficarra et al., 2009; Van Kampen et al., 2000) and between 31.1% and 86.39% after robot-assisted laparoscopic prostatectomy (Ficarra et al., 2009; Joseph et al., 2006; Menon et al., 2007; Tewari et al., 2003). One year after radical prostatectomy, several reports from prestigious academic centres claimed that only 5% of patients were still incontinent (Anderson et al., 2015; Myers, 1995; Poon et al., 2000; Walsh et al., 1994). However, other studies cast a rather more pessimistic light on the problem. They reported that 20% to 40% of the patients were wearing an incontinence pad 1 year or more after surgery (Bishoff et al., 1998; Boccon-Gibod, 1997; Braslis et al., 1995; Carlsson et al., 2016). Twelve months after surgery, 2% to 39% (open) (Coehlo et al., 2010; Ficarra et al., 2012), 3% to 31% (robot) (Coehlo et al., 2010; Ficarra et al., 2012) and 5% to 52% (laparoscopic) (Coehlo et al., 2010) of patients did not regain continence (Cao et al., 2019; Coughlin et al., 2018; Haglind et al., 2015; Ong et al., 2016).

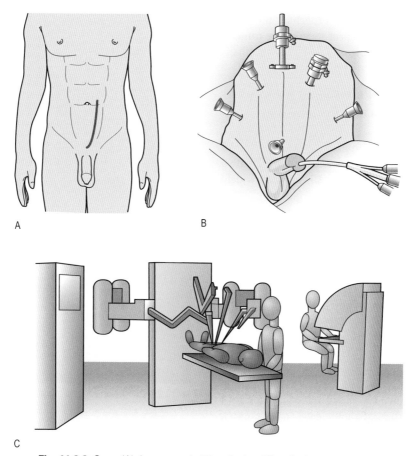

Fig. 11.2.3 Open (A), laparoscopic (B) and robot (C) radical prostatectomy.

Several studies compared UI after open and robot radical prostatectomy. Different studies found that patients achieved continence much earlier after robot than after open radical prostatectomy (Ficarra et al., 2009), but other studies could not confirm this (Seo et al., 2016). Variation in reported frequency of incontinence depends on the definition of incontinence, the difference in outcome measures, various follow-up periods and the person (patient, physician, urologist or therapist) performing the surgical procedure and/or the assessments afterwards (Donnellan et al., 1997; Fowler et al., 1995, Moore et al., 1999).

Incontinence after adenectomy for prostate hyperplasia is thought most likely to be due to pre-existing abnormalities of bladder function, as bladder overactivity or poor compliance, more than sphincter injury (Anderson et al., 2015). After radical prostatectomy, intrinsic sphincter deficiency is the primary cause of

incontinence and ranges from 60% to 97% (Baert et al., 1996; Groutz et al., 2000; Hoyland et al., 2014). An overlooked cause is detrusor overactivity. Outlet obstruction that results in overflow incontinence is rare (Baert et al., 1996; Foote et al., 1991; Grise and Thurman, 2001; Gudziak et al., 1996; Haab et al., 1996).

A small group of patients reported terminal and post-micturition dribble in the early postoperative period (Chang et al., 1998; Porru et al., 2001; Yang and Lee, 2019). This is due to urethral dysfunction because of decreased or absent post-void urethral milking resulting in residual unexpelled urine in the bulbous urethra (Bader et al., 2001; Wille et al., 2000; Yang and Lee, 2019).

Many risk factors were described that increase the possibility of UI after radical prostatectomy: previous transurethral resection, pre-existing abnormalities of detrusor contractility, preoperative radiotherapy, shortened functional urethral length, no preservation of the bladder neck, no preservation of the neurovascular bundles, higher age, less surgical expertise, and more advanced clinical and pathological stage of the tumour (Aboseif et al., 1994; Anderson et al., 2015; Eastham et al., 1996; Van Kampen et al., 1998).

Evidence for Effect of Pelvic Floor Muscle Training in Prevention and Treatment of Urinary Incontinence

We analysed literature on UI in males to generate clinical recommendations. Overall effectiveness of conservative management of post-prostatectomy UI has been widely investigated (Anderson et al., 2015; Burgio et al., 1989; Ceresoli et al., 1995; Dorey, 2000; Meaglia et al., 1990; Moul, 1998). Symptoms of incontinence after prostatectomy tend to improve over time without intervention. The *specific* effectiveness of a physical therapeutic approach for incontinence after prostatectomy can only be evaluated in randomized controlled studies. Different types of intervention are described. PFMT involves any method of training the pelvic floor muscles, including pelvic floor muscle exercises (PFMEs), BF and ES. BF involves the use of a device to provide visual or auditory feedback. ES involves any type of stimulation by using an anal probe or transcutaneous electrodes (Fig. 11.2.4). This method has been reported to facilitate awareness of contraction of the pelvic floor muscles or to inhibit detrusor contraction (Jezernik et al., 2002; Zaidan and Bezerra da Silva, 2016).

Due to increasing research in the domain of chronic pelvic pain and male sexual dysfunction, more focus is currently being applied to the fact that relaxation of the pelvic floor muscles is as important as contraction. In particular, it is hypothesized that high-tone pelvic floor muscles and/or chronic pain is a distraction to effective and sustained corporal smooth muscle relaxation (Cohen et al., 2016).

Anderson et al. (2015), Campbell et al. (2012), Hunter et al. (2004, 2007), and Moore et al. (2001) have carried out Cochrane reviews concerning conservative management for post-prostatectomy UI. Clinical guidelines on UI were published by Nambiar et al. (2018). There was a wide variation in outcome measures of incontinence. Assessment of incontinence was mostly based on the number of pads, where 0 and 1 pad were defined as continent (Holze et al., 2019). Different pad tests (20-, 45-, 60-minute and 24-, 48- and 72-hour pad tests) were used to assess incontinence objectively (Hunter et al., 2004; Moore et al., 2001; Yamanishi et al., 2010). Other assessments were voiding diaries for voiding frequency,

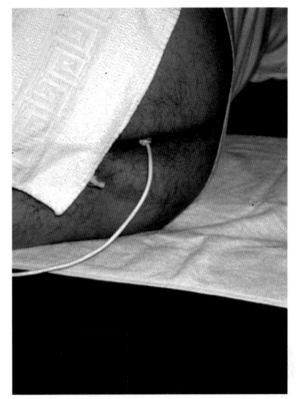

Fig. 11.2.4 Biofeedback and electrical stimulation of the pelvic floor with an anal probe prostatectomy.

incontinent episodes and number of pads, strength of the pelvic floor by digital test/perineometry, visual analogue scale (VAS) for the subjective bother regarding incontinence, and several questionnaires regarding urinary/bowel/sexual/pelvic floor symptoms (the Expanded Prostate Cancer Index Composite [EPIC], the International Consultation on Incontinence Questionnaire [ICIQ], the International Continence Society short form [ICSmaleSF], the Incontinence Impact Questionnaire [IIQ], the Just Culture Assessment Tool [JCAT], the Pelvic Floor Inventories Leiden [PeLFIs], the St George UI score) and quality-of-life (QoL) questionnaires (the European Organization for the Research and Treatment of Cancer Quality of Life Questionnaire [EORTC-QLQ C30], the Functional Assessment of Cancer Therapy–Prostate [FACT-P], the King's Health Questionnaire [KHQ], the Patient-Oriented Prostate Utility Scale [PORPUS], RAND-36, the 12- and 36-item Short Form Health Survey Questionnaires [SF-12 and SF-36], and the University of California at Los Angeles

Prostate Cancer Index [UCLA-PCI]) (Anderson et al., 2015; Herr, 1994; Laycock, 1994). The American Urological Association (AUA) Symptom Score, the International Prostate Symptom Score (IPSS) and the Danish Prostatic Symptom Score (DAN-PSS-1) assess lower urinary tract symptoms (Barry et al., 1992; Hald et al., 1991). Regarding the assessment of incontinence, a standardized definition for continence would be desirable, as it is one of the most important preconditions to guarantee sound comparison of continence rates. Since there are enough other factors that make comparison difficult, we suggest using a voiding diary including a 72-hour pad test. The patient can easily measure his urine loss objectively at home, it leaves no room for interpretation and it is able to clearly indicate progress towards continence.

Research Methods

The search was updated from the cut-off date of the previous update (July 2015) to June 2020 and included PubMed, the Cochrane Library and PEDro. Only English language articles and randomized controlled trials were considered. No abstracts were included. For post-prostatectomy incontinence, 1021 articles were identified and screened by two independent reviewers. Data extraction was then carried out for the relevant studies by screening by title (phase I), by abstract (phase II) and by full text (phase III), resulting in 53 articles in total (5 on physical therapy and incontinence after TURP/HoLEP, 46 on physical therapy and incontinence after radical prostatectomy, and 2 on physical therapy and incontinence after transurethral resection and radical prostatectomy [without data of the different subgroups]) (Ip, 2004; Joseph et al., 2000) (Table 11.2.1). For terminal and post-void dribble, 16 articles were identified and screened, resulting in 3 articles.

The methodological quality of all identified studies concerning incontinence after prostatectomy based on PEDro ranged between 1 and 8 out of 10 (Table 11.2.2).

TABLE 11.2.1	**Randomized Controlled Studies of Physical Therapy for Incontinence After Prostatectomy**
Author	**Ahmed et al., 2012**
Design	E[1]: ES, E[2]: BFB + ES
	C: information
Sample size	90 men after RP (E1=30, E2=30, C=30)
Diagnosis	24h pad test, IIQ-7
Training protocol	Start one week after catheter removal
	E[1]: 15 min ES, E[2]: 15 min BFB + 15 min ES (2×/week (12 weeks)
	C: verbal+written info (Kegel-exercises [3× 15-20 contractions/day])
Drop-out	10/90 (11.1%) (E1:4, E2: 2, C:4)
Results	Mean leakage weight significantly lower in E2 than in E1 and C at 6, 12 and 24 weeks, significant different continence rates for respectively E2, E1 and C at 12 and 24 weeks (71%, 54%, 35% and 96%, 77%, 65%)
Author	**Anan et al., 2020**
Design	E: instructions for PFME preop + postop
	C: instructions for PFME postop
Sample size	72 men before HoLEP (E=36, C=36)
Diagnosis	Number of pads/day, ICIQ-SF
Training protocol	E: instructions for PFME (at least 3 min 3×/d) from 28d preop + postop after catheter withdrawal)
	C: instructions for PFME postop (at least 3 min 3×/d)
Drop-out	2/72 (2.7%) (E:1, C:1)
Results	At 3 months: significant lower incontinence rate in E (3% vs 26%), at 3d, 1M and 6M no significant difference
	No significant difference in ICIQ-SF at 1M, 3M or 6M
Author	**Au et al., 2020**
Design	E: PFME+pfilates+hypopressives
	C: PFME
Sample size	50 men after RP (E=25, C=25)

Continued

TABLE 11.2.1	**Randomized Controlled Studies of Physical Therapy for Incontinence After Prostatectomy—cont'd**
Diagnosis	24-h pad test, number of pads, 3d-bladder diary (number/voids), Modified Oxford Scale, HRQoL (FACT-P, PORPUS), IPSS
Training protocol	E: PFME+pfilates+hypopressives (30 contractions/d during weeks 1–2 up to 180 contr/d for weeks 7–26)
	C: PFME (comparable volume of exercises)
Drop-out	13/50 (26%) (E:7, C:6)
Results	At 26W, E had less total leakage and day leakage, no other significant differences between groups
Author	**Aydin Sayilan, 2018**
Design	E: PFME
	C: no therapy
Sample size	60 men after RP (E=30, C=30)
Diagnosis	Number of pads, ICIQ-UI score
Training protocol	E: PFME (5 sessions with PT (from 1 week before surgery until cathether removal (10 days postop)); home exercise program (60 contractions:d)
	C: No PFME
Drop-out	0/60
Results	C used significant more pads in month 1 and 6
	ICIQ-UI score of C was significantly higher at 3 and 6 months
Author	**Bales et al., 2000**
Design	E: preoperative PFMT + EMG BF
	C: preoperative information about PFMT
Sample size	100 men (E = 50, C = 50)
Diagnosis	Questionnaire UI, number of pads
Training protocol	E: one treatment 45 min preoperatively BF with surface electrodes + home exercises pre- and postoperatively
	C: information (written and brief verbal information) pre- and postoperatively + same home exercises as E
	Home: 10–15 contractions of 5–10 s, 4×/day
Drop-out	3%
Results	No significant difference in pad usage between E and C group at 1–6 months after surgery
Author	**Burgio et al., 2006**
Design	E: preoperative PFMT + EMG BF
	C: postoperative verbal information of surgeon
Sample size	125 men (E = 63, C = 62)
Diagnosis	Number of leakage (diary), pad use, IIQ, QoL questionnaires
Training protocol	E: one treatment preoperatively BF with rectal probe + home exercises pre- and postoperatively
	Home: 15 contractions of 2–10 s, 3×/day
	C: brief verbal information to interrupt urine stream postoperatively once a day
Drop-out	10% after surgery; 18% after 6 months
Results	Significant difference in duration of incontinence (number of leakage) between E and C group at 6 months after surgery (p = 0.04); number of patients wearing pads (p < 0.05)
Author	**Centemero et al., 2010**
Design	E: preoperative and postoperative PFME
	C: postoperative PFME
Sample size	118 men (E = 59, C = 59)
Diagnosis	Self-reported continence, ICS male SF score, 24-h pad-test

TABLE 11.2.1   Randomized Controlled Studies of Physical Therapy for Incontinence After Prostatectomy—cont'd

Training protocol	E: 8 guided PFME preoperatively + 30 days home exercises preoperatively and 8 guided PFME during 1 month after catheter removal, at home; PFME postoperatively till continence, 30 min daily
	C: same postoperative programme
Drop-out	0%
Results	Significant difference in incontinence between E and C group: at 1 and 3 months after surgery (p = 0.018/0.028) for self-reported continence
	at 1 and 3 months after surgery (p = 0.002/0.002) for ICS male SF score
	at 1 and 3 months after surgery (p = 0.040/0.033) for 24-h pad-test
Author	**De Lira et al., 2019**
Design	E: 2 preoperative sessions (PFMT+BF) + home exercises preop and postop
	C: usual post-RP care
Sample size	31 men before RP (E=16, C=15)
Diagnosis	Number of pads/day, ICIQ-SF, IIEF-5 until 3 months after RP
Training protocol	E: 2 pre-RP PFMT +BF sessions + home exercises (3×/day at progressively higher intensity) until surgery + advice to resume after catheter withdrawal
	C: usual post-RP care
Drop-out	0/31
Results	No significant UI rate at three months after RP, (73% in the Control Group and 70.0% in the Physical Therapy Group). No significant difference in ICIQ-SF scores.
Author	**Dijkstra-Eshuis et al., 2015**
Design	E: preoperative PFMT + BFB
	C: preoperative no treatment
Sample size	121 men after laparoscopic RP
Diagnosis	PeLFIs, KHQ, IPSS, bladder diary, 24hr pad test, PF examination
Training protocol	E: preoperative: 1×/week 30′ PFMT +BFB during 4 weeks + home ex (2×30 contractions/day); postoperative: home ex (2×30 contractions/day) until 6 weeks after RP
	C: preoperative no treatment, postoperative written info regarding PFMT
	At 6 weeks postoperative: E+C: PFMT + BFB and/or ES if they were still incontinent
Drop-out	19/121 (15,7%) (E: 9, C:10)
Results	No significant difference of incidence of SUI and Qol between groups
	77.2% achieved continence at 1 year postoperative
Author	**Dubbelman et al., 2010**
Design	E: information and guided PFME
	C: verbal instructions and information folder PFME
Sample size	79 men (E = 35, C = 44)
Diagnosis	24-h pad-test (< 4 g = continent) and 1-h pad-test (< 1 g = continent)
Training protocol	E: maximum 9 guided PFME 30 min sessions postoperatively at week 2, 3, 4, 6, 8, 12, 16, 20 and 26 + 150 home exercises daily
	C: verbal instructions and information folder of PFME
Drop-out	13/79
Results	No significant difference in incontinence between E and C group:
	- at 1, 4, 8, 12 and 26 weeks after catheter removal for 24-h pad test
	- at 1, 12 and 26 weeks for 1-h pad-test
Author	**Filocamo et al., 2005**
Design	E: PFME programme
	C: no instructions in PFME
Sample size	300 men after RP (E = 150, C = 150)
Diagnosis	1-h pad-test, 24-h pad test, number/pads daily, ICS-male questionnaire

Continued

TABLE 11.2.1   Randomized Controlled Studies of Physical Therapy for Incontinence After Prostatectomy—cont'd

Training protocol	PFME started after catheter removal (Kegel exercises only, no rectal ES or BF). Contractions were evaluated by digital anal control. At home (10 contractions of 5 s and 10 s rest in between). PFME in all positions, PFME before any effort or activity that might induce UI
Drop-out	2/300 (1%)
Results	Significantly more patients in the E group were continent at 1 and 6 months after surgery compared to the C group. Patient age correlated with continence in the E group, but not in the C group. 93.3% of the total population achieved continence after 1 year
Author	**Floratos et al., 2002**
Design	E: PFMT + EMG BF
	C: verbal instructions about PFMT
Sample size	42 men (E = 28, C = 14)
Diagnosis	ICS 1-h pad-test and questionnaire
Training protocol	E: 15 sessions EMG BF with surface electrodes, 3×/week, 30 min, at home: 50 to 100 contractions/day
	C: verbal instructions on PFMT, 1 session anal control; at home: 80–100 contractions/day 3–5 s with submaximal strength of 70%
Drop-out	0%
Results	No significant difference in incontinence (ICS 1-h pad-test and number of pads) between E and C group at baseline 1, 2, 3 and 6 months after surgery (p > 0.05)
Author	**Franke et al., 2000**
Design	E: PFMT + BF
	C: no treatment
Sample size	30 men (E = 15, C = 15)
Diagnosis	Voiding diary, 48-hour pad-test
Training protocol	Experimental: 5 sessions of 45 min BF behavioural therapy
	C: no therapy
Drop-out	6 at 6 weeks, 7 at 12 weeks, 15 at 24 weeks
Results	No significant difference E and C group in pad-test and incontinence episodes at 6 weeks, 3 and 6 months
Author	**Geraerts et al., 2013**
Design	E: pre- and postoperative PFME + BF
	C: postoperative PFME + BF
Sample size	180 men (E = 91, C = 89)
Diagnosis	Test 24 h (0 g 3 days = continent) and 1-h pad-test, VAS, IPSS, KHQ
Training protocol	E: preop: 3 guided PFME + BF preoperatively + 21 days home: 60 exercises/day preoperatively; postoperative after catheter removal: weekly guided PFME + BF till continence
	Home: PFME 10 contractions 1 s, 10 contractions 10 s, 3× daily
	C: same postoperative programme
Drop-out	5%
Results	No significant difference E and C group in time to continence by pad-test, and incontinence episodes at 1, 3, 6 and 12 months after catheter removal
Author	**Glazener et al., 2011**
Design	Trial 1: men after RP; trial 2: men after TURP
	E: 4 PFMT sessions with a therapist (over 3 months)
	C: standard care and lifestyle advice
Sample size	Men incontinent after RP (trial 1), TURP (trial 2)
	Trial 1: n = 411/1158 (E = 205, C = 206)
	Trial 2: n = 442/5986 (E = 220, C = 222)
Diagnosis	ICIQ-UI SF questionnaire, measure of cost-effectiveness (QALY), use of pads and catheters, day and night urinary frequency and UI, EQ-5D and SF-12 (QoL)

TABLE 11.2.1 Randomized Controlled Studies of Physical Therapy for Incontinence After Prostatectomy—cont'd

Training protocol	E: one-to-one therapy sessions including PFMT and BT if OAB/urgency symptoms + PFMT and lifestyle leaflet (4 treatment sessions in 3 months starting 6 weeks after surgery) C: standard care + lifestyle leaflet only, no individual PFMT instruction or sessions
Drop-out	Trial 1: 20/411 (5%); trial 2: 45/442 (10%)
Results	Trial 1: the rate of UI did not significantly differ between E and C at 12 months after surgery. There were no significant differences in the prevalence of UI or the mean ICIQ score between the groups at any of the time points Trial 2: identical results to trial 1
Author	**Gomes et al., 2018**
Design	E^1: Pilates protocol, E^2: PFMT with ES C: no treatment
Sample size	110 men after RP with complaint of PPUI (E^1=36, E^2=38, C=36)
Diagnosis	Voiding diary, 24h pad test, ICIQ-SF, number of pads/day at 4 months after RP
Training protocol	E^1: Pilates 10 weeks during 45 min + daily exercises at home E^2: PFMT 10 weeks during 45min + ES + contractions every day at home C: no treatment
Drop-out	6 (5%) (E1: 2, E2: 3, C: 1)
Results	Significant reduction in pad usage in all groups No significant difference between E^1 and E^2 in improvements in 24h pad test E^1 and E^2 had a higher proportion of continents (no pads/day) than C after treatment Significant improvements in the ICIQ-SF scores in E^1, E^2 and C after 4 months
Author	**Goode et al., 2011**
Design	E^1: 8 weeks of behavioural therapy (PFMT, bladder control strategies) E^2: behavioural therapy plus in-office, dual-channel EMG BF and daily home PF ES (20 Hz, current up to 100 mA) C: delayed treatment
Sample size	208 men with UI, 1–17 years after RP
Diagnosis	Percentage reduction in mean number of UI episodes after 8 weeks of treatment (7-day bladder diaries), AUA-7 symptom index, IPSS-QoL question, IIQ, EPIC, SF-36, global perception of improvement and the patient satisfaction question
Training protocol	The *behavioural therapy* (PFMT, bladder control strategies) consisted of (4 visits, ± 2 weeks apart): explanation of anatomy and PFME (anal palpation); home exercises (3 daily sessions (lying, sitting and standing position) with 15 repetitions of a 2–10 s contraction and an equal relaxation period). The contraction and relaxation duration was advanced by 1 second each week to a max of 10–20 s. Once-daily participants had to interrupt voiding for the first 2 weeks. Participants kept daily bladder diaries and exercise logs during 8 weeks of treatment. Patients received a fluid management handout. Strategies to avoid stress and urge urinary incontinence were clarified Behavioural therapy plus BF and ES (*behaviour plus*) was similarly conducted with the addition of in-office, dual-channel BF and daily home pelvic floor ES (with an anal probe, 20 Hz, pulse width 1 msec, 5 s on and 15 s off, current up to 100 mA, during 15 min) + additional 2 daily sessions of PFME Participants in the delayed-treatment group kept daily bladder diaries, which were reviewed during their clinic visits every 2 weeks. After 8 weeks, they were offered off-protocol treatment with their choice of behavioural therapy with or without BF and ES
Drop-out	32/208 (15%)
Results	Mean incontinence episodes decreased significantly more in E^1 and E^2 compared to C. There was no significant difference in incontinence reduction between treatment groups. Improvements were durable to 12 months in the active treatment groups

Continued

TABLE 11.2.1 Randomized Controlled Studies of Physical Therapy for Incontinence After Prostatectomy—cont'd

Author	**Heydenreich et al., 2020**
Design	E: standard PFMT and oscillating rod therapy
	C: standard PFMT and relaxation therapy
Sample size	184 men with UI after RP (E=93, C= 91)
Diagnosis	24h pad test, 1h pad test, HRQL, FACT-P at 3 weeks after surgery
Training protocol	E: daily supervised PFMT and coordination training for the PF using an oscillating rod (30 min), 3 weeks
	C: daily supervised PFMT and 30 min listening to relaxation music, 3 weeks
Drop-out	0/184
Results	E: significant reduction in UI (24h pad test, 1h pad test), significant improvement HRQL
	Continence significantly improved in both groups (24h pad test E: 243–127 g vs C 238–181g, 1h pad test E: 23–8.5g vs 23–18g)
Author	**Hou et al., 2013**
Design	E: daily postoperative PFMT
	C: no treatment
Sample size	66 men after TURP (E=33, C=33)
Diagnosis	IPSS, uroflowmetry, SF-36 before surgery, at 1, 4, 8 and 12 weeks after surgery
Training protocol	E: 5 min PFMT (5 s contraction, 10 s relaxation), 3 times/day, 12 weeks
	C: no treatment
Drop-out	5/66 (E=1, C=4)
Results	At 12 weeks postoperative E had significantly better maximal urinary flow rate, greater decrease in IPSS-scores (only concerning storage [not voiding] symptom scores [urgency, frequency, nocturia]) and higher SF-36 subscores. No significant differences in postvoiding residual volume.
Author	**Ip et al., 2004**
Design	E: PFMT with information on a refrigerator magnet
	C: PFMT with information on a paper copy
Sample size	16 men with UI after TURP or RP
Diagnosis	Self-developed questionnaire and St George Urinary Incontinence Score
	Pre-admission, 2 weeks and 3 months postoperative
Training protocol	E: non-guided PFMT with information on a refrigerator magnet. PFMT: 6 contractions of 5 s contraction, 5 s rest; 6 times a day
	C: non-guided PFMT with information on a paper copy, same E
	Duration of treatment: 3 months
Drop-out	2/16 after 2 weeks; 0/16 after 3 months
Results	Unable to conclude that men in magnet group had a higher compliance with PFMT when compared with the paper copy group
Author	**Jalalinia et al., 2020**
Design	E: PFMT
	C: ward's patient education training
Sample size	68 men with UI after RP (E=34, C=34)
Diagnosis	ICIQ-UI SF, I-QOL
Training protocol	E: 100 contractions/day over 3 times/day (from 3 s/contraction gradually increasing to 10 s/contraction), during 3 months
	C: ward's patient education training
Drop-out	8/68 (E=4, C=4)
Results	E had significantly less UI and better Qol at 1, 2 and 3 months after surgery compared to C
Author	**Joseph et al., 2000**
Design	E: verbal feedback (N=5)
	C: biofeedback therapy (N= 6)
Sample size	11 patients (N=4 after RRP, N=6 after RPP, N=1 after TURP), at least 6 months after surgery
Diagnosis	VUD-testing, pad test, Joseph Continence Assessment Tool (JCAT), bladder diary, subjective estimation of degree of UI at 3, 6 and 12 months

TABLE 11.2.1   Randomized Controlled Studies of Physical Therapy for Incontinence After Prostatectomy—cont'd

Training protocol	E: verbal feedback during digital rectal examination (15 min/week, 4 visits)
	C: verbal feedback during digital rectal examination + visual confirmation (15 min/week, 4 visits)
Drop-out	0/11
Results	No significant differences between both groups
Author	**Kongtragul et al., 2014**
Design	E: Kegel exercise + concentration therapy
	C: Kegel exercise
Sample size	135 men after RP
Diagnosis	1h pad test (≥2 gram UI), evaluated by phone visit at 3,4,5,6,8,10 and 12 weeks after surgery
Training protocol	E: ≥ 240 contractions/day, while specifically concentrating on the exercise, from 3 weeks to 3 months
	C: ≥ 240 contractions/day, from 3 weeks to 3 months
Drop-out	3/138
Results	Significant difference in continence rate at 3 months (96% (E) vs 72% (C)).
	Adherence to exercises differed significantly between both groups (E: 97% vs C:51%)
Author	**Laurienzo et al., 2013**
Design	E[1]: preoperative PFMT
	E[2]: preoperative PFMT+ES
	C: verbal instructions to contract the perineum
Sample size	58 men before RP
Diagnosis	1h pad test, ICIQ-SF, SF-36
Training protocol	E[1]: Kegel exercises (10 preoperative sessions)
	E[2]: Kegel exercises + ES (20Hz, 700 μsec, 10 min + 65Hz, 150 μsec, 5min) (10 preoperative sessions)
	C: only verbal instructions to contract the perineum
Drop-out	9/58 (15.5%)
Results	No significant difference in the 1h pad test, ICIQ-SF and SF-36 between the 3 groups at 1, 3 and 6 months
Author	**Laurienzo et al., 2018**
Design	E[1]: home PFMT
	E[2]: home PFMT + ES
	C: no treatment
Sample size	123 men after RP (>2g UI at 1h pad test, at 1 month after surgery) (E1=44, E2= 45, C=43)
Diagnosis	1h pad test, ICIQ-SF, IIEF-5, IPSS, perineometry
Training protocol	E[1]: three types of home PFM exercises, two to three x/day until 6 months postoperative
	E[2]: same home exercises as E[1] + ES 2×/week for 7 weeks with a physiotherapist
	C: no treatment
Drop-out	9/123 (7.3%) (E1:3, E2: 3, C:3)
Results	No statistical difference in 1h pad test, ICIQ-SF, IIEF-5, IPSS and muscle strength between E1, E2 and C at 1, 3 and 6 months postoperative
Author	**Manassero et al., 2007**
Design	Experimental E: an intensive PFMT programme
	C: no instructions
Sample size	107 incontinent (24-h pad-test > 2 g) men after retropubic RP with bladder neck preservation (E = 54, C = 53)
Diagnosis	24-h pad-test, VAS, a single question of QoL
Training protocol	E: PFMT (active PFE with verbal feedback) as long as any degree of UI persisted (within a 1-year period). In case of weak PFM, home ES with an anal probe. Home exercises: 45 contractions (3 sessions of 15) per day at home, progressively increasing until 90 per day
	C: no treatment

Continued

TABLE 11.2.1   Randomized Controlled Studies of Physical Therapy for Incontinence After Prostatectomy—cont'd

Drop-out	13/107 (12%)
Results	The overall spontaneous continence rate after catheter removal was 23.6%. The proportion of men still incontinent was significantly higher in C compared to E at 1, 3, 6 and 12 months after surgery. VAS and QoL also significantly differed between E and C at 12 months after RP
Author	**Marchiori et al., 2010**
Design	E: intensive daily PFMT + BF + ES for 2–3 weeks C: Advice to perform 3*30 contractions/day
Sample size	332 incontinent (> 1 pad/daily) men at 30 days after radical prostatectomy (E = 166, C = 166)
Diagnosis	ICIQ-male, RAND 36-item health survey, use of pads
Training protocol	E: intensive daily PFMT + BF teaching of correct contraction, 10 sets of ES of 15 minutes each; for 2–3 weeks on daily basis
	C: Advice to perform 3*30 contractions/day at home
Drop-out	Not mentioned
Results	Patients enrolled in the E group achieved continence earlier than the C group (44±2 days versus 76±4 days)
Author	**Mariotti et al., 2009**
Design	E: information and guided PFMT
	C: verbal instructions and information folder PFMT
Sample size	60 men (E = 30, C = 30)
Diagnosis	24-h pad-test (2 g or less = continent), number of pads
Training protocol	E: BF (15 min) and ES (20 min: 30 Hz 10 min and 50 Hz 10 min) 12 sessions 2×/week, start 7 days postoperatively home exercises daily
	C: verbal instructions and written examples of PFMT
Drop-out	No
Results	Significant difference in UI between E and C: at 2, 4 weeks and 2, 3, 4, 5, 6 months after catheter removal for 24h pad test and number of pads
Author	**Mathewson-Chapman et al., 1997**
Design	E: 30 min preoperative information about PFMT and perineal muscle evaluation (not defined), post-operatively home exercises with BF
	C: 30 min preoperative information about PFMT and perineal muscle evaluation (not defined)
Sample size	53 men (E = 27, C = 26)
Diagnosis	Voiding diary, perineal muscle strength; number of pads
Training protocol	E: information preoperatively PFME, home exercises with BF
	C: information preoperatively PFME
	Home: 15 contractions of few seconds daily increasing by 10 contractions every 4 weeks
Drop-out	4%
Results	No significant difference between E and C group in number of pads
Author	**Milios et al., 2019**
Design	E: 6*20 contractions/day (fast [1 s] and slow [10 s])
	C: usual care (3*10 contractions/day [slow [10 s]])
	From 5 weeks preoperative until 12 weeks postoperative
Sample size	101 (E=51, C=50)
Diagnosis	24h pad test, IPSS, EPIC-CP, RTUS
Training protocol	Both groups 2 preoperative sessions (30 min, with written and verbal instructions regarding PFMT) at 5 weeks before surgery; afterwards:
	E: 6*20 contractions/day (fast [1 s] and slow [10 s])
	C: usual care (3*10 contractions/day [slow [10 s]])
	Until 12 weeks after surgery
Drop-out	4/101 (E=1, C=3)
Results	E scored significantly better than C regarding PFM function, UI and Qol. At 2, 6 and 12 weeks, respectively 14% vs 4%, 32 vs 11% and 74% vs 43% were continent in the E and C group.

TABLE 11.2.1   Randomized Controlled Studies of Physical Therapy for Incontinence After Prostatectomy—cont'd

Author	Moore et al., 1999
Design	E^1: PFMT E^2: PFMT + ES C: verbal and written information about PFMT
Sample size	63 men (E^1 = 21, E^2 = 21, C = 21)
Diagnosis	24-hour pad-test ($\leq$ 8 g = continent) and questionnaires (IIQ7 and EORTC QLQ C30) at 12, 16 and 24 weeks after enrollment (8 weeks after surgery)
Training protocol	E^1: information (written and brief verbal information) pre- and postoperatively + treatment 30 min PFMT in outpatient clinic 2×/week for 12 weeks + home exercises E^2: idem E^1 + ES: surface anal electrode, 50 Hz, biphasic pulse shape with 1s bursts, a 1 s pulse width and 1s pulse trains + home exercises C: information (written and brief verbal information) pre- and postoperatively + same home exercises Home exercises: 12–20 contractions of 5–10 s, 8–10 contractions of 20–30 s and repetitive contractions in 10 s 3×/day
Drop-out	8%
Results	No significant difference in incontinence between E^1, E^2 and C group for all assessments
Author	Moore et al., 2008
Design	Experimental group E: PFMT and BF C: telephone contact about PFMT
Sample size	205 men (E = 106, C = 99)
Diagnosis	24h pad test ($\leq$ 8 g = continent) and questionnaires (Incontinence Impact Questionnaire IIQ7 and IPSS) and perception of urine loss as a problem preoperatively and at week 4, 8, 12, 16, 28, 52 after surgery
Training protocol	E: information (written and verbal information) 4 weeks postoperatively; treatment 30 min PFMT and BF in outpatient clinic weekly till continence (maximum 24 weeks) + home exercises C: written and brief verbal information + same home exercises Home exercises: 10–12 contractions 3×/day
Drop-out	8%
Results	No significant difference in incontinence between E and C group for all assessments
Author	Nilssen et al., 2012
Design	same study as Overgard E: information and guided PFME or DVD C: verbal instructions and information on PFME
Sample size	85 men (E = 42, C = 43)
Diagnosis	QoL: UCLA-PCI, SF-12
Training protocol	E: guided PFME 45 min session, once weekly starting immediately after catheter withdrawal till continence; contractions of 6–8 s; 30 home exercises daily. Training recorded in training diary C: verbal instructions and written information on PFME
Drop-out	5.9%
Results	No significant difference in HR QoL between E and C group at 6 weeks, 3, 6 and 12 months after surgery
Author	Ocampo-Trujillo et al., 2014
Design	16 men before RP (E=8, C=8)
Sample size	E: PFMT starting 30 days before RP C: standard preoperative management
Diagnosis	Number of pads/day, UCLA-PCI, SF-12 at day of catheter removal
Training protocol	E: intensive PFMT, with biofeedback (3×/day, starting 30 days before RP) C: routine hygienic-dietary education

Continued

TABLE 11.2.1   Randomized Controlled Studies of Physical Therapy for Incontinence After Prostatectomy—cont'd

Drop-out	0/16
Results	Proportion of continent patients and number of pads/day was not significantly different between respectively E and C (after catheter removal 62% vs 37% continent and 75% vs 25% no pad). No differences in HRQol between both groups.
Author	**Oh et al., 2020**
Design	84 men after RARP (E=42, C=42)
Sample size	E: BF-PFMT and verbal and written instructions regarding PFMT
	C: verbal and written instructions
Diagnosis	24h pad test, IPSS at 1, 2, 3 months
Training protocol	E: extracorporeal BF-PFMT and verbal and written instructions regarding PFMT (4×/day, 10 min/session, 10 s/contraction)
	C: verbal and written instructions regarding PFMT
Drop-out	2/84 (E=2, C=0)
Results	E had significantly less UI than C at 1 month (24h pad test), E had significantly lower IPSS scores at 1 month, no significant differences from 2 months onwards. At 3 months, 67.5% in E vs 61.9% in C were continent
Author	**Overgard et al., 2008**
Design	Experimental group E: information and guided PFME or DVD
	C: verbal instructions and information on PFME
Sample size	85 men (E = 42, C = 43)
Diagnosis	Number of pads (0 = continent), self-reported continence, 24-h pad-test (< 2 g = continent) and muscle strength by anal pressure (cmH$_2$O)
Training protocol	E: guided PFME 45 min session, 1×/week, starting immediately after catheter withdrawal till continence; contractions of 6–8 s; 30 home exercises daily. Training recorded in training diary.
	C: verbal instructions and written information on PFME
Drop-out	5/85
Results	No significant difference in incontinence between E and C group: at 1, 4, 8, 12 and 26 weeks after catheter removal for number of pads and self-report, 24h pad test, strength; at 1 year, significant difference in incontinence between E and C group only on number of pads and self-report (92% vs 72%)
Author	**Parekh et al., 2003**
Design	Experimental group E: preoperative and postoperative PFMT + BF
	C: no formal PFE instructions
Sample size	38 men (E = 19, C = 19)
Diagnosis	Number of pads/day at 6, 12, 16, 20, 28 and 52 weeks
Training protocol	E: two treatments pre- and postoperatively 1×/3 weeks for 3 months PFME (+ BF depending the patient), exercises described
	C: no formal education on PFMT
	Home: 6 months or longer functional re-training (2×/d)
Drop-out	5%
Results	Significant difference in achievement of continence between E and C group at week 12, but not at 1 year
	Significant difference in median time to regain continence between E (12 weeks) and C group (16 weeks)
Author	**Park et al., 2012**
Design	E: combined exercise treatment of PFME + general exercises of resistance and flexibility of whole body
	C: PFME
Sample size	66 men (E = 33, C = 33)

TABLE 11.2.1   Randomized Controlled Studies of Physical Therapy for Incontinence After Prostatectomy—cont'd

Diagnosis	Physical function (functional fitness: sit-ups, grip strength, flexibility and balance ability: chair stand); continence and QoL (24-hour pad-test (< 1 g = continent), continence rate, ICIQ, Beck Depression Inventory, SF-36
	Assessment: preoperatively, at start of treatment and after 12 weeks
Training protocol	Starting at week 3 postop, 2×/week for 12 weeks
	E: combined exercise treatment of PFME + general exercises of resistance and flexibility of whole body with a ball and elastic band
	C: PFME (no details)
	Home: 60 min total exercise time/day
Drop-out	17/66 (25%)
Results	Significant difference in functional physical fitness, flexibility, balance ability. NS for grip strength.
	Significant difference in 24h pad test in favour of E group at week 12 and ICIQ
	Significant difference in SF-36 in favour of E group
Author	**Pedriali et al., 2016**
Design	E[1]: Pilates
	E[2]: PFME+ES
	C: no treatment
Sample size	90 men 4 weeks after RP; (E[1]=28, E[2]=31, C=31)
Diagnosis	24h pad test, bladder diary, ICIQ-SF at 4 months after RP (0 pads= continent)
Training protocol	E[1]: Pilates, 1×/week, 45 minutes, 10 weeks + written info regarding daily home exercises
	E[2]: PFME+ES, 1×/week, 40–50 minutes (20 min ES and 3×10 contractions), 10 weeks + written info regarding daily home exercises
	C: no treatment
Drop-out	5/90 (5.5%) (E[1]=2, E[2]=3, C=0)
Results	Significant improvements in nocturia, pad usage, 24h pad test and Qol in all groups at 4 months. No significant difference between groups at 4 months in nocturia, daily urinary frequency, pad weight. E[1] had a significantly better result in daily pad usage and ICIQ-SF score at 4 months.
Author	**Porru et al., 2001**
Design	E: PFMT + BF
	C: information (written and verbal information) postoperatively + same home exercises
Sample size	58 men after TURP (E = 30, C = 28)
Diagnosis	Questionnaires of LUTS (AUA) and QoL, voiding diary and post-micturition dribble, digital test for strength/PFM
Training protocol	E: 4 treatments postoperatively 1×/week PFMT + home exercises
	C: information (written and verbal information) postoperatively + same home exercises
	Home: 15 contractions on strength and endurance, 3×/day
Drop-out	3/58 (5%)
Results	AUA: both significantly improved pre- compared to 4 weeks postoperatively, no significant difference between E and C group
	QoL and PFM-strength: significant difference in E group only between preoperatively and week 4 postoperatively
	Incontinent episodes and post-micturition dribble: significant difference between E and C group at 1,2 and 3 weeks
Author	**Ribeiro et al., 2010**
Design	E: PFMT and BF
	C: usual care
Sample size	73 men after RP (E = 36, C = 37)
Diagnosis	24h pad test, ICS male SF, IIQ, PFM strength (Oxford scale) at 1, 3, 6 and 12 months after RP (≤1 pad/day= continent)

Continued

TABLE 11.2.1 Randomized Controlled Studies of Physical Therapy for Incontinence After Prostatectomy—cont'd

Training protocol	E: written and verbal information 4 weeks after RP; treatment 30 min PFMT and BF in outpatient clinic from postop day 15, weekly till continence (maximum of 3 months) + home exercises (3×10 rapid contractions, 3× contractions of 5, 7 or 10 s; supine position: 10 contractions during prolonged expiration) Home exercises: 10–12 contractions 3×/day while lying, sitting and standing C: verbal information from the urologist to contract PF
Drop-out	19/73 (26%)
Results	Significant difference in incontinence between E and C group for all incontinence assessments and strength. For QoL only significant difference at 1 month.
Author	**Robinson et al., 2008**
Design	E: one preoperative and one session of PFMT at 1 month after surgery + 4 BF-sessions immediately after catheter withdrawal C: idem E without 4 BF-sessions
Size of sample	126 men planned for RP (E = 62, C = 64)
Diagnosis	LUTS intensity, LUTS distress and HRQol at 3, 6 and 12 months after RP
Training protocol	E: brief verbal instruction in PFMT before surgery and one BF session at 2 months after surgery plus PFMT for 4 weeks with BF immediately after catheter withdrawal C: brief verbal instruction in PFMT before surgery and one BF session at 2 months after surgery
Drop-out	Not mentioned
Results	Decrease in LUTS-intensity and -distress in both groups, but no between-group differences. No between-group differences in HRQol.
Author	**Santos et al., 2017**
Design	E: PFME + BF C: PFME
Size of sample	16 men with UI (>2g) after RRP/LRP (E=8, C=8)
Diagnosis	1h pad test,
Training protocol	All patients, oral and written information regarding home exercises E: PFME + BF (1×/week, 8 weeks, 20 minutes BF + active exercises) C: PFME (1×/week, 8 weeks, active exercises)
Drop-out	3/16 (E=1, C=2)
Results	At 8 weeks, 69% of patients were continent with a significant difference between pre- and post-treatment in both groups. Nocturia decreased significantly from pre to post in E. Pad usage significantly decreased in both groups. There were no significant differences between both groups regarding severity and duration of UI.
Author	**Sueppel et al., 2001**
Design	E: preoperative (instructions about PFMT and one session [PFMT + BF]) + 6 weeks postop (PFMT + BF) and 3, 6, 9, 12 months after surgery + home exercises C: 6 weeks postop (PFMT + BF) and 3, 6, 9 12 months after surgery + home exercises
Sample size	16 men (E = 8, C = 8)
Diagnosis	Pad-test 45 min, bladder diary, number of incontinence episodes, number of pads/day, QoL, AUA and leakage index before surgery and at 6 weeks, 3, 6, 9, 12 months after surgery
Training protocol	E: information on PFMT (written and brief verbal information) and PFMT + BF with rectal pressure probe pre- and postoperatively 6 weeks, 3, 6, 9, 12 months after surgery + home exercises C: PFMT + BF with rectal pressure probe 6 weeks, 3, 6, 9, 12 months after surgery + same home exercises Home: ? contractions, 3×/day
Drop-out	Not reported
Results	Only descriptive statistics but better improvement in incontinence in E group

TABLE 11.2.1 Randomized Controlled Studies of Physical Therapy for Incontinence After Prostatectomy—cont'd

Author	Tantawy et al., 2019
Design	E: PFMT + whole body vibration C: PFMT
Sample size	64 men with mild SUI after RP (E=32, C=32)
Diagnosis	I-VAS, ICIQ-UI-SF, 24h pad test
Training protocol	E: PFMT + whole body vibration, 3×/week, 4 weeks C: PFMT, 3×/week, 4 weeks Home exercises: daily (15× 10 s, 20× 1 s), 2–4 sessions
Drop-out	3/64 (E=2, C=1)
Results	I-VAS, ICIQ-UI-SF and 24h pad test significantly changed between baseline and 4 weeks and between 4 weeks and 2 months (except for I-VAS between baseline and 4 weeks) I-VAS, ICIQ-UI-SF and 24h pad test were significantly better in E at 4 weeks and 2 months
Author	**Tibaek et al., 2007**
Design	E: preoperative PFMT C: no training
Sample size	58 men with BPH planned for TURP
Diagnosis	Danish Prostate Symptom Score (DAN-PSS-1), voiding diary, pad usage, 24h pad test, PFM assessment at 2 weeks, 4 weeks and 3 months
Training protocol	E: preoperative: 1h individual information, 3×1h group lesson (PFMT) + home training program (force/endurance PFME, 6–10× supine/sitting/standing, 1–2×/day), continuing until 4 weeks after surgery C: preoperative: no info, postoperative: brief verbal info regarding PFMT
Drop-out	9/58
Results	No between-group differences at 2 weeks, 4 weeks or 3 months. E had significantly better endurance than C at 4 weeks.
Author	**Tienforti et al., 2012**
Design	E: 1 preoperative PFMT + BF C: pre- and postoperative verbal information
Sample size	34 men (E = 17, C = 17)
Diagnosis	ICIQ-UI; incontinence episodes, pad use; ICIQ-OAB, IPSS-QoL
Training protocol	E: one treatment session preoperatively PFME + BF + home exercises pre- and postoperatively Home: 15 contractions of 2–10 s, 3×/day Postop: monthly treatment session + home exercises C: oral and written instructions for PFME
Drop-out	5.8%
Results	Significant difference in UI between E and C group at 1, 3 and 6 months after catheter removal for ICIQ-UI; at 3 and 6 months after catheter removal for UI episodes, pad use, ICIQ-OAB No significant difference in QoL between E and C group at 1, 3 and 6 months after catheter removal
Author	**Van Kampen et al., 2000**
Design	E: PFMT + BF C: placebo treatment
Sample size	102 men (E = 50, C = 52)
Diagnosis	24h and 1h pad test, VAS, voiding volume charts, IPSS, number of pads/day (0 pads = continent)

Continued

TABLE 11.2.1   Randomized Controlled Studies of Physical Therapy for Incontinence After Prostatectomy—cont'd

Training protocol	E: 30 min PFME and BF 1×/week till continence + home exercises
	C: 30 min placebo ES, 1×/week till continence
	Home: total of 90 contractions/day: 40 contractions of 1s and 50 contractions of 10 s/day in supine, sitting or standing position
Drop-out	4%
Results	Significant difference between E and C group in duration and degree of UI at 1, 6 and 12 months after RP
Author	**Wille et al., 2003**
Design	E^1: information + PFMT and ES
	E^2: information + PFMT + ES + BF
	C: information about PFME
Sample size	139 men (E1 = 46, E2 = 46, C = 47)
Diagnosis	20-min pad-test, diary with number of pads/day (≤1 pad/day = continent) and urine symptom inventory at baseline, 3,12 months
Training protocol	Started after catheter withdrawal, duration: 3 months
	E^1: PFMT + ES: ES = surface electrodes, 27 Hz, biphasic 1 s bursts, 5 s pulse width and 2 s pulse trains, 15 min 2×/day home device
	E^2: PFMT, ES (5 s stimulation time, 5 s contracting and 15 s relaxing), BF: 15 min 2×/day same home device
	C: information (written and brief verbal information) and 3 days therapy 20–30 min + home exercises (2×/day for 3 months)
Drop-out	Not specified
Results	No significant difference between E^1, E^2 and C group in UI at 3 and 12 months
Author	**Yamanishi et al., 2010**
Design	E: PFMT + ES
	C: PFMT + sham ES
Sample size	56 men with severe UI after RP
Diagnosis	3-day pad-test, ICIQ-SF, KHQ
Training protocol	E: standard PFMT + ES (50 Hz square waves with a 300 µs pulse duration and a maximum output of 70 mA (5 s on, 5 s off))
	C: standard PFMT + sham ES (50 Hz square waves with a 300 µs pulse duration and a output of 3 mA (2 s on, 13 s off)
Drop-out	9/56 (16%)
Results	Significant difference in the number of continent patients between both groups at 1, 3 and 6 months. The time to achieve continence was significantly shorter in E than in C (2.7 ± 2.6 months vs 6.8 ± 3.9 months)
	Significantly larger changes in the amount of leakage, the ICIQ-SF and the KHQ score in E than in C at 1 month. No differences at 12 months.
Author	**Yokoyama et al., 2004**
Design	E1: FES
	E2: ExMI
	C: PFMT
Sample size	36 (12 patients each in the FES, ExMI and PFMT group)
Diagnosis	Bladder diaries, 24h pad test, a validated QoL survey

TABLE 11.2.1   Randomized Controlled Studies of Physical Therapy for Incontinence After Prostatectomy—cont'd

Training protocol	E1: FES with an anal probe, 20 Hz square waves (300 μs pulse duration and a maximal output current of 24 mA), 15 min, 2×/day for 1 month
	E2: 10 Hz, intermittently for 10 min, rest of 2 min, and a 2nd treatment at 50 Hz intermittently for 10 min. Treatment session duration was 20 min, 2×/week for 2 months
	C: PFMT with anal digital palpation, verbal and written instructions for home practice of PFME
Drop-out	Not reported
Results	The leakage weight during the 24 hours after removing the catheter was not significantly different between groups
	At 1 month, the leakage weight significantly differed between E^1 and C and at 2 months between E^2 and C. At 6 months after surgery the average 24-h leakage weight was < 10 g in all groups. QoL measures decreased after surgery, but gradually improved over time in all groups
Author	**Zachovajeviene et al., 2019**
Design	E^1: Diaphragm muscle training
	E^2: Abdominal muscle training
	C: PFMT
Sample size	148 men with UI after RP (E1=50, E2=49, C= 49)
Diagnosis	PFM strength and endurance, UI-level (8h pad test)
Training protocol	E^1: Diaphragm muscle training, breathing exercises with resistance (2 sets of 6–8 repetitions, 2×/day, 30 min)
	E^2: Abdominal muscle training (2×/day, 30 min)
	C: PFMT (short contractions, 2×/day, 30 min)
	Training duration: 6 months
Drop-out	21/148 (14.2%) (E^1=7, E^2=7, C=7)
Results	PFM strength increased significantly more in C than in E1, PFM endurance increased significantly more in E1 than in C
	UI-level: no significant differences between groups
	Increase in PFM strength correlated better with UI than PFME
Author	**Zhang et al., 2007**
Design	E: PFME + BF (1× 45 min), home PFME + group meetings
	C: PFME + BF (1×45 min), home PFME
Sample size	29 men with UI >6 months (average 18-21 months after RP) (E = 14, C = 15)
Diagnosis	VAS and use of pads; Prostate Cancer Index and AUASI, Illness Intrusiveness Rating Scale (IIRS) at start and after 3 months
Training protocol	E: postoperative PFME + BF (1× 45 min), 6 biweekly meetings over 3 months by psychologist + home exercises 2–3 times a day for 5–10 min
	C: postoperative PFME + BF (1× 45 min) + home exercises same as E group
Drop-out	2/29 (6%)
Results	Significant difference in continence VAS and Qol in favour of E group after 3 months
	Borderline significant difference in use of pads between E and C group
	Compliance of PFME: 86% in E group, 46% in C group

For abbreviations, see text.

TABLE 11.2.2 PEDro Quality Score of Randomized Controlled Trials in Systematic Review of Physical Therapy for Incontinence After Prostatectomy

E – Eligibility criteria specified
1 – Subjects randomly allocated to groups
2 – Allocation concealed
3 – Groups similar at baseline
4 – Subjects blinded
5 – Therapist administering treatment blinded
6 – Assessors blinded
7 – Measures of key outcomes obtained from > 85% of subjects
8 – Data analysed by intention to treat
9 – Statistical comparison between groups conducted
10 – Point measures and measures of variability provided

Study	E	1	2	3	4	5	6	7	8	9	10	Total score
Ahmed, 2012	+	+	+	+	–	–	–	+	–	+	+	6
Anan, 2020	+	+	–	+	–	–	–	+	–	+	+	5
Au, 2020	–	+	+	+	–	–	–	–	+	+	+	6
Aydin Sayilan, 2018	+	+	–	+	–	–	–	+	+	+	+	6
Bales, 2000	+	+	–	–	–	–	+	+	+	+	–	5
Burgio, 2006	+	+	–	+	–	–	+	+	+	+	+	7
Centemero, 2010	+	+	+	+	–	–	–	+	–	+	+	6
De Lira, 2019	–	+	–	+	–	–	+	+	+	+	+	7
Dijkstra-Eshuis, 2015	–	+	–	–	–	–	–	+	+	+	+	4
Dubbelman, 2010	+	+	+	+	–	–	–	–	–	+	+	5
Filocamo, 2005	+	+	–	+	–	–	–	+	–	+	+	5
Floratos, 2002	+	+	–	–	–	–	–	+	+	+	+	5
Franke, 2000	+	+	–	+	–	–	–	–	–	+	+	4
Geraerts, 2013	+	+	+	+	–	–	+	+	+	+	+	8
Glazener, 2011	+	+	+	+	–	–	–	+	+	+	+	7
Gomes, 2018	+	+	+	+	–	–	+	+	–	+	+	7
Goode, 2011	+	+	+	+	–	–	–	–	+	+	+	6
Heydenreich, 2020	+	+	+	–	–	–	+	+	+	+	+	7
Hou, 2013	+	+	–	+	–	–	–	+	–	+	+	5
Ip, 2004	–	+	–	+	–	–	–	–	–	–	+	3
Jalalinia 2020	+	+	–	+	–	–	–	+	–	+	+	5
Joseph, 2000	–	+	–	–	–	–	–	–	–	–	–	1
Kongtragul, 2014	+	+	–	+	–	–	–	+	–	+	+	5
Laurienzo, 2018	+	+	+	+	–	–	+	+	–	+	–	6
Laurienzo, 2013	+	+	–	+	–	–	–	–	–	+	+	4
Manassero, 2007	+	+	–	+	–	–	+	+	–	+	+	6
Marchiori, 2010	+	+	–	–	–	–	–	–	–	+	+	3
Mariotti, 2009	+	+	–	+	–	–	–	+	–	+	+	5
Mathewson-Chapman, 1997	–	+	–	–	–	–	–	+	–	+	+	4
Milios, 2019	+	+	–	+	–	–	–	+	–	+	+	5
Moore, 1999	+	+	+	–	–	–	–	+	–	+	+	5
Moore, 2008	+	+	+	–	–	–	–	+	+	+	+	6
Nilssen, 2012	+	+	–	+	–	–	–	+	–	+	+	5
Ocampo-Trujillo, 2014	–	+	+	+	–	–	–	–	+	+	+	6
Oh, 2020	+	+	–	+	–	–	–	+	+	+	+	6
Overgard, 2008	+	+	–	+	–	–	–	+	–	+	+	5
Parekh, 2003	+	+	–	–	–	–	–	+	+	+	+	5
Park, 2012	–	+	+	+	–	–	–	–	–	+	–	4

TABLE 11.2.2 PEDro Quality Score of Randomized Controlled Trials in Systematic Review of Physical Therapy for Incontinence After Prostatectomy—cont'd

												Total
Pedriali, 2016	+	+	+	+	−	−	+	+	−	+	+	7
Porru, 2001	+	+	−	+	−	−	+	+	−	+	+	6
Ribeiro, 2010	−	+	−	+	−	−	−	−	−	+	−	3
Robinson, 2008	+	+	+	+	−	−	−	+	+	+	+	7
Santos, 2017	+	+	−	+	−	−	−	−	−	−	+	3
Sueppel, 2001	+	−	−	+	−	−	−	+	−	−	−	2
Tantawy, 2019	+	+	−	+	−	−	−	+	−	+	+	5
Tibaek, 2007	+	+	+	+	−	−	+	−	−	+	+	6
Tienforti, 2012	+	+	−	−	−	−	−	+	−	+	+	4
Van Kampen, 2000	+	+	+	+	−	−	−	+	+	+	+	7
Wille, 2003	+	+	−	+	−	−	−	+	−	+	+	5
Yamanishi, 2010	+	+	+	+	+	−	+	+	−	+	+	8
Yokoyama, 2004	−	+	−	+	−	−	−	−	−	+	−	3
Zachovajeviene, 2019	−	+	+	+	−	−	−	+	+	+	+	7
Zhang, 2007	+	+	−	+	−	−	−	+	−	+	−	4

+, Criterion is clearly satisfied; −, criterion is not satisfied. Total score is determined by counting the number of criteria that are satisfied, except that 'eligibility criteria specified' score is not used to generate the total score. Total scores are out of 10.

Results

The following hypotheses were tested for the role of PFMT in alleviating UI after adenectomy or radical prostatectomy.

Pelvic Floor Muscle Training Is Better Than No Treatment or Placebo (10 Trials)

In seven trials (Aydin Sayilan, 2018; Filocamo et al., 2005; Goode et al., 2011; Hou et al., 2013; Jalalinia et al., 2020; Manassero et al., 2007; Van Kampen et al., 2000), a significant difference in incontinence was found between the experimental and control group. Hou et al. (2013) provided treatment after TURP, and the other studies showed a significant difference after radical prostatectomy. In five studies, pelvic floor exercises were started within 7 days after catheter withdrawal (Filocamo et al., 2005; Hou et al., 2013; Jalalinia et al., 2020; Manassero et al., 2007, Van Kampen et al., 2000). Goode et al. (2011) included patients with persistent UI 1 to 17 months after radical prostatectomy. The treatment of Goode et al. (2011), Hou et al. (2013) and Jalalinia et al. (2020) took 8 weeks, 12 weeks and 3 months, respectively. In the studies of Van Kampen et al. (2000), Manassero et al. (2007) and Filocamo et al. (2005), patients were treated as long as any degree of incontinence persisted, with a time frame of 1 year. Aydin Sayilan (2018) provided five sessions, starting 1 week before surgery and continuing until the day of catheter withdrawal.

In three trials (Franke et al., 2000; Glazener et al., 2011; Laurienzo et al., 2018), no significant difference between the experimental and control group was found. Franke et al. (2000) started 6 weeks postoperatively with pelvic floor exercises and BF, and five sessions were given. The high rate of drop-outs in this study was remarkable. Glazener et al. (2011) included one group after TURP and one group after radical prostatectomy. The authors gave one to four sessions spread over 3 months with a therapist to the patients in the experimental group, starting at 6 weeks after radical prostatectomy. In the study of Laurienzo et al. (2018), patients performed home exercises from 1 month until 6 months after radical prostatectomy. As the most progress in achieving urinary continence is to be expected in the first weeks after catheter removal (Geraerts et al., 2013; Van Kampen et al., 2000), it seems of general interest to start PFMT as soon as possible after radical prostatectomy. Nevertheless, there is no consensus on this matter yet, as several authors are convinced that due to spontaneous recuperation in approximately 50% of patients in the first month, postponed treatment is acceptable.

Preoperative and Postoperative Pelvic Floor Muscle Training Is Better Than Only Postoperative Pelvic Floor Muscle Training (Nine Trials)

Eight studies attempted to investigate the effect of preoperative PFMT on the duration, and in some studies on the severity, of UI after radical prostatectomy. One study

(Anan et al., 2020) investigated the aforementioned in patients after HoLEP. Four studies found positive results of preoperative PFMT (Burgio et al., 2006; Centemero et al., 2010; Sueppel et al., 2001; Tienforti et al., 2012). Two studies (Anan et al., 2020; Parekh et al., 2003) found a significant difference in incontinence at 3 months after radical prostatectomy/HoLEP in favour of the early start of PFMT but not at respectively 1 year (Parekh et al., 2003) and 3 days, 1 month and 6 months after HoLEP. Three studies (De Lira et al., 2019; Dijkstra-Eshuis et al., 2015; Geraerts et al. 2013) could not find any favour of early PFMT. However, due to the multitude of existing bias, results must be interpreted with caution. Parekh et al. (2003), Burgio et al. (2006), Tienforti et al. (2012) and De Lira et al. (2019) altered both pre- and postoperative treatment, which made defining the effect of preoperative PFMT impossible. Sueppel et al. (2001) compared only one preoperative session (written and brief verbal information and PFMT and BF with a rectal probe) with a control group who completed PFMT 6 weeks after surgery and only included 16 patients. Furthermore, follow-up was usually only 3 or 6 months. Finally, a wide range of continence criteria was used among studies, which made it difficult to compare results.

Only Centemero et al. (2010), Geraerts et al. (2013) and Anan et al. (2020) gave the control and the experimental group exactly the same postoperative therapy. Centemero et al. (2010) found a positive effect in favour of the experimental group and Geraerts et al. (2013) found no significant difference when three preoperative sessions were given to the experimental group. Anan et al. (2020) only found a significant difference between both groups at 3 months after HoLEP. All three studies started postoperative training directly after catheter removal. Dijkstra-Eshuis et al. (2015) offered 4 weeks of preoperative training and home exercises to the experimental group and no training to the control group. After surgery, the experimental group was encouraged to resume the home exercises, whereas the control group received written information regarding PFMT. Only at 6 weeks after radical prostatectomy, both groups received guided PFMT and BF/ES if they were still incontinent.

Preoperative Pelvic Floor Muscle Training and Biofeedback Is Better Than Only Preoperative/No Information About Pelvic Floor Muscle Training (Four Trials)

In all four trials (Bales et al., 2000; Laurienzo et al., 2013; Ocampo-Trujillo et al., 2014; Tibaek et al., 2007), no significant difference in incontinence could be found between the experimental and control groups. Tibaek et al. (2007) was the only study including patients planned for TURP. Bales et al. (2000) added one session of electromyography BF 2 to 4 weeks before surgery; Laurienzo et al. (2013) offered 10 preoperative sessions of PFMT (+ ES); Ocampo-Trujillo et al. (2014) preoperatively provided 30 daily PFMT + BF sessions; and Tibaek et al. (2007) provided an individual information session, three group lessons regarding PFMT and home exercises. In the control group, no or brief information on PFMT was given. In two studies, both groups had to perform postoperative home exercises (Bales et al. 2000; Tibaek et al. 2007). Bales et al. (2000) suggested that more intensive BF training instead of one training might have led to a better outcome.

Postoperative Pelvic Floor Muscle Training Is Better Than Only Information About Pelvic Floor Muscle Training Before and After Surgery (Eight Trials)

In one study (Porru et al., 2001), one group received guided PFMT combined with home exercises after TURP for 4 weeks. The control group was only given information and home exercises about PFMT before and after surgery. A significant difference in incontinence episodes was found between the experimental and control group at 1, 2 and 3 weeks after surgery, but not at 4 weeks. The authors concluded that early PFMT should be recommended to all cooperative patients after TURP.

Three trials could not find results in favour of a training programme compared with information (Dubbelman et al., 2010; Moore et al., 1999, 2008). On the contrary, Overgard et al. (2008) and Oh et al. (2020) did find a beneficial effect of PFMT. In particular, Oh et al. (2020) indicated a beneficial effect of PFMT for the recovery of continence in the early period after catheter removal (at 1 month). Overgard et al. (2008) could not find a positive effect in the short term, but only at 12 months after radical prostatectomy. In addition, Nilssen et al. (2012) investigated the effect of PFMT compared to information on QoL in the same population as Overgard et al. (2008). As a result, QoL was not affected by guided exercises in the short nor long term. One study (Ribeiro et al., 2010) proved that a structured programme (guided PFMT and BF once weekly, combined with home exercises) decreased the duration of incontinence significantly compared to offering only postoperative information.

Adding Biofeedback to Pelvic Floor Muscle Training Is Better Than Pelvic Floor Muscle Training Alone or Information Alone (Five Trials)

Five trials (Floratos et al., 2002; Joseph et al., 2000; Mathewson-Chapman, 1997; Robinson et al., 2008; Santos et al., 2017) could not prove an additional effect by adding BF to exercises alone or verbal instructions only concerning treatment for incontinence after radical prostatectomy or TURP. As in all included studies, it is important to mention that participants with and without awareness on how to contract or relax the pelvic floor muscles were included. To a certain extent, this could have influenced the results of the studies.

Adding Rectal Stimulation to Pelvic Floor Muscle Training Is Better Than Pelvic Floor Muscle Training Alone or Information Alone (Five Trials)

Two trials (Moore et al., 1999; Wille et al., 2003) could not prove any additional effect by adding ES to exercises alone or instructions only. Two trials (Ahmed et al., 2012; Yamanishi et al., 2010) could not confirm this result and demonstrated a shorter time to continence in the experimental group at 1, 3 and 6 months. According to Yamanishi et al. (2010), this difference between both groups disappeared at 12 months. In all trials, ES was offered to all patients of the experimental group. Some guidelines, however, indicated before that ES should preferably be preserved for patients who cannot actively contract the pelvic floor muscles (National Institute for Health and Care Excellence, 2019). One trial (Yokoyama et al., 2004) examined the effect of extracorporeal magnetic innervation (ExMI) compared to functional electrostimulation (FES) and/or standard PFMT. The authors indicated a significant effect of FES and ExMI, at respectively 1 and 2 months after surgery, compared to standard PFMT, but not between FES and ExMI.

Pelvic Floor Muscle Training With Adherence Strategies Gives Better Continence Results (Two Trials)

Methods to increase adherence/compliance with the exercises in male patients are rarely described. Only two studies compared two different methods to improve compliance (Ip, 2004; Kongtragul et al., 2014). The purpose of the work of Ip (2004) was to validate a new education tool (a refrigerator magnet) in comparison to a paper copy with the same information to determine if patient compliance with the exercises increased. Results

of this study made it unable to conclude that men in the magnet group had a higher compliance with PFMT when compared to the paper copy group. The patient group was quite small, no statistical data were available and the methodological quality of the study was quite low. Kongtragul et al. (2014) offered PFMT to both groups, but the experimental group was asked to concentrate on the exercise and to eliminate other subjects or issues (concentration therapy). A significant difference in continence rate was found at 3 months between both groups. In addition, adherence to exercises was much higher for the PFMT + concentration group than for the PFMT group.

Adding Biofeedback and Electrostimulation to Pelvic Floor Muscle Training Gives Better Results Than Pelvic Floor Muscle Exercises Alone or Information Alone (Five Trials)

Three studies (Ahmed et al., 2012; Marchiori et al., 2010; Mariotti et al., 2009) exclusively gave information to the control group. All three studies found a significant difference in favour of the PFMT + BF + ES group concerning the continence duration/severity. This result could not be confirmed by Wille et al. (2003); however, the control group not only received information but also three PFMT sessions. Goode et al. (2011) found a significant difference in the mean incontinence episodes between the PFMT + BF + ES group and the control group but could not demonstrate an effect of supplementary BF and ES to PFMT concerning the reduction of incontinence. The rating of specific effects of BF alone or ES alone was not possible in these trials, as both techniques were combined.

Adding General Exercises to Pelvic Floor Muscle Training for Incontinence After Surgery Is Better Than Pelvic Floor Muscle Training Alone (Five Trials)

Four studies (Au et al., 2020; Heydenreich et al., 2020; Park et al., 2012; Tantawy et al., 2019) added general exercises (respectively resistance and flexibility exercises, Pilates and hypopressive exercises, stabilizing exercises with an oscillating rod, and whole-body vibration therapy). All four studies found a significant effect of adding general exercises to standard PFMT regarding severity of incontinence at respectively 12 weeks (Park et al., 2012), 26 weeks (Au et al., 2020), 3 weeks (Heydenreich et al., 2020) and 4 weeks and 2 months (Tantawy et al., 2019). Zachovajeviene et al. (2019) compared two experimental groups, respectively diaphragm muscle training (DMT) and abdominal muscle training, to a control group, who followed PFMT. The duration of treatment was 6 months. Pelvic floor muscle strength increased significantly more in the PFMT group than in the DMT group; endurance, on the contrary, increased significantly more in the DMT group. Regarding the incontinence level, no significant differences were found.

Guided Pelvic Floor Muscle Training for Incontinence for an Average of 18 Months After Surgery Is Better Than Pelvic Floor Muscle Training Alone (One Trial)

Zhang et al. (2007) investigated the efficacy of guided PFMT compared to a group receiving only one session of PFMT and additional home exercises for an average of 18 months after surgery. The continence rate and QoL were significantly better in the experimental group.

Pilates for Incontinence After Surgery Is Better Than No Treatment (Two Trials)

Two studies (Gomes et al., 2018; Pedriali et al., 2016) compared 10 weeks of Pilates training with a control group without treatment. Both studies found a significant effect on pad usage, but not regarding frequency, nocturia and pad weight. Pedriali et al. (2016) also mentioned a significant better ICIQ score than the control group. Pilates training comprises exercises that are focused on pelvic stability, mobility and body alignment. PFMEs are performed in coordination with breathing, with concomitant recruitment of the trunk muscles in various positions (Gomes et al., 2018; Pedriali et al., 2016).

Adding Electrostimulation to Pelvic Floor Muscle Training for Incontinence After Surgery Is Better Than No Treatment (Two Trials)

Two studies (Gomes et al., 2018; Pedriali et al., 2016) compared PFMT combined with ES, over 10 weeks, with a control group receiving no treatment. Both studies reported a significantly reduced pad usage and 24-hour pad test in the experimental and control group at 4 months after treatment compared to immediately after radical prostatectomy. However, only Gomes et al. (2018) reported a higher proportion of continent patients (no pads over 24 hours) for the PFMT + ES group.

Intensity of Pelvic Floor Muscle Training

The study of Milios et al. (2019) is the only one that investigated the effect of increasing the intensity of treatment for UI at 12 weeks after radical prostatectomy.

Both groups received two preoperative PFMT sessions 5 weeks before surgery. After radical prostatectomy, the experimental group had to perform 120 contractions a day (focused on strength and endurance) and the control group 30 contractions a day (only focused on endurance) until 12 weeks after surgery. As a result, the experimental group scored significantly better than the control group regarding pelvic floor muscle function, incontinence (24-hour pad test) and QoL.

Adverse Effects

In one study (Moore et al., 1999), one patient complained of rectal pain by contracting the pelvic floor muscles and discontinued the therapy. No other authors described adverse effects of PFMT after prostatectomy.

Health Economics

Information on the total costs of the intervention of physical therapy after prostatectomy was never given. One study (Wille et al., 2003) gave details of the costs of a home BF and ES device. In another study (Van Kampen et al., 2000), the number of physical therapy sessions (an average of 8 in the experimental group and 16 in the control group) were calculated, and the authors concluded that the costs of treatment were low.

Discussion

UI is a common problem after radical prostatectomy or TURP, and the role of physical therapy as a first-line treatment option provides only a small base for evidence because of the different results in the studies.

Only seven studies are available to determine the effect of pelvic floor training after TURP. However, several studies have poor methodological quality (cfr. PEDro scores) Three studies described a clear benefit on the recovery of incontinence with PFMT (Anan et al., 2020; Hou et al., 2013; Porru et al., 2001). However, Glazener et al. (2011) found no beneficial effect of one to four sessions of PFMT compared to standard care and lifestyle advice. Furthermore, incontinence rates were much higher in this study at 12 months after surgery compared to other studies described in the literature.

After radical prostatectomy, conclusions about physical therapy for incontinence are difficult to make because of the heterogeneity of the results (continence definitions, methods used, etc.) Six of the eight trials showed that PFMT was significantly more effective than no treatment or sham treatment in the immediate postoperative period (Aydin Sayilan, 2018; Filocamo et al.,

2005; Goode et al., 2011; Jalalinia et al., 2020; Manassero et al., 2007; Van Kampen et al., 2000). The results of preoperative PFMT on incontinence were positive in five of the eight trials (Burgio et al., 2006; Centemero et al., 2010; Parekh et al., 2003; Sueppel et al., 2001; Tienforti et al., 2012). None of the studies could indicate an additional effect of preoperative PFMT + BF compared to preoperative/no information (Bales et al., 2000; Laurienzo et al., 2013; Ocampo-Trujillo et al., 2014; Tibaek et al., 2007). Three of seven studies (Oh et al., 2020; Overgard et al., 2008; Ribeiro et al., 2010) proved that a structured programme decreased the duration of incontinence significantly in comparison with information only. No additional effect of BF was found in males undergoing a radical prostatectomy in four studies (Floratos et al., 2002; Mathewson-Chapman, 1997; Robinson et al., 2008; Wille et al., 2003). The role of ES and ExMI compared to regular PFMT or information was confirmed in three of the five studies (Ahmed et al., 2012; Yamanishi et al., 2010; Yokoyama et al., 2004). Adding adherence strategies to regular PFMT, such as concentration therapy, was beneficial in one trial (Kongtragul et al., 2014). Four of five studies demonstrated a positive effect of the combination of PFMT, BF and ES (Ahmed et al., 2012; Goode et al., 2011; Marchiori et al., 2010; Mariotti et al., 2009). Combining PFMT with general exercises, such as stabilizing exercises, whole-body vibration and Pilates, seemed to be beneficial for incontinence outcomes according to four studies (Au et al., 2020; Heydenreich et al., 2020; Park et al., 2012; Tantawy et al., 2019). Consequently, the efficacy of guided PFMT even 18 months after radical prostatectomy has been proved in one study (Zhang et al., 2007). Lastly, the role of Pilates and of PFMT combined with ES versus no treatment was confirmed in two studies (Gomes et al., 2018; Pedriali et al., 2016).

Several limitations should be considered in the different studies. A variety of outcome measurements were used to assess UI. The most widely used assessment is the number of pads (Anan et al., 2020; Aydin Sayilan, 2018; Bales et al., 2000; Floratos et al., 2002; Ocampo-Trujillo et al., 2014). In most studies, no pad or one pad per 24 hours is defined as continent. Clinical experience revealed that some men wear one pad but have a urine loss greater than 10 g, whereas other men wear a pad just for safety reasons. The severity of incontinence was objectively assessed by the International Continence Society 1-hour pad test (Floratos et al., 2002, Kongtragul et al., 2014; Van Kampen et al., 2000) or during 24 hours

(Au et al., 2020; Geraerts et al., 2013; Moore et al., 1999; Van Kampen et al., 2000). In rather few studies, an effort was made to assess pelvic floor muscle strength prior to surgery (De Lira et al., 2019; Dijkstra-Eshuis et al., 2015; Geraerts et al., 2013). Geraerts et al. (2013) mentioned that patients with stronger pelvic floor muscles before surgery tended to need less time to become continent compared to patients with a weaker pelvic floor (Oxford scale 0–3). However, currently we do not know whether these patients would also benefit more from having BF and ES in addition to regular PFMT in the preoperative phase. Furthermore, no data are currently available regarding the possible benefit of using wireless BF. This would allow patients and therapists to use this device in more functional circumstances. Some studies described a limited number of treatments. However, only one study investigated the effect of a more intensive treatment regarding continence outcomes. Milios et al. (2019) found a beneficial effect of 120 contractions a day against only 30 contractions a day in the control group. The instruction was formulated as follows: 'Stop the flow of urine and shorten the penis while continuing to breathe'. Only one study focused on the gain in pelvic floor muscle strength and endurance (Zachovajeviene et al., 2019). As a result, endurance increased more after DMT than after PFMT; strength, on the contrary, improved significantly more after PFMT than after DMT. A possible explication for this could be that during DMT, the pubococcygeus muscle ensures postural control of the pelvic floor. As a result, concentric contraction of this muscle causes ascension and descension during the eccentric contraction. This could be the reason DMT had a significantly higher impact on PFMEs compared to PFMT. However, no differences were seen regarding the effect on the UI level.

Nevertheless, pelvic floor muscle maximal strength correlated better with UI than endurance.

Many hypotheses were not investigated or were poorly investigated, and as a result, conclusions on male incontinence after prostatectomy are limited. The effect of lifestyle changes such as weight loss, smoking cessation, adequate fluid intake and regular bowel movements on incontinence after prostatectomy remain undetermined, as no trial involved these interventions. Other questions are the competence level of the physical therapist, the (intensity of the) programme of training, the motivation and the adherence to the programme of the patient. No studies were found to investigate these questions.

Summary and Clinical Recommendations

The value of PFMT for the treatment of incontinence after prostatectomy remains inconclusive. There may be some benefit to offering PFMT preoperatively or PFMT immediately after catheter withdrawal after prostatectomy. The therapy is non-invasive and avoids the side effects that can occur with medical or surgical treatments. There is no consensus on the efficacy of information on PFMT in comparison with effective treatment. The efficacy of additional BF training has not been proved. Similarly, some studies have shown a positive effect in adding ES, extracorporeal magnetic stimulation or general exercises, without drawing definite conclusions on this matter. Finally, a more intensive therapy seems to offer the best results.

TERMINAL AND POST-VOID DRIBBLE

A prolonged final part of micturition when the flow has slowed to a dribble is a troublesome and common problem in older men. In an Australian survey, 12% of older men reported frequent terminal dribble (Sladden et al., 2000), mostly associated with obstruction of the urethra. Post-voiding dribble is the involuntary loss of urine, usually after leaving the toilet (D'Ancona et al., 2019). Some authors suggested that the condition is caused by pooling of urine in the bulbar urethra for unknown reasons (Denning, 1996; Millard, 1989) or because of failure of the bulbocavernosus muscle to empty the urethra (Dorey et al., 2002; Dorey, 2008). A small group of patients reported post-micturition dribble in the early postoperative period after prostatectomy because of urethral dysfunction (Wille et al., 2000). A decreased or absent post-void urethral milking results in residual unexpelled urine in the bulbar urethra (Wille et al., 2000).

Bulbar urethral massage, with the finger behind the scrotum and moving in a forward and upward direction to evacuate the remaining urine from the urethra, is not perceived as the optimal long-term treatment strategy by many men. PFMT can eliminate the urine left in the bulbar urethra after voiding and provide men with a more acceptable option for management (Dorey et al., 2004; Paterson et al., 1997).

Evidence for Effect of Pelvic Floor Muscle Training for Treatment of Post-Micturition Dribble

A systematic review of treatment of post-micturition dribble in males was done by Dorey (2008). The

effectiveness of a physical therapy approach for terminal and post-micturition dribble is only investigated in three randomized controlled studies (Dorey et al., 2004; Paterson et al., 1997; Porru et al., 2001). One study (Paterson et al., 1997) recruited participants with pure post-micturition dribble without history of surgery of bladder, prostate or urethra nor a history of urgency or stress incontinence. Two other studies investigated the efficacy of PFMEs after TURP on post-micturition dribble (Porru et al., 2001; Dorey et al., 2004) (Table 11.2.3). One study investigated post-micturition dribble in patients with erectile dysfunction (Dorey et al., 2004). The methodological quality of all identified studies concerning post-micturition dribble based on PEDro was rather low and ranged between 3 and 6 out of 10 (Table 11.2.4).

Paterson et al. (1997) compared PFMT and bulbar urethral massage with only counselling on drinking and toileting. Assessment was done by a pad test of less than 4 hours stored in two sealed plastic bags over 72 hours, and improvement in pad weight gain was measured. The best results were obtained by PFMT, eliminating an average of 4.9 g of urine, whereas the effect of urethral massage was 2.9 g. The counselling group showed no improvement. The outcome measure was significantly influenced by the degree of urine loss at the start of the study; if the initial urine loss was too small, then it would not be possible to detect a treatment effect.

Porru et al. (2001) investigated the efficacy of PFMT after TURP for 4 weeks. The control group was only given information about PFMT before and after surgery. This study has already been discussed in the preceding section on post-prostatectomy. A significant difference for post-micturition dribble was found in favour of the experimental group at 1, 2 and 3 weeks after surgery. For that reason, early PFMT should be considered in alleviating the problem of post-micturition dribble after TURP.

Dorey et al. (2004) concluded that PFMT including a post-void 'squeeze out' pelvic floor muscle contraction is an effective treatment for post-micturition dribble in males with erectile dysfunction.

Summary and Clinical Recommendations

The evaluation of the efficacy of physical therapy for men with post-void dribble was hampered by the paucity and the methodological quality of published reports in the field. At the present time we can consider that PFMT is effective for post-micturition dribble based on three studies reporting positive results of PFMT in

TABLE 11.2.3 Randomized Controlled Studies of Physical Therapy for Incontinence for Terminal and Post-Micturition Dribble

Author	Dorey et al., 2004
Design	E: PFMT including a strong post-void 'squeeze out' pelvic floor muscle contraction, BF, suggestions for lifestyle changes
	C: suggestions for lifestyle changes
Sample size	55 men (E = 28, C = 27)
Diagnosis	Interview, digital anal measurements, anal manometric measurements
Training protocol	E: education of the anatomy of the pelvic floor, PFMT with BF + post-void 'squeeze out' pelvic floor muscle contraction. Five 30-minute periods in consecutive weeks. Advice on lifestyle changes and a list of home exercises
	C: advice on lifestyle changes only in five 30-minute periods in consecutive weeks. These men were offered to cross over to the intervention group at 3 months
Drop-out	13.9%
Results	36 (65.5%) of 55 subjects reported post-micturition dribble (PMD) at baseline. At 3 months, there was significant reduction in PMD after intervention compared to C. In both groups combined after 3 months of PFMT, 75% became asymptomatic, 8.3% improved and 2.8% still reported PMD
Author	**Paterson et al., 1997**
Design	E[1]: PFMT
	E[2]: urethral milking by bulbar massage
	C: counselling about drinking and toileting, relaxation therapy
Sample size	49 men (E[1] = 14, E[2] = 15, C = 15)
Diagnosis	Pad-test, pelvic muscle strength by Oxford Grading System from 0 to 4, bladder chart
Training protocol	E[1]: PFMT for 12 weeks with control at 5, 7, 13 weeks
	Home exercises: 5 contractions of 1 s, contractions of endurance gradually extending the number of repetitions, spread exercise sessions throughout the day in lying, sitting and standing position
	E[2]: urethral milking by bulbar massage
	C: counselling about drinking and toileting, relaxation therapy
Drop-out	12%
Results	Significant difference in incontinence between E[1] and C group for pad test, significant difference in incontinence between E[2] and C group for pad test
Author	**Porru et al., 2001**
Design	E: PFMT + BF
	C: preoperative information about PFMT
Sample size	58 men after TURP (E = 30, C = 28)
Diagnosis	Voiding diary
Training protocol	E: 4 treatments postoperatively 1×/week PFMT + home exercises
	C: information (written and verbal information) postoperatively + same home exercises
	Home: 15 contractions on strength and endurance, 3×/day
Drop-out	3/58 (5%)
Results	Post-micturition dribble significant difference between E and C group

For abbreviations, see text

comparison with information only. Bulbar massage can give an additional effect to PFMT for post-micturition dribble, as shown in one study.

CONCLUSION

Many male patients with incontinence and lower urinary tract symptoms are referred for physical therapy based on the results of pelvic physical therapy in women. Despite the high number of referrals, evidence for physical therapy in males is focused only on incontinence after prostatectomy and post-void dribble. Physical therapy is a non-invasive treatment modality, and adverse effects or complications of physical therapy are rare in contrast to pharmacological treatment and surgery (Glazener et al., 2011).

TABLE 11.2.4   PEDro Quality Score of Randomized Controlled Trials in Systematic Review of Physical Therapy for Post-Micturition Dribble

E – Eligibility criteria specified
1 – Subjects randomly allocated to groups
2 – Allocation concealed
3 – Groups similar at baseline
4 – Subjects blinded
5 – Therapist administering treatment blinded
6 – Assessors blinded
7 – Measures of key outcomes obtained from > 85% of subjects
8 – Data analysed by intention to treat
9 – Statistical comparison between groups conducted
10 – Point measures and measures of variability provided

Study	E	1	2	3	4	5	6	7	8	9	10	Total score
Dorey, 2004	–	+	+	+	–	–	+	+	–	–	+	6
Paterson, 1997	+	+	–	–	–	–	+	+	–	+	+	5
Porru, 2001	+	+	–	+	–	–	+	+	–	+	+	6

+, Criterion is clearly satisfied; –, criterion is not satisfied. Total score is determined by counting the number of criteria that are satisfied, except that 'eligibility criteria specified' score is not used to generate the total score. Total scores are out of 10.

Concerning incontinence and physical therapy after TURP, conclusions are limited because of the lack of a sufficient number of studies. However, two studies described a positive effect on incontinence when patients were treated with PFMT over 3 months postoperatively (Anan et al., 2020; Hou et al., 2013).

Concerning physical therapy after radical prostatectomy, there was quite some evidence (7 of 10 trials) that PFMT was significantly more effective than no treatment or sham treatment preoperatively or in the immediate postoperative period. Regarding the need of preoperative training added to postoperative PFMT before radical prostatectomy/HoLEP, 6 of 9 studies indicated a positive effect, although several studies were rather small. Only offering preoperative PFMT without postoperative treatment to patients after radical prostatectomy had no added value over preoperative information. A treatment programme of additional BF-enhanced PFMT did not affect continence after radical prostatectomy. Conclusions on the efficacy of information on PFMT in comparison with guided PFMT or the efficacy of ES cannot be drawn because of the heterogeneity of the studies. Adding general exercises or Pilates (with specific attention towards the pelvic floor muscles) to PFMT could, however, enhance continence results.

For post-micturition dribble, physical therapy is effective, as shown in three studies. All reported the positive results of PFMT in comparison with bulbar massage, lifestyle changes or no treatment.

Due to heterogeneity of available studies, the current knowledge on the biological rationale and effects of physical therapy for UI and lower urinary tract dysfunction is increasing but remains limited. Considering the absence of side effects, the low costs and risks, pelvic floor re-education as an option in alleviating the problem of incontinence after prostatectomy remains debated. Future high-quality research is required to determine at what time and which men are most likely to benefit from which treatment modality of physical therapy.

REFERENCES

Aboseif, S. R., Konety, B., Schmidt, R. A., et al. (1994). Preoperative urodynamic evaluation: Does it predict the degree of urinary continence after radical retropubic prostatectomy? *Urologia Internationalis, 53*, 68–73.

Abrams, P., Cardozo, L., Fall, M., et al. (2003). The standardisation of terminology in lower urinary function: Report from the standardisation sub-committee of the International continence society. *Urology, 61*(1), 37–49.

Ahmed, M. T., Mohammed, A. H., Amansour, A., et al. (2012). Effect of pelvic floor electrical stimulation and biofeedback on the recovery of urinary continence after radical prostatectomy. *Turkish Journal of Physical Medicine and Rehabilitation, 58*, 170–176.

Anan, G., Kaiho, Y., Iwamura, H., et al. (2020). Preoperative pelvic floor muscle exercise for early continence after holmium laser enucleation of the prostate: A randomized controlled study. *BMC Urology, 20*, 3–9.

Anderson, C. A., Omar, M. I., Campbell, S. E., et al. (2015). Conservative management for postprostatectomy urinary incontinence. *Cochrane Database of Systematic Reviews 20*, CD001843.

Au, D., Matthew, A. G., Alibhai, S. M. H., et al. (2020). Pfilates and hypopressives for the treatment of urinary incontinence after radical prostatectomy: Results of a feasibility randomized controlled trial. *Pharmacy Management R, 12*, 55–63.

Aydin Sayilan, A., & Ozbas, A. (2018). The effect of pelvic floor muscle training on incontinence problems after radical prostatectomy. *American Journal of Men's Health, 12*, 1007–1015.

Bader, P., Hugonnet, C. L., Burkhard, F. C., et al. (2001). Inefficient urethral milking secondary to urethral dysfunction as an additional risk factor for incontinence after radical prostatectomy. *Journal of Urology, 166*, 2247–2252.

Baert, L., Elgamal, A. A., & Van Poppel, H. (1996). Complications of radical prostatectomy. In Z. Petrovich, L. Baert, & L. W. Brady (Eds.), *Carcinoma of the prostate* (pp. 139–156). Berlin: Springer Verlag.

Bales, G. T., Gerber, G. S., Minor, T. X., et al. (2000). Effect of preoperative biofeedback/pelvic floor training on continence in men undergoing radical prostatectomy. *Urology, 56*, 627–630.

Barry, M. J., Fowler, F. J., O'Leary, M. P., et al. (1992). The American urological association symptom index for benign prostatic hyperplasia. The measurement committee of the American urological association. *Journal of Urology, 148*, 1549–1557.

Berghmans, B., van Waalwijk van Doorn, E., Nieman, F., et al. (2002). Efficacy of physical therapeutic modalities in women with proven bladder overactivity. *European Urology, 4*, 581–587.

Berghmans, L. C., Hendriks, H. J., Bo, K., et al. (1998). Conservative treatment of stress urinary incontinence in women: A systematic review of randomised clinical trials. *British Journal of Urology, 82*(2), 181–191.

Bishoff, J. T., Motley, G., Optenberg, S. A., et al. (1998). Incidence of fecal and urinary incontinence following radical perineal and retropubic prostatectomy in a national population. *Journal of Urology, 160*(2), 454–458.

Boccon-Gibod, L. (1997). Urinary incontinence after radical prostatectomy. *European Urology, 6*, 112–116.

Braslis, K. G., Santa-Cruz, C., Brickman, A. L., et al. (1995). Quality of life 12 months after radical prostatectomy. *British Journal of Urology, 75*, 48–53.

Burgio, K. L., Goode, P. S., Urban, D. A., et al. (2006). Preoperative biofeedback assisted behavioral training to decrease post-prostatectomy incontinence: A randomized, controlled trial. *Journal of Urology, 175*(1), 196–201.

Burgio, K. L., Stutzman, R. E., & Engel, B. T. (1989). Behavioral training for post-prostatectomy urinary incontinence. *Journal of Urology, 141*, 303–306.

Cao, L., Yang, Z., Qi, L., et al. (2019). Robot-assisted and laparoscopic vs open radical prostatectomy in clinically localized prostate cancer: Perioperative, functional, and oncological outcomes. A systematic review and meta-analysis. *Medicine, 98*, 22.

Campbell, S. E., Glazener, C. M., Hunter, K. F., et al. (2012). Conservative management for postprostatectomy urinary incontinence. *Cochrane Database of Systematic Reviews 1*, CD001843.

Carlsson, S., Jäderling, F., Wallerstedt, A., et al. (2016). Oncologic and functional outcomes one year after radical prostatectomy for very low risk prostate cancer. Results from the prospective LAPPRO trial. *BJU International, 118*, 205–212.

Centemero, A., Rigatti, L., Giraudo, D., et al. (2010). Preoperative pelvic floor muscle exercise for early continence after radical prostatectomy: A randomised controlled study. *European Urology, 57*(6), 1039–1044.

Ceresoli, A., Zanetti, G., Trinchieri, A., et al. (1995). Stress urinary incontinence after perineal radical prostatectomy [in Italian]. *Archivio Italiano di Urologia, Andrologia, 67*, 207–210.

Chang, P. L., Tsai, T. H., Huang, S. T., et al. (1998). The early effect of pelvic floor muscle exercise after transurethral prostatectomy. *Journal of Urology, 160*, 402–405.

Coehlo, R., Rocco, B., Patel, H. R. H., et al. (2010). Retropubic, laparoscopic, and robot-assisted radical prostatectomy: A critical review of outcomes reported by high-volume centers. *Journal of Endourology, 24*(12), 2003–2015.

Cohen, D., Gonzalez, J., & Goldstein, I. (2016). The role of pelvic floor muscles in male sexual dysfunction and pelvic pain. *The Journal of Sexual Medicine, 4*, 53–62.

Cornu, J. N., Ahyai, S., Bachmann, A., et al. (2015). A systematic review and meta-analysis of functional outcomes and complications following transurethral procedures for lower urinary tract symptoms resulting from benign prostatic obstruction: An update. *European Urology, 67*, 1066–1096.

Coughlin, G. D., Yaxley, J. W., Chambers, S. K., et al. (2018). Robot-assisted laparoscopic prostatectomy versus open radical retropubic prostatectomy: 24-month outcomes from a randomised controlled study. *The Lancet Oncology, 19*, 1051–1060.

D'Ancona, C., Haylen, B., Oelke, M., et al. (2019). The International Continence Society (ICS) report on the terminology for adult male lower urinary tract and pelvic floor symptoms and dysfunction. *Neurourology and Urodynamics, 38*, 433–477.

De Lira, G. H. S., Fornari, A., Cardoso, L. F., et al. (2019). Effects of perioperative pelvic floor muscle training on early recovery of urinary continence and erectile function in men undergoing radical prostatectomy: A randomized clinical trial. *International Brazilian Journal of Urology*, 45, 1196–1203.

Denning, J. (1996). Male urinary incontinence. In C. Norton (Ed.), *Nursing for continence* (2nd ed.) (p. 163). Beaconsfield, UK: Beaconsfield Publishers.

Dijkstra-Eshuis, J., Van den Bos, T. W., Splinter, R., et al. (2015). Effect of preoperative pelvic floor muscle therapy with biofeedback versus standard care on stress urinary incontinence and quality of life in men undergoing laparoscopic radical prostatectomy: A randomized control trial. *Neurourology and Urodynamics*, 34, 144–150.

Diokno, A. C. (1998). Post prostatectomy urinary incontinence. *Ostomy Wound Manage*, 44(6), 54–60.

Donnellan, S. M., Duncan, H. J., MacGregor, R. J., et al. (1997). Prospective assessment of incontinence after radical retropubic prostatectomy: Objective and subjective analysis. *Urology*, 49, 225–230.

Dorey, G. (2000). Male patients with lower urinary tract symptom: Treatment. *British Journal of Nursing*, 9(9), 553–558.

Dorey, G. (2001). *Conservative treatment of male urinary incontinence and erectile dysfunction*. London: Whurr Publishers.

Dorey, G. (2002). Prevalence, aetiology and treatment of post-micturition dribble in men: Literature review. *Physiotherapy*, 88, 225–234.

Dorey, G. (2008). Post-micturition dribble: Aetiology and treatment. *Nursing Times*, 104, 46–47.

Dorey, G., Speakman, M., Feneley, R., et al. (2004). Pelvic floor exercises for treating post-micturition dribble in men with erectile dysfunction: A randomized controlled trial. *Urologic Nursing*, 24(6), 490–497.

Dubbelman, Y., Groen, J., Wildhagen, M., et al. (2010). The recovery of urinary continence after radical retropubic prostatectomy: A randomized trial comparing the effect of physical therapist-guided pelvic floor muscle exercises with guidance by an instruction folder only. *BJU International*, 106, 515–522.

Eastham, J. A., Kattan, M. W., Rogers, E., et al. (1996). Risk factors for urinary incontinence after radical prostatectomy. *Journal of Urology*, 156, 1707–1713.

Ficarra, V., Novara, G., Fracalanza, S., et al. (2009). A prospective, non-randomized trial comparing robot-assisted laparoscopic and retropubic radical prostatectomy in one European institution. *BJU International*, 104, 534–539.

Ficarra, V., Novara, G., Rosen, R. C., et al. (2012). Systematic review and meta-analysis of studies reporting urinary continence recovery after robot-assisted radical prostatectomy. *European Urology*, 62, 405–417.

Filocamo, M. T., Li Marzi, V., Del Popolo, G., et al. (2005). Effectiveness of early pelvic floor rehabilitation treatment for post-prostatectomy incontinence. *European Urology*, 48, 734–738.

Floratos, D. L., Sonke, G. S., Rapidou, C. A., et al. (2002). Biofeedback versus verbal feedback as learning tools for pelvic muscle exercises in the early management of urinary incontinence after radical prostatectomy. *BJU International*, 89, 714–719.

Foote, J., Yun, S., & Leach, G. E. (1991). Postprostatectomy incontinence. Pathophysiology, evaluation and management. *Urology Clinical North American*, 18(2), 229–241.

Fowler, F. J., Barry, M. J., Lu-Yao, G., et al. (1995). Effects of radical prostatectomy for prostate cancer on patient quality of life: Results from a medicare survey. *Urology*, 45, 1007–1014.

Franke, J. J., Gilbert, W. B., Grier, J., et al. (2000). Early post prostatectomy pelvic floor biofeedback. *Journal of Urology*, 163, 191–193.

Geraerts, I., Van Poppel, H., Devoogdt, N., et al. (2013). Influence of preoperative and postoperative pelvic floor muscle training (PFMT) compared with postoperative PFMT on urinary incontinence after radical prostatectomy: A randomized controlled trial. *European Urology*, 64(5), 766–772.

Glazener, C., Boachie, C., Buckley, B., et al. (2011). Urinary incontinence in men after formal one-to-one pelvic-floor muscle training following radical prostatectomy or transurethral resection of the prostate (MAPS): Two parallel randomised controlled trials. *Lancet*, 378, 328–337.

Gomes, C. S., Pedriali, F. R., Urabano, M. R., et al. (2018). The effects of Pilates method on pelvic floor muscle strength in patients with post-prostatectomy urinary incontinence: A randomized clinical trial. *Neurourology and Urodynamics*, 37, 346–353.

Goode, P. S., Burgio, K. L., Johnson, T. M., et al. (2011). Behavioral therapy with or without biofeedback and pelvic floor electrical stimulation for persistent postprostatectomy incontinence: A randomised controlled trial. *JAMA*, 305, 151–159.

Grise, P., & Thurman, S. (2001). Urinary incontinence following treatment of localized prostate cancer. *Cancer Control*, 8(6), 532–539.

Groutz, A., Blaivas, J. G., Chaikin, D. C., et al. (2000). The pathophysiology of post-radical prostatectomy incontinence: A clinical and video urodynamic study. *Journal of Urology*, 163, 1767–1770.

Gudziak, M. R., McGuire, E. J., & Gormley, E. A. (1996). Urodynamic assessment of urethral sphincter function in post-prostatectomy incontinence. *Journal of Urology*, 156, 1131–1135.

Haab, F., Yamaguchi, R., & Leach, G. E. (1996). Postprostatectomy incontinence. *Urology Clinical North American*, 23, 447–457.

Haglind, E., Carlsson, S., Stranne, J., et al. (2015). Urinary incontinence and erectile dysfunction after robotic versus open radical prostatectomy: A prospective, controlled, non-randomised trial. *European Urology*, 68, 216–225.

Hald, T., Nordling, J., Andersen, J. T., et al. (1991). A patient weighted symptom score system in the evaluation of uncomplicated benign prostatic hyperplasia. *Scandinavian Journal of Urology & Nephrology - Supplementum, 138*, 59–62.

Herr, H. W. (1994). Quality of life of incontinent men after radical prostatectomy. *Journal of Urology, 151*, 652–654.

Heydenreich, M., Puta, C., Gabriel, H. H., et al. (2020). Does trunk muscle training with an oscillating rod improve urinary incontinence after radical prostatectomy? A prospective randomized controlled trial. *Clinical Rehabilitation, 34*, 320–333.

Holze, S., Mende, M., Healy, K. V., et al. (2019). Comparison of various continence definitions in a large group of patients undergoing radical prostatectomy: A multicenter, prospective study. *BMC Urology, 19*, 70.

Hou, C. P., Chen, T. Y., Chang, C. C., et al. (2013). Use of the SF-36 quality of life scale to assess the effect of pelvic floor muscle exercise on aging males who received transurethral prostate surgery. *Clinical Interventions in Aging, 8*, 667–673.

Hoyland, K., Vasdev, N., Abrof, A., et al. (2014). Post-radical prostatectomy incontinence: Etiology and prevention. *Reviews in Urology, 16*, 181–188.

Hunter, K. F., Moore, K. N., Cody, D. J., et al. (2004). Conservative management for post prostatectomy urinary incontinence. *Cochrane Database of Systematic Reviews* 2, CD001843.

Hunter, K. F., Moore, K. N., Cody, D. J., et al. (2007). Conservative management for post prostatectomy urinary incontinence. *Cochrane Database of Systematic Reviews* 1, CD001843.

Ip, V. (2004). Evaluation of a patient education tool to reduce the incidence of incontinence post-prostate surgery. *Urologic Nursing, 24*(5), 401–407.

Jalalinia, S. F., Raei, M., Naseri-Alahshour, V., et al. (2020). The effect of pelvic floor muscle strengthening exercise on urinary incontinence and quality of life in patients after prostatectomy: A randomized clinical trial. *Journal of Caring Sciences, 9*, 33–38.

Jezernik, S., Craggs, M., Grill, W. M., et al. (2002). Electrical stimulation for the treatment of bladder dysfunction: Current status and future possibilities. *Neurological Research, 24*, 5.

Joseph, A. C., & Chang, M. K. (2000). Comparison of behavior therapy methods for urinary incontinence following prostate surgery: a pilot study. *Urol Nurs, 20*(3), 203–204.

Joseph, J. V., Rosenbaum, R., Madeb, R., et al. (2006). Robotic extraperitoneal radical prostatectomy: An alternative approach. *Journal of Urology, 175*, 945–951.

Ko, Y. W. F., & Sawatzky, J. A. (2008). Understanding urinary incontinence after radical prostatectomy: A nursing framework. *Clinical Journal of Oncology Nursing, 12*, 647–654.

Kongtragul, J., Tukhanon, W., Tudpudsa, P., et al. (2014). Effect of adding concentration therapy to Kegel exercise to improve continence after radical prostatectomy, randomized control. *Medical Journal of the Medical Association of Thailand, 97*, 513–517.

Laurienzo, C. E., Magnabosco, W. J., Jabur, F., et al. (2018). Pelvic floor muscle training and electrical stimulation as rehabilitation after radical prostatectomy: A randomized controlled trial. *Journal of Physical Therapy Science, 30*, 825–831.

Laurienzo, C. E., Sacomani, C. A., Rodrigues, T. R., et al. (2013). Results of preoperative electrical stimulation of pelvic floor muscles in the continence status following radical retropubic prostatectomy. *International Brazilian Journal of Urology, 39*, 182–188.

Laycock, J. (1994). Clinical evaluation of the pelvic floor. In B. Schüssler, J. Laycock, P. Norton, et al. (Eds.), *Pelvic floor Re-education* (pp. 42–48). London: Springer Verlag.

Lourenco, T., Armstrong, N., Nabi, G., et al. (2008). Systematic review and economic modelling of effectiveness and cost utility of surgical treatments for men with benign prostatic enlargement (BPE). *Health Technology Assessment, 12*(35) ix–x, 1–146, 169–515.

Lucas, M. G., Bosch, J. L. H. R., Cruz, F. R., et al. (2012). EAU guidelines on assessment and nonsurgical management of urinary incontinence. *European Urology, 62*(6), 1130–1142.

Manassero, F., Traversi, C., Ales, V., et al. (2007). Contribution of early intensive prolonged pelvic floor exercises on urinary continence recovery after bladder neck-sparing radical prostatectomy: Results of a prospective controlled randomized trial. *Neurourology and Urodynamics, 26*, 985–989.

Marchiori, D., Bertaccini, A., Manferrari, F., et al. (2010). Pelvic floor rehabilitation for continence recovery after radical prostatectomy: Role of a personal training re-educational program. *Anticancer Research, 30*, 553–556.

Mariotti, G., Sciarra, A., Gentilucci, A., et al. (2009). Early recovery of urinary continence after radical prostatectomy using early pelvic floor electrical stimulation and biofeedback associated treatment. *Journal of Urology, 181*, 1788–1793.

Mathewson-Chapman, M. (1997). Pelvic floor exercise/biofeedback for urinary incontinence after prostatectomy. *Journal of Cancer Education, 12*, 218–223.

Meaglia, J. P., Joseph, A. C., Chang, M., et al. (1990). Post-prostatectomy urinary incontinence: Response to behavioral training. *Journal of Urology, 144*, 674–676.

Menon, M., Shrivastava, A., & Kaul, S. (2007). Vattikuti Institute prostatectomy: Contemporary technique and analysis of results. *European Urology, 51*, 648–657.

Milios, J. E., Ackland, T. R., & Green, D. J. (2019). Pelvic floor muscle training in radical prostatectomy: A randomized controlled trial of the impacts on pelvic floor muscle function and urinary incontinence. *BMC Urology, 19*, 116–126.

Millard, R. J. (1989). After dribble. In *Bladder control: A simple self-help guide* (pp. 89–90). Sydney, Australia: William & Wilkins.

Milsom, I., Altman, D., Lapitan, M. C., et al. (2009). Epidemiology of urinary (UI) and faecal (FI) incontinence and pelvic organ prolapse (POP). In P. Abrams, L. Cardozo, S. Khoury, et al. (Eds.), *Fourth international consultation on incontinence. Recommendations of the international scientific committee: Evaluation and treatment of urinary incontinence, pelvic organ prolapse and faecal incontinence* (pp. 35–111). Paris: Health Publication/Editions 21.

Moore, K. N., Cody, D. J., & Glazener, C. M. A. (2001). *Conservative management for post prostatectomy urinary incontinence. The Cochrane Database of Systematic Reviews,* (2), CD 001843.

Moore, K. N., Griffiths, D., & Hughton, A. (1999). Urinary incontinence after radical prostatectomy: A randomised controlled trial comparing pelvic muscle exercises with or without electrical stimulation. *BJU International, 83,* 57–65.

Moore, K. N., Valiquette, L., Chetner, M. P., et al. (2008). Return to continence after radical retropubic prostatectomy: A randomized trial of verbal and written instructions versus therapist-directed pelvic floor muscle therapy. *Urology, 72,* 1280–1286.

Mottet, N., Bellmunt, J., Bolla, M., et al. (2017). EAU-ESTRO-SIOG guidelines on prostate cancer. Part 1: Screening, diagnosis, and local treatment with curative intent. *European Urology, 71,* 618–629.

Moul, J. W. (1998). Pelvic muscle rehabilitation in males following prostatectomy. *Urologic Nursing, 18,* 296–300.

Myers, R. P. (1995). Radical retropubic prostatectomy: Balance between preserving urinary continence and achievement of negative margins. *European Urology, 27,* 32–33.

Nambiar, A. K., Bosch, R., Cruz, F., et al. (2018). EAU guidelines on assessment and nonsurgical management of urinary incontinence. *European Urology, 73,* 596–609.

National Institute for Health and Care Excellence. (2019). *Urinary incontinence and pelvic organ prolapse in women: Management.* London: National Institute for Health and Care Excellence.

Nilssen, S. R., Mørkved, S., Overgard, M., et al. (2012). Does physical therapist–guided pelvic floor muscle training increase the quality of life in patients after radical prostatectomy? A randomized clinical study. *Scandinavian Journal of Urology and Nephrology, 46,* 397–404.

Ocampo-Trujillo, A., Carbonell-Gonzalez, J., Martinez-Blanco, A., et al. (2014). Pre-operative training induces changes in histomorphometry and muscle function of the pelvic floor in patients with indication of radical prostatectomy. *Actas Urológicas Españolas, 38,* 378–384.

Oh, J. J., Kim, J. K., Lee, H., et al. (2020). Effect of personalized extracorporeal biofeedback device for pelvic floor muscle training on urinary incontinence after robot-assisted radical prostatectomy: A randomized controlled trial. *Neurourology and Urodynamics, 39,* 674–681.

Ong, W. L., Evans, S. M., Spelman, T., et al. (2016). Comparison of oncological and health-related quality of life outcomes between open and robot-assisted radical prostatectomy for localised prostate cancer—findings from the population-based Victorian Prostate Cancer Registry. *BJU International, 118,* 563–569.

Overgard, M., Angelsen, A., Lydersen, S., et al. (2008). Does physical therapist–guided pelvic floor muscle training reduce urinary incontinence after radical prostatectomy? A randomised controlled trial. *European Urology, 54,* 438–448.

Parekh, A. R., Feng, M. I., Kirages, D., et al. (2003). The role of pelvic floor exercises on post-prostatectomy incontinence. *Journal of Urology, 170,* 130–133.

Park, S. W., Kim, T. N., Nam, J. K., et al. (2012). Recovery of overall exercise ability, quality of life, and continence after 12-week combined exercise intervention in elderly patients who underwent radical prostatectomy: A randomized controlled study. *Urology, 80,* 299–305.

Paterson, J., Pinnock, C. B., & Marshall, V. R. (1997). Pelvic floor exercises as a treatment for post-micturition dribble. *British Journal of Urology, 79,* 892–897.

Pedriali, F. R., Gomes, C. S., Soares, L., et al. (2016). Is Pilates as effective as conventional pelvic floor muscle exercises in the conservative treatment of post-prostatectomy urinary incontinence? A randomised controlled trial. *Neurourology and Urodynamics, 35,* 615–621.

Peyromaure, M., Ravery, V., & Boccon-Gibod, L. (2002). The management of stress urinary incontinence after radical prostatectomy. *BJU International, 90,* 155–161.

Poon, M., Ruckle, H., Bamshad, B. R., et al. (2000). Radical retropubic prostatectomy: Bladder neck preservation versus reconstruction. *Journal of Urology, 163*(1), 194–198.

Porru, D., Campus, G., Caria, A., et al. (2001). Impact of early pelvic floor rehabilitation after transurethral resection of the prostate. *Neurourology and Urodynamics, 20,* 53–59.

Ribeiro, L. H., Prota, C., Gomes, C. M., et al. (2010). Long-term effect of early postoperative pelvic floor biofeedback on continence in men undergoing radical prostatectomy: A prospective, randomized, controlled trial. *Journal of Urology, 184,* 1034–1039.

Robinson, J. P., Bradway, C. W., Nuamah, I., et al. (2008). Systematic pelvic floor training for lower urinary tract symptoms post-prostatectomy: A randomized clinical trial. *International Journal of Urological Nursing, 2*(1), 3–13.

Santos, N. A., Saintrain, M. V., Regadas, R. P., et al. (2017). Assessment of physical therapy strategies for recovery of urinary continence after prostatectomy. *Asian Pacific Journal of Cancer Prevention, 18,* 81–86.

Seo, H. J., Na, R. L., Soo, K. S., et al. (2016). Comparison of robot-assisted radical prostatectomy and open radical prostatectomy outcomes: A systematic review and meta-analysis. *Yonsei Medical Journal, 57,* 1165–1177.

Sladden, M. J., Hughes, A. M., Hirst, G. H., et al. (2000). A community study of lower urinary tract symptoms in older men in Sydney, Australia. *Australian and New Zealand Journal of Surgery, 70,* 322–328.

Sueppel, C., Kreder, K., & See, W. (2001). Improved continence outcomes with preoperative pelvic floor muscle exercises. *Urologic Nursing, 21,* 201–210.

Tantawy, S. A., Elgohary, H. M. I., Abdelbasset, W. K., et al. (2019). Assessment of physical therapy strategies for recovery of urinary continence after prostatectomy. *Physiotherapy, 105,* 338–345.

Tewari, A., Srivasatava, A., Menon, M., et al. (2003). A prospective comparison of radical retropubic and robot-assisted prostatectomy: Experience in one institution. *BJU International, 92,* 205–210.

Tibaek, S., Klarskov, P., Lund Hansen, B., et al. (2007). Pelvic floor muscle training before transurethral resection of the prostate: A randomized, controlled, blinded study. *Scandinavian Journal of Urology and Nephrology, 41,* 329–334.

Tienforti, D., Sacco, E., Marangi, F., et al. (2012). Efficacy of an assisted low-intensity programme of perioperative pelvic floor muscle training in improving the recovery of continence after radical prostatectomy: A randomized controlled trial. *BJU International, 110,* 1004–1010.

Tienza, A., Robles, J. E., Hevia, M., et al. (2018). Prevalence analysis of urinary incontinence after radical prostatectomy and influential preoperative factors in a single institution. *The Aging Male, 21,* 24–30.

Van Kampen, M., De Weerdt, W., Van Poppel, H., et al. (1997). Urinary incontinence following transurethral, transvesical and radical prostatectomy. Retrospective study of 489 patients. *Acta Urologica Belgica, 65,* 1–7.

Van Kampen, M., De Weerdt, W., Van Poppel, H., et al. (1998). Prediction of urinary incontinence following radical prostatectomy. *Urologia Internationalis, 60,* 80–84.

Van Kampen, M., De Weerdt, W., Van Poppel, H., et al. (2000). Effect of pelvic-floor re-education on duration

and degree of incontinence after radical prostatectomy: A randomised controlled trial. *Lancet, 355,* 98–102.

Walsh, P. C., Partin, A. W., & Epstein, J. I. (1994). Cancer control and quality of life following anatomical radical retropubic prostatectomy: Results at 10 years. *Journal of Urology, 152,* 1831–1836.

Wille, S., Mills, R. D., & Studer, U. E. (2000). Absence of urethral post-void milking: An additional cause of incontinence after radical prostatectomy? *European Urology, 37*(6), 665–669.

Wille, S., Sobotta, A., Heidenrich, A., et al. (2003). Pelvic floor exercises, electrical stimulation and biofeedback after radical prostatectomy: Results of a prospective randomized trial. *Journal of Urology, 170,* 490–493.

Yamanishi, T., Mizuno, T., Watanabe, M., et al. (2010). Randomized, placebo controlled study of electrical stimulation with pelvic floor muscle training for severe urinary incontinence after radical prostatectomy. *Journal of Urology, 184,* 2007–2012.

Yang, D. Y., & Lee, W. K. (2019). A current perspective on post-micturition dribble in males. *Investigative and Clinical Urology, 60,* 142–147.

Yokoyama, T., Nishiguchi, J., Watanabe, T., et al. (2004). Comparative study of effects of extracorporeal magnetic innervation versus electrical stimulation for urinary incontinence after radical prostatectomy. *Urology, 63,* 264–267.

Zachovajeviene, B., Siupsinskas, L., Zachovajevas, P., et al. (2019). Effect of diaphragm and abdominal muscle training on pelvic floor strength and endurance: Results of a prospective randomized trial. *Scientific Reports, 9,* 19192–19202.

Zaidan, P., & Bezerra da Silva, E. (2016). Pelvic floor muscle exercises with or without electric stimulation and post-prostectomy urinary incontinence: A systematic review. *Fisioter Movement Curitiba, 29,* 635–649.

Zhang, A. Y., Strauss, G. J., Siminoff, L. A., et al. (2007). Effects of combined pelvic floor muscle exercise and a support group on urinary incontinence and quality of life of post-prostatectomy patients. *Oncology Nursing Forum, 34,* 47–53.

11.3 Pelvic Floor Muscle Training and Male Sexual Dysfunction

Marijke Van Kampen, Inge Geraerts and Anne Asnong

INTRODUCTION

This chapter provides a summary of the current evidence for the physiotherapeutic treatment of erectile dysfunction (ED) and premature ejaculation. The *Diagnostic and Statistical Manual of Mental Disorders, Fifth*

Edition (DSM-5) classifies erectile disorder as belonging to a group of sexual dysfunction disorders typically characterized by a clinically significant inability to respond sexually or to experience sexual pleasure. Premature ejaculation is a sexual dysfunction in which ejaculation takes place with minimal sexual stimulation, before, on or shortly after penetration, or simply earlier than desired (American Psychiatric Association, 2013).

The DSM-5 classification categorizes male sexual dysfunction in four items: erectile disorders, male hypoactive sexual desire disorders, premature (early) ejaculation and delayed ejaculation.

The specific DSM-5 criteria for erectile disorder (a) and premature (early) ejaculation (b) are as follows (American Psychiatric Association, 2013):

- In almost all or all (75%–100%) sexual activity, the experience of at least one of the following three symptoms: (1) marked difficulty in obtaining an erection during sexual activity, (2) marked difficulty in maintaining an erection until the completion of sexual activity or (3) marked decrease in erectile rigidity;
- In almost all or all (75%–100%) sexual activity, the experience of a pattern of ejaculation occurring during partnered sexual activity within 1 minute after vaginal penetration and before the individual wishes it;
- (a)+(b) The preceding symptoms have persisted for approximately 6 months;
- (a)+(b) The preceding symptoms cause significant distress to the individual;
- (a)+(b) The dysfunction cannot be better explained by non-sexual mental disorder, a medical condition, the effects of a drug or medication, or severe relationship distress or other significant stressors.

Randomized controlled studies considering physical therapy for men with ED have been published since 1993 (Claes and Baert, 1993; Dorey et al., 2004; Lin et al., 2012; Prota et al., 2012; Nilssen et al., 2012; Geraerts et al., 2016; Carboni et al., 2018; de Lira et al., 2019; Milios et al., 2020). A recent review has described the evidence for physical therapy for erectile disorders and premature ejaculation (Myers and Smith, 2019). Clinical guidelines regarding erectile disorders mostly consist of medicamentous (phosphodiesterase-5 inhibitors [PDE-5-I], testosterone therapy, intra-urethral alprostadil, intra-cavernosal injection) and surgical treatments (penile prosthesis implantation, penile arterial reconstruction, intra-cavernosal stem cell therapy) and psychosexual counseling (Hatzimouratidis, 2016; Burnett et al., 2018; Hackett et al., 2018). With reference to premature ejaculation, clinical guidelines recommend patient counselling/education, pharmacotherapy (recommended as a first-line treatment option in case of lifelong premature ejaculation) and behavioural therapy (Salonia et al., 2020).

According to the literature, physical therapy should have the potential to alleviate some erectile and ejaculation disorders. Nevertheless, the number of studies regarding these symptoms is scarce. The efficacy of pelvic floor muscle training (PFMT) for ED in the general population and after radical prostatectomy is investigated in three (Claes and Baert, 1993; Dorey et al., 2004; Carboni et al., 2018) and six randomized controlled trials (Lin et al., 2012; Nilssen et al., 2012; Prota et al., 2012; Geraerts et al., 2016; de Lira et al., 2019; Milios et al., 2020). The efficacy of low-intensity extracorporeal shockwave treatment (Li-ESWT) for ED is evaluated in 10 randomized controlled trials (Vardi et al., 2012; Yee et al., 2014; Olsen et al., 2015; Srini et al., 2015; Kalyvianakis and Hatzichristou, 2017; Fojecki et al., 2017, 2018; Zewin et al., 2018; Baccaglini et al., 2020; Sramkova et al., 2020). The efficacy of PFMT for premature ejaculation is studied in two trials (Pastore et al., 2012; Jiang et al., 2020).

Finally, we will also briefly discuss climacturia or orgasm-related incontinence at the end of this chapter.

RESEARCH METHODS

The search was updated from the cut-off date of the previous update (July 2015) to June 2020 and included PubMed, the Cochrane Library and PEDro. Only English language articles and randomized controlled trials were considered. No abstracts were included. For ED, 890 articles were identified and screened by two independent reviewers. Data extraction was then carried out for the relevant studies by screening by title (phase I), by abstract (phase II) and by full text (phase III), resulting in 21 articles in total: 9 regarding PFMT for ED (Table 11.3.1), 10 regarding Li-ESWT for ED (Table 11.3.2) and 2 regarding physical therapy for premature ejaculation (Table 11.3.3).

The methodological quality of all identified studies concerning PFMT for ED and premature ejaculation based on PEDro ranged between 3 and 9 out of 10 (Tables 11.3.4 and 11.3.5).

ERECTILE DISORDERS

For a full understanding of the changes in erectile function occurring after radical prostatectomy, a basic knowledge of the anatomy and physiology of erection is essential (Fig. 11.3.1). Erection is a complex neurovascular phenomenon under hormonal control. The penis

Text continued on page 578

TABLE 11.3.1	Randomized Controlled Studies of Physical Therapy for Erectile Dysfunction
Author	**Carboni et al. (2018)**
Design	E group: ES
	C group: placebo ES
Sample size	22 men with known ED (IIEF-5 score <22) (E: 11, C: 11)
Diagnosis	IIEF, EHS, WHOQOL-BREF at 4 weeks after start/treatment
Training protocol	E group: functional ES (50 Hz, 500 μs), intensity lower than motor threshold, 15 min 2×/week for 4 weeks
	C group: placebo functional ES, same routine
Drop-out	0
Results	IIEF, EHS and WHOQOL-BREF scores (except for environment) showed significant differences between E and C groups
	In the E group, all scores (except for the environment domain of WHOQOL-BREF) showed significant differences pre- and post-treatment; in the C group, only psychological and personal relationship domains of WHOQOL-BREF improved
Author	**Claes and Baert (1993)**
Design	E group: surgery of deep dorsal vein
	C group: PFMT
Sample size	150 men with venogenic ED (E: 72, C: 78)
Diagnosis	Venogenic ED
	Digital anal assessment at baseline, 4 and 12 months; 40 mg of papaverine + needle, electromyography of ischiocavernosus muscle + max pelvic floor muscle contraction
Training protocol	E group: surgery of deep dorsal vein
	C group: 5 weekly PFME + home exercises
Drop-out	Not reported
Results	At 4 months:
	E group: 44 (61%) cured; 17 (23.6%) improved; 11 (15.2%) failed
	C group: 36 (46%) cured; 22 (28%) improved; 20 (25.6%) failed
	At 12 months:
	E group: 30 (42%) cured; 23 (32%) improved
	C group: 33 (42%) cured; 24 (31%) improved; 45 (58%) refused surgery
Author	**De Lira et al. (2019)**
Design	E group: perioperative PFMT
	C group: usual care
Sample size	31 men undergoing open retropubic RP (E: 16, C: 15)
Diagnosis	ICIQ-SF, IIEF-5 at baseline and 3 months after RP
Training protocol	E group: 2 × pre-RP PFMT sessions: exercises, BF, verbal and written instructions to continue PFMT until RP and to resume it after urethral catheter removal (3×/day)
	C group: usual post-RP care
Drop-out	0
Results	3 months post-RP, there was no significant improvement in urinary incontinence or erectile function
Author	**Dorey et al. (2004)**
Design	E group: (home) PFMT + BF + advice on lifestyle changes
	C group: advice on lifestyle changes
Sample size	55 men with ED (E: 28, C: 27)
Diagnosis	IIEF, PIIEF, ED-EQoL, anal manometry at baseline, 3 months and 6 months
Training protocol	E group: patient education, PFME and anal pressure BF, 30 min, 1×/week for 5 weeks, home exercises, lifestyle changes
	C group: 5× weekly lifestyle changes and transfer to active arm at 3 months
Drop-out	5/55 (9%)
Results	The E group significantly improved on the erectile function domain of the IIEF as well as anal pressure at 3 months, and all showed further improvements (the C group was transferred to the active arm after 3 months) at 6 months

Continued

TABLE 11.3.1   Randomized Controlled Studies of Physical Therapy for Erectile Dysfunction—cont'd

Author	**Geraerts et al. (2016)**
Design	E group: (home) PFMT at 12 months
	C group: (home) PFMT at 15 months
Sample size	33 men with ED (E: 16, C: 17), minimum 12 months after RP
Diagnosis	IIEF at 12, 15, 18 and 21 (only C group) months after RP
Training protocol	E group: PFMT (exercises supported with ES for 10 min) starting 12 months postoperatively, 1×/week (first 6 weeks) and 1×/2 weeks (next 6 weeks), for 3 months + home PFMT program (60 contractions/day)
	C group: between 12 and 15 months, no treatment, PFMT starting 15 months postoperatively (analogue to the E group)
Drop-out	3/33 (9%)
Results	At 15 months post-RP, the E group had significantly better erectile function (better hardness, length, tumescence and elevation) than the C group and significantly higher improvement of climacturia (other subdomains of the IIEF were not significant), and the effects were maintained during follow-up (at 18 months)
Author	**Lin et al. (2012)**
Design	E group: PFME after catheter removal post-RP
	C group: PFME at 3 months post-RP
Sample size	72 patients with ED after RP (E: 41, C: 31)
Diagnosis	IIEF at baseline, 3, 6, 9 and 12 months
Training protocol	E group: 3× 10-s strength contractions + 3× 10-s relaxation, 2×/day in 3 positions + PFME DVD + BF at first visit
	C group: same intervention as the E group, starting at 3 months
Drop-out	10/72 (14%)
Results	Significant differences in IIEF scores at 6 and 12 months between the E and C groups; sexual function of the E group was better than that of the C group
Author	**Milios et al. (2020)**
Design	E group: 6 sets of PFME/day in standing position
	C group: 'usual care' (3 sets of PFME/day)
Sample size	101 men undergoing RP (E: 50, C: 47)
Diagnosis	EPIC-CP, IIEF, ultrasound at 2, 6 and 12 weeks after RP
Training protocol	E group: PT-directed PFMT for 2 × 30-min sessions, 5 weeks pre-RP, then daily PFMT programme: 6 sets/day, 10 fast (1-s) + 10 slow (10-s) contractions/set, with equal rest time in a standing position (120 contractions/day in total)
	C group: PT-directed PFMT for 2 × 30-min sessions, 5 weeks pre-RP, then daily PFMT programme: 3 sets/day (in supine/sitting/standing position), 10 contractions/set, 10-s contraction with equal rest time (30 contractions/day in total)
Drop-out	4/101 (0.01%)
Results	At 2, 6 and 12 weeks after RP, no significant group differences regarding EPIC-CP EF score and IIEF-EF score at any of the time points
Author	**Nilssen et al. (2012)**
Design	E group: PT-guided PFMT (in groups or by DVD)
	C group: home training
Sample size	85 men undergoing RP (E: 42, C: 43)
Diagnosis	UCLA-PCI, SF-12 at 6 weeks, 6 months and 12 months
Training protocol	E group: PT-guided PFMT, 45 min, 1×/week, starting immediately after catheter removal for as long as the patient used pads or chose to continue + home programme of 3 × 10 contractions/day (supine, sitting, standing), 6–8 s, 3–4 fast contractions at the end of each contraction (if unable to attend hospital sessions: DVD) + oral and written instructions
	C group: oral and written instructions on postoperative training programme (3 × 10 PFME/day)

TABLE 11.3.1   Randomized Controlled Studies of Physical Therapy for Erectile Dysfunction—cont'd

Drop-out	5/85 (6%)
Results	UCLA-PCI scores for sexual function and SF-12 scores showed a statistically significant effect of time over 12 months in the E and C groups, but no statistically significant difference in HRQoL between the E and C groups was found
Author	**Prota et al. (2012)**
Design	E group: PFMT + BF + home programme C group: verbal instructions to contract the pelvic floor
Sample size	52 men with post-RP ED (E: 26, C: 26)
Diagnosis	IIEF at baseline, 1, 3, 6 and 12 months after catheter removal
Training protocol	E group: starting at 15 days after catheter removal, PFMT + BF for 30 min, 1×/week for 12 weeks + home programme (with verbal + written instructions) C group: verbal instructions to contract the pelvic floor
Drop-out	19/52 (37%) (before treatment/first month of evaluation)
Results	Patients in the E group showed superior results in terms of duration and severity of ED after 12 months, and a strong association was found between potency and urinary continence in the E and C groups

BF, Biofeedback; *ED,* erectile dysfunction; *ED-EQoL,* Erectile Dysfunction-Effect on Quality of Life; *EHS,* Erectile Hardness Scale; *EPIC-CP,* Expanded Prostate Cancer Index Composite for Clinical Practice; *EPIC-CP EF,* Expanded Prostate Cancer Index Composite for Clinical Practice Erectile Function domain; *ES,* electrical stimulation; *ICIQ-SF,* International Consultation on Incontinence Questionnaire - Short Form; *IIEF,* International Index of Erectile Function; *IIEF-EF,* International Index of Erectile Function-Erectile Dysfunction domain; *PFME,* pelvic floor muscle exercise; *PFMT,* pelvic floor muscle training; *PIIEF,* Partner's International Index of Erectile Function; *PT,* physical therapist; *RP,* radical prostatectomy; *SF-12,* Short Form (12) Health Survey; *UCLA-PCI,* University of California at Los Angeles Prostate Cancer Index; *WHOQOL-BREF,* World Health Organization Quality of Life Brief Version.

TABLE 11.3.2   Randomized Controlled Studies of Shockwave Therapy for Erectile Dysfunction

Author	**Baccaglini (2020)**
Design	E group: tadalafil 5 mg/day + 2400 shocks/session (1×/week) C group: tadalafil 5 mg/day
Sample size	77 men after radical prostatectomy (E: 36, C: 41)
Diagnosis	Vasculogenic ED IIEF-5 (≥4-point difference = significant)
Training protocol	E group: tadalafil 5 mg/day + 2400 shocks/session (1×/week), distributed on 4 different penile regions, 8 weeks in total C group: tadalafil 5 mg/day, 8 weeks in total
Drop-out	0
Results	At 8 weeks after catheter withdrawal, no significant difference between the E and C groups
Author	**Fojecki et al. (2017)**
Design	E group: Li-ESWT (1×/week, 5 weeks), 4-week break, Li-ESWT (1×/week, 5 weeks) C group: sham (1×/week, 5 weeks), 4-week break, Li-ESWT (1×/week, 5 weeks)
Sample size	126 men with an IIEF-EF score <25
Diagnosis	IIEF (increase of ≥5 points), EHS (increase to at least score 3), Sexual QoL-men, EDITS at baseline, after 9 and 18 weeks
Training protocol	E group: Li-ESWT (1×/week, 5 weeks), 4-week break, Li-ESWT (1×/week, 5 weeks); 600 shockwaves/session C group: sham (1×/week, 5 weeks, gel pad preventing passage of energy), 4-week break, Li-ESWT (1×/week, 5 weeks)
Drop-out	3% (E: 3, C: 1)
Results	No clinically relevant effect of Li-ESWT in the short term (9 and 18 weeks) found

Continued

TABLE 11.3.2   Randomized Controlled Studies of Shockwave Therapy for Erectile Dysfunction—cont'd

Author	Fojecki et al. (2018)
Design	E group: Li-ESWT (1×/week, 5 weeks), 4-week break, Li-ESWT (1×/week, 5 weeks)
	C group: sham (1×/week, 5 weeks), 4-week break, Li-ESWT (1×/week, 5 weeks)
Sample size	95 men with an IIEF-EF score <25
Diagnosis	IIEF (increase of ≥5 points), EHS (increase to at least a score of 3), Sexual QoL-men, EDITS at baseline, after 6 and 12 months
Training protocol	E group: Li-ESWT (1×/week, 5 weeks), 4-week break, Li-ESWT (1×/week, 5 weeks); 600 shockwaves/session
	C group: sham (1×/week, 5 weeks, gel pad preventing passage of energy), 4-week break, Li-ESWT (1×/week, 5 weeks)
Drop-out	25% (E: 11, C: 20)
Results	No clinically relevant effect of Li-ESWT in the long term (6 and 12 months) found
Author	**Kalyvianakis and Hatzichristou (2017)**
Design	E group: 12 sessions of Li-ESWT
	C group: sham procedure
Sample size	46 men with ED (E: 30, C: 16)
Diagnosis	Penile triplex ultrasonography before and 3 months after treatment
	IIEF-EF minimal clinically important difference at baseline, 1, 3, 6, 9 and 12 months after treatment
Training protocol	E group: 1500 shocks (5 locations) per session of 20 min, 12 sessions (biweekly) at weeks 1, 2, 3, 7, 8 and 9 after washout period
	C group: sham shockwave applicator (that blocked delivery of shockwaves), equal times as the E group
Drop-out	0
Results	IIEF-EF minimal clinically important differences for the E group vs the C group were observed for 57% vs 12% at 1 month, 57% vs 12% at 3 months, 63% vs 19% at 6 months, 67% vs 31% at 9 months and 75% vs 25% at 12 months
Author	**Olsen (2015)**
Design	E group: Li-ESWT (5 sessions/5 weeks)
	C group: placebo (after 10 weeks, also 5 sessions/5 weeks)
Sample size	112 men unable to have intercourse with/without medication
Diagnosis	EHS, IIEF-15 at screening, 5, 12 and 24 weeks after treatment
Training protocol	E group: Li-ESWT (5 sessions/5 weeks, total 3000 impulses, 6 locations/penis)
	C group: placebo (after 10 weeks, also 5 sessions/5 weeks)
Drop-out	7
Results	Significant difference in EHS score at 5 weeks of FU between E and C groups (57% [E] had EHS 3–4 vs 9% [C]); no significant difference between E and C groups in IIEF-EF after week 5.
Author	**Sramkova et al. (2020)**
Design	E group: Li-ESWT, 4 sessions
	C group: placebo, 4 sessions
	After washout period of 4 weeks
Sample size	60 men with mild to severe vasculogenic ED ≥6 months; all patients were at least partial responders to PDI-5-i
Diagnosis	IIEF-5, EHS, SEP2, SEP3, GAQ at baseline, 4 and 12 weeks after treatment
Training protocol	E group: Li-ESWT, tailored treatment (on average 6000 shocks/session (4 sessions)
	C group: placebo, special applicator probe blocking shockwaves (4 sessions)
Drop-out	0
Results	Significant difference between E and C groups regarding quality of erection (IIEF-5 [at 4 and 12 weeks] and EHS [at 12 weeks]); significant increase in EHS (at weeks 4 and 12), at week 12 in GAQ, SEP2, SEP3, patient's and partner's satisfaction

TABLE 11.3.2 Randomized Controlled Studies of Shockwave Therapy for Erectile Dysfunction—cont'd

Author	Srini et al. (2015)
Design	E group: 12 sessions of Li-ESWT C group: placebo ESWT
Sample size	135 men (E: 95, C: 40)
Diagnosis	Vasculogenic ED, EHS, IIEF-EF, CGIC at 1, 3, 6, 9 and 12 months post-treatment
Training protocol	E group: Li-ESWT: 2 sessions/week (3 weeks), 3-week break, 2 sessions/week (3 weeks), 1500 shocks/session C group: placebo/sham ESWT After a 1-month PDE-5-I washout period
Drop-out	35/95 (37%, E), 23/40 (58%, C)
Results	Significant increase in EHS and IIEF-EF from 1 month to 12 months after treatment for the E group compared to the C group; 78% of men at 1 month and 71% of men at 12 months after treatment, who had an initial EHS score ≤2, had an erection hard enough for penetration compared to none in the placebo group
Author	**Vardi et al. (2012)**
Design	E group: Li-ESWT, 12 sessions C group: sham, 12 sessions After a 1-month PDE-5-I washout period
Sample size	67 men (E: 46, C: 21) with an IIEF-EF ≥19 while on PDE-5-I
Diagnosis	IIEF-EF, EHS at 1 month after the final treatment (=FU1)
Training protocol	E group: Li-ESWT, 9 weeks (1500 shocks/session [5 locations], 15 min) (weeks 1–3: 2×/week, weeks 4–6: none, weeks 7–9: 2×/week) C group: sham shockwave applicator (that blocked delivery of shockwaves), equal times as the E group
Drop-out	7 (E: 6, C: 1)
Results	The E group had a significantly higher IIEF-EF score at FU1 than the C group; at FU1, 19 men in the E group, with initial EHS score ≤2, had an erection sufficiently firm for penetration compared to none of the C group
Author	**Yee et al. (2014)**
Design	E group: Li-ESWT, 9 weeks (12 sessions) C group: sham After a 2-week PDE-5-I washout period
Sample size	70 men with ED, SHIM ≤21, ED ≥6 months
Diagnosis	SHIM, IIEF-EF, EHS at 4 weeks after the last treatment
Training protocol	E group: Li-ESWT, 9 weeks (1500 shocks/session [5 locations], 20 min) (weeks 1–3: 2×/week, weeks 4–6: none, weeks 7–9: 2×/week) C group: sham shockwave applicator (that blocked delivery of shockwaves), equal times as the E group After a 2-week PDE-5-I washout period
Drop-out	12 (E: 6, C: 6)
Results	No significant differences between E and C groups at week 13 regarding IIEF-EF and EHS; stratification into SHIM subgroups indicated a significant difference between E and C groups for the severe ED group regarding IIEF-EF
Author	**Zewin et al. (2018)**
Design	E[1] group: Li-ESWT (N = 42) E[2] group: PDE-5-I (N = 43) C group: FU without therapy (N = 43)
Sample size	152 sexually active men after bilateral nerve-sparing radical cystoprostatectomy for muscle invasive bladder cancer

Continued

TABLE 11.3.2   Randomized Controlled Studies of Shockwave Therapy for Erectile Dysfunction—cont'd

Diagnosis	IIEF-15, EHS, penile Doppler ultrasound, before surgery, at 1, 3, 6 and 9 months postoperatively
Training protocol	E^1 group: Li-ESWT, 12 sessions (2×/week for 3 weeks), 3 weeks rest, 2×/week for 3weeks), 1500 shocks/session (5 locations), 15 min/treatment
	E^2 group: PDE-5-I, oral sildenafil (50 mg daily for 6 months)
	C group: FU without therapy
Drop-out	24 (E1: 7, E2: 7, C: 10)
Results	Potency recovery rates at 9 months were 76.2%, 79.1% and 60.5% in E1, E2 and C groups; statistically significant increase in IIEF-EF and EHS scores during all FU periods in all groups, but no significant differences between groups

CGIC, Clinical Global Impression of Change; *ED,* erectile dysfunction; *EDITS,* Erectile Dysfunction Inventory of Treatment Satisfaction; *EHS,* Erectile Hardness Scale; *ESWT,* extracorporeal shockwave treatment; *FU,* follow-up; *GAQ,* Global Assessment Question; *IIEF,* International Index of Erectile Function; *IIEF-EF,* International Index of Erectile Function-Erectile Dysfunction domain; *Li-ESWT,* low-intensity extracorporeal shockwave treatment; *PDE-5-I,* phosphodiesterase-5 inhibitor; *QoL,* quality of life; *SEP2,* Sexual Encounter Profile, Q2: Were you able to insert your penis into your partner's vagina?; *SEP3,* Sexual Encounter Profile, Q3: Did your erection last long enough for you to have successful intercourse?; *SHIM,* Sexual Health Inventory for Men.

TABLE 11.3.3   Randomized Controlled Studies of Physical Therapy for Premature Ejaculation

Author	**Jiang et al. (2020)**
Design	E group: penis-root masturbation
	C group: Kegel exercise
Sample size	44 heterosexual males with primary premature ejaculation (E: 22, C: 22)
Diagnosis	IELT, PEDT
Training protocol	E group: 10–15 min of penis-root masturbation (circular massage of the penis root or along the proximal end, without ejaculation), 3×/week for 3 months
	C group: contraction of pelvic floor muscles for 3–5 s, 3×/day, 50–100 repetitions each time
Drop-out	7/44 (16%)
Results	IELT was significantly longer and PEDT scores were significantly lower in both E and C groups, but the effect was more significant in the E group ($p < 0.05$)
Author	**Pastore et al. (2012)**
Design	E group: PFMT
	C group: 30 or 60 mg of on-demand dapoxetine
Sample size	40 men with lifelong premature ejaculation (E: 19, C: 21)
Diagnosis	IELT
Training protocol	E group: PFMT + electrical stimulation + biofeedback, 3 × 60-min session/week, during which these 3 techniques were applied for 20 min each
	C group: 30 or 60 mg of dapoxetine (random) 1–3 h before sexual intercourse
Drop-out	6/21 (29%) (E: 0, C: 6)
Results	Overall mean IELT increased significantly after 12 weeks in the E and C groups; the increase was significantly greater in the C groups compared with the E group ($p < 0.05$)

IELT, Intra-vaginal ejaculatory latency time; *PEDT,* Premature Ejaculation Diagnostic Tool; *PFMT,* pelvic floor muscle training.

consists of two corpora cavernosa and one corpus spongiosum, surrounding the urethra. These corpora are connected via minuscule blood vessels and surrounded by smooth muscle tissue.

On sexual stimulation, erection is initiated by the parasympathetic part of the autonomic nervous system. Parasympathetic branches extend from the sacral plexus into the arteries supplying the erectile tissue. On sexual stimulation, nerve impulses cause the release of nitric oxide. This in turn results in the conversion of guanosine monophosphate to cyclic guanosine monophospate. The release of cyclic guanosine monophospate results in

TABLE 11.3.4   PEDro Quality Score of Randomized Controlled Trials in Systematic Review of Pelvic Floor Physical Therapy for Erectile Dysfunction

E – Eligibility criteria specified
1 – Subjects randomly allocated to groups
2 – Allocation concealed
3 – Groups similar at baseline
4 – Subjects blinded
5 – Therapist administering treatment blinded
6 – Assessors blinded
7 – Measures of key outcomes obtained from >85% of subjects
8 – Data analysed by intention to treat
9 – Statistical comparison between groups conducted
10 – Point measures and measures of variability provided

Study	E	1	2	3	4	5	6	7	8	9	10	Total Score
Carboni et al. (2018)	−	+	+	+	+	−	+	+	+	+	+	9/10
Claes and Baert (1993)	−	+	−	+	−	−	−	+	−	+	+	5/10
De Lira et al. (2019)	−	+	−	+	−	−	+	+	+	+	+	7/10
Dorey et al. (2004)	+	+	+	−	−	−	−	+	+	+	+	6/10
Geraerts et al. (2016)	−	+	−	+	−	−	−	+	−	+	+	5/10
Lin et al. (2012)	+	+	+	+	−	−	−	+	−	+	+	6/10
Milios et al. (2020)	+	+	−	+	−	−	−	+	−	+	−	4/10
Nilssen et al. (2012)	+	+	−	+	−	−	−	+	−	+	+	5/10
Prota et al. (2012)	+	+	−	+	−	−	−	−	−	+	+	4/10

TABLE 11.3.5   PEDro Quality Score of Randomized Controlled Trials in Systematic Review of Pelvic Floor Physical Therapy for Premature Ejaculation

E – Eligibility criteria specified
1 – Subjects randomly allocated to groups
2 – Allocation concealed
3 – Groups similar at baseline
4 – Subjects blinded
5 – Therapist administering treatment blinded
6 – Assessors blinded
7 – Measures of key outcomes obtained from >85% of subjects
8 – Data analysed by intention to treat
9 – Statistical comparison between groups conducted
10 – Point measures and measures of variability provided

Study	E	1	2	3	4	5	6	7	8	9	10	Total Score
Jiang et al. (2020)						Currently being rated						
Pastore et al. (2012)	−	+	−	−	−	−	−	+	−	−	+	3/10

relaxation of the smooth muscle cells in the corpus cavernosa and in the walls of the supplying arteries. This results in an increased arterial blood flow, penile tumescence and compression of the venular plexuses, resulting in almost total occlusion of venous outflow (Lue, 2000; Albersen et al., 2010). The ischiocavernosus and bulbospongiosus muscles also compress the veins of the corpora cavernosa, limiting the venous drainage of blood.

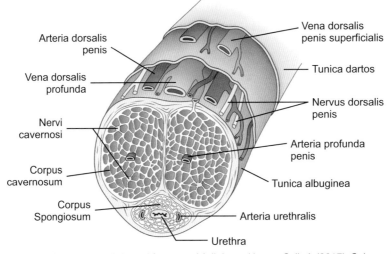

Fig. 11.3.1 Anatomy of the penis. *(Adapted from van Muilekom, H., van Spil, J. (2017). Seksueel disfunctioneren. In: Handboek prostaatcarcinoom. Bohn Stafleu van Loghum, Houten.)*

ED is defined by the International Continence Society as the complaint of inability to achieve and sustain an erection firm enough for satisfactory sexual performance (D'Ancona et al., 2019). It is highly prevalent in males, increasing with age. It affects 50% of men older than 40 years (Lopushnyan and Chitaley, 2012) and generally increases by 10% each decade of life (Cohen et al., 2016). In addition, ED tends to exert substantial effects on quality of life (Latini et al., 2003). Risk factors for erectile disorders are cardiovascular disease, lack of exercise, obesity, smoking, hypercholesterolaemia, metabolic syndrome and radical prostatectomy (Hatzimouratidis et al., 2016). After radical prostatectomy, large ranges of potency rates among various groups have been revealed in different studies (Ficarra et al., 2012). The variation in potency rates is probably due to patient selection, the proportion of nerve-sparing procedures, surgeon and hospital volume. However, different methods of data collection, the assessment method, and the definitions of ED and potency also influence the outcome. A systematic review by Ficarra et al. (2012) indicated 12-month potency rates between 26% and 63% after open, 32% and 78% for laparoscopic, and 55% and 81% for robot-assisted radical prostatectomy (Ficarra et al., 2012).

Assessment of Erectile Function/Hardness

Assessment of erectile function/hardness is mostly done by questionnaires such as the International Index of Erectile Function (IIEF), Sexual Health Inventory for Men (SHIM), Erectile Dysfunction Inventory of Treatment Satisfaction (EDITS), Erectile Hardness Scale (EHS) and Sexual Encounter Profile (SEP). The IIEF is, by far, the most commonly used questionnaire in research. Some researchers defined an International Index of Erectile Function–Erectile Dysfunction domain (IIEF-EF) difference of 6 points as the minimal clinically important difference (MCID) (Goldstein et al., 1998; Padma-Nathan et al., 2008). A more recent study by Rosen et al. (2011) indicated that the receiver operating characteristic (ROC)-based MCID is only 4 points.

Evidence for the Effect of Pelvic Floor Muscle Training in the Treatment of Erectile Disorders

Literature regarding male erectile disorders was analysed to generate clinical recommendations. Several efficacy studies were performed in the pre-Viagra era (Mamberti-Dias and Bonierbale-Branchereau, 1991; Schouman, 1991; Colpi et al., 1994; Claes et al., 1995; Stief et al., 1996; Derouet et al., 1998; van Kampen et al., 2003). The majority of these studies showed beneficial results after a pelvic floor muscle exercise (PFME) programme for men with ED of different causes. Different types of intervention were described. PFMT involves any method of training the pelvic floor muscles, including PFMEs, biofeedback (BF) and electrical stimulation (ES). BF involves the use of a device to provide visual or auditory feedback. ES involves any type of stimulation by using a rectal probe or transcutaneous electrodes (see Chapter 11.2). This method is used to facilitate awareness of contraction of the pelvic floor muscles or to inhibit detrusor contraction. However, the largest effect regarding the treatment of erectile disorders was seen in trials combining PFMEs and electrostimulation.

Consequently, the specific effectiveness of a physical therapeutic approach for erectile disorders can only be evaluated in randomized controlled studies. Currently, nine randomized controlled trials are present regarding the effectiveness of PFMT in treating erectile disorders (Claes and Baert, 1993; Dorey et al., 2004; Lin et al., 2012; Nilssen et al., 2012; Prota et al., 2012; Geraerts et al., 2016; Carboni et al., 2018; de Lira et al., 2019; Milios et al., 2020) (see Table 11.3.1).

In three trials (Claes and Baert, 1993; Dorey et al., 2004; Carboni et al., 2018), men with known ED for at least 6 months were studied. Dorey et al. (2004) and Carboni et al. (2018) respectively offered the patients once or twice per week PFME + BF or functional ES. Training respectively lasted for 5 and 4 weeks. The control group was offered placebo ES (Carboni et al.) or lifestyle changes advice (Dorey et al.). As a result, both studies found a significant result after treatment regarding the IIEF-EF. Dorey et al. (2004) indicated that a total of 22 (40%) participants attained normal function, 19 (34.5%) participants had improved erectile function and 14 (25.5%) participants failed to improve. On the contrary, Claes and Baert (1993) randomized patients with ED of vasculogenic origin into a surgery group (deep dorsal vein) or a PFMT group (five weekly PFME sessions + home exercises). Surgery was not superior to the pelvic floor training programme either subjectively or objectively. Moreover, a significant improvement was found following the training programme; 42% of the patients were satisfied with the outcome and refused surgery (Claes and Baert, 1993).

Six trials studied the effect of PFMT for ED in patients scheduled for radical prostatectomy (Lin et al., 2012; Nilssen et al., 2012; Prota et al., 2012; Geraerts et al., 2016; de Lira et al., 2019; Milios et al., 2020). Two trials started training preoperatively (De Lira et al., 2019; Milios et al., 2020), one trial 12 months after radical prostatectomy (Geraerts et al., 2016) and three trials immediately after catheter withdrawal (Lin et al., 2012; Nilssen et al., 2012; Prota et al., 2012). Most treatments had a duration of 3 months; only the study of Nilssen et al. (2012) indicated that patients could continue training as long as they had any pad usage. Milios et al. (2020)

focused on the intensity of PFMT (see below). Four (Lin et al., 2012; Nilssen et al., 2012; Prota et al., 2012; Geraerts et al., 2016) of the remaining five studies found a significant result in favour of the PFMT group. Only de Lira et al. (2019) could not confirm these findings.

Geraerts et al. (2016) was the only trial restarting intensive PFMT specifically for ED at 12 months after radical prostatectomy. At the time of inclusion, all patients had to be continent (except for possibly existing climacturia or orgasm-associated incontinence [cfr. infra]).

The rationale behind the success of PFMT can be found in the decrease of venous outflow. Contraction of the pelvic floor muscles results in a higher pressure at the base of the penis; in particular, the bulbocavernosus and the ischiocavernosus muscles encircle 33% to 50% of the base of the penis and are responsible for preventing blood from escaping during an erection by exerting pressure on the deep dorsal vein (Geraerts et al., 2016). Furthermore, physical therapy interventions offer non-invasive methods that are painless, inexpensive and easy to perform (Carboni et al., 2018).

Intensity of Pelvic Floor Muscle Training Treatment

Milios et al. (2020) studied the effect of intensifying treatment on the potency outcome at 12 weeks after radical prostatectomy. Both groups received two preoperative PFMT sessions 5 weeks before surgery. After radical prostatectomy, the experimental group had to perform 120 contractions per day (focus on strength and endurance) and the control group 30 contractions per day (only focus on endurance) until 12 weeks after surgery. As a result, the experimental group scored significantly better than the control group regarding the incontinence domains, but not regarding the erectile function domains (EPIC-CF EF [Expanded Prostate Cancer Index Composite for Clinical Practice Erectile Function domain], IIEF-EF).

Adverse Effects

No adverse effects were mentioned.

Evidence for the Effect of Low-Intensity Extracorporeal Shockwave Therapy in the Treatment of Erectile Disorders

Apart from PFMT, the use of Li-ESWT is gaining increasing interest. Shockwave therapy is a non-invasive treatment that uses the passage of acoustic waves through tissue (Sokolakis et al., 2019). Results from basic science experiments have provided evidence that Li-ESWT induces cellular microtrauma, which in turn stimulates the release of angiogenic factors and the subsequent neovascularization of the treated tissue (Gruenwald et al., 2013). It was originally used in the treatment of kidney stones and has since been used in the management of many other conditions, including bone fractures, musculoskeletal disorders, wound healing, Peyronie disease and ischemic cardiovascular disorders. Observational trials indicated beneficial effects of Li-ESWT. Chung and Cartmill (2015) demonstrated that Li-ESWT during 6 weeks in patients, who tried and failed oral PDE-5-I, resulted in an improvement in IIEF-5 scores by 5 points (60%) and EDITS index score by greater than 50% (70%). Consequently, most patients were satisfied (scoring 4/5; 67%). Ayala et al. (2017) studied 710 males with ED of more than 3 months. All patients received five shockwave sessions. After the last session, the EHS score improved in 43% of patients and the ability to penetrate increased from 27% to 44%. Since 2010, several randomized controlled trials tried to demonstrate an improvement of erectile function in patients with vasculogenic ED after Li-ESWT. We identified 10 randomized controlled trials (Vardi et al., 2012; Yee et al., 2014; Olsen et al., 2015; Srini et al., 2015; Kalyvianakis and Hatzichristou, 2017; Fojecki et al., 2017, 2018; Zewin et al., 2018; Baccaglini et al., 2020; Sramkova et al., 2020) (see Table 11.3.2). Most trials described patients with ED of vasculogenic origin, and two trials indicated the effect of Li-ESWT after radical (cysto) prostatectomy (Zewin et al., 2018; Baccaglini et al., 2020). A systematic review and meta-analysis described the effects of Li-ESWT on ED (Clavijo et al., 2017).

Five studies offered Li-ESWT at a frequency of once a week (Olsen et al., 2015; Fojecki et al., 2017, 2018; Baccaglini et al., 2020; Sramkova et al., 2020) and five studies twice a week (Vardi et al., 2012; Yee et al., 2014; Srini et al., 2015; Kalyvianakis and Hatzichristou, 2017; Zewin et al., 2018). Duration of the treatment varied between 4 and 14 weeks. The most frequently used treatment programme was to offer Li-ESWT for 3 to 5 weeks, followed by a break of 3 to 4 weeks, ended by again Li-ESWT for 3 to 5 weeks (Vardi et al., 2012; Yee et al., 2014; Srini et al., 2015; Kalyvianakis and Hatzichristou, 2017; Fojecki et al., 2017, 2018; Zewin et al., 2018). The number of shocks per session differed a lot between the studies: 600 shocks per session (Olsen et al., 2015; Fojecki et al., 2017, 2018), 1500 shocks per session (Vardi et al., 2012; Yee et al., 2014; Srini et al., 2015; Kalyvianakis and

Hatzichristou, 2017; Zewin et al., 2018), 2400 shocks per session (Baccaglini et al., 2020) and 6000 shocks per session (Sramkova et al., 2020).

Only one study (Baccaglini et al., 2020) investigated the additional effect of Li-ESWT over 8 weeks, once a week to daily tadalafil 5 mg (Cialis) in males after radical prostatectomy. The authors found no significant difference in the IIEF score.

Zewin et al. (2018) studied men after cystoprostatectomy for bladder cancer, offering one group Li-ESWT (two times/week for 3 weeks, 3-week break, two times/week for 3 weeks), one group daily sildenafil 50 mg (Viagra) for 6 months and one group (control) follow-up without therapy. IIEF-EF and EHS scores significantly increased during all follow-up periods in the three groups, but no significant differences could be identified between the groups.

In all other studies, men with ED without surgical intervention in the medical history were included. Five of eight studies found a statistically significant result regarding erectile function in favour of Li-ESWT (Vardi et al., 2012; Olsen et al., 2015; Srini et al., 2015; Kalyvianakis and Hatzichristou, 2017; Sramkova et al., 2020). In the studies of Olsen et al. (2015), Srini et al. (2015) and Vardi et al. (2012), 57% versus 9%, 78% versus 0% and 47.5% versus 0%, respectively, were able to penetrate during sexual intercourse (EHS score 3–4) at 1 month after treatment. Kalyvianakis and Hatzichristou (2017) observed an MCID in the IIEF-EF score between the Li-ESWT group and the sham group at every time point (1, 3, 6, 9 and 12 months after treatment). Sramkova et al. (2020) only offered four sessions of Li-ESWT, but with 6000 shocks per session. Nevertheless, they indicated that the IIEF score differed significantly at 4 and 12 weeks after treatment between the Li-ESWT group and the sham group. In addition, the EHS significantly differed between both groups at 12 weeks.

Three studies (Yee et al., 2014; Fojecki et al., 2017, 2018) could not support these findings. Fojecki et al. (2017, 2018) could not find a significant difference between the Li-ESWT group (one time/week for 5 weeks, 4-week break, one time/week for 5 weeks) and the control group at 9 and 18 weeks (Fojecki et al., 2017) and 6 and 12 months (Fojecki et al., 2018). Yee et al. (2014) could not demonstrate a significant difference in IIEF-EF and EHS scores between the Li-ESWT group and the sham group, except in the severe ED subgroup.

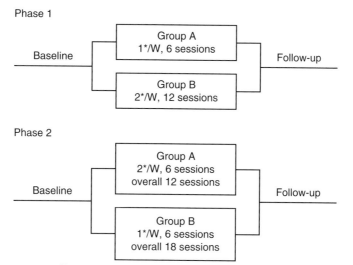

Fig. 11.3.2 Kalyvianakis et al. (2018) study design.

Intensity of Treatment

Kalyvianakis et al. (2018) studied the effect of intensifying Li-ESWT treatment on the potency outcomes after treatment. Patients with vasculogenic ED that responded to PDE-5-I were randomized into two groups: low-intensity shockwave therapy sessions once (group A) or twice (group B) per week for 6 consecutive weeks (phase 1). Patients who completed 6-month follow-up were offered six additional sessions (phase 2), with two sessions per week for group A and 1 session per week for group B. Patients were then again followed for 6 months (Fig. 11.3.2).

In phase 1, groups A and B showed improvement in the IIEF-EF score, MCID and SEP3 score ('Did your erection last long enough for you to have sexual intercourse?'). There was a trend towards improved MCID results in patients receiving 12 sessions compared to those receiving 6 sessions, but this did not reach statistical significance. In the second phase, group A showed a greater increase in the percentage of yes responses to SEP3. However, MCIDs in the IIEF-EF score from baseline were achieved in 62%, 74% and 83% of patients after 6, 12 and 18 sessions, respectively (Kalyvianakis et al., 2018).

Adverse Events

No treatment-related side effects were reported.

Discussion

ED is a common problem in the general population and certainly after radical prostatectomy. The role for physical therapy as a part of the conservative management strategies is not well known among physicians.

Except for some older efficacy studies from the pre-Viagra era, only three randomized controlled trials are available to demonstrate the effect of PFMT for ED caused by venous leakage and six randomized controlled trials for ED after radical prostatectomy. Seven of these studies compared PFMT and/or ES with usual care/placebo (Dorey et al., 2004; Lin et al., 2012; Nilssen et al., 2012; Prota et al., 2012; Geraerts et al., 2016; Carboni et al., 2018; de Lira et al., 2019). Consequently, all but one (De Lira et al., 2019) found a beneficial effect of therapy for ED.

In males with ED (mostly due to venous leakage) in the general population, two studies indicated a significant effect of PFMT/ES on erectile function (Dorey et al., 2004; Carboni et al., 2018). Quality of life also improved in both studies, but only in the study of Carboni et al. (2018) was a significant difference between the experimental and control group seen. The third study of Claes and Baert (1993) compared PFMT with surgery of the deep dorsal vein. Comparison of both treatments indicated that at 12 months in both groups, 42% of patients were cured. Consequently, PFMT can be seen as a realistic alternative to surgery in patients with mild degrees of venous leakage (Claes and Baert, 1993).

In the past, ED was considered, in most cases, to be a purely psychogenic disorder, but current evidence suggests that more than 80% of cases have an organic aetiology. Causes of organic ED can now be broadly divided into non-endocrine and endocrine. Of the non-endocrine aetiologies, vasculogenic (affecting blood supply) is the most common and can involve arterial inflow disorders and abnormalities of venous outflow (corporeal veno-occlusion); there are also neurogenic (affecting innervation and nervous function) and iatrogenic (relating to a medical or surgical treatment) aetiologies. In terms of endocrine factors leading to ED, reduced serum testosterone levels have been implicated, but the exact mechanism has not been fully elucidated. Often, organic ED involves a psychological component—that is, regardless of the precipitating event, ED imposes negative effects on interpersonal relationships, mood and quality of life (Yafi et al., 2016).

In males with ED after radical prostatectomy, four of five studies demonstrated a positive effect of PFMT (Lin et al., 2012, Nilssen et al., 2012; Prota et al., 2012; Geraerts et al., 2016). De Lira et al. (2019), on the contrary, concluded that at 3 months after surgery, no significant improvement existed between the experimental group and the control group. However, patients were only offered two preoperative sessions and after catheter withdrawal were encouraged to resume these exercises without extra guidance of a therapist (De Lira et al., 2019).

Finally, Milios et al. (2020) concluded that offering a more intense PFMT programme (120 contractions/day vs only 30 contractions/day) resulted in significantly better continence outcomes but made no difference regarding the recovery of erectile function. Nevertheless, they mentioned that the more intense PFMT group had a faster uptake of traditional penile rehabilitation, with a faster return to sexual activity. This association is most likely related to earlier continence recovery (Milios et al., 2020).

Li-ESWT has been proposed as a treatment option for ED with no to minimal side effects (Clavijo et al., 2017).

Most studies used a similar study design, with Li-ESWT for 3 to 5 weeks, followed by a break of 3 to 4 weeks, and ended by again Li-ESWT for 3 to 5 weeks (Vardi et al., 2012; Yee et al., 2014; Srini et al., 2015; Kalyvianakis and Hatzichristou, 2017; Fojecki et al., 2017, 2018; Zewin et al., 2018). All studies except Zewin et al. (2018) compared Li-ESWT with sham Li-ESWT (the sham shockwave applicator contained an element that blocked delivery of shockwaves) at equal moments.

Half of the studies found a beneficial effect for the Li-ESWT group (Vardi et al., 2012; Srini et al., 2015; Kalyvianakis and Hatzichristou, 2017), and the other three studies could not support these findings (Yee et al., 2014; Fojecki et al., 2017, 2018). Zewin et al. (2018) could not demonstrate a superior effect of Li-ESWT compared to 6 months of sildenafil. Baccaglini et al. (2020) studied the additional effect of Li-ESWT to daily tadalafil over 8 weeks but could not find a significant difference between both groups regarding the IIEF-5 score.

Finally, Olsen et al. (2015) and Sramkova et al. (2020) both offered only four to five sessions of Li-ESWT at a frequency of once a week to their experimental group. However, both studies differed a lot in the number of shocks per session, respectively 600 versus 6000 shocks per session. Nevertheless, both studies found a significant change in EHS after treatment (Olsen et al., 2015; Sramkova et al., 2020).

Kalyvianakis et al. (2018) demonstrated that the total number of Li-ESWT sessions affects the efficacy of ED treatment, as patients can benefit more in sexual performance from 12 sessions twice per week compared with 6 sessions once a week. In addition, Li-ESWT can be safely repeated up to a total of 18 sessions. Furthermore, a 3-week break period (as performed in most studies) to offer 12 sessions does not seem necessary.

It has been determined that a change of 4 points in the IIEF-EF score is the MCID, which indicates a difference that could be clinically meaningful to the patients (Clavijo et al., 2017). However, using the mean change in the erectile function domain for all patients who showed improvement is rather conservative in estimating the MCID. In contract, the ROC-based approach is used to identify an MCID that provides optimal classification of responders and non-responders regardless of the initial treatment condition. In this approach, the MCID was defined as a change in the IIEF-EF score equal to or greater than 2, 5 and 7 points for mild, moderate and severe ED, respectively. Analysis demonstrated that 73% of patients were correctly classified as having improved using the ROC approach compared to only 47% of the patients using the other method (ANOVA) (Rosen et al., 2011; Clavijo et al., 2017; Kalyvianakis and Hatzichristou, 2017).

Summary and Clinical Recommendations

In the general population, several efficacy studies and later also some randomized controlled trials have been performed regarding the effect of PFMT on ED. Three of the four randomized controlled trials indicated a positive effect. In addition, most studies in males after radical prostatectomy could also indicate a beneficial effect of PFMT to potency outcomes. However, it was of tremendous importance to offer sufficiently guided PFMT sessions to the patients. More intense PFMT programmes led directly to better continence outcomes. This was not confirmed related to the recovery of erectile function. However, it was mentioned that the more intense PFMT group had a faster uptake of traditional penile rehabilitation, with a faster return to sexual activity—probably due to an earlier continence recovery (Milios et al., 2020).

Comparison of the different studies regarding the effect of Li-ESWT on ED could not define a unanimous conclusion, although several studies found a statistically significant improvement in the IIEF-EF score for men who underwent Li-ESWT compared with those who underwent sham therapy. More stringent randomized controlled trials are warranted before there will be widespread acceptance of this treatment (Clavijo et al., 2017).

EJACULATION DISORDERS

Premature ejaculation is a common male sexual dysfunction, with prevalence rates of 20% to 30% (Hatzimouratidis et al., 2016). The severity of premature (early) ejaculation is specified as follows: mild (occurring within approximately 30 seconds to 1 minute of vaginal penetration), moderate (occurring within approximately 15–30 seconds of vaginal penetration) or severe (occurring before sexual activity, at the start of sexual activity or within approximately 15 seconds of vaginal penetration). The duration of the dysfunction is subdivided into lifelong (present since first sexual experience) or acquired (developing after a period of relative normal sexual functioning) (American Psychiatric Association, 2013).

The aetiology of premature ejaculation is unknown, with scarce data to support the suggested biological and psychological hypotheses, including anxiety, penile hypersensitivity and serotonin receptor dysfunction (Hatzimouratidis et al., 2016).

Assessment of Premature Ejaculation

Measurement of clinical response to therapy regarding premature ejaculation is often performed via assessment of the intra-vaginal ejaculatory latency time (IELT).

IELT is defined as the time from vaginal intromission to intra-vaginal ejaculation (Waldinger et al., 2005) and can be used as a standardized method to compare different treatments in clinical trials, next to questionnaires such as the Premature Ejaculation Diagnostic Tool (PEDT) (Pastore et al., 2012).

Evidence for the Effect of Pelvic Floor Muscle Training in the Treatment of Premature Ejaculation

Myers and Smith (2019) gave an overview of the efficacy of PFMT in the course of treatment of premature ejaculation. They concluded that PFMT could be effective in treating ED. However, PFMT as a treatment for premature ejaculation has only been scarcely investigated, and most of the studies had methodological limitations. Reported treatment effects were measured through patient-reported response, IELT or the PEDT. PFMT protocols (with ES and most with BF) were implemented two to three times per week, lasted between 4 weeks to 3 months and varied in the amount of therapist intervention (Myers and Smith, 2019).

Notwithstanding the lack of knowledge about premature ejaculation aetiology, a possible explanation for the effectivity of PFMT in treating premature ejaculation could be the increased control over ejaculation (La Pera and Nicastro, 1996). Seeing that the involuntary contraction of the bulbospongiosus muscle is responsible for expelling ejaculate (Dorey et al., 2004; Siegel, 2014), improving control over this muscle's contraction and relaxation (together with the rest of the pelvic floor) could influence control over IELT (La Pera and Nicastro, 1996; Pastore et al., 2012).

Only two randomized controlled trials investigated the effect of PFMT on premature ejaculation (Pastore et al., 2012; Jiang et al., 2020) (see Table 11.3.3). Jiang et al. (2020) compared daily Kegel exercises (three times/day, 50–100 repetitions) with penis root masturbation (PRM; three times/week, 10–15 minutes) for 3 months in 44 men with lifelong premature ejaculation. The other study (Pastore et al., 2012) investigated the effect of 12 weeks of PFMT with ES and BF three times per week compared to on-demand use of dapoxetine in 40 men with lifelong premature ejaculation. Both investigations showed increased IELT after all treatments, with significantly greater improvement after PRM or dapoxetine. Jiang et al. (2020) also reported significantly lower PEDT scores in the PRM group.

Discussion

To date, the effect of PFMT on premature ejaculation has only been studied scarcely, with studies reporting multiple methodological limitations. Nonetheless, the aforementioned randomized controlled trials (Pastore et al., 2012; Jiang et al., 2020) showed promising results regarding PFMT as a possible treatment for premature ejaculation. This type of exercises leads to an improvement of body awareness and could thereby influence the sense of control as well as the ejaculation reflex (Pastore et al., 2012). Additionally, PFMT is a treatment option without any side effects, as opposed to medication, which has been reported to be a reason for discontinuing treatment due to the undesirable sexual side effects, cost and limited long-term or unsatisfactory efficacy (Pastore et al., 2012; Jiang et al., 2020).

Summary and Clinical Recommendations

PFMT seems to have merit as a treatment option for premature ejaculation, with or without supplemental treatment. However, more randomized controlled trials with a focus on PFMT-programmes and longer follow-up are necessary before drawing conclusions.

CLIMACTURIA

Climacturia or orgasm-associated incontinence occurs in 22%–43% of post-prostatectomy patients, which often causes embarrassment and avoidance of sexual activity (Choi et al., 2007; Guay and Seftel, 2008; Tsivian et al., 2009; Kannan et al., 2019; Milios et al., 2020). Only one case report (Sighinolfi et al., 2009) and one randomized controlled trial (Geraerts et al., 2016) investigated the effect of PFMT for climacturia. Both studies found a beneficial effect of 3–4 months of PFMT combined with electrostimulation (once/week) + home exercises.

CONCLUSION

Affecting 50% of men older than 40 years (Lopushnyan and Chitaley, 2012), and generally increasing by 10% each decade in life (Cohen et al., 2016), the treatment of ED remains a challenging matter. The effectiveness of PFMT has already been discussed for several years. In the general population and after radical prostatectomy, the majority of the available studies indicated a beneficial effect of PFMT on potency outcomes. Of clinical importance was the guidance of the exercises by a therapist. The link between a higher intensity of exercises and a faster return to sexual activity was probably rather indirect. In particular, more intense exercises led to better continence outcomes, which in turn led to a faster uptake of penile rehabilitation.

Consequently, comparison of the different studies regarding the effect of Li-ESWT on ED, could not define a unanimous conclusion, although several studies found a statistically significant improvement in IIEF-EF score for men who underwent Li-ESWT compared with those who underwent sham therapy.

In addition, premature ejaculation is a common male sexual dysfunction with prevalence rates of 20% to 30% (Hatzimouratidis et al., 2016). To date, only two randomized controlled trials investigated the effect of PFMT on (lifelong) premature ejaculation. Both studies (Pastore et al., 2012; Jiang et al., 2020) showed promising results regarding PFMT as a possible treatment for premature ejaculation, although the results were not superior over PRM or dapoxetine. Nevertheless, more randomized controlled trials with a focus on PFMT programmes and longer follow-up are necessary to draw definitive conclusions. Finally, climacturia or orgasm-associated incontinence is only scarcely investigated in the literature, although it is a rather frequent and bothersome problem in post-prostatectomy patients. Nevertheless, there certainly is a role for PFMT in this group of patients.

REFERENCES

Albaugh, J., & Lewis, J. H. (1999). Insights into the management of erectile dysfunction: Part I. *Urologic Nursing*, *19*(4), 241–247.

Albersen, M., Shindel, A. W., Mwamukonda, K. B., et al. (2010). The future is today: Emerging drugs for the treatment of erectile dysfunction. *Expert Opinion on Emerging Drugs*, *15*, 467–480.

American Psychiatric Association. (2013). Chapter Sexual dysfunctions. In *Diagnostic and statistical manual of mental disorders* (5th ed.) (pp. 426–429). Arlington, VA: American Psychiatric Association. Arlington, VA.

Ayala, H. A. C., Cuartas, J. P. S., & Cleves, D. C. (2017). Impact on the quality of erections after completing a low-intensity extracorporeal shock wave treatment cycle on a group of 710 patients. *Advancement Urology*, 2017 1843687.

Baccaglini, W., Pazeto, C. L., Correa Barros, E. A., et al. (2020). The role of low-intensity extracorporeal shock-wave therapy on penile rehabilitation after radical prostatectomy: A randomized clinical trial. *The Journal of Sexual Medicine*, *17*, 688–694.

Burnett, A. L., Nehra, A., Breau, R. H., et al. (2018). Erectile dysfunction: AUA guideline. *Journal of Urology, 200,* 633–641.

Carboni, C., Fornari, A., Bragante, K. C., et al. (2018). An initial study on the effect of functional electrical stimulation in erectile dysfunction: A randomized controlled trial. *International Journal of Impotence Research, 30,* 97–101.

Choi, J. M., Nelson, C. J., Stasi, J., et al. (2007). Orgasm associated incontinence (climacturia) following radical pelvic surgery: Rates of occurrence and predictors. *Journal of Urology, 177,* 2223–2226.

Chung, E., & Cartmill, R. (2015). Evaluation of clinical efficacy, safety and patient satisfaction rate after low-intensity extracorporeal shockwave therapy for the treatment of male erectile dysfunction: An Australian first open-label single-arm prospective clinical trial. *BJU International, 115,* 46–49.

Claes, H., & Baert, L. (1993). Pelvic floor exercise versus surgery in the treatment of impotence. *British Journal of Urology, 71,* 52–57.

Claes, H., Van Kampen, M., Lysens, R., et al. (1995). Pelvic floor exercises in the treatment of impotence. *European Journal of Physical Medicine and Rehabilitation, 5,* 135–140.

Clavijo, R. R., Kohn, T. P., Kohn, J. R., et al. (2017). Effects of low-intensity extracorporeal shockwave therapy on erectile dysfunction: A systematic review and meta-analysis. *The Journal of Sexual Medicine, 14,* 27–35.

Cohen, D., Gonzalez, J., & Goldstein, I. (2016). The role of pelvic floor muscles in male sexual dysfunction and pelvic pain. *Sex Medicine Review, 4,* 53–62.

Colpi, G. M., Negri, L., Scroppo, F. I., et al. (1994). Perineal floor rehabilitation: A new treatment for venogenic impotence. *Journal of Endocrinological Investigation, 17,* 34.

D'Ancona, C. D., Haylen, B. T., Oelke, M., et al. (2019). An International Continence Society (ICS) report on the terminology for adult male lower urinary tract and pelvic floor symptoms and dysfunction. *Neurourology and Urodynamics, 38,* 433–477.

De Lira, G. H. S., Fornari, A., Cardoso, L. F., et al. (2019). Effects of perioperative pelvic floor muscle training on early recovery of urinary continence and erectile function in men undergoing radical prostatectomy: A randomized clinical trial. *International Braz J Urol, 6,* 1196–1203.

Derouet, H., Nolden, W., Jost, W. H., et al. (1998). Treatment of erectile dysfunction by an external ischiocavernosus muscle stimulator. *European Urology, 34*(4), 355–359.

Dorey, G., Speakman, M., Feneley, R., et al. (2004). Randomised controlled trial of pelvic floor muscle exercises and manometric biofeedback for erectile dysfunction. *British Journal of General Practice, 54*(508), 819–825.

Ficarra, V., Novara, G., Ahlering, T. E., et al. (2012). Systematic review and meta-analysis of studies reporting potency rates after robot-assisted radical prostatectomy. *European Urology, 62,* 418–430.

Fojecki, G. L., Tiessen, S., Osther, P. J., et al. (2017). Effect of low-energy linear shockwave therapy on erectile dysfunction—a double-blinded, sham-controlled, randomized clinical trial. *The Journal of Sexual Medicine, 14,* 106–112.

Fojecki, G. L., Tiessen, S., & Osther, P. J. S. (2018). Effect of linear low-intensity extracorporeal shockwave therapy for erectile dysfunction—12-month follow-up of a randomized, double-blinded, sham-controlled study. *Sexual Medicine, 6,* 1–7.

Geraerts, I., Van Poppel, H., Devoogdt, N., et al. (2016). Pelvic floor muscle training for erectile dysfunction and climacturia 1 year after nerve sparing radical prostatectomy: A randomized controlled trial. *International Journal of Impotence Research, 28,* 9–13.

Goldstein, I., Lue, T. F., Padma-Nathan, H., et al. (1998). Oral sildenafil in the treatment of erectile dysfunction. *New England Journal of Medicine, 338,* 1397–1404.

Gruenwald, I., Appel, B., Kitrey, N. D., et al. (2013). Shockwave treatment of erectile dysfunction. *Theraphy Advancement Urology, 5,* 95–99.

Guay, A., & Seftel, A. D. (2008). Sexual foreplay incontinence in men with erectile dysfunction after radical prostatectomy: A clinical observation. *International Journal of Impotence Research, 20,* 199–201.

Hackett, G., Kirby, M., Wylie, K., et al. (2018). British Society for Sexual Medicine guidelines on the management of erectile dysfunction in men—2017. *The Journal of Sexual Medicine, 15,* 430–457.

Hatzimouratidis, K., Giuliano, F., Moncada, A., et al. (2016). *Guidelines on erectile dysfunction, premature ejaculation, penile curvature and priapism.* Arnhem, Netherlands: EAU Guidelines Office.

Jiang, M., Yan, G., Deng, H., et al. (2020). The efficacy of regular penis-root masturbation, versus Kegel exercise in the treatment of primary premature ejaculation: A quasi-randomised controlled trial. *Andrologia, 52,* e13473.

Kalyvianakis, D., & Hatzichristou, D. (2017). Low-intensity shockwave therapy improves hemodynamic parameters in patients with vasculogenic erectile dysfunction: A triplex ultrasonography-based sham-controlled trial. *The Journal of Sexual Medicine, 7,* 891–897.

Kalyvianakis, D., Memmos, E., & Mykoniatis, I. (2018). Low-intensity shockwave therapy for erectile dysfunction: A randomized clinical trial comparing 2 treatment protocols and the impact of repeating treatment. *The Journal of Sexual Medicine, 15,* 334–345.

Kannan, P., Winser, S. J., Ho, L. C., et al. (2019). Effectiveness of physiotherapy interventions for improving erectile function and climacturia in men after prostatectomy: A systematic review and meta-analysis of randomized controlled trials. *Clinical Rehabilitation, 33,* 1298–1309.

Kirby, R., Carson, C., & Goldstein, I. (1999). Anatomy, physiology and pathophysiology. In R. Kirby (Ed.), *Erectile dysfunction: A clinical guide* (pp. 11–28). Oxford: Isis Medical Media.

La Pera, G., & Nicastro, A. (1996). A new treatment for premature ejaculation: The rehabilitation of the pelvic floor. *Journal of Sex & Marital Therapy, 22*(1), 22–26.

Latini, D. M., Penson, D. F., Lubeck, D. P., et al. (2003). Longitudinal differences in disease specific quality of life in men with erectile dysfunction: Results from the exploratory comprehensive evaluation of erectile dysfunction study. *Journal of Urology, 169,* 1437–1442.

Lin, Y. H., Yu, T. J., Lin, V. C. -H., et al. (2012). Effects of early pelvic-floor muscle exercise for sexual dysfunction in radical prostatectomy recipients. *Cancer Nursing, 35,* 106–114.

Lopushnyan, N. A., & Chitaley, K. (2012). Genetics of erectile dysfunction. *Journal of Urology, 188,* 1676–1683.

Lue, T. F. (2000). Erectile dysfunction. *New England Journal of Medicine, 342,* 1802–1813.

Mamberti-Dias, A., & Bonierbale-Branchereau, M. (1991). Therapy for dysfunctioning erections: Four years later, how do things stand? *Sexologique, 1,* 24–25.

Milios, J. E., Ackland, T. R., & Green, D. J. (2020). Pelvic floor muscle training and erectile dysfunction in radical prostatectomy: A randomized controlled trial investigating a non-invasive addition to penile rehabilitation. *Sexual Medicine, 8*(3), 414–421.

Myers, C., & Smith, M. (2019). Pelvic floor muscle training improves erectile dysfunction and premature ejaculation: A systematic review. *Physiotherapy, 105,* 235–243.

Nilssen, S. R., Mørkved, S., Overgard, M., et al. (2012). Does physiotherapist-guided pelvic floor muscle training increase the quality of life in patients after radical prostatectomy? A randomized clinical study. *Scandinavian Journal of Urology and Nephrology, 46,* 397–404.

Olsen, A. B., Persiani, M., Boie, S., et al. (2015). Can low-intensity extracorporeal shockwave therapy improve erectile dysfunction? A prospective, randomized, double-blind, placebo-controlled study. *Scandinavian Journal of Urology, 49,* 329–333.

Padma-Nathan, H., McCullough, A. R., Levine, L. A., et al. (2008). Randomized, double-blind, placebo-controlled study of postoperative nightly sildenafil citrate for the prevention of erectile dysfunction after bilateral nerve-sparing radical prostatectomy. *International Journal of Impotence Research, 20,* 479–486.

Pastore, A. L., Palleschi, G., Leto, A., et al. (2012). A prospective randomized study to compare pelvic floor

rehabilitation and dapoxetine for treatment of lifelong premature ejaculation. *International Journal of Andrology, 35,* 528–533.

Prota, C., Gomes, C. M., Ribeiro, L. H. S., et al. (2012). Early postoperative pelvic-floor biofeedback improves erectile function in men undergoing radical prostatectomy: A prospective, randomized, controlled trial. *International Journal of Impotence Research, 24,* 174–178.

Rosen, R. C., Allen, K. R., Ni, X., et al. (2011). Minimal clinically important differences in the erectile function domain of the International Index of Erectile Function scale. *European Urology, 60,* 1010–1016.

Schouman, M., & Lacroix, P. (1991). Apport de la rééducation pelvi-périnéale au traitement des fuites veino-caverneuses. *Ann. Urol., 25,* 92–93.

Salonia, A., Bettocchi, C., Carvalho, J., et al. (2020). *EAU guidelines on sexual and reproductive Health.* Arnhem, Netherlands: European Association of Urology.

Siegel, A. L. (2014). Pelvic floor muscle training in males: Practical applications. *Urology, 84*(1), 1–7.

Sighinolfi, M. C., Rivalta, M., Mofferdin, A., et al. (2009). Potential effectiveness of pelvic floor rehabilitation treatment for postradical prostatectomy incontinence, climacturia, and erectile dysfunction: A case series. *The Journal of Sexual Medicine, 6,* 3496–3499.

Sokolakis, I., Dimitriadis, F., Pearline, T., et al. (2019). The basic science behind low-intensity extracorporeal shockwave therapy for erectile dysfunction: A systematic scoping review of pre-clinical studies. *The Journal of Sexual Medicine, 16,* 168–194.

Sramkova, T., Motil, I., Jarkovsky, J., et al. (2020). Erectile dysfunction treatment using focused linear low-intensity extracorporeal shockwaves: Single-blind, sham-controlled, randomized clinical trial. *Urologia Internationalis, 104*(5–6), 417–424.

Srini, V. S., Reddy, R. K., Shultz, T., et al. (2015). Low intensity extracorporeal shockwave therapy for erectile dysfunction: A study in an Indian population. *The Canadian Journal of Urology, 22,* 7614–7622.

Stief, C. G., Weller, E., Noack, T., et al. (1996). Functional electromyostimulation of the penile corpus cavernosum (FEMCC). Initial results of a new therapeutic option of erectile dysfunction. *Der Urologe. Ausg. A, 35*(4), 321–325.

Tsivian, M., Mayes, J. M., Krupski, T. L., et al. (2009). Altered male physiologic function after surgery for prostate cancer: Couple perspective. *International Brazilian Journal of Urology, 35,* 673–682.

Van Kampen, M., De Weerdt, W., Claes, H., et al. (2003). Treatment of erectile dysfunction by perineal exercises, electromyographic biofeedback and electrical stimulation. *Physical Therapy, 83*(6), 536–543.

Vardi, Y., Appel, B., Kilchevsky, A., et al. (2012). Does low intensity extracorporeal shock wave therapy have a physiological effect on erectile function? Short-term results of a randomized, double-blind, sham controlled study. *Journal of Urology, 187,* 1769–1775.

Waldinger, M. D., Zwinderman, A. H., Olivier, B., et al. (2005). Proposal for a definition of lifelong premature ejaculation based on epidemiological stopwatch data. *The Journal of Sexual Medicine, 2*(4), 498–507.

World Health Organization. (1992). *International statistical classification of diseases and related Health problems. 1989 revision.* Geneva: World Health Organization.

Yafi, F. A., Jenkins, L., Albersen, M., et al. (2016). Erectile dysfunction. *Nature Reviews Disease Primers, 2,* 16003.

Yee, C. H., Chan, E. S., Hou, S. S., et al. (2014). Extracorporeal shockwave therapy in the treatment of erectile dysfunction: A prospective, randomized, double-blinded, placebo controlled study. *International Journal of Urology, 21,* 1041–1045.

Zewin, T. S., El-Assmy, A., Harraz, A. M., et al. (2018). Efficacy and safety of low-intensity shock wave therapy in penile rehabilitation post nerve-sparing radical cystoprostatectomy: A randomized controlled trial. *International Urology and Nephrology, 50,* 2007–2014.

12

Evidence for Pelvic Floor Physical Therapy in Childhood

Janet Walker Chase and
Marieke van Engelenburg- van Lonkhuyzen

INTRODUCTION

Bladder or bowel dysfunction (BBD), or both, formerly known as dysfunctional elimination syndrome, in neurologically normal and otherwise healthy children (i.e., functional BBD) is common in all age groups (Wright, 2015). Terminology used aligns with International Children's Continence Society definitions (Austin et al., 2016) or Rome IV criteria (Hyams et al., 2016). Table 12.1 shows the symptoms and signs of the most common childhood BBDs encountered in physiotherapy practice. Less common bladder problems, such as urethrovaginal reflux, extraordinary daytime urinary only frequency, giggle incontinence and stress urinary incontinence, have been excluded.

Bladder Dysfunctions

Children with bladder dysfunction generally present with daytime urinary incontinence (DUI), enuresis (bedwetting) (both from the age of 5 years), and symptoms of urinary urgency and frequency.

DUI is defined as the leakage of urine in discrete amounts that occurs while awake. Exclusively during sleeping periods, it is termed *enuresis*. Increased urinary frequency describes children who void more than eight times per day; voiding on less than three occasions does not have a formal diagnostic label but is of clinical importance. Urinary urgency refers to the sudden and unexpected experience of an immediate and compelling need to void. The term is not applicable before the attainment of bladder control (Austin et al., 2016).

Nocturnal enuresis (NE) or enuresis (bedwetting) is bladder emptying during sleep in a child who is 5 years or older. It is due to a mismatch between the rate of urine production, habitual bladder storage and the child's ability to wake to the sensation of a full bladder. NE is often regarded as a benign condition in primary healthcare;

TABLE 12.1   Childhood Bladder and Bowel Dysfunctions

Type	Symptoms	Signs	Potential Psychological Aspects
Overactive bladder[a]	Detrusor overactivity (cystometry), urinary urgency, frequency, incontinence, constipation, enuresis	'Tower' or normal flow pattern, low-volume voids, thickened bladder wall, posturing to control urge	May be associated with dysfunctional voiding Subclinical symptoms: sadness, social withdrawal, anxiety, reduced self-esteem and QoL Externalising disorders (ADHD, ODD, conduct disorders) and internalising disorders (separation anxiety)
Dysfunctional voiding[a]	Incomplete sphincter/ pelvic floor muscle relaxation during voiding, variable micturition frequency, urinary urgency, incontinence, constipation, UTIs, enuresis	'Staccato' or interrupted flow pattern, post-void residual urine, thickened bladder wall	May be associated with overactive bladder Externalising disorders as above
Voiding postponement[a]	Low micturition frequency, urinary urgency, incontinence, constipation	Normal flow pattern, holding manoeuvres	Externalising disorders as above (especially ODD)
Underactive bladder[a]	Unsustained detrusor contractions (cystometry), low micturition frequency, straining to void, incontinence, constipation, UTIs	Interrupted flow pattern, large-volume voids, post-void residual urine	Low micturition frequency, straining to void, incontinence, constipation, UTIs May be the consequence of dysfunctional voiding No known studies, but assume as above
Enuresis[a]	Primary: never been dry at night Secondary: wetting after over 6 months no symptoms; both a symptom and a condition of intermittent incontinence that occurs during periods of sleep from 5 years		
	Monosymptomatic enuresis, no day symptoms	Nocturnal polyuria, arousal dysfunction, less ladder storage	Constipation, sleep-disordered breathing, neurodevelopmental disorder (e.g., ADHD), low self-esteem, other psychiatric disorders
	Non-monosymptomatic enuresis, day symptoms present	Less bladder storage, nocturnal polyuria, arousal dysfunction	Constipation, UTIs daytime urinary incontinence, urgency, voiding difficulties, high or low daytime voiding frequency (<4 or >8/day)

Continued

TABLE 12.1 Childhood Bladder and Bowel Dysfunctions—cont'd

Type	Symptoms	Signs	Potential Psychological Aspects
Functional constipation[b]	**Infants and Toddlers** Must have ≥2 of following criteria for ≥1 month: • ≤2 defaecations/week • History of painful or hard bowel movements • History of excessive stool retention • History of large-diameter stools • Presence of a large faecal mass in rectum • ≥1 episode of faecal incontinence/week (in toilet-trained children) • History of large-diameter stools that can obstruct toilet **Children and Adolescents** Must include ≥2 of following in child with developmental age ≥4 years: • ≤2 defaecations in toilet/week • ≥1 episode of faecal incontinence/week • History of retentive posturing or excessive volitional stool retention • History of painful or hard bowel movements • Presence of large faecal mass in rectum • History of large-diameter stools that may obstruct toilet *Criteria fulfilled ≥1×/week for ≥1 month prior to diagnosis, with insufficient criteria for diagnosis of irritable bowel syndrome*		Abdominal pain, flatulence, no appetite, bloated belly, failure to thrive; sadness, social withdrawal, anxiety, reduced self-esteem and QoL Internalising and externalising Separation anxiety, specific phobias, generalized anxiety, ADHD, ODD QoL severely reduced with combined bladder and/or bowel dysfunction and failed treatment
Functional non-retentive faecal incontinence[b]	Child >3 years, must include all criteria: • Defaecation in inappropriate places • No evidence of other processes that explain symptoms • No evidence of faecal retention • Reduced perception of urge to defaecate • Normal consistency and frequency bowel actions • Faecal incontinence, often late in day • Laxatives worsen soiling		As for functional constipation

[a]Terminology of bladder function in children and adolescents (International Children's Continence Society).
[b]Rome IV criteria.
ADHD, Attention-deficit/hyperactivity disorder; *ODD*, oppositional defiant disorder; *QoL*, quality of life; *UTI*, urinary tract infection.

however, if left untreated, it may result in poor self-esteem, avoidance of social activities and parental stress (Collis et al., 2019). Furthermore, there are data suggesting that enuresis is linked to chronically disturbed sleep, and successful treatment can lead to improved daytime behaviour and executive function (Van Herzeele et al., 2016). For these reasons, treatment is recommended, particularly after the age of 6 years. Spontaneous resolution of NE after the age of 9 years is unlikely.

Bowel Dysfunctions

Bowel disorders include constipation and faecal incontinence, abdominal pain, and pain during defaecation (Hyams et al., 2016). Symptoms of bowel dysfunctions were formulated by paediatric gastroenterologists in 2016 and included in the Rome IV criteria (Hyams et al., 2016). Definitions relate to symptoms from the age of 4 years onwards.

Chronic constipation is categorised into separate groups, subclassified as:
• normal proximal transit but hold-up at the anorectum and
• delayed colonic transit (slow transit constipation) (Vriesman, et al. 2020).

The age of onset of functional constipation in children is usually around the time of toilet training, likely related to behavioural factors associated with distress around defaecation. Triggers of functional constipation include hard painful stools, anal fissures, or experiences that induced or caused fear or anxiety. The resultant stool withholding is considered the most common cause of constipation in children; if left untreated, it can lead to secondary problems related to faecal impaction. The sequelae include rectal hyposensitivity, overflow faecal incontinence, development of a megarectum and subsequent loss of the urge to defaecate. The behavioural, emotional and social consequences of this cascade of events profoundly impact a child's quality of life.

Faecal incontinence in children is defined as either voluntary or involuntary passage of faeces in inappropriate places and at unacceptable times, from the age of 4 years onwards. Organic causes must have been excluded. Faecal incontinence is differentiated into retentive faecal incontinence (also known 'overflow faecal incontinence' in constipation) and non-retentive faecal incontinence (NRFI; no concomitant other bowel symptoms).

NRFI refers to defaecation into places inappropriate to the sociocultural context when there is no evidence of faecal retention, and after appropriate medical evaluation, the faecal incontinence cannot be explained by another medical condition. These children have normal bowel motility and frequency of defaecation, so laxative medication is not useful. For both functional constipation and NRFI, there are negative consequences on self-esteem and well-being. Early intervention from the age of 2.5 to 3 years onwards will prevent the secondary consequences.

Childhood Bladder and Bowel Dysfunction

Bladder dysfunction often coexists with bowel dysfunction (Burgers et al., 2013a). The association between childhood and adult BBD is well established, with risk factors being multifactorial and complex (Fitzgerald et al., 2006). Genetic, familial, environmental, demographic, behavioural, physical factors and more recently neurobiological factors may be involved, lending weight to the argument for a biopsychosocial interdisciplinary model of care (Vriesman et al., 2020). Children with at least one elimination disorder had significantly higher values on the 'anxious/depressed' items of the Child Behaviour Checklist (CBCL) than controls who were continent (Nevéus et al., 2020a; van Dijk et al., 2010; von Gontard et al., 2011; von Gontard et al., 2019). Neurodevelopmental disorders such as attention-deficit/hyperactivity disorder are associated with higher rates of incontinence in children and adolescents, including

NE, DUI, faecal incontinence and constipation (Von Gontard et al., 2022).

Observational studies using longitudinal latent class analysis modelling provide trajectories of normal and atypical development. The most recent is the Avon Longitudinal Study of Parents and Children (ALSPAC) from the UK in which children were surveyed at 4.5 and 9 years. Four trajectories were found for each of DUI, faecal incontinence and NE, normative, delayed, persistent and relapsing, with the latter two being more severe and unlikely to spontaneously improve. When compared to data of the same children at 14 years (without treatment), it was apparent that the younger children with DUI alone, NE alone, DUI and NE, and delayed attainment were all more likely to have difficulties at age 14 years (Heron et al., 2008; Heron et al., 2017). On initial presentation of the young child we do not know into which trajectory a child will fall; however, because of the potential negative effects on self-esteem, behaviour, quality of life, learning, socialisation and long-term effects on renal and gastrointestinal tract function, every child with BBD should be assessed and managed.

Prevalence rates of functional BBD have been described in children. The pooled prevalence of constipation is 9.5% as compared to estimates of constipation in the general paediatric population, which range from 0.3% to 8% (Koppen et al., 2018). Faecal incontinence occurs in 0.8% to 7.8% of children in Western societies (Hyams et al., 2016). The overall prevalence of DUI on meta-analysis is 6.4% (Franco et al., 2015). NE is found in 5% to 10% of 7-year-old children (Nevéus et al., 2020b). Childhood BBD is often accompanied by urinary tract infections and abdominal pain (Heron et al., 2008).

ASSESSMENT AND MANAGEMENT OF CHILDHOOD BLADDER OR BOWEL DYSFUNCTION

In addition to taking a medical history to quantify symptoms, tools such as bladder and bowel diaries, standardised pad tests, pain measures, stool consistency descriptors (Bristol stool form scale) and urine flow (uroflowmetry) are used. Questionnaires, pelvic ultrasound and abdominal radiography also aid in the evaluation of childhood BBD.

Physical therapy, as a discipline, differs from other health professionals as the primary focus is (dys)functions of the musculoskeletal system (posture, core stability, movements and bodily awareness) and the interaction between control of smooth muscle and striated muscle.

Urotherapy is defined as 'a conservative-based therapy and treatment of lower urinary tract dysfunction that rehabilitates the lower urinary tract'. Urotherapy uses non-pharmacological, non-surgical methods and behavioral interventions. Standard urotherapy comprises components such as provision of information, instructions, lifestyle advice, counselling and documentation of symptoms. Specific urotherapy is tailored towards specific disorders and includes alarm treatment, pelvic floor muscle training (± biofeedback), neurostimulation and other interventions. Physical therapy can be considered as a specialised form of urotherapy.

Health professionals involved in the management of children with BBD require competency in the principles of urotherapy, particularly when seeing children as first-contact practitioners with responsiblity for aspects of assessment and diagnosis. The International Children's Continence Society has developed position statement documents relating to DUI, NE, dysfunctional voiding, behavioural comorbidities, outcome measurements, bowel dysfunction related to the lower urinary tract neurobiological disorders and BBD (Franco, 2012; Heron et al. 2008; Koppen et al., 2015).

INTERVENTIONS IN CHILDHOOD BLADDER OR BOWEL DYSFUNCTION

Standard Medical Care

Standard medical care for childhood BBD in routine practice is provided by general practitioners or paediatricians. When needed, medication or laxatives are prescribed.

Interventions include education of parents and child, demystification by addressing their beliefs and fears, dietary advice (adequate fibre and fluid intake), regulation of the toilet regime, and normalising withholding behaviour (including posture). When necessary, a toilet seat or footstool, or both, are advised (Chase et al., 2010; Hodges et al., 2007). Children are engaged in toileting regimes, attention to toilet posture, core stability, sensory integration and directed pelvic floor muscle relaxation to facilitate complete bladder and bowel emptying (Beaudry-Bellefeuille and Lane, 2017; Beaudry-Bellefeuille et al., 2019; Chase et al., 2009; Hodges et al., 2007; Sapsford and Hodges, 2001). Intervention is

supported by diaries, charts and pictures such as those of the Bristol stool form scale (Riegler and Esposito, 2001).

Physical Therapy

A generally accepted explanation of the aetiology of functional BBD in children is a lack of coordination between the pelvic floor muscles and visceral smooth muscles which are important in urination and defaecation (Burgers et al., 2013b). The treatment of this as a dysfunction of motor control, coordination and timing by a physical therapist is logical.

Education, information, documentation, and supporting the children and their parents are important parts of therapy. The aim is to inform and support both the child and the parents with:

- education and demystification (using explanatory materials, charts, pictures, and bladder and bowel diaries);
- dietary advice regarding fluid and fibre intake (supported by fluid and fibre-rich food lists);
- patient-centred instructions to institute an appropriate bladder and bowel regime and to normalise bladder and bowel emptying mechanics (normalising toilet habits with an agreed-on toilet regime, avoidance of withholding to urinate and defaecate);
- documentation of symptoms and toilet habits using bladder and bowel diaries or frequency–volume charts; and
- continuous support of the family and encouragement of the child.

Motor control interventions are implemented by physical therapists. Motor control exercises help maintain an adequate posture on the toilet, and functional training optimises the timing of emptying efforts (Chase et al., 2009; Ladi-Seyedian et al., 2014; Pollock, 2012; Sapsford, 2004; van Engelenburg–van Lonkhuyzen et al., 2013; van Engelenburg–van Lonkhuyzen et al., 2017b).

Other strategies include:

- sensory processing techniques, such as filtering, organizing and integrating sensory information to become aware of the urge to urinate and defaecate (Beaudry-Bellefeuille et al., 2019; van Engelenburg–van Lonkhuyzen et al., 2013; van Engelenburg–van Lonkhuyzen et al., 2017b);
- relaxation and breathing exercises to teach adequate abdominal breathing and targeted straining while defaecating (Hodges et al., 2007; Sapsford and Hodges, 2001; Silva and Motta, 2013); and

- pelvic floor and abdominal muscle training (aware-ness, relaxation and functional training) (De Paepe et al., 1998; de Paepe et al., 2002; de Paepe et al., 2000; Hoebeke et al., 1996; van Engelenburg–van Lonkhuyzen et al., 2013; van Engelenburg–van Lonkhuyzen et al., 2017b; van Summeren et al., 2018).

Manual therapy techniques such as abdominal massage have not been adequately studied.

Biofeedback is an adjunctive tool to support motor control interventions (Abd El-Moghny et al., 2018; Buckley et al., 2019; Chase et al., 2005; de Jong et al., 2007; Kajbafzadeh et al., 2011; Ladi-Seyedian et al., 2014; Ladi-Seyedian et al., 2015; Ladi-Seyedian et al., 2019; Ladi-Seyedian et al., 2020; Sharifi-Rad et al., 2018; van Engelenburg–van Lonkhuyzen et al., 2013; van Engelen-burg–van Lonkhuyzen et al., 2017b; Vasconcelos et al., 2006). Relevant forms include:

- uroflowmetry,
- electromyography (EMG),
- anorectal manometry,
- rectal balloon training, and
- real-time transabdominal ultrasound.

Overall, due to the breadth of the term *biofeedback*, there is no consistency in applied interventions and equipment used. An added limitation is the diversity of BBD (DUI, constipation, faecal incontinence, con-comitant chronic constipation, faecal incontinence and abnormal defaecation dynamics, faecal incontinence and pelvic floor dyssynergia).

Electrical therapy is an adjunctive intervention (Buckley et al., 2019; Chase et al., 2005; Kajbafzadeh et al., 2015; Ladi-Seyedian et al., 2019; Ladi-Seyedian et al., 2020; Sharifi-Rad et al., 2018):

- Functional electrical stimulation
- Interferential
- Transcutaneous electrical nerve stimulation (TENS)
- Percutaneous electrical nerve stimulation

The use of electrical therapy in children with BBD is not easy. Different modes of application have been trialled in mostly small series of children. There is minimal standardisation of populations, application parameters or outcome measures, and short periods of follow-up. Thus, evidence is largely drawn from low-quality studies with considerable risk of bias (Tables 12.2 and 12.3). A recent Cochrane review found that when comparing TENS versus sham, more children with day wetting receiving active TENS may achieve continence, but there is low-certainty evidence (Buck-ley et al., 2019).

Biofeedback and electrical therapy are adjunctive treatments that form part of a 'package' of prescribed interventions rather than being provided as stand-alone interventions. Clearly, biofeedback and electrical therapy in physical therapy practice warrants large, con-trolled and randomised studies.

EVIDENCE OF PHYSICAL THERAPY IN CHILDREN

A large variation of applied physical therapeutic inter-ventions has been published across a heterogeneous group of childhood BBD dysfunctions. Evidence was gathered from randomised controlled trials (RCTs). The PubMed, Cochrane Library and PEDro databases were searched from inception to 1 October 2020 with the following keywords (MeSH and free-text words): *(day/night time urinary/f(a)ecal) incontinence, enuresis, bedwetting, constipation, dysfunctional elimination syn-drome, (dyssynergic/dyssynergia micturition/def(a)eca-tion), encopresis, anismus, biofeedback, electrical (nerve) stimulation, electrotherapy, manometry, physiotherapy/ physical therapy, core stability, musculoskeletal, massage, myofeedback, pelvic floor (muscles) (training), exercises, sensory processing, toilet training, child(ren), childhood and p(a)ediatric.*

We included all RCTs or quasi-RCTs where physical therapists were involved in the study and assessed in at least one trial arm the effect of (a form) of physical ther-apy. Other trial arms must include one of the following: another form of physical therapy, 'no intervention', addi-tional motor control–related intervention, sham or pla-cebo intervention, or medication in children (aged 4–18 years) presenting with a history of BBD (as defined by the trial authors). All languages were eligible for inclusion.

We excluded studies on adults and neurological, psy-chological, psychiatric, congenital, surgery, drug, non childhood BBD studies, and complementary and alter-native medicine.

Table 12.2 shows data of 14 RCTs, and Table 12.3 presents the PEDro quality scores of the trials.

When possible, we pooled outcome data from rele-vant studies that were sufficiently similar in interven-tions and length (6 and 12 months) of follow-up. The following conclusions were drawn:

TABLE 12.2	Characteristics of Included Studies
	STANDARD MEDICAL CARE VS PHYSICAL THERAPY
Author	**Kajbafzadeh et al. (2011)**
Design	2-arm RCT
N	80
Diagnosis	Dysfunctional elimination syndrome
Protocol	SMC vs PT
Completed	100% at 6 months and 1 year following treatment
Results	No data on number of children cured from, their initial choice of inclusion, dysfunctional voiding and simultaneous constipation and/or faecal soiling available
Author	**Vesna et al. (2011)**
Design	2-arm RCT
N	86
Diagnosis	Dysfunctional voiding
Protocol	SMC vs PT
Completed	87.2% at 12 months after start of study
Results	No prespecified primary outcomes on dysfunctional voiding reported
Author	**Ladi-Seyedian et al. (2014)**
Design	2-arm RCT
N	60
Diagnosis	Dysfunctional voiding
Protocol	SMC (standard urotherapy) vs PT
Completed	98.3% at 12 months
Results	No data on number of children cured from, their initial choice of inclusion or dysfunctional voiding, available
Author	**Ladi-Seyedian et al. (2015)**
Design	2-arm RCT
N	50
Diagnosis	Non-neuropathic UAB
Protocol	SMC vs PT, uroflowmetry and EMG BF
Completed	100% at 12 months
Results	No data on number of children cured from, their initial choice of inclusion or non-neuropathic UAB available
Author	**Kajbafzadeh et al. (2015)**
Design	2-arm RCT
N	36
Diagnosis	Non-neuropathic UAB
Protocol	PT vs PT IF-FES
Completed	36 (100%) at 12 months
Results	No data on number of children cured from, their initial choice of inclusion or UAB available
Author	**Van Engelenburg–van Lonkhuyzen et al. (2016)**
Design	2-arm RCT
N	53
Diagnosis	Constipation (Rome III)

TABLE 12.2 Characteristics of Included Studies—cont'd

STANDARD MEDICAL CARE VS PHYSICAL THERAPY

Protocol	SMC vs PT
Completed	92.5% at 6 months
Results	Significantly more children receiving PT cured (observed) (odds ratio: 7.1, 95% CI: 1.4–36.4, p = 0.02)
Author	**Van Summeren et al. (2019)**
Design	2-arm RCT
N	134
Diagnosis	Constipation (Rome III)
Protocol	SMC vs PT
Completed	83.6% at 4 months; 76.1% at 8 months
Results	No significant differences found at 8 months (adjusted RR: 0.8, 95% CI: 0.44–1.3, p = 0.4 NS; no ITT)

PT vs any other form of PT

Author	**Vasconcelos et al. (2006)**
Design	2-arm RCT
N	59 at 12 months
Diagnosis	Dysfunctional elimination syndrome
Protocol	PT over 3-month period vs PT + BF (EMG) over 2-month period
Completed	94.9%
Results	No prespecified primary outcomes on dysfunctional elimination syndrome reported
Author	**Van Kampen et al. (2009)**
Design	2-arm RCT
N	63
Diagnosis	Enuresis
Protocol	PT vs PT + BF (BF: unclear)
Completed	93.7% at 6 months
Results	No significant differences found at 6 months (RR: 1.29, 95% CI: 0.31–5.31, p = 0.72) and at 18 months (RR: 0.36, 95% CI: 0.08–1.62, p = 0.18; no ITT)
Author	**Abd El-Moghny et al., 2018**
Design	3-arm RCT
N	90
Diagnosis	Monosymptomatic enuresis
Protocol	PT vs PT + BF; anal pressure probe vs PT + FES; endoanal probe
Completed	100% at 3 months
Results	No significant differences found at 6 months (RR: 0.78, 95% CI: 0.75–1.01, p = 0.07
Author	**Sharifi-Rad et al. (2018)**
Design	2-arm RCT
N	90
Diagnosis	Functional constipation (Rome III)
Protocol	PT + sham IF vs PT + IF
Completed	98.9% at 6 months

Continued

TABLE 12.2	**Characteristics of Included Studies—cont'd**
	STANDARD MEDICAL CARE VS PHYSICAL THERAPY
Results	Significant differences found at 6 months in favour of PT + IF (RR: 0.45, 95% CI: 0.27–0.76, p = 0.002
Author	**Ladi-Seyedian et al. (2019)**
Design	2-arm RCT
N	46
Diagnosis	Urinary incontinence
Protocol	PT vs PT + IF electrical stimulation (transcutaneous)
Completed	100% at 6 and 12 months
Results	At 6-month follow-up, urinary incontinence significantly reduced in favour of PT + IF (PT: 13/23 [56.5%] vs PT + IF: 19/23 [82%], p < 0.04; at 12 months, respectively 6/23 [26%] and 13/23 [56.5%], p = 0.5)
Author	**Ladi-Seyedian et al. (2020)**
Design	2-arm RCT
N	34
Diagnosis	Bladder and bowel dysfunction
Protocol	PT vs PT + IF electrical stimulation (transcutaneous)
Completed	100% after 10 treatment sessions
Results	Significantly more children receiving PT + IF (11/17 [64.7%]) had full response (100% reduction of bladder and bowel dysfunction symptoms) vs PT (5/15 [29.4%], p = <0.03)
PT vs medical treatment	
Author	**Campos et al. (2013)**
Design	2-arm RCT
N	47
Diagnosis	Non-monosymptomatic enuresis
Protocol	Antimuscarinic treatment vs PT: pelvic floor muscle training and diaphragmatic breathing
Completed	93.6% at 3 months
Results	No significant differences found (RR: 0.61, 95% CI: 0.35–1.06, p = 0.008; no ITT)

BF, Biofeedback; *EMG*, electromyography; *FES*, functional electrical stimulation; *IF*, interferential; *ITT*, intention to treat; *PT*, physiotherapy/physical therapy; *NS*, not statistically significant; *RCT*, randomized controlled trial; *RR*, relative risk; *SMC*, standard medical care; *UAB*, underactive bladder.

- DUI: No significant differences between the effect of the interventions at 6 months and at 12 months were found, although at 12 months there was a trend towards improvement in incontinent children receiving physical therapy.
- Nocturnal enuresis: Pooling the results of these studies, at 6 months, no differences were shown between the effect of the interventions, although there was a trend towards improvement in enuretic children receiving physical therapy. Statistically significantly more children receiving physical therapy were cured at 12 months.
- Constipation: At 6 and at 12 months, significant differences occurred in favour of physical therapy.
- Faecal incontinence: At 6 and at 12 months, no significant difference in the effect of the interventions was shown, although there was a trend towards improvement in the groups of children receiving physical therapy at 6 and 12 months.

TABLE 12.3 **PEDro quality score of randomised trials of physiotherapy for childhood bladder and/or bowel dysfunctions**

Study	BBD*	E	1	2	3	4	5	6	7	8	9	10	Total
Campos 2013 (Campos, et al. 2013)	Non monosymptomatic enuresis	?	+	+	+	-	-	?	+	-	?	?	4
Kajbafzadeh 2011 (Kajbafzadeh, et al. 2011)	Dysfunctional elimination syndrome (bowel and voiding dysfunction)	?	?	?	?	-	-	?	+	+	?	+	3
Kajbafzadeh 2015 (Kajbafzadeh, et al. 2015)	Non-neuropathic underactive bladder in children with voiding dysfunction	+	+	+	+	-	-	?	+	+	?	?	5
Ladi-Seyedian 2014 (Ladi-Seyedian, et al. 2014)	Dysfunctional voiding	-	+	+	+	-	-	?	+	+	+	+	7
Ladi-Seyedian 2015 (Ladi-Seyedian, et al. 2015)	Non-neuropathic underactive bladder in children with voiding dysfunction	+	+	+	+	-	-	?	+	+	?	?	5
Ladi-Seyedian 2019 (Ladi-Seyedian, et al. 2019)	Urinary incontinence	?	+	+	+	-	-	?	+	+	+	+	7
Ladi-Seyedian 2020 (Ladi-Seyedian, et al. 2020)	Bladder Bowel Dysfunction	+	+	?	+	-	-	?	+	+	?	?	4
Sharifi-Rad 2018 (Sharifi-Rad, et al. 2018)	Constipation (Rome III)	+	+	+	+	-	-	+	+	-	+	+	7
van Engelenburg-van Lonkhuyzen 2017 (van Engelenburg-van Lonkhuyzen, et al. 2017)	Constipation (Rome III)	+	+	+	+	-	-	+	+	+	+	+	8
van Kampen 2009 (Van Kampen, et al. 2009)	Nocturnal enuresis	-	+	+	+	-	-	-	+	-	?	+	5
van Summeren 2019 (van Summeren, et al. 2019)	Constipation (Rome III)	?	+	+	?	-	-	+	-	-	-	-	3
Vasconcelos 2006 (Vasconcelos, et al. 2006)	Dysfunctional elimination syndrome	?	+	+	?	-	-	?	+	-	-	-	3
Zivcovic 2011 (Zivkovic, et al. 2011)	Dysfunctional voiding	?	+	+	?	-	-	?	+	-	-	-	3

* BBD Included bladder and bowel dysfunctions as defined by the authors
E= Eligibility criteria specified; 1 = Random allocation; 2 = Concealed allocation; 3 = Groups similar at baseline; 4 = Subjects blinded; 5 = herapists administering treatment blinded; 6 = Assessors blinded; 7 = Measures of at least one primary key outcome obtained from >85% of subjects; 8 = Data analysed by tension to treat; 9 = Statistical comparisons between groups conducted; 10 = Both point measures and measures of variability provided.
+: criterion is clearly satisfied; –: criterion is not satisfied; ?: not clear if the criterion was satisfied. Total scores are out of 10.

TOOLS UTILIZED TO DIAGNOSE AND EVALUATE CHILDHOOD BLADDER OR BOWEL DYSFUNCTION

Measurement instruments applied to diagnose and further evaluate childhood BBD in clinical practice were identified. The PubMed and COSMIN (COnsensus-based Standards for the selection of health Measurement Instruments) databases were searched on questionnaires, health-related patient-reported outcomes and quality of life measures, developed for children (aged 4–18 years) presenting with a history of BBD. Having been published in English (preferably translated to other languages), easy to obtain and suitable for use in physical therapy practice were other conditions. The quality of measurements instrument is crucial (De Vet et al., 2011), and description of the development and testing the psychometric qualities (validation, reliability, responsiveness and interpretability) should be published (Mokkink et al., 2010a; Mokkink et al., 2010b; Mokkink et al., 2016). Therefore we excluded instruments that did not meet this last condition.

Overall, five health-related patient-reported outcomes were identified. The questionnaires were ranked by year of publication and are described in Table 12.4. One quality-of-life questionnaire was included (Paediatric Incontinence Quality of Life [PinQ]) (Bower et al., 2006b), because it is disease specific for childhood lower urinary tract symptoms.

Dysfunctional Voiding Scoring System

Farhat et al., 2000) developed the Dysfunctional Voiding Scoring System (DVSS), a 10-item parent-completed questionnaire, with seven items pertaining to bladder symptoms, two related to bowel symptoms and one addressing quality of life. A Turkish version (Kaya Narter et al., 2017) and a Brazilian version (Rizzini et al., 2009) were identified. Criterion validity was reported, and the cut-off score was 6.026 for females (sensitivity 92.77% and specificity 87.09%) and 9.02 for males (sensitivity of 80.95% and specificity of 91.3%).

Vancouver Symptom Score for Dysfunctional Elimination Syndrome

The Vancouver Symptom Score for Dysfunctional Elimination Syndrome (VSSDES), originally the Vancouver-NULTD/DES questionnaire (Afshar et al., 2009), was developed by Afshar et al. (2009) and primarily has a diagnostic purpose. Factor analysis of the Vancouver-NULTD/DES showed loading on four factors, corresponding to UI, urgency (of urine), obstruction (of urine) and constipation/faecal incontinence. The receiver operating characteristic curve showed a score of 11 as the optimum threshold with an area under the curve of 0.903 (95% CI: 0.814–0.948). Test–retest reliability was good ($r = 0.845$, $p < 0.001$). Cronbach's α total score was 0.445, and Cronbach's α's of subscales were not reported.

Childhood Bladder and Bowel Dysfunction Questionnaire

With the close cooperation of parents of children aged 5 to 15 years, both with and without childhood BBD, Van Engelenburg–van Lonkhuyzen et al. (2017a) developed an 18-item instrument. For use among children aged 5 to 12 years, the Childhood Bladder and Bowel Dysfunction Questionnaire (CBBDQ5-12y) is feasible, and it demonstrates content and structural validity and good internal consistency and test–retest reliability (bladder: Cronbach's α: 0.74, intra-class correlation [ICC]: 0.95 (95% CI 0.93-0.96); bowel: Cronbach's α: 0.71, ICC: 0.94 (95% CI: 0.91-0.96)) (Van Engelenburg–van Lonkhuyzen et al., 2017a).

Iowa Pediatric Bladder and Bowel Dysfunction Questionnaire

Anwar et al., 2019 developed the Iowa Pediatric Bladder and Bowel Dysfunction (Iowa Ped BBD) questionnaire, an 18-item, 5-point Likert scale, diagnostic questionnaire for those aged 3 to 19 years (mean age 9.5 years) capturing bladder (11 items) and bowel (6 items) dysfunction and QoL (1 item). Content and structural validity were reported. The internal consistency of the enuresis and lower urinary tract symptoms subscales was good (Cronbach's α: 0.81 and 0.74, respectively) and acceptable for the bowel symptoms subscale (Cronbach's α: 0.62). Test–retest demonstrated a strong correlation between the number of subjective symptoms reported by patients and the total questionnaire score. The Pearson correlation coefficient was 0.81. Sensitivity (83.4%) and specificity (87.6), as well as area under the curve (0.935, $p < 0.001$), were reported.

Paediatric Incontinence Quality of Life

Bower et al. (2006b, 2006c) described the development and the validation process of the PinQ. The instrument was valid. Test–retest reliability was reported: ICC total score 0.88 (95% CI: 0.79–0.94, $p < 0.0001$), ICC intrinsic subscale

TABLE 12.4 Childhood Bladder or Bowel Dysfunction Questionnaires

Questionnaire (Author), Abbreviation and Age Children (Years)	Number of Items, Scale/Subscales	Psychometric Qualities According to COSMIN
Dysfunctional voiding scoring system (Farhat et al., 2000) DVSS 3–10	Total: 10 (scores: 0–30) Bladder: 7 Bowel: 2 QoL: 1	Validity: criterion ROC, females cut of 6.03 (sensitivity: 92.77%, specificity: 87.09%); males 9.02 (sensitivity: 80.95%, specificity: 91.3%) Reliability: ICC children 0.41 (95% CI: 0.07–0.66); ICC parents 0.41 (95% CI: 0.07–0.67) Responsiveness: NR
Vancouver NULTD/DES questionnaire (Afshar et al., 2009) VSSDES 4–16	Total: 14 (scores: 0–72), 5-point Likert scale Bladder: 10 Bowel: 3 Feasibility: 1	Validity: construct ICC agreement; 0.67 95%CI(0.18–0.84) (External criterium VSSDES) Criterion validity: AUC 0.98 95% CI(0.96–0.99) Reliability: Bladder: Cronbach's α = 0.74; ICC: 0.80 95%CI(0.74–0.86), Bowel: Cronbach's α = 0.71 test/retest: ICC agreement 0.94 (95%CI:0.91–0.96) Responsiveness: NR
Childhood Bladder and Bowel Dysfunction Questionnaire (Van Engelenburg–van Lonkhuyzen et al. 2017a) CBBDQ5-12y 5–12	Total: 18 (scores: 0–72), 5-point Likert scale Bladder: 10 (0–40) Bowel: 8 (0–32)	Validity: content and structural Reliability: bladder (Cronbach's α = 0.74, ICC: 0.80, 95% CI: 0.74–0.86; bowel (Cronbach's α = 0.71, ICC: 0.79, 95% CI: 0.70–0.85) Responsiveness: under study
Iowa Pediatric Bladder and Bowel Dysfunction Questionnaire (Anwar et al., 2019) Iowa Ped BBD 3–19[a]	Total: 18 (scores: 0–72), 5-point Likert scale Bladder: 11 Bowel: 6 QoL: 1	Validity: criterion ROC (sensitivity: 83.4%, specificity: 87.6%, AUC: 0.935, p < 0.001) Reliability: LUTS Cronbach's α = 0.74; enuresis Cronbach's α = 0.81, urinary holding Cronbach's α = NR; bowel symptoms Cronbach's α = 0.62; DUI Cronbach's α = NR; bother associated with BBD Cronbach's α = NR; test–retest reliability (r = 0.81); 40 patients Responsiveness: NR
Paediatric Incontinence Quality of Life (Bower et al., 2006b) PinQ-p****; PinQ 6–17	Total: 20 (scores: 0–80), 5-point Likert scale	Validity: structural, Rasch: 110–199 subjects (adequate) Reliability: intrinsic factors Cronbach's α = 0.91, ICC: 0.86, 95% CI: 0.75–0.93, p < 0.0001; extrinsic factors Cronbach's α = 0.72, ICC: 0.88, 95% CI: 0.78–0.93, p < 0.0001 Responsiveness: NR

[a]Answered by child > 8 years: [b]: proxy version, parents to answer
AUC, Area under the curve; *BBD*, bladder or bowel dysfunction; *COSMIN*, COnsensus-based Standards for the selection of health Measurement Instruments; *DUI*, daytime urinary incontinence; *ICC*, intra-class correlation; *LUTS*, lower urinary tract symptoms; *QoL*, quality of life; *NR*, not reported; *ROC*, receiver operating characteristic.
ICC: two-way mixed, 0.81–1 ('almost perfect'), 0.61–0.8 ('good'), 41–0.6 ('acceptable'), 0.21–0.4 ('moderate'), 0–0.2 ('hardly'), <0 ('poor'); Cronbach's α: 0.7–0.89 ('good'), 0.6–0.69 ('acceptable'), ≤0.59 ('poor').
Rasch: ≥200 subjects (very good), 100 to 199 subjects (adequate), 50 to 99 subjects (doubtful), <50 subjects (inadequate).
Pearson's correlation coefficient (r): 0.90 > r ≤ 1.00 'very high (positive)'; 0.70 > r ≤ 0.90 'high (positive)'; 0.50 > r < 0.70 'average'; 30 > r ≤ 0.50 'poor' 0.00 > r ≤ 0.30 'hardly or no correlation'.

score 0.86 (95% CI: 0.75–0.93, p < 0.0001) and ICC extrinsic subscale 0.88 (95% CI: 0.78–0.93, p < 0.0001). Cronbach's α's for intrinsic and extrinsic factors were 0.91 and 0.72, respectively. PinQ was able to detect clinically important changes over time (Bower et al., 2006b).

Behavioural Comorbidities

Behavioural comorbidities can be assessed using the Short Screening Instrument for Psychological Problems in Enuresis (SSIPPE) (Van Hoeck et al., 2007), Strengths and Difficulties Questionnaire (SDQ) (Muris et al., 2003;

Muris et al., 2004), the parental Child Behavior Checklist (CBCL/6-18) or the Pediatric Quality of Life Inventory (PedsQL) (Varni et al., 2011) among others.

RECOMMENDATIONS AND DISCUSSION

To date, the evidence for physical therapy as a separate modality in the management of childhood BBD is limited by lack of higher-quality research. Regarding pelvic floor muscle training, efficacy measurement strategy must be non-invasive and specific to what is being measured. To date, secondary measures have been used, such as uroflow, post-void residual and severity of incontinence. Measurement of muscle function is problematic; a gold standard methodology is warranted. Both transabdominal and transperineal ultrasound hold promise, having been validated for this purpose in adults and shown to be useful in children (Bower et al., 2006a).

Clinicians and researchers need to be vigilant about confounders of measurement. Kinesiological electromyography (EMG) is used in biofeedback (flowmetry, EMG feedback, etc.) and is an indicator of the absence/presence of striated muscle activity, but care needs to be taken if measuring the effects of training (Bø, 2015). An EMG reading alone is not comparable on two different occasions. Pelvic floor muscle EMG and pressure measurements can be affected by contact of electrodes, posture, talking, breathing and especially 'cross-talk' from surrounding muscles. Muscle measurement needs to be done in a standardised position before and after intervention and confounders controlled.

It is necessary to acknowledge the distinct age-related differences in children to make informed decisions about optimal clinical interventions. Developmental maturation of the child, and individual biomechanical and musculoskeletal status will inform each clinician's approach to providing a part or whole solution for children with continence difficulties. Children are physically different and changing over time, and under the influence of rapidly altering cognitive function and abilities. Cognitive ability and motor performance go hand in hand to develop functional outcomes in children (Chase and Schrale, 2017), whereas in adults there are demarcations in some research (e.g., childbearing years, postmenopause, etc.) interventions for BBD in childhood do not yet take age and development into account.

Without a complete published description of interventions, clinicians and patients cannot reliably implement interventions that are shown to be useful, and other researchers cannot replicate or build on research findings. In physical therapy, consensus-based approaches to pelvic floor muscle exercises as Slade et al. (2021) described are of use, as are available published study protocols (van Engelenburg–van Lonkhuyzen et al., 2013; van Summeren et al., 2018). The Template for Intervention Description and Replication (TIDieR) checklist and guide has been developed, and it is recommended that future studies should adhere to the 12 items (Hoffmann et al., 2014).

The future aim is to bring the level of evidence for physical therapy working with children to the same level as exists in adults with incontinence. Evidence-based practice involves not only scientific evidence from systematic research but also the physical therapist's expertise and judgement combined with the values and preferences of the child and family.

ACKNOWLEDGEMENT

We thank Wendy Bower for reading and approving the content of this chapter.

REFERENCES

Abd El-Moghny, S. M., El-Din, M. S., & El Shemy, S. A. (2018). Effectiveness of intra-anal biofeedback and electrical stimulation in the treatment of children with refractory monosymptomatic nocturnal enuresis: A comparative randomized controlled trial. *International Neurourology Journal*, 22(4), 295–304.

Afshar, K., Mirbagheri, A., Scott, H., et al. (2009). Development of a symptom score for dysfunctional elimination syndrome. *Journal of Urology*, 182(Suppl. 4), 1939–1943.

Anwar, T., Cooper, C. S., Lockwood, G., et al. (2019). Assessment and validation of a screening questionnaire for the diagnosis of pediatric bladder and bowel dysfunction. *Journal of Pediatric Urology*, 15(5), 528.e1–528.e8.

Austin, P. F., Bauer, S. B., Bower, W., et al. (2016). The standardization of terminology of lower urinary tract function in children and adolescents: Update report from the standardization committee of the international children's continence society. *Neurourology and Urodynamics*, 35(4), 471–481.

Beaudry-Bellefeuille, I., & Lane, S. J. (2017). Examining sensory overresponsiveness in preshcool children with retentive fecal incontinence. *American Journal of Occupational Therapy*, 71(5), 1–8.

Beaudry-Bellefeuille, I., Lane, S. J., & Lane, A. E. (2019). Sensory integration concerns in children with functional defecation disorders: A scoping review. *American Journal of Occupational Therapy, 73*(3), 1–13.

Bø, K. (2015). Measurements of pelvic floor muscle function and strengths, and pelvic organ prolapse. In K. Bø, B. Berghmans, S. Mørkved, et al. (Eds.), *Evidence-based physical therapy for the pelvic floor* (2nd ed.) (pp. 44–109). Edinburgh: Churchill Livingstone/Elsevier.

Bower, W. F., Chase, J. W., & Stillman, B. C. (2006a). Normative pelvic floor parameters in children assessed by transabdominal ultrasound. *Journal of Urology, 176*(1), 337–341.

Bower, W. F., Sit, F. K. Y., Bluyssen, N., et al. (2006b). PinQ: A valid, reliable and reproducible quality-of-life measure in children with bladder dysfunction. *Journal of Pediatric Urology, 2*(3), 185–189.

Bower, W. F., Wong, E. M., & Yeung, C. K. (2006c). Development of a validated quality of life tool specific to children with bladder dysfunction. *Neurourology and Urodynamics, 25*(3), 221–227.

Buckley, B. S., Sanders, C. D., Spineli, L., et al. (2019). Conservative interventions for treating functional daytime urinary incontinence in children. *Cochrane Database of Systematic Reviews, 9,* CD012367.

Burgers, R., de Jong, T. P. V. M., Visser, M., et al. (2013a). Functional defecation disorders in children with lower urinary tract symptoms. *Journal of Urology, 189*(5), 1886–1891.

Burgers, R. E., Mugie, S. M., Chase, J., et al. (2013b). Management of functional constipation in children with lower urinary tract symptoms: Report from the standardization committee of the international children's continence society. *Journal of Urology, 190*(1), 29–36.

Campos, R. M., Gugliotta, A., Ikari, O., et al. (2013). Comparative, prospective, and randomized study between urotherapy and the pharmacological treatment of children with urinary incontinence. *Einstein (Sao Paulo), 11*(2), 203–208.

Chase, J., Austin, P., Hoebeke, P., et al. (2010). The management of dysfunctional voiding in children: A report from the standardisation committee of the international children's continence society. *Journal of Urology, 183*(4), 1296–1302.

Chase, J., Robertson, V. J., Southwell, B., et al. (2005). Pilot study using transcutaneous electrical stimulation (interferential current) to treat chronic treatment-resistant constipation and soiling in children. *Journal of Gastroenterology and Hepatology, 20*(7), 1054–1061.

Chase, J., & Schrale, L. (2017). Childhood incontinence and pelvic floor muscle function: Can we learn from adult research? *Journal of Pediatric Urology, 13,* 94–101.

Chase, J. W., Stillman, B. C., Gibb, S. M., et al. (2009). Trunk strength and mobility changes in children with slow transit constipation. *Journal of Gastroenterology and Hepatology, 24*(12), 1876–1884.

Collis, D., Kennedy-Behr, A., & Kearney, L. (2019). The impact of bowel and bladder problems on children's quality of life and their parents: A scoping review. *Child: Care, Health and Development, 45*(1), 1–14.

De Jong, T. P. V. M., Klijn, A. J., Vijverberg, M. A. W., et al. (2007). Effect of biofeedback training on paradoxical pelvic floor movement in children with dysfunctional voiding. *Urology, 70*(4), 790–793.

De Paepe, H., Hoebeke, P., Renson, C., et al. (1998). Pelvic-floor therapy in girls with recurrent urinary tract infections and dysfunctional voiding. *British Journal of Urology, 81*(Suppl. 3), 109–113.

De Paepe, H., Renson, C., Hoebeke, P., et al. (2002). The role of pelvic-floor therapy in the treatment of lower urinary tract dysfunctions in children. *Scandinavian Journal of Urology and Nephrology, 36*(4), 260–267.

De Paepe, H., Renson, C., Van Laecke, E., et al. (2000). Pelvic-floor therapy and toilet training in young children with dysfunctional voiding and obstipation. *BJU International, 85*(7), 889–893.

De Vet, H. C. W., Terwee, C. B., Mokkink, L. B., et al. (2011). *Measurement in medicine: A practical guide. Practical guides to Biostatistics and Epidemiology.* Cambridge: Cambridge University Press.

Farhat, W., Bagli, D. J., Capolicchio, G., et al. (2000). The dysfunctional voiding scoring system: Quantitative standardization of dysfunctional voiding symptoms in children. *Journal of Urology, 164*(3 Pt. 2), 1011–1015.

Fitzgerald, M. P., Thom, D. H., Wassel-Fyr, C., et al. (2006). Childhood urinary symptoms predict adult overactive bladder symptoms. *Journal of Urology, 175*(3 Pt. 1), 989–993.

Franco, I. (2012). Functional bladder problems in children: Pathophysiology, diagnosis, and treatment. *Pediatric Clinics of North America, 59*(4), 783–817.

Franco, I., Austin, P., Bauer, S., et al. (Eds.). (2015). *Pediatric incontinence: Evaluation and clinical management.* Oxford: Wiley Blackwell.

Heron, J., Grzeda, M. T., von Gontard, A., et al. (2017). Trajectories of urinary incontinence in childhood and bladder and bowel symptoms in adolescence: Prospective cohort study. *BMJ Open, 7*(3), e014238.

Heron, J., Joinson, C., Croudace, T., et al. (2008). Trajectories of daytime wetting and soiling in a United Kingdom 4 to 9-year-old population birth cohort study. *Journal of Urology, 179*(5), 1970–1975.

Hodges, P. W., Sapsford, R., & Pengel, L. H. (2007). Postural and respiratory functions of the pelvic floor muscles. *Neurourology and Urodynamics, 26*(3), 362–371.

Hoebeke, P., Vande Walle, J., Theunis, M., et al. (1996). Outpatient pelvic-floor therapy in girls with daytime incontinence and dysfunctional voiding. *Urology, 48*(6), 923–927.

Hoffmann, T. C., Glasziou, P. P., Milne, R., et al. (2014). Better reporting of interventions: Template for intervention description and replication (TIDieR) checklist and guide. *British Medical Journal*, 7(348), g1687.

Hyams, J. S., Di Lorenzo, C., Saps, M., et al. (2016). Childhood functional gastrointestinal disorders: Child/adolescent. *Gastroenterology*, 150, 1456–1468.

Kajbafzadeh, A. M., Sharifi-Rad, L., Ghahestani, S. M., et al. (2011). Animated biofeedback: An ideal treatment for children with dysfunctional elimination syndrome. *Journal of Urology*, 186(6), 2379–2384.

Kajbafzadeh, A. M., Sharifi-Rad, L., Mozafarpour, S., et al. (2015). Efficacy of transcutaneous interferential electrical stimulation in treatment of children with primary nocturnal enuresis: A randomized clinical trial. *Pediatric Nephrology*, 30(7), 1139–1145.

Kaya Narter, F., Tarhan, F., Narter, K. F., et al. (2017). Reliability and validity of the bladder and bowel dysfunction questionnaire among Turkish children. *Turkish Journal of Medical Sciences*, 47(6), 1765–1769.

Koppen, I. J., Lammers, L. A., Benninga, M. A., et al. (2015). Management of functional constipation in children: Therapy in practice. *Paediatric Drugs*, 17, 349–360.

Koppen, I. J. N. (2018). Prevalence of functional defecation disorders in children: a systematic review and meta-analysis. *J Pediatr.*, 198, 121–130.

Ladi-Seyedian, S. S., Kajbafzadeh, A.-M., Sharifi-Rad, L., et al. (2015). Management of non-neuropathic underactive bladder in children with voiding dysfunction by animated biofeedback: A randomized clinical trial. *Urology*, 85(1), 205–210.

Ladi-Seyedian, S. S., Sharifi-Rad, L., Ebadi, M., et al. (2014). Combined functional pelvic floor muscle exercises with Swiss ball and urotherapy for management of dysfunctional voiding in children: A randomized clinical trial. *European Journal of Pediatrics*, 173(10), 1347–1353.

Ladi-Seyedian, S. S., Sharifi-Rad, L., & Kajbafzadeh, A.-M. (2019). Pelvic floor electrical stimulation and muscles training: A combined rehabilitative approach for management of non-neuropathic urinary incontinence in children. *Journal of Pediatric Surgery*, 54(4), 825–830.

Ladi-Seyedian, S. S., Sharifi-Rad, L., & Kajbafzadeh, A.-M. (2020). Management of bladder bowel dysfunction in children by pelvic floor interferential electrical stimulation and muscle exercises: A randomized clinical trial. *Urology*, 144, 182–187.

Mokkink, L. B., Prinsen, C. A. C., Bouter, L. M., et al. (2016). The COnsensus-based Standards for the selection of health Measurement INstruments (COSMIN) and how to select an outcome measurement instrument. *Brazilian Journal of Physical Therapy*, 20(2), 105–113.

Mokkink, L. B., Terwee, C. B., Patrick, D. L., et al. (2010a). The COSMIN checklist for assessing the methodological quality of studies on measurement properties of health status measurement instruments: An international delphi study. *Quality of Life Research*, 19(4), 539–549.

Mokkink, L. B., Terwee, C. B., Patrick, D. L., et al. (2010b). The COSMIN study reached international consensus on taxonomy, terminology, and definitions of measurement properties for health-related patient-reported outcomes. *Journal of Clinical Epidemiology*, 63(7), 737–745.

Muris, P., Meesters, C., Eijkelenboom, A., et al. (2004). The self-report version of the strengths and difficulties questionnaire: Its psychometric properties in 8- to 13-year-old non-clinical children. *British Journal of Clinical Psychology*, 43(Pt. 4), 437–448.

Muris, P., Meesters, C., & van den Berg, F. (2003). The Strengths and Difficulties Questionnaire (SDQ)—further evidence for its reliability and validity in a community sample of Dutch children and adolescents. *European Child & Adolescent Psychiatry*, 12(1), 1–8.

Nevéus, T., Fonseca, E., Franco, I., et al. (2020a). Management and treatment of nocturnal enuresis—an updated standardization document from the International Children's Continence Society. *Journal of Pediatric Urology*, 16(1), 10–19.

Nevéus, T., Eggert, P., Evans, J., et al. (2020b). Evaluation of and treatment for monosymptomatic enuresis: A standardization document from the international children's continence society. *Journal of Urology*, 183(2), 441–447.

Pollock, M. R. (2012). *The association between sensory processing disorder and dysfunctional elimination syndrome in children*. Department of Rehabilitation Sciences, University of Toledo.

Riegler, G., & Esposito, I. (2001). Bristol scale stool form. A still valid help in medical practice and clinical research. *Techniques in Coloproctology*, 5(3), 163–164.

Rizzini, M., Donatti, T. L., Bergamaschi, D. P., et al. (2009). [Conceptual, item, and semantic equivalence of the Brazilian version of the Dysfunctional Voiding Scoring System (DVSS) instrument for evaluating lower urinary tract dysfunction in children]. *Cadernos de Saúde Pública*, 25(8), 1743–1755.

Sapsford, R. (2004). Rehabilitation of pelvic floor muscles utilizing trunk stabilization. *Manual Therapy*, 9(1), 3–12.

Sapsford, R. R., & Hodges, P. W. (2001). Contraction of the pelvic floor muscles during abdominal maneuvers. *Archives of Physical Medicine and Rehabilitation*, 82(8), 1081–1088.

Sharifi-Rad, L., Ladi-Seyedian, S. S., Manouchehri, N., et al. (2018). Effects of interferential electrical stimulation plus pelvic floor muscles exercises on functional constipation in children: A randomized clinical trial. *American Journal of Gastroenterology*, 112(2), 295–302.

Silva, C. A., & Motta, M. E. (2013). The use of abdominal muscle training, breathing exercises and abdominal massage to treat paediatric chronic functional constipation. *Colorectal Disease*, 15(5), e250–e255.

Slade, S. C., Morris, M. E., Frawley, H., et al. (2021). Comprehensive reporting of pelvic floor muscle training for urinary incontinence: CERT-PFMT. *Physiotherapy*, 112, 103–112.

Van Dijk, M., Benninga, M. A., Grootenhuis, M. A., et al. (2010). Prevalence and associated clinical characteristics of behavior problems in constipated children. *Pediatrics*, 125(2), e309–e317.

Van Engelenburg–van Lonkhuyzen, M. L., Bols, E. M. J., Bastiaenen, C. H. G., et al. (2017a). Childhood bladder and bowel dysfunction questionnaire: Development, feasibility and aspects of validity and reliability. *Journal of Pediatric Gastroenterology and Nutrition*, 64(6), 911–917.

Van Engelenburg–van Lonkhuyzen, M. L., Bols, E. M. J., Benninga, M. A., et al. (2013). The effect of pelvic physiotherapy on reduction of functional constipation in children: Design of a multicentre randomised controlled trial. *BMC Pediatrics*, 13(1), 112.

Van Engelenburg–van Lonkhuyzen, M. L., Bols, E. M. J., Benninga, M. A., et al. (2016). Physiotherapy interventions for functional bladder and bowel dysfunctions in neurologically normal and otherwise healthy children (Protocol). *Cochrane Database of Systematic Reviews*, 11, CD012434.

Van Engelenburg–van Lonkhuyzen, M. L., Bols, E. M. J., Benninga, M. A., et al. (2017b). Effectiveness of pelvic physiotherapy in children with functional constipation, compared with standard medical care. *Gastroenterology*, 152(152), 82–91.

Van Herzeele, C., Dhondt, K., Roles, S. P., et al. (2016). Desmopressin (melt) therapy in children with monosymptomatic nocturnal enuresis and nocturnal polyuria results in improved neuropsychological functioning and sleep. *Pediatric Nephrology*, 31(9), 1477–1484.

Van Hoeck, K. J., Bael, A., Van Dessel, E., et al. (2007). Do holding exercises or antimuscarinics increase maximum voided volume in monosymptomatic nocturnal enuresis? A randomized controlled trial in children. *Journal of Urology*, 178(5), 2132–2136.

Van Kampen, M., Lemkens, H., Deschamps, A., et al. (2009). Influence of pelvic floor muscle exercises on full spectrum therapy for nocturnal enuresis. *Journal of Urology*, 182(Suppl. 4), 2067–2071.

Van Summeren, J. J. G. T., Holtman, G. A., Kollen, B. J., et al. (2019). Physiotherapy for children with functional constipation: A pragmatic randomized controlled trial in primary care. *Journal Pediatric*, 216, 25–31.

Van Summeren, J. J. G. T., Holtman, G. A., Lisman–van Leeuwen, Y., et al. (2018). Physiotherapy plus conventional treatment versus conventional treatment only in the treatment of functional constipation in children: Design of a randomized controlled trial and cost-effectiveness study in primary care. *BMC Pediatrics*, 18(1), 249.

Varni, J. W., Limbers, C. A., Neighbors, K., et al. (2011). The PedsQL™ infant scales: Feasibility, internal consistency reliability, and validity in healthy and ill infants. *Quality of Life Research*, 20(1), 45–55.

Vasconcelos, M., Lima, E., Caiafa, L., et al. (2006). Voiding dysfunction in children. Pelvic-Floor exercises or biofeedback therapy: A randomized study. *Pediatric Nephrology*, 21(12), 1858–1864.

Vesna, Z. D., Milica, L., Stankovic, I., et al. (2011). The evaluation of combined standard urotherapy, abdominal and pelvic floor retraining in children with dysfunctional voiding. *Journal of Pediatric Urology*, 7(3), 336–341.

Von Gontard, A., Baeyens, D., Van Hoecke, E., et al. (2011). Psychological and psychiatric issues in urinary and fecal incontinence. *Journal of Urology*, 185(4), 1432–1436.

Von Gontard, A., Hussong, J., Yang, S. S., et al. (2022). Neurodevelopmental disorders and incontinence in children and adolescents: Attention-deficit/hyperactivity disorder, autism spectrum disorder, and intellectual disability—a consensus document of the international children's continence society. *Neurourology and Urodynamics*, 41(1), 102–114.

Von Gontard, A., Vrijens, D., Selai, C., et al. (2019). Are psychological comorbidities important in the aetiology of lower urinary tract dysfunction-ICI-RS 2018? *Neurourology and Urodynamics*, 38(Suppl. 5), 8–17.

Vriesman, M. H., Koppen, I. J. N., Camilleri, M., et al. (2020). Management of functional constipation in children and adults. *Nature Reviews Gastroenterology & Hepatology*, 17(1), 21–39.

Wright, A. (2015). The epidemiology of childhood incontinence. In I. Franco, P. Austin, S. Bauer, et al. (Eds.), *Pediatric incontinence: Evaluation and clinical management* (pp. 37–60). Oxford: Wiley Blackwell.

13

Gynaecological Cancer and Pelvic Floor Dysfunction

Helena Frawley and Robyn Brennen

OUTLINE

GYNAECOLOGICAL CANCER PREVALENCE

Gynaecological cancers include cancers of the uterus, ovaries, cervix, vagina, vulva and fallopian tubes and make up 16.5% of all cancers diagnosed in women worldwide (World Cancer Research Fund [WCRF], n.d.). The most common gynaecological cancers are cervical, endometrial and ovarian. In 2018 there were 569,847 cases of cervical cancer diagnosed worldwide (WCRF, n.d.); however, in many high-income countries the number of women diagnosed with cervical cancer has decreased over the past 10 to 30 years due to improved screening and prevention (Arbyn et al., 2020; Organisation for Economic Co-operation and Development, n.d.). In contrast, there has been a global increase in the number of new cases of endometrial and ovarian cancer, linked to increasing population growth, obesity and age (Coburn et al., 2017; Lortet-Tieulent et al., 2018; Zhang et al., 2019). With increasing prevalence and survival rates (Allemani et al., 2018; Zhang et al., 2019), substantially more women are living with the sequelae of gynaecological cancer and cancer treatments.

GYNAECOLOGICAL CANCER TREATMENTS

Treatments for gynaecological cancer include surgery, radiation therapy and pharmacological therapies, including traditional chemotherapy, targeted therapies and hormone therapy (Cancer Australia, 2012). These treatments may impact on pelvic floor (PF) structures, which may contribute to increased prevalence of PF dysfunction in women who have undergone these treatments.

PATHOPHYSIOLOGY AND AETIOLOGY OF PELVIC FLOOR DYSFUNCTION AFTER GYNAECOLOGICAL CANCER

Gynaecological cancer variables that may impact on PF dysfunction include the size, stage and aggressiveness of the tumour, and the type and extent of treatment (Cancer Australia, 2012; Cancer Council, 2016a, 2016b). With advanced size or stage of the tumour, more tissues are affected directly by tumour invasion and indirectly by physical pressure or distortion, which can cause pain, obstruction and necrosis (Jin et al., 2020; Pawlik et al., 2006). The greater the stage and aggressiveness of the

cancer, the more aggressive the treatment, with more extensive surgery and adjuvant therapy (radiotherapy or chemotherapy) required (Ang et al., 2014). These treatments can contribute to PF dysfunction via direct or indirect mechanisms, with possible mechanisms of action shown in Fig. 13.1.

MECHANISMS OF PELVIC FLOOR DYSFUNCTION FOLLOWING GYNAECOLOGICAL CANCER TREATMENT

Two of the most common surgical treatment combinations for gynaecological cancer are total hysterectomy and bilateral salpingo-oophorectomy, and radical hysterectomy and bilateral salpingo-oophorectomy (Cancer Australia, 2012). Radical hysterectomy involves removing additional surrounding tissues, especially the vesicouterine and cardinal ligaments, through which run neurovascular structures that supply the bladder, such as the cervicovesical blood vessels and the inferior hypogastric nerve plexus (Fujii et al., 2007; Jarruwale et al., 2013). Although nerve-sparing radical hysterectomy can be attempted, and may reduce postoperative voiding dysfunction (Bogani et al., 2018; Novackova et al., 2020), outcomes may depend on the extent of the

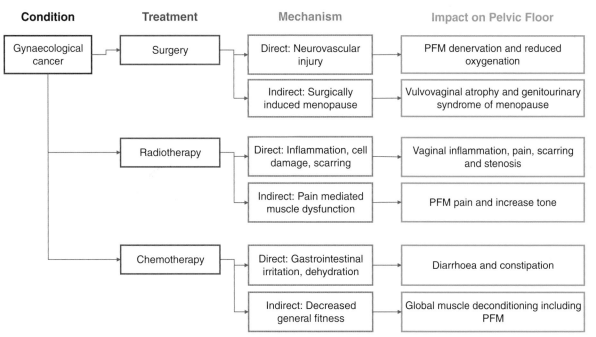

Fig. 13.1 Effect of cancer treatment on the pelvic floor. *PFM*, Pelvic floor muscle.

cancer and surgical skill. Not only can surgery contribute to the morbidity of PF dysfunction through such neural, structural, muscular and vascular damage (Ang et al., 2014; Bernard et al., 2017; Chuang et al., 2003), but the removal of the ovaries can cause surgically induced menopause, or worsen menopause symptoms in postmenopausal women (Faubion et al., 2015). This can contribute to vulvovaginal atrophy and genitourinary syndrome of menopause (Crean-Tate et al., 2020). In women who have retained their ovaries, radiotherapy and chemotherapy can also contribute to ovarian insufficiency and genitourinary syndrome of menopause (American Cancer Society, 2020a, 2020b; Crean-Tate et al., 2020).

Surgery with or without radiotherapy may impact on pelvic floor muscle (PFM) function and morphometry. Increased tone, increased stiffness, reduced flexibility, lower coordination and endurance in the PFMs, measured with an intra-vaginal dynamometric speculum, have been observed in women with urinary incontinence and dyspareunia following hysterectomy with or without adjuvant therapy for endometrial or cervical cancer compared to a control group (Cyr et al., 2021). Similar findings, plus a reduction in PFM strength, have been observed in women with urinary incontinence after hysterectomy and radiotherapy for endometrial cancer (Bernard et al., 2017).

Radiotherapy is delivered via pelvic external-beam radiotherapy (EBRT) or internal vaginal radiotherapy (brachytherapy), with brachytherapy resulting in more localized irradiation than EBRT (American Cancer Society, 2020b). Radiotherapy, especially pelvic EBRT, can result in irradiation of the PFMs as well as the bladder and bowel, which is likely to contribute to morphological and functional changes in these structures (Bernard et al., 2016; Bernard et al., 2017). Irradiated tissues will be affected by inflammation and cell destruction, causing side effects such as radiation cystitis, resulting in urinary urgency, frequency and incontinence; vaginal scarring and stenosis, interfering with sexual function; gastrointestinal inflammation and fibrosis, resulting in diarrhoea and faecal incontinence; and pain (Hofsjö et al., 2017; Hofsjö et al., 2018; Lawrie et al., 2018; Pascoe et al., 2019).

Common side effects of chemotherapy include physical fatigue, reduced physical function and gastrointestinal irritation resulting in diarrhoea (Prue et al., 2010; Shabaruddin et al., 2013). Cancer-related fatigue has

been associated with reduced voluntary muscle fibre recruitment, muscle mass and strength (Kilgour et al., 2010; Yavuzsen et al., 2009); these same effects may occur in the PFMs. Diarrhoea can contribute to faecal incontinence (Milsom et al., 2017), and constipation can be caused by anti-diarrhoeal medication; together with PFM fatigue, these sequalae may be risk factors for developing faecal or urinary incontinence (Dumoulin et al., 2017; Milsom et al., 2017).

PREVALENCE OF PELVIC FLOOR DYSFUNCTION AFTER GYNAECOLOGICAL CANCER

A 2018 systematic review investigated the prevalence of PF dysfunction before and after treatment for gynaecological cancer (Ramaseshan et al., 2018). We ran the same search strategy in June 2020, including articles published between May 2017 and June 2020; this revealed 31 new studies reporting on the prevalence of PF symptoms in women before and after treatment for gynaecological cancer. Of these 31 studies, most reported on cervical cancer (n = 19) (Campbell et al., 2017; Fokdal et al., 2018; Hofsjö et al., 2018; Jensen et al., 2018; Jiang et al., 2019; Lucidi et al., 2017; Miguel et al., 2020; Nantasupha and Charoenkwan, 2018; Novackova et al., 2020; Plotti et al., 2018; Raspagliesi et al., 2017; Shankar et al., 2020; Sun et al., 2018; Wang et al., 2019; Wenzel et al., 2020; Wu et al., 2019; Yang et al., 2020; Yuan et al., 2019; Zhao et al., 2020), whereas the remainder reported on endometrial cancer (n = 3) (Lipetskaia et al., 2019; Segal et al., 2017; Soisson et al., 2018) or on mixed cohorts with different gynaecological cancers (n = 9) (Gressel et al., 2019; Guner et al., 2018; Lindgren et al., 2020; Liu et al., 2020; Ribas et al., 2020; Stabile et al., 2017; Wang et al., 2018; White et al., 2018; Yeung et al., 2020). Combined results of rates of prevalence of PF dysfunction from Ramaseshan et al. (2018) plus our recent search are shown in Table 13.1.

The broad range of prevalence data reported is likely to reflect heterogeneity of type and stage of cancer, type of treatment and time after treatment when symptoms were reported, as well as study design, methods and tools used to collect the prevalence data. Overall, higher rates of urgency urinary incontinence and dyspareunia were present in studies that included radiotherapy with or without other treatments (Gressel et al., 2019; Guner et al., 2018; Hofsjö et al., 2018;

TABLE 13.1 Prevalence of Pelvic Floor Dysfunction in Women Before and After Gynaecological Cancer Treatment

UPDATED SEARCH 2020, INCLUDING RESULTS OF RAMASESHAN ET AL. (2018)										
Cancer	**No. of Patients**	**Cancer Treatment Status**	**Prevalence %**							
			UI	**SUI**	**UUI**	**UR**	**FI**	**FU**	**Dys**	**POP**
Cervical	6898	Before	NR	16–44	8–18	NR	0–6	0–11	NR	16
		After	1–55	4–76	3–59	0–49	2–34	0–52	12–58	NR
Uterine/ endometrial	5912	Before	28	29–36	15–25	NR	3	NR	NR	7
		After	15–74	69–84	67–80	1	11–46	32–55	7–39	5–44
Ovarian	375	Before	NR	32–42	15–39	NR	4	NR	NR	17
		After	NR	NR	NR	NR	7	NR	62	NR
Vulvar	604	Before	NR	44	22	NR	7	NR	62	NR
		After	4–32	6–20	NR	NR	1–20	NR	NR	1–16
Mixed cohorts	1476	Before	NR	5	4	NR	0	48	11–35	NR
		After	NR	8–25	45	NR	3–53	27–41	24–39	NR

Dys, Dyspareunia; *FI*, faecal incontinence; *FU*, faecal urgency; *NR*, not reported; *POP*, pelvic organ prolapse; *SUI*, stress urinary incontinence; *UI*, urinary incontinence; *UR*, urinary retention; *UUI*, urgency urinary incontinence.

Lindgren et al., 2020; Miguel et al., 2020; Segal et al., 2017; Stabile et al., 2017) compared to those that did not (Lucidi et al., 2017; Wang et al., 2018; Wang et al., 2019), whereas rates of faecal urgency were higher in studies that provided radiotherapy only (Jensen et al., 2018; Ribas et al., 2020). Many of the published rates indicate a much higher prevalence of PF symptoms compared to community-dwelling women with no history of gynaecological cancer treatment, who have rates of urinary incontinence of 5% to 69%, stress urinary incontinence of 2% to 29%, urgency urinary incontinence of 1% to 20% and faecal incontinence of 2% to 11% (Milsom et al., 2017). These differences highlight the magnitude of the problem of PF dysfunction in women following treatment for gynaecological cancer.

BURDEN OF PELVIC FLOOR DYSFUNCTION ON GYNAECOLOGICAL CANCER SURVIVORS

The burden of PF dysfunction on women and society is well documented (Lee and Hirayama, 2012; Wagner et al., 2017; Yaakobi et al., 2017). PF symptom distress has been found to be higher in gynaecological cancer survivors than in non-cancer populations (Hazewinkel et al., 2010b; Hazewinkel et al., 2012), with these symptoms remaining distressing over time (Ntinga and Maree, 2015; Sabulei and Maree, 2019). Gynaecological cancer treatments affect not only physiological fertility and physical capacity for penetrative sexual intercourse but also can affect sexual self-image (Sekse et al., 2019). Dyspareunia inhibits sexual function and affects relationships, self-identity and role function (Afiyanti et al., 2020; Fischer et al., 2019). The findings from an integrative review highlight that women needed support from health professionals related to coping with physical, mental and psychosocial well-being including intimate and sensitive issues (Sekse et al., 2019).

Studies have identified positive correlations between PF dysfunction and reduced physical activity in individuals without cancer (Dakic et al., 2021; Lee and Hirayama, 2012). Increased severity of PF symptoms has been associated with reduced physical activity and more sedentary time in women with advanced ovarian cancer (Schofield et al., 2018), and faecal incontinence has been associated with reduced frequency of physical activity in female pelvic cancer survivors (Lindgren et al., 2020). Exercise is established as a safe and effective intervention to counteract many of the adverse physical and psychological effects of cancer and its treatment and is recommended during and after cancer treatment (Cormie et al., 2018; Rock

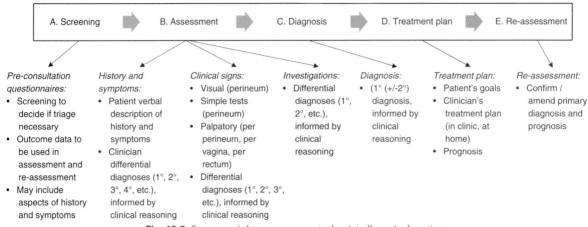

Fig. 13.2 Framework for management of pelvic floor dysfunction.

et al., 2012). The possibility that PF dysfunction may present a barrier to physical activity in the survivorship phase is important to consider.

Women with gynaecological cancer may not seek care for their PF symptoms for the same reasons as women without cancer (Howard and Steggall, 2010; Toye and Barker, 2020; Vethanayagam et al., 2017), in addition to cancer-related reasons. These include lack of information (Hay et al., 2018; Lindgren et al., 2017; Sekse et al., 2019), feeling too overwhelmed with their medical situation and believing that their oncology care would cure their PF dysfunction (Doyle et al., 2017), and a belief that their PF symptoms were bearable in light of their cancer diagnosis (Hazewinkel et al., 2010a). Nevertheless, many women with symptoms of PF dysfunction stated interest in a timely referral to a PF specialist (Doyle et al., 2017) and expressed a positive attitude towards trying pelvic floor muscle training (PFMT) (Lindgren et al., 2017).

Given the magnitude of impact from both prevalence and burden of PF dysfunction on gynaecological cancer survivors, healthcare providers should consider referral for PF assessment, with a view to appropriate and evidence-based management to improve quality of life (QoL) in survivors.

MANAGEMENT OF PELVIC FLOOR DYSFUNCTION AFTER GYNAECOLOGICAL CANCER TREATMENT

Physical therapy management of the woman presenting with symptoms of PF dysfunction after treatment for gynaecological cancer includes assessment (history,

physical examination and investigations), diagnosis, formulation of a treatment plan and prognosis, and ongoing re-assessment, as illustrated in Fig. 13.2. Management should be undertaken by a physical therapist who is competent in PF physical therapy, include informed consent, and adhere to local policies and procedures that govern infection control and intimate assessment procedures (Frawley et al., 2019). The physical therapist needs to appreciate the biopsychosocial effects of gynaecological cancer and cancer treatment, be sensitive to the individual woman's experience of cancer and current well-being, and practise within a biopsychosocial framework to ensure the process is patient centred. A woman may present with symptoms of bladder, bowel, sexual dysfunction or pelvic pain. Physical therapists should be guided by evidence-based clinical practice guidelines for PF dysfunction (Dumoulin et al., 2017; National Institute for Health and Care Excellence, 2014, 2019):

A. Screening: A clinician may ask a patient to complete pre-attendance questionnaires for the purpose of triaging a referral or collecting patient-reported data.

B. Assessment:
1. Symptoms: This includes current PF symptoms, noting any PF symptoms pre-dating cancer diagnosis, treatment sought and response to treatment. Include relevant patient-reported outcome measures to use in re-assessment.
2. Details of current general health (including exercise participation, nutrition, fatigue, sleep), medical history and current medications, psychological well-being, social situation, details of cancer diagnosis, cancer treatment to date, and any planned future cancer treatment should be obtained.

3. Clinical signs: Care should be taken to ensure that the woman fully understands the components of the physical examination. Digital palpation must be performed gently, due to possible scarring, vaginal stricture, pain and patient apprehension which may limit assessment. Aspects of PFM function to assess include resting tone, tenderness, contractility (strength, endurance), relaxation ability and organ support. Include relevant clinician-reported outcome measures to use in re-assessment.

4. Investigations: These may include assessment of the bladder and bowel where indicated or tolerated, and assessment of PFM function using manometry, dynamometry, myotonometry, electromyography, ultrasound imaging or algometry, as indicated or tolerated. Include relevant instrumented outcome measures to use in re-assessment.

C. Diagnosis: This may include a biomedical disorder, as well as a psychosocial condition, depending on patient presentation.

D. Treatment plan: Evidence to inform choice of PFM therapies to treat PF dysfunction following treatment for gynaecological cancer from randomized controlled trials (RCTs) is emerging (see the section on physical therapy for PF dysfunction after gynaecological cancer treatment), although many uncertainties remain. There is not yet evidence to customize treatment according to cancer type and cancer treatment type. PFM therapies (non-surgical, non-pharmacological therapies aimed at changing the structure or function of the PFMs) may be combined with behaviour change techniques, with the aim to enhance patient commitment and adherence (Frawley et al., 2017). A collaborative approach will incorporate patient preferences and, for the individual woman, will engender a sense of control over her own health.

E. Re-assessment: A slow or non-response should trigger a re-assessment, and an alternative treatment plan may be required. In-clinic re-assessment frequency and length of supervised treatment will be determined by individual patient, therapist and health system factors.

PHYSICAL THERAPY FOR PELVIC FLOOR DYSFUNCTION AFTER GYNAECOLOGICAL CANCER TREATMENT

PFM therapies do not carry the risks associated with pharmacological and surgical interventions for PF dysfunction, an important consideration in women who have already undergone cancer treatments which themselves carry morbidity. These include therapies aimed at changing the structure or function of the PFMs such as PFM exercise, relaxation training, dilator therapy, electrical stimulation and manual muscle release techniques.

Evidence for Effectiveness of Pelvic Floor Physical Therapy

A recent systematic review evaluated physical therapy for symptoms of PF dysfunction in women after gynaecological cancer treatment (Brennen et al., 2020). Five RCTs with 412 participants were identified, with two of these investigating a combination of PFMT plus yoga or core exercises (Li et al., 2016; Rutledge et al., 2014). The review found moderate-level evidence that PFMT with yoga or core exercises improved QoL and sexual function, and insufficient data to evaluate the impact of PFMT on bladder and bowel symptoms. An update of this systematic review, using the same search strategy as Brennen et al. (2020), was undertaken in October 2020. Only randomized trials were included, with full articles in English reporting on PFMT, vaginal dilator therapy or electrical stimulation in adult women after gynaecological cancer treatment. The characteristics of the seven included RCTs—five from Brennen et al. (2020) and two published since—are detailed in Table 13.2.

Methodological Quality

The PEDro rating score was used to classify the methodological quality of the included trials (Table 13.3), resulting in low (3 of 10) to high (7 of 10) methodological quality.

Interventions Provided
Pelvic Floor Muscle Training

Rutledge et al. (2014) found that PFMT improved Patient Global Impression of Improvement compared to no treatment; however, they did not find between-group differences in incontinence-specific impact and severity measures and PFM strength. This intervention included only one in-person training session and one reminder phone call, with a 12-week unsupervised home exercise program forming the bulk of the intervention.

Pelvic Floor Muscle Training and Yoga or Core Exercises

Li et al. (2016) found improvements in sexual function and QoL; however, physical function decreased.

TABLE 13.2   Characteristics of Included Randomized Controlled Trials of Pelvic Physical Therapy for Pelvic Floor Dysfunction in Women With Gynaecological Cancer

Author	Cerentini et al. (2019)
Study design	RCT
Study population	88 women, mean age 44 years, during or post brachytherapy ± chemotherapy and/or surgery for cervical cancer stages IB–IVA
Intervention	Intervention group 1: individually sized vaginal dilator + advice + 3-month dilator home program of 10–15-min dilator use 4×/week, starting during brachytherapy Intervention group 2: individually sized vaginal dilator + advice + 3-month dilator home program of 10–15-min dilator use 4×/week, starting 4 weeks after brachytherapy Control group: standard care
Drop-out/adherence	Drop-out at 3 months: intervention group 69.6%, control group 71.9% Adherence not reported
Outcome (measure)	CRO: Vaginal length (hysterometer), width (number of half-turns of screw on gynaecological speculum) and area (cross-sectional area of dilator cm^3); PFM contractility (bi-digital vaginal palpation) PRO: QoL and function (EORTC QLQ-C30)
Results (between-group analyses)	Results reported for intervention groups 1 and 2 combined because no difference between these groups Vaginal length, width and area: no difference between intervention and control groups (respectively 6.9 ± 0.31 vs 7.2 ± 0.3 cm, p = 0.111; 8.5 ± 0.8 vs 7.3 ± 0.7, p = 0.484; 41 ± 6.9 vs 41 ± 6.8 cm^2, p = 0.743) PFM contractility: no difference between intervention and control group classifications hypoactive (59% vs 78%), normal (24% vs 22%) or hyperactive (18% vs 0%), p = 0.210 EORTC QLQ-C30 Global, Functional and Symptom scales: no difference between intervention and control groups (80 ± 4.1 vs 79 ± 5.1, p = 0.936, 74 ± 4.6 vs 74 ± 6.6, p = 0.967; 24 ± 3.6 vs 24 ± 4.5, p = 0.666)
Author	Li et al. (2019)
Study design	RCT
Study population	91 women, 11 days post radical hysterectomy and pelvic lymph node dissection for cervical cancer stages IA2–IB2
Intervention	Intervention subgroup 1: bladder function training over 3 days; 8 am to 10 pm catheter opened every 2 hours for 15 min, 10 pm to 8 am catheter opened continuously + external pubic ES of 15–20 min twice a day frequency 35 Hz, pulse width 200 μs Intervention subgroup 2: bladder function training over 3 days, 8 am to 10 pm catheter opened every 2 hours for 15 min, 10 pm to 8 am catheter opened continuously + external pubic ES of 15–20 min twice a day frequency 1 Hz, pulse width 270 μs Control group: bladder function training
Drop-out/adherence	Drop-out rate: 0% Adherence not reported
Outcome (measure)	CRO: PVR bladder volume on ultrasound (cm^3); PFM contractility (measured using a 0–V-point sustained strength scale and a 0–V-point repeated rapid strength scale) of deep PFMs (vaginal palpation 1.5 cm from vaginal fornix) and superficial PFMs (vaginal palpation at perineum); postoperative fever (days); antibiotic use (days of antibiotic use); urine test for infection (leukocyte count on urine test) PRO: nil

TABLE 13.2 Characteristics of Included Randomized Controlled Trials of Pelvic Physical Therapy for Pelvic Floor Dysfunction in Women With Gynaecological Cancer—cont'd

Results (between-group analyses)	PVR bladder volume: difference in favour of intervention (56.85 ± 29.44 vs 95.79 ± 24.07, p = 0) Urinary retention incidence: difference in favour of intervention (10.41% vs 46.51%, p = 0); no difference in incidence of urinary retention between intervention subgroups 1 and 2 (11.54% vs 9.09%, p = 0.782) Deep PFM sustained strength: difference in favour of intervention (2.98 ± 0.56 vs 1.88 ± 0.63, p = 0), yet groups different at baseline (2.06 ± 0.67 vs 1.93 ± 0.63, p = 0.039) Deep PFM strength on repeated rapid contraction: difference in favour of intervention (3.08 ± 0.58 vs 1.98 ± 0.6, p = 0) Superficial PFM sustained strength: difference in favour of intervention (2.92 ± 0.58 vs 2.05 ± 0.58, p = 0) Superficial PFM strength on repeated rapid contraction: difference in favour of intervention (2.75 ± 0.6 vs 2 ± 0.58, p = 0), yet groups different at baseline (2 ± 0.74 vs 2.05 ± 0.53, p = 0.036) No difference between intervention and control groups in postoperative fever (2 vs 2, p = 0.667), antibiotic use (3 vs 3, p = 0.728), urine infection (3 vs 3, p = 0.911)
Author	**Li et al. (2016)**
Study design	RCT
Study population	226 women, mean age 46 years prior to discharge from hospital after surgery for cervical cancer stages IA–IIA
Intervention	Intervention group: 1x supervised PFMT session (no further details reported) + 1x supervised yoga session + instructional yoga CD + education + online communication platform + PFMT home exercise for 6 months, 1 set of 10 contractions of 10-s each 3–5x/day Control group: standard care
Drop-out/adherence	Drop-out rate: 0% Adherence not reported
Outcome (measure)	CRO: nil PRO: QoL and function (FACT-Cx), sexual function (FSFI), adaptability and emotional bonding (cohesion) within family of patient with cancer (FACES-II)
Results (between-group analyses)	At 6 months: FACT-Cx QoL, emotional, social and cervical change scores: difference in favour of intervention (respectively 33.3 vs 1.94, p = 0; 2.95 vs 0.56, p = 0; 1.18 vs 0.28, p = 0; 6.7 vs 0.84, p = 0) FSFI: difference in favour of intervention (2.57 vs –2.32, p = 0) No difference in FACT-Cx physical function change scores (0.21 vs –0.12, p = 0.583) FACT-Cx functional scale change scores: difference in favour of control group (–0.69 vs 0.72, p = 0) FACES-II adaptability score: difference in favour of intervention (3.19, 95% CI: 2.78–3.6 vs 0.15, 95% CI: –0.28 to 0.58, p = 0). FACES-II cohesion score: difference in favour of intervention (3.24, 95% CI: 2.72–3.77 vs –0.15, 95% CI: –0.71 to 0.4, p = 0)
Author	**Zhu et al. (2016)**
Study design	RCT
Study population	86 women, mean age 49 years, 3 months after surgery for stage I–II cervical cancer
Intervention	Intervention group: 1x PFMT training session (no further details reported) + vaginal ES + EMG BF + education + patient service hotline + PFMT home exercise (details not reported) Control group: no intervention
Drop-out/adherence	Drop-out rate: 0% Adherence not reported

Continued

TABLE 13.2 **Characteristics of Included Randomized Controlled Trials of Pelvic Physical Therapy for Pelvic Floor Dysfunction in Women With Gynaecological Cancer—cont'd**

Outcome (measure)	CRO: nil PRO: QoL (WHOQOL-100), pelvic floor dysfunction symptoms and bother (PFDI-SF)
Results (between-group analyses)	WHOQOL-100 scores: difference in favour of intervention group compared to control group in post-treatment social relations score (48.84 ± 4.63, p < 0.05), psychological field score (73.72 ± 2.84 vs 64.07 ± 4.06, p < 0.05), environmental field score (64.07 ± 4.08 vs 55.7 ± 4.86, p < 0.05), physiological index score (44.77 ± 4.22 vs 36.53 ± 4.29, p < 0.05), independence score (64.81 ± 5.85 vs 53.95 ± 5.91, p < 0.05) and QoL score (88.30 ± 5.75 vs 76.65 ± 5.21, p < 0.05) PFDI-SF: not measured at baseline
Author	**Rutledge et al. (2014)**
Study design	RCT
Study population	40 women, mean age 57 years, 1–5 years after surgery, radiotherapy, chemotherapy or combinations of therapy for uterine, ovarian, cervical or other gynaecological cancer
Intervention	Intervention group: 1x supervised PFMT session, 10x 5-s PFM contractions + behavioural management instruction + PFMT home exercise for 12 weeks, 1 set of 10 contractions of 5 s 3x/day Control group: no intervention
Drop-out/adherence	Drop-out rate: 15% in control group, 5% in intervention group Adherence: intervention group self-reported adherence 75% 'excellent' or 'good', 20% 'poor', 5% did not perform exercises at all
Outcome (measure)	CRO: PFM strength (digital palpation) PRO: urinary incontinence severity (ISI), type of urinary incontinence (QUID), distress from urinary incontinence (UDI-6 [% reporting bother from their urinary incontinence]), impact of urinary incontinence (IIQ-7), improvement in urinary incontinence (PGII % improved ['much better' or 'very much better'] and % not improved ['no change' or 'much worse'])
Results (between-group analyses)	At 3 months: PFM strength and QUID: between-group analysis not reported UDI-6: no difference (70% vs 50%, p = 0.62) IIQ-7: no difference, details not reported ISI: between-group analysis not reported PGII: difference in favour of intervention (80% vs 40% improved, 20% vs 60% not improved, p = 0.025)
Author	**Yang et al., (2012)**
Study design	RCT
Study population	28 women, mean age 52 years, 1–5 years after surgery ± radiotherapy and/or chemotherapy for cervical and endometrial cancer stages I–III
Intervention	Intervention group: 4x supervised PFMT sessions with 40 contractions of 10 s each using BF with intra-vaginal pressure BF and abdominal EMG BF + core exercises + PFMT home exercise for 4 weeks, 1 set of 10 contractions of 10-s ply 10 'fast contractions' a day + phone support line Control group: PFMT instruction leaflet + phone support line
Drop-out/adherence	Drop-out rate: 14.3% Adherence not reported
Outcome (measure)	CRO: PFM strength (manometer), MEP of PFMs during sacral stimulation, cranial stimulation and PFM rest, and cranial stimulation and PFM MVC PRO: pelvic floor symptoms (APFQ), QoL and function (EORTC-QLQ-30, EORTC QLQ-CX24)

TABLE 13.2   Characteristics of Included Randomized Controlled Trials of Pelvic Physical Therapy for Pelvic Floor Dysfunction in Women With Gynaecological Cancer—cont'd

Results (between-group analyses)	At 4 weeks: PFM strength: difference in favour of intervention (MD between groups: 14.22, p = 0.036) MEP of PFMs during sacral stimulation: difference in favour of intervention (MD between groups: –0.49, p = 0.014) All other MEP tests: no difference between groups; PFM nerve latency (MD: 1.90, p = 0.569) and amplitude (MD: 0.25, p = 0.273) with sacral stimulation; PFM nerve latency (MD: –4.08, p = 0.385), amplitude (MD: –0.05, p = 0.880), threshold (–0.43, p = 0.235) with cranial stimulation with PFMs at rest; PFM nerve latency (MD: –0.10, p = 0.74), amplitude (MD: –0.05, p = 0.865), threshold (–0.14, p = 0.715) with cranial stimulation and PFM MVC APFQ bladder function score, APFQ bowel function score: no difference (MD between groups: 0, p = 0.452; –0.16, p = 0.497) APFQ sexual function score: difference in favour of intervention (MD between groups: –0.55, p = 0.048) EORTC QLQ-30 and EORTC QLQ-CX2 subscales: between-group analysis not reported
Author	**Robinson et al. (1999)**
Study design	RCT
Study population	32 women, mean age 47 years, after start of radiotherapy ± surgery and/or chemotherapy for cervical or endometrial cancer stages I–II
Intervention	Intervention group: 2 motivational group psychoeducational group sessions + instruction booklet, PFMT home exercise and dilator, home protocol not specified Control group: advice + instruction booklet
Drop-out/adherence	Drop-out rate not reported Adherence: 30.5% of control group and 46.7% of intervention group reported using their dilator or having sexual intercourse ≥3×/week
Outcome (measure)	CRO: nil PRO: sexual function (SHF), sexual health knowledge (SKQ), fears about cancer and sexuality (FACS)
Results (between-group analyses)	SHF scores: no difference, details not reported SKQ: difference in favour of intervention for subjects >41.5 years (2.31 points, 95% CI: 1.18–3.04, p ≤ 0.0001); no significant difference for subjects ≤41.5 years (0.26 points, p = 0.53) FACS: difference in favour of intervention (MD: –0.33, 95% CI: 0.051–0.615, p = 0.01)

APFQ, Australian Pelvic Floor Questionnaire; *BF*, biofeedback; *CRO*, clinician-reported outcome; *EMG*, electromyography; *EORTC QLQ-C30*, European Organization for the Research and Treatment of Cancer Quality of Life Questionnaire–Core 30; *EORTC QLQ-CX24*, European Organization for the Research and Treatment of Cancer Quality of Life Questionnaire–Cervical Cancer Module; *ES*, electrical stimulation; *FACES-II*, Family Adaptability and Cohesion Scale, Second Edition; *FACS*, Fears About Cancer and Sexuality questionnaire; *FACT-Cx*, Functional Assessment of Cancer Therapy for Cervical Cancer questionnaire; *FSFI*, Female Sexual Function Index; *IIQ-7*, Incontinence Impact Questionnaire–Short Form; *ISI*, Incontinence Severity Index; *MD*, mean difference; *MEP*, motor evoked potential; *MVC*, maximum voluntary contraction; *PFDI-SF*, Pelvic Floor Distress Inventory–Short Form; *PFMT*, pelvic floor muscle training; *PGII*, Patient Global Impression of Improvement; *PFM*, pelvic floor muscle; *PRO*, patient-reported outcome; *PVR*, post-void residual; *QoL*, quality of life; *QUID*, Questionnaire for Urinary Incontinence Diagnosis; *RCT*, randomized controlled trial; *SHF*, Sexual History Form; *SKQ*, Sexual Knowledge Questionnaire; *UDI-6*, Urinary Distress Inventory–Short Form; *WHOQOL-100*, World Health Organization Quality of Life 100.

TABLE 13.3 PEDro Quality Score of Randomized Controlled Trials in Systematic Review

E – Eligibility criteria specified
1 – Subjects randomly allocated to groups
2 – Allocation concealed
3 – Groups similar at baseline
4 – Subjects blinded
5 – Therapists administering treatment blinded
6 – Assessors blinded
7 – Measures of key outcomes obtained from >85% of subjects
8 – Data analysed by intention to treat
9 – Statistical comparison between groups conducted
10 – Point measures and measures of variability provided

Study	E	1	2	3	4	5	6	7	8	9	10	Total Score
Cerentini et al. (2019)	+	+	?	+	−	−	−	−	+	+	+	5
Li et al. (2019)	+	+	+	+	−	−	+	+	?	+	+	7
Li et al. (2016)	+	+	?	+	?	−	?	+	+	+	+	6
Zhu et al. (2016)	+	+	−	+	−	−	−	+	−	+	+	5
Rutledge et al. (2014)	+	+	+	?	−	−	?	+	+	+	+	6
Yang et al. (2012)	+	+	−	+	−	−	+	−	−	+	+	5
Robinson et al. (1999)	+	+	?	−	−	−	?	?	?	+	+	3

+, Criterion is clearly satisfied; −, criterion is not satisfied; ?, not clear if the criterion was satisfied.
The total score is determined by counting the number of criteria that are satisfied, except the 'eligibility criteria specified 'score is not used to generate the total score. Total scores are out of 10.

This intervention included only one in-person training session for each of PFMT and yoga, ongoing unspecified follow-up by phone and home visits every two or three months supporting a 6-month unsupervised home exercise program. These authors intended the yoga exercises to improve psychosocial well-being, indirectly contributing to improved sexual function and QoL. Yang et al. (2012) found improvements in sexual function and PFM strength, but not in bladder or bowel function. This intervention included four in-person treatment sessions and four supervised core exercise sessions, with assessments completed at the end of the 4-week intervention period. These authors proposed that integrating core stabilizing exercises would enhance the benefit of PFMT; however, this proposal has not been supported by evidence (Bø and Herbert, 2013; Kruger et al., 2019).

Pelvic Floor Muscle Training and Vaginal Dilators

Robinson et al. (1999) found decreased fears about cancer and sexuality, but no difference in sexual function, after two group sessions that included dilator and PFMT instruction.

Pelvic Floor Muscle Training and Electrical Stimulation

Zhu et al. (2016) found improved QoL after one in-person session of PFMT with vaginal electrical stimulation and electromyography biofeedback and an unsupervised home exercise program.

Vaginal Dilators

Cerentini et al. (2019) found no improvements in vaginal dimensions, PFM function or QoL with one session of individual instruction with individually sized vaginal dilators compared to standard care.

Electrical Stimulation

Li et al. (2019) found improved bladder function and PFM strength after external pubic area electrical stimulation occurring prior to postoperative removal of an indwelling catheter.

Quality of the Intervention: Dose–Response Issues

Pelvic Floor Muscle Training

There was large variation of PFMT parameters in the six studies that included PFMT. All studies used protocols for strength training of the PFMs. Correct contraction was not confirmed in one study (Robinson et al., 1999), confirmed in two (Rutledge et al., 2014; Yang et al., 2012) and unclear in two (Li et al., 2016; Zhu et al., 2016). Two studies reported that PFMT was taught individually (Rutledge et al., 2014; Yang et al., 2012), one in a group setting (Robinson et al., 1999) and two were unclear (Li et al., 2016; Zhu et al., 2016). The training period varied from 4 weeks (Yang et al., 2012) to 6 months (Li et al., 2016). In one study the training period was not reported (Robinson et al., 1999).

Three studies reported details of the PFMT home programme, and these included 10 contractions of 5 to 10 seconds each, repeated between one and five times per day (Li et al., 2016; Rutledge et al., 2014; Yang et al., 2012). The programme that included only one session per day included a second set of 20 to 30 seconds of fast PFM contractions (Yang et al., 2012). Only one study reported the body position for the PFMT home programme (Yang et al., 2012).

Drop-out rates ranged from 0% to 14.3%. Adherence to the PFMT home programme was reported in only one study, in which most intervention group participants reported good to excellent adherence (Rutledge et al., 2014). Motivational strategies used were social support, self-monitoring of behaviour and action planning (Rutledge et al., 2014; Robinson et al., 1999; Yang et al., 2012).

Considerable variation was reported in the use of outcomes measures, combinations with other treatments, and detail regarding PFMT parameters and adherence; this variation makes it difficult to directly compare results of PFMT based on dose–response outcomes. In light of evidence for supervision of PFMT in general female populations (Hay-Smith et al., 2011), the level of supervision in the included studies was suboptimal and may have reduced the potential clinical impact of the interventions.

Vaginal Dilators

Neither study that included vaginal dilator training observed correct use of the vaginal dilators. The home program was specified in only one study: four 10- to 15-minute sessions per week (Cerentini et al., 2019), whereas a frequency of three times a week was used as the threshold

for adherence in the other study (Robinson et al., 1999). Drop-out rates were high in one study (Cerentini et al., 2019) and adherence rates low in the other (Robinson et al., 1999). Motivational strategies included socialization, normalization of feelings, social support, handling of dilators and action planning (Robinson et al., 1999).

The variation in the use of different outcomes measures, and the combination of vaginal dilator therapy with other treatments, makes it difficult to compare results based on dilator dose–response outcomes.

Electrical Stimulation

Variation was reported in electrode type and location, with one study using an intra-vaginal electrode (Zhu et al., 2016) and the other using extra-vaginal electrodes (Li et al., 2019). The intervention periods were 3 days (Li et al., 2019) and 3 months (Yang et al., 2012). There were no drop-outs, but adherence was not reported. The number of sessions in the 3-day intervention was six, with 15 to 30 minutes per session (Li et al., 2019). Participants were allocated to electrical parameters of 35-Hz frequency and 200-μs pulse width or 1-Hz frequency and 270-μs pulse width (Li et al., 2019). As one article was available in Chinese only, we were unable to extract details about the number of electrical stimulation sessions and electrical parameters (Zhu et al., 2016).

Due to the scarcity of studies, the lack of information on treatment parameters, the use of different outcome measures and the combination with other treatments in one study, it is not possible to compare dose–response outcomes between studies. In the study that compared electrical stimulation protocols with different electrical parameters, there was no between-group difference in results (Li et al., 2019). Furthermore, the safety of applying electrical stimulation in the region of known or suspected cancer is unknown, and therefore current guidelines recommend that local application of electrical stimulation is contraindicated when malignancy is present (Houghton et al., 2010). There are no guidelines regarding the application of electrical stimulation in a body region with a past history but no evidence of current malignancy.

CONCLUSION

The prevalence of PF dysfunction is higher in women after gynaecological cancer than in non-cancer populations. The impact of PF dysfunction on a woman's life appears to be significant. Women presenting with symptoms of PF dysfunction require careful and thorough assessment to guide treatment decisions. Evidence from RCTs for PFM therapies to treat PF dysfunction following treatment for gynaecological cancer is limited. There is moderate-level evidence that PFMT and yoga or core exercises improve sexual function and QoL after gynaecological cancer. Insufficient evidence exists for the effect of PFMT on bladder or bowel function. There is no evidence from RCTs for the impact of vaginal dilators on PF function. There is emerging evidence that electrical stimulation may reduce voiding dysfunction; however, the safety of electrical stimulation in patients with a history of cancer is unknown. The quality of the evidence from RCTs is varied, and several intervention protocols have been applied with suboptimal dosage or insufficient reporting to allow evaluation of therapy dosage. Due to the effects of cancer treatments on PF tissues, more intensive PFM therapies with supervision of correct contraction and progression may be required to achieve more effective outcomes. A recent study suggests that PF therapies delivered at therapeutic dosages are feasible and well accepted in gynaecological cancer survivors with dyspareunia (Cyr et al., 2020).

CLINICAL RECOMMENDATIONS

- Assessment of PF symptoms needs to consider the potential biopsychosocial sequalae of gynaecological cancer. Treatments should be directed to the symptom the patient is most bothered by.
- PFMT and yoga or core exercises could be considered for treating sexual dysfunction in women who have had gynaecological cancer.
- Due to a paucity of evidence from RCTs for symptoms of bladder and bowel dysfunction, clinicians should apply physical therapy interventions judiciously and reassess regularly to ensure that patient response to therapy is optimal.

FUTURE RESEARCH DIRECTIONS

- Large well-designed RCTs that test interventions delivered at effective dosage and supervision levels to meet current recommendations for PFMT in the general population, report adherence and provide long-term follow-up are needed in this population.
- To minimize patient burden, it is important to test the effectiveness of single interventions; however,

combinations of therapies may provide more time-efficient improvement in symptoms in patients with complex PF dysfunction; these comparisons require testing.
- Cost of treatment information should be included in future studies to allow for cost–benefit analyses.

REFERENCES

Afiyanti, Y., Setyowati, Milanti, A., et al. (2020). 'Finally, I get to a climax': The experiences of sexual relationships after a psychosexual intervention for Indonesian cervical cancer survivors and the husbands. *Journal of Psychosocial Oncology*, 38, 293–309.

Allemani, C., Matsuda, T., Di Carlo, V., et al. (2018). Global surveillance of trends in cancer survival 2000–14 (CONCORD-3): Analysis of individual records for 37,513,025 patients diagnosed with one of 18 cancers from 322 population-based registries in 71 countries. *Lancet*, 391, 1023–1075.

American Cancer Society. (2020a). Chemotherapy Side Effects [Online]. Available: https://www.cancer.org/treatment/treatments-and-side-effects/treatment-types/chemotherapy/chemotherapy-side-effects.html. (Accessed 10.11.20).

American Cancer Society. (2020b). Radiation Therapy for Cervical Cancer [Online]. Available: https://www.cancer.org/cancer/cervical-cancer/treating/radiation.html. (Accessed 10.11.20).

Ang, C., Bryant, A., Barton, D. P. J., et al. (2014). Exenterative surgery for recurrent gynaecological malignancies. *Cochrane Database of Systematic Reviews*, 2, CD010449.

Arbyn, M., Weiderpass, E., Bruni, L., et al. (2020). Estimates of incidence and mortality of cervical cancer in 2018: A worldwide analysis. *Lancet Glob Health*, 8, e191–e203.

Bernard, S., Moffet, H., Dumoulin, C., et al. (2016). Pelvic floor properties of women with urinary incontinence after endometrial cancer: Canadian physiotherapy association national congress 2016 may 26–28 victoria BC. *Physiotherapie Canada*, 68, 34.

Bernard, S., Moffet, H., Plante, M., et al. (2017). Pelvic-floor properties in women reporting urinary incontinence after surgery and radiotherapy for endometrial cancer. *Physical Therapy*, 97, 438–448.

Bogani, G., Rossetti, D. O., Ditto, A., et al. (2018). Nerve-sparing approach improves outcomes of patients undergoing minimally invasive radical hysterectomy: A systematic review and meta-analysis. *Journal of Minimally Invasive Gynecology*, 25, 402–410.

Bø, K., & Herbert, R. D. (2013). There is not yet strong evidence that exercise regimens other than pelvic floor muscle training can reduce stress urinary incontinence in women: A systematic review. *Journal of Physiotherapy, 59*, 159–168.

Brennen, R., Lin, K.-Y., Denehy, L., et al. (2020). The effect of pelvic floor muscle interventions on pelvic floor dysfunction after gynecological cancer treatment: A systematic review. *Physical Therapy, 100*, 1357–1371.

Campbell, P., Casement, M., Addley, S., et al. (2017). Early catheter removal following laparoscopic radical hysterectomy for cervical cancer: Assessment of a new bladder care protocol. *Journal Obstetrics and Gynaecology, 37*, 970–972.

Cancer Australia. (2012). *Gynaecological cancers in Australia: An overview. Cancer series.* Cranberra: Australian Institute of Health and Welfare.

Cancer Council. (2016a). *Optimal care pathways for women with endometrial cancer.* Melbourne: Cancer Council Victoria.

Cancer Council. (2016b). *Optimal care pathways for women with ovarian cancer.* Melbourne: Cancer Council Victoria.

Cerentini, T. M., Schlöttgen, J., Viana Da Rosa, P., et al. (2019). Clinical and psychological outcomes of the use of vaginal dilators after gynaecological brachytherapy: A randomized clinical trial. *Advances in Therapy, 36*, 1936–1949.

Chuang, T.-Y., Yu, K.-J., Penn, I. W., et al. (2003). Neurourological changes before and after radical hysterectomy in patients with cervical cancer. *Acta Obstetricia et Gynecologica Scandinavica, 82*, 954–959.

Coburn, S. B., Bray, F., Sherman, M. E., et al. (2017). International patterns and trends in ovarian cancer incidence, overall and by histologic subtype. *International Journal of Cancer, 140*, 2451–2460.

Cormie, P., Atkinson, M., Bucci, L., et al. (2018). Clinical Oncology Society of Australia position statement on exercise in cancer care. *Medical Journal of Australia, 209*, 184–187.

Crean-Tate, K. K., Faubion, S. S., Pederson, H. J., et al. (2020). Management of genitourinary syndrome of menopause in female cancer patients: A focus on vaginal hormonal therapy. *American Journal of Obstetrics and Gynecology, 222*, 103–113.

Cyr, M.-P., Dumoulin, C., Bessette, P., et al. (2020). Feasibility, acceptability and effects of multimodal pelvic floor physical therapy for gynecological cancer survivors suffering from painful sexual intercourse: A multicenter prospective interventional study. *Gynecologic Oncology, 159*(3), 778–784.

Cyr, M.-P., Dumoulin, C., Bessette, P., et al. (2021). Characterizing pelvic floor muscle function and morphometry in survivors of gynecological cancer who have dyspareunia: A comparative cross-sectional study. *Physical Therapy, 101*(4), pzab042.

Dakic, J., Hay-Smith, J., Cook, J., et al. (2021). Effect of pelvic floor symptoms on women's participation in exercise: A mixed-methods systematic review with meta-analysis. *Journal of Orthopaedic & Sports Physical Therapy, 51*(7), 345–361.

Doyle, P. J., Thomas, S. G., & Buchsbaum, G. M. (2017). Barriers to urogynecological care in a population of gynecological oncology patients. *international Urology journal, 28*, 913–916.

Dumoulin, C., Adewuyi, T., Booth, J., et al. (2017). Adult conservative management. In P. Abrams, L. Cardozo, A. Wagg, et al. (Eds.), *Incontinence* (6th ed.) (pp. 1176–1180). Bristol, UK: International Continence Society.

Faubion, S. S., MacLaughlin, K. L., Long, M. E., et al. (2015). Surveillance and care of the gynecologic cancer survivor. *J. Womens Health (Larchmt.), 24*, 899–906.

Fischer, O. J., Marguerie, M., & Brotto, L. A. (2019). Sexual function, quality of life, and experiences of women with ovarian cancer: A mixed-methods study. *The Journal of Sexual Medicine, 7*, 530–539.

Fokdal, L., Pötter, R., Kirchheiner, K., et al. (2018). Physician assessed and patient reported urinary morbidity after radio-chemotherapy and image guided adaptive brachytherapy for locally advanced cervical cancer. *Radiotherapy & Oncology, 127*, 423–430.

Frawley, H. C., Dean, S. G., Slade, S. C., et al. (2017). Is pelvic-floor muscle training a physical therapy or a behavioral therapy? A call to name and report the physical, cognitive, and behavioral elements. *Physical Therapy, 97*, 425–437.

Frawley, H. C., Neumann, P., & Delany, C. (2019). An argument for competency-based training in pelvic floor physiotherapy practice. *Physiotherapy Theory and Practice, 35*, 1117–1130.

Fujii, S., Takakura, K., Matsumura, N., et al. (2007). Precise anatomy of the vesico-uterine ligament for radical hysterectomy. *Gynecologic Oncology, 104*, 186–191.

Gressel, G. M., Dioun, S. M., Richley, M., et al. (2019). Utilizing the patient reported outcomes measurement information system (PROMIS®) to increase referral to ancillary support services for severely symptomatic patients with gynecologic cancer. *Gynecologic Oncology, 152*, 509–513.

Guner, O., Gumussoy, S., Celik, N., et al. (2018). An examination of the sexual functions of patients who underwent a gynecologic cancer operation and received brachytherapy. *Pakistan Journal of Medicine & Science in Sports, 34*, 15–19.

Hay-Smith, E. J. C., Herderschee, R., Dumoulin, C., et al. (2011). Comparisons of approaches to pelvic floor muscle training for urinary incontinence in women. *Cochrane Database of Systematic Reviews, 12*, CD009508.

Hay, C. M., Donovan, H. S., Hartnett, E. G., et al. (2018). Sexual health as part of gynecologic cancer care: What do patients want? *International Journal of Gynecological Cancer, 28*, 1737–1742.

Hazewinkel, M. H., Sprangers, M. A., Taminiau-Bloem, E. F., et al. (2010a). Reasons for not seeking medical help for severe pelvic floor symptoms: A qualitative study in survivors of gynaecological cancer. *British Journal of Obstetrics and Gynaecology, 117*, 39–46.

Hazewinkel, M. H., Sprangers, M. A., Van Der Velden, J., et al. (2010b). Long-term cervical cancer survivors suffer from pelvic floor symptoms: A cross-sectional matched cohort study. *Gynecologic Oncology, 117*, 281–286.

Hazewinkel, M. H., Sprangers, M. A., Velden, J., et al. (2012). Severe pelvic floor symptoms after cervical cancer treatment are predominantly associated with mental and physical well-being and body image: A cross-sectional study. *International Journal of Gynecological Cancer, 22*, 154–160.

Hofsjö, A., Bergmark, K., Blomgren, B., et al. (2018). Radiotherapy for cervical cancer—impact on the vaginal epithelium and sexual function. *Acta Oncologica, 57*, 338–345.

Hofsjö, A., Bohm-Starke, N., Blomgren, B., et al. (2017). Radiotherapy-induced vaginal fibrosis in cervical cancer survivors. *Acta Oncologica, 56*, 661–666.

Houghton, P., Nussbaum, E., & Hoens, A. (2010). Electrophysical agents—contraindications and precautions: An evidence-based approach to clinical decision making in physical therapy. *Physiotherapie Canada, 62*(5), 1–80.

Howard, F., & Steggall, M. (2010). Urinary incontinence in women: Quality of life and help-seeking. *British Journal of Nursing, 19*, 742–749.

Jarruwale, P., Huang, K.-G., Benavides, D. R., et al. (2013). Nerve-sparing radical hysterectomy in cervical cancer. *Gynecology Minimally Invasive Therapy, 2*, 42–47.

Jensen, N. B. K., Pötter, R., Kirchheiner, K., et al. (2018). Bowel morbidity following radiochemotherapy and image-guided adaptive brachytherapy for cervical cancer: Physician- and patient reported outcome from the embrace study. *Radiotherapy & Oncology, 127*, 431–439.

Jiang, W., Liang, M., Han, D., et al. (2019). A modification of laparoscopic type C1 hysterectomy to reduce postoperative bladder dysfunction: A retrospective study. *Journal of Investigative Surgery, 32*, 272–280.

Jin, M., Shen, F., Li, M., et al. (2020). Palliative treatment for bowel obstruction in ovarian cancer: A meta-analysis. *Archives of Gynecology and Obstetrics, 302*, 241–248.

Kilgour, R. D., Vigano, A., Trutschnigg, B., et al. (2010). Cancer–related fatigue: The impact of skeletal muscle mass and strength in patients with advanced cancer. *Journal Cachexia Sarcopenia Muscle, 1*, 177–185.

Kruger, J., Budgett, D., Goodman, J., et al. (2019). Can you train the pelvic floor muscles by contracting other related muscles? *Neurourology and Urodynamics, 38*, 677–683.

Lawrie, T. A., Green, J. T., Beresford, M., et al. (2018). Interventions to reduce acute and late adverse gastrointestinal effects of pelvic radiotherapy for primary pelvic cancers. *Cochrane Database of Systematic Reviews, 1*, CD012529.

Lee, A. H., & Hirayama, F. (2012). Physical activity and urinary incontinence in older adults: A community-based study. *Current Aging Science, 5*(1), 35–40.

Li, J., Huang, J., Zhang, J., et al. (2016). A home-based, nurse-led health program for postoperative patients with early-stage cervical cancer: A randomized controlled trial. *European Journal of Oncology Nursing, 21*, 174–180.

Lindgren, A., Dunberger, G., & Enblom, A. (2017). Experiences of incontinence and pelvic floor muscle training after gynaecologic cancer treatment. *Supportive Care in Cancer, 25*, 157–166.

Lindgren, A., Dunberger, G., Steineck, G., et al. (2020). Identifying female pelvic cancer survivors with low levels of physical activity after radiotherapy: Women with fecal and urinary leakage need additional support. *Supportive Care in Cancer, 28*, 2669–2681.

Lipetskaia, L., Sharma, S., Johnson, M. S., et al. (2019). Urinary incontinence and quality of life in endometrial cancer patients after robotic-assisted laparoscopic hysterectomy with lymph node dissection. *Journal Obstetrics and Gynaecology, 39*, 986–990.

Liu, Q., Li, P., Sun, Y., et al. (2020). Effect of laparoscopic nerve-sparing radical hysterectomy on bladder function recovery. *Journal of Investigative Surgery, 33*, 381–386.

Li, H., Zhou, C.-K., Song, J., et al. (2019). Curative efficacy of low frequency electrical stimulation in preventing urinary retention after cervical cancer operation. *World Journal of Surgical Oncology, 17*, 141.

Lortet-Tieulent, J., Ferlay, J., Bray, F., et al. (2018). International patterns and trends in endometrial cancer incidence, 1978–2013. *Journal of the National Cancer Institute, 110*(4), 354.

Lucidi, A., Windemut, S., Petrillo, M., et al. (2017). Self-reported long-term autonomic function after laparoscopic total mesometrial resection for early-stage cervical cancer: A multicentric study. *International Journal of Gynecological Cancer, 27*, 1501–1507.

Miguel, T. P., Laurienzo, C. E., Faria, E. F., et al. (2020). Chemoradiation for cervical cancer treatment portends high risk of pelvic floor dysfunction. *PLoS One, 15*, e0234389.

Milsom, I., Altman, D., Cartwright, R., et al. (2017). Epidemiology of urinary incontinence (UI), and other lower urinary tract symptoms (LUTS), pelvic organ prolapse (POP) and anal incontinence (AI). In P. Abrams, L. Cardozo,

A. Wagg, et al. (Eds.), *Incontinence* (6th ed.) (pp. 1–142). Bristol, UK: International Continence Society.

Nantasupha, C., & Charoenkwan, K. (2018). Predicting factors for resumption of spontaneous voiding following nerve-sparing radical hysterectomy. *Journal Gynecologic Oncology, 29*, e59.

National Institute for Health and Care Excellence. (2014). *Faecal incontinence in adults [Online]*. Available: https://www.nice.org.uk/guidance/qs54. (Accessed 27.11.20).

National Institute for Health and Care Excellence. (2019). *Urinary incontinence and pelvic organ prolapse in women: Management*. [Online]. Available: https://www.nice.org.uk/guidance/ng123. (Accessed 7.10.20).

Novackova, M., Pastor, Z., Chmel, R., Jr., et al. (2020). Urinary tract morbidity after nerve-sparing radical hysterectomy in women with cervical cancer. *International Urology Journal, 31*, 981–987.

Ntinga, S. N., & Maree, J. E. (2015). Living with the late effects of cervical cancer treatment: A descriptive qualitative study at an academic hospital in gauteng. *South African Journal of Obstetrics and Gynaecology, 7*, 21–26.

Organisation for Economic Co-operation and Development, n.d. Health Status [Online]. Available: https://stats.oecd.org/index.aspx?datasetcode=health_stat#. (Accessed 23.11.20).

Pascoe, C., Duncan, C., Lamb, B. W., et al. (2019). Current management of radiation cystitis: A review and practical guide to clinical management. *BJU International, 123*, 585–594.

Pawlik, T., Skibber, J., & Rodriguez-Bigas, M. (2006). Pelvic exenteration for advanced pelvic malignancies. *Annals of Surgical Oncology, 13*, 612–623.

Plotti, F., Terranova, C., Capriglione, S., et al. (2018). Assessment of quality of life and urinary and sexual function after radical hysterectomy in long-term cervical cancer survivors. *International Journal of Gynecological Cancer, 28*, 818–823.

Prue, G., Allen, J., Gracey, J., et al. (2010). Fatigue in gynecological cancer patients during and after anticancer treatment. *Journal of Pain and Symptom Management, 39*, 197–210.

Ramaseshan, A. S., Felton, J., Roque, D., et al. (2018). Pelvic floor disorders in women with gynecologic malignancies: A systematic review. *International Urology Journal, 29*, 459–476.

Raspagliesi, F., Bogani, G., Spinillo, A., et al. (2017). Introducing nerve-sparing approach during minimally invasive radical hysterectomy for locally-advanced cervical cancer: A multi-institutional experience. *European Journal of Surgical Oncology, 43*, 2150–2156.

Ribas, Y., Bonet, M., Torres, L., et al. (2020). Bowel dysfunction in survivors of gynecologic malignancies. *Supportive Care in Cancer, 28*, 5501–5510.

Robinson, J. W., Faris, P. D., & Scott, C. B. (1999). Psycho-educational group increases vaginal dilation for younger women and reduces sexual fears for women of all ages with gynecological carcinoma treated with radiotherapy. *International Journal of Radiation Oncology, Biology, Physics, 44*, 497–506.

Rock, C. L., Doyle, C., Demark-Wahnefried, W., et al. (2012). Nutrition and physical activity guidelines for cancer survivors. *CA: A Cancer Journal for Clinicians, 62*, 242–274.

Rutledge, T. L., Rogers, R., Lee, S. J., et al. (2014). A pilot randomized control trial to evaluate pelvic floor muscle training for urinary incontinence among gynecologic cancer survivors. *Gynecologic Oncology, 132*, 154–158.

Sabulei, C., & Maree, J. E. (2019). An exploration into the quality of life of women treated for cervical cancer. *Curationis, 42*, e1–e9.

Schofield, C., Newton, R. U., Cohen, P. A., et al. (2018). Health-related quality of life and pelvic floor dysfunction in advanced-stage ovarian cancer survivors: Associations with objective activity behaviors and physiological characteristics. *Supportive Care in Cancer, 26*(7), 2239–2246.

Segal, S., John, G., Sammel, M., et al. (2017). Urinary incontinence and other pelvic floor disorders after radiation therapy in endometrial cancer survivors. *Maturitas, 105*, 83–88.

Sekse, R. J. T., Dunberger, G., Olesen, M. L., et al. (2019). Lived experiences and quality of life after gynaecological cancer—an integrative review. *Journal of Clinical Nursing, 28*, 1393–1421.

Shabaruddin, F. H., Chen, L.-C., Elliott, R. A., et al. (2013). A systematic review of utility values for chemotherapy-related adverse events. *PharmacoEconomics, 31*, 277–288.

Shankar, A., Patil, J., Luther, A., et al. (2020). Sexual dysfunction in carcinoma cervix: Assessment in post treated cases by LENTSOMA scale. *Asian Pacific Journal of Cancer Prevention, 21*(2), 349–354.

Soisson, S., Ganz, P. A., Gaffney, D., et al. (2018). Long-term, adverse genitourinary outcomes among endometrial cancer survivors in a large, population-based cohort study. *Gynecologic Oncology, 148*, 499–506.

Stabile, C., Goldfarb, S., Baser, R. E., et al. (2017). Sexual health needs and educational intervention preferences for women with cancer. *Breast Cancer Research and Treatment, 165*(1), 77–84.

Sun, H., Cao, D., Shen, K., et al. (2018). Piver type II vs. type III hysterectomy in the treatment of early-stage cervical cancer: Midterm follow-up results of a randomized controlled trial. *Front Oncology, 8*, 568.

Toye, F., & Barker, K. (2020). A meta-ethnography to understand the experience of living with urinary incontinence: 'is it just part and parcel of life?' *BMC Urology, 20*, 1–25.

Vethanayagam, N., Orrell, A., Dahlberg, L., et al. (2017). Understanding help-seeking in older people with urinary incontinence: An interview study. *Health and Social Care in the Community*, 25, 1061–1069.

Wagner, T., Moore, K., Subak, L., et al. (2017). Economics of urinary and faecal incontinence, and prolapse. In P. Abrams, L. Cardozo, A. Wagg, et al. (Eds.), *Incontinence* (6th ed.) (pp. 2479–2512). Bristol, UK: International Continence Society.

Wang, X., Chen, C., Liu, P., et al. (2018). The morbidity of sexual dysfunction of 125 Chinese women following different types of radical hysterectomy for gynaecological malignancies. *Archives of Gynecology and Obstetrics*, 297, 459–466.

Wang, Z., Huang, J., Zeng, A., et al. (2019). Vaginoplasty with acellular dermal matrix after radical resection for carcinoma of the uterine cervix. *Journal of Investigative Surgery*, 32, 180–185.

Wenzel, H. H. B., Kruitwagen, R., Nijman, H. W., et al. (2020). Short-term surgical complications after radical hysterectomy—a nationwide cohort study. *Acta Obstetricia et Gynecologica Scandinavica*, 99, 925–932.

White, K. L., Varrassi, E., Routledge, J. A., et al. (2018). Does the use of volumetric modulated arc therapy reduce gastrointestinal symptoms after pelvic radiotherapy? *Clinical Oncology*, 30, e22–e28.

World Cancer Research Fund, n.d. Worldwide Cancer Data: Global Cancer Statistics for the Most Common Cancers in the World [Online]. Available: https://www.wcrf.org/dietandcancer/cancer-trends/worldwide-cancer-data. (Accessed 4.11.20).

Wu, J., Ye, T., Lv, J., et al. (2019). Laparoscopic nerve-sparing radical hysterectomy vs laparoscopic radical hysterectomy in cervical cancer: A systematic review and meta-analysis of clinical efficacy and bladder dysfunction. *Journal of Minimally Invasive Gynecology*, 26, 417–426.e6.

Yaakobi, T. M. A., Handelzalts, J. E. P., Peled, Y. M. D., et al. (2017). Direct and indirect effects of personality traits on psychological distress in women with pelvic floor disorders. *Female Pelvic Medicine & Reconstructive Surgery*, 23(6), 412–416.

Yang, E. J., Lim, J.-Y., Rah, U. W., et al. (2012). Effect of a pelvic floor muscle training program on gynecologic cancer survivors with pelvic floor dysfunction: A randomized controlled trial. *Gynecologic Oncology*, 125, 705–711.

Yang, L., Yuan, J., Zeng, X., et al. (2020). The outcomes and quality of life of young patients undergoing adjuvant radiotherapy versus non-radiotherapy following surgery treating early FIGO stage cervical squamous cell cancer in southwestern China. *Scientific Reports*, 10, 9583.

Yavuzsen, T., Davis, M. P., Ranganathan, V. K., et al. (2009). Cancer-related fatigue: Central or peripheral? *Journal of Pain and Symptom Management*, 38, 587–596.

Yeung, A. R., Pugh, S. L., Klopp, A. H., et al. (2020). Improvement in patient-reported outcomes with intensity-modulated radiotherapy (RT) compared with standard RT: A report from the NRG oncology RTOG 1203 study. *Journal of Clinical Oncology*, 38(15), 1685–1692.

Yuan, Z., Cao, D., Yang, J., et al. (2019). Laparoscopic vs. open abdominal radical hysterectomy for cervical cancer: A single-institution, propensity score matching study in China. *Front Oncology*, 9, 1107.

Zhang, S., Gong, T.-T., Liu, F.-H., et al. (2019). Global, regional, and national burden of endometrial cancer, 1990–2017: Results from the Global Burden of Disease study, 2017. *Front Oncology*, 9, 1440.

Zhao, D., Li, B., Wang, Y., et al. (2020). Clinical outcomes in early cervical cancer patients treated with nerve plane-sparing laparoscopic radical hysterectomy. *Journal of Minimally Invasive Gynecology*, 27(3), 687–696.

Zhu, G., Li, X., & Yang, S. (2016). [Effect of postoperative intervention on the quality of life of patients with cervical cancer]. *Cancer Research Clinical*, 28, 819–822.

14

Aetiology of Incontinence in Older Adults

Adrian Wagg

OUTLINE

INTRODUCTION

An increasing number of countries face profound demographic change due to a decrease in birth rates and an increase in the proportion of people surviving into very late life. The greatest expansion will be in the proportion of the oldest old in the population, those in their ninth decade of life (Kinsella and He, 2009). For many developed countries, the number of people older than 65 years outnumbers those younger than 20 years. Whereas approximately 50% of people may age without significant comorbidity, physical or cognitive impairment, the proportion of those living with coexisting non-communicable disease, medical complexity or frailty increases rapidly after the age of 75 years (Divo

et al, 2014). Research into, and the development of, age-appropriate interventions is required to meet the needs of older adults. The major focus of healthcare delivery in this sector of the population should be to ensure an integrated and comprehensive approach to the needs of older people and their care partners. The quest for adequate and cost-effective healthcare for the growing number of older adults has received increased attention from health service providers, national governments and international organizations as the need to improve quality of services and at the same time constrain healthcare spending becomes paramount. Of particular relevance to continence in older people, the International Consultation on Urological Diseases, in conjunction with the European Association of Urology, has taken the lead on developing evidence-based guidelines into the causes and management of incontinence in older adults and those living with frailty through the International Consultation on Incontinence (Gibson et al., 2021)

PREVALENCE

The prevalence of urinary incontinence (UI) increases with increasing age, affects women more than men, and is associated with significant personal stress, shame and social stigma (Irwin et al., 2006), considerable morbidity (Coyne et al., 2012; Milsom et al., 2012), and cost (Milsom et al., 2013; Stothers et al., 2005; Thom et al., 2005). The social and psychological consequences associated with incontinence are such that sufferers become less socially and less physically active (Coyne et al., 2013). Social isolation and physical deconditioning themselves lead to further morbidity and poor health outcomes such as falls and depression, and social isolation is a risk factor for intellectual decline.

The presence of comorbidities and functional impairment in older adults may lead clinicians to overlook incontinence and thus leave it untreated, and merely contained by continence products. The influence of coexisting diseases on the impact of incontinence in older people has been well described; however, there are few data that describe the treatment of these coexisting comorbidities in terms of the impact on lower urinary tract symptoms or incontinence. Data that do exist cover the management of obesity, sleep apnoea and Parkinson's disease (but not reported separately in older adults). One area that has received attention is the effect of exercise, either as musculoskeletal exercises to increase gait speed and stamina alone or combined with pelvic floor muscle (PFM) re-education, in a variety of older people, from those who are community dwelling to nursing home residents. Physical exercise interventions not only have a positive impact on incontinence and nocturia but also ameliorate fall risk and reduce cardiovascular risk, with underlying weight loss probably accounting for some of this effect. This impact on incontinence may be simply that, by improving gait speed and stamina, urinary urgency can be better controlled with a reduced likelihood of incontinence but also might be conveyed by a reduction in the metabolic risk factors which are associated with overactive bladder and urgency incontinence and the mass effect on the pelvic floor, reducing the likelihood of exertional incontinence (Kim et al., 2010, Kim et al., 2011; Sugaya et al., 2007; van Houten et al., 2007).

Classification of Incontinence

The prevalence of different types of incontinence alters in association with increasing age. Storage symptoms, such as nocturia, nocturnal polyuria, urinary urgency, frequency, and urgency and stress (exertional) incontinence, become more common, as do voiding symptoms (Irwin et al., 2006). Voiding symptoms are more common in men, probably due to the increased prevalence of bladder outflow tract obstruction, but this difference is less than is traditionally taught, largely due to the influence of reduced bladder contractile efficiency. In addition to the 'classical' subtypes of UI, functional incontinence, now termed *disability-associated incontinence*, occurs more frequently in older than young people; this is where the incontinence is not necessarily due to a lower urinary tract disorder but is a reflection of either physical or cognitive disability such that the affected individual fails to maintain continence or voids in an inappropriate place or at a socially inappropriate time, so-called unsuccessful toileting as a result of toileting disability.

Who Are the Elderly and 'Frail' Elderly?

Societal ageing has been described as one of the greatest challenges of the 21st century. Whereas *ageing* for many is characterized as 'a progressive, generalized impairment of function resulting in a loss of adaptive response to stress (loss of biological reserve) and in a growing risk of age-associated disease' (Kirkwood, 1995), there has been a change in the physical wellness of older people in the 'baby boomer' generation, which has led to reductions in late life disability (Martin et al., 2010) but with disparity between the sexes, women living longer but with more disability associated life years than men (Carmel, 2019). To label all older adults over the age of 65 years together is far too simple. A helpful distinction might be drawn between the *robust* and medically complex or *frail* elderly. Frailty has a number of definitions that centre around the concept of biological reserve. The frailty phenotype combines impaired physical activity, mobility, balance, muscle strength, motor processing, cognition, nutrition and endurance (Ferrucci et al., 2004; Fried et al., 2001). It is not identical to disability and the presence of coexisting disease (comorbidity). In a study of older people meeting strict 'phenotypic' criteria for frailty, only 22% of the sample also had both comorbidity and disability, 46% had comorbidity without disability, 6% had disability without comorbidity, and 27% had neither (Fried et al., 2001). Frailty may also be defined in a more mechanistic fashion, by adding up the total number of pre-existing biomedical and social comorbidities to create a frailty index expressed as the number of impairments divided by the total number counted, originally derived from the comprehensive geriatric assessment; frail people, however defined, do have a higher risk of intercurrent disease, increased disability, hospitalization and death than those without frailty (Lacas and Rockwood, 2012). Definitions of old age often reflect the theory of ageing that each definition is attempting to explain, or, occasionally, merely convenience. A balanced approach to understanding the ageing process includes not only the understanding of the physiological changes that occur but also the social context in which they occur and the attitudinal changes of ageing persons themselves (Stein and Moritz, 1999). The 'life course' conceptual framework considers the influence of modifiable factors of lifestyle, such as not smoking or abusing alcohol, regular exercise and good social supports, and of non-modifiable factors such as economic circumstances and depressive disorders—all of which are independently predictive of healthy ageing in a 50-year prospective cohort study (Vaillant and Mukamal, 2001). Functional status of an individual therefore depends on the interaction of all of an individual's life course events and is independent of chronological age.

Chronological age is in fact a very poor indicator of functional status. Individuals of the same age show great variability in social, psychological and physical changes. However, the chronological age of retirement, commonly 65 years in many nations (although this is changing as a result of population-wide pension burdens), is the age when 'old age' becomes operationalized. The World Health Organization (Stein and Moritz, 1999) uses the 'life course' framework to define *ageing* as 'the process of progressive change in the biological, psychological and social structure of individuals' without prescribing any chronological ages associated with this process. When ages are, however, superimposed on this definition, 'mid-life' is defined as beginning at 50 years or after menopause in women, 'young old' at 60 years and 'very old' at 80-plus years.

'Incontinence' as a diagnosis or as a symptom fits well into the life course model, where comorbidities or life events have an impact on the course of the disease process or symptoms, and chronological age may not be a significant factor in either symptom presence or severity, although age is an immutable risk factor associated with UI.

The first general assumption, made by the committee on the frail elderly for the Sixth International Consultation on Incontinence, is that there is no reason to suspect that interventions proven to be effective in the management of community-dwelling older people should not be effective in frail older adults and that such interventions should not be withheld for reasons of age alone. However, due regard should be given to remaining life expectancy, the wishes of the patient and care partner, and the potential for benefits and harms of the proposed treatment (Gibson et al., 2021). Incontinence in older people most often has multiple underlying causes and, as such, forms a true geriatric syndrome in a similar fashion to falls and delirium. Cure, as defined by total absence of symptoms, as for most other chronic conditions, is the exception rather than the rule when dealing with frail older people, but there is great opportunity to relieve the burden of symptoms and greatly improve quality of well-being for most older people affected by incontinence (Ouslander, 2000)

Prevalence of Incontinence in the Elderly

Estimates of the prevalence of UI vary widely, depending upon the definition used in the study (the International Continence Society definition stating 'any involuntary loss of urine' says nothing of severity, frequency, duration or impact) and the setting in which the study took place. Generally, the more functionally dependent the study population, the higher the prevalence of UI such that the highest prevalence occurs in frail older people in residential long-term care (nursing homes). Crude prevalence estimates for the most inclusive definitions of UI in women ('ever', 'any' or 'at least once in the past 12 months') range from 5% to 69%, with most studies reporting a prevalence of any UI in the range of 25% to 45% (Abrams et al., 2018). There are, however, still gaps in our knowledge; for instance, in a systematic review of incontinence in people with a dementia diagnosis living at home, rates of incontinence varied between 1.1% in a general community population to 38% in those receiving homecare services (Drennan et al., 2013). Men overall appear to have half the prevalence of UI than women. The increasing prevalence in association with age is largely due to the contribution of urgency urinary incontinence (UUI) rather than exertional or stress urinary incontinence (SUI). One study demonstrated an increasing rate of UUI from 0.7% between ages 50 and 59 years to 3.4% for 70 years and older men. SUI prevalence was steady at 0.5% and 0.1%, respectively (Ueda et al., 2000). A similar trend of increasing proportions of urgency and UI with increasing age was shown in the United States and smaller population-based Canadian studies (Diokno et al., 2007; Finkelstein, 2002). Conversely, Maral et al. (2001) showed increasing prevalence of SUI with age, from 0.9% between ages 35 and 44 years to 4.9% at age 65 and older.

Faecal incontinence is also more prevalent in older adults, although more difficult to measure due to a lack of standard definitions. Prevalence rates were reported to vary between 5% and 10% in community-dwelling adults older than 60 years in the Netherlands (88% response rate) (Teunissen et al., 2004). In a single, relatively bias-free study using a standardized instrument to ascertain faecal incontinence, rates varied between 11% and 15% (Macmillan et al., 2004). Faecal incontinence rates show no sex difference and increase in association with increasing age for both men and women.

Regarding older adults seeking assistance for symptoms of incontinence, rates of the use of health services have been shown to be consistently low. Andersson et al. (2004) investigated by questionnaire how UI affects daily activities and help-seeking behaviours in a Swedish regional population (n = 2129) and found that only 18% of those aged 65 to 79 years requested treatment—those with the worst leakage and level of distress. Hannestad et al. (2000) found that only 25% of symptomatic older Norwegian women sought help—again, those who were older and with worse symptoms. In the UK, a similar mailed questionnaire to an older regional population (n = 915) found that 15% of those with incontinence had used continence services. The most significant factor for continence service usage was being asked about their symptoms by a health professional (OR: 15.7, 95% CI: 7.3–33.9). Other significant factors were more severe and bothersome symptoms, as well as worse general health (Peters et al., 2004). These figures were similar to another UK study, in which only 9% of all adults with severe symptoms sought a consultation, which the authors found was associated with an acceptance of incontinence as normal in older women (McGrother et al., 2004). However, in an Australian study, 73% of women aged 70 to 75 years had sought help or advice about their incontinence, and these were women with more severe symptoms (Miller et al., 2003). There is a general lack of understanding or awareness of pelvic floor disorders which may exacerbate the lack of healthcare seeking. In a survey of 346 community-dwelling women, a lack of knowledge reached 72% for incontinence and 53.6% for prolapse. On multivariate analysis, lower educational attainment, being unaware of incontinence or prolapse as medical conditions, and having no history of care seeking for these conditions were significantly associated with this lack of knowledge (Chen et al., 2019). Regarding the impression that incontinence is normal for being older is commonly held, a recent Canadian study found that two-thirds of more than 4000 women older than 65 years felt this to be the case (Shaw et al., 2019).

Although UI is widely purported to be a predictor of nursing home admission, data supporting this assertion are few (Thom et al., 1997). Holroyd-Leduc et al. (2004) investigated the relationship of UI to key adverse outcomes (death, nursing home admission, functional decline) in 5500 community-dwelling elderly with a mean age of 77 years (range: 69–103 years) and concluded that UI was not an independent risk factor for these adverse outcomes, but higher levels of illness severity and functional impairment were.

AETIOLOGY AND PATHOPHYSIOLOGY

In older adults, UI may be associated with reversible factors. These can be remembered using the mnemonic 'DIPPERS' (Gibson et al., 2021) (Box 14.1). These factors are useful to consider in the initial assessment of an older person with recent-onset UI and describe those areas to which attention might be paid, leading to an amelioration of symptoms without any intervention aimed specifically at the lower urinary tract. UI in an older person forms a geriatric syndrome, with a complex interaction of underlying pathophysiological changes, risk factors and modifying factors. Addressing incontinence in frail or medical complex older adults then usually requires a multifactorial intervention to achieve benefit.

BOX 14.1 Associated Factors in Urinary Incontinence: DIPPERS

D – Delirium
I – Infection
P – Pharmaceuticals
P – Psychological
E – Excess fluid intake
R – Restricted mobility
S – Stool impaction (and other factors)

Central Neurological Factors Affecting Control of Continence

1. Diseases that affect central neurological control include stroke, brain tumour, Parkinson's disease, multiple sclerosis, diabetes mellitus, cerebral atrophy, multisystem atrophy, normal pressure hydrocephalus, dementia and depression (De Ridder et al., 1998; Gariballa, 2003).

2. Neurological disorders that affect suprasacral spinal cord pathways, with deficits affecting both somatic and autonomic nervous systems, include multiple sclerosis, dorsal column neuropathies, spinal cord injury (Blok et al., 1997) leading to sphincter dyssynergia through upper motor neuron damage or conversely sphincter underactivity via sympathetic dysfunction (Corcos and Schick, 2001).

3. Progressive sympathetic nervous system activation occurs in older age and may be a causal component in urinary tract pathophysiology, although the underlying central nervous system mechanisms mediating this increase in activity are unknown (Esler et al., 2002).

4. Peripheral nerve root compression (S2–S4) from musculoskeletal injury or degeneration can lead to decreased lower limb mobility, impaired sensation and reflexes, and PFM and striated sphincter weakness (Corcos and Schick, 2001).

Non-Neurological Disease
Ageing Urinary Tract

Physiological changes in the lower urinary tract of men and women in association with age have been well described but are limited by their cross-sectional nature and in that most studies have been done in people with pre-existing lower urinary tract symptoms (Collas and Malone-Lee, 1996; Malone-Lee and Wahedna, 1993; Pfisterer et al., 2006a; Pfisterer et al., 2006b; Resnick et al., 1995). Urodynamic changes associated with age have typically included smaller voided volume, increased residual volume, smaller bladder capacity and increased rates of detrusor overactivity. Reported age-related changes in the lower urinary tract are shown in Table 14.1 and detailed in the following. Urodynamic

TABLE 14.1   Reported Age-Related Changes in the Lower Urinary Tract Likely to Increase the Chance of Urinary Incontinence

Age-Related Change	Potential Effects on Continence
Bladder overactivity and urgency UI	Impaired bladder contractile function, increased residual urine, and decreased bladder capacity
Bladder function: Decreased capacity Decreased sensation of filling Increased detrusor overactivity Decreased bladder contractile function Increased residual urine	Increased likelihood of urinary symptoms and UI
Urethra: Decreased closure pressure in women and men	Increased likelihood of stress and urgency UI
Prostate: Increased incidence of benign prostatic obstruction Increased incidence of prostate cancer	Increased likelihood of urinary symptoms and UI
Decreased oestrogen (women)	Increased incidence of genitourinary syndrome of menopause and related symptoms Increased incidence of recurrent urinary tract infections
Increased night-time urine production	Increased likelihood of nocturia and night-time UI
Altered central and peripheral neurotransmitter concentrations and actions	Increased likelihood of lower urinary tract dysfunction
Altered immune function	Increased likelihood of recurrent urinary tract infections
Increased prevalence of white matter hyperintensities in brain	Increased prevalence of severe urge/urgency, link to cognitive impairment and impaired mobility

UI, Urinary incontinence.

findings may not relate to symptoms: in a urodynamic study of community-based healthy persons older than 55 years, detrusor overactivity was found in 42% of continent women, one-third of whom were totally free of lower urinary tract symptoms (Resnick et al., 1995). Nevertheless, in a cross-sectional study involving ambulatory, cognitively intact, community-dwelling older female volunteers, maximum urethral closure pressure, detrusor contraction strength and urine flow rate all declined significantly with age, regardless of whether detrusor overactivity was present or not (Pfisterer et al., 2006a):

1. Bladder: Yoshida et al. (2001, 2004) investigated changes to detrusor neurotransmitters with increasing age. They showed that purinergic neurotransmission increased with age, whereas cholinergic transmission decreased with age, most likely as a result of decreased release of acetylcholine from parasympathetic nerves supplying the detrusor and from the urothelium (non-neuronal acetylcholine). Conversely, the bladder becomes stiffer with ageing due to an accumulation of connective and fibrous tissue. This leads to a slower speed of detrusor contraction, and a low flow rate is the result during voiding (Schafer, 1999). Detrusor smooth muscle contractility itself appears to be unaffected by age in the absence of bladder dysfunction. The observation of impaired emptying appears to be the result of a dampening of generated contractile force by the accumulated connective tissue (Susset et al., 1978). However, where there is detrusor overactivity, a reduction in detrusor contractility can be demonstrated, in line with the observed reduction in acetylcholine release from nerve stimulation (Fry et al., 2011; Yoshida et al., 2004).

2. Sphincter integrity: In an intraurethral ultrasound investigation, Klauser et al. (2004) found that with increasing age, the striated urethral sphincter showed a linear decline in thickness and ability to produce urethral closure pressure. Based on a sample of 82 women aged 20 to 70 years, urethral closure pressure was found to decrease by 15 cmH$_2$O per decade (Trowbridge et al., 2007). In ageing paraurethral tissue, the connective tissue component has been shown to increase, altering in composition to be more fibrous relative to other components, and show a decrease in the vascularity of the mucosa and urethral nerve supply (Verelst et al., 2002). Regarding decreased urethral muscle function, Perucchini et al.

(2002a, 2002b) showed a decline in the number of striated muscle fibres, fibre density and total cross-sectional area of striated muscle in a dissection study of the anterior and posterior walls of the urethra in 25 female cadavers aged 15 to 80 years. A sevenfold variance was seen, however, between the specimens with the most and fewest muscle fibres anteriorly, and localized losses were found in the proximal posterior striated sphincter muscles (Perucchini et al., 2002a; Perucchini et al., 2002b). Similarly, an age-related apoptosis of human rhabdosphincter myocytes has been described (Strasser et al., 2000).

3. PFM ageing: Despite the relatively high prevalence of pelvic floor disorders in older women, the underlying pathophysiology of age-related PFM dysfunction remains poorly understood. Many studies are cross-sectional in nature rather than longitudinal, focus on symptomatic women and are hampered by small samples with inadequate controls, particularly for parity—a major influencing factor (Hwang et al., 2019). PFM isometric strength measured by maximum volitional vaginal closure force in the mid-sagittal plane shows no significant decline with increasing age (Trowbridge et al., 2007). This is somewhat unexpected, as a 30% to 40% loss of skeletal muscle volume and cross-sectional area is the usual finding in striated muscle with advancing age. Changes in skeletal muscle occur with age in endocrine, neural, enzymatic and energy systems, partially genetically driven, and result in a decrease in muscle mass by fibre, vascular and mitochondrial degradation and loss associated with the sarcopenia of ageing (Powers and Howley, 2001). A small cadaveric study revealed that the PFMs were disproportionately affected by age-related fibrotic degeneration compared to comparator muscles of the obturator internus and vastus lateralis (Rieger et al., 2021). This is in direct contradiction to the earlier magnetic resonance imaging (MRI) study comparing nulliparous young and old women, where no change in volume of the levator ani in association with age could be demonstrated, whereas the obturator internus, used as a comparator, did demonstrate such an effect (Morris et al., 2012). Furthering this investigation, a case–control study comparing two groups of nulliparous women younger than 40 years (n = 12) and 70 years or older (n = 9), using clinical assessment and MRI, found a similar preservation of PFM strength in the older

group not seen using hand grip strength, and levator bowl volume at rest was greater than 80% among older women compared to the younger group, indicating posterior distension with age (Swenson et al., 2020). Dimpfl et al. (1998) showed histomorphological changes in the PFMs in older women compared to women younger than 40 years, such as decreased fibre circumference and fibrosis. In a more recent study on the biomechanical properties of PFMs from younger (43.4 ± 11.6 years, n = 5) versus older (74.9 ± 11.9 years, n = 10) women, an increase in stiffness in the passive phase not shown in non-PFMs was reported (Burnett et al., 2020). Gunnarsson and Mattiasson (1999), using surface electromyography (EMG), showed that older women without incontinence did not show as much of a decline in PFM strength as women with SUI, UUI or mixed incontinence. In this study, the investigators hypothesized that neuromuscular changes in the pelvic floor were progressive and present for a long time before symptoms appeared. This finding was confirmed in a study of 70 nulliparous women (age range: 18–69 years) using clinical assessment and surface EMG, where no significant differences were observed between the different age groups in PFM digital palpation, manometry values and surface EMG (Bocardi et al., 2018). However, Constantinou et al. (2002), using MRI, showed that older women displaced the pelvic floor significantly less than younger women on voluntary contraction. A computed tomography study comparing pelvic floor variables in the standing and supine position using 139 volunteers (70 men, mean 46.7 years; 69 women, mean 47.3 years) showed that the bladder neck (men, 22.2 ± 4.9 mm vs 28.3 ± 5.3 mm; women, 9 ± 5.1 mm vs 19 ± 4 mm) and anorectal junction (men, −18.8 ± 5.5 mm vs −12.1 ± 5.1 mm; women, −20 ± 4.7 mm vs −11.2 ± 4.3 mm) were significantly lower when in a standing position than when lying. Differences in all variables between standing and lying were larger in women than in men. Descent of the anorectal junction was greater in older women (Narita et al., 2020). In men, reduction in puborectalis and ischiocavernosus muscles thickness was studied using MRI reconstruction, and in younger men, older men and post-prostatectomy men with erectile dysfunction and UI. There was a significant reduction in puborectalis and ischiocavernosus muscle and thickness in older men, hypothesized to be due to age-related atrophy. There were no non-PFM controls for comparison (Tai et al., 2020). A larger cross-sectional, blinded MRI study of both men and women (163 men, 206 women; median age 58 years [range: 17–92 years]) reported thinning and increased concavity of the levator ani associated with increasing age. There was no control for parity in women (Komemushi et al., 2019).

4. Ageing changes in the fascial supports of the urinary tract: Ageing connective tissue shows evidence of fewer and more immature collagen cross-linkages, resulting in a two- to threefold reduction in the maximum load to failure, decreased plasticity and elasticity, but this does not imply a direct causative effect of 'ageing' (Frankel and Nordin, 1980).

Other Aetiologies

1. Side effects: This includes side effects from prescription and over-the-counter drugs.
2. Social and environmental status: This relates to the characteristics of the living environment (ease of access to washroom), mobility, and need for social support of care from either a formal or informal (friend or family) care partner.
3. Disturbance of the vasopressin system, or diseases causing a shift in diuresis: This includes diseases such as diabetes mellitus, congestive heart failure, dependent oedema and sleep apnoea cause a shift in diuresis from daytime to night-time (i.e., nocturnal polyuria; Asplund 2004).
4. Functional impairment: This is described as the difference between environmental demand and functional capability (Eekhof et al., 1996) and can be modified by treatable factors such as intercurrent illnesses, medications, nutritional status, vision and hearing status, mobility and dexterity, pain, anxiety, and depression (Harari et al., 2003). Within functional impairment, strength impairment and mobility are the critical domains (Jenkins and Fultz, 2005) for predicting UI. In stroke, functional impairment, particularly needing help to access the toilet, is the strongest independent factor associated with new-onset faecal incontinence after a stroke (Harari et al., 2003). Addressing mobility and physical impairment may be more important than intervention for cognitive dysfunction (Su et al., 2020).
5. Obesity: Obesity is a risk factor, more for SUI than for UUI, but is increasingly important as the

proportion of either very overweight or obese people in the population of developed countries increases. The mechanism behind the increased risk may be simply mechanical but may also reflect the influence of metabolic syndrome on the development of incontinence in later life (Chu et al., 2013). Central obesity in women appears to be a significant risk factor over and above that attributable to increased body mass index (Krause et al., 2010).

Factors in Females

Factors in females are:
- becoming oestrogen deficient postmenopausally (Davila et al., 2003; Schaffer and Fantl, 1996);
- high parity (Simeonova et al., 1999);
- certain types of intrapelvic surgery, including hysterectomy (Sherburn et al., 2001); and
- female circumcision (Stein and Moritz, 1999).
Becoming oestrogen deficient leads to:
- loss of collagen, thinning epithelium in vagina, caused by decreased collagen synthesis (Falconer et al., 1996) and increased collagenase activity (Kushner et al., 1999);
- decreased vascular plexi in the submucosa of the urethra—this submucosal vascular bed gives passive urethral control and loss can lead to a loss of up to 30% of urethral closure pressure (Corcos and Schick, 2001); and
- less acidic urethral and vaginal environments (increased pH), leading to changes in the vaginal flora and more risk of colonization with gram-negative bacteria, which in turn leads to a higher risk of genitourinary syndrome of menopause and urinary tract infections (Bachmann and Nevadunsky, 2000; Nilsson et al., 1995; Notelovitz, 1995; Samsioe. 1998).

Factors in Males

Factors in males are increased prostatic size in:
- benign prostatic enlargement (Blanker et al., 2000; Madersbacher et al., 1999) and
- prostatic carcinoma.

In benign prostatic enlargement the outer zones of the prostate progressively atrophy while the inner zones begin to grow again until death. In carcinoma the outer glandular epithelium enlarges. This leads to:
- impaired urinary flow,
- obstruction of the urethra,
- urinary retention,
- urinary frequency,
- detrusor overactivity, and
- incomplete emptying and retrograde filling of the ureters (Timiras and Leary, 2003).

Treatment of these disorders by prostatectomy, whether simple, radical or transurethral, carries a risk of urethral vascular bed destruction and nerve damage, even in 'nerve-sparing' surgery (Corcos and Schick, 2001), although robot-assisted prostatectomy appears to be associated with a small reduction in the rate of incontinence compared to laparoscopic and conventional approaches (Basiri et al., 2018; Carbonara et al., 2021).

Faecal Incontinence and Constipation

Faecal incontinence and constipation in older adults has many risk factors. Age has been established as a risk factor for faecal incontinence in many population-based studies (Nelson, 2004; Quander et al., 2005; Roberts et al., 1999; Whitehead et al., 2009). Other factors that have been associated include female sex, coexistent UI, poor general health, physical limitations, cognitive impairment, stool consistency, prior colorectal surgery and high body mass index (Abramov et al., 2005; Goode et al., 2005; Khullar et al., 1998; Nelson et al., 1998; Varma et al., 2006). However, among population-based studies among older adults, when controlled for, risk factors related to birth are no longer significantly associated with faecal incontinence (Bharucha et al., 2010; Whitehead et al., 2009). Many diseases and comorbid disorders are also associated with faecal incontinence and include diabetes, dementia-related incontinence, irritable bowel syndrome, inflammatory bowel disease, systemic sclerosis and neurological diseases such as cerebrovascular disease (Bytzer et al., 2001; Harari et al., 2003; Quander et al., 2005; Rey et al., 2010; Thoua et al., 2011; Varma et al., 2006; Wald, 1995; Wang et al., 2010). The association between faecal incontinence and loose stool consistency (diarrhoea) is robust in community-dwelling populations and nursing home studies (Bharucha et al., 2010; Johanson et al., 1997; Markland et al., 2010; Nelson et al., 1998; Rey et al., 2010; Whitehead et al., 2009). The aetiology of faecal incontinence, in a similar fashion to UI, remains multifactorial and treatment depends on the underlying mechanisms or specific comorbid disorders, as well as the overall burden of multimorbidity including medications used to manage multiple chronic disorders.

Ageing changes of increased fibrous connective tissue within the gut wall and a decreased neural supply to the colon are likely causes of constipation (Camilleri et al., 2000). On high spatial resolution endoanal MRI in normal ageing in continent elderly (Rociu et al., 2000), there was a thinning of the external anal sphincter and longitudinal muscle of the anus, and compensatory thickening of the internal anal sphincter. Likewise, ageing was associated with a thickening of the internal anal sphincter. Older, faecally incontinent women had a thinner external anal sphincter, had decreased maximum squeeze pressures, and were hypersensitive to rectal distension with decreased tolerable rectal volumes and urge to defaecate at lower volumes (Lewicky-Gaupp et al., 2009). In older men and women with faecal incontinence, studies have reported an age-related increase in pudendal neuropathy in incontinent women that may be unrelated to squeeze pressures (Van Meegdenburg et al., 2015; Vernava et al., 1993). Anorectal function in older incontinent patients and continent age- and sex-matched controls showed that individuals with faecal incontinence had reduced anal resting pressures (Barrett et al., 1989; Lewicky-Gaupp, et al. 2009). One study comparing eight older incontinent women (mean age: 71.6 years, SD: 7.5) with nine older continent women (mean age: 71.6 years, SD: 7.5) and nine younger continent women (mean age: 28.7, SD: 7.3) found that women with faecal incontinence were more likely to have decreased maximum squeeze pressures and levator ani defects (Lewicky-Gaupp et al., 2010). Older faecally incontinent females tolerated lower balloon anorectal manometry volumes before the urge to defaecate, which was indicative of rectal hypersensitivity (Lewicky-Gaupp et al., 2009).

REFERENCES

Abramov, Y., Sand, P. K., Botros, S. M., et al. (2005). Risk factors for female anal incontinence: New insight through the evanston–northwestern twin sisters study. *Obstetrics & Gynecology, 106*(4), 726–732.

Abrams, P., Andersson, K. E., Apostolidis, A., et al. (2018). 6th International Consultation on Incontinence. Recommendations of the international scientific committee: Evaluation and treatment of urinary incontinence, pelvic organ prolapse and faecal incontinence. *Neurourology and Urodynamics, 37*(7), 2271–2272.

Andersson, G., Johansson, J. E., Garpenholt, O., et al. (2004). Urinary incontinence—prevalence, impact on daily living and desire for treatment: A population-based study. *Scandinavian Journal of Urology and Nephrology, 38*(2), 125–130.

Asplund, R. (2004). Nocturia, nocturnal polyuria, and sleep quality in the elderly. *Journal of Psychosomatic Research, 56*(5), 517–525.

Bachmann, G. A., & Nevadunsky, N. S. (2000). Diagnosis and treatment of atrophic vaginitis. *American Family Physician, 61*(10), 3090–3096.

Barrett, J. A., Brocklehurst, J. C., Kiff, E. S., et al. (1989). Anal function in geriatric patients with faecal incontinence. *Gut, 30*(9), 1244–1251.

Basiri, A., de la Rosette, J. J., Tabatabaei, S., et al. (2018). Comparison of retropubic, laparoscopic and robotic radical prostatectomy: Who is the winner? *World Journal of Urology, 36*(4), 609–621.

Bharucha, A. E., Zinsmeister, A. R., Schleck, C. D., et al. (2010). Bowel disturbances are the most important risk factors for late onset fecal incontinence: A population-based case–control study in women. *Gastroenterology, 139*(5), 1559–1566.

Blanker, M. H., Bohnen, A. M., Groeneveld, F. P., et al. (2000). Normal voiding patterns and determinants of increased diurnal and nocturnal voiding frequency in elderly men. *Journal of Urology, 164*(4), 1201–1205.

Blok, B. F. M., Sturms, L. M., & Holstege, G. (1997). A PET study on cortical and subcortical control of pelvic floor musculature in women. *The Journal of Comparative Neurology, 389*, 535–544.

Bocardi, D. A. S., Pereira-Baldon, V. S., Ferreira, C. H. J., et al. (2018). Pelvic floor muscle function and EMG in nulliparous women of different ages: A cross-sectional study. *Climacteric, 21*(5), 462–466.

Burnett, L. A., Cook, M., Shah, S., et al. (2020). Age-associated changes in the mechanical properties of human cadaveric pelvic floor muscles. *Journal of Biomechanics, 98*, 109436.

Bytzer, P., Talley, N. J., Leemon, M., et al. (2001). Prevalence of gastrointestinal symptoms associated with diabetes mellitus: A population-based survey of 15,000 adults. *Archives of Internal Medicine, 161*(16), 1989–1996.

Camilleri, M., Lee, J. S., Viramontes, B., et al. (2000). Insights into the pathophysiology and mechanisms of constipation, irritable bowel syndrome, and diverticulosis in older people. *Journal of the American Geriatrics Society, 48*(9), 1142–1150.

Carbonara, U., Srinath, M., Crocerossa, F., et al. (2021). Robot-assisted radical prostatectomy versus standard laparoscopic radical prostatectomy: An evidence-based analysis of comparative outcomes. *World Journal of Urology, 39*(10), 3721–3732.

Carmel, S. (2019). Health and well-being in late life: Gender differences worldwide. *Frontiers of Medicine, 6*, 218.

Chen, C. C. G., Cox, J. T., Yuan, C., et al. (2019). Knowledge of pelvic floor disorders in women seeking primary care: A cross-sectional study. *BMC Family Practice, 20*(1), 70.

Chu, K. F., Rotker, K., & Ellsworth, P. (2013). The impact of obesity on benign and malignant urologic conditions. *Postgraduate Medical Journal, 125*(4), 53–69.

Collas, D., & Malone-Lee, J. G. (1996). Age associated changes in detrusor sensory function in patients with lower urinary tract symptoms. *International Urogynecology Journal and Pelvic Floor Dysfunction, 7*, 24–29.

Constantinou, C. E., Hvistendahl, G., Ryhammer, A., et al. (2002). Determining the displacement of the pelvic floor and pelvic organs during voluntary contractions using magnetic resonance imaging in younger and older women. *BJU International, 90*(4), 408–414.

Corcos, J., & Schick, E. (Eds.). (2001). *The urinary sphincter.* New York: Marcel Dekker.

Coyne, K. S., Kvasz, M., Ireland, A. M., et al. (2012). Urinary incontinence and its relationship to mental health and health-related quality of life in men and women in Sweden, the United Kingdom, and the United States. *European Urology, 61*(1), 88–95.

Coyne, K. S., Wein, A., Nicholson, S., et al. (2013). Comorbidities and personal burden of urgency urinary incontinence: A systematic review. *International Journal of Clinical Practice, 67*(10), 1015–1033.

Davila, G. W., Singh, A., Karapanagiotou, I., et al. (2003). Are women with urogenital atrophy symptomatic? *American Journal of Obstetrics and Gynecology, 188*(2), 382–388.

De Ridder, D., Vermeulen, C., De Smet, E., et al. (1998). Clinical assessment of pelvic floor dysfunction in multiple sclerosis: Urodynamic and neurological correlates. *Neurourology and Urodynamics, 17*(5), 537–542.

Dimpfl, T., Jaeger, C., Mueller-Felber, W., et al. (1998). Myogenic changes of the levator ani muscle in premenopausal women: The impact of delivery and age. *Neurourology and Urodynamics, 17*, 197–205.

Diokno, A. C., Estanol, M. V., Ibrahim, I. A., et al. (2007). Prevalence of urinary incontinence in community dwelling men: A cross sectional nationwide epidemiological survey. *International Urology and Nephrology, 39*(1), 129–136.

Divo, M. J., Martinez, C. H., Mannino, D. M. (2014). Ageing and the epidemiology of multimorbidity. *Respir J., 44*(4), 1055–1068.

Drennan, V. M., Rait, G., Cole, L., et al. (2013). The prevalence of incontinence in people with cognitive impairment or dementia living at home: A systematic review. *Neurourology and Urodynamics, 32*(4), 314–324.

Eekhof, J. A., De Bock, G. H., Schaapveld, K., et al. (1996). [Potential role for family physicians in pushing back age-related impairment: Hearing and vision disorders, incontinence and arthrosis]. *Nederlands Tijdschrift Voor Geneeskunde, 140*(48), 2402–2406.

Esler, M., Lambert, G., Kaye, D., et al. (2002). Influence of aging on the sympathetic nervous system and adrenal medulla at rest and during stress. *Biogerontology, 3*, 45–49.

Falconer, C., Ekman-Ordeberg, G., & Ulmsten, U. (1996). Changes in para-urethral connective tissue at menopause are counteracted by oestrogen. *Maturitas, 24*, 197–204.

Ferrucci, L., Guralnik, J. M., Studenski, S., et al. (2004). Designing randomized, controlled trials aimed at preventing or delaying functional decline and disability in frail, older persons: A consensus report. *Journal of the American Geriatrics Society, 52*(4), 625–634.

Finkelstein, M. M. (2002). Medical conditions, medications, and urinary incontinence. Analysis of a population-based survey. *Canadian Family Physician, 48*, 96–101.

Frankel, V. H., & Nordin, M. (1980). *Basic biomechanics of the skeletal system.* Philadelphia: Lea & Febiger.

Fried, L. P., Tangen, C. M., Walston, J., et al. (2001). Frailty in older adults: Evidence for a phenotype. *The Journals of Gerontology. Series A, Biological Sciences and Medical Sciences, 56*(3), M146–M156.

Fry, C. H., Bayliss, M., Young, J. S., et al. (2011). Influence of age and bladder dysfunction on the contractile properties of isolated human detrusor smooth muscle. *BJU International, 108*(2 Pt. 2), e91–e96.

Gariballa, S. E. (2003). Potentially treatable causes of poor outcome in acute stroke patients with urinary incontinence. *Acta Neurologica Scandinavica, 107*(5), 336–340.

Gibson, W., Johnson, T., Kirschner-Hermanns, R., et al. (2021). Incontinence in frail elderly persons: Report of the 6th International Consultation on Incontinence. *Neurourology and Urodynamics, 40*(1), 38–54.

Goode, P. S., Burgio, K. L., Halli, A. D., et al. (2005). Prevalence and correlates of fecal incontinence in community-dwelling older adults. *Journal of the American Geriatrics Society, 53*(4), 629–635.

Gunnarsson, M., & Mattiasson, A. (1999). Female stress, urge, and mixed urinary incontinence are associated with a chronic and progressive pelvic floor/vaginal neuromuscular disorder: An investigation of 317 healthy and incontinent women using vaginal surface electromyography. *Neurourology and Urodynamics, 18*(6), 613–621.

Hannestad, Y. S., Rortveit, G., Sandvik, H., et al. (2000). A community-based epidemiological survey of female urinary incontinence: The Norwegian EPINCONT study. Epidemiology of incontinence in the county of nord-trondelag. *Journal of Clinical Epidemiology, 53*(11), 1150–1157.

Harari, D., Coshall, C., Rudd, A. G., et al. (2003). New-onset fecal incontinence after stroke: Prevalence, natural history, risk factors, and impact. *Stroke, 34*(1), 144–150.

Holroyd-Leduc, J. M., Mehta, K. M., & Covinsky, K. E. (2004). Urinary incontinence and its association with death, nursing home admission, and functional decline. *Journal of the American Geriatrics Society, 52*(5), 712–718.

Hwang, J. Y., Kim, B. I., & Song, S. H. (2019). Parity: A risk factor for decreased pelvic floor muscle strength and endurance in middle-aged women. *International Urogynecology Journal*, *30*(6), 933–938.

Irwin, D. E., Milsom, I., Hunskaar, S., et al. (2006). Population-based survey of urinary incontinence, overactive bladder, and other lower urinary tract symptoms in five countries: Results of the EPIC study. *European Urology*, *50*(6), 1306–1314; discussion 1314–1305.

Jenkins, K. R., & Fultz, N. H. (2005). Functional impairment as a risk factor for urinary incontinence among older Americans. *Neurourology and Urodynamics*, *24*, 51–55.

Johanson, J. F., Irizarry, F., & Doughty, A. (1997). Risk factors for fecal incontinence in a nursing home population. *Journal of Clinical Gastroenterology*, *24*(3), 156–160.

Khullar, V., Damiano, R., Toozs-Hobson, P., et al. (1998). Prevalence of faecal incontinence among women with urinary incontinence. *British Journal of Obstetrics and Gynaecology*, *105*(11), 1211–1213.

Kim, H., Yoshida, H., & Suzuki, T. (2010). The effects of multidimensional exercise treatment on community-dwelling elderly Japanese women with stress, urge, and mixed urinary incontinence: A randomized controlled trial. *International Journal of Nursing Studies*, *48*(10), 1165–1172.

Kim, H., Yoshida, H., & Suzuki, T. (2011). The effects of multidimensional exercise on functional decline, urinary incontinence, and fear of falling in community-dwelling elderly women with multiple symptoms of geriatric syndrome: A randomized controlled and 6-month follow-up trial. *Archives of Gerontology and Geriatrics*, *52*(1), 99–105.

Kinsella, K. W., & He, W. (2009). *An aging World: 2008*. Washington, DC: US Census Bureau.

Kirkwood, T. B. L. (1995). The evolution of ageing. *Reviews in Clinical Gerontology*, *5*, 3–9.

Klauser, A., Frauscher, F., Strasser, H., et al. (2004). Age-related rhabdosphincter function in female urinary stress incontinence: Assessment of intraurethral sonography. *Journal of Ultrasound in Medicine*, *23*(5), 631–637; quiz 638–639.

Komemushi, Y., Komemushi, A., Morimoto, K., et al. (2019). Quantitative evaluation of age-related changes to pelvic floor muscles in magnetic resonance images from 369 patients. *Geriatrics and Gerontology International*, *19*(8), 834–837.

Krause, M. P., Albert, S. M., Elsangedy, H. M., et al. (2010). Urinary incontinence and waist circumference in older women. *Age and Ageing*, *39*(1), 69–73.

Kushner, L., Chen, Y., Desautel, M., et al. (1999). Collagenase activity is elevated in conditioned media from fibroblasts of women with pelvic floor weakening. *International Urogynecology Journal and Pelvic Floor Dysfunction*, *10*(Suppl. 1), 34.

Lacas, A., & Rockwood, K. (2012). Frailty in primary care: A review of its conceptualization and implications for practice. *BMC Medicine*, *10*, 4.

Lewicky-Gaupp, C., Brincat, C., Yousuf, A., et al. (2010). Fecal incontinence in older women: Are levator ani defects a factor? *American Journal of Obstetrics and Gynecology*, *202*(5), 491.e1–491.e6.

Lewicky-Gaupp, C., Hamilton, Q., Ashton-Miller, J., et al. (2009). Anal sphincter structure and function relationships in aging and fecal incontinence. *American Journal of Obstetrics and Gynecology*, *200*(5), 559.e1–559.e5.

Macmillan, A. K., Merrie, A. E., Marshall, R. J., et al. (2004). The prevalence of fecal incontinence in community-dwelling adults: A systematic review of the literature. *Diseases of the Colon & Rectum*, *47*(8), 1341–1349.

Madersbacher, S., Pycha, A., Klingler, C. H., et al. (1999). Interrelationships of bladder compliance with age, detrusor instability, and obstruction in elderly men with lower urinary tract symptoms. *Neurourology and Urodynamics*, *18*(1), 3–15.

Malone-Lee, J., & Wahedna, I. (1993). Characterisation of detrusor contractile function in relation to old-age. *British Journal of Urology*, *72*, 873–880.

Maral, I., Ozkardes, H., Peskircioglu, L., et al. (2001). Prevalence of stress urinary incontinence in both sexes at or after age 15 years: A cross-sectional study. *Journal of Urology*, *165*(2), 408–412.

Markland, A. D., Goode, P. S., Burgio, K. L., et al. (2010). Incidence and risk factors for fecal incontinence in black and white older adults: A population-based study. *Journal of the American Geriatrics Society*, *58*(7), 1341–1346.

Martin, L. G., Schoeni, R. F., & Andreski, P. F. (2010). Trends in health of older adults in the United States: Past, present, future. *Demography*, *47*(Suppl. 1), 17–40.

McGrother, C. W., Donaldson, M. M., Shaw, C., et al. (2004). Storage symptoms of the bladder: Prevalence, incidence and need for services in the UK. *BJU International*, *93*(6), 763–769.

Miller, Y. D., Brown, W. J., Smith, N., et al. (2003). Managing urinary incontinence across the lifespan. *International Journal of Behavioral Medicine*, *10*(2), 143–161.

Milsom, I., Coyne, K. S., Nicholson, S., et al. (2013). Global prevalence and economic burden of urgency urinary incontinence: A systematic review. *European Urology*, *65*(1), 79–95.

Milsom, I., Kaplan, S. A., Coyne, K. S., et al. (2012). Effect of bothersome overactive bladder symptoms on health-related quality of life, anxiety, depression, and treatment seeking in the United States: Results from EpiLUTS. *Urology*, *80*(1), 90–96.

Morris, V. C., Murray, M. P., Delancey, J. O., et al. (2012). A comparison of the effect of age on levator ani and obturator internus muscle cross-sectional areas and volumes in nulliparous women. *Neurourology and Urodynamics, 31*(4), 481–486.

Narita, K., Yamada, Y., Yamada, M., et al. (2020). Pelvic floor morphology in the standing position using upright computed tomography: Age and sex differences. *International Urogynecology Journal, 31*(11), 2387–2393.

Nelson, R. (2004). Epidemiology of fecal incontinence. *Gastroenterology, 126*(1 Suppl. 1), 3–7.

Nelson, R., Furner, S., & Jesudason, V. (1998). Fecal incontinence in Wisconsin nursing homes: Prevalence and associations. *Diseases of the Colon & Rectum, 41*(10), 1226–1229.

Nilsson, K., Risberg, B., & Heimer, G. (1995). The vaginal epithelium in the postmenopause—cytology, histology and pH as methods of assessment. *Maturitas, 21*(1), 51–56.

Notelovitz, M. (1995). Estrogen therapy in the management of problems associated with urogenital ageing: A simple diagnostic test and the effect of the route of hormone administration. *Maturitas, 22*(Suppl. l), 31–33.

Ouslander, J. G. (2000). Intractable incontinence in the elderly. *BJU International, 85*(Suppl. 3), 72–78; discussion 81–72.

Perucchini, D., DeLancey, J. O., Ashton-Miller, J. A., et al. (2002a). Age effects on urethral striated muscle. I. Changes in number and diameter of striated muscle fibers in the ventral urethra. *American Journal of Obstetrics and Gynecology, 186*(3), 351–355.

Perucchini, D., DeLancey, J. O., Ashton-Miller, J. A., et al. (2002b). Age effects on urethral striated muscle. II. Anatomic location of muscle loss. *American Journal of Obstetrics and Gynecology, 186*(3), 356–360.

Peters, T. J., Horrocks, S., Stoddart, H., et al. (2004). Factors associated with variations in older people's use of community-based continence services. *Health and Social Care in the Community, 12*(1), 53–62.

Pfisterer, M. H., Griffiths, D. J., Rosenberg, L., et al. (2006a). The impact of detrusor overactivity on bladder function in younger and older women. *Journal of Urology, 175*(5), 1777–1783; discussion 1783.

Pfisterer, M. H., Griffiths, D. J., Schaefer, W., et al. (2006b). The effect of age on lower urinary tract function: A study in women. *Journal of the American Geriatrics Society, 54*(3), 405–412.

Powers, S. K., & Howley, E. T. (2001). *Exercise physiology and application to fitness and performance.* New York: McGraw Hill.

Quander, C. R., Morris, M. C., Melson, J., et al. (2005). Prevalence of and factors associated with fecal incontinence in a large community study of older individuals. *American Journal of Gastroenterology, 100*(4), 905–909.

Resnick, N. M., Elbadawi, A. E., & Yalla, S. V. (1995). Age and the lower urinary tract: What is normal? *Neurourology and Urodynamics, 14*, 1647.

Rey, E., Choung, R. S., Schleck, C. D., et al. (2010). Onset and risk factors for fecal incontinence in a US community. *American Journal of Gastroenterology, 105*(2), 412–419.

Rieger, M., Duran, P., Cook, M., et al. (2021). Quantifying the effects of aging on morphological and cellular properties of human female pelvic floor muscles. *Annals of Biomedical Engineering, 49*(8), 1836–1847.

Roberts, R. O., Jacobsen, S. J., Reilly, W. T., et al. (1999). Prevalence of combined fecal and urinary incontinence: A community-based study. *Journal of the American Geriatrics Society, 47*(7), 837–841.

Rociu, E., Stoker, J., Eijkemans, M. J., et al. (2000). Normal anal sphincter anatomy and age- and sex-related variations at high-spatial-resolution endoanal MR imaging. *Radiology, 217*(2), 395–401.

Samsioe, G. (1998). Urogenital aging—a hidden problem. *American Journal of Obstetrics and Gynecology, 178*(5), S245–S249.

Schafer, W. (1999). Urodynamics of micturition. *Current Opinion in Urology, 2*, 252–256.

Schaffer, J., & Fantl, J. A. (1996). Urogenital effects of the menopause. *Baillieres Clinical Obstetrics & Gynaecology, 10*(3), 401–417.

Shaw, C., Rajabali, S., Tannenbaum, C., et al. (2019). Is the belief that urinary incontinence is normal for ageing related to older Canadian women's experience of urinary incontinence? *International Urogynecology Journal, 30*(12), 2157–2160.

Sherburn, M., Guthrie, J. R., Dudley, E. C., et al. (2001). Is incontinence associated with menopause? *Obstetrics & Gynecology, 98*(4), 628–633.

Simeonova, Z., Milsom, I., Kullendorff, A. M., et al. (1999). The prevalence of urinary incontinence and its influence on the quality of life in women from an urban Swedish population. *Acta Obstetricia et Gynecologica Scandinavica, 78*(6), 546–551.

Stein, C., & Moritz, I. (1999). *A life course perspective of maintaining independence in older age.* Geneva: World Health Organization.

Stothers, L., Thom, D., & Calhoun, E. (2005). Urologic diseases in America project: Urinary incontinence in males—demographics and economic burden. *Journal of Urology, 173*(4), 1302–1308.

Strasser, H., Tiefenthaler, M., Steinlechner, M., et al. (2000). Age dependent apoptosis and loss of rhabdosphincter cells. *Journal of Urology, 164*(5), 1781–1785.

Sugaya, K., Nishijima, S., Owan, T., et al. (2007). Effects of walking exercise on nocturia in the elderly. *Biomedical Research, 28*(2), 101–105.

Susset, J. G., Servot-Viguier, D., Lamy, F., et al. (1978). Collagen in 155 human bladders. *Investigative Urology, 16*(3), 204–206.

Su, Y. Y., Tsai, Y. Y., Chu, C. L., et al. (2020). Exploring a path model of cognitive impairment, functional disability, and incontinence among male veteran home residents in southern Taiwan. *Scientific Reports, 10*(1), 5553.

Swenson, C. W., Masteling, M., DeLancey, J. O., et al. (2020). Aging effects on pelvic floor support: A pilot study comparing young versus older nulliparous women. *International Urogynecology Journal, 31*(3), 535–543.

Tai, J. W., Sorkhi, S. R., Trivedi, I., et al. (2020). Evaluation of age- and radical-prostatectomy related changes in male pelvic floor anatomy based on magnetic resonance imaging and 3-dimensional reconstruction. *World Journal Mens Health, 39*(3), 566–575.

Teunissen, T. A., van den Bosch, W. J., van den Hoogen, H. J., et al. (2004). Prevalence of urinary, fecal and double incontinence in the elderly living at home. *International Urogynecology Journal and Pelvic Floor Dysfunction, 15*(1), 10–13; discussion 13.

Thom, D. H., Haan, M. N., & Van Den Eeden, S. K. (1997). Medically recognized urinary incontinence and risks of hospitalization, nursing home admission and mortality. *Age and Ageing, 26*(5), 367–374.

Thom, D. H., Nygaard, I. E., & Calhoun, E. A. (2005). Urologic diseases in America project: Urinary incontinence in women—national trends in hospitalizations, office visits, treatment and economic impact. *Journal of Urology, 173*(4), 1295–1301.

Thoua, N. M., Abdel-Halim, M., Forbes, A., et al. (2011). Fecal incontinence in systemic sclerosis is secondary to neuropathy. *American Journal of Gastroenterology, 107*(4), 597–603.

Timiras, M. L., & Leary, J. (2003). The kidney, the lower urinary tract, body fluids and the prostate. In P. S. Timiras (Ed.), *Physiological basis of aging and geriatrics* (3rd ed.) (pp. 347–351). Boca Raton, FL: CRC Press.

Trowbridge, E. R., Wei, J. T., Fenner, D. E., et al. (2007). Effects of aging on lower urinary tract and pelvic floor function in nulliparous women. *Obstetrics & Gynecology, 109*(3), 715–720.

Ueda, T., Tamaki, M., Kageyama, S., et al. (2000). Urinary incontinence among community-dwelling people aged 40 years or older in Japan: Prevalence, risk factors, knowledge and self-perception. *International Journal of Urology, 7*(3), 95–103.

Vaillant, G. E., & Mukamal, K. (2001). Successful aging. *The American Journal of Psychiatry, 158*(6), 839–847.

Van Houten, P., Achterberg, W., & Ribbe, M. (2007). Urinary incontinence in disabled elderly women: A randomized clinical trial on the effect of training mobility and toileting skills to achieve independent toileting. *Gerontology, 53*(4), 205–210.

Van Meegdenburg, M. M., Heineman, E., & Broens, P. M. (2015). Pudendal neuropathy alone results in urge incontinence rather than in complete fecal incontinence. *Diseases of the Colon & Rectum, 58*(12), 1186–1193.

Varma, M., Brown, J., Creasman, J., et al. (2006). Fecal incontinence in females older than aged 40 years: Who is at risk? *Diseases of the Colon & Rectum, 49*(6), 841–851.

Verelst, M., Maltau, J. M., & Orbo, A. (2002). Computerised morphometric study of the paraurethral tissue in young and elderly women. *Neurourology and Urodynamics, 21*(6), 529–533.

Vernava, A. M., 3rd, Longo, W. E., & Daniel, G. L. (1993). Pudendal neuropathy and the importance of EMG evaluation of fecal incontinence. *Diseases of the Colon & Rectum, 36*(1), 23–27.

Wald, A. (1995). Systemic diseases causing disorders of defecation and continence. *Seminars in Gastrointestinal Disease, 6*(4), 194–202.

Wang, J., Varma, M. G., Creasman, J. M., et al. (2010). Pelvic floor disorders and quality of life in women with self-reported irritable bowel syndrome. *Alimentary Pharmacology & Therapeutics, 31*(3), 424–431.

Whitehead, W. E., Borrud, L., & Goode, P. S. (2009). Fecal incontinence in US adults: Epidemiology and risk factors. *Gastroenterology, 137*(2), 512–517, 517.e1–517.e2.

World Health Organization. (2011). Global Health and Ageing [Online]. Available: https://www.who.int/ageing/publications/global_health/en/ (Accessed 21.4.21).

Yoshida, M., Homma, Y., Inadome, A., et al. (2001). Age-related changes in cholinergic and purinergic neurotransmission in human isolated bladder smooth muscles. *Experimental Gerontology, 36*(1), 99–109.

Yoshida, M., Miyamae, K., Iwashita, H., et al. (2004). Management of detrusor dysfunction in the elderly: Changes in acetylcholine and adenosine triphosphate release during aging. *Urology, 63*(3 Suppl. 1), 17–23.

14.1 Pelvic Floor Muscle Training for Older Women With Urinary Incontinence

Chantale Dumoulin

INTRODUCTION

Urinary incontinence (UI) is caused by a greater and more diverse range of factors in older women than younger women, including ageing; hormonal changes; comorbidities; and deficits in strength, mobility and cognition (Gibson et al., 2020). Previous systematic reviews of randomized controlled trials (RCTs) have examined and supported the efficacy of UI interventions in women as a general population (Dumoulin et al. 2017; Dumoulin et al., 2018). However, this raises valid questions about the generalizability of existing RCTs to older women with UI: treatments that are effective in younger and middle-aged women may not be as effective or appropriate in older women. Thus the effects of UI treatments in older women must be addressed separately, as this distinct subpopulation of women may respond differently to specific interventions or experience adverse effects that differ in type and prevalence compared to younger women. Therefore, this chapter presents pelvic floor muscle training (PFMT) for older women with UI.

METHODS

Two systematic reviews (published in 2012 and 2015) identified five RCTs investigating the effect of PFMT on UI symptoms and quality of life (QOL) in older women (Pereira et al., 2012; Stenzelius et al., 2015). Using the same strategies as the 2015 review, we conducted a literature search up to September 2020. The search comprised all trials that included women 60 years and older, which generated seven additional RCTs. Details on each of the 12 trials can be found in Tables 14.1.1 and 14.1.2. Although some RCTs from the literature were titled 'PFMT in *older women*', they sometimes included perimenopausal or menopausal women 45 years and older (Alves et al., 2015; Burns et al., 1990; Burns et al., 1993; Dougherty et al., 2002; Pereira et al., 2013; Wells et al., 1991; Wyman et al., 1998). We decided not to include this age group and only consider studies with

female participants 60 years and older or studies that randomized and/or analysed this subgroup separately, in line with the definition of older age by Gorman and Randel (1999). The World Health Organization further separates old age into categories of elderly (those ≥65 years or sometimes ≥60 years) and the oldest old (≥80 years) (World Health Organization, 2007), and therefore we aim to document RCTs for each subgroup of elderly women.

EVIDENCE FOR PELVIC FLOOR MUSCLE TRAINING TO TREAT URINARY INCONTINENCE IN OLDER WOMEN

Participants

In the 12 PFMT studies included in the literature search, participants were healthy community-dwelling women aged 60 to 82 years. The mean age of participants was in the mid-60s. No RCT was found in the 'oldest-old' women category. Study participants had symptoms of stress urinary incontinence (SUI) in six trials, SUI or mixed urinary incontinence (MUI) in one trial, and all UI types in the five remaining trials. The sample size was small (<50 participants) in two trials, moderate (between 50 and 100 participants) in five trials and large (>100 participants) in five trials (see Tables 14.1.1 and 14.1.2).

Outcome Measures

Outcomes of interest included patient-reported cure; UI episodes on the bladder diary; percentage reduction in UI episodes; UI-specific symptoms questionnaires; UI-specific QoL questionnaires; leakage amount on the paper towel test; Patient Global Impression of Improvement (PGII); and to other lower urinary tract symptoms questionnaires such as frequency, nocturia and urgency. Secondary outcomes included pelvic floor muscle (PFM) morphometry and PFM function, gait speed and lower limb muscle strength, among others (see Tables 14.1.1 and 14.1.2).

TABLE 14.1.1   Review of Randomized Control Trials on Pelvic Floor Muscle Training for Urinary Incontinence in Older Women

Author	**Karger Jahromi et al. (2015)**
Design	RCT
Study population	50 community-dwelling women with SUI, aged 60–74 years (mean age: group 1, 67.15; group 2, 68.05) UI severity: ≥2 episodes/week for 90% in group 1 and 93.3% in group 2
Methods	Group 1: PFMT in group + education + body awareness, breathing, relaxation, strength training + home-based exercises Group 2: no intervention
Intervention	45-min session, 1×/week for 8 weeks PFMT: 8–12 maximal contractions of 6–8 s in lying, standing and sitting positions Home-based exercises: 8–12 high-intensity (close to maximum) contractions 3×/day
Drop-out/adherence	Drop-out: group 1, n = 1; group 2, n = 1 Adherence not reported
Outcomes/results	Significantly lower scores on ICIQ-UI SF at 2 months in group 1 (mean: 9.07, SD: 2.33) vs group 2 (mean: 12.30, SD: 3.6)
Author	**Leong and Mok (2015)**
Design	RCT
Study population	55 community-dwelling women with SUI, MUI or UUI, aged >65 years (mean age: group 1, 73; group 2, 75.4 UI severity: group 1, mean of 11 UI episodes/week; group 2, mean of 8 UI episodes/week
Methods	Group 1: PFMT with individual session + education + bladder training Group 2: education pamphlet with information about UI management
Intervention	30-min session, 1×/week for 4 weeks and 2×/week for 8 weeks PFMT: 10–35 submaximal contractions of 5–10 s, 5–10 fast maximal contractions; Knack lying, sitting and standing positions
Drop-out/adherence	Drop-out: group 1, n = 0; group 2, n = 0 Adherence not reported
Outcomes/results	Significant reduction in number of UI episodes at 3 months in group 1 (mean: 1, SD: 1.9) vs group 2 (mean: 7.4, SD: 6.2) Significant improvement in quality of life at 3 months in group 1 (mean: 1.1, SD: 1.2) vs group 2 (mean: 5, SD: 2.8)
Author	**McFall et al. (2000a, 2000b)**
Design	RCT
Study population	145 community-dwelling women with UI, aged ≥65 years (mean age: group 1, 73.9; group 2, 75.6) UI severity: not reported
Methods	Group 1: PFMT in group + education + bladder training + relaxation + social support Group 2: no intervention
Intervention	2×/week for 5 weeks PFMT: parameters not reported
Drop-out/adherence	Drop-out: group 1, n = 23; group 2, n = 14 Adherence not reported
Outcomes/results	Significantly higher improvement of symptoms in group 1 vs group 2 (change in number of incontinent episodes at 3 months) Significantly decreased impact of UI on sexual intercourse, relationships with family and relationships with spouses in group 1 vs group 2

Continued

TABLE 14.1.1 **Review of Randomized Control Trials on Pelvic Floor Muscle Training for Urinary Incontinence in Older Women—cont'd**

Author	Miller et al. (1998)
Design	RCT
Study population	27 community-dwelling women with SUI, aged ≥60 years (mean age: 68.4) UI severity: ≥1 and ≤5 leaks/day; mean urine leakage episodes/day, 1.36
Methods	Group 1: individual assessment/consultation and education with nurse to ensure adequate pelvic floor contraction Group 2: no intervention
Intervention:	Practice Knack at home for 1 week
Drop-out/adherence	Drop-out: group 1, n = 0; group 2, n = 0 Adherence not reported
Outcomes/results	Significantly reduced urine loss on medium and deep cough, paper towel test at 1 week: mean cm^2 of wetness area (SD), group 1, 0.4 (1.04) with Knack and group 2, 23.8 (46.5); group 1, 5.4 (15.3) with Knack and group 2, 26.8 (46.7), respectively
Author	**Radzimińska et al. (2018)**
Design	RCT
Study population	84 community-dwelling women with SUI, aged ≥60 years (median age: group 1, 69.5; group 2, 69.5) UI severity: not reported
Methods	Group 1: PFMT in group + education Group 2: no intervention
Intervention	45-min session, 3×/week for 4 weeks PFMT: exercise type and difficulty individually adjusted to psychophysical fitness of participants; vaginal digital palpation
Drop-out/adherence	Drop-out: group 1, n = 4; group 2, n = 6 Adherence not reported
Outcomes/results	Significant improvement in SUI severity at 4 weeks in group 1 vs group 2 (Revised Urinary Incontinence Scale score (0–13), median): group 1, 6; group 2, 9
Author	**Sherburn et al. (2011)**
Design	RCT
Study population	83 community-dwelling women with urodynamic verified SUI, aged ≥65 years (mean age: group 1, 71.6; group 2, 72) UI severity: group 1, median of 8.5 episodes/week; group 2, median of 15 episodes/week
Methods	Group 1: PFMT in group + education + home-based exercises Group 2: general muscle training in group + education + home-based bladder training programme
Intervention	Group 1: 1-h session, 1×/week for 5 months; PFMT: 8–12 maximal contractions of 6–8 s with 3–4 added contractions in lying, standing, kneeling and sitting positions; home-based exercises 7×/week: 8–12 high-intensity (close to maximum) contractions 3×/day; individual assessment/ consultation with physiotherapist (0–4 times) to ensure adequate pelvic floor contraction Group 2: 1-h session, 1×/week for 5 months; training: gentle exercise class including stretches, with breath awareness and relaxation (no PFMT), bladder training (without PFM contractions) and group discussions; exercises parameters not reported; individual assessment/consultation with physiotherapist (0–4 times) to ensure adequate pelvic floor contraction
Drop-out/adherence	Drop-out: group 1, n = 2; group 2, n = 5 Adherence to home exercise routine: group 1, 96.8%; group 2: 93.1%

TABLE 14.1.1	Review of Randomized Control Trials on Pelvic Floor Muscle Training for Urinary Incontinence in Older Women—cont'd
Outcomes/results	Significantly lower amounts of leakage during cough test at 5 months in both groups, with significantly lower leakage in group 1 vs group 2 (g of urine loss median): group 1, 0.1; group 2, 0.5 Significantly more improvement in ICIQ-UI SF scores at 5 months in group 1 (mean: 5.9, SD: 3.3) vs group 2 (mean: 8.5, SD: 4.4) Significantly higher global perception of change at 5 months in group 1 vs group 2 Significantly lower number of weekly UI at 5 months in group 1 (median: 4) vs group 2 (median: 9.5) Significantly improved quality of life in both groups at 5 months, mean Assessment of Quality of Life total score (SD): group 1, 8.7 (4.8); group 2, 8.9 (5.2)

ICIQ-UI SF, International Consultation on Incontinence Questionnaire -Urinary Incontinence Short Form; *MUI,* mixed urinary incontinence; *PFMT,* pelvic floor muscle training; *RCT,* randomized controlled trial; *SD,* standard deviation; *SUI,* stress urinary incontinence; *UI,* urinary incontinence; *UUI,* urgency urinary incontinence.

TABLE 14.1.2	Randomized Controlled Trials on PFMT+ in Older Women With Urinary Incontinence
Author	**Kim et al. (2007)**
Design	RCT
Study population	70 community-dwelling women with SUI, aged ≥70 years (mean age: group 1, 76.6; group 2, 76.6 UI severity: UI ≥1×/month
Methods	Group 1: PFMT in group + fitness exercises + home-based exercises Group 2: no intervention
Intervention	1-h session, 2×/week for 12 weeks, then 1×/month for 1 year PFMT: 10 fast contractions (3 s) and 10 maximal contractions (6–8 s) in sitting, lying and standing positions with legs apart Stretching exercises: 10–15 min warm-up and global stretching exercises Fitness exercises: body awareness; breathing; relaxation; strength training of thigh, abdominal and back muscles; use of training balls Home-based exercises after intensive 12-week programme: 30-min session, 2×/week Parameters not reported
Drop-out/adherence	Drop-out: group 1, n = 4; group 2, n = 3 Adherence to exercise frequency at follow-up found in 30.3% of participants
Outcomes/results	Significant decrease in mean urine leakage frequency score at 3 months (0–5 with 0 = no urine leakage and 5 = everyday leakage) in group 1 (mean: 1.5, SD: 1.8) but not in group 2 (mean: 2.4, SD: 1.4) Cure rate at 3 months: group 1, 54.5%; group 2, 9.4%
Author	**Kim et al. (2011b)**
Design	RCT
Study population	147 community-dwelling women with SUI, MUI or UUI, aged >70 years (mean age: group 1, 75.7; group 2, 76.7; group 3, 75.8) UI severity: UI ≥1×/month
Methods	Group 1: PFMT and fitness exercises in group + bladder training + general education on health topics once per month Group 2: PFMT and fitness exercises in group + bladder training + general education on health topics once per month + daily heat and steam–generating sheet application on lower back Group 3: general education on health topics once per month + daily heat and steam–generating sheet application on lower back

Continued

TABLE 14.1.2   Randomized Controlled Trials on PFMT+ in Older Women With Urinary Incontinence—cont'd

Intervention	2×/week for 12 weeks PFMT: 10 fast contractions (3 s) and 10 maximal contractions (6–8 s) in sitting, lying and standing positions with legs apart Stretching exercises: 5–10 min of warm-up and global stretching exercises Fitness exercises: strength training of thigh and abdominal muscles including chair exercises, weight-bearing exercises, ball exercises and others
Drop-out/adherence	Drop-out: group 1, n = 0; group 2: n = 2; group 3: n = 2 Adherence not reported
Outcomes/results	Significant improvement in groups 1 and 2, but not in group 3; cure rate at 3 months: group 1, 53.8% for SUI, 16.7% for UUI, 30% for MUI; group 2, 61.5% for SUI, 50% for UUI, 40% for MUI; group 3, 9.1% for SUI, 0% for UUI, 0% for MUI Significantly lower frequency of urine leakage for SUI and UUI in groups 1 and 2, but not in group 3
Author	**Kim et al. (2011a)**
Design	RCT
Study population	127 community-dwelling women SUI, MUI or UUI, aged ≥70 years (mean age: group 1, 76.1; group 2, 75.7 UI severity: UI ≥1/month
Methods	Group 1: PFMT in group + stretching and fitness exercises + home-based exercises Group 2: general education on health topics
Intervention	Group 1: 1×/week for 12 weeks, then 1×/month for 7 months PFMT: 10 fast contractions (3 s) and 10 maximal contractions (6–8 s) in sitting, lying and standing positions with legs apart Stretching and fitness exercises: 10 min of warm-up and stretching exercises, including shoulder rotation, waist rotation and others; strength training of thigh and abdominal muscles, use of exercises balls Home-based exercises after intensive 12-week programme: 30-min session, 3×/week; 2–3 sets of 13 fitness exercises and PFM exercises learned during group exercise sessions Group 2: 1×/month for 12 weeks
Drop-out/adherence	Drop-out: group 1, n = 4; group 2, n = 3 Adherence to exercise frequency during follow-up in group 1: every day in 35.7% of participants
Outcomes/results	Significantly higher cure rate in group 1 (44.1%) vs group 2 (1.6%) at 3 months and in group 1 (39.3%) and group 2 (1.6%) at 7 months Significant decrease in urine leakage frequency score (0–5 with 0 = no urine leakage and 5 = everyday leakage) in group 1 vs group 2 at 3 and 7 months
Author	**Virtuoso et al. (2019)**
Design	RCT
Study population	32 community-dwelling women with SUI, aged ≥60 years (mean age: group 1, 64.8; group 2, 66.5) UI severity: UI ≥2/week
Methods	Group 1: PFMT + weight training + home-based exercises Group 2: PFMT + home-based exercises

TABLE 14.1.2 Randomized Controlled Trials on PFMT+ in Older Women With Urinary Incontinence—cont'd

Intervention	Group 1: PFMT: 30-min session, 2×/week for 12 weeks; 8–12 repetitions of 6–10 s sustained contractions + 3–5 fast contractions, Knack manoeuvre; lying down, sitting and standing Weight training: 50-min session, 2×/week for 12 weeks; 3 sets of 15 repetitions of maximal contractions of pectoral, gluteus, quadriceps, hamstrings, latissimus dorsi, adductor, triceps brachii, biceps brachii and rectus abdominis; 3 different weights used during programme and PFMs engaged during exercises Home based exercises: suggested intensity of 30 contractions/day Group 2: 30-min session, 2×/week for 12 weeks. PFMT: 8–12 repetitions of 6-10 s sustained contractions + 3–5 fast contractions, Knack manoeuvre; lying down, sitting and standing Home based exercises: suggested intensity of 30 contractions/day
Drop-out/adherence	Drop-out: group 1, n = 2; group 2, n = 4 Adherence for home exercise: group 1, 9/10; group 2: 8/10
Outcomes/results	Significantly higher rate of absence of symptoms at 4 weeks in group 1 (58.3%) vs group 2 (14.8%) No significant differences in reduction in ICIQ-UI SF scores at 1-month follow-up, mean differences (SD): group 1, 8 (5.6); group 2, 9.1 (5) Similar decrease in UI with sneezing, coughing and laughing in both groups
Author	**Wagg et al. (2019)**
Design	RCT
Study population	625 community-dwelling women with SUI, MUI or UUI, aged 60–75 years (mean age: group 1, 64.5; group 2, 64.7) UI severity: group 1, mean of 12.6 UI episodes over 3 days; group 2, mean of 11.3 UI episodes over 3 days
Methods	Group 1: PFMT and general exercises in group + education + brisk walking Group 2: educational classes
Intervention	Group 1: 1-h session for group sessions and 30-min session for brisk walking, 2×/week for 12 weeks PFMT: 4 sets of 3–10 quick contractions, 4 repetitions of 4–10 s maximal contractions; half strength hold for 20–30 s, 4 Knack manoeuvres; in lying sitting and standing positions General exercises: 5–10 min of warm-up and stretching exercises including exercises of body awareness; breathing; relaxation; strengthening of thigh, abdominal and back muscles; and balance training Group 2: 1-h session, 2×/week for 12 weeks
Drop-out/adherence	Drop-out: group 1, n = 37; group 2, n = 9 Adherence not reported
Outcomes/results	Significantly lower number of leakage episodes over 3 days at 24 weeks in group 1 (mean: 1.7, SD: 1) vs group 2 (mean: 8.2, SD: 2.4)
Author	**Dumoulin et al. (2020)**
Design	RCT
Study population	362 community-dwelling women with SUI and MUI, aged ≥60 years (mean age: group 1, 68; group 2, 67.9) UI severity (median UI episodes/day): group 1, 1.43 (0.86–2.14); group 2, 1.57 (0.86–2.71)
Methods	Group 1: PFMT in group of 8 women (targeting PFMs and integrating into daily living activities) + education + home-based exercises Group 2: individual PFMT (targeting PFMs and integrating into daily living activities) + education + intra-vaginal electromyographic biofeedback + home-based exercises

Continued

TABLE 14.1.2 **Randomized Controlled Trials on PFMT+ in Older Women With Urinary Incontinence—cont'd**	
Intervention	Groups 1 and 2:
	1-h session included 15-min educational period and 45-min exercise component, 1×/week for 12 weeks
	PFMT: 3 sets of 6–10 repetitions of 6–10 maximal voluntary contractions, 3 sets of 6–10 repetitions of fast contractions, 3 sets of 3 podium (6–10 s/steps), 3 Knack manoeuvres with 1–3 coughs; in lying, sitting and standing positions; PFM contraction during dance virtual reality game
	Home-based exercises: 5 days/week during progressive 12-week physiotherapy programme (lying, sitting, standing) and subsequently 3 days/week for 9 months
Drop-out/adherence	Drop-out: group 1, n = 24; group 2, n = 19
	Adherence to home PFM exercises during 12-week intervention: group 1, 89%; group 2, 86%
Outcomes/results	At 1 year, median % reduction in UI episodes on 7-day bladder diary was 74% group 1 (95% CI: 46%–86%) vs 70% for group 2 (95% CI: 44%– 89%); difference: −4%, 95% CI: −10% to 7%, p = 0.58

ICIQ-UI SF, International Consultation on Incontinence Questionnaire -Urinary Incontinence Short Form; *MUI,* mixed urinary incontinence; *PFM,* pelvic floor muscle; *PFMT,* pelvic floor muscle training; *PFMT+,* pelvic floor muscle training plus a more general exercise programme; *RCT,* randomized controlled trial; *SD,* standard deviation; *SUI,* stress urinary incontinence; *UI,* urinary incontinence; *UUI,* urgency urinary incontinence.

Trial Quality

The trials scored between 4 of 10 and 8 of 10 on the PEDro scale (PEDro Partnership, 2020). Details on each of the 12 trials can be found in Table 14.1.3. Overall, eligibility criteria were specified in all but 1 trial, and subjects were randomly allocated to intervention groups in all 12 trials. Allocation was concealed in 4 of 12 trials, unclear in 6 trials and not concealed in 2 trials. Groups were similar at baseline regarding the most important prognostic indicators in 10 of 12 trials. None of the study trials included blinding of the study subjects or the therapists who administered the therapy. Only 4 of 12 trials reported blinding of all assessors who measured at least one key outcome. Measures of at least one key outcome were obtained from more than 85% of the subjects, who were initially allocated to groups in 10 of 12 trials. All subjects for whom outcome measures were available received the treatment or the control condition as allocated. Where this was not the case, data for at least one key outcome was analysed by 'intention to treat' in only 2 of 12 trials. The results of between-group statistical comparisons were reported for at least one key outcome in all 12 trials. Both point measures and measures of variability were provided for at least one key outcome in all 12 trials. All trials therefore had sufficient statistical information to make their results interpretable.

Results

Based on the intervention components, two subgroups were identified: studies with PFMT as the main comparator and studies with PFMT plus a more general exercise programme (PFMT+) as the main comparator. This systematic review presents results of the trials for each subgroup.

Pelvic Floor Muscle Training Trials

Six trials were categorized as PFMT trials: four trials compared PFMT to a control group (Karger Jahromi et al., 2015; Leong and Mok, 2015; Miller et al., 1998; Radzimińska et al., 2018), one trial compared PFMT plus bladder training (patient education programme and scheduled voiding regimen with gradually adjusted voiding interval) (Haylen et al., 2010) to a control intervention (McFall et al., 2000a; McFall et al., 2000b), and one trial compared PFMT to bladder training (Sherburn et al., 2011) (see Table 14.1.1). RCTs comparing PFMT to no treatment or a control group were favourable to PFMT and showed significantly higher improvement of UI symptoms, significantly lower impact of UI on QoL and an overall significantly higher satisfaction. In the trial of McFall et al. (2000a, 2000b) the active treatment arm (PFMT + bladder training) was more effective than the absence of treatment to reduce frequency of UI episodes and decrease its impact on QoL. Finally, the

TABLE 14.1.3 PEDro Quality Score of Randomized Controlled Trials on PFMT and PFMT+ for Urinary Incontinence in Older Women

E – Eligibility criteria specified
1 – Random allocation
2 – Allocation concealed
3 – Group similar at baseline
4 – Subject blinded
5 – Therapist administering treatment blinded
6 – Assessor blinded
7 – Measure of key outcome obtained from 85% of subjects
8 – Intention to treat
9 – Comparison between group conducted
10 – Point measure and measure of variability provided

Study	E	1	2	3	4	5	6	7	8	9	10	Total Score
Karger Jahromi et al. (2015)	+	+	?	+	−	−	?	+	−	+	+	5
Leong and Mok (2015)	+	+	+	?	−	−	?	+	−	+	+	5
McFall et al. (2000a, 2000b)	+	+	?	+	−	−	?	−	−	+	+	4
Miller et al. (1998)	+	+	−	−	−	−	?	+	−	+	+	4
Radzimińska et al. (2018)	+	+	−	+	−	−	?	+	−	+	+	5
Sherburn et al. (2011)	+	+	+	+	−	−	+	+	+	+	+	8
Kim et al. (2007)	+	+	?	+	−	−	?	+	−	+	+	5
Kim et al. (2011a)	+	+	?	+	−	−	+	+	−	+	+	6
Kim et al. (2011b)	+	+	?	+	−	−	?	+	−	+	+	5
Virtuoso et al. (2019)	−	+	?	+	−	−	+	−	−	+	+	5
Wagg et al. (2019)	+	+	+	+	−	−	−	+	−	+	+	6
Dumoulin et al. (2020)	+	+	+	+	−	−	+	+	+	+	+	8

+, Criterion is clearly satisfied; −, criterion is not satisfied; ?, not clear if the criterion was satisfied.
The total score is determined by counting the number of criteria that are satisfied, except the 'eligibility criteria specified' score is not used to generate the total score. Total scores are out of 10.

trial comparing PFMT plus bladder training to bladder training alone (Sherburn et al. 2011) favoured PFMT plus bladder training with significantly less leakage during the cough test, significantly fewer weekly urine leakage episodes, significantly greater improvement of UI-specific symptoms and QoL scores, and significantly higher global perception of change.

Pelvic Floor Muscle Training Plus Other Intervention Trials

Six trials were consistent with this category: two trials compared PFMT plus general fitness exercises to a control group (Kim et al. 2007; Kim et al., 2011a), one trial compared PFMT plus walking to a control group (Wagg et al., 2019), one trial compared PFMT plus weight training to PFMT alone (Virtuoso et al., 2019), one compared PFMT plus general fitness exercises to PFMT plus general fitness exercises plus local heat (Kim et al., 2011b) and one compared individual PFMT plus functional training (PFMT during a dancing exergame) to group-based PFMT plus functional training (Dumoulin et al., 2020) (see Table 14.1.2).

Both RCTs on PFMT plus general fitness (body awareness, breathing, relaxation and strength training for the trunk and lower extremities) proved to be significantly more effective than the control condition for UI frequency score and UI cure after intervention and at follow-up, for all types of UI and with greater effect on SUI (Kim et al., 2007; Kim et al., 2011a). In the PFMT plus brisk walking trial, improvement of UI symptoms was found in both treatment arms, but patients in the PFMT plus brisk walking group had significantly fewer leakage episodes than the education-only group 3 months after treatment (Wagg et al., 2019). In the PFMT plus weight training trial, the rate of urinary continence was significantly higher in the PFMT plus weight training group after 4 weeks of treatment compared to PFMT alone. However, there was no difference between the interventions for the rate of UI or UI-specific symptoms and QoL questionnaire scores at the 1-month follow-up. Therefore, the combination of weight training and PFMT provided earlier improvement of UI than PFMT alone in elderly women (Virtuoso et al., 2019). In another trial, PFMT plus general fitness exercise and PFMT plus general fitness exercise plus local heat demonstrated significant improvements in UI cure rate and significant improvement in urine leakage frequency compared to the education group (Kim et al., 2011b). Finally, in the trial comparing group-based PFMT to individual PFMT, average percentage reduction in UI episodes at 1 year was high but not significantly different between groups, with 70% (95% CI: 44%–89%) in individual PFMT versus 74% (95% CI: 46%–86%) in group-based PFMT 89% (Dumoulin et al., 2020).

QUALITY OF THE INTERVENTIONS

PFMT and PFMT+ programmes varied in duration from 1 week to 5 months, with most lasting 12 weeks (7 of 12 trials). Participants had between one and three physical therapy sessions per week, and 6 of 12 trials prescribed home PFM exercises in addition to physical therapy. Six of 12 trials confirmed that participants were performing correct PFM contractions with intra-vaginal evaluations prior to training (Dumoulin et al., 2020; Karger Jahromi et al., 2015; Leong and Mok, 2015; Miller et al., 1998; Radzimińska et al., 2018; Sherburn et al., 2011), and 1 of 12 trials confirmed correct PFM contractions upon request (Wagg et al., 2019). As for the PFM exercise programme itself, 6 of 12 trials included the 'Knack' manoeuvre and 10 of 12 included maximum voluntary contraction; in addition, 9 of 12 added rapid and endurance exercises and 9 of 12 progressed their PFMT programme from lying to standing. More details on the PFMT and PFMT+ programmes can be found in Tables 14.1.1 and 14.1.2.

DISCUSSION

Despite unfavourable conditions for older women such as longer duration and more severe UI symptoms, higher prevalence of urgency urinary incontinence (UUI) and MUI (which are more difficult to treat) and potential comorbidities, our review shows that PFMT (alone or with the addition of bladder training) or PFMT+ (PFMT + general exercises) reduces UI symptoms immediately after treatment and for up to 1 year in older women. These findings suggest that older women are able to integrate motor learning strategies like the Knack (Miller et al., 1998), as well as improve PFM morphometry and function to reduce urinary leakage. To this end, the secondary analysis of Cacciari et al. (2020) of group-based PFMT vs individual PFMT (Dumoulin et al., 2020) found that both interventions resulted in comparable improvements in overall PFM function and pelvic floor morphometry during coughs in older women with SUI or MUI, which were sustained at 1 year. More specifically, when participants coughed, pelvic floor structures were better supported (reflected by less caudal movement of the puborectalis sling and a smaller opening of the levator hiatus on 3D perineal ultrasound) in a pattern consistent with the Knack strategy, which has been shown to reduce bladder neck mobility (Peschers et al., 2001). Furthermore, both interventions resulted in stronger, faster, more coordinated and endurant PFMs, as measured with PFM dynamometry (Cacciari et al., 2020). Finally, in the RCT of Radzimińska et al. (2018) comparing PFMT with a control group in older women, biochemical changes post-intervention were assessed alongside incontinence severity. Significantly lower myostatin concentration and lower severity of UI were observed post-treatment in the PFMT group compared to the control group. As the inhibition of serum myostatin increases muscle strength and mass, it appears that PFMT caused a downregulation of myostatin concentrations, which further supports the increase in muscle morphometry and function observed after PFMT by Cacciari et al. (2020).

Of great interest, a large number of RCTs (see Table 14.1.2) compared PFMT+ to an inactive/active control group (Dumoulin et al., 2020; Kim et al., 2007; Kim et al., 2011a; Kim et al., 2011b; Virtuoso et al., 2019; Wagg et al., 2019). This UI treatment approach is based on the increasing knowledge of concurrent gait, balance and cognitive deficits in older women with UI, particularly those with MUI and UUI (Berre et al. 2019; Lussier et al., 2009; Paquin et al., 2020). To this end, some of these trials measured the impact of PFMT+ on outcomes other than UI. Kim et al. (2007, 2011a) demonstrated that PFMT plus general fitness (which included body awareness, breathing, relaxation and strength training for the trunk and lower extremities) proved to be more effective than the control condition for increasing walking speed and adductor muscle strength, both after intervention and at follow-up. In the work of Kim et al. (2011a), PFMT plus general fitness exercise and PFMT plus general fitness exercise plus local heat demonstrated significant improvements in muscle strength and walking speed compared to the education group. Finally, Dumoulin et al. (2020) used individualized and group-based PFMT plus functional training (PFMT during a dancing exergame). Although all secondary outcomes of this trial have not yet been published, earlier pilot study results from the same group support the value of this approach to improve gait stability and cognitive performance during dual tasks (Fraser et al., 2014).

A PFMT+ approach consisting of PFMT plus lower extremity strength, mobility and cognitive training may have potential advantages over PFMT alone to treat UI signs and symptoms in older incontinent women with concomitant gait, balance and cognitive problems. Increasing walking speed and improving balance can be quite helpful to reach the toilet on time for those with UUI or MUI and also to keep continence during abrupt movement for those with SUI. However, there is currently no RCT comparing standard PFMT to PFMT+. Further high-quality trials are needed to validate these new PFMT+ approaches on multifactorial aspects of UI in older women using validated outcomes for UI, gait, balance and cognition.

CONCLUSION

UI in older women is specific to the complexity of its pathophysiology. Evidence to date suggests that healthy elderly women aged 60 to 80 years with UI benefit from PFMT and PFMT+ up to 1 year post-treatment. The benefits of PFMT are shown across all types of UI (mostly SUI and MUI), using different PFMT regimens (mostly maximal voluntary contractions) and assessed by multiple outcomes. PFMT should therefore be promoted as first-line treatment to all older women with

UI. As for the oldest old, although high-level evidence is not available, preliminary results from a good-quality cohort study on 10 older women with UI (all types) (Perrin et al., 2005) demonstrate that those women are good candidates to undertake physical therapies for UI, follow study demands and reduce symptoms.

CLINICAL RECOMMENDATIONS

- Teach the patient about the PFMs and lower urinary tract function using diagrams, drawings and models.
- Discuss the impact of ageing and hormonal changes on the PFMs and genitourinary symptoms (Dumoulin et al., 2019).
- Explain a correct PFM contraction. Allow the patient to practise before checking the ability to contract.
- Assess PFM contraction. Take special care when conducting a digital examination, as older women may suffer from the genitourinary syndrome of menopause.
- If the woman is able to contract, set up an individual training programme to be conducted at home in addition to individual or group physiotherapy treatment.
- Aim for close to maximum contraction, building up to three sets of 8 to 12 contractions per day in addition to rapid and endurance contractions.
- In addition to a PFMT regimen, ask the patient to precontract and hold the contraction before and during coughing, laughing, sneezing and lifting (conscious precontraction, the Knack).
- Ask the patient to suggest where and when exercises should be performed.
- Supply the patient with an exercise diary.
- If available, discuss whether the use of biofeedback could motivate the patient to exercise.
- If the woman is unable to contract, try manual techniques, pressure/electromyography biofeedback or electrical stimulation.
- Follow up with weekly or bi-weekly supervised progressive training. Supervised training can be conducted individually or in groups.
- Assess/address other lower urinary tract symptoms such as urgency and frequency.
- Assess/address gait, balance and overall cognitive function, as they can impact PFMT progress.
- Asses/address risk factors (i.e., constipation, obesity, chronic cough) and comorbidities (i.e., diabetes), as they can impact PFMT progress.

- Follow development in PFM function closely, using responsive, reliable and valid assessment tools.
- Suggested assessment of urinary leakage and QoL before and after treatment using reliable and valid assessment tools such as:
  - UI-specific symptoms questionnaires (i.e., International Consultation on Incontinence Questionnaire–Urinary Incontinence [ICIQ-UI]);
  - 3- or 7-day bladder diaries (leakage episodes);
  - pad tests (48-, 24-, 1-hour and short tests with standardized bladder volume); and
  - general and disease-specific QoL questionnaires (37-item Short Form Health Survey Questionnaire [SF-37], International Consultation on Incontinence Questionnaire–Urinary Incontinence Short Form [ICIQ-UI SF]).

REFERENCES

Alves, F. K., Riccetto, C., Adami, D. B. V., et al. (2015). A pelvic floor muscle training program in postmenopausal women: A randomized controlled trial. *Maturitas, 81,* 300–305.

Berre, M. L., Morin, M., Corriveau, H., et al. (2019). Characteristics of lower limb muscle strength, balance, mobility, and function in older women with urge and mixed urinary incontinence: An observational pilot study. *Physiotherapie Canada, 71,* 250–260.

Burns, P. A., Pranikoff, K., Nochajski, T., et al. (1990). Treatment of stress incontinence with pelvic floor exercises and biofeedback. *Journal of the American Geriatrics Society, 38,* 341–344.

Burns, P. A., Pranikoff, K., Nochajski, T. H., et al. (1993). A comparison of effectiveness of biofeedback and pelvic muscle exercise treatment of stress incontinence in older community-dwelling women. *Journal of Gerontology, 48,* M167–M174.

Cacciari, L. P., Morin, M., Mayrand, M.-H., et al. (2020). Pelvic floor morphometrical and functional changes immediately after pelvic floor muscle training and at 1-year follow-up, in older incontinent women. *Neurourology and Urodynamics, 40*(1), 245–255.

Dougherty, M. C., Dwyer, J. W., Pendergast, J. F., et al. (2002). A randomized trial of behavioral management for continence with older rural women. *Research in Nursing & Health, 25,* 3–13.

Dumoulin, C., Adewuyi, T., Booth, J., et al. (2017). Adult conservative management. In P. H. Abrams, L. Cardoza, A. E. Khoury, et al. (Eds.), *Incontinence: Sixth international consultation on urinary incontinence.* Plymouth, UK: Health Publication/Plymbridge Distributors pp. 1443–1628.

Dumoulin, C., Cacciari, L. P., & Hay-Smith, E. J. C. (2018). Pelvic floor muscle training versus no treatment, or inactive control treatments, for urinary incontinence in women. *Cochrane Database of Systematic Reviews, 10,* CD005654.

Dumoulin, C., Morin, M., Danieli, C., et al. (2020). Group-based vs individual pelvic floor muscle training to treat urinary incontinence in older women: A randomized clinical trial. *JAMA Internal Medicine, 180,* 1284–1293.

Dumoulin, C., Pazzoto Cacciari, L., & Mercier, J. (2019). Keeping the pelvic floor healthy. *Climacteric, 22,* 257–262.

Fraser, S. A., Elliott, V., de Bruin, E. D., et al. (2014). The effects of combining videogame dancing and pelvic floor training to improve dual-task gait and cognition in women with mixed-urinary incontinence. *Games Health Journal, 3,* 172–178.

Gibson, W., Johnson, T., Kirschner-Hermanns, R., et al. (2020). Incontinence in frail elderly persons: Report of the 6th International Consultation on Incontinence. *Neurourology and Urodynamics, 40*(1), 38–54.

Gorman, M., & Randel, J. (1999). *The ageing and development report: Poverty, independence and the world's older people.* London: Earthscan Publications.

Haylen, B. T., de Ridder, D., Freeman, R. M., et al. (2010). An International Urogynecological Association (IUGA)/ International Continence Society (ICS) joint report on the terminology for female pelvic floor dysfunction. *Neurourology and Urodynamics, 29,* 4–20.

Karger Jahromi, M., Talebizadeh, M., & Mirzaei, M. (2015). The effect of pelvic muscle exercises on urinary incontinency and self-esteem of elderly females with stress urinary incontinency, 2013. *Global Journal Health Science, 7,* 71–79.

Kim, H., Suzuki, T., Yoshida, Y., et al. (2007). Effectiveness of multidimensional exercises for the treatment of stress urinary incontinence in elderly community-dwelling Japanese women: A randomized, controlled, crossover trial. *Journal of the American Geriatrics Society, 55,* 1932–1939.

Kim, H., Yoshida, H., & Suzuki, T. (2011a). The effects of multidimensional exercise treatment on community-dwelling elderly Japanese women with stress, urge, and mixed urinary incontinence: A randomized controlled trial. *International Journal of Nursing Studies, 48,* 1165–1172.

Kim, H., Yoshida, H., & Suzuki, T. (2011b). Effects of exercise treatment with or without heat and steam generating sheet on urine loss in community-dwelling Japanese elderly women with urinary incontinence. *Geriatrics and Gerontology International, 11,* 452–459.

Leong, B. S., & Mok, N. W. (2015). Effectiveness of a new standardised Urinary Continence Physiotherapy Programme for community-dwelling older women in Hong Kong. *Hong Kong Medical Journal, 21,* 30–37.

Lose, G., Fantl, J. A., Victor, A., et al. (1998). Outcome measures for research in adult women with symptoms of lower urinary tract dysfunction. , *17*, 255–262.

Lussier, M., Renaud, M., Chiva-Razavi, S., et al. (2009). *L'incontinence urinaire mixte est associée à des déficits cognitifs chez la femme âgée. Annual Conference of the Réseau Québécois de Recherche sur le Vieillissement (RQRV), FRQS, Quebec City, Quebec.* Canada.

McFall, S. L., Yerkes, A. M., & Cowan, L. D. (2000a). Outcomes of a small group educational intervention for urinary incontinence: Episodes of incontinence and other urinary symptoms. *Journal of Aging and Health, 12,* 250–267.

McFall, S. L., Yerkes, A. M., & Cowan, L. D. (2000b). Outcomes of a small group educational intervention for urinary incontinence: Health-related quality of life. *Journal of Aging and Health, 12,* 301–317.

Miller, J. M., Ashton-Miller, J. A., & DeLancey, J. O. L. (1998). A pelvic muscle precontraction can reduce cough-related urine loss in selected women with mild SUI. *Journal of the American Geriatrics Society, 46,* 870–874.

Paquin, M.-H., Duclos, C., Lapierre, N., et al. (2020). The effects of a strong desire to void on gait for incontinent and continent older community-dwelling women at risk of falls. *Neurourology and Urodynamics, 39,* 642–649.

PEDro Partnership. (2020). PEDro: Physiotherapy Evidence Database [Online]. Available: https://pedro.org.au/. (Accessed 03.08.20).

Pereira, V. S., de Melo, M. V., Correia, G. N., et al. (2013). Long-term effects of pelvic floor muscle training with vaginal cone in post-menopausal women with urinary incontinence: A randomized controlled trial. *Neurourology and Urodynamics, 32,* 48–52.

Pereira, V. S., Escobar, A. C., & Driusso, P. (2012). Effects of physical therapy in older women with urinary incontinence: A systematic review. *Brazilian Journal of Physical Therapy, 16,* 463–468.

Perrin, L., Wood Dauphinée, S., Corcos, J., et al. (2005). Pelvic floor muscle training with biofeedback and bladder training in elderly women: A feasibility study. *Journal of Wound, Ostomy and Continence Nursing, 32*(3), 186–199.

Peschers, U. M., Fanger, G., Schaer, G. N., et al. (2001). Bladder neck mobility in continent nulliparous women. *British Journal of Obstetrics and Gynaecology, 108,* 320–324.

Radzimińska, A., Weber-Rajek, M., Strączyńska, A., et al. (2018). The impact of pelvic floor muscle training on the myostatin concentration and severity of urinary incontinence in elderly women with stress urinary incontinence—a pilot study. *Clinical Interventions in Aging, 13,* 1893–1898.

Sherburn, M., Bird, M., Carey, M., et al. (2011). Incontinence improves in older women after intensive pelvic floor muscle training: An assessor-blinded randomized controlled trial. *Neurourology and Urodynamics, 30,* 317–324.

Stenzelius, K., Molander, U., Odeberg, J., et al. (2015). The effect of conservative treatment of urinary incontinence among older and frail older people: A systematic review. *Age and Ageing, 44,* 736–744.

Virtuoso, J. F., Menezes, E. N., & Mazo, G. Z. (2019). Effect of weight training with pelvic floor muscle training in elderly women with urinary incontinence. *Research Quarterly for Exercise & Sport, 90,* 141–150.

Wagg, A., Chowdhury, Z., Galarneau, J.-M., et al. (2019). Exercise intervention in the management of urinary incontinence in older women in villages in Bangladesh: A cluster randomised trial. *Lancet Global Health, 7,* e923–e931.

Wells, T. J., Brink, C. A., Diokno, A. C., et al. (1991). Pelvic muscle exercise for stress urinary incontinence in elderly women. *Journal of the American Geriatrics Society, 39,* 785–791.

World Health Organization. (2007). *Women, ageing and health: A framework for action. Focus on gender.* Geneva: WHO Press.

Wyman, J. F., Fantl, J. A., McClish, D. K., et al. (1998). Comparative efficacy of behavioral interventions in the management of female urinary incontinence. *American Journal of Obstetrics and Gynecology, 179,* 999–1007.

15

Evidence for Pelvic Floor Physical Therapy for Neurological Diseases

Marijke Van Kampen, Inge Geraerts and Anne Asnong

OUTLINE

INTRODUCTION

Several neurological disease processes can cause changes in bladder and bowel function. Bladder and bowel problems cause much anxiety and may reduce quality of life (QoL) (Coggrave et al., 2014; Corcos and Przydacz, 2018). Treatment procedures of neurological patients with genitourinary and bowel problems are largely based on empirical evidence with a limited research base (Blok et al., 2018; Coggrave et al., 2014; Corcos and Przydacz, 2018; International Continence Society, 2019). An assessment of the patient's physical, psychological, cognitive and emotional limitations may influence the treatment strategy. Although many options exist for therapy, a stepwise approach with initially non-invasive

treatment is important considering the course of the disease (Panicker et al., 2015; Phé et al., 2016).

The role of pelvic floor physical therapy for bladder and bowel problems in specific neurological diseases is actually more and more investigated. Twenty-three randomized controlled studies of pelvic floor physical therapy for stroke (Dong and Shi., 2019; Guo et al., 2014; Guo and Kang, 2018; Liu et al., 2016; Monteiro et al., 2014; Shin et al., 2016; Tibaek et al., 2004, 2005, 2007, 2016) and multiple sclerosis (MS) patients (Khan et al., 2010; Klarskov et al., 1994; Lúcio et al., 2010, 2011, 2016; McClurg et al., 2006, 2008, 2011, 2018; Pérez et al., 2020; Prasad et al., 2003; Silva Ferreira et al., 2019; Vahtera et al., 1997) with bladder and bowel problems are published. Other neurological pathologies like Parkinson's disease, spina bifida, syringomyelia, peripheral neuropathies, Huntington's disease, multiple system atrophy, dementia, spinal cord injuries, disc prolapse and tumours of the spinal cord might also be responsible for the development of neurogenic bladder and bowel dysfunctions.

This chapter is limited to treatment of stroke and MS patients with genitourinary and/or bowel problems.

RESEARCH METHODS

The search was updated from the cut-off date of the previous update (July 2015) to June 2020 and included PubMed, the Cochrane Library and PEDro. Only English language articles and randomized controlled trials were considered. No abstracts were included. For stroke, 25 articles were identified and screened by two independent reviewers. Data extraction was then carried out for the relevant studies, by screening by title (phase I), by abstract (phase II) and by full-text (phase III), resulting in 10 articles in total (Table 15.1). For MS, 25 articles were identified and 13 were included (Table 15.2).

The methodological quality of all identified studies concerning PFMT for neurological diseases based on PEDro scores ranged between 3 and 9 out of 10 (Table 15.3).

TABLE 15.1 Randomized Controlled Studies of Physical Therapy for Bladder and Bowel Dysfunctions in Stroke Patients

Author	Dong and Shi (2019)
Design	E group: PFMT + acupuncture C group: PFMT
Sample size	112 stroke patients with UI (E: 56, C: 56)
Diagnosis	Effective rate ([markedly effective cases + effective cases]/total number of cases × 100%), muscle potential test, urodynamic parameters (total urine leakage, Valsalva leak point pressure, maximum urethral closure pressure), ICIQ-SF, SF-36 at baseline and 1 month
Training protocol	E group: PFMT by a rehabilitation expert, with PFM contraction for 3–5 s, followed by relaxation for 10 s, 20–30 times, 3 sets/day for 1 month + acupuncture C group: PFMT
Drop-out	Not reported
Results	Effective rate significantly better in E group and myoelectric potentials significantly higher than those before treatment in both groups and higher in E than C Urodynamic parameters, ICIQ-SF scores and SF-36 scores were better in E than C
Author	Guo et al. (2014)
Design	E group: TENS C group: basic therapy
Sample size	61 patients with poststroke UI (E: 32, C: 29)
Diagnosis	OABSS, BI, urodynamics examination at baseline and after 60 days
Training protocol	E group: TENS 30 min/day for 60 days, pulse duration of 70 μs, frequency of 75 Hz in form of unidirectional square wave, maximum therapeutic current 16 mA (1 kΩ) Positive electrode on second lumbar spinous process, 2 negative electrodes on inside of middle and lower third of junction between posterior superior iliac spine and ischia node C group: basic therapy
Drop-out	Not reported
Results	Daily micturition, nocturia, urinary urgency, and UUI in E group improved more obviously than in C group; OABSSs significantly lower in E; patients in E were superior in the self-care ability of daily living and urodynamic indexes were better
Author	Guo and Kang (2018)
Design	E group: NMES C group: sham therapy
Sample size	82 patients with UI after stroke (E: 41, C: 41)

Continued

TABLE 15.1   Randomized Controlled Studies of Physical Therapy for Bladder and Bowel Dysfunctions in Stroke Patients—cont'd

Diagnosis	OABSS, BI, urodynamic values, ICIQ-SF at baseline and after 10 weeks
Training protocol	E group: NMES 30 min/day for 10 weeks, pulse duration of 250 μs, frequency of 50 Hz, 10-s on/30-s off; positive pad at region of second sacral level on opposite sides of vertebral column, and negative pad placed at inside of middle and lower third of junction between posterior superior iliac spine and ischial node C group: same protocol but without an active probe
Drop-out	8/82 (10%)
Results	Patients treated with NMES showed better outcomes for urodynamic values, OABSSs, ICIQ-SF and BI than patients in sham group
Author	Liu et al. (2016)
Design	E^1 group: TENS (20 Hz) E^2 group: TENS (75 Hz) C group: no treatment
Sample size	81 patients with UI after stroke (E^1: 27, E^2: 27, C: 27)
Diagnosis	OABSS, BI, urodynamic values, voiding diary parameters at baseline and after 90 days
Training protocol	E^1 group: TENS 30 min/day for 90 days, pulse duration of 150 μs, frequency of 20 Hz; positive electrodes placed in region of second sacral level on opposite sides of vertebral column, and negative electrodes placed on inside of the middle and lower third of junction between posterior superior iliac spine and ischial node E^2 group: analogue to E^1, but 75 Hz C group: no treatment
Drop-out	0
Results	E^1 patients had significantly better OABSSs, BI scores, urodynamic values and voiding diary parameters than E^2, but E^2 also scored significantly better compared to C
Author	Monteiro et al. (2014)
Design	E group: ES C group: general advice
Sample size	24 men with neurogenic OAB secondary to ischemic stroke (E: 12, C: 12)
Diagnosis	3-day voiding diary, subjective assessment of symptoms at baseline, after 12 sessions (45 days) and 12 months
Training protocol	E group: 30-min ES of posterior tibialis nerve, 2×/week for 6 weeks, pulse duration of 200 μs, frequency of 10 Hz, continuous mode; negative electrode on medial malleolus, and positive electrode 10 cm above negative electrode, also on medial side C group: general advice, 12 stretching sessions (30 min) and home exercises, over 6 weeks
Drop-out	1/24 (4%)
Results	Patients in E group experienced significant improvement in urinary symptoms (urgency, incontinence and nocturia) and daytime frequency. and reported subjective improvement after treatment and at 12-month follow-up (except for UUI), in relation to baseline In relation to C group, daytime frequency significantly better after treatment and nocturia, frequency and subjective improvement at 12-month follow-up
Author	Shin et al. (2016)
Design	E group: PFMT + general rehabilitation C group: general rehabilitation
Sample size	35 female patients with post-stroke SUI (E: 18, C: 17)
Diagnosis	Perineometer, intra-vaginal electromyography, Bristol Female Lower Urinary Tract Symptoms (B-FLUTS) questionnaire at baseline and after 6 weeks

TABLE 15.1 Randomized Controlled Studies of Physical Therapy for Bladder and Bowel Dysfunctions in Stroke Patients—cont'd

Training protocol	E group: general rehabilitation with 50 min of gait training and stretching, 3×/week for 6 weeks + PFMT 50 min, 3×/week for 6 weeks; education, recognition training, training in a range of respiratory conditions, resistance training C group: general rehabilitation
Drop-out	4/35 (11%)
Results	In E group, maximal vaginal squeeze pressure and activity of PFMs showed a significant increase and LUTS scores were significantly lower (for daily living inconvenience and urinary symptoms)
Author	**Tibaek et al. (2004)**
Design	E group: PFMT C group: standard programme of general rehabilitation
Sample size	26 women with UI after ischemic stroke (E: 14, C: 12)
Diagnosis	SF-36, IIQ-7 at baseline and 12 weeks
Training protocol	E group: PFMT 6-s contraction, 6-s rest, 3-s contraction, 3-s rest, 30-s contraction, 30-s rest; every contraction 4–8 times in different positions; group treatment (6–8 patients) 60 min/week over 12 weeks as outpatient; individuals did vaginal palpation 2–3 times over 12 weeks; home exercises 1–2×/day C group: no treatment for UI but normal standard programme for rehabilitation
Drop-out	2/24 (8%)
Results	No significant difference between E and C groups in SF-36 and IIQ-7
Author	**Tibaek et al. (2005)**
Design	E group: PFMT C group: standard programme of general rehabilitation
Sample size	26 women with UI after ischemic stroke (E: 14, C: 12)
Diagnosis	Voiding diary, UI, number of pads, 24-h pad test, digital palpation of pelvic floor muscles at baseline and 12 weeks
Training protocol	Identical to Tibaek et al. (2004)
Drop-out	2/24 (8%)
Results	Significant difference between E and C groups in frequency of voiding, 24-h home pad test and endurance of PFMs
Author	**Tibaek et al. (2007)**
Design	E group: PFMT C group: standard programme of general rehabilitation
Sample size	24 women (E: 12, C: 12)
Diagnosis	SF-36, IIQ-7 at baseline and 6 months
Training protocol	Identical to Tibaek et al. (2004, 2005)
Drop-out	2/24 (8%)
Results	No significant difference between E and C groups in SF-36 and IIQ-7; only trend
Author	**Tibaek et al. (2016)**
Design	E group: PFMT C group: standard programme of general rehabilitation
Sample size	31 men with post-stroke LUTS (E: 16, C: 15)
Diagnosis	SF-36, N-QoL at baseline, 12 weeks and 6 months
Training protocol	E group: theory, home exercises, group treatment and digital anal palpation of PFMs C group: standard programme of general rehabilitation with no specific LUTS treatment
Drop-out	1/30 (0.03%)
Results	No significant difference between E and C groups in SF-36 and N-QoL

BI, Barthel Index; *C*, control; *E*, experimental; *ES*, electrical stimulation; *ICIQ-SF*, International Consultation on Incontinence Questionnaire - Short Form; *IIQ-7*, Incontinence Impact Questionnaire -Short Form; *LUTS*, lower urinary tract symptoms; *NMES*, neuromuscular electrical stimulation; *N-QoL*, Nocturia Quality of Life; *OABSS*, Overactive Bladder Symptom Score; *PFM*, pelvic floor muscle; *PFMT*, pelvic floor muscle training; *SF-36*, Short Form 36 Health Survey Questionnaire; *SUI*, stress urinary incontinence; *TENS*, transcutaneous electrical nerve stimulation; *UI*, urinary incontinence; *UUI*, urgency urinary incontinence.

TABLE 15.2   Randomized Controlled Studies of Physical Therapy for Bladder and Bowel Dysfunctions in Patients With Multiple Sclerosis

Author	**Khan et al. (2010)**
Design	E group: individualized bladder rehabilitation programme C group: wait-list group
Sample size	74 patients with MS and bladder issues (E: 40, C: 34)
Diagnosis	UDI-16, NDS, AUA, IIQ-7 at baseline and 12 months
Training protocol	E group: Multidisciplinary bladder rehabilitation programme over 1 year: individualized inpatient (3 h/day over 6 weeks) or outpatient (30 min, 2–3×/week) programme Therapy: individual, assessment of bladder type, diary with strict fluid, PFMT, timed voiding C group: wait-list group with usual care
Drop-out	16/74 (22%)
Results	Significant difference between E and C groups in all questionnaires, improvement in bladder function, overactivity and QoL at 12 months
Author	**Klarskov et al. (1994)**
Design	E group: PFMT + BF C group: PFMT
Sample size	15 women and 5 men with MS and bladder dysfunction (E: ?, C: ?)
Diagnosis	VAS (incontinence and voiding symptoms), voiding diary on weekends, 1-h pad test, urodynamics at baseline and after treatment
Training protocol	E group: behavioural modification, pharmacological adjustment, PFMT (40 min, 2×/week, median of 6 sessions) and BF C group: behavioural modification, pharmacological adjustment and PFMT (40 min, 2×/week, median of 6 sessions)
Drop-out	Not reported
Results	Both groups improved, but no differences between groups
Author	**Lúcio et al. (2010)**
Design	E group: PFMT with assistance of vaginal perineometer C group: sham treatment with vaginal perineometer
Sample size	27 women with MS and LUTD complaints (E: 13, C: 14)
Diagnosis	Urodynamics, 24-h pad test, voiding diary, pelvic floor assessment (PERFECT scheme) at baseline and 12 weeks
Training protocol	E group: PFMT with perineometer, 30 slow contractions and 3 min of fast contractions in supine position Treatment: 30 min, 2×/week for 12 weeks (outpatient) Home exercises: 3×/day 30 slow contractions, 3 min of fast contractions C group: introduction of perineometer inside vagina without contraction over 30 min
Drop-out	Not reported
Results	Significant difference between E and C groups in 24-h pad test, number of pads, nocturia and improvement of pelvic floor muscle power, endurance, resistance and fast contractions, no significant difference in urodynamics
Author	**Lúcio et al. (2011)**
Design	E group: PFMT with assistance of vaginal perineometer C group: sham treatment with vaginal perineometer
Sample size	35 women with MS and LUTD complaints (E: 18, C: 17)
Diagnosis	OAB questionnaire, SF-36, ICIQ-SF, Qualiveen questionnaire at baseline and 12 weeks

TABLE 15.2 Randomized Controlled Studies of Physical Therapy for Bladder and Bowel Dysfunctions in Patients With Multiple Sclerosis—cont'd

Training protocol	Identical to Lúcio et al. (2010)
Drop-out	8/35 (23%)
Results	Significant difference between E and C groups in all questionnaires
Author	**Lúcio et al. (2016)**
Design	E[1] group: PFMT + BF + NMES E[2] group: PFMT + BF + TTNS C group: PFMT + BF + sham NMES
Sample size	30 women with MS and LUTS (E[1]: 10, E[2]: 10, C: 10)
Diagnosis	24-hour pad test, 3-day bladder diary, assessment of PFM function (strength and muscle tone), urodynamic studies, OAB-v8, ICIQ-SF and Qualiveen questionnaire at baseline and 12 weeks
Training protocol	E[1] group: PFMT (see C group) + BF + NMES (pulse width of 200 µs, 10-Hz frequency, for 30 min) E[2] group: PFMT (see C group) + BF + TTNS (1 electrode below left medial malleolus and other located 5 cm cephalad to distal electrode; pulse width of 200 µs, 10-Hz frequency, for 30 min) C group: PFMT (30 slow contractions and 3 min of fast contractions) + BF + sham NMES (surface electrodes over sacrum, pulse width of 50 ms, 2-Hz frequency for 2 s, 60-s rest, for 30 min)
Drop-out	5/30 (17%)
Results	All groups showed significant reductions in pad weight, urgency, urgency urinary incontinence and improvement in all PFM functions E[1] group: PFM function (tone, flexibility, ability to relax pelvic floor) and OAB-v8 scores significantly more improved compared to E[2] and C groups
Author	**McClurg et al. (2006)**
Design	E[1] group: PFMT + advice + BF E[2] group: PFMT + advice + BF + NMES C group: PFMT + advice
Sample size	30 women with MS and bladder dysfunction (E[1]: 10, E[2]: 10, C: 10)
Diagnosis	Leakages on voiding diary, 24-h pad test, uroflowmetry, pelvic floor assessment (PERFECT scheme), IIQ, UDI, KHQ, MSQoL-54 at baseline and after 9, 16 and 24 weeks
Training protocol	C group: advice + PFMT gradually, 5×/day for 9 weeks (E[1]: + BF, E[2]: + BF + NMES) ES = biphasic CC, 2 parameter settings: pulse duration of 250 µs, 40-Hz frequency, 5-s on/10-s off and 450 µs, 10-Hz frequency, 10-s on/3-s off; duration of 5–30 min/day
Drop-out	2/30 (7%)
Results	Significant difference in favour of E[2] compared with C at 9, 16 and 24 weeks for leakages, 24-h pad test, digital assessment in some parts of questionnaires Significant difference in favour of E[1] compared with C for leakages, 24-h pad test, digital assessment in some parts of questionnaires at 16 and 24 weeks
Author	**McClurg et al. (2008)**
Design	E group: PFMT + advice + BF + active NMES C group: PFMT + advice + BF + placebo NMES
Sample size	74 women with MS and LUTD (E: 37, C: 37)
Diagnosis	Leakages on voiding diary, 24-h pad test, uroflowmetry, pelvic floor assessment (PERFECT scheme), EMG BF, VAS, IIQ, UDI, IPSS at baseline and after 9, 16 and 24 weeks
Training protocol	E group: PFMT + BF + active NMES ES = biphasic CC, 2 parameter settings: pulse duration of 250 µs, 40-Hz frequency, 5-s on/10-s off and 450 µs (at clinic), 10-Hz frequency, 10-s on/3-s off (at home); duration of 5–30 min/day C group: PFMT + BF + placebo NMES ES = biphasic CC, 2 parameter settings: pulse duration of 50 µs, 2-Hz frequency, 2-s on/60-s off; duration of 5–30 min/day

Continued

TABLE 15.2 Randomized Controlled Studies of Physical Therapy for Bladder and Bowel Dysfunctions in Patients With Multiple Sclerosis—cont'd

Drop-out	2/74 (3%)
Results	Significant difference in favour of E group compared with C for leakages, 24-h pad test, digital assessment and in some parts of questionnaires
Author	McClurg et al. (2011)
Design	E group: advice on bowel management + massage C group: advice on bowel management
Sample size	30 women with MS and constipation (E: 15, C: 15)
Diagnosis	CSS, NBDS, bowel diary at baseline and after 4 and 8 weeks
Training protocol	E group: advice on bowel management (good defaecation posture, adequate fluid intake, importance of diet and exercise) + abdominal massage daily for 4 weeks C group: advice only
Drop-out	1/30 (3%)
Results	Significant difference in favour of E group compared with C for constipation symptoms (CSS) and frequency of defaecation at 4 weeks and NBDS at 8 weeks
Author	McClurg et al. (2018)
Design	E group: advice on bowel management + massage C group: advice on bowel management
Sample size	189 patients with MS (E: 90, C: 99)
Diagnosis	NBDS (primary), bowel diary, adherence diary, CSS, patient resource questionnaire, EQ-5D-5L (secondary) at baseline and after 24 weeks
Training protocol	E group: advice on bowel management (good defaecation posture, adequate fluid intake, importance of diet and exercise) + abdominal massage (DVD, booklet, demonstration, practice) daily for 6 weeks C group: advice only
Drop-out	20/189 (11%)
Results	NBDS showed slight improvement in E group but not statistically significant; participants in E showed significant improvement in frequency of stool evacuation/week and number of times/week they felt bowels were completely emptied
Author	Pérez et al. (2020)
Design	E group: physical therapist–guided PFMT C group: PFMT
Sample size	48 patients with relapsing-remitting MS and urinary incontinence (E: 24, C: 24)
Diagnosis	3-day bladder diary (number of leakages), second part of OAB-q SF, third question of ICIQ-SF scale (QoL), questions 1–3 of ICIQ-SF scale (urinary incontinence severity), first part of OAB-q SF (LUTS), exercise diary (treatment adherence) at baseline and after 12 weeks
Training protocol	E group: 12-week PFMT program with physiotherapist guidance, home training program 3×/day (8–12 contractions for 6–8 s + 3–4 fast contractions) (in writing) + 30-min appointment/week (internal palpation and guidance on proper exercise technique) C: 12-week PFMT program without physiotherapist guidance, home training program 3×/day (in writing, with verbal explanation)
Drop-out	8/48 (17%)
Results	At 12 weeks, E and C groups reported significantly reduced number of leakages but no significant differences between groups; adherence to PFMT might be better under guidance
Author	Prasad et al. (2003)
Design	E[1] group: abdominal pressure E[2] group: abdominal vibration C group: no treatment

TABLE 15.2 Randomized Controlled Studies of Physical Therapy for Bladder and Bowel Dysfunctions in Patients With Multiple Sclerosis—cont'd

Sample size	28 patients with MS and post-void residual bladder volumes
Diagnosis	Post-void residual bladder volumes after each 2-week period
Training protocol	E^1 group: lower abdominal pressure (Crede's manoeuvre) over 2 weeks E^2 group: bladder stimulation with bladder stimulator over 2 weeks; 1 min after voiding C group: no treatment
Drop-out	2/30 (7%)
Results	No significant difference between E^1 and E^2 groups, but trend in favour of vibration Significant difference between E^2 and C groups in residual volumes
Author	**Silva Ferreira et al. (2019)**
Design	E group: PFMT + ES C group: PFMT
Sample size	30 women in moderate stage of recurring-remitting MS (E: 16, C: 15)
Diagnosis	OAB assessment questionnaire, PERFECT scheme, Qualiveen questionnaire at baseline and after 6 months
Training protocol	E group: pelvic floor exercise programme (3 sets of 8–10 contractions of 10 s) + intra-vaginal ES (pulse duration of 1 µs, 2-Hz frequency, 30 min, 20 fast + slow contractions during stimulation) (2×/week, 6 months) C group: home pelvic floor exercise programme (same programme) (2×/week, 6 months)
Drop-out	1/31 (3%)
Results	Significant difference for repetitions between groups (E > C) and both groups showed significant improvement for OAB, but results from E group significantly better
Author	**Vahtera et al. (1997)**
Design	E group: PFMT C group: no treatment
Sample size	50 women and 30 men with MS (E: 40, C: 40)
Diagnosis	LUTS by self-administered questionnaire, muscle activity by surface EMG BF at baseline and after 2 and 6 months
Training protocol	E group: PFMT: 3-s contraction, 3-s rest (10 times) 5-s contraction, 3-s rest (5 times) 15-s contraction, 30-s rest (5 times), others: 5 times in different positions ES: interferential currents carrier frequency of 2000-Hz treatment frequency of 5–10 Hz, 10–50 Hz and 50 Hz, 10 min of each frequency, 3-min rest, 6 sessions over 21 days (outpatient) BF: same PFMT after ES during 2 sessions; home exercises: 20 contractions 3–5×/week over 6 months in sitting and standing positions C group: no treatment
Drop-out	At 2 months 2/40 (5%), at 6 months 3/40 (8%) in E group; not mentioned in C group
Results	Significant difference between E and C groups in LUTS (incontinence, nocturia, urge), QoL (travelling, social shame and need of pads), muscle activity

AUA, American Urological Association; *BF*, biofeedback; *C*, control; *CC*, constant current; *CSS*, Constipation Scoring System; *E*, experimental; *EMG*, electromyography; *EQ-5D-5L*, 5-level EuroQOL Health-Related Quality of Life; *ES*, electrical stimulation; *ICIQ-SF*, International Consultation on Incontinence Questionnaire -Short Form; *IIQ*, Incontinence Impact Questionnaire; *IIQ-7*, Incontinence Impact Questionnaire -Short Form; *IPSS*, International Prostate Symptom Score; *KHQ*, King's Health Questionnaire; *LUTD*, lower urinary tract dysfunction; *LUTS*, lower urinary tract symptoms; *MS*, multiple sclerosis; *MSQoL-54*, 54-item Multiple Sclerosis Quality of Life; *NBDS*, Neurogenic Bowel Dysfunction Score; *NDS*, Neurological Disability Scale; *NMES*, neuromuscular electrostimulation; *OAB*, overactive bladder; *OAB-q SF*, Overactive Bladder Questionnaire -Short Form; *OAB-v8*, 8-item Overactive Bladder Questionnaire; *PFM*, pelvic floor muscle; *PFMT*, pelvic floor muscle training; *QoL*, quality of life; *SF-36*, Short Form 36 Health Survey Questionnaire; *TTNS*, transcutaneous tibial nerve stimulation; *UDI*, Urogenital Distress Inventory; *UDI-16*, 16-item Urinary Distress Inventory; *VAS*, visual analogue score.

TABLE 15.3   PEDro Quality Score of Randomized Controlled Trials in Systematic Review of Pelvic Floor Physical Therapy for Neurological Diseases

E – Eligibility criteria specified
1 – Subjects randomly allocated to groups
2 – Allocation concealed
3 – Groups similar at baseline
4 – Subjects blinded
5 – Therapist administering treatment blinded
6 – Assessors blinded
7 – Measures of key outcomes obtained from >85% of subjects
8 – Data analysed by intention to treat
9 – Statistical comparison between groups conducted
10 – Point measures and measures of variability provided

Study	E	1	2	3	4	5	6	7	8	9	10	Total Score
Stroke												
Dong and Shi (2019)	+	+	−	−	−	−	−	−	−	+	+	3/10
Guo et al. (2014)	+	+	−	+	−	−	−	−	−	+	+	4/10
Guo and Kang (2018)	+	+	+	+	+	−	+	+	+	+	+	9/10
Liu et al. (2016)	+	+	+	+	−	−	+	+	−	+	+	7/10
Monteiro et al. (2014)	+	+	−	+	−	−	−	+	−	+	+	5/10
Shin et al. (2016)	+	+	−	+	−	−	+	+	−	+	+	6/10
Tibaek et al. (2004)	+	+	−	+	?	−	−	+	−	+	+	5/10
Tibaek et al. (2005)	+	+	−	+	?	−	−	+	−	+	+	5/10
Tibaek et al. (2007)	+	+	−	+	−	−	+	−	−	+	+	5/10
Tibaek et al. (2016)	+	+	+	+	−	−	+	−	−	+	+	6/10
Multiple Sclerosis												
Khan et al. (2010)	+	+	+	+	−	−	−	+	+	+	+	7/10
Klarskov et al. (1994)	−	+	+	−	−	−	−	+	−	−	−	3/10
Lúcio et al. (2010)	−	+	−	+	−	−	+	+	−	+	+	6/10
Lúcio et al. (2011)	−	+	−	+	−	−	+	+	−	+	+	6/10
Lúcio et al. (2016)	+	+	−	+	−	−	+	−	−	+	+	5/10
McClurg et al. (2006)	+	+	−	+	−	−	+	+	+	+	+	6/10
McClurg et al. (2008)	+	+	+	+	+	−	+	+	+	+	+	9/10
McClurg et al. (2011)	+	+	−	+	−	−	+	+	−	+	+	6/10
McClurg et al. (2018)	+	+	+	+	−	−	+	+	+	+	+	8/10
Pérez et al. (2020)	+	+	−	+	−	−	−	−	−	+	+	4/10
Prasad et al. (2003)	+	−	−	−	−	−	+	−	+	+	+	4/10
Silva Ferreira et al. (2019)	−	+	−	+	−	−	−	+	−	+	+	5/10
Vahtera et al. (1997)	+	+	−	+	−	−	−	−	−	+	+	4/10

+, Criterion is clearly satisfied; −, criterion is not satisfied; ?, not clear if the criterion was satisfied.
The total score is determined by counting the number of criteria that are satisfied, except the 'eligibility criteria specified' score is not used to generate the total score. Total scores are out of 10.

STROKE

Definition

Over the years, the definition of stroke has shifted. During the 1970s the World Health Organization (1978) description described *stroke* as 'rapidly developed clinical signs of focal (or global) disturbance of cerebral function, lasting more than 24 hours or leading to death, with no apparent cause other than of vascular origin'. In 2013 the definition was updated to one that includes silent infarctions (inclusive of cerebral, spinal and retinal) and silent haemorrhages by the American Heart Association/American Stroke Association (Sacco et al., 2013).

Incidence and Prevalence

The Global Burden of Disease Study showed that the worldwide prevalence of stroke is high, with more than 80 million survivors in 2016, and close to 14 million new stroke cases and 5.5 million deaths due to stroke in 2016. Even though the age-standardized disability-adjusted life-years have been declining since 1990, the absolute amount of disability-adjusted life-years increased due to a growing and ageing population, keeping the global stroke burden high (Johnson et al., 2019).

Urological and Bowel Symptoms

A systematic review of urological symptoms after stroke showed that the prevalence of these symptoms widely varies due to inconsistent use of terminology. This variation can also be explained by the fact that the progression of urological symptoms is determined by the nature and extent of the stroke incident itself (Ruffion et al., 2013).

In the early period after stroke, different studies have shown that urinary incontinence (UI) rates vary between 32% and 79% (Mehdi et al., 2013). At least 3 months post-stroke, UI was still prevalent in 10% to 51% of post-stroke patients (Ruffion et al., 2013). Patel et al. (2001b) investigated the natural history of UI following stroke and found that it shows a gradual, spontaneous improvement from 19% at 3 months to 15% at 1 year and 10% at 2 years. More recent studies, however, showed varying rates for persistent UI 1 year after stroke, between 9% and 38% (Rotar et al., 2011; Williams et al., 2012).

Next to UI, patients also report other urinary symptoms after stroke. At least 1 month after stroke, the most frequently occurring urological symptom is nocturia (36%–79%), followed by urgency (19%–70%) and daytime frequency (15%–59%) (Brittain et al., 1998; Sakakibara et al., 1996; Tibaek et al., 2008; Williams et al., 2012).

UI is predicted by female sex, pre-stroke UI, increasing age, leg weakness, severity of stroke, depressive symptoms and lower cognitive function (Jørgensen et al., 2005; Patel et al., 2001a; Williams et al., 2012). UI in the acute stage is a predictor of survival and closely associated with disability severity (Kolominski-Rabas et al., 2003; Patel et al., 2001a). Furthermore, UI emerged as a risk factor for nursing home replacement (Kolominsky-Rabas et al., 2003; Patel et al., 2001a; Pettersen et al., 2002).

Post-stroke anal incontinence for stool was prevalent in 8% to 56% shortly after the incident and decreased to 11% to 21% around 3 months post-stroke (Baztán et al., 2003; Harari et al., 2004; Kovindha et al., 2009). Older age is a risk factor for faecal incontinence, and faecal incontinence is associated with a poor long-term prognosis for functional recovery (Baztán et al., 2003; Jacob and Kostev, 2020).

Pathophysiology

Urodynamic investigation shows that initially after stroke the bladder is often areflexic (Flisser and Blaivas, 2004). Detrusor hyperreflexia and urgency incontinence generally follow. Sphincteric incontinence in the recovery phase is normally not a consequence of the stroke but is almost always a premorbid condition (Flisser and Blaivas, 2004).

Not all incontinence after stroke is directly related to neurological injury of the micturition pathways. Other mechanisms are general impairment, cognitive deficits and overflow incontinence unrelated to stroke (Flisser and Blaivas, 2004). The neurophysiological explanation for detrusor areflexia in the initial phase after stroke is unknown. Detrusor hyperreflexia was noted in lesions of the frontal lobe as well as the basal ganglia. Uninhibited sphincter relaxation is typical for frontal lobe lesions, and detrusor sphincter dyssynergia is common in basal ganglia lesions (Sakakibara et al., 1996). The location of the injury, the extent of the damage and the role of the affected area determine the precise urological impact (Flisser and Blaivas, 2004; Ruffion et al., 2013). Rationale for physical therapy after stroke can be explained because patients have problems of urgency, stress and urge incontinence. The aim of physical therapy is to strengthen or to relax the pelvic floor muscles and to reduce frequency, urgency and nocturia.

Evidence-Based Medicine on Stroke and Pelvic Floor Physical Therapy

The effect of pelvic floor muscle training (PFMT) (Dong and Shi, 2019; Shin et al., 2016; Tibaek et al., 2004; Tibaek et al., 2005; Tibaek et al., 2007; Tibaek et al., 2016) or electrical stimulation (ES) (Guo and Kang, 2018; Guo et al., 2014; Liu et al., 2016; Monteiro et al., 2014) on lower urinary tract symptoms (LUTS) in stroke patients was evaluated in 10 randomized controlled studies.

Pelvic Floor Muscle Training

Tibaek et al. (2004, 2005) investigated the effect of PFMT in 26 incontinent women, which resulted in two publications because two different assessment tools were used. A third study investigated the 6-month long-term effect of 24 of these women on QoL (Tibaek et al., 2007), and in a fourth study the influence of PFMT on QoL was also investigated in 31 men (Tibaek et al., 2016). Shin et al. (2016) researched the additional effect of PFMT next to general rehabilitation as well in 35 female patients with and Dong and Shi (2019) examined whether acupuncture had an added effect on UI in a mixed population of 112 subjects.

The effect of pelvic floor exercises in women with UI after stroke was measured by QoL parameters (Tibaek et al., 2004, 2007); by diary for the frequency of voiding, incontinence episodes and number of pads, 24-hour home pad test, and vaginal palpation of pelvic floor muscles (Tibaek et al., 2005); and by a perineometer, intra-vaginal electromyography and the Bristol Female Lower Urinary Tract Symptoms (B-FLUTS) questionnaire (Shin et al., 2016).

In the research of Tibaek et al. (2004, 2005, 2007), the intervention included group treatment over 12 weeks that included 12 to 24 standardized pelvic floor exercises. The control group followed the normal standard programme of stroke rehabilitation without specific treatment of UI. The protocol of Shin et al. (2016) consisted of 6 weeks of general rehabilitation, supplemented with a PFMT programme for the intervention group.

QoL, measured with the Short Form 36 Health Survey Questionnaire (SF-36) and Incontinence Impact Questionnaire–Short Form (IIQ-7) did not show significant difference between the two groups after 12 weeks (Tibaek et al., 2004) or after 6 months (Tibaek et al., 2007). However, a trend to a long-lasting effect regarding role limitations because of emotional problems (SF-36) and a tendency to a decreased impact of UI compared with the control group (IIQ-7) were found in the long term (Tibaek et al., 2007).

Regarding the parameters specifically related to UI, Tibaek et al. (2005) showed a significant improvement in frequency of voiding, 24-hour home pad test and endurance of pelvic floor muscles in the treatment group compared with the control group. Shin et al. (2016) demonstrated that 6 weeks of PFMT resulted in a significant increase in the maximal vaginal squeeze pressure and activity of the pelvic floor muscles, as well as significantly lower B-FLUTS scores.

In men with post-stroke LUTS, 12 weeks of PFMT compared to a standard rehabilitation programme did not result in a significant difference between groups in terms of QoL measured with the SF-36 and Nocturia Quality of Life (N-QoL) questionnaires (Tibaek et al., 2016). Lastly, Dong and Shi (2019) analysed the added effect of acupuncture on 1 month of PFMT by measuring the effective rate, myoelectric potentials, urodynamic parameters and questionnaires (International Consultation on Incontinence Questionnaire–Short Form [ICIQ-SF], SF-36) in a mixed population with UI. Between both groups, the intervention group scored significantly better on all outcome measures.

Methodological specifications are presented in Table 15.3 by PEDro scores. A limitation to bear in mind was the small sample size in all of these randomized controlled trials except for the one of Dong and Shi (2019). Furthermore, the use of the SF-36 and IIQ-7 to document the effect on QoL is not the optimal choice because the SF-36 gives an indication of general health (Dong and Shi, 2019; Tibaek et al., 2004, 2007, 2016) and the IIQ-7 turned out to be rather insensitive towards women with urge UI (Tibaek et al., 2004, 2007).

Electrical Stimulation

The effect of transcutaneous electrical stimulation (TENS) was investigated in 82 patients (Guo and Kang, 2018), 61 patients (Guo et al., 2014) and 81 patients (Liu et al., 2016) with post-stroke UI and in 24 men with neurogenic overactive bladder (OAB) after ischemic stroke (Monteiro et al., 2014). In each study, different parameters for ES were used (Table 15.4).

TABLE 15.4	Overview of Electrical Stimulation Parameters			
Author	**Amount of Time**	**Treatment Duration**	**Pulse Duration**	**Frequency**
Guo et al. (2014)	30 min/day	60 days	70 µs	75 Hz
Guo and Kang (2018)	30 min/day	10 weeks	250 µs	50 Hz
Liu et al. (2016)	30 min/day	90 days	150 µs	20/75 Hz
Monteiro et al. (2014)	30 min, 2×/week	45 days	200 µs	10 Hz

The treatment effect on disability was quantified by the Barthel Index (BI) (Guo and Kang, 2018; Guo et al., 2014; Liu et al., 2016). The Overactive Bladder Symptom Score (OABSS) and urodynamics were used to represent the influence on urological symptoms (Guo and Kang, 2018; Guo et al., 2014; Liu et al., 2016), as well as a voiding diary (Liu et al., 2016; Monteiro et al., 2014) and the ICIQ-SF (Guo and Kang, 2018). Furthermore, Monteiro et al. (2014) questioned the subjective assessment of symptoms.

Regarding TENS, Guo et al. (2014) demonstrated a significant treatment effect on urgency, frequency, nocturia and urgency UI, as well as significantly reduced OABSS scores and better self-care ability of daily living (BI scores) after 60 days compared to basic therapy. Along the same line, after 90 days of TENS, patients reported significantly better OABSS scores, BI scores, urodynamic values and voiding diary parameters when TENS was applied at 20 Hz in comparison to no treatment. These effects were even more prominent when a frequency of 75 Hz was used (Liu et al., 2016). Furthermore, Monteiro et al. (2014) established that the treatment effect could continue up to 12 months after treatment in relation to daytime frequency, nocturia and subjective improvement of symptoms.

Lastly, Guo and Kang (2018) presented a significantly better treatment effect after 10 weeks of ES, compared to sham therapy. Patients in the intervention group scored better on all outcome measures related to urodynamic values, OAB and QoL.

Again, methodological specifications are presented in Table 15.3 by PEDro scores. The main limitation of studies on ES for LUTS in stroke patients was the relatively short follow-up period (Guo and Kang, 2018; Guo et al., 2014; Liu et al., 2016; Monteiro et al., 2014).

Clinical Recommendations

Clinical recommendations are based on current evidence to promote 6 to 12 weeks of PFMT to reduce urological symptoms, with special attention to education, improvement of physical functions and social interaction. Conclusions have to be drawn cautiously because of limited research with large sample sizes. Regarding ES, TENS and neuromuscular electrical stimulation (NMES) have been proven effective in reducing LUTS.

MULTIPLE SCLEROSIS

Definition

MS is caused by tissue damage that is a result of a complex interplay between the immune system, glia and neurons. The lesions can show up throughout the central nervous system and are characterized by areas of demyelination, glial reaction and inflammation of the white matter. This leads to a wide variety of neurological deficits (Reich et al., 2018).

Incidence and Prevalence

MS is not common, but nevertheless it is a potentially severe cause of neurological disability. In 2016, there were 2.2 million prevalent cases of MS and approximately 19,000 deaths due to MS according to the Global Burden of Disease Study. There is a substantial difference in global prevalence of MS by sex. Around the age of 60 years, the ratio is 2:1 in favour of women (Wallin et al., 2019).

Urological and Bowel Symptoms

LUTS are common in patients with MS. At first presentation of MS, the presence of urological symptoms is rare (10% of patients). However, on an average of 6 years after disease onset, these symptoms start to appear, and after 10 years, almost every patient with MS presents with some form of LUTS (De Sèze et al., 2007). Storage symptoms are most frequently reported, with increased urinary urgency (38%–99%) and urinary frequency (26%–85%) as the most predominant symptoms (Al Dandan et al., 2020; Phé et al., 2016). Voiding symptoms

(6%–79%) and post-micturition symptoms (60%–61%) are also prevalent, and different manifestations of the aforementioned LUTS often coexist (50%–59%) (Al Dandan et al., 2020; de Sèze et al., 2007; Phé et al., 2016).

Bladder symptoms, as well as bowel symptoms, can have a significant negative impact on health-related QoL (Khalaf et al., 2016; Preziosi et al., 2018; Vitkova et al., 2014), notwithstanding that bowel symptoms have only been scarcely investigated in patients with MS. Constipation was found in 49% of MS patients, whereas 14% to 32% experienced faecal incontinence (Khan et al., 2009; Lin et al., 2019).

Prevalence of both urological and bowel symptoms correlate to an increasing disease duration and higher levels of disability (Lin et al., 2019; Mahajan et al., 2010), but the clinical presentation (subjective symptoms) does not offer a lot of information on detrusor sphincter disorders shown by urodynamic evaluations (objective symptoms) (De Sèze et al., 2007).

Pathophysiology

Using urodynamic observations, detrusor sphincter disorders can present in different patterns due to damage to the innervation of the lower urinary tract. The following patterns can be distinguished:

- detrusor overactivity (31%–99%) and/or decreased bladder sensation (2%–35%) (storage symptoms);
- detrusor sphincter dyssynergia (5%–83%) and/or detrusor underactivity (0%–48%) (voiding symptoms); and
- post-void residue (13%–16%) (post-micturition symptoms) (Al Dandan et al., 2020; de Sèze et al., 2007).

Regarding bowel dysfunction in MS, the neuropathological mechanisms are not yet defined completely, but involvement of the spinal cord seems to play a central role in the pathophysiology. Constipation may involve different neurological mechanisms which influence anorectal sensation, colonic motility and pelvic floor muscles. Analogously, faecal incontinence could find its origin in an altered anorectal sensation, pelvic floor muscle weakness or uncontrolled colonic contractions (Preziosi et al., 2018).

Evidence-Based Medicine on Multiple Sclerosis and Pelvic Floor Physical Therapy

Evidence-based medicine on pelvic floor physical therapy for MS was researched in 13 randomized controlled trials (see Table 15.2): 5 studies described the efficacy of physical therapy to reduce urgency, frequency, incontinence, nocturia and bladder emptying (Khan et al., 2010; Klarskov et al., 1994; Lúcio et al., 2010; Lúcio et al., 2011; Pérez et al., 2020); 6 studies investigated the added effect of ES (Lúcio et al., 2016; McClurg et al., 2006; McClurg et al., 2008; Prasad et al., 2003; Silva Ferreira et al., 2019; Vahtera et al., 1997); and 2 studies researched massage in the context of bowel dysfunction (McClurg et al., 2011; McClurg et al., 2018).

Pelvic Floor Muscle Training as a Treatment for Urological Symptoms

Klarskov et al. (1994) demonstrated a significant improvement in incontinence episodes and pad usage after PFMT with behavioural modification in 20 MS patients and found no added effect of biofeedback (BF). Lúcio et al. (2010) randomized 27 female MS patients in a group that received PFMT with a vaginal perineometer and a sham group where the perineometer was introduced but no contractions were requested. They concluded that PFMT is an effective approach to treat lower urinary tract dysfunction in MS. In a second study of 35 MS patients, Lúcio et al. (2011) assessed QoL and again found results in favour of PFMT compared to sham therapy. Khan et al. (2010) assessed the effectiveness of a 6-week bladder rehabilitation programme in 40 persons with MS with a control wait-list group. A multifaceted, individualized rehabilitation programme reduced disability and improved QoL in MS patients compared with no intervention after 12 months of follow-up. Lastly, Pérez et al. (2020) investigated the effect of physiotherapist-guided PFMT versus a PFMT programme without guidance in 48 patients with relapsing-remitting MS. PFMT with and without guidance resulted in a significantly reduced number of leakages, but there was no difference between groups.

Pelvic Floor Muscle Training and Electrical Stimulation as a Treatment for Urological Symptoms

Vahtera et al. (1997) investigated the effect of ES and pelvic floor muscle exercises on LUTS in MS patients. ES with interferential currents in combination with regular pelvic floor exercises improved urgency, frequency, incontinence, nocturia and bladder emptying significantly in comparison with a control group without treatment. The therapy significantly improved the maximal strength and endurance of the pelvic floor muscles.

Compliance with the pelvic floor muscle exercises was 62.5% after 6 months; others trained irregularly. In another study, which compared PFMT associated or not with ES in 30 women with MS, OAB symptoms and pelvic floor muscle function also showed significant improvement. Adding ES to PFMT seemed to potentiate the benefits (Silva Ferreira et al., 2019).

McClurg et al. (2006) compared three treatment modalities in 30 women with MS: PFMT and advice; PFMT, advice and electromyography BF; and another group adding NMES. They found a statistically significant difference between groups 1 and 3 for the number of leaks and pad test, and a statistical benefit for group 2 compared with group 1 for the pad test. In a second study, they found a statistical superior benefit by adding NMES to a programme of PFMT and electromyography BF on lower urinary tract dysfunction in 74 female MS patients (McClurg et al., 2008). Lúcio et al. (2016) compared three groups; all of them received PFMT and BF, supplemented with (sham) NMES or transcutaneous tibial nerve stimulation. They further demonstrated the advantage of adding NMES to PFMT with BF in reducing pelvic floor muscle tone and OAB symptoms in 30 women experiencing LUTS (Lúcio et al., 2016).

Prasad et al. (2003) compared, in 28 MS patients with post-void residual volumes, lower abdominal pressure with external bladder stimulation and no therapy to aid bladder emptying. All patients received all therapies during 2 weeks but were randomized in the sequence of therapy. Analysis was only done after 6 weeks for the whole group. The difference between abdominal pressure and vibration just failed to reach significance, but both therapies were more effective than no treatment. There was no significant reduction in either the frequency of micturition or episodes of incontinence.

Massage as a Treatment for Bowel Dysfunction

McClurg et al. (2011) investigated the effect of abdominal massage compared to advice on bowel management for the alleviation of constipation in 30 patients with MS and found a significant difference after 4 weeks in favour of massage for constipation symptoms and frequency of defaecation and after 8 weeks in the Neurogenic Bowel Dysfunction Score. In a larger (n = 189) second study, no significant difference in the Neurogenic Bowel Dysfunction Score could be demonstrated at 24 weeks, but daily massage for 6 weeks resulted in a significant improvement in frequency of defaecation and the number of times patients felt that their bowels were completely emptied (McClurg et al., 2018).

Clinical Recommendations

Based on current evidence, PFMT—whether or not complemented with ES to potentiate the effects—decreases urgency, frequency, incontinence and nocturia and improves bladder emptying and pelvic muscle activity in MS patients. Abdominal massage is effective to reduce constipation in the short term and provide improvement in the frequency of stool evacuation.

CONCLUSION

Conclusions and clinical recommendations on the role of pelvic floor physical therapy for genitourinary and bowel problems in specific neurological diseases, such as stroke, have to be taken with care because of the lack of randomized controlled trials with a sufficient number of patients. Pelvic floor physical therapy does not result in significant short-term differences in QoL in men and women with UI after stroke, but in the long term, a positive effect could be possible. Concerning urological symptoms, a 6- to 12-week PFMT programme results in better function of the pelvic floor, as well as reduced LUTS in women. Adding ES can provide improvements in urological symptoms, urodynamics and disability in the short term, which could be maintained in the long term.

For MS patients, a significant difference in LUTS and pelvic floor muscle activity was found after ES, BF and pelvic floor muscle exercises or bladder training compared with a control group without specific treatment or with one modality of treatment. Abdominal massage has a positive effect on the symptoms of constipation.

For patients with other neurological disorders, the efficacy of physical therapy is not yet investigated.

Research on efficacy and selection criteria for pelvic floor physical therapy is necessary to help neurological patients to prevent urological and bowel complications and to improve QoL. Future research, with larger sample sizes and longer follow-up, has to be undertaken not only on stroke and MS but also on other neurological diseases.

REFERENCES

Al Dandan, H. B., Coote, S., & McClurg, D. (2020). Prevalence of lower urinary tract symptoms in people with multiple sclerosis: A systematic review and meta-analysis. *International Journal MS Care, 22*(2), 91–99.

Baztán, J. J., Domenech, J. R., & González, M. (2003). New-onset fecal incontinence after stroke: Risk factor or consequence of poor outcomes after rehabilitation? *Stroke, 34*(8), e101–e102.

Blok, B., Castro-Diaz, D., Del Popolo, G., et al. (2018). *EAU guidelines*. Copenhagen: EAU Annual Congress.

Brittain, K., Peet, S. M., Castleden, C. M., et al. (1998). Stroke and incontinence. *Stroke, 29*, 524–528.

Coggrave, M., Norton, C., & Cody, J. D. (2014). Management of faecal incontinence and constipation in adults with central neurological diseases. *Cochrane Database of Systematic Reviews, 2*, CD002115.

Corcos, J., Przydacz, M. (Eds.). 2018. Pathologies responsible for the development of the neurogenic bladder. *Consultation in neurourology: A private evidence-based guide* (pp. 17–36). Cham: Springer.

De Sèze, M., Ruffion, A., Denys, P., et al. (2007). The neurogenic bladder in multiple sclerosis: Review of the literature and proposal of management guidelines. *Multiple Sclerosis, 13*(7), 915–928.

Dong, R., & Shi, Z. (2019). Pelvic floor muscle training combined acupuncture for treatment of urinary incontinence after stroke. *International Journal of Clinical and Experimental Medicine, 12*(3), 2704–2709.

Flisser, J. A., & Blaivas, J. G. (2004). Cerebrovascular accidents, intracranial tumors and urologic consequences. In J. Corcos, & E. Schick (Eds.), *Textbook of the neurogenic bladder: Adults and children* (pp. 305–313). London: Martin Dunitz/Taylor & Francis Group.

Guo, G. Y., & Kang, Y. G. (2018). Effectiveness of neuromuscular electrical stimulation therapy in patients with urinary incontinence after stroke: A randomized sham controlled trial. *Medicine, 97*(52), e13702.

Guo, Z. F., Liu, Y., Hu, G. H., et al. (2014). Transcutaneous electrical nerve stimulation in the treatment of patients with poststroke urinary incontinence. *Clinical Interventions in Aging, 9*, 851–856.

Harari, D., Norton, C., Lockwood, L., et al. (2004). Treatment of constipation and fecal incontinence in stroke patients: Randomized controlled trial. *Stroke, 35*(11), 2549–2555.

International Continence Society. (2019). *ICS Standards 2019*, (Vol. 1). Bristol, UK: International Continence Society.

Jacob, L., & Kostev, K. (2020). Urinary and fecal incontinence in stroke survivors followed in general practice: A retrospective cohort study. *Annals Physiology Rehabilitation Medicine, 63*(6), 488–494.

Johnson, C. O., Nguyen, M., Roth, G. A., et al. (2019). Global, regional, and national burden of stroke, 1990–2016: A systematic analysis for the global burden of disease study 2016. *The Lancet Neurology, 18*(5), 439–458.

Jørgensen, L., Engstad, T., & Jacobsen, B. K. (2005). Self-reported urinary incontinence in noninstitutionalized long-term stroke survivors: A population-based study. *Archives of Physical Medicine and Rehabilitation, 86*, 416–420.

Khalaf, K. M., Coyne, K. S., Globe, D. R., et al. (2016). The impact of lower urinary tract symptoms on health-related quality of life among patients with multiple sclerosis. *Neurourology and Urodynamics, 35*, 48–54.

Khan, F., Pallant, J. F., Pallant, J. I., et al. (2010). A randomised controlled trial: Outcomes of bladder rehabilitation in persons with multiple sclerosis. *Journal of Neurology Neurosurgery and Psychiatry, 81*(9), 1033–1038.

Khan, F., Pallant, J. F., Shea, T. L., et al. (2009). Multiple sclerosis: Prevalence and factors impacting bladder and bowel function in an Australian community cohort. *Disability & Rehabilitation, 31*(19), 1567–1576.

Klarskov, P., Heely, E., Nyholdt, I., et al. (1994). Biofeedback treatment of bladder dysfunction in multiple sclerosis: A randomized trial. *Scandinavian Journal of Urology & Nephrology - Supplementum, 157*, 61–65.

Kolominsky–Rabas, P. L., Hilz, M. J., Neundoerfer, B., et al. (2003). Impact of urinary incontinence after stroke: Results from a prospective population–based stroke register. *Neurourology and Urodynamics, 22*(4), 322–327.

Kovindha, A., Wattanapan, P., Dejpratham, P., et al. (2009). Prevalence of incontinence in patients after stroke during rehabilitation: A multi-centre study. *Journal of Rehabilitation Medicine, 41*(6), 489–491.

Lin, S. D., Butler, J. E., Boswell-Ruys, C. L., et al. (2019). The frequency of bowel and bladder problems in multiple sclerosis and its relation to fatigue: A single centre experience. *PLoS One, 14*(9), e0222731.

Liu, Y., Xu, G., Luo, M., et al. (2016). Effects of transcutaneous electrical nerve stimulation at two frequencies on urinary incontinence in poststroke patients: A randomized controlled trial. *American Journal of Physical Medicine & Rehabilitation, 95*(3), 183–193.

Lúcio, A. C., Campos, R. M., Perissinotto, M. C., et al. (2010). Pelvic floor muscle training in the treatment of lower urinary tract dysfunction in women with multiple sclerosis. *Neurourology and Urodynamics, 29*(8), 1410–1413.

Lúcio, A. C., D'Ancona, C. A. L., Perissinotto, M. C., et al. (2016). Pelvic floor muscle training with and without electrical stimulation in the treatment of lower urinary tract symptoms in women with multiple sclerosis. *Journal Wound Ostomy Continence Nurs., 43*(4), 414–419.

Lúcio, A. C., Perissinoto, M. C., Natalin, R. A., et al. (2011). A comparative study of pelvic floor muscle training in women with multiple sclerosis: Its impact on lower urinary tract symptoms and quality of life. *Clinics*, 66(9), 1563–1568.

Mahajan, S. T., Patel, P. B., & Marrie, R. A. (2010). Under treatment of overactive bladder symptoms in patients with multiple sclerosis: An ancillary analysis of the NARCOMS patient registry. *Journal of Urology*, 183(4), 1432–1437.

McClurg, D., Ashe, R. G., & Lowe–Strong, A. S. (2008). Neuromuscular electrical stimulation and the treatment of lower urinary tract dysfunction in multiple sclerosis—a double blind, placebo controlled, randomised clinical trial. *Neurourology and Urodynamics*, 27(3), 231–237.

McClurg, D., Ashe, R. G., Marshall, K., et al. (2006). Comparison of pelvic floor muscle training, electromyography biofeedback, and neuromuscular electrical stimulation for bladder dysfunction in people with multiple sclerosis: A randomized pilot study. *Neurourology and Urodynamics*, 25(4), 337–348.

McClurg, D., Hagen, S., Hawkins, S., et al. (2011). Abdominal massage for the alleviation of constipation symptoms in people with multiple sclerosis: A randomized controlled feasibility study. *Multiple Sclerosis*, 17(2), 223–233.

McClurg, D., Harris, F., Goodman, K., et al. (2018). Abdominal massage plus advice, compared with advice only, for neurogenic bowel dysfunction in MS: A RCT. *Health Technology Assessment*, 22(58), 1–134.

Mehdi, Z., Birns, J., & Bhalla, A. (2013). Post–stroke urinary incontinence. *International Journal of Clinical Practice*, 67(11), 1128–1137.

Monteiro, É. S., de Carvalho, L. B. C., Fukujima, M. M., et al. (2014). Electrical stimulation of the posterior tibialis nerve improves symptoms of poststroke neurogenic overactive bladder in men: A randomized controlled trial. *Urology*, 84(3), 509–514.

Panicker, J. N., Fowler, C. J., & Kessler, T. M. (2015). Lower urinary tract dysfunction in the neurological patient: Clinical assessment and management. *The Lancet Neurology*, 14(7), 720–732.

Patel, M., Coshall, C., Lawrence, E., et al. (2001a). Recovery from poststroke urinary incontinence: Associated factors and impact on outcome. *Journal of the American Geriatrics Society*, 49, 1229–1233.

Patel, M., Coshall, C., Rudd, A. G., et al. (2001b). Natural history and effects on 2-year outcomes of urinary incontinence after stroke. *Stroke*, 32, 122–127.

Pérez, D. C., Chao, C. W., Jiménez, L. L., et al. (2020). Pelvic floor muscle training adapted for urinary incontinence in multiple sclerosis: A randomized clinical trial. *International Urology Journal*, 31(2), 267–275.

Pettersen, R., Dahl, T., & Wyller, T. B. (2002). Prediction of long-term functional outcome after stroke rehabilitation. *Clinical Rehabilitation*, 16, 149–159.

Phé, V., Chartier–Kastler, E., & Panicker, J. N. (2016). Management of neurogenic bladder in patients with multiple sclerosis. *Nature Reviews Urology*, 13(5), 275–288.

Prasad, R. S., Smith, S. J., & Wright, H. (2003). Lower abdominal pressure versus external bladder stimulation to aid bladder emptying in multiple sclerosis: A randomized controlled study. *Clinical Rehabilitation*, 17(1), 42–47.

Preziosi, G., Gordon-Dixon, A., & Emmanuel, A. (2018). Neurogenic bowel dysfunction in patients with multiple sclerosis: Prevalence, impact, and management strategies. *Degenerative Neurological and Neuromuscular Disease*, 8, 79–90.

Reich, D. S., Lucchinetti, C. F., & Calabresi, P. A. (2018). Multiple sclerosis. *New England Journal of Medicine*, 378(2), 169–180.

Rotar, M., Blagus, R., Jeromel, M., et al. (2011). Stroke patients who regain urinary continence in the first week after acute first–ever stroke have better prognosis than patients with persistent lower urinary tract dysfunction. *Neurourology and Urodynamics*, 30(7), 1315–1318.

Ruffion, A., Castro-Diaz, D., Patel, H., et al. (2013). Systematic review of the epidemiology of urinary incontinence and detrusor overactivity among patients with neurogenic overactive bladder. *Neuroepidemiology*, 41(3–4), 146–155.

Sacco, R. L., Kasner, S. E., Broderick, J. P., et al. (2013). An updated definition of stroke for the 21st century: A statement for healthcare professionals from the American Heart Association/American Stroke Association. *Stroke*, 44(7), 2064–2089.

Sakakibara, R., Hattori, T., Yasuda, K., et al. (1996). Micturitional disturbance after acute hemispheric stroke: Analysis of the lesion site by CT and MRI. *Journal of Neurological Sciences*, 137, 47–56.

Shin, D. C., Shin, S. H., Lee, M. M., et al. (2016). Pelvic floor muscle training for urinary incontinence in female stroke patients: A randomized, controlled and blinded trial. *Clinical Rehabilitation*, 30(3), 259–267.

Silva Ferreira, A. P., de Souza Pegorare, A. B. G., Junior, A. M., et al. (2019). A controlled clinical trial on the effects of exercise on lower urinary tract symptoms in women with multiple sclerosis. *American Journal of Physical Medicine & Rehabilitation*, 98(9), 777–782.

Tibaek, S., Gard, G., Dehlendorff, C., et al. (2016). Can pelvic floor muscle training improve quality of life in men with mild to moderate post-stroke and lower urinary tract symptoms? A randomised, controlled and single-blinded trial. *European Journal of Physical and Rehabilitation Medicine*, 53, 416–425.

Tibaek, S., Gard, G., & Jensen, R. (2005). Pelvic floor muscle training is effective in women with urinary incontinence after stroke: A randomised, controlled and blinded study. *Neurourology and Urodynamics*, 24(4), 348–357.

Tibaek, S., Gard, G., & Jensen, R. (2007). Is there a long-lasting effect of pelvic floor muscle training in women with urinary incontinence after ischemic stroke? *International Urology Journal, 18*(3), 281–287.

Tibaek, S., Gard, G., Klarskov, P., et al. (2008). Prevalence of lower urinary tract symptoms (LUTS) in stroke patients: A cross–sectional, clinical survey. *Neurourology and Urodynamics, 27*(8), 763–771.

Tibaek, S., Jensen, R., Lindskov, G., et al. (2004). Can quality of life be improved by pelvic floor muscle training in women with urinary incontinence after ischemic stroke? A randomised, controlled and blinded study. *International Urology Journal, 15*(2), 117–123.

Vahtera, T., Haaranen, M., Viramo-Koskela, A. L., et al. (1997). Pelvic floor rehabilitation is effective in patients with multiple sclerosis. *Clinical Rehabilitation, 11*(3), 211–219.

Vitkova, M., Rosenberger, J., Krokavcova, M., et al. (2014). Health-related quality of life in multiple sclerosis patients with bladder, bowel and sexual dysfunction. *Disability & Rehabilitation, 36*, 987–992.

Wallin, M. T., Culpepper, W. J., Nichols, E., et al. (2019). Global, regional, and national burden of multiple sclerosis 1990–2016: A systematic analysis for the global burden of disease study 2016. *The Lancet Neurology, 18*(3), 269–285.

Williams, M. P., Srikanth, V., Bird, M., et al. (2012). Urinary symptoms and natural history of urinary continence after first-ever stroke—a longitudinal population-based study. *Age and Ageing, 41*(3), 371–376.

World Health Organization. (1978). *The WHO medium-term mental health programme 1975–1982, interim report 1978.* Geneva: World Health Organization. (No. WHO/MNH/78.1).

16

Physical Activity, Elite Athletes and the Pelvic Floor

Kari Bø

INTRODUCTION

Physical activity is defined as 'any bodily movement produced by the skeletal muscles that results in a substantial increase over the resting energy expenditure' (Bouchard et al., 1993) and is an important and modifiable health factor for all age groups. To date, there is evidence that 'exercise is medicine' for a wide range of diseases and conditions (Pedersen and Saltin, 2015; World Health Organization [WHO], 2002). Physical activity can be performed in different domains such as during work/school hours, commuting, household or other cores, and leisure time activity including exercise or sport. *Exercise training* is defined as 'one form of physical activity usually performed on a repeated basis over an extended period of time with a specific external objective such as improvement of fitness, physical performance or health' (Bouchard et al., 1993). The report of the Physical Activity Guidelines Advisory Committee (2018) concludes that regular physical activity lowers the risk of all-cause mortality; cardiovascular disease mortality; cardiovascular disease; hypertension; type 2 diabetes; adverse blood lipid profile; cancers of bladder, breast, colon, endometrium, esophagus, kidney, lung and stomach; dementia; anxiety and depression; and falls and fall-related injuries. It improves cognition, quality of life (QoL), sleep, bone health and physical function; slows or reduces weight gain or weight loss; and prevents weight regain. In addition, for the large number of adults who already have a chronic disease or condition, there is a reduced risk of developing a new chronic condition and reduced risk of progression of the condition they already have, as well as improvements in QoL and physical function. Hence to stay physically active throughout the lifespan is of great importance for health and well-being (WHO, 2002).

The pelvic floor may be the only part of the body where there is a debate whether physical activity and specifically strenuous exercise training is good or bad.

Bø (2004a) described the two opposite hypotheses of physical activity/exercise and the pelvic floor, and this was further elaborated by Bø and Nygaard (2019) in a follow-up review. The two hypotheses and possible consequences are presented next.

Hypothesis 1 is that general exercise training strengthens the pelvic floor. This is based on a theory that impacts occurring during physical activity may stretch and fatigue the pelvic floor muscles (PFMs), leading to a training effect. Furthermore, impacts during the actual movements could lead to a co-contraction of the PFMs, creating an acute indirect training effect. This may reduce the levator hiatus area by causing hypertrophy and shortening of the surrounding muscles, thereby lifting the pelvic floor and internal organs into a higher pelvic location. Theoretically, such morphological changes could reduce the risk of urinary incontinence (UI), anal incontinence (AI) and pelvic organ prolapse (POP). However, it is also theoretically possible that these changes could negatively impact labor and childbirth by making it more difficult for the foetus to descend with pushing.

Hypothesis 2 is that general exercise training overloads, stretches and weakens the pelvic floor. This hypothesis is based on the fact that physical activity increases both intra-abdominal pressure (IAP) and ground reaction forces, and if the PFMs and connective tissue are not strong enough to withstand these forces, the levator hiatus could become wider and the PFMs stretched and weakened. According to this theory, overload of the PFMs may increase the risk of UI, AI and POP but could also result in easier childbirth. For a more detailed discussion on the evidence for each of these hypotheses, see the work of Bø (2004a) and Bø and Nygaard (2019).

The aim of this chapter is to give a systematic review of the literature on UI, AI and POP in connection with participation in sport and fitness activities with a special emphasis on prevalence and treatment of stress urinary incontinence (SUI) in female elite athletes.

METHODS

This is a systematic review of the literature covering incidence, prevalence, treatment and prevention of female pelvic floor dysfunction in sport and fitness activities, with a focus on SUI. For epidemiological studies, a computerized search on Sport and PubMed was done. Mesh words of *urinary incontinence* or *pelvic organ prolapse* or *anal incontinence* combined with *exercise*,

fitness, *physical activity* and *sport* were used. In addition, the chapter on epidemiology from the Sixth International Consultation on Incontinence (Milsom et al., 2017) and systematic reviews (Bø and Nygaard, 2019; De Mattos Lourenco et al., 2018; Teixeira et al., 2018) were consulted. For treatment, the same computerized search was conducted, together with a manual search of systematic reviews reported in the Cochrane Library (Dumoulin et al., 2018; Hay-Smith et al., 2011; Herderschee et al., 2011), the International Consultation on Incontinence (Dumoulin et al., 2017), and the National Institute for Health and Care Excellence (NICE) guidelines (NICE, 2019).

IMPACT OF EXERCISE ON THE PELVIC FLOOR

Bø and Nygaard (2019) reviewed studies on impact of movements and exercises on the pelvic floor. Two exercise modalities may increase IAP to a greater extent than others and thus possibly affect the pelvic floor; strength training and weightlifting are characterized by short-duration bursts of impact with possible high increases in IAP but low ground reaction forces (Fig. 16.1).

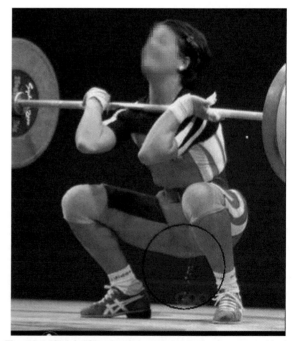

Fig. 16.1 Weightlifting increases abdominal pressure, and leakage may occur.

High-impact activities are associated with a high number of impacts from both ground reaction forces and (probably smaller) increases of IAP. Fig. 16.3 shows a gymnast performing a jump. The results of published studies differ both between studies and between women during the same exercises. An interesting study challenged the widely held belief that there are some pelvic floor 'safe' exercises that generate lower IAPs than corresponding conventional exercises; no differences in IAPs were found between the recommended and discouraged versions of half the exercises, including ball rotations, lunges, core, push-ups and squats (Tian et al., 2018). Others have also pointed out that activities generally restricted after surgery may generate lower IAPs than unrestricted activities. For example, mean maximal IAP was greater when standing up from a chair than it was for abdominal crunches, climbing stairs, sit-ups and many lifting activities (O'Dell et al., 2007; Weir et al 2006). Similarly, lifting 9.08 kg generated less IAP than standing up from a chair (Yamasato et al., 2014). In general, coughing generates higher IAP than most exercises (Bø and Nygaard, 2019).

In addition, ground reaction forces must be withstood by the pelvic floor. Hay (1993) estimated maximum vertical ground reaction forces during different activities and reported those during running to be 3 to 4 times the body weight, 5 to 12 times for jumping, 9 times for landing from a front summersault, 14 times for landing from double back summersault, and 16 times for long jumps. Seegmiller and McCraw (2003) studied ground reaction forces in drop landings in 10 competitive gymnasts. They reported that the first peak vertical force magnitudes ranged from 9.5 N/kg at 30-cm height to 32.8 N/kg at 90-cm height, whereas the second much greater peak vertical force magnitudes ranged from 27.1 at 30-cm height to 56 N/kg at 90 cm. For example, artistic gymnasts may experience these forces during the landing phases of many of their routines.

Unfortunately, studies that attempt to measure the PFMs during physical activity may be flawed by measurement errors such as movement of the measuring device, impossibility to separate IAP and PFM response (pressure measurement), and cross-talk from surrounding muscles (surface electromyography) (Bø and Nygaard, 2019). Two studies were found measuring the acute effect of one bout of exercise. In a short-term experimental crossover study of young nulliparous women with symptoms of SUI, there was a 17% reduction of maximum voluntary PFM contraction after a

90-minute session that included strenuous high-impact endurance and strength training but no change in vaginal resting pressure or muscular endurance (Ree et al., 2007). In contrast, immediately after one bout of strenuous exercise in women who habitually performed CrossFit and one bout of non-strenuous exercise in recreational controls, there was no change in maximum PFM contraction, but there was a decrease in vaginal resting pressure in both groups, as well as slightly worse vaginal support (Middlekauff et al., 2016). To date, there is inconclusive evidence whether female athletes have stronger or weaker PFMs. Borin et al. (2013) compared PFM strength in 10 handball players, 10 volleyball players, 10 basketball players and a non-exercising control group, finding weaker muscles in the volleyball and basketball players compared with controls. They also found that lower strength correlated with increased symptoms of UI. On the contrary, de Araujo et al. (2015) found that 49 high-impact athletes had stronger PFMs than controls (70.1 cm H_2O ± 2.4 vs 34.3 ± 1.7, p < 0.001). Most studies do not find differences in PFM strength between exercisers and non-exercisers (Bø and Nygaard, 2019). There is an urgent need to study mechanisms of physical activity on the pelvic floor, including responses of the pelvic floor to increased IAP and ground reaction forces in women with no pelvic floor dysfunction symptoms.

PREVALENCE OF URINARY INCONTINENCE IN WOMEN PARTICIPATING IN FITNESS ACTIVITIES

The very definition of SUI implies that urine loss occurs during physical exertion (Haylen et al., 2010). If SUI is present, it is therefore likely that urine loss will occur during physical activity. Thus sedentary women who are less exposed to physical exertion may not manifest SUI, although the underlying condition may be present. SUI has shown to lead to withdrawal from participation in sport and fitness activities (Bø et al., 1989a; Nygaard et al., 1990) and may be considered a barrier for lifelong participation in health and fitness activities in women (Brown and Miller, 2001). Although UI itself does not cause significant morbidity or mortality, it may lead to inactivity. A sedentary lifestyle is an independent risk factor for several diseases and conditions (Pedersen and Saltin, 2015; WHO, 2002), and preventing and treating UI therefore becomes an important health issue. Cross-sectional studies in the general female population reporting that physically active women have less incontinence compared to their sedentary counterparts are difficult to interpret, which may be because women with incontinence have stopped exercising (Brown et al., 1996; Danforth et al., 2007; Hannestad et al., 2003; Kikuchi et al., 2007; Østbye et al., 2004; Townsend et al., 2008; Van Oyen and Van Oyen, 2002; Zhu et al., 2008). Contradictory to these studies, Fozzatti et al. (2012) found that 24.6% of nulliparous women attending gyms compared to 14.3% in a group not attending gyms or doing high-impact activities (except running) reported UI (p = 0.006). This supports the results from a study on group fitness instructors, showing a prevalence of 26%, and with the same prevalence in those teaching yoga and Pilates (Bø et al., 2011). Hence general physical activity cannot be used as a treatment for UI. A randomized controlled trial (RCT) of high methodological quality compared PFMT with PFMT plus general physical activity consisting of running and jumping. There was no effect of adding running and jumping to PFMT alone (Luginbuehl et al., 2019).

Prevalence of Urinary Incontinence in High-Impact Female Athletes

There is a high prevalence of symptoms of both SUI and urgency urinary incontinence (UUI) in young nulliparous as well as parous elite athletes participating in high-impact sports (sports including running and jumping activities) (Bø and Nygaard, 2019; Bø et al., 1989b; de Mattos Lourenco et al., 2018; Eliasson et al., 2002; Nygaard et al., 1994; Teixeira et al., 2018; Thyssen et al., 2002). Seven studies compared the prevalence of incontinence in elite athletes with that of a non-exercising or less exercising control group (Almeida et al., 2016; Bø and Borgen, 2001; Carvalhais et al., 2018; Caylet et al., 2006; Dockter et al., 2007; Fernandes et al., 2014; Figueres et al., 2008). All but two of these studies (Bø and Borgen, 2001; Dockter et al., 2007) found a higher prevalence in the athletes compared to control groups. Systematic reviews have concluded that the odds of UI in athletes and exercising women may be 3.5 times that of controls (De Mattos Lourenco et al., 2018; Teixeira et al., 2018).

None of the listed studies characterized incontinence with urodynamic testing (simultaneous measurement of urethral and bladder pressures during an increase in abdominal pressure). However, in a study by Sandvik et al. (1993), questions used in a survey were validated against the diagnosis made by a gynaecologist after urodynamic evaluation. The diagnosis of SUI increased from 51% to 77%, mixed urinary incontinence (MUI) decreased from 39% to 11% and UUI increased from 10% to 12% after urodynamic assessment. In another study of nulliparous physical education students, six of seven students who underwent ambulatory urodynamic assessment showed evidence of urodynamic SUI (Bø et al., 1994).

Eliasson et al. (2002) was the only research group adding clinical measurements to the study. They measured urinary leakage in all elite trampolinists who reported the leakage to be a problem during trampoline training. The leakage was verified in all participants with a mean leakage of 28 g (range: 9–56) in a 15-minute test on the trampoline. PFM function was measured in a subgroup of 10 women. They were all classified as having strong voluntary contractions by vaginal palpation.

A high proportion of athletes report that the leakage is embarrassing, affects their sport performance, or is a social or hygienic problem (Caylet et al., 2006; Eliasson et al., 2008; Gram and Bø, 2020; Skaug et al., 2020). Caylet et al. (2006) found that even small quantities of urine loss caused embarrassment and that 84% of the athletes had never spoken to anyone about the condition.

There is limited knowledge about associated factors. In a study of college athletes, Nygaard et al. (1994) found no significant association between incontinence and amenorrhoea, weight, hormonal therapy or duration of athletic activity. In a study of former Olympians, they found that among factors such as age, body mass index, parity, Olympic sport group and incontinence during Olympic sport 20 years ago, only current body mass index was significantly associated with regular SUI or UUI symptoms (Nygaard, 1997). Bø and Borgen (2001) reported that significantly more elite athletes with eating disorders had symptoms of both SUI and and Eliasson et al. (2002) showed that incontinent trampolinists were significantly older (16 vs 13 years), had been training longer and more frequently, and were less able to interrupt the urine flow stream by voluntarily contracting the PFMs than the non-leaking group.

Prevalence of Urinary Incontinence in Female Strength Athletes

So far, there have been few studies on the prevalence of UI in women participating in weightlifting and strength sports. Wikander et al. (2019) found a prevalence of lifting-related UI in Australian female powerlifters of 37%, but only 11% leaked during daily activities. In another study, all athletes 18 years and older competing in one or more national championships in powerlifting or Olympic weightlifting in 2018 and 2019 in Norway were studied (Skaug et al., 2020). The prevalence of symptoms of UI was 50%. SUI was reported by 41.7% of the females, and 87.8% of those reported a negative influence on sports performance. Rohde et al. (2020) studied 342 female members of USA Weightlifting, USA Powerlifting (USAPL) and/or US CrossFit affiliates and found that 44.8% reported leakage during physical activity and exercise. Qualitative reports demonstrated feelings of embarrassment, frustration and hopelessness with UI during and outside of exercise. Women reported double-unders, deadlift, running/jumping, front squats, cleans and push press as the primarily offending movements that cause leakage during exercise. Main barriers to QoL included adjustments to or elimination of training exercises, as well as feelings of annoyance/irritation, but also that UI is an acceptable side effect of training. Some of the preceding cited studies are limited with low response rates and therefore should be interpreted with caution.

PREVALENCE OF ANAL INCONTINENCE IN FEMALE ELITE ATHLETES

There are fewer studies on AI than UI in female elite athletes. The prevalence of AI among athletes aged 18 to 40 years was 14.8% in 169 intensive sport athletes compared to 4.9% in 224 non-intensive active women. For most, the reported AI was categorized as flatus (Vitton et al., 2011). In an Internet survey of 311 female triathletes, 28% reported AI (Yi et al., 2016). Almeida et al. (2016) found a prevalence of AI of 64.6% among 67 members of a Brazilian sport club, with no difference between athletes and controls, and in a study of strength and Olympic weightlifters, 80% reported AI; more than 70% reported leaking gas only (Skaug et al., 2020).

PREVALENCE OF PELVIC ORGAN PROLAPSE IN FEMALE ELITE ATHLETES

In the general population, Danish nursing assistants were 1.6 times more likely to undergo surgery for genital prolapse and incontinence than women in the general population (Jørgensen et al., 1994). However, the study did not control for parity. Hence it is difficult to conclude whether heavy lifting is an aetiological factor. In a study of women undergoing surgery for POP, 56 women agreed to admit to the ward 1 day before and participate in 1 hour of prescribed physical activities (walking for 45 minutes, including going up and down one flight of stairs, standing up from sitting 5 times, bending down to pick up something off the floor 10 times and jogging/stamping briskly on the spot for 1 minute), and then to remain mostly mobile for 4 to 6 hours after a Pelvic Organ Prolapse Quantification (POP-Q) test. The POP-Q test was repeated the next morning with the same examiner. A total of 70% maintained the same POP-Q stage, 4% had a lower stage and 26% increased the stage (Ali-Ross et al., 2009). Although there is a theoretical risk for and anecdotal reports of POP in young, nulliparous marathon runners and weightlifters, there are very few studies on this condition in exercising women. In a study comparing nulliparous women before and after 6 weeks of summer military training, women attending paratrooper training were significantly more likely to have stage 3 prolapse (Relative risk (RR) = 2.72, 1.37 < relative risk < 5.40, p = 0.003) after the camp. They were also significantly more likely to have worsening in their pelvic support regardless of initial POP stage (Larsen and Yavorek, 2007) (Fig. 16.2).

Yi et al. (2016) found that 5% of 311 female triathletes reported POP symptoms, but no POP symptoms were reported in 67 athletes in Brazil (Almeida et al., 2016). Among female powerlifters and Olympic weightlifters, Skaug et al. (2020) found that 23.3% of the participants reported the feeling of a bulge inside or outside the vagina. There is an urgent need for further studies on mechanisms, risk factors and preventive strategies for POP in female exercisers and athletes.

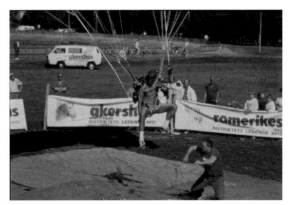

Fig. 16.2 The reaction force during landing in parachute jumping must be counteracted by the pelvic floor.

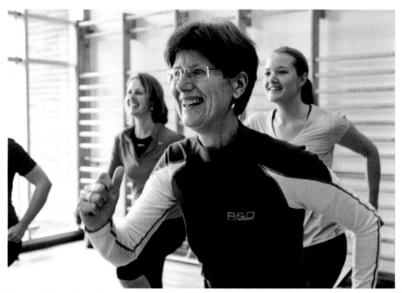

Fig. 16.3 Stress urinary incontinence is common during high-impact activities (e.g., jumping and running).

PREVALENCE OF URINARY INCONTINENCE AND ANAL INCONTINENCE IN MALE ATHLETES

There are almost no studies on male athletes. This may indicate that UI and AI have not been reported as a problem among men or that this may still be more of a taboo area among them than among women. In a study by Bø et al. (2011), 3 of 152 male group instructors (2%) reported UI, but this leakage was not related to physical activity. Only one study was found including male athletes (Skaug et al., 2020). In a Norwegian study of 204 males participating in one or more national championships in powerlifting or Olympic weightlifting in 2018 and 2019, the prevalence of UI and AI was 9.3% and 61.8%, respectively (Skaug et al., 2020). AI was mostly reported as gas, and the men were only minimally bothered by the condition.

Although the prevalence of pelvic floor dysfunction is high in female athletes, many athletes have no problems during strenuous activities and high increases in IAP. From a theoretical understanding of functional anatomy and biomechanics, it is likely that heavy lifting and strenuous activity may promote these conditions, especially in women already at risk (e.g., those with benign hypermobility joint syndrome). There is a need for further basic science studies to understand the mechanisms of exercise on the pelvic floor.

PREVENTION

There are no studies applying pelvic floor muscle training (PFMT) for primary prevention of UI, AI or POP. Theoretically, one could argue that strengthening the PFMs by specific training would have the potential to prevent pelvic floor dysfunction in general. Strength training of the PFMs has been shown to increase the thickness of the muscles, reduce muscle length, reduce the levator hiatus area and lift the levator plate to a more cranial level inside the pelvis in women with POP (Brækken et al., 2010). If the pelvic floor possesses a certain 'stiffness', 'tone' or 'tightness' (Ashton-Miller et al., 2001; Haderer et al., 2002), it is likely that this would prevent excessive downward movement and opening of the levator hiatus and the urethra, vagina and rectum. This could also allow the PFMs to pre- or co-contract with IAP rise and/or stabilize the whole pelvic floor during movements created by the ground reaction forces. However, most likely, such contractions may not be necessary if the pelvic floor is situated in an optimal location and the levator hiatus remains closed. More studies are needed to understand the mechanisms for continence during strenuous work or physical exertion.

Preventive Devices

Devices that involve external urinary collection, intravaginal support of the bladder neck or blockage of urinary leakage by occlusion are available, and some have been shown to be effective in preventing leakage during physical activity. A vaginal tampon can be such a simple device. In a study by Glavind (1997), six women with SUI demonstrated total dryness when using a vaginal device during 30 minutes of aerobics. For smaller leakage, specially designed protecting pads can be used during training and competition.

TREATMENT OF STRESS URINARY INCONTINENCE IN ELITE ATHLETES

SUI can be treated with bladder training, PFMT with or without resistance devices, vaginal cones or biofeedback, electrical stimulation, drug therapy or surgery (Dumoulin et al., 2017; Dumoulin et al., 2018; Hay-Smith et al., 2011; Herderschee et al., 2011). One would assume that female elite athletes would respond in the same way to treatment as other women do. However, given the high impact on their pelvic floor, they may need stronger and tighter PFMs than non-athletes.

To date, there are methodological problems assessing bladder and urethral function during physical activity before and after treatment (Flury et al., 2017; James, 1978; Kulseng-Hanssen and Klevmark, 1988).

Surgery

Elite athletes are young and mostly nulliparous, and it is therefore recommended that PFMT should be the first choice of treatment, and always tried before surgery (Dumoulin et al., 2017; Dumoulin et al., 2018; NICE, 2019). The leakage in athletes seems to be related to strenuous high-impact activity, and elite athletes do not seem to have more UI than others later in life when the activity is reduced (Nygaard, 1997; Bø and Sundgot-Borgen, 2010). Therefore, surgery seems inappropriate in young, elite athletes.

Bladder Training

Anecdotally, most elite athletes empty their bladder before practice and competition, which was also reported to be common in young nulliparous women attending gyms (Fozzatti et al., 2012) and in elite strength athletes (Skaug et al., 2020). Therefore it is unlikely that any of them would exercise with a high bladder volume. However, as with the rest of the population, elite athletes may have a non-optimal toilet behaviour and the use of a frequency–volume chart may be an important first step to improve this.

Oestrogen

The role of oestrogen in incidence, prevalence and treatment of SUI is controversial. Meta-analyses of the effect have concluded that local oestrogen therapy for UI may be beneficial, although there was little evidence for a long-term effect (Andersson et al., 2017). Systematic hormone replacement using conjugated equine oestrogens may actually make UI worse. In addition, there are few data on the dose type of oestrogen and route of administration (Andersson et al., 2017). Oestrogen given alone therefore does not seem to be an effective treatment for SUI. There is a higher prevalence of eating disorders in athletes compared to non-athletes, and these athletes may be low in oestrogen (Bø and Borgen, 2001). However, most amenorrhoeic elite athletes would be on oestrogen replacement therapy because of the risk of osteoporosis. Oestrogen may have adverse effects such as a higher risk of coronary heart disease and cancer (Andersson et al., 2017).

Pelvic Floor Muscle Training

Based on systematic reviews and meta-analysis of RCTs, it has been stated that conservative treatment should be first-line treatment for SUI (Dumoulin et al., 2017). Cochrane reviews conclude that PFMT is an effective treatment for adult women with SUI or MUI, and consistently better than no treatment or placebo treatments (Dumoulin et al., 2018; Hay-Smith et al., 2011; Herderschee et al., 2011). Subjective cure and improvement rates after PFMT for SUI or MUI was reported in RCTs to be up to 70% (Dumoulin et al., 2017; Dumoulin et al., 2018). Cure rates, defined as 2 g or less leakage on pad tests, vary between 44% and 70% in SUI (Bø et al., 1999; Dumoulin et al., 2004; Mørkved et al., 2002). Adverse effects are rare and minor (Dumoulin et al., 2017; Dumoulin et al., 2018; NICE, 2019). Bø et al. (1990, 1999) and Mørkved et al. (2002) used tests involving high-impact exercise (running and jumping) before and after treatment and showed that it is possible to cure or reduce urinary leakage that occurs during physical activity. Bø et al. (1989a) demonstrated that after specific strength training of the PFMs, 17 of 23 women reported improvement during jumping and running, and 15 during lifting. Significant improvement was also obtained while dancing or hiking, during general group exercise and in an overall score on ability to participate in different activities. Measured with a pad test with standardized bladder volume during activities including running, jumping jacks and sit-ups, there was a significant reduction in urine loss from a mean of 27 g (95% CI: 8.8–45.1, range: 0–168) to 7.1 g (95% CI: 0.8–12.4, range: 0–58.3), p < 0.01 (Bø et al., 1990). Mørkved et al. (2002) demonstrated a 67% cure rate in a test involving physical activity after individual biofeedback-assisted strength training of the PFMs.

Several small uncontrolled studies have suggested that athletes and soldiers demonstrate improvements of symptoms in PFM strength after PFMT (Da Roza et al., 2012; Rivalta et al., 2010; Sherman et al., 1997). In the only found RCT evaluating the effect of PFMT on SUI in 32 volleyball players, PFMT improved UI in more women than in those given written information (Ferreira et al., 2014). However, athletes have a low level of knowledge of the pelvic floor and how to train the PFMs (Cardoso et al., 2018; Gram and Bø, 2020; Skaug et al., 2020).

Elite athletes are accustomed to regular training and are highly motivated for exercise. Adding three sets of 8 to 12 close-to-maximum contractions of the PFMs three to four times a week (Garber et al., 2011) to their regular strength-training programme does not seem to be a big task. However, there is no reason to believe that they are more able than the general population to perform a correct PFM contraction. Therefore thorough instruction and assessment of ability to contract is mandatory. Because most elite athletes are nulliparous, there are no ruptures of ligaments, fascias, muscle fibres, or peripheral nerve damage. As such, it is expected that the effect would be equal or even better in this specific group of girls and women. However, the impact and increase in abdominal pressure that must be counteracted by the PFMs in athletes performing high-impact activities is much higher than what is required in the sedentary population. The pelvic floor therefore probably needs to be better positioned, tighter and 'fitter' in elite athletes.

There are two different theoretical rationales for the effect of PFMT (Bø, 2004b). Miller et al. (1998) found that a voluntary contraction of the PFMs before and during cough ('the Knack') reduced leakage by 98% and 73% during a medium and deep cough, respectively. In a more recent study, performing the Knack during several daily activities causing leakage in women with both SUI and MUI, a statistically significant improvement was found in the intervention group compared to the control group (Miller et al., 2018). Kegel (1948) first described the PFMT method in 1948 as 'tightening' of the pelvic floor. The rationale behind a strength-training regimen is to increase muscle tone and cross-sectional area of the muscles and increase stiffness of connective tissue within the muscle, thereby lifting the pelvic floor into a higher pelvic position. Such changes have been found after PFMT (Brækken et al., 2010).

It is unlikely that continent elite athletes or participants in fitness activities think about the PFMs or pre-contract them voluntarily. A contraction of the PFMs most likely occurs automatically and simultaneously or even before the impact or abdominal pressure increase (Constantinou and Govan, 1981). It seems impossible to voluntarily pre-contract the PFMs before and during every increase in abdominal pressure while participating in sport and leisure activities (Fig. 16.4). The aim of the training programme therefore would be to build up the PFMs to a firm structural base where there is no need for such contractions or where such contractions occur automatically.

Given that few athletes know about the PFMs or have trained these muscles regularly (Gram and Bø, 2019; Skaug et al., 2020), the potential for improvement in function and strength may be huge. PFMT has proved to be effective when conducted intensively and with a close follow-up in the general female population (Dumoulin et al., 2017). It is a functional and physiological non-invasive treatment with no known serious adverse effects, and it is cost effective compared to other treatment modalities (Imamura et al., 2010). However, there is a need for further high-quality RCTs to evaluate the effect of PFM strength training in different elite sports.

CONCLUSION

SUI may be a barrier to women's participation in sport and fitness activities and may therefore be a threat to women's health, self-esteem and well-being. Its prevalence among young, nulliparous elite athletes is high, with the highest prevalence found in those involved in high-impact activities such as gymnastics, track and field, and some ball games. There are few studies on AI and POP and in male athletes. One RCT was found on PFMT in female elite athletes which showed significant reduction of SUI compared to the control. There is a need for more basic research on the pelvic floor and PFM function during physical activity; the effect of PFMT on UI, AI and POP in female elite athletes; and AI in male athletes.

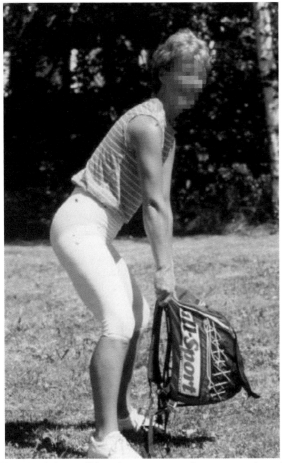

Fig. 16.4 It is possible to learn to pre- and co-contract the pelvic floor muscles before and during single-task activities such as lifting.

CLINICAL RECOMMENDATIONS

- Give information on the pelvic floor, pelvic floor dysfunction and PFMT to instructors of fitness activities and athletic coaches.
- Suggest the use of preventive devices or tampons to prevent leakage during physical activity.
- Follow general recommendations for PFMT for SUI and POP for female elite athletes.

REFERENCES

Ali-Ross, N. S., Smith, A. R., & Hosker, G. (2009). The effect of physical activity on pelvic organ prolapse. *British Journal of Obstetrics and Gynaecology, 116*(6), 824–828.

Almeida, M. B. A., Barra, A. A., Saltiel, F., et al. (2016). Urinary incontinence and other pelvic floor dysfunctions in female athletes in Brazil: A cross-sectional study. *Scandinavian Journal of Medicine & Science in Sports, 26,* 1109–1116.

Andersson, K.-E., Cardozo, L., Cruz, F., et al. (2017). Committee 8: Pharmacological treatment of urinary incontinence. In P. Abrams, L. Cardozo, A. Wagg, et al. (Eds.), *Incontinence: Sixth international consultation on urinary incontinence* (pp. 805–957). Plymouth, UK: Health Publication/Plymbridge Distributors.

Ashton-Miller, J., Howard, D., & DeLancey, J. (2001). The functional anatomy of the female pelvic floor and stress continence control system. *Scandinavian Journal of Urology & Nephrology - Supplementum, 207,* 1–7; discussion 106–125.

Bø, K. (2004a). Urinary incontinence, pelvic floor dysfunction, exercise and sport. *Sports Medicine, 34*(7), 451–464.

Bø, K. (2004b). Pelvic floor muscle training is effective in treatment of stress urinary incontinence, but how does it work? *International Urogynecology Journal and Pelvic Floor Dysfunction, 15,* 76–84.

Bø, K., & Borgen, J. (2001). Prevalence of stress and urge urinary incontinence in elite athletes and controls. *Medicine & Science in Sports & Exercise, 33,* 1797–1802.

Bø, K., Bratland-Sanda, S., & Sundgot-Borgen, J. (2011). Urinary incontinence among fitness instructors including yoga and Pilates instructors. *Neurourology and Urodynamics, 30,* 370–373.

Bø, K., Hagen, R., Kvarstein, B., et al. (1989a). Female stress urinary incontinence and participation in different sport and social activities. *Scandinavian Journal of Sports Sciences, 11*(3), 117–121.

Bø, K., Hagen, R., Kvarstein, B., et al. (1990). Pelvic floor muscle exercise for the treatment of female stress urinary incontinence: III. Effects of two different degrees of pelvic floor muscle exercise. *Neurourology and Urodynamics, 9,* 489–502.

Bø, K., Mæhlum, S., Oseid, S., et al. (1989b). Prevalence of stress urinary incontinence among physically active and sedentary female students. *Scandinavian Journal of Sports Sciences, 11*(3), 113–116.

Bø, K., & Nygaard, I. E. (2019). Is physical activity good or bad for the female pelvic floor? A narrative review. *Sports Medicine, 50*(3), 471–484.

Bø, K., Stien, R., Kulseng-Hanssen, S., et al. (1994). Clinical and urodynamic assessment of nulliparous young women with and without stress incontinence symptoms: A case control study. *Obstetrics & Gynecology, 84,* 1028–1032.

Bø, K., & Sundgot-Borgen, J. (2010). Are former female elite athletes more likely to experience urinary incontinence later in life than non-athletes? *Scandinavian Journal of Medicine & Science in Sports, 20,* 100–104.

Bø, K., Talseth, T., & Holme, I. (1999). Single blind, randomised controlled trial of pelvic floor exercises, electrical stimulation, vaginal cones, and no treatment in management of genuine stress incontinence in women. *British Medical Journal, 318,* 487–493.

Borin, L. C. M. S., Nunes, F. R., & Guirro, E. C. O. G. (2013). Assessment of pelvic floor muscle pressure in female athletes. *Physical Medicine and Rehabilitation, 5,* 189–193.

Bouchard, C., Shephard, R. J., & Stephens, T. (1993). *Physical activity, fitness and health. Consensus statement.* Champaign, IL: Human Kinetics Publishers.

Brækken, I. H., Maijida, M., Engh, M. E., et al. (2010). Morphological changes after pelvic floor muscle training measured by 3-dimensional ultrasonography. A randomized controlled trial. *Obstetrics & Gynecology, 115*(2), 317–324.

Brown, W. J., & Miller, Y. D. (2001). Too wet to exercise? Leaking urine as a barrier to physical activity in women. *Journal of Science and Medicine in Sport, 4*(4), 373–378.

Brown, J. S., Seeley, D. G., Fong, J., et al. (1996). Urinary incontinence in older women: Who is at risk? Study of osteoporotic fractures research group. *Obstetrics & Gynecology, 87,* 715–721.

Cardoso, A. M. B., de Paiva Lima, C. R. O., & Ferreira, C. W. S. (2018). Prevalence of urinary incontinence in high-impact sport athletes and their association with knowledge, attitude and practice about this dysfunction. *European Journal of Sports Sciences, 18*(10), 1405–1412.

Carvalhais, A., Natal, R. J., & Bø, K. (2018). Performing high-level sport is strongly associated with urinary incontinence in elite athletes: A comparative study of 372 elite female athletes and 372 controls. *British Journal of Sports Medicine, 52*(24), 1586–1590.

Caylet, N., Fabbro-Peray, P., Mares, P., et al. (2006). Prevalence and occurrence of stress urinary incontinence in elite women athletes. *The Canadian Journal of Urology, 13*(4), 3174–3179.

Constantinou, C. E., & Govan, D. E. (1981). Contribution and timing of transmitted and generated pressure components in the female urethra. In *Female incontinence* (pp. 113–120). New York: Allan R. Liss.

Da Roza, T., Araujo, M. P., Viana, R., et al. (2012). Pelvic floor muscle training to improve urinary incontinence in young, nulliparous sport students: A pilot study. *International Urology Journal, 23,* 1069–1073.

Danforth, K. N., Shah, A. D., Townsend, M. K., et al. (2007). Physical activity and urinary incontinence among healthy, older women. *Obstetrics & Gynecology, 109,* 721–727.

De Araujo, M., Parmigiano, T., Della Negra, L., et al. (2015). Evaluation of athletes' pelvic floor: Is there a relation with urinary incontinence? *Revista Brasileira Medicine Esporte, 21,* 442–446.

De Mattos Lourenco, T. H., Matsuoka, P. K., Baracat, E. C., et al. (2018). Urinary incontinence in female athletes: Systematic review. *International Urology Journal, 29,* 1757–1763.

Dockter, M., Kolstad, A. M., Martin, K., et al. (2007). Prevalence of urinary incontinence: A comparative study of collegiate female athletes and non-athletic controls. *Journal Womens Health Physical Therapy, 31,* 12–17.

Dumoulin, C., Adewuyi, T., Booth, J., et al. (2017). Adult conservative management. In P. Abrams, L. Cardozo, A. Wagg, et al. (Eds.), *Incontinence* (6th ed.) (Vol. 2)(pp. 1443–1628). Bristol, UK: International Continence Society.

Dumoulin, C., Cacciari, L. P., & Hay-Smith, E. J. C. (2018). Pelvic floor muscle training versus no treatment, or inactive control treatments, for urinary incontinence in women. *Cochrane Database of Systematic Reviews, 10,* CD005654.

Dumoulin, C., Lemieux, M., Bourbonnais, D., et al. (2004). Physiotherapy for persistent postnatal stress urinary incontinence: A randomized controlled trial. *Obstetrics & Gynecology, 104,* 504–510.

Eliasson, K., Edner, A., & Mattsson, E. (2008). Urinary incontinence in very young and mostly nulliparous women with a history of regular organized high-impact trampoline training: Occurrence and risk factors. *International Urology Journal, 19,* 687–696.

Eliasson, K., Larsson, T., & Mattson, E. (2002). Prevalence of stress incontinence in nulliparous elite trampolinists. *Scandinavian Journal of Medicine & Science in Sports, 12,* 106–110.

Fernandes, A., Fitz, F., Silva, A., et al. (2014). Evaluation of the prevalence of urinary incontinence symptoms in adolescent female soccer players and their impact on quality of life. *Occupational and Environmental Medicine, 71*(Suppl. 1), A1–A132.

Ferreira, S., Ferreira, M., Carvalhais, A., et al. (2014). Reeducation of pelvic floor muscles in volleyball athletes. *Revista da Associação Médica Brasileira, 60,* 428–433.

Figueres, C. C., Boyle, K. L., Caprio, K. M., et al. (2008). Pelvic floor muscle activity and urinary incontinence in weight-bearing female athletes vs non-athletes. *Journal Womens Health Physical Therapy, 32,* 7–11.

Flury, N., Koenig, I., & Radlinger, L. (2017). Crosstalk considerations in studies evaluating pelvic floor muscles using surface electromyography in women: A scoping review. *Archives of Gynecology and Obstetrics, 295*(4), 799–809.

Fozzatti, C., Riccetto, C., Herrmann, V., et al. (2012). Prevalence study of stress urinary incontinence in women who perform high-impact exercises. *International Urology Journal, 23,* 1687–1691.

Garber, C. E., Blissmer, B., Deschenes, M. R., et al. (2011). American college of sports medicine position stand. Quantity and quality of exercise for developing and maintaining cardiorespiratory, musculoskeletal, and neuromotor fitness in apparently healthy adults: Guidance for prescribing exercise. *Medicine & Science in Sports & Exercise, 43*(7), 1334–1359.

Glavind, K. (1997). Use of a vaginal sponge during aerobic exercises in patients with stress urinary incontinence. *International Urogynecology Journal and Pelvic Floor Dysfunction, 8*, 351–353.

Gram, M. C. D., & Bø, K. (2020). High level rhythmic gymnasts and urinary incontinence: Prevalence, risk factors, and influence on performance. *Scandinavian Journal of Medicine & Science in Sports, 30*, 159–165.

Haderer, J., Pannu, H., Genadry, R., et al. (2002). Controversies in female urethral anatomy and their significance for understanding urinary continence: Observations and literature review. *International Urogynecology Journal and Pelvic Floor Dysfunction, 13*, 236–252.

Hannestad, I., Rortveit, G., Daltveit, A. K., et al. (2003). Are smoking and other lifestyle factors associated with female urinary incontinence? The Norwegian EPINCONT study. *British Journal Obstetrics and Gynecology, 110*, 247–254.

Hay, J. (1993). Citius, altius, longius (faster, higher, longer): The biomechanics of jumping for distance. *Journal of Biomechanics, 26*(Suppl. 1), 7–21.

Hay-Smith, E. J. C., Herderschee, R., Dumoulin, C., et al. (2011). Comparisons of approaches to pelvic floor muscle training for urinary incontinence in women. *Cochrane Database of Systematic Reviews, 12*, CD009508.

Haylen, B. T., de Ridder, D., Freeman, R. M., et al. (2010). An International Urogynecological Association (IUGA)/International Continence Society (ICS) joint report on the terminology for female pelvic floor dysfunction. *International Urology Journal, 21*, 15–26.

Herderschee, R., Hay-Smith, E. J. C., Herbison, G. P., et al. (2011). Feedback or biofeedback to augment pelvic floor muscle training for urinary incontinence in women. *Cochrane Database of Systematic Reviews, 7*, CD009252.

Imamura, M., Abrams, P., Bain, C., et al. (2010). Systematic review and economic modelling of the effectiveness and cost-effectiveness of non-surgical treatments for women with stress urinary incontinence. *Health Technology Assessment, 14*(40), 1–188, iii–iv.

James, E. D. (1978). The behaviour of the bladder during physical activity. *British Journal of Urology, 50*, 387–394.

Jørgensen, S., Hein, H., & Gyntelberg, F. (1994). Heavy lifting at work and risk of genital prolapse and herniated lumbar disc in assistant nurses. *Occupational Medicine (Oxford), 44*(1), 47–49.

Kegel, A. H. (1948). Progressive resistance exercise in the functional restoration of the perineal muscles. *American Journal of Obstetrics and Gynecology, 56*, 238–249.

Kikuchi, A., Niu, K., Ikeda, Y., et al. (2007). Association between physical activity and urinary incontinence in a community-based elderly population aged 70 years and over. *European Urology, 2*, 868–875.

Kulseng-Hanssen, S., & Klevmark, B. (1988). Ambulatory urethrocystorectometry: A new technique. *Neurourology and Urodynamics, 7*, 119–130.

Larsen, W. I., & Yavorek, T. (2007). Pelvic prolapse and urinary incontinence in nulliparous college women in relation to paratrooper training. *International Urology Journal, 18*, 769–771.

Luginbuehl, H., Lehmann, C., Koenig, I., et al. (2019). Involuntary reflexive pelvic floor muscle training in addition to standard training versus standard training alone for women with stress urinary incontinence: A randomized controlled trial. *International Urology Journal, 33*(3), 531–540.

Middlekauff, M. L., Egger, M. J., Nygaard, I. E., et al. (2016). The impact of acute and chronic strenuous exercise on pelvic floor muscle strength and support in nulliparous healthy women. *American Journal of Obstetrics and Gynecology, 215*(3), 316.e1–316.e7.

Miller, J., Ashton-Miller, J., & DeLancey, J. (1998). A pelvic muscle precontraction can reduce cough-related urine loss in selected women with mild SUI. *Journal of the American Geriatrics Society, 46*, 870–874.

Miller, J., Hawthorne, K., Park, L., et al. (2018). Self-perceived improvement in bladder health after viewing a novel tutorial on Knack use: A randomized controlled trial pilot study. *Journal Womens Health (Larchmt.), 29*(10), 1319–1327.

Milsom, I., Altman, D., Cartwright, R., et al. (2017). Committee 1: Epidemiology of urinary incontinence (UI) and other lower urinary tract symptoms (LUTS), pelvic organ prolapse (POP) and anal incontinence. In P. Abrams, L. Cardozo, A. Wagg, et al. (Eds.), *Incontinence: Sixth international consultation on urinary incontinence* (pp. 1–141). Plymouth, UK: Health Publication/Plymbridge Distributors.

Mørkved, S., Bø, K., & Fjørtoft, T. (2002). Is there any additional effect of adding biofeedback to pelvic floor muscle training? A single-blind randomized controlled trial. *Obstetrics & Gynecology, 100*(4), 730–739.

National Institute for Health and Care Excellence. (2019). *Urinary incontinence and pelvic organ prolapse in women: Management.* London: National Institute for Health and Care Excellence.

Nygaard, I. (1997). Does prolonged high-impact activity contribute to later urinary incontinence? A retrospective cohort study of female Olympians. *Obstetrics & Gynecology, 90*, 718–722.

Nygaard, I., DeLancey, J. O. L., Arnsdorf, L., et al. (1990). Exercise and incontinence. *Obstetrics & Gynecology, 75*, 848–851.

Nygaard, I., Thompson, F. L., Svengalis, S. L., et al. (1994). Urinary incontinence in elite nulliparous athletes. *Obstetrics & Gynecology, 84*, 183–187.

O'Dell, K. K., Morse, A. N., Crawford, S. L., et al. (2007). Vaginal pressure during lifting, floor exercises, jogging, and use of hydraulic exercise machines. *International Urology Journal, 18*, 1481–1489.

Østbye, T., Seim, A., Krause, K. M., et al. (2004). A 10-year follow-up of urinary and fecal incontinence among the oldest old in the community: The Canadian study of health and aging. *Canadian Journal on Aging, 23*(4), 319–331.

Pedersen, B. K., & Saltin, B. (2015). Exercise as medicine—evidence for prescribing exercise as therapy in 26 different chronic diseases. *Scandinavian Journal of Medicine & Science in Sports, 25*(Suppl. 3), 1–72.

Physical Activity Guidelines Advisory Committee. (2018). *Physical activity guidelines advisory committee scientific report.* Washington, DC: US Department of Health and Human Services.

Ree, M. L., Nygaard, I., & Bø, K. (2007). Muscular fatigue in the pelvic floor muscles after strenuous physical activity. *Acta Obstetricia et Gynecologica Scandinavica, 86*, 870–876.

Rivalta, M., Sighinolfi, M. C., Micali, S., et al. (2010). Urinary incontinence and sport: First and preliminary experience with a combined pelvic floor rehabilitation program in three female athletes. *Health Care for Women International, 31*(5), 435–443.

Rohde, M., Brumitt, J., Sandvik, J., et al. (2020). *Prevalence, risk factors, and quality of life concerning stress urinary incontinence in US female athletes.* Participating in Strength Sports (Abstract 507) [Online]. Available: https://www.ics.org/2020/abstract/507. (Accessed 04.08.22).

Sandvik, H., Hunskaar, S., Seim, A., et al. (1993). Validation of a severity index in female urinary incontinence and its implementation in an epidemiological survey. *Journal of Epidemiology & Community Health, 47*, 497–499.

Seegmiller, J. G., & McCraw, S. T. (2003). Ground reaction forces among gymnasts and recreational athletes in drop landings. *Journal of Athletic Training, 38*, 311–314.

Sherman, R. A., Wong, M. F., & Davis, G. D. (1997). Behavioral treatment of exercise induced urinary incontinence among female soldiers. *Military Medicine, 162*(10), 690–694.

Skaug, K. L., Frawley, H., Engh, M. E., et al. (2020). Prevalence of pelvic floor dysfunction, bother and risk factors and knowledge of the pelvic floor in Norwegian male and female powerlifters and Olympic weightlifters. *Journal of Strength and Conditioning Research, 36*(10), 2800–2807.

Teixeira, R. V., Cola, C., Sbruzzi, G., et al. (2018). Prevalence of urinary incontinence in female athletes: A systematic review with meta-analysis. *International Urology Journal, 29*, 1717–1725.

Thyssen, H. H., Clevin, L., Olesen, S., et al. (2002). Urinary incontinence in elite female athletes and dancers. *International Urogynecology Journal and Pelvic Floor Dysfunction, 13*, 15–17.

Tian, T., Budgett, S., Smalldridge, J., et al. (2018). Assessing exercises recommended for women at risk of pelvic floor disorders using multivariate statistical techniques. *International Urology Journal, 29*, 1447–1454.

Townsend, M. K., Danforth, K. N., Rosner, B., et al. (2008). Physical activity and incident urinary incontinence in middle-aged women. *Journal of Urology, 179*(3), 1012–1017.

Van Oyen, H., & Van Oyen, P. (2002). Urinary incontinence in Belgium: Prevalence, correlates and psychosocial consequences. *Acta Clinica Belgica, 57*, 207–218.

Vitton, V., Baumstarck-Barrau, K., Brardjanian, S., et al. (2011). Impact of high-level sport practice on anal incontinence in a healthy young female population. *Journal Womens Health, 20*(5), 757–763.

Weir, L. F., Nygaard, I. E., Wilken, J., et al. (2006). Postoperative activity restrictions. *Obstetrics & Gynecology, 107*, 305–309.

Wikander, L., Cross, D., & Gahreman, D. E. (2019). Prevalence of urinary incontinence in women powerlifters: A pilot study. *International Urology Journal, 30*, 2031–2039.

World Health Organization. (2002). *Physical inactivity a leading cause of disease and disability.* Warns WHO [Online]. Available: https://www.who.int/news/item/04-04-2020-physical-inactivity-a-leading-cause-of-disease-and--disability-warns-who. (Accessed 04.08.22).

Yamasato, K. S., Oyama, I. A., & Kaneshiro, B. (2014). Intraabdominal pressure with pelvic floor dysfunction: Do postoperative restrictions make sense? *Journal of Reproductive Medicine, 59*(7–8), 409–413.

Yi, J., Tenfelde, S., Tell, D., et al. (2016). Triathlete risk of pelvic floor disorders, pelvic girdle pain, and female athlete triad. *Female Pelvic Medicine & Reconstructive Surgery, 22*(5), 373–376.

Zhu, L., Lang, J., Wang, H., et al. (2008). The prevalence of and potential risk factors for female urinary incontinence in Beijing, China. *Menopause, 15*, 566–569.

17

Evidence for Mobile Apps: Where Do We Stand and Where Should We Go?

Bary Berghmans

INTRODUCTION

Although there are positive reports of short-term (Kaya et al., 2015) and long-term effects (Bø and Hilde, 2013) for practically every kind of treatment for pelvic floor dysfunction (Dumoulin et al., 2014; Dumoulin et al., 2015c; Dumoulin et al., 2016), there remains doubt especially related to long-term effects (Bø and Hilde, 2013; Pereira et al., 2013). Success of pelvic floor muscle training (PFMT) is broadly threatened by insufficient adherence to the required pelvic floor muscle (PFM) exercise program. Only 64% of patients adhere to PFMT in the short term and, even worse, only 23% in the long term (Dumoulin et al., 2015b). Certainly, adherence is a major cornerstone of an adequate and effective PFMT program (Dumoulin et al., 2015b; McClurg et al., 2015). Therefore, strategies to increase adherence need more attention among clinicians and researchers (Dumoulin et al., 2016).

Adherence can be defined as 'the extent to [which] a patient's behavior matches agreed recommendations/ instructions from the prescriber; it is intended to be non-judgmental, a statement of fact, rather than to ascribe blame to the patient, prescriber, or treatment method' (Haynes et al., 2015). Adherence is crucial during the supervised clinical phase of PFMT (short term) and during the home maintenance phase after ending the physiotherapy sessions (long term) (McClurg et al., 2015). Several strategies to increase adherence short term as well as long term have been reported (Frawley et al., 2015), although long-term adherence is the more problematic (Dumoulin et al., 2015a; Dumoulin et al., 2015b). Adherence is associated with better education and information about the importance of the pelvic floor and PFM skills for urinary incontinence (UI) cure; with the patient's positive feelings regarding PFMT (Sluijs et al., 1991); and with an individualized approach, matching age, gender, and ethnicity (Frawley et al., 2015). Prioritization and integration of PFMT into daily activities (Frawley et al., 2015) have been strongly recommended (Dumoulin et al., 2015a). Unfortunately, adherence remains a weak point in PFMT programs. However, the rapid advance of Internet, e-health and telemedia empowers interpersonal communication more and more. Social media is now a reality, reachable for virtually every citizen in the world, and in 2014, Internet access by mobile phone overtook fixed Internet access (Chaffey et al., 2021). For instance, in 2017, worldwide there were an estimated 3.7 billion mobile health app downloads (https://www.statista.com/ statistics/625034/mobile-health-app-downloads/). In fact, interconnection has been improved daily.

The development of increasing use of social media facilitates a new horizon for (home) training and adherence science, as new devices can be developed utilizing the environment of Internet and social media, allowing new ways of contact between patient and therapist. Surfing on the Internet, dozens of applications 'training' the PFMs by smartphone are available for the general public. For instance, using the keyword *pelvic floor*, a quick search in Google Play Store, an engine for downloading Android mobile applications (mApps), showed 45 free download applications and 16 for purchase (Google Play Store, 2016), whereas Apple Store returned 10 apps, with 9 of them for purchase (Apple Store, 2016).

So far, there is sparse literature about the use of those applications by the general population (Latorre et al., 2018). However, Latorre et al. (2018) reported that Google Play Store keeps a record of the total number of downloads of each application. They stated that their quick search revealed that 3 applications had been downloaded more than 100,000 times, with 13 of them more than 10,000 times. Only 30 were downloaded less than 1000 times. The mean of downloads by application was nearly 7000, and the total count for all applications exceeds more than half a million downloads, which shows the population's huge interest in mApps for PFMT (Latorre et al., 2018). However, very little relevant literature related to concepts, methodology, effects or use of PFMT applications were found (Latorre et al., 2018). In most cases, the applications use simple instruction protocols, showing the patient images and/or sounds representing the time to contract and relax the PFMs. No real feedback is offered, as there is no physical link between the mobile phone and the patient's body: those applications work in the same way as simple verbal instructions. Moreover, 33% do not specifically train the PFMs but are a mix of PFMT with other general gymnastics.

Almost all relevant e-health systems lack evidence related to protocol and content (Latorre et al., 2018), and procedures are not based on physiological training principles (Bø et al., 2015). For instance, many applications did not use maximal PFM contractions during strength training. Others present endurance training, violating solid principles of exercise physiology (McCardle et al., 2014) and the International Urogynecological Association (IUGA)/International Continence Society (ICS)-validated protocol for PFM endurance training (Berghmans, 2017; McCardle et al., 2014). Another issue is the lack of specificity: protocols often are similar for all patients. Men or women, elderly or young, pregnant, mother or nulliparous—everyone will perform the same training program even though each patient population requires different needs of PFMT (Berghmans, 2017; Bø et al., 2015). Only two mApps take notice of a referral by a healthcare professional, but the literature shows that one-third of women are unable to contract the PFMs (Henderson et al., 2013), often pushing down instead of lifting the PFMs inwards during the contraction. Considering this situation as a whole, an mApp for PFMT could be useful as an option before any surgery and urodynamic examinations, given that 80% of patients could be cured by physiotherapy (Bø et al., 2015). But such a mApp should be built respecting the modern and validated scheme of physiotherapeutic treatment, already proved to be efficient and effective (Bø et al., 2015), and/or based on relevant international guidelines for treating UI (Bernards et al., 2014; Loohuis et al., 2021).

An mApp that delivers advice, training and motivation for managing UI in isolation or supporting supervised treatment as a new and modern tool would be quite useful for maintaining motivation when performing a PFMT program.

In this chapter, based on systematic review and randomized controlled trial (RCT) evidence, the effect and clinical practical value of current mApps are evaluated and discussed. Does current available literature verify and/or justify the introduction of an optimal Web-based platform for PFMT (home) training and adherence to this training? It has been suggested that such a platform should include an especially designed website, use of social media and a specifically designed mApp to log data collection and communication between the healthcare provider and the patient, aiming to establish long-term results, reinforcing adherence and motivation (Latorre et al., 2018). Therefore, current scientific evidence, experience, considerations and recommendations from relevant research should be taken into account.

SCIENTIFIC EVIDENCE

So far, only a few RCTs have been published in the field of mApps for pelvic floor dysfunctions (Table 17.1 and Table 17.2).

Asklund et al. (2017), a Swedish study group of general practitioners (GPs), demonstrated mApp efficacy regarding symptoms, quality of life and urinary leakage in an RCT of 123 women with a mean age of 44.7 years

TABLE 17.1	Randomized Controlled Trials to Evaluate the Effect of Mobile Applications
Author	**Asklund et al. (2017)**
Design	2-arm RCT: mApp group: Tät (n = 62) Control group: postponed treatment (n = 61)
Sample size and age (years)	123 women; mean age 44.7 (SD: 9.4, range: 27–72)
Diagnosis	SUI (slight [2.4%, 3/123], moderate [63.4%, 78/123] or severe [34.1%, 42/123]), with ≥1 episode/week for the last 6 months based on website questionnaire
Training protocol	mApp (designed for iOS or Android devices) with treatment program for SUI, focused on PFMT: treatment program based on experiences reported by researchers, clinicians and users with a previous Internet program (Sjöström et al., 2013); PFMT program, with 6 basic and 6 advanced levels, 3×/day during treatment; at end treatment, instructions to continue PFMT 2 or 3×/week for maintenance training Control group: no intervention
Drop-out	2/123
Adherence	Of all women assigned to mApp who completed follow-up (n = 61), 83.6% (51/61) used app reminder setting and 86.9% (53/61) used statistics function and registered a mean of 141 exercises/person during study; at follow-up, during last 4 weeks, 41% (25/61) performed PFMT daily, 42.6% (26/61) performed PFMT weekly but not daily and 14.8% (9/61) performed PFMT more sporadically Control group: 26.7% (16/60) did not perform any PFMT; 56.7% (34/60) performed PFMT sporadically
Results	Primary outcome: mApp group: symptom severity Mean ICIQ-UI SF score reduction: 3.9, 95% CI: 3–4.7 Condition-specific quality of life, mean ICIQ-LUTSqol score reduction: 4.8, 95% CI: 3.4–6.2 Control group: symptom severity (mean ICIQ-UI SF score reduction: 0.9, 95% CI: 0.1–1.6), but not in condition-specific quality of life (mean ICIQ-LUTSqol score reduction: 0.7, 95% CI: −0.5 to 1.8) Groups significantly different for both outcome measures at follow-up Secondary outcomes: Patient Global Impression of Improvement (PGII), weekly leakage episodes, use of incontinence aids: mApp significant better than control 66.7% (40/60) satisfied with treatment outcome, and 21.7% (13/60) planned to seek additional treatment for UI
Author	**Sjöström et al. (2017)**
Design	2-arm RCT on cost-effectiveness: mApp group: Tät (n = 62) Control group: postponed treatment (n = 61)
Sample size and age (years)	123 women; mean age 44.7 (SD: 9.4, range: 27–72)
Diagnosis	SUI (slight [2.4%, 3/123], moderate [63.4%, 78/123] or severe [34.1%, 42/123]), with ≥1 episode/week for the last 6 months based on website questionnaire
Training protocol	mApp (designed for iOS or Android devices) with treatment program for SUI, focused on PFMT: treatment program based on experiences reported by researchers, clinicians and users with a previous internet program (Sjöström et al., 2013); PFMT program, with 6 basic and 6 advanced levels, 3×/day during treatment; at end treatment, instructions to continue PFMT 2 or 3×/week for maintenance training. Control group: no intervention

Continued

TABLE 17.1   Randomized Controlled Trials to Evaluate the Effect of Mobile Applications—cont'd

Drop-out	2/123
Adherence	Of all women assigned to mApp who completed follow-up (n = 61), 83.6% (51/61) used app reminder setting and 86.9% (53/61) used statistics function and registered a mean of 141 exercises/person during study; at follow-up, during last 4 weeks, 41% (25/61) performed PFMT daily, 42.6% (26/61) performed PFMT weekly but not daily and 14.8% (9/61) performed PFMT more sporadically Control group: 26.7% (16/60) did not perform any PFMT; 56.7% (34/60) performed PFMT sporadically
Results	Cost-effectiveness: costs from a 1-year societal perspective; costs included mailing of 2-day leakage diary, estimated time spent by study administrator emailing each participant link to Web-based questionnaire, incontinence aids and any extra laundry due to leakage, cost of individual's time (time spent on PFMT during last 4 weeks); all costs represented total societal cost; all costs in euro, based on 2013 year-end prices Main outcome incremental cost-effectiveness ratio, defined as difference in cost-effectiveness between mApp group and control group Total cost/participant: mApp €547, control €482.4
Author	**Hoffman et al. (2017)**
Design	2 years of follow-up for 2-arm RCT: mApp group: Tät (n = 62) Control group: postponed treatment (n = 61)
Sample size and age (years)	123 women; mean age 44.7 (SD: 9.4, range: 27–72)
Diagnosis	SUI (slight [2.4%, 3/123], moderate [63.4%, 78/123] or severe [34.1%, 42/123]), with ≥1 episode/week for the last 6 months based on website questionnaire
Study protocol	121/123 participants of 3-month follow-up for RCT (Asklund et al., 2017) received email with link to web survey; emails sent approximately 18–32 months after inclusion in RCT of Asklund et al. (2017) (average 24 months); 2-year follow-up by web-based questionnaires as outcome
Drop-out	15/61 (24.6%)
Adherence	46/61 women responded at 2 years; all 46 women reported downloading mApp and using it; eight women (17.4%) were still using it at the two-year follow-up
Results	Eight women (17.4%) were still using it at the two-year follow-up 12 (26%) did not perform PFMT, 21 (46%) performed it sporadically and 13 (28%) performed it regularly in the previous 4 weeks Symptom severity score (ICIQ-UI SF) decreased significantly from baseline to 2-year follow-up, mean decrease 3.1 (95% CI: 2–4.2); for condition-specific quality of life (ICIQ-LUTSqol), mean decrease 4 (95% CI: 2.1–5.9); 21.7% (10/46) sought other treatment for their SUI since beginning study, and 4.3% (2/46) had surgery
Author	**Araujo et al. (2020)**
Design	2-arm RCT: mApp group: EMG BF guide for home PFMT (n = 17) Control group: written instructions without EMG BF (n = 16)
Sample size and age (years)	33 women; mean age: mApp 47.2 (SD: ±10.6), control 53.3 (SD: ±13.2)
Diagnosis	Self-reported SUI symptoms based on demonstration of urinary leakage on straining or coughing; mixed UI was predominant type of SUI, based on self-reported symptoms using Questionnaire for Urinary Incontinence Diagnosis (QUID)

TABLE 17.1 Randomized Controlled Trials to Evaluate the Effect of Mobile Applications—cont'd

Training protocol	Exercises 2×/day; re-evaluation repeated at 1, 2 and 3 months after initial evaluation; changes in urinary and vaginal symptoms evaluated using questionnaires, and Oxford modified scale was determined through digital palpation
	Surface EMG used to improve women's comprehension about their contraction by visualizing muscle activity signals through device's screen; correct pelvic floor muscle contraction assured by PT, who explained performance appropriately
	Exercise protocol same in mApp and control groups
	Each completed protocol comprising 8-s hold/8-s relaxation followed by 3 phasic contractions, repeated 8 times, with total 32 contractions and 152 s; PT recommended patient to do completed protocol 2×/day (sitting, lying down or standing) for 3 months
Drop-out	12/33 (36.3%)
Adherence	After 3 months of adherence to home PFMT: mApp 43.8 ± 8.7, control 17.7 ± 6.3 (between groups p <0.001)
Results	Adherence (number of repetitions) higher in mApp group at 2 and 3 months after PFMT (p < 0.001), but adherence decreased, especially in control group, at 1, 2 and 3 months
	Vaginal symptoms (p < 0.001), quality of life (p = 0.003), urinary symptoms (p < 0.001) and SUI symptoms (p < 0.001) improvement comparing baseline and during treatment, no difference between mApp and control groups (p-values 0.887, 0.817, 0.573, and 0.825, respectively)
	No significant differences between groups in either symptom severity or quality of life
Author	**Loohuis et al. (2021)**
Design	Pragmatic, non-inferiority trial in Dutch primary care 2-arm RCT: mApp group: UrinControl (n = 131) Control group: care-as-usual (n = 131)
Sample size and age (years)	262 women; mean age: mApp 53.2 (SD: ±12.8), control 51.3 (SD: ±10.3)
Diagnosis	SUI, ≥2 UI episodes/week
Training protocol	UrinControl step-by-step program for self-management of UI based on relevant Dutch general practitioners and international guidance for treating UI; details available in the work of Loohuis et al. (2018)
Drop-out	61/262 (23.2%)
Adherence	Not measured
Results	195 patients attended follow-up
	Change in symptom severity with mApp group (–2.16; 95% CI: –2.67 to –1.65) non-inferior compared to control group (–2.56; 95% CI: –3.28 to –1.84), with mean difference 0.058 points (95% CI: –0.776 to 0.891) between groups
	Neither treatment superior to other; both groups showed improvements in outcome measures after treatment

BF, Biofeedback; *EMG,* electromyography; *ICIQ-LUTSqol,* International Consultation on Incontinence Questionnaire -Lower Urinary Tract Symptoms Quality of Life; *ICIQ-UI SF,* International Consultation on Incontinence Questionnaire -Urinary Incontinence Short Form; *mApp,* mobile application; *PFMT,* pelvic floor muscle training; *PT,* physical therapist; *RCT,* randomized controlled trial; *SUI,* stress urinary incontinence; *UI,* urinary incontinence.

(range: 27–72). They included community-dwelling adult women with one or more stress urinary incontinence (SUI) episodes per week, who were recruited through their website and randomized to an app treatment (mApp Tät, n = 62) or a control group (postponed treatment, n = 61). The mApp contains a treatment program focused on PFMT, as well as information about SUI and lifestyle factors. Primary outcomes were 3 months after randomization: symptom severity (International Consultation on Incontinence Questionnaire–Urinary Incontinence Short Form [ICIQ-UI SF]) and condition-specific quality of life (International Consultation on Incontinence–Lower Urinary

TABLE 17.2   PEDro Quality Score of Randomized Controlled Trials in Systematic Review of Mobile Applications for Urinary Incontinence

E – Eligibility criteria specified
1 – Subjects randomly allocated to groups
2 – Allocation concealed
3 – Groups similar at baseline
4 – Subjects blinded
5 – Therapist administering treatment blinded
6 – Assessors blinded
7 – Measures of key outcomes obtained from >85% of subjects
8 – Data analysed by intention to treat
9 – Statistical comparison between groups conducted
10 – Point measures and measures of variability provided

Study	E	1	2	3	4	5	6	7	8	9	10	Total Score
Asklund et al. (2017)	+	+	+	+	−	−	+	+	+	+	+	8
Sjöström et al. (2017)	+	+	+	+	−	−	+	+	+	+	+	8
Hoffman et al. (2017)	+	+	+	+	−	−	+	+	+	+	+	8
Araujo et al. (2020)	+	+	+	−	−	−	+	−	−	+	+	5
Loohuis et al. (2021)	+	+	+	+	−	−	+	−	+	+	+	7

+, Criterion is clearly satisfied; −, criterion is not satisfied; ?, not clear if the criterion was satisfied.
The total score is determined by counting the number of criteria that are satisfied, except the 'eligibility criteria specified' score is not used to generate the total score. Total scores are out of 10.

Tract Symptoms Quality of Life [ICIQ-LUTSqol]). A total of 120 of the 123 included patients had moderate/severe SUI (97.5%). Their mean baseline score of the ICIQ-UI SF was 11.1 (SD: 2.8), and that of the ICIQ-LUTSqol was 34.4 (SD: 6.1). At follow-up, the app group reported improvements in symptom severity (mean ICIQ-UI SF score reduction: 3.9, 95% CI: 3–4.7) and condition-specific quality of life (mean ICIQ-LUTSqol score reduction: 4.8, 95% CI: 3.4–6.2), and the groups were significantly different (mean ICIQ-UI SF score difference: −3.2, 95% CI: −4.3 to −2.1; mean ICIQ-LUTSqol score difference: −4.6, 95% CI: −7.8 to −1.4). In the app group, 98.4% (60 of 61) performed PFMT at follow-up, and 41% (25 of 61) performed it daily. Asklund et al. (2017) concluded that the mApp was effective for women with SUI and yielded clinically relevant improvements, and that this mApp may increase access to first-line treatment and adherence to PFMT.

Sjöström et al. (2017) analysed the cost-effectiveness of the mApp Tät. They stated that this mApp for treating SUI is a cost-effective, first-line treatment with potential for increasing access to care in a sustainable way for this patient group.

Hoffman et al. (2017) published long-term effects of the previous RCT reporting that 3 months of self-managing SUI with support from the mApp Tät was effective. The authors followed up with the women in the app group (n = 62) 2 years after the initial RCT using again the same primary outcomes for symptom severity (ICIQ-UI SF) and condition-specific quality of life (ICIQ-LUTSqol) and compared the scores with those at baseline. Of the women, 61 and 46 (75.4%), respectively, participated in 3-month and 2-year follow-ups. Baseline data did not differ between responders and non-responders at follow-up. The mean decreases in ICIQ-UI SF and ICIQ-LUTSqol scores after 2 years were 3.1 (95% CI: 2–4.2) and 4 (95% CI: 2.1–5.9), respectively. Of the 46 participants, 4 women (8.7%) rated themselves as very much better, 9 (19.6%) as much better, and 16 (34.8%) as a little better. The use of incontinence protection products decreased significantly (p = 0.04), and the proportion of women who felt that they could contract their pelvic muscles correctly increased from 14 of 46 (30.4%) at baseline to 31 of 46 (67.4%) at follow-up (p < 0.001). Hoffman et al. (2017) concluded that self-management of SUI support from the mApp Tät had significant and clinically relevant long-term effects and may serve as first-line treatment.

Araujo et al. (2020) evaluated in a small, prospective randomized study of 21 women the use of an mApp using the same visual component of electromyography as a guide for PFMT and following exercises shown on the screen for the treatment of SUI (mApp: n = 12) compared to controls (n = 9), who received written instructions with the same protocol as mApp but without the dynamic sequence of PFMT images, through adherence to home PFMT and its impact on urinary symptoms. Changes in urinary and vaginal symptoms were evaluated using questionnaires, and the Oxford modified scale was determined through digital palpation. Adherence (number of repetitions) was higher in the mApp group at 2 and 3 months after PFMT (p < 0.001), but adherence decreased, especially in the control group at 1, 2 and 3 months. Vaginal symptoms (p < 0.001), quality of life (p = 0.003), urinary symptoms (p < 0.001) and SUI symptoms (p < 0.001) showed improvement comparing the baseline and during treatment, but there was no difference between mApp and control groups (p-values of 0.887, 0.817, 0.573 and 0.825, respectively). The authors concluded that using the app increased adherence to PFMT in women with UI symptoms and improved subjective perception.

In a pragmatic, randomized, controlled, non-inferiority trial in Dutch primary care, Loohuis et al. (2021) included 262 eligible adult women with two or more episodes of UI per week comparing a stand-alone app-based treatment with both PFMT and bladder training (mApp UrinControl) with care-as-usual provided by GPs according to the Dutch GP guideline for UI treatment. The primary outcome was the difference between groups in the change of UI severity from baseline to 4 months, assessed by the ICIQ-UI SF. As secondary outcomes, differences in effect between groups in the change in the ICIQ-LUTSqol and the change in the of number of UI episodes per day from baseline to 4 months were assessed with a frequency–volume chart and the Patient Global Impression of Improvement (PGII) of incontinence at 4 months were measured. Non-inferiority (<1.5 points) was analysed by linear regression. A total of 195 patients attended follow-up. The change in symptom severity with the mApp (–2.16, 95% CI: –2.67 to –1.65) was non-inferior compared to care-as-usual (–2.56, 95% CI: –3.28 to –1.84), with a mean difference of 0.058 points (95% CI: –0.776 to 0.891) between groups. Neither treatment was superior to the other, and both groups showed improvements in outcome measures after treatment. The authors concluded that the mApp was at least as effective as

care-as-usual in primary care. As such, app-based treatments may provide women with a good alternative for consultation (Loohuis et al., 2021).

Although there was positive effectiveness (also with regard to cost), the authors publishing on the mApp Tät reported some consideration ns.

The study of Hoffman et al. (2017) yielded promising long-term effects. The mApp is non-invasive and can be used without seeking medical care, and it may serve as first-line treatment for women who feel confident in managing the consequences of their health problem with SUI independently. The original study of Asklund et al. (2017) came from the field of GPs. Hoffman et al. (2017) reported that the long-term effects were at the same level as in studies of supervised PFMT (by a physical therapist). In cases where self-management is not successful, the next step may be to seek care from a health provider. The app may also be used as a complement to other healthcare treatments for those who want it.

The conclusion of Hoffman et al. (2019) that the long-term effects were at the same level as supervised PFMT should be viewed cautiously. A limitation of this study is the absence of a control group given that the original control group of the Asklund et al. (2017) study could access the mApp after their first follow-up at 3 months. Another limitation may be that the participants in the mApp Tät study may not be representative of the general population. Approximately 80% had studied at university level; in the general Swedish population, approximately 25% of women aged 25 years and older had some university education. New technology generally attracts highly educated individuals.

As part of the evaluation of an mApp-based treatment, the user's experiences of using such an mApp and engaging in the PFMT program is important to determine how and why app-based treatment could be effective. Asklund et al. (2019) explored women's experiences of using the Tät program for SUI and reported that most participants found PFMT difficult and challenging, but at the same time they felt confident that they could master it well on their own. Some did not feel completely sure that they were doing the PFM contractions correctly, even though they could feel that their PFM strength improved and their incontinence symptoms reduced.

Considerations related to the mApp UrinControl were that among women with stress, urgency and mixed UI, this stand-alone intervention was at least as effective after 4 months as guideline-based care provided by GPs. In this study, PFMT for SUI with bladder training for urgency and mixed UI was combined, whereas others have focused on SUI alone, excluding in that way most women with symptomatic UI (Loohuis et al., 2021). The symptom scores in the Loohuis et al. (2021) reductions were slightly smaller compared to other studies. One of the reasons for this may be that the participants in this study relied on self-motivation or on the reminder function within the mApp, whereas in other studies participants received reminder emails from the researcher or physical therapist. Loohuis et al. (2021) focused on the change of effect on UI severity and did not measure adherence, which might have offered new ways to track adherence to treatment by self-registration within the mApp logging data automatically.

In a qualitative study, Wessels et al. (2020) showed that women tended to appreciate the mApp UrinControl for treating UI. They stated that the use of this app may lower barriers to seeking treatment, increase self-awareness and support treatment adherence. However, some women in the study wanted more information about new therapies, more variety in the distraction games, contact with care providers, improved feedback and simplification of some areas (e.g., text with less detail and complexity and more understandable graphs). Notably, several women experienced a negative impact as awareness of their symptoms increased. The authors concluded that these points of improvement need to be taken into account with further development of an mApp. Furthermore, they stated that experiences and recommendations outlined in this quality study can be used to optimize the implementation of apps in the future.

Difficulties in understanding how to do the exercises and knowledge of whether they are done correctly are known barriers to adherence to PFMT. Enablers related to these difficulties are feedback, affirmation of progress and professional involvement (supervision by a specialized physical therapist) (French et al., 2017). However, most women can correctly perform PFM contractions after a simple verbal cue (Henderson et al., 2013). Certainly, the conclusions of Asklund et al. (2019) that women using Tät enabled them to self-manage an up-to-date treatment for their condition may be valid for their study population, but more high-quality, well-designed studies are needed to assess the effects of new apps in a more critical light (Byambasuren et al., 2018). In doing so, Loohuis et al. (2021) stated that one may find that the purported positive effects of many apps are smaller in clinical settings.

Future research should clarify the long-term outcomes, as well as the barriers and facilitators to the use and implementation of app-based treatment, and develop an optimal mApp taking into account different patient populations and their needs (Alves et al., 2015; Latorre et al., 2018).

So far, mApps for PFMT work better for those who are interested in them and have high expectations about them (Nyström et al., 2018). In addition, it is justified to consider mApps related to PFMT as a first-line cost-effective treatment with the potential to increase access to care (Asklund et al., 2017; Sjöström et al., 2017).

This in the light of the nuanced and complex ways in which potential users engage with and contribute to online sources of information and use these sources together with face-to-face encounters with doctors and other healthcare professionals, such as physical therapists (Lupton and Maslen, 2019). After all, when digital health technologies like the mApp fail to work as expected, these agential (including the capacity to seek and generate information and create a better sense of understanding and performing [home] PFMT) capacities are not realized. Lupton and Maslen (2019) found that women responded with feelings of frustration, disappointment and annoyance, leading them to become disenchanted with the possibilities of the digital technologies they had tried.

CONSTRUCTION OF A MOBILE APPLICATION FOR PELVIC FLOOR MUSCLE TRAINING USED BY PHYSIOTHERAPISTS

In a systematic review, Latorre et al. (2018) identified and analysed current mApps available to the public. Inclusion criteria were apps which contain exercises for UI or the pelvic floor. Their methodology has been described elsewhere (Latorre et al., 2018). Thirteen variables relative to the construct and content were identified and organized in tables. In doing so, straight comparison between the mApps and the identification of lacks was realized (Latorre et al., 2018). It appeared that, so far, none of the mApps had all 13 variables (Latorre et al., 2018). To create an adequate and optimal mApp, the authors described several sequential phases of methodological development from face validity up to implementation (Latorre et al., 2018).

Today, 12 theories or models related to behavioural changes, PFMT training and adherence can be identified (Dumoulin et al., 2015a; Hay-Smith et al., 2016; Latorre et al., 2018). The new mApp should be constructed taking into consideration all of these theories and models.

Another condition sine qua non is that the new mApp should be built on the base of the Bø et al. (2015) PFMT protocol, considering that PFMT currently has level 1 evidence and grade A recommendation (Berghmans, 2017; Berghmans and Seleme, 2020). In their review, Latorre et al. (2018) suggested 12 variables as necessary conditions helping to create the ideal mApp for PFMT.

VALIDITY OF THE NEW DEVELOPED MOBILE APPLICATION

To investigate its usefulness and validity, clinical studies regarding face validity, content validity and construct validity of the mApp need to be executed. Latorre et al. (2018) showed that none of all mApps available to download incorporate all of the parameters the literature has pointed out as fundamental for an ideal mApp for PFMT adherence. The challenge for the development of an ideal mApp is to combine all of those parameters into a single mApp.

Effects of the optimally designed mApp should then be investigated in high-quality, well-designed RCTs.

CONCLUSION

Currently, lack of adherence is a major drawback to PFMT success. Current literature shows guidance to improve PFMT and adherence, and the increasing use of social media opens the way for mApps helping to improve (home) PFMT and adherence. There are dozens of PFMT mApps available, but almost none have all of the evidence-based parameters for correct PFMT.

RCT evidence suggests that mApps are effective for women with UI, who yielded clinically relevant improvements in the short term, and that mApps may increase access to first-line treatment and adherence to PFMT. Although some positive results in the long-term have been published, up to now the effect over the long term remains inconclusive.

So far, mApps for PFMT work better in those who are interested in and have high expectations about it, and they are a first-line cost-effective treatment with the potential to increase access to care.

Current evidence of adherence to PFMT together with a PFMT evidence-based level 1, grade A protocol may facilitate construction of an optimal mApp.

RECOMMENDATIONS FOR CLINICAL PRACTICE

The use of evidence-based mApps for PFMT to improve training in and adherence to pelvic physiotherapy and to improve access to UI care is recommended.

RECOMMENDATIONS FOR RESEARCH

Observational studies on validity and RCTs on efficacy (over the long term) and effectiveness (including that associated with cost) of mApps for PFMT are needed.

REFERENCES

Alves, F. K., Riccetto, C., Adami, D. B., et al. (2015). A pelvic floor muscle training program in postmenopausal women: A randomized controlled trial. *Maturitas, 81*, 300–305.

Apple Store. (2016). *Engine for mobile applications download [online]*. https://www.apple.com/us/search/pelvic-floor?src=globalnav. (Accessed 16.11.16).

Araujo, C. C., Marques, A. A., & Juliato, C. R. (2020). The adherence of home pelvic floor muscles training using a mobile device application for women with urinary incontinence: A randomized controlled trial. *Female Pelvic Medicine & Reconstructive Surgery, 26*(11), 697–703.

Asklund, I., Nyström, E., Sjöström, M., et al. (2017). Mobile app for treatment of stress urinary incontinence: A randomized controlled trial. *Neurourology and Urodynamics, 36*(5), 1369–1376.

Asklund, I., Samuelsson, E., Hamberg, K., et al. (2019). User experience of an app-based treatment for stress urinary incontinence: Qualitative interview study. *Journal of Medical Internet Research, 21*(3), e11296.

Berghmans, B. (2017). Pelvic floor muscle training: What is important? A mini-review. *Obstetrics & Gynecology International Journal, 6*(4), 00214.

Berghmans, B., & Seleme, M. (2020). The '5 F's concept for pelvic floor muscle training: From finding the pelvic floor to functional use. *Journal Womens Health Developmental, 3*(2), 142–145.

Bernards, A. T. M., Berghmans, B. C. M., Slieker-Ten Hove, M. C. P., et al. (2014). Dutch guidelines for physiotherapy in patients with stress urinary incontinence: An update. *International Urology Journal, 25*, 171–179.

Bø, K., Berghmans, B., Mørkved, S., et al. (Eds.). (2015). Overview of physical therapy for pelvic floor dysfunction. In: *Evidence-based physical therapy for the pelvic floor: Bridging science and clinical Practice* (2nd ed.) London: Churchill Livingstone, 1–8.

Bø, K., & Hilde, G. (2013). Does it work in the long term? A systematic review on pelvic floor muscle training for female stress urinary incontinence. *Neurourology and Urodynamics, 32*, 215–223.

Byambasuren, O., Sanders, S., Beller, E., et al. (2018). Prescribable mHealth apps identified from an overview of systematic reviews. *Nature Partner Journals Digital Medicine, 1*, 12.

Chaffey, D. (2021). *Mobile marketing statistics compilation 2021*. Available: https://www.smartinsights.com/mobile-marketing/mobile-marketing-analytics/mobile-marketing-statistics/. (Accessed 04.08.22).

Dumoulin, C., Adewuyi, T., & Booth, J. (2016). Adult conservative management. In P. Abrams, L. Cardozo, A. Wagg, et al. (Eds.), *Incontinence: Sixth international consultation on urinary incontinence*. Plymouth, UK: Health Publication/Plymbridge Distributors. 1443–1628.

Dumoulin, C., Alewijnse, D., Bo, K., et al. (2015a). Pelvic floor muscle training adherence: Tools, measurements and strategies—2011 ICS state-of-the-science seminar research paper II of IV. *Neurourology and Urodynamics, 34*, 615–621.

Dumoulin, C., Hay-Smith, J., Frawley, H., et al. (2015b). Consensus statement on improving pelvic floor muscle training adherence: International Continence Society 2011 state-of-the-science seminar. *Neurourology and Urodynamics, 34*, 600–605.

Dumoulin, C., Hay-Smith, J., Habée-Séguin, G. M., et al. (2015c). Pelvic floor muscle training versus no treatment, or inactive control treatments, for urinary incontinence in women: A short version cochrane systematic review with meta-analysis. *Neurourology and Urodynamics, 34*, 300–308.

Dumoulin, C., Hay-Smith, E. C., & Mac Habée-Séguin, G. (2014). Pelvic floor muscle training versus no treatment, or inactive control treatments, for urinary incontinence in women. *Cochrane Database of Systematic Reviews* Issue 14, Art. No. CD005654.

Frawley, H. C., McClurg, D., Mahfooza, A., et al. (2015). Health professionals' and patients' perspectives on pelvic floor muscle training adherence—2011 ICS state-of-the-science seminar research paper IV of IV. *Neurourology and Urodynamics, 34*, 632–639.

French, B., Thomas, L., Harrison, J., et al. (2017). Client and clinical staff perceptions of barriers to and enablers of the uptake and delivery of behavioural interventions for urinary incontinence: Qualitative evidence synthesis. *Journal of Advanced Nursing, 73*(1), 21–38.

Google Play Store. (2016). *Engine for mobile applications download*. Available: https://play.google.com/store/search?q=pelvic%20floor&c=apps&hl=nl (Accessed 16.11.16).

Hay-Smith, E. J., McClurg, D., Frawley, H., et al. (2016). Exercise adherence: Integrating theory, evidence and behaviour change techniques. *Physiotherapy, 102*, 7–9.

Haynes, R. B., Ackloo, E., Sahota, N., et al. (2015). Scoping review of adherence promotion theories in pelvic floor muscle training—2011 ICS state-of-the-science seminar research paper I of IV. *Neurourology and Urodynamics, 34*, 606–614.

Henderson, J. W., Wang, S., Egger, M. J., et al. (2013). Can women correctly contract their pelvic floor muscles without formal instruction? *Female Pelvic Medicine & Reconstructive Surgery, 19*(1), 8–12.

Hoffman, V., Söderström, L., & Samuelsson, E. (2017). Self-management of stress urinary incontinence via a mobile app: Two-year follow-up of a randomized controlled trial. *Acta Obstetricia et Gynecologica Scandinavica, 96*(10), 1180–1187.

Kaya, S., Akbayrak, T., Gursen, C., et al. (2015). Short-term effect of adding pelvic floor muscle exercise to bladder training for female incontinence: A randomized controlled trial. *International Urology Journal, 26*, 285–293.

Latorre, G. F., de Fraga, R., Seleme, M. R., et al. (2018). An ideal e-health system for pelvic floor muscle training adherence: Systematic review. *Neurourology and Urodynamics, 38*(1), 63–80.

Loohuis, A. M., Wessels, N. J., Dekker, J. H., et al. (2021). App-based treatment in primary care for urinary incontinence: A pragmatic, randomized controlled trial. *The Annals of Family Medicine, 19*(2), 102–109.

Loohuis, A. M., Wessels, N. J., Jellema, P., et al. (2018). The impact of a mobile application-based treatment for urinary incontinence in adult women: Design of a mixed-methods randomized controlled trial in a primary care setting. *Neurourology and Urodynamics, 37*, 2167–2176.

Lupton, D., & Maslen, S. (2019). How women use digital technologies for health: Qualitative interview and focus group study. *Journal of Medical Internet Research, 21*(1), e11481.

McCardle, W., Katch, F. I., & Katch, V. L. (2014). *Exercise physiology: Energy, nutrition, and human performance*. New York: Wolters Kluwer.

McClurg, D., Frawley, H., Hay-Smith, J., et al. (2015). Scoping review of adherence promotion theories in pelvic floor muscle training—2011 ICS state-of-the-science seminar research paper I of IV. *Neurourology and Urodynamics, 34*, 606–614.

Nyström, E., Asklund, I., Sjöström, M., et al. (2018). Treatment of stress urinary incontinence with a mobile app: Factors associated with success. *International Urology Journal, 29*(9), 1325–1333.

Pereira, V. S., de Melo, M. V., Correia, G. N., et al. (2013). Long-term effects of pelvic floor muscle training with vaginal cone in postmenopausal women with urinary incontinence: A randomized controlled trial. *Neurourology and Urodynamics, 32,* 48–52.

Sjöström, M., Lindholm, L., & Samuelsson, E. (2017). Mobile app for treatment of stress urinary incontinence: A cost-effectiveness analysis. *Journal of Medical Internet Research, 19*(5), e154.

Sjöström, M., Umefjord, G., Carlbring, P., et al. (2013). Internet-based treatment of stress urinary incontinence. A randomised controlled study with focus on pelvic floor muscle training. *BJU International, 112,* 362–372.

Sluijs, E. M., & Knibbe, J. J. (1991). Patient compliance with exercise: Different theoretical approaches to short-term and long-term compliance. *Patient Education and Counseling, 11,* 191–204.

Wessels, N. J., Hulshof, L., & Loohuis, A. M. (2020). User experiences and preferences regarding an app for the treatment of urinary incontinence in adult women: Qualitative study. *JMIR Mhealth Uhealth, 8*(6), e17114.

Selection and Goal-Oriented Application of Measurement Instruments in Pelvic Physical Therapy

Esther Bols, Anna Beurskens and Bary Berghmans

OUTLINE

RELEVANCE OF USING MEASUREMENT INSTRUMENTS FOR THE (PELVIC) PHYSICAL THERAPIST AND PATIENT

The use of measurement instruments in healthcare is increasing, as healthcare professionals are challenged to offer affordable care that is evidence based and at the same time meets the needs of patients (Black, 2013). Measurement instruments support (pelvic) physical therapists with clinical reasoning by providing them with an overview of clinical phenomena or helping them to objectify and quantify them. Frequently used measurement instruments are patient-reported outcome measures (PROMs), which are questionnaires that capture aspects of a patient's health status directly reported by the patient (Van der Wees et al., 2019). Other types of measurement instruments are performance or function tests, as well as observation lists (Walton et al., 2015). Measurements can illustrate and evaluate one's own actions and at the same time standardize communication with colleagues, doctors or insurance representatives. Measurement results can be used to better inform patients about their situation and to involve them more easily in therapy decisions (shared decision making) (Stevens, 2017). Shared decision making is increasingly being recognized as part of client-centered care, as well as value-based healthcare, which essentially means that (policy) choices and reimbursements for healthcare are guided by outcomes in terms of patient-reported experiences regarding the quality of care (Hoffmann et al., 2020; Porter and Teisberg, 2006). Furthermore, measurements on a group level are carried out to provide insight into the quality of care (performance feedback), for external accountability (e.g., health insurance companies) and scientific research. The use of measurement instruments fits well into evidence-based practice. Evidence-based products (EBPs) function as the cornerstone in (pelvic) physical therapy (Braun et al., 2018). Important facets of these EBPs are the use of measurement instruments. Although these instruments can support clinical practice, different studies show that the implementation of measurement instruments recommended in these EBPs is challenging (Braun et al., 2018; Foster et al., 2018). Reasons for these implementation problems are, among others, the extensive number instruments, their diversity, and the way in which the results can be interpreted and presented.

Moreover, the use of measurement instruments should not be viewed in isolation. Physical therapists should always try to integrate them into their process of methodical reasoning and use it as part of their intervention. But how do you choose the right instrument in view of the impressive number of measurement instruments and how do you embed measurement results in practice? The answer to this question can be found in the use of a 10-step plan [(Beurskens et al., 2020)]. With its help, physical therapists can integrate the use of measurement instruments into their daily practice (Fig. 18.1). The first two, and most important, steps are to systematically and critically determine why you want to measure (step 1) and what you want to measure (step 2) so that you will truly use the results and can justify why measuring is useful. Measurement results only become meaningful for patients and healthcare professionals if words translate the number into what the patient and his environment perceive as really important. After you have completed all steps of the step-by-step plan, you will have a complete picture of the most suitable measurement instrument for your patient and how you can interpret and use the results.

STEP-BY-STEP PLAN: TOOL FOR SELECTION OF AN ADEQUATE MEASUREMENT INSTRUMENT

The step-by-step plan will help select measurement instruments and as such represents a tool to support clinical reasoning in individual patients (Beurskens et al., 2020). The steps are inter-related, and sometimes it is necessary to reconsider former steps (see Fig. 18.1).

Step 1: Why do you want to measure? The first step is about *why* you want to measure. From the perspective of patients, healthcare professionals, colleagues, referrers and other stakeholders, various reasons exist for why it makes sense to use measurement instruments to determine (clinical) symptoms, experiences or outcomes in clinical practice. Measurement results can support in making a (physiotherapeutic) *diagnosis*, to determine

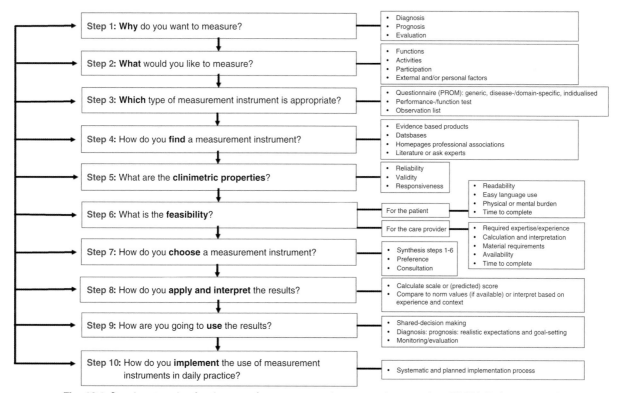

Fig. 18.1 Step-by-step plan for the use of measurement instrument into practice. *PROM,* Patient-reported outcome measure *(Beurskens et al., 2020).*

the *prognosis* or to *monitor or evaluate* interventions/ treatments.

Step 2: What would you like to measure? The second step is about *what* you want to measure, also called a *construct* or *domain*. This concerns which aspects of health or functioning you want to measure, such as (pelvic) pain, severity of urinary incontinence or quality of life. Several reasons determine what you want to measure, always based on the patient's request for help. Different formats and models of clinical reasoning can help with this, such as the frequently used International Classification of Functioning, Disability and Health (ICF; with the domain problems in functions and anatomical properties, limitations in activities, participation problems, and external and personal factors) (World Health Organization, 2001). Huber et al. (2011, 2016) introduced the concept of positive health, which consists of overlapping dimensions (bodily functions, mental functions and perception, spiritual/existential dimension, quality of life, social and societal participation, and daily functioning) compared to the ICF. Moreover, the purpose of the measurement (diagnostic, prognostic or evaluative), the target group and the context/setting also determine what you want to measure.

Step 3: Which type of measurement instrument is appropriate? The third step describes which *type* of measurement instrument is appropriate. There are several ways of classifying types of instruments:

- If types of instruments are categorized based on *method*, we can distinguish observation and performance tests and PROMs. In observation and performance tests, we observe a patient or ask a patient to perform a certain activity. PROMs (e.g., questionnaires or diaries) provide insight into how someone assesses their own health and well-being. PROMs differ in complexity (single item vs multi-item) and mode of administration (paper, digital, telephone or face to face).
- PROMS can be classified based on *types* of measurements, consisting of generic instruments (measuring health-related quality of life on a broad scale, useful for many disorders), such as the 36-item Short Form Health Survey Questionnaire (SF-36) (Ware and Sherbourne, 1992); disease/condition-specific instruments (specifically developed to measure the diagnosis or outcomes related to a certain disorder), such as the International Consultation on Incontinence Questionnaire–Urinary Incontinence Short Form

(ICIQ-UI SF) (Avery et al., 2004); domain-specific instruments (measuring only one domain of quality of life, e.g., depression, pain or participation), such as the Numeric Pain Rating Scale (NPRS) (Farrar et al., 2001); and individualized instruments (instruments that take into account individual or environmental differences in relation to quality of life. Every patient selects relevant activities or problems which are scored subsequently, such as the Patient-Specific Functioning Scale (PSFS) (Stratford, 1995), which has been further developed into a six-step method— the so-called Patient Specific Goal-setting method (Stevens et al., 2017). Patient-reported experience measures measure the patient-reported experiences of the healthcare process and quality (Whelan et al., 2011); they are mostly used on a group level.
- If types of instruments are categorized based on *goal*, we can distinguish diagnostic, prognostic and evaluative measures.
- In addition, many apps, devices and wearables are available to measure (Dunn et al., 2018; Latorre et al., 2019), although they can vary in comprehensiveness and quality (Wallace et al., 2019).

Every type of instrument has (dis)advantages, such as degree of specificity and generalizability. The selection of a particular type of instrument is mainly dependent on the goal of measurement.

Step 4: How do you find a measurement instrument? The next step is about *where* to look for measurement instruments. In mono- or multidisciplinary expert-based products and/or EBPs, such as guidelines, evidence statements (Berghmans et al., 2015), consensus publications (Bordeianou et al., 2020; Bosch et al., 2017), books (Moore and Karantanis, 2008), (quality) standards or protocols, measurement instruments are often recommended or published. The guidelines, standards or original versions of the measurement instruments can often be accessed via the home pages of pelvic physical therapy professional associations. Many measurement instruments are freely available or available for a fee. A widely used source of measurement instruments is the Rehabilitation Measures Database (https://www. sralab.org/rehabilitation-measures), the Dutch website https://meetinstrumentenzorg.nl and the PROQOLID database (https://eprovide.mapi-trust.org/about/about-proqolid). In addition, modules of the International Consultation on Incontinence Questionnaire (ICIQ), assessing pelvic problems, are available on request

(Bosch et al., 2017; International Consultation on Incontinence, 2020). Most ICIQ modules are available in different languages. Sometimes measurement instruments are incorporated in electronic patient records.

The application of apps and wearables in healthcare is developing rapidly. There are currently a huge number of healthcare apps and websites. In a recent review, 61 mobile applications have been identified for pelvic floor muscle training adherence alone (Latorre et al., 2019). It is difficult for healthcare professionals and healthcare users to determine which applications are reliable and user-friendly and which respect privacy. If you have not found any measurement instruments via EBPs or freely accessible databases, you can search the literature (e.g., PubMed, PEDro) or ask experts for advice. Systematic reviews of outcome measurement instruments (summarizing the evidence on measurement properties) are accessible through the COnsensus-based Standards for the selection of health Measurement INstruments (COSMIN) database (https://database.cosmin.nl).

Step 5: What are the clinimetric properties? Various aspects of the *clinimetric properties* are of great importance for the selection of an adequate measurement instrument. Some methodological knowledge is required for this (Bosch et al., 2017; De Vet et al., 2011). It must be clear what is meant by the concepts of *validity* (the degree to which an outcome measure measures the construct it purports to measure), *reliability* (the degree to which the measurement is free from measurement error) and *responsiveness* (the ability of an outcome measure to detect change over time in the construct to be measured) and how they must be assessed. Content validity is especially important for daily practice, which means that you need to look closely whether the domains and items in the measurement instrument match with the domain(s)/construct(s) you intend to measure. On the COSMIN website (https://www.cosmin.nl), you can find up-to-date information on checklists, criteria and guidelines in relation to the selection of measurement instruments.

When measuring in practice, the patient's request for help will give direction to why and what you want to measure. The measurement goal (diagnostic, prognostic or evaluative) determines which clinimetric properties are especially important. For a diagnostic and prognostic goal, a measurement instrument needs to be able to distinguish individuals (e.g., on health status), whereas for an evaluative goal, a measurement instrument needs to demonstrate change over time.

Step 6: What is the feasibility? The next step is the *feasibility* of the measurement instrument. This is of great importance for individual patient care, because patients and therapists should be able to use the instruments and they must fit into the flow of daily practice. One of the ways to classify feasibility is to make a distinction between objective and the more subjective aspects (Stevens et al., 2013). *Objective feasibility* is related to the measurement instrument itself and includes, among others, obtainability, material requirements, time to complete, availability, calculation and interpretation. *Subjective feasibility* is described from the perspective of both the patient (e.g., readability, easy language use, physical or mental burden, relevance, information and communications technology [ICT] skills) and the healthcare professional (required expertise, time to complete). Special attention should be paid to the group of people who have low literacy and/or communication deficits.

Step 7: How do you choose a measurement instrument? Based on the knowledge from the previous steps, one or more measurement instrument is *selected*. This is illustrated on the basis of the case study presented in this chapter. The most important aspects are that the content of a measurement instrument (what it measures) matches the purpose of the measurement, the aspects and domains that you want to measure and the target group. You ultimately make a selection based on the clinimetric quality, feasibility, consultation with colleagues and patient, or own preference. EBPs (Berghmans et al., 2015) or other literature sources (Bosch et al., 2017) often provide recommendations on measurement instruments for the assessment or evaluation of pelvic floor dysfunctions in which steps 1 through 6 are already considered and taken into account.

Step 8: How do you apply and interpret the results? After the selection, it is important that you know how to apply the measurement instrument in practice and how to interpret the results. Patients can complete questionnaires at home or before and after treatment. This can be done in practice, on paper, via the computer, or with the aid of all kinds of devices and wearables. Each method has (dis)advantages regarding efficiency, risk of non-response, missing values, logistics, costs, required ICT or interview skills, perception of non-verbal signals, privacy, in-depth information and validity of information (e.g., in those who have low literacy and/or communication deficits).

Measuring is only meaningful and useful when it adds value to the clinical reasoning process, communication or provision of insight. Requirements for adequate interpretation of measurement results are as follows:

- Scores should be calculated according to guidelines.
- The meaning of scores should be clear (e.g., a higher score on the ICIQ-UI SF means more severity and impact in patients with UI).
- Scores should be clinically relevant–that is, based on (often available) norm values, they should provide guidance for the treatment plan/clinical reasoning process. For example, the Pelvic Organ Prolapse Quantification (POP-Q) is a classification system that records pelvic organ prolapse and provides stages for compartments based on measurement of anatomical locations (Bump et al., 1996).

Interpretation of a *single score* (for the purpose of diagnosis or prognosis, when distinguishing individuals on health status is of relevance) can be done by using a single valid cut-off score or norm values (assessed on a group level with healthy/diseased persons). When cut-off or norm values are unavailable, professionals should trust in their own experience in relation to a target group and take the context into account.

Interpretation of *repeated measurements* (change scores in case of evaluation) requires information on the clinical relevance of the change score (smallest detectable change and minimally important change). Real change has occurred when the a change in score is larger than both the smallest detectable change and minimally important change (De Vet et al., 2011).

Step 9: How are you going to use the results? The next step is to *use* the results in the care and treatment process—how you can really use the data for the goals you formulated in steps 1 and 2. You can use results to clarify the request for help, to (better) make a diagnosis, to jointly decide on treatments, and to monitor and evaluate care.

- Diagnostic use of measurement results: Measuring becomes useful when measurement results are used to gain insight into personal goals and actions that inspire and motivate the patient (customized care). Measuring may clarify the request for help and may support the process of shared decision making—for example, social and emotional problems are better identified and discussed more often when the results of PROMs are brought in. Discussing important results also reduces insecurity and negative feelings about the disease (e.g., worrying thoughts or fear).

Positive expectations may improve motivation and treatment results. Moreover, measurement results can improve communication with the caregiver at home and between professionals.

- Prognostic use of measurement results: Based on PROMs, it is often possible to predict whether clinically relevant improvement is likely, for example, after a certain treatment option (Hendriks et al., 2010; Labrie et al., 2014). This information may also improve illness insight and assists in formulating realistic treatment goals.
- Evaluative use of measurement results: A repeated measurement provides quantitative feedback. The healthcare professional translates this feedback into qualitative feedback by inviting the patient to describe the experienced change ('What do these scores mean to you'?). The context and treatment process should always be kept in mind. To improve self-empowerment, it is important to clarify what the actual (feedback) and desired (feed-up) situation is. The patient and healthcare provider together discuss what is necessary to achieve the desired situation (feed forward).

Measurement results can be presented in different forms to the patient: numbers, words, pictures or graphs. The patient prefers simple graphs without statistical information and a clear legend (Snyder et al., 2019). Text is preferred over numbers (e.g., mild, severe, very severe). Moreover, results are easier to interpret when a higher score also means a better score. When scores deviate from normal, an exclamation mark or colours are useful to mark them. Professionals have similar preferences, although they value norm scores and statistical information.

Effective learning strategies to learn to communicate appropriately about measurement results with patients, which ask for new attitudes and skills, are critical self-reflection or peer review (Santana et al., 2015).

Step 10: How do you implement the use of measurement instruments in daily practice? In this last step, the emphasis is on how to implement the measurement process in daily practice (Damschroder et al., 2009; Foster et al., 2018). Successful implementation of measurement requires more than just the selection of measurement instruments. For example, attention is needed for the knowledge and skills of healthcare professionals and patients, the support of management, the embedding in ICT systems and the organization of the practice.

In the implementation process, choosing a measurement instrument is an important first step. To use it correctly in practice, the therapist needs customization and experience. It is therefore advisable to start with a manageable number of simple measurement instruments and to gain experience in handling them before moving on to more complex ones. The more familiar a therapist is with the use of a test, the more reliably the results can be interpreted later.

APPLICATION OF THE STEP-BY-STEP PLAN FOR A PATIENT WITH ANAL INCONTINENCE (CASE STUDY)

Reason for meeting Mrs. Smith: Resume social activities and return to work.

History taking: Mrs. Smith, 33 years old, experiences daily flatus incontinence without conscious control, occurring after her first delivery 6 weeks ago. She had a total sphincter rupture, which was not surgically repaired. Other comorbidities or urogynaecological complaints are absent; however, she has fear of returning to work (sedentary work, accountant's office) due to her symptoms. Her husband is very supportive in the household, care of the baby and discussing her symptoms.

Additional examination: Anal endo-ultrasound revealed an external and internal anal sphincter defect at 11-1 hours.

Mrs. Smith is referred to the pelvic physical therapist.

Based on this case study, Table 18.1 summarizes the decisions for all steps of the step-by-step plan. Fig. 18.2 specifically provides an overview of steps 1 through 3 according to the ICF model (World Health Organization, 2001).

Step 1. In the diagnostic process, the pelvic physical therapist would like to examine the nature, severity and

TABLE 18.1	Decisions for All Steps of the Step-by-Step Plan
Reason for Encounter	• Resume social activities • Return to work
Diagnostic Process	• History taking/examination: daily flatus incontinence postpartum • Use of measurement instruments: step-by-step plan as supportive tool
Step 1 Why do you want to measure?	• For diagnostic purposes: frequency/severity of AI, muscle and reservoir function, reflexes, consistency of stool, social support, awareness and acknowledgement of health problem, knowledge on health problem AI/coping • For evaluative purposes: frequency/severity of AI, muscle and reservoir function, reflexes, consistency of stool, limitations in activities, participation problems, quality of life
Step 2 What would you like to measure?	• Problems in functions and anatomical properties: frequency/severity of AI, muscle and reservoir function, reflexes, consistency of stool • Activities and participation: limitations in activities, participation problems • External factors: social support • Personal factors: awareness and acknowledgement of health problem, knowledge on health problem/coping, quality of life
Step 3 Which type of measurement instrument is appropriate?	• Questionnaires (PROMs): • Frequency/severity of AI: defaecation diary, Wexner score, GPE • Consistency of stool: BSFS • Limitations in activities, participation problems, impact on quality of life: ICIQ-B, FIQL • Performance/function test: • Muscle and reservoir function, reflexes (RAIR and SRSR): manometry (rectal balloon), anorectal palpation, EMG BF (probe)
Step 4 How do you find a measurement instrument?	• Wexner score: PROQOLID database, literature (Jorge and Wexner, 1993; Vaizey et al., 1999), https://www.meetinstrumentenzorg.nl • ICIQ-B: PROQOLID database, https://www.iciq.net • FIQL: PROQOLID database, literature (Rockwood et al., 2000), https://www.meetinstrumentenzorg.nl

Continued

TABLE 18.1	**Decisions for All Steps of the Step-by-Step Plan—cont'd**	
Step 5 What are the clinimetric properties?	Wexner/ICIQ-B/FIQL: validity, reliability and responsiveness: sufficient
Step 6 What is the feasibility?	Wexner/ICIQ-B/FIQL: minimal burden, no specific expertise/equipment Wexner: short time to complete, ICIQ-B/FIQL: lengthy
Step 7 How do you choose a measurement instrument?	Synthesis steps 1–6
Step 8 How do you apply and interpret the results?	Calculation sum scores and own experience
Step 9 How are you going to use the results?	Diagnostic use: shared decision making, realistic expectations Evaluative use: monitoring and evaluation of treatment, adaptation treatment plan
Step 10 How do you implement the use of measurement instruments in daily practice?	Discussion in (multidisciplinary) team meeting

AI, Anal incontinence; *BF*, biofeedback; *BSFS*, Bristol Stool Form Scale; *EMG*, electromyography; *FIQL*, Fecal Incontinence Quality of Life Scale; *GPE*, Global Perceived Effect; *ICIQ-B*, International Consultation on Incontinence Questionnaire -Anal Incontinence Symptoms and Quality of Life Module; *PROMs*, patient-reported outcome measures; *RAIR*, rectoanal inhibitory reflex; *SRSR*, striated rectosphincter reflex.

degree of modifiability of the patient's AI and evaluate the therapy progress. Therefore, the pelvic physical therapist would like to measure for diagnostic and evaluative purposes.

Steps 2 and 3. The selected constructs to be measured capture all domains of the ICF model, and reflect questionnaires/PROMs and performance/function tests. For the purposes of clarity and deepening in subject, steps 4 to 10 are only elaborated for the underlined measurement instruments in step 3 (see Table 18.1).

Step 4. The original versions of the Wexner (Cleveland Clinic) score (Jorge and Wexner, 1993), International Consultation on Incontinence Questionnaire–Anal Incontinence Symptoms and Quality of Life Module (ICIQ-B) (Cotterill et al., 2011), and Fecal Incontinence Quality of Life Scale (FIQL) (Rockwood et al., 2000) can be accessed through different sources, although they may have specific conditions of use, such as the ICIQ modules or PROQOL database.

Step 5. The Wexner score assesses the frequency and severity of AI, pad use and lifestyle restrictions, consists of only 5 items and ranges from 0 to 20. The FIQL measures specifically the impact of AI, contains 29 items (reflecting four subscales: Lifestyle, Coping/behaviour,

Depression and Embarrassment), and scoring ranges from 4 to 16. The ICIQ-B evaluates symptoms of AI and impact on quality of life. It has 20 items, each consisting of 2 items (symptoms and degree of bother). Scores range from 1 to 21 for bowel pattern, 0 to 28 for bowel control and 0 to 26 for impact on quality of life associated with AI symptoms. Current measurement instruments available for evaluating severity and quality of life in AI do not yet attain the highest levels of clinimetric soundness; however, aspects of validity, reliability or responsiveness have been established with rigour or are indicated. Therefore, the three questionnaires of interest have been recommended for use (Avery et al., 2007), although the ICIQ-B is preferred (grade A+, highly recommended with additional evidence of published content validity) compared to the FIQL (grade A, highly recommended) (Bosch et al., 2017).

Step 6. All questionnaires have a minimal burden and do not require specific equipment or expertise. The Wexner score is easy and quick to complete, whereas the FIQL and ICIQ-B need more time to complete.

Step 7. Based on the reason for encounter and knowledge from the previous steps, three questionnaires are under consideration. They all match the aspects that

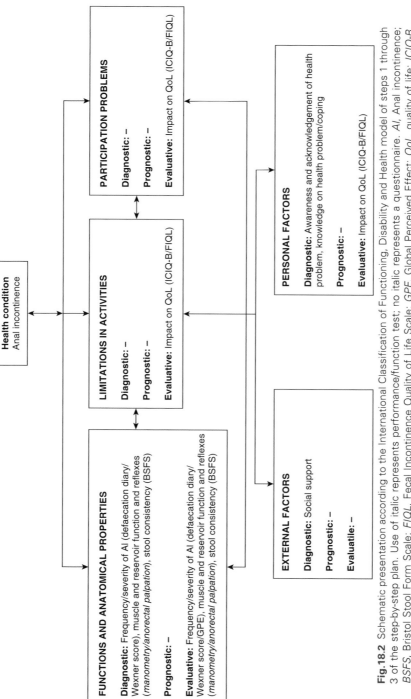

Fig.18.2 Schematic presentation according to the International Classification of Functioning, Disability and Health model of steps 1 through 3 of the step-by-step plan. Use of italic represents performance/function test; no italic represents a questionnaire. *AI*, Anal incontinence; *BSFS*, Bristol Stool Form Scale; *FIQL*, Fecal Incontinence Quality of Life Scale; *GPE*, Global Perceived Effect; *QoL*, quality of life; *ICIQ-B*, International Consultation on Incontinence Questionnaire -Anal Incontinence Symptoms and Quality of Life Module.

are indicated to be measured and the purpose of the measurement. The pelvic physical therapist is aware of a quality-of-life questionnaire specific for postpartum women with AI (the Postpartum Flatal and Faecal Incontinence Quality-of-Life Scale [Cockell et al., 2003]). This questionnaire better reflects the target group and is an adaptation of the FIQL for postpartum women. However, it is even more lengthy (68 items) and not recommended or graded, as insufficient data is available on clinimetric properties. The ICIQ-B seems more adequate to choose compared to the FIQL for measuring quality of life, as it has comparable feasibility; a higher recommendation grade (Bosch et al., 2017); incorporation of questions on bother in relation to AI, an aspect which adds valuable information for the therapist—besides presence of symptoms—on impact on daily life (Moossdorff-Steinhauser et al., 2020); and incorporation of the Bristol Stool Form Scale (BSFS), which assesses stool consistency, a parameter in which the pelvic physical therapist is also interested (step 2) (Lewis and Heaton, 1997).

Although the Wexner score is appealing for assessing the type and severity of AI when considering completion time and burden, the therapist decides to use the ICIQ-B for this purpose, as this measure also captures the domains of bowel symptoms and control, next to quality of life.

Mrs. Smith agrees with applying the ICIQ-B.

Step 8. The ICIQ-B sum scores for bowel pattern (score: 4 [range: 1–21]), bowel control (score: 12 [range: 0–28]) and quality of life (score: 20 [range: 0–26]) are calculated according to the guidelines. A higher score means more severe symptoms or more impact on quality of life. No norm values are available; however, considering the range of possible scores and own experience, the pelvic physical therapist concludes that Mrs. Smith experiences a high impact on quality of life and symptoms mainly relate to flatus incontinence, caused by a sphincter defect.

Step 9. The pelvic physical therapist discusses the results with Mrs. Smith and explains that many postpartum women experience AI, which often has a major impact, and that treatment options are available. They jointly decide on a treatment plan which will reduce symptoms and experienced bother and increase participation in social life and work. Mrs. Smith feels less insecure and has positive expectations of the treatment process. The pelvic physical therapist applies the ICIQ-B

again after 3 and 6 weeks to monitor and evaluate the treatment and adjust it in consultation with Mrs. Smith when necessary.

Step 10. The pelvic physical therapist introduces the step-by-step plan in a (multidisciplinary) team meeting. Together they discuss their current use of measurement instrument and what is necessary to obtain optimal implementation of goal-oriented selection and use of measurement instruments in their practice.

REFERENCES

Avery, K., Bosch, J. L., Gotoh, M., et al. (2007). Questionnaires to assess urinary and anal incontinence: Review and recommendations. *Journal of Urology, 177*(1), 39–49.

Avery, K., Donovan, J., Peters, T. J., et al. (2004). Iciq: A brief and robust measure for evaluating the symptoms and impact of urinary incontinence. *Neurourology and Urodynamics, 23*(4), 322–330.

Berghmans, L. C., Groot, J. A., van Heeswijk-Faase, I. C., et al. (2015). Dutch evidence statement for pelvic physical therapy in patients with anal incontinence. *International Urogynecology Journal, 26*(4), 487–496.

Beurskens, S., van Peppen, R., Swinkels, R., et al. (2020). *Meten in de praktijk. Stappenplan voor het gebruik van meetinstrumenten in de gezondheidszorg.* Houten, Netherlands: Bohn Stafleu Van Loghum.

Black, N. (2013). Patient reported outcome measures could help transform healthcare. *British Medical Journal, 346,* f167.

Bordeianou, L. G., Anger, J. T., Boutros, M., et al. (2020). Measuring pelvic floor disorder symptoms using patient-reported instruments: Proceedings of the consensus meeting of the pelvic floor consortium of the American Society of Colon and Rectal Surgeons, the International Continence Society, the American Urogynecologic Society, and the Society of Urodynamics, Female Pelvic Medicine and Urogenital Reconstruction. *Female Pelvic Medicine & Reconstructive Surgery, 26*(1), 1–15.

Bosch, R., Castro Diaz, D., Costantiini, E., et al. (2017). Committee 5B: Patient-reported outcome assessment. In *Incontinence* (6th ed.). Bristol, UK: International Continence Society. 541–598.

Braun, T., Rieckmann, A., Weber, F., et al. (2018). Current use of measurement instruments by physiotherapists working in Germany: A cross-sectional online survey. *BMC Health Services Research, 18,* 810.

Bump, R. C., Mattiasson, A., & Bø, K. (1996). The standardization of terminology of female pelvic organ prolapse and pelvic floor dysfunction. *American Journal of Obstetrics and Gynecology, 175*(1), 10–17.

Cockell, S. J., Oates-Johnson, T., Gilmour, D. T., et al. (2003). Postpartum flatal and fecal incontinence quality-of-life scale: A disease- and population-specific measure. *Qualitative Health Research*, 13(8), 1132–1144.

Cotterill, N., Norton, C., Avery, K., et al. (2011). Psychometric evaluation of a new patient-completed questionnaire for evaluating anal incontinence symptoms and impact on quality of life: The ICIQ-B. *Diseases of the Colon & Rectum*, 54(10), 1235–1250.

Damschroder, L. J., Aron, D. C., Keith, R. E., et al. (2009). Fostering implementation of health services research findings into practice: A consolidated framework for advancing implementation science. *Implementation Science*, 4, 50.

De Vet, H., Terwee, C., Knol, D., et al. (2011). *Measurement in Medicine: A practical guide*. New York: Cambridge University Press.

Dunn, J., Runge, R., & Snyder, M. (2018). Wearables and the medical revolution. *Per Medicine*, 15(5), 429–448.

Farrar, J., Young, J. J., LaMoureaux, L., et al. (2001). Clinical importance of changes in chronic pain intensity measured on an 11-point numerical pain rating scale. *Pain*, 94(2), 149–158.

Foster, A., Croot, L., Brazier, J., et al. (2018). The facilitators and barriers to implementing patient reported outcome measures in organisations delivering health related services: A systematic review of reviews. *Journal Patient Report Outcomes*, 2, 46.

Hendriks, E. J., Kessels, A. G., de Vet, H. C. W., et al. (2010). Prognostic indicators of poor short-term outcome of physiotherapy intervention in women with stress urinary incontinence. *Neurourology and Urodynamics*, 29(3), 336–343.

Hoffmann, T., Lewis, J., & Maher, C. (2020). Shared decision making should be an integral part of physiotherapy practice. *Physiotherapy*, 107, 43–49.

Huber, M., Knottnerus, J., Green, L., et al. (2011). How should we define health? *British Medical Journal*, 343, d4163.

Huber, M., van Vliet, M., Giezenberg, M., et al. (2016). Towards a 'patient-centred' operationalisation of the new dynamic concept of health: A mixed methods study. *BMJ Open*, 6(1), e010091.

International Consultation on Incontinence. (2020). *The international consultation on incontinence questionnaire (ICIQ)*. Available: https://iciq.net (Accessed 08 August, 2022).

Jorge, J. M., & Wexner, S. D. (1993). Etiology and management of fecal incontinence. *Diseases of the Colon & Rectum*, 36(1), 77–97.

Labrie, J., Lagro-Janssen, A., Fischer, K., et al. (2014). Predicting who will undergo surgery after physiotherapy for female stress urinary incontinence. *International Urogynecology Journal*, 26, 329–334.

Latorre, G. F. S., de Fraga, R., & Seleme, M. R. (2019). An ideal e-health system for pelvic floor muscle training adherence: Systematic review. *Neurourology and Urodynamics*, 38(1), 63–80.

Lewis, S. J., & Heaton, K. W. (1997). Stool form scale as a useful guide to intestinal transit time. *Scandinavian Journal of Gastroenterology*, 32(9), 920–924.

Moore, K. H., & Karantanis, E. (2008). Outcome measures in pelvic floor rehabilitation. In K. Baessler, K. L. Burgio, P. A. Norton, et al. (Eds.), *Pelvic floor Re-education: Principles and practice* (pp. 162–174). London: Springer.

Moossdorff-Steinhauser, H., Berghmans, L. C. M., Spaanderman, M. E. A., et al. (2020). Urinary incontinence during pregnancy: Prevalence, experience of bother, beliefs, and help-seeking behavior. *International Urogynecology Journal*, 32(3), 695–701.

Porter, M., & Teisberg, E. (2006). *Redefining health care: Creating value-base competition on results*. Boston: Harvard Business Review Press.

Rockwood, T. H., Church, J. M., Fleshman, J. W., et al. (2000). Fecal incontinence quality of life scale: Quality of life instrument for patients with fecal incontinence. *Diseases of the Colon & Rectum*, 43(1), 9–16; discussion 16–17.

Santana, M. J., Haverman, L., Absolom, K., et al. (2015). Training clinicians in how to use patient-reported outcome measures in routine clinical practice. *Quality of Life Research*, 24(7), 1707–1718.

Snyder, C., Smith, K., Holzner, B., et al. (2019). Making a picture worth a thousand numbers: Recommendations for graphically displaying patient-reported outcomes data. *Quality of Life Research*, 28(2), 345–356.

Stevens, A. (2017). The use and perceived usefulness of a patient-specific measurement instrument in physiotherapy goal setting. A qualitative study. *Musculoskelet Science Practice*, 27, 23–31.

Stevens, A., Beurskens, A., Köke, A., et al. (2013). The use of patient-specific measurement instruments in the process of goal-setting: A systematic review of available instruments and their feasibility. *Clinical Rehabilitation*, 27(11), 1005–1019.

Stevens, A., Köke, A., van der Weijden, T., et al. (2017). Ready for goal setting? Process evaluation of a patient-specific goal-setting method in physiotherapy. *BMC Health Services Research*, 17(1), 618.

Stratford, P. (1995). Assessing disability and change on individual patients: A report of a patient specific measure. *Physiotherapie Canada*, 47(4), 258–263.

Vaizey, C. J., Carapeti, E., Cahill, J. A., et al. (1999). Prospective comparison of faecal incontinence grading systems. *Gut*, 44(1), 77–80.

Van der Wees, P., Verkerk, E., Verbiest, M., et al. (2019). Development of a framework with tools to support the selection and implementation of patient-reported outcome measures. *Journal Patient Report Outcomes*, 30(1), 75.

Wallace, S. L., Mehta, S., Farag, S., et al. (2019). In search of mobile applications for urogynecology providers. *Female Pelvic Medicine & Reconstructive Surgery, 25*(6), 439–442.

Walton, M. K., Powers, J. H., Hobart, J., et al. (2015). Clinical outcome assessments: Conceptual foundation—report of the ISPOR clinical outcomes assessment—emerging good practices for outcomes research task force. *Value in Health, 18*(6), 741–752.

Ware, J., & Sherbourne, C. (1992). The MOS 36-item short form health survey (SF-36). I. Conceptual framework and item selection. *Medical Care, 30*(6), 473–483.

Whelan, P., Reddy, L., & Andrews, T. (2011). Patient satisfaction rating scales v. patient-related outcome and experience measures. *Psychiatrist, 35*(1), 32–33.

World Health Organization. (2001). *International classification of functioning, disability and health (ICF)*. Geneva: World Health Organization.

The Development of Clinical Practice Guidelines

Bary Berghmans, Nol Bernards and Rob de Bie

INTRODUCTION

Quality assurance and cost-effectiveness are, worldwide, issues of great concern in modern-day healthcare. The development of clinical practice guidelines (CPGs) can be considered a strategy to guarantee and improve the quality and efficiency of care.

A useful working definition of CPGs is derived from the Institute of Medicine (Field and Lohr, 1992). *Clinical practice guidelines* are defined as 'systematically, on the basis of (best) evidence and consensus developed recommendations, drafted by experts, field-tested, and directed at performing diagnostic and therapeutic interventions in persons with definitive, suspected or health-threatening conditions, or directed at areas which have to do with good management and administration of the profession(al)' (Field and Lohr, 1992; Grol et al., 2005; Hendriks et al., 1995; Hendriks et al., 1996; Hendriks et al., 1998a; Hendriks et al., 1998b).

A shorter and more modern definition states *guidelines* to be 'statements that include recommendations, intended to optimize patient care, that are informed by a systematic review of evidence and an assessment of the benefits and harms of alternative care options' (Institute of Medicine, 2011).

The Institute of Medicine further specifies, 'Rather than dictating a one-size-fits-all approach to patient care, CPGs offer an evaluation of the quality of the relevant scientific literature and an assessment of the likely benefits and harms of a particular treatment' (American Physical Therapy Association, 2020).

For both national and international physical therapy (physiotherapy) associations, the development and the implementation of CPGs constitute an important part of the quality of physical therapy care (policy) (Schünemann et al., 2014; Van der Wees et al., 2003). Increasing pressure from society (policy makers, healthcare managers, financiers and patients) on physical therapists (PTs) to ensure quality of care and to justify their position in the healthcare system (Hendriks et al., 2000b; Schünemann et al., 2014) and from PTs and their professional bodies necessitated this to embed evidence-based practice into their profession (American Physical Therapy Association, 2020; Van der Wees et al., 2003).

At the beginning of the 21st century, the European Region of the World Confederation for Physical Therapy

(WCPT) developed a framework for the development of CPGs (Van der Wees and Mead, 2004). By 2010, eight European countries had physical therapy–specific guideline programmes (WCPT, 2010). In this chapter the ongoing process and development of the CPGs of the Royal Dutch Society for Physical Therapy (Koninklijk Nederlands Genootschap voor Fysiotherapie [KNGF]) are described.

Methods for guideline development have been harmonized to a certain degree (Burgers et al., 2003; Van der Wees et al., 2007b), for which the AGREE (Appraisal of Guidelines, Research and Evaluation) instrument provides an important framework (Brouwers et al., 2010).

Every few years the whole method is updated and synchronized with appraisal and assessment techniques of evidence. In addition, new and shorter variants of CPGs have emerged (evidence statements and standards) (KNGF, 2019).

The latest 'KNGF guideline methodology' came into force in 2017. Every year, this methodology is adjusted where necessary on the basis of experience gained with the application of the methodology, and (legal) requirements and criteria regarding the development and content of quality standards, including guidelines (World Health Organization [WHO], 2018). The KNGF guideline methodology is therefore a 'living' document.

The AGREE instrument can be used to assess the quality of CPGs and helps guideline developers structure and improve the process of guideline development (Table 19.1).

TABLE 19.1 The 23 Key Items of the AGREE Instrument

AGREE II consists of 23 key items organized within six domains followed by two global rating items ('Overall Assessment'). Each domain captures a unique dimension of guideline quality.

Domain 1: Scope and purpose

1. The overall objective(s) of the guideline is (are) specifically described.
2. The health question(s) covered by the guideline is (are) specifically described.
3. The population (patients, public, etc.) to whom the guideline is meant to apply is specifically described.

Domain 2: Stakeholder involvement

1. The guideline development group includes individuals from all relevant professional groups.
2. The views and preferences of the target population (patients, public, etc.) have been sought.
3. The target users of the guideline are clearly defined.

Domain 3: Rigour of development

1. Systematic methods were used to search for evidence.
2. The criteria for selecting the evidence are clearly described.
3. The strengths and limitations of the body of evidence are clearly described.
4. The methods for formulating the recommendations are clearly described.
5. The health benefits, side effects and risks have been considered in formulating the recommendations.
6. There is an explicit link between the recommendations and the supporting evidence.
7. The guideline has been externally reviewed by experts prior to its publication.
8. A procedure for updating the guideline is provided.

Domain 4: Clarity of presentation

1. The recommendations are specific and unambiguous.
2. The different options for management of the condition or health issue are clearly presented.
3. Key recommendations are easily identifiable.

Domain 5: Applicability

1. The guideline describes facilitators and barriers to its application.
2. The guideline provides advice and/or tools on how the recommendations can be put into practice.
3. The potential resource implications of applying the recommendations have been considered.
4. The guideline presents monitoring and/or auditing criteria.

Domain 6: Editorial independence

1. The views of the funding body have not influenced the content of the guideline.
2. Competing interests of guideline development group members have been recorded and addressed.

The Dutch programme for guideline development in physical therapy was critically reviewed and evaluated using the AGREE instrument (Van der Wees et al., 2007a). Identification of weaknesses was subsequently used to update the programme.

The framework of the updated Dutch guideline programme is shown in Table 19.2.

Today, Dutch CPG programmes comply with almost all AGREE criteria including piloting of the CPGs among target users.

CPGs can be considered as important state-of-the-art documents, which can guide professionals in their daily practice and make explicit what professionals can do in a certain situation or with a specific condition, and why they do it. CPGs should not be applied rigidly but are intended to be more flexible; however, in most cases they can and should be followed. Yet it is important to realize that CPGs only reflect the current state of knowledge, at the time of publication, and expertise on effective and appropriate care with respect to a certain health problem. They are subject to a continuous process of integration of new views, based on inevitable changes in the state of scientific information and technology. New evidence is mostly gathered in systematic reviews. However, this kind of research is not a panacea for the problems associated with reviews of the literature. Due to its non-experimental nature, it is prone to the flaws that apply to all non-experimental research (De Bie, 1996; Shaneyfelt and Centor, 2009).

Thus readers should always keep these facts in mind while studying both systematic reviews and CPGs and must be critical in their appraisal of the information. In particular, statements about efficacy and efficiency of interventions, only based on clinical practice or experience or reflecting opinions of so-called experts in the field, might be biased and the real value discussed.

TABLE 19.2	**Updated Dutch Programme for Guideline Development in Physical Therapy**
Section	**Description**
1. Structure and organization	Central professional organization in collaboration with other institutes; monodisciplinary development group (5–10 members); small group (2–3) of employed staff within development group responsible for review of literature and actual writing of guideline; patients involved in external review group and focus groups
2. Preparation/ initiation	Special interest groups can propose topics using application form; procedure is described for prioritizing topics; guideline committee selects; KNGF board makes final decision; literature orientation on subject; barriers and needs of physical therapists and patients described in application form
3. Development	Literature search using systematic strategy; systematic review or meta-analysis if no (recent) review available; quality of studies assessed using different tools for diagnosis, intervention and systematic reviews; hierarchy of evidence described in four levels according to Dutch consensus; grading of recommendations in four levels; standardized formulation of recommendations according to grading; Outline of guideline divided in physical therapy diagnosis and treatment based on clinical reasoning process; use of International Classification of Functioning, Disability and Health as nomenclature
4. Validation	Draft guideline sent to group of peers to test practicality, clarity and acceptability; draft guideline discussed in external review group (relevant healthcare professionals, patients, stakeholders); separate check by patient advisory board; final draft checked by Guideline Committee; endorsement by KNGF; test piloting after endorsement
5. Dissemination and implementation	Four products: practice guideline, review of evidence, summary (in flow chart), patient version; publication as supplement of *Dutch Journal for Physical Therapy*; sent to all members of KNGF; translated into English; publication on website; implementation plan with every guideline
6. Evaluation and update	No later than 5 years after publication, decision about update, based on new evidence, results from pilot, professional developments and developments in guideline methodology; additional (systematic) review of literature; weighing of evidence and recommendations adjusted or added if necessary

KNFG, Koninklijk Nederlands Genootschap voor Fysiotherapie (Royal Dutch Society for Physical Therapy).

GUIDING PRINCIPLES IN THE DEVELOPMENT OF CLINICAL PRACTICE GUIDELINES

Important guiding principles in the development of CPGs include the following (Hendriks et al., 1998c; Hendriks et al., 2000a):

- The subject matter is clearly delineated based on a clear medical diagnosis of health problems and related conditions that can be addressed by physical therapy.
- CPGs should be structured according to the phases of the physical therapy process (Fig. 19.1; see Table 19.1)

as laid down in CPGs by the professional organization (Heerkens et al., 2003; KNGF, 1993).

- A uniform professional language is used. Whenever indicated, use is made of available (international) classifications and accepted terminology, particularly the International Classification of Functioning, Disability and Health (WHO, 2018), but also the International Classification of Diseases (WHO, 2014), the Dutch Classification of Procedures (Heerkens et al., 1995) and Medical Terms for Health Professionals (Heerkens et al., 1998) (see Fig. 19.1). The last two are specific for the Dutch situation.

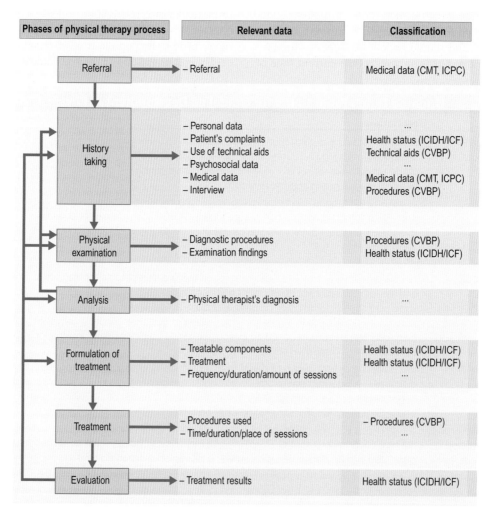

Fig. 19.1 The physical therapy process, relevant data and necessary classifications. *CMT,* Classification of medical terms; *CVBP,* Classification of Interventions and Procedures (for the allied health professions); *ICF,* International Classification of Functioning, Disability and Health; *ICIDH,* International Classification of Impairments, Disabilities and Handicaps; *ICPC,* International Classification of Primary Care.

- Uniform and valid diagnostic and responsive outcome measurements are used.
- CPGs should be based on the best available clinical evidence, and on consensus between experts if no evidence is available.
- Clinical considerations have priority over cost-effectiveness.
- CPGs should be consistent with CPGs produced by other professions or groups of professions.
- CPGs should be based on integration and coherence of care. Physical therapy may be one of the possible interventions in the total care of a patient. It should be evident at which point and why physical therapy is appropriate.
- CPGs should be patient orientated and in agreement with the policies of patient organizations. Individual patients also need to have a voice in determining care (Hartford Kvael et al., 2019). Are the expectations and treatment goals of patients the same as those of PTs?
- The necessary expertise and knowledge required of PTs should be made clear.

Currently, the KNGF has added the following criteria for the development of a *new* CPG:

- the need for the field;
- the prevalence of the health problem in everyday practise;
- the extent of the health problem, where it is plausible that physical therapy leads to health gains;
- the degree of scientific evidence;
- the degree of variation in physical therapeutic action;
- the possibility to limit the subject;
- whether it is realistic for the relevant parties to reach consensus;
- whether the directive can be incorporated into or linked to an external body in the short term, directive or standard of care; and
- the importance of the CPG for the positioning of physical therapy.

In case of *revision* of a CPG, additional criteria apply (KNGF, 2019):

- the age of the directive or module;
- the degree and relevance of new insights and/or scientific evidence;
- the extent to which the directive is used in everyday practice;
- the seriousness of the bottlenecks identified in the application of the guideline or module;
- a new external directive on the subject has been published, changing the (organization of) physical therapeutic care.

THE DEVELOPMENT PROCESS OF CLINICAL PRACTICE GUIDELINES

CPGs should be based on the different stages of the physical therapy cure and care process, such as diagnosis, therapy and prognosis (Bernards et al., 2011; Hendriks et al., 2000a; Hendriks et al., 2000b); the available clinical evidence; and expert consensus. Priority is given to a cost-effective approach and multidisciplinary consensus on diagnosis, intervention and secondary prevention. Recommendations are based on the results of new or recorded systematic reviews or meta-analysis.

As an example, five groups contributed to the development of the Dutch CPGs (Fig. 19.2):

1. The KNGF and four collaborating partners (the Dutch Institute of Allied Health Care [NPi], the Center for Evidence-Based Physiotherapy [CEBP], the Department of Epidemiology at Maastricht University, and the Dutch Organization for Quality Assurance [CBO] which initiates and eventually endorses the CPGs)
2. The steering group which plans and coordinates the activities
3. The working group which develops the CPGs
4. A group of clinical experts in the subject matter of the CPGs who comment on the guidelines or parts of it during the development
5. A randomly selected group of PTs who pilot test the guidelines in clinical practice.

The workflow of the development process consists of formulation of clinical questions and patient-relevant outcomes, systematic identification and summarizing of relevant evidence, synthesis of the evidence by grading its quality, and formulation of recommendations for daily practice (Van der Wees et al., 2007a; van der Wees et al., 2011). The different elements in guideline development are described in Table 19.1.

Phases in the Development of Clinical Practice Guidelines

There are four important phases in the development of CPGs:

1. The preparatory phase
2. The design phase, encompassing the draft guidelines and the authorization phase
3. The implementation phase
4. The evaluation and updating phase.

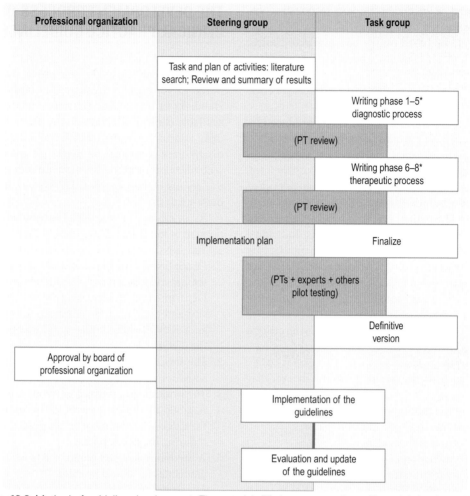

Fig. 19.2 Method of guideline development. The asterisk (*) denotes to refer to Box 19.2 for the writing phases. *PT,* Physical therapist.

Method of the Development of Clinical Practice Guidelines

The Preparatory Phase

This phase involves the selection of a topic based on certain criteria (Field and Lohr, 1992; Grimshaw et al., 1995a; Grol et al., 2005; van der Wees et al., 2011; van Everdingen et al., 2004) (Box 19.1).

The scope and objectives of the guideline are defined. The clinical questions and patient-important outcomes are formulated.

The Design Phase

This phase should guide the working group in the development of the guidelines and is, for educational reasons,

based on the different stages of the physical therapy process (Box 19.2; see Fig. 19.1). In the process of physical therapy practice, several inter-related stages can be distinguished (Heerkens et al., 2003; Hendriks et al., 2000b): a PT sees a patient, depending on the actual national situation with or without a medical referral and a request for professional help. The PT takes the patient's history, examines the patient, draws conclusions, and finally informs the patient about the findings and conclusions. After this diagnostic phase, the PT formulates together with the patient a treatment plan and treatment goals.

Following the formulation of a plan of activities and basic algorithms, systematic literature searches, reviews

BOX 19.1 Possible Criteria to Select a Subject for the Development of Clinical Practice Guidelines

- The subject concerns a problem or controversy in healthcare for which healthcare providers are seeking a solution.
- It is anticipated that consensus about the procedure/intervention is possible.
- Healthcare providers are awaiting guidelines because they need a state-of-the-art document about a subject/topic.
- The subject is relevant because it has an impact on the costs of healthcare in terms of prevention of health problems or saving of costs.
- There is enough scientific evidence.
- There is a genuine expectation that the guidelines fit within existing norms, values and routines.
- The subject matter can be reasonably delineated.
- It is possible to collect data about the care.

BOX 19.2 Different Phases of the Process of Physical Therapy Practice

1. Examination of the referral data
2. History taking
3. Physical examination and evaluation of the patient's (functional) status
4. Formulating the physical therapist's diagnosis and deciding whether or not physical therapy is indicated
5. Formulating the treatment plan
6. Providing the treatment
7. Evaluating the (changes in) a patient's (functional) status and one's own course of action
8. Concluding the treatment period and reporting to the referring discipline

BOX 19.3 Guidelines for Selecting Articles That Are Most Likely to Provide Valid Results

Therapy
- Was the assignment of patients to treatments randomized?
- Were all of the patients who entered the trial properly accounted for and attributed at its conclusion?

Diagnosis
- Was there an independent, blind comparison with a reference standard?
- Did the patient sample include an appropriate spectrum of the sort of patients to whom the diagnostic test will be applied in clinical practice?

Harm
- Were there clearly identified comparison groups that were similar with respect to important determinations of outcome (other than the one of interest)?
- Were outcomes and exposures measured in the same way in groups being compared?

Prognosis
- Was there a representative patient sample at a well-defined point in the course of disease?
- Was the follow-up sufficiently long and complete?

Describing the quality of the evidence is important so that users of the guidelines can interpret the relative importance of the evidence. Each type of evidence (e.g., risk factors, diagnostic testing, prognosis, prevention, treatment) should be reviewed against a set of methodological criteria and systematically applied within study types. For evidence on interventions, high-quality randomized clinical trials are considered to provide the strongest evidence, followed by cohort studies, case–control studies and non-analytic studies such as case reports or case series. Based on the quality of individual studies, an overall synthesis of the evidence will result in evidence statements expressed in levels of evidence. The PEDro scale was used in the updated SUI guidelines to study the internal validity of clinical trials, where high scores on the 11-item quality scale indicate a low risk of bias (Bernards et al., 2011; Maher et al., 2004).

When scientific evidence from systematic reviews or primary trials is not available, the working group and the clinical experts formulate the CPGs on the basis of consensus. The working group first develops the diagnostic

and/or meta-analyses are conducted into the efficacy of diagnostic procedures, possible interventions, measurement instruments, prognosis, prevention, patient preferences and current practice (Grol et al., 2005; van Everdingen et al., 2004). The strategy described in Box 19.3 is used. The purpose of these rigorous literature reviews is to document the evidence to justify the recommendations and to minimize the potential for any bias (Van der Wees et al., 2011; van Tulder et al., 2003). For an example on stress urinary incontinence (SUI), see the work of Dumoulin et al. (2016), Dumoulin et al. (2018) or Hay-Smith and Dumoulin, (2006).

part of the CPGs that may include an algorithm of the process of care and clinical decision making to formulate the management goals and an intervention plan. Twenty-five practicing PTs with special interest and expertise in the problem area review this part of the CPGs.

Following the plan of activities, the working group continues with the therapeutic part of the guidelines that, if indicated and possible, should include the recommended intensity, frequency and duration of the intervention(s). The same group of therapists who were consulted in the previous phase review this part.

When both diagnostic and therapeutic parts of the guidelines are completed, the first draft is sent to randomly selected specialized therapists for pilot testing and comments. Additional comments are obtained from clinical experts in relevant professions. Based on the comments and experiences of the PTs and the clinical experts, the draft is rewritten. The modified draft is then discussed by the 'Authorization Committee' (see Fig. 19.2). Following approval of this committee, the guidelines are published in a scientific journal and introduced and implemented in the field.

The final product consists of four parts:
- The practice guidelines themselves
- A summary or algorithm, digital and/or on an A4 laminated quick reference card
- A scientific justification with references
- A specific strategy and instruments for implementation of the guidelines (e.g., a knowledge check to test for discrepancies between the actual and the recommended practice as stated in the guidelines)
- In some cases, educational materials that are developed or outlines for these, to be developed by third parties.

During and after the course of treatment, the therapeutic process and results are evaluated. Data obtained during the care process are recorded according to the CPGs for documentation that have been developed to ensure systematic and uniform record keeping (ADAPTE Collaboration, 2010; Heerkens et al., 2003; Hendriks et al., 1998b; Hendriks et al., 1998c; KNGF, 1993).

The Implementation Phase

To be successful, a CPG has to be developed, disseminated to the right target audience and finally be implemented. This phase comprises the dissemination of specific strategies to implement the developed CPGs, according to the general method of implementation (Hendriks et al., 1998c; Hendriks et al., 2000a; Hendriks et al., 2000c).

The concept of implementation is complex. If not adopted in daily practice, even the highest quality guideline is useless (Rauh et al., 2018). Some studies have raised substantial doubt about guideline implementation. It is estimated that 30% to 40% of all medical patients may receive treatments not based on guidelines. What is worse, 15% to 20% may receive unnecessary or even harmful treatment (Grol and Grimshaw, 2003). Rauh et al. (2018) stated that barriers to guideline implementation have been well identified and can be divided into the PT's personal factors (knowledge and attitude), guideline-related factors and external factors (lack of resources, organizational constraints, heavy workload, social norms and so on [Baiardini et al., 2009]). Guideline-related barriers may be the easiest to resolve but need to be identified: poor layout, too high complexity or poor access to guidelines are rather easily tackled. Personal factors (of the applying PT) need more complex interventions. Even concerning the most pertinent guidelines, guideline compliance and adherence may vary and may be substantially lower than expected. One of the impeding factors is that PTs do not hold realistic perceptions of their adherence to CPGs (Maas et al., 2015). PTs have to be motivated to use guidelines.

Lack of knowledge or skills can be tackled with ongoing education, certification, registration and audits. Adequate discussion platforms, communication and key opinion leadership will support and stimulate the professional attitude towards using guidelines and performance. Exchange and cooperation with other relevant disciplines will serve to reach optimal consensus, upgrading CPGs from a general healthcare problem focus to an applied decision on the individual level. The barriers mentioned so far need to be overcome, and for this a good strategy seems to be to develop a guidelines checklist to be considered in any treated patient with functional problems of the pelvic floor, regardless of the type of dysfunction.

Checklists have been identified as one tool to raise CPG adherence (Fischer et al., 2016). A checklist has a didactic role in recalling standard procedures, but it also is useful to document and better structure the mandatory information needed to perform a society board decision, in line with international CPGs. As a society board decision should be a mainstay in pelvic physiotherapy decision making for every patient, the checklist will also underline its necessity to come to a therapeutic decision for any individual patient.

A checklist could be helpful to encourage CPG use and adaptation and application to local needs and standards towards state-of-the art needs (Rauh et al., 2018). Based on the experience of (barriers of) implementation of other CPGs in the allied health or medical field, here we introduce the idea of developing such a checklist as one of the strategies for better adherence to and application of CPGs.

Another strategy is peer assessment. Peer assessment is an implementation strategy for CPGs within existing communities of practice. It is the process in which professionals evaluate or are being evaluated by their peers and provide each other with performance feedback. In doing so, it aims to improve guideline adherence by enhancing reflective practice, awareness of professional performance and attainment of personal goals (Maas et al., 2015). This strategy appeared to be more effective than the usual care discussion strategy on adherence to CPGs for PT management. The main difference between peer assessment and usual care discussion is that in the peer assessment approach, the tasks are structured, with a focus on performance rather than discussion, and participant roles are pre-defined. The effectiveness of peer assessment can be attributed to the structured and performance-based design of such a programme. Maas et al. (2015) recommended a shift in the feedback culture of PTs in primary care, from avoiding performance feedback to actively seeking feedback.

In addition, a structured and well-organized peer group training has been developed as a tailored implementation strategy aiming at improving healthcare provider adherence to guidelines (Joosen et al., 2019). This kind of training is held in small interactive peer sessions over a long interval. Joosen et al. (2019) showed this training to be effective in implementing guidelines, but the authors stated that this has limited impact if external barriers continue to hinder guideline adherence. This implementation strategy is useful as a generic approach to address key barriers for change (Joosen et al., 2019).

Finally, without the clinical input of the PT, it is unlikely that whatever implementation strategy is used will be effective and sustainable. The informed PT can and should be an integral part of sustaining new, effective clinical care and conducting ongoing evaluation to monitor its impact over time.

The Evaluation and Updating Phase

The effectiveness of the guidelines needs to be evaluated at the level of professionals and patients (see Fig. 19.2). The CPGs should be updated every 3 to 5 years after the guidelines are put into practice, or whenever new scientific insights make an update necessary.

DISCUSSION

The Dutch CPGs for physiotherapists' diagnosis and management of SUI in adult women (Berghmans et al., 1998a; Berghmans et al., 1998b) were the first to be developed for the diagnosis and management by PTs of SUI (in adult women). At the time of publication, the guidelines provided up-to-date information on diagnosis, intervention, consultation and education on this specific health problem, information that the profession generally accepts as representing the state of the art (Grol et al., 2005; Hendriks et al., 1996; Hendriks et al., 1998a; Hendriks et al., 1998b; Hendriks et al., 2000a; van Everdingen et al., 2004).

However, subsequent developments led to improvements in the application of physical therapy in this group of patients and had an impact on the information contained in these guidelines. The CPGs mentioned previously have been updated and extended also to adult men, and the revised version was published in 2011 (Bernards et al., 2011). The latest revision took place in 2017 (KNGF, 2017) and was published electronically. The update of the guideline is in line with the structure and methods for guideline development, implementation and updating of KNGF guidelines which offers practical recommendations for a strategy to collect the relevant literature, including the selection of search terms, sources to be consulted and the period covered by the search (Hendriks et al., 1998a; Hendriks et al., 2000a; van der Wees et al., 2007a; van der Wees 2007b; van der Wees et al., 2011). The CPG is available in Dutch and English and can be downloaded at the website https://www.fysionet-evidencebased.nl.

Changing Practice

As stated before, an important strategy to improve the quality of physical therapy and to minimize undesirable variability in clinical practice is the development and implementation of evidence-based CPGs. In general, it can be concluded that the provision of explicit CPGs, supported by reinforcement strategies, will improve the PT's performance and, in certain situations as a main goal, the patients' health outcomes.

It is clear that just the developing and disseminating of CPGs is not sufficient. Even well-established guidelines, like the example of the updated guidelines for SUI (Bernards et al., 2011, revised September 2017), will not contribute to an improved quality unless they are embedded in effective implementation programme (Grol and Grimshaw, 2003; Grol and Wensing, 2006; Grol et al., 2005; van der Wees et al., 2011). Implementation implies the introduction of a change or innovation such that it becomes a normal component of clinical practice for individual PTs and is no longer considered as new. In other words, a vital element of successful CPG implementation is changing the individual PTs' behavioral process that has to take place in the constantly changing environment of evidence-based practice and lifelong learning.

CPG implementation is often laborious and has proved to be the weakest link in the whole process (Grol et al., 2005). Therefore, next to publication, dissemination and implementation of the CPGs, a set of (postgraduate) courses and tools were developed and published to facilitate and promote practical use of the guidelines in clinical practice (Bekkering et al., 2005; Van Ettekoven and Hendriks, 1998). The GuideLine Implementability Appraisal (GLIA) can be of assistance in formulating actionable and precisely defined recommendations, with the aim of improving the applicability of guidelines (Shiffman et al., 2005).

Following a standard implementation procedure, the CPGs for the Physiotherapy of Patients with Stress Urinary Incontinence have been successfully implemented in the Netherlands.

Several systematic reviews by Grimshaw et al. (1995a, 1995b) described 91 studies and showed that the effect of introducing guidelines, especially in terms of their impact on clinical practice, is greater than had been previously assumed. In addition, on the basis of several studies (Davis and Taylor-Vaisey, 1997; Grimshaw and Russell, 1993; Grimshaw et al., 1995a; Grimshaw et al., 1995b; van der Wees et al., 2011), it can be concluded that thoroughly developed guidelines can alter clinical practice patterns and can lead to positive changes in patient outcomes. However, the studies also showed that the acceptance and use of guidelines are closely connected with the way in which they are developed and introduced. These findings were confirmed by the reviews of Grimshaw et al. (2001) and Grol and Grimshaw (2003).

The CPGs on SUI were developed by an independent multidisciplinary group of experts who represented all concerned professional organizations. The CPGs were based on the results of systematic reviews or meta-analyses (e.g., Berghmans et al., 1998c; Dumoulin et al., 2016; Hay-Smith and Dumoulin, 2006; Hendriks et al., 1998c; Hendriks et al., 2000c), because CPGs should provide clear clinical recommendations based on scientific and clinical evidence.

To optimize the development of CPGs, it is recommended that future users are involved as much as possible in the developmental process (Grol et al., 1994; Grol et al., 2005; Grimshaw et al., 2001; National Institute for Health and Care Excellence, 2019; van Everdingen et al., 2004; van der Wees et al., 2008) and that PTs are able to exert a great deal of influence on guideline implementation. The use of a top-down approach will engender resistance and thus have an adverse effect. However, adopting a bottom-up approach is often inefficient in terms of making the best use of the time invested and of avoiding ambiguity. To increase the acceptance and use of CPGs, it might therefore be helpful to adapt centrally produced guidelines, with the help of a local team, to deal specifically with the local situation or to add a number of complementary agreements or criteria if necessary.

Although guidelines can immediately be put into practice, they may also be adapted to individual situations. Converting guidelines into a locally used protocol is possible and, at times, desirable. The conversion of centrally produced guidelines into a local protocol ensures that there is a local investment in, or 'buying into', the guidelines. This will speed up acceptance and thus implementation of the guidelines.

THE FUTURE

Evaluation of the effect of the implementation process of CPGs is needed to draw conclusions about how CPGs can be effectively and efficiently implemented in the future. Only by evaluating carefully the effect of developing and implementing the centrally produced guidelines is it possible to identify specific barriers and impediments that need to be overcome in the successful implementation of guidelines, or to identify innovations.

Besides the Dutch CPGs for SUI, an evidence-based statement for anal incontinence has been published (Bols et al., 2013). The development of this evidence-based statement was in line with the proposal of van der Wees et al. (2011) to establish a collaborative for the production of international evidence statements for PT practice. The purpose of these evidence statements is to provide a universal starting point for further specification and contextualization of recommendations for PT practice at a national level. Tailoring of recommendations at a national level is important to enhance implementation and may be related to characteristics of PT service, available resources and patients (Van der Wees et al., 2011). The statements aim to provide a basis for PT diagnosis and treatment in terms of function, activities, and participation, based on the International Classification of Functioning, Disability and Health (WHO, 2018).

REFERENCES

ADAPTE Collaboration. (2010). *The ADAPTE process: Resource toolkit for guideline adaptation*. Version 2.0 [Online]. Available: http://www.g-i-n.net (Guidelines International Network [G-I-N]). (Accessed 05.08.22).

American Physical Therapy Association. (2020). *APTA clinical practice guideline process manual, revised*. Alexandria, VA: American Physical Therapy Association.

Baiardini, I., Braido, F., Bonini, M., et al. (2009). Why do doctors and patients not follow guidelines? *Current Opinion in Allergy and Clinical Immunology, 9*, 228–233.

Bekkering, G. E., van Tulder, M. W., Hendriks, E. J., et al. (2005). Implementation of clinical guidelines on physical therapy for patients with low back pain: Randomized trial comparing patient outcomes after a standard and active implementation strategy. *Physical Therapy, 85*(6), 544–555.

Berghmans, L. C., Bernards, A. T., Bluyssens, A. M., et al. (1998a). KNGF–Richtlijn stress urine-incontinentie. *Nederlands Tijdschrift voor Fysiotherapie, 108*(Suppl. 4).

Berghmans, L. C., Bernards, A. T., Hendriks, H. J., et al. (1998b). Physiotherapeutic management for genuine stress incontinence. *Physical Therapy Reviews, 3*, 133–147.

Berghmans, L. C., Hendriks, H. J., Bø, K., et al. (1998c). Conservative treatment of stress urinary incontinence in women. A systematic review of randomized controlled trials. *British Journal of Urology, 82*, 181–191.

Bernards, A. T., Berghmans, L. C., Van Heeswijk-Faase, I. C., et al. (2011). Clinical practice guidelines for physiotherapists for physical therapy in patients with stress urinary incontinence. *Nederlands Tijdschrift voor Fysiotherapie, 121*(Suppl. 3).

Bols, E. M., Groot, J. A., van Heeswijk-Faase, I. C., et al. (2013). *KNGF evidence statement*. Anale Incontinentie [Online]. Available: https://www.fysionet-evidencebased.nl. (Accessed 05.08.22).

Brouwers, M. C., Kho, M. E., Browman, G. P., et al. (2010). Development of the AGREE II, part 2: Assessment of validity of items and tools to support application. *Canadian Medical Association Journal, 182*, e472–e478.

Burgers, J. S., Grol, R., Klazinga, N. S., et al. (2003). Towards evidence-based clinical practice: An international survey of 18 clinical guideline programs. *International Journal for Quality in Health Care, 15*, 31–45.

Davis, D. A., & Taylor-Vaisey, A. (1997). Translating guidelines into practice. A systematic review of theoretic concepts, practical experience and research evidence in the adoption of clinical practice guidelines. *Canadian Medical Association Journal, 157*, 408–416.

De Bie, R. A. (1996). Methodology of systematic reviews: An introduction. *Physical Therapy Reviews, 1*, 47.

Dumoulin, C., Adewuyi, T., & Booth, J. (2016). Adult conservative management. In P. Abrams, L. Cardozo, A. Wagg, et al. (Eds.), *Incontinence: Sixth international consultation on incontinence*. Bristol, UK: ICUD. 1443–1628.

Dumoulin, C., Cacciari, L. P., & Hay-Smith, E. J. C. (2018). Pelvic floor muscle training versus no treatment, or inactive control treatments, for urinary incontinence in women. *Cochrane Database of Systematic Reviews, 10*, CD005654.

Field, M. J., & Lohr, K. N. (Eds.). (1992). *Guidelines for clinical practice: From development to use*. Washington, DC: National Academies Press.

Fischer, F., Lange, K., Klose, K., et al. (2016). Barriers and strategies in guideline implementation—a scoping review. *Healthcare (Basel), 4*(3), 36.

Grimshaw, J., Eccles, M., & Russell, I. (1995a). Developing clinically valid practice guidelines. *Journal of Evaluation in Clinical Practice, 1*(1), 37–48.

Grimshaw, J., Freemantle, N., Wallace, S., et al. (1995b). Developing and implementing clinical practice guidelines. *Quality and Safety in Health Care, 4*(1), 55–64.

Grimshaw, J., & Russell, I. T. (1993). Effect of clinical guidelines on medical practice: A systematic review of rigorous evaluations. *Lancet, 342*, 1317–1322.

Grimshaw, J., Shirran, L., Thomas, R., et al. (2001). Changing provider behavior. An overview of systematic reviews of interventions. *Medical Care, 39*(8 Suppl. 2) II-2–II-45.

Grol, R., & Grimshaw, J. (2003). From best evidence to best practice: Effective implementation of change in patient's care. *Lancet, 362*, 1225–1230.

Grol, R., van Everdingen, J. J., & Casparie, A. P. (1994). *Invoering van richtlijnen en veranderingen. Een handleiding voor de medische, paramedische en verpleegkundige praktijk*. Utrecht: De Tijdstroom.

Grol, R., & Wensing, M. (2006). *Implementatie: Effectieve verbetering van de patientenzorg*. Maarssen, Netherlands: Elsevier.

Grol, R., Wensing, M., & Eccles, M. (2005). *Improving patient care: The implementation of change in clinical practice.* London: Elsevier Butterworth-Heinemann.

Hartford Kvael, L. A., Debesay, J., & Bye, A. (2019). Health–care professionals' experiences of patient participation among older patients in intermediate care—at the intersection between profession, market and bureaucracy. *Health Expectations, 22*, 921–930.

Hay-Smith, E. J., & Dumoulin, C. (2006). Pelvic floor muscle training versus no treatment, or inactive control treatments, for urinary incontinence in women. *Cochrane Database of Systematic Reviews*, 1, CD005654.

Heerkens, Y. F., Lakerveld-Heijl, K., Verhoeven, A., et al. (2003). Herziening Richtlijn voor de fysiotherapeutische Verslaglegging. *Ned Tijdschr Fysiother, 113*(Suppl. 1), 1–36.

Heerkens, Y. F., van den Heuvel, J., van Klaveren, A. A., et al. (Eds.). (1995). *Voorlopige WCC–Standaard CVPB. Vaste Commissie voor Classificaties en Definities* Zoetermeer.

Heerkens, Y. F., van den Heuvel, J., van Klaveren, A. A., et al. (1998). *Ontwerp classificatie 'medische' termen (CMT) voor paramedische beroepen.* Amersfoort: Nederlands Paramedisch Instituut.

Hendriks, H. J., Bekkering, G. E., van Ettekoven, H., et al. (2000a). Development and implementation of national practice guidelines: A prospect for continuous quality improvement in physiotherapy. *Physiotherapy, 86*(10), 535–547.

Hendriks, H. J., Oostendorp, R. A., Bernards, A. T., et al. (2000b). The diagnostic process and indication for physiotherapy: A prerequisite for treatment and outcome evaluation. *Physical Therapy Reviews, 5*, 29–47.

Hendriks, H. J., van Ettekoven, H., Bekkering, G. E., et al. (2000c). Implementatie van KNGF–Richtlijnen. *FysioPraxis, 2*, 9–13.

Hendriks, H. J., Reitsma, E., & van Ettekoven, H. (1995). Improving the quality of physical therapy by national (central) guidelines: Introduction of a method of guideline development and implementation, Proceedings of the World Confederation for Physical Therapy Congress, Washington DC, June 25–30.

Hendriks, H. J., Reitsma, E., & van Ettekoven, H. (1996). Centrale Richtlijnen in de fysiotherapie. Nederlands Tijdschrift voor Fysiotherapie1:2–11.

Hendriks, H. J., van Ettekoven, H., Reitsma, E., et al. (1998a). *Methode voor Centrale Richtlijnontwikkeling en implementatie in de fysiotherapie.* Amersfoort: KNGF/NPi/CBO.

Hendriks, H. J., van Ettekoven, H., & van der Wees, P. J. (1998b). *Eindverslag van het Project Centrale Richtlijnen in de fysiotherapie. Deel I. Achtergronden en evaluatie van het project.* Amersfoort: KNGF/NPi/CBO.

Hendriks, H. J., van Ettekoven, H., & van der Wees, P. J. (1998c). *Eindverslag van het project Centrale Richtlijnen in de fysiotherapie. Deel II. Producten van het project.* Amersfoort: KNGF/NPi/CBO.

Institute of Medicine (US). (2011). Committee on standards for developing trustworthy clinical practice guidelines. In R. Graham, M. Mancher, D. M. Wolman, et al. (Eds.), *Clinical practice guidelines we can trust.* Washington, DC: National Academies Press.

Joosen, M. C., Beurden van, K. M., Rebergen, D. S., et al. (2019). Effectiveness of a tailored implementation strategy to improve adherence to a guideline on mental health problems in occupational health care. *BMC Health Services Research, 19*, 281.

Koninklijk Genootschap voor Fysiotherapie (KNGF). (2017). KNGF-richtlijn Stress (urine-)incontinentie. Supplement bij het Nederlands Tijdschrift voor Fysiotherapie Jaargang 121 · Nummer 3 · 2011 Update klinimetrie 2017.

Koninklijk Nederlands Genootschap voor Fysiotherapie (KNGF). (1993). *Richtlijnen voor de Fysiotherapeutische verslaglegging.* Amersfoort: KNGF.

Koninklijk Nederlands Genootschap voor Fysiotherapie (KNGF). (2019). *KNGF-richtlijnenmethodiek.* Amersfoort: KNGF.

Maas, M. J. M., van der Wees, P. J., Braam, C., et al. (2015). An innovative peer assessment approach to enhance guideline adherence in physical therapy: Single-masked, cluster-randomized controlled trial. *Physical Therapy, 95*, 600–612.

Maher, C. G., Sherrington, C., Elkins, M., et al. (2004). Challenges for evidence-based physical therapy: Accessing and interpreting high quality evidence on therapy. *Physical Therapy, 84*, 644–654.

National Institute for Health and Care Excellence. (2019). *Urinary incontinence and pelvic organ prolapse in women: Management.* NICE Guideline [NG123] [Online]. Available: https://www.nice.org.uk/guidance/ng123. (Accessed 05.08.22).

Rauh, S., Arnold, D., Braga, S., et al. (2018). Challenge of implementing clinical practice guidelines. Getting ESMO's guidelines even closer to the bedside: introducing the ESMO Practising Oncologists' checklists and knowledge and practice questions. *ESMO Open, 3*, e000385. doi:10.1136/esmoopen-2018-000385

Schünemann, H. J., Wierchioch, W., Etxeandia, I., et al. (2014). Guidelines 2.0: Systematic development of a comprehensive checklist for a successful guideline enterprise. *Canadian Medical Association Journal, 186*(3), e123–e142.

Shaneyfelt, T. M., & Centor, R. M. (2009). Reassessment of clinical practice guidelines: Go gently into that good night. *JAMA, 301*, 868–869.

Shiffman, R. N., Dixon, J., Brandt, C., et al. (2005). The Guide-Line Implementability Appraisal (GLIA): Development of an instrument to identify obstacles to guideline implementation. *BMC Medical Informatics and Decision Making, 5*, 23.

Van Ettekoven, H., & Hendriks, H. J. (1998). *Specifiek Implementatieplan en implementatie-instrumenten voor het invoeren van de centrale richtlijn 'Stress Urine-incontinentie'.* Amersfoort/Utrecht: KNGF/CBO/NPi.

Van Everdingen, J. J., Burgers, J. S., Assendelft, W. J., et al. (2004). *Evidence-based richtlijnontwikkeling. Een leidraad voor de praktijk.* Houten: Bohn, Stafleu van Loghum.

Van Tulder, M., Furlan, A., Bombadier, C., et al. (2003). Updated method guidelines for sytematic reviews in the Cochrane Collaboration Group. *Spine, 28,* 1290–1299.

Van der Wees, P. J., Hendriks, E. J., Custers, J. W., et al. (2007a). Comparison of international guideline programs to evaluate and update the Dutch program for clinical guideline development in physical therapy. *BMC Health Services Research, 7,* 191.

Van der Wees, P. J., Hendriks, H. J., Heldoorn, M., et al. (2007b). *Methode voor ontwikkeling, implementatie en bijstelling van KNGF Richtlijnen. Methode versie 2.5.* Amersfoort/Maastricht: KNGF.

Van der Wees, P. J., Hendriks, H. J., & Veldhuizen, R. J. (2003). Quality assurance in The Netherlands: From development to implementation and evaluation. *Dutch Journal Physical Therapy, 3,* 3–6.

Van der Wees, P. J., Jamtvedt, G., Rebbeck, T., et al. (2008). Multifaceted strategies may increase implementation of physiotherapy clinical guidelines: A systematic review. *Australian Journal of Physiotherapy, 54*(4), 233–241.

Van der Wees, P. J., & Mead, J. (2004). *Framework for clinical guideline development in physiotherapy.* Brussels: European Region of World Confederation for Physical Therapy.

Van der Wees, P. J., Moore, A. P., Powers, C. M., et al. (2011). Development of clinical guidelines in physical therapy: Perspective for international collaboration. *Physical Therapy, 91,* 1551–1563.

World Confederation for Physical Therapy (WCPT). (2010). *Clinical guideline development programmes in the European region of WCPT.* Berlin: World Confederation for Physical Therapy.

World Health Organization. (2014). *International statistical classification of disease and related health problems (ICD-11).* Geneva: World Health Organization.

World Health Organization. (2018). *International classification of functioning, disability and health.* Geneva: World Health Organization.

Note: Page numbers followed by 'b' indicate boxes, 'f' indicate figures and 't' indicate tables.